Capute & Accardo's
Neurodevelopmental Disabilities
in Infancy and Childhood

THIRD EDITION

Volume I:
Neurodevelopmental
Diagnosis and Treatment

Capute & Accardo's
Neurodevelopmental Disabilities
in Infancy and Childhood

THIRD EDITION

Volume I:
Neurodevelopmental
Diagnosis and Treatment

Edited by

Pasquale J. Accardo, M.D.

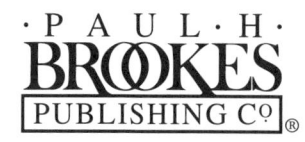
·P A U L·H·
BROOKES
PUBLISHING CO.®

Baltimore • London • Sydney

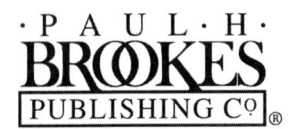

Paul H. Brookes Publishing Co.
Post Office Box 10624
Baltimore, Maryland 21285-0624

www.brookespublishing.com

Typeset by Maryland Composition Company, Laurel, Maryland.
Manufactured in the United States of America by
The Maple-Vail Book Manufacturing Group, York, Pennsylvania.

**Capute & Accardo's Neurodevelopmental Disabilities in Infancy and Childhood,
Third Edition,** is a two-volume set:
Volume I: *Neurodevelopmental Diagnosis and Treatment*
Volume II: *The Spectrum of Neurodevelopmental Disabilities*

Clinical vignettes are derived from the authors' actual experiences. Pseudonyms have been used
and identifying details have been changed to protect confidentiality.

Library of Congress Cataloging-in-Publication Data

Capute & Accardo's neurodevelopmental disabilities in infancy and childhood / edited by Pasquale
J. Accardo. — 3rd ed.
   p.;   cm.
   Rev. ed. of: Developmental disabilities in infancy and childhood / edited by Arnold J. Capute
and Pasquale J. Accardo. 2nd ed. c1996.
   Includes bibliographical references and index.
   ISBN-13: 978-1-55766-756-4 (hardcover)
   ISBN-10: 1-55766-756-X (hardcover)
   ISBN-13: 978-1-55766-758-8 (hardcover)
   ISBN-10: 1-55766-758-6 (hardcover)
   1. Developmental disabilities.   I. Accardo, Pasquale J.   II. Capute, Arnold J., 1923-   III.
Developmental disabilities in infancy and childhood.   IV. Title: Capute and Accardo's
neurodevelopmental disabilities in infancy and childhood. V. Title: Neurodevelopmental
disabilities in infancy and childhood.
   [DNLM: 1. Developmental Disabilities. WS 350.6 D48884 2008]
   RJ135.D476 2008
   618.92'85889—dc22   2007032278

British Library Cataloguing in Publication data are available from the British Library.

Contents

Volume I

Contents

Volume II

Editorial Board

Contributors

Volume I

Jennifer A. Accardo, M.D.
Sleep Fellow
Children's Hospital of Philadelphia
34th Street and Civic Center Boulevard
Philadelphia, Pennsylvania 19104

Pasquale J. Accardo, M.D.
James H. Franklin Professor of Developmental
    Research in Pediatrics
Virginia Commonwealth University
Stony Point Pediatrics
9000 Stony Point Parkway
Richmond, Virginia 23235

Marilee C. Allen, M.D.
Professor of Pediatrics
The Johns Hopkins University School of
    Medicine
Co-director, NICU Developmental Clinic
The Johns Hopkins Hospital
600 North Wolfe Street
Nelson 2-133
Baltimore, Maryland 21287

Claudine Amiel-Tison, M.D.
Professor Emerita of Pediatrics
Hôpital Saint-Vincent de Paul
82, Avenue Denfert-Rochereau
75674 Paris
Cedex 14 France

Harolyn M.E. Belcher, M.D., M.H.S.
Associate Professor of Pediatrics
The Johns Hopkins University School of
    Medicine
Director of Research
Kennedy Krieger Institute Family Center
2911 East Biddle Street
Baltimore, Maryland 21213

Peter A. Blasco, M.D.
Associate Professor of Pediatrics
Oregon Health and Science University
Director, Neurodevelopmental Programs
Child Development and Rehabilitation Center
707 Southwest Gaines Road
Portland, Oregon 97239

Joann N. Bodurtha, M.D., MPH
Professor of Human Genetics, Pediatrics,
    Obstetrics and Gynecology, Preventive
    Medicine and Community Health
Virginia Commonwealth University
Campus Box 980033
Richmond, Virginia 23298

Colleen Boyle, Ph.D.
Associate Director for Science and Public Health
Centers for Disease Control and Prevention
National Center on Birth Defects and
    Developmental Disabilities
Mail Stop E-87
1600 Clifton Road
Atlanta, Georgia 30333

Ewa Brandys, M.D.
Instructor of Physical Medicine and
    Rehabilitation
The Johns Hopkins University School of
    Medicine
Physician, Pediatric Rehabilitation and Spinal
    Cord Injury
Kennedy Krieger Institute
707 North Broadway
Baltimore, Maryland 21205

Errol J. Candy, M.B., Ch.B
Neuroradiologist
Presbyterian Hospital of Dallas
8440 Walnut Hill Lane, Suite 510
Dallas, Texas 75231

George T. Capone, M.D.
Associate Professor of Pediatrics
The Johns Hopkins University School of
    Medicine
Research Scientist
Center for Genetic Disorders of Cognition and
    Behavior
Kennedy Krieger Institute
1750 East Fairmount Avenue
Baltimore, Maryland 21231

John C. Carter, B.A.
Research Assistant and Study Coordinator
Center for Genetic Disorders of Cognition and
    Behavior
Kennedy Krieger Institute
3901 Greenspring Avenue
Baltimore, Maryland 21211

Thomas D. Challman, M.D.
Assistant Professor of Pediatrics
Jefferson Medical College
Neurodevelopmental Pediatrics
Janet Weis Children's Hospital
Geisinger Health System
100 North Academy Avenue
Danville, Pennsylvania 17822

James Christensen, M.D.
Associate Professor of Physical Medicine &
    Rehabilitation and Pediatrics
The Johns Hopkins University School of
    Medicine
Director of Pediatric Rehabilitation
Kennedy Krieger Institute
707 North Broadway
Baltimore, Maryland 21205

Ann W. Cox, Ph.D., RN
Former Associate Director and Director of
    Preservice Training
Virginia Institute for Developmental Disabilities
Virginia Commonwealth University
Richmond, Virginia
Retired
3001 Jones Ferry Road
Chapel Hill, North Carolina 27516

Cecilia T. Davoli, M.D., MPH
Medical Director, Outpatient Services
Kennedy Krieger Institute
707 North Broadway
Baltimore, Maryland 21205

Iser G. DeLeon, Ph.D.
Assistant Professor of Psychiatry
The Johns Hopkins University School of
    Medicine
Director of Research Development for the
    Department of Behavioral Psychology
Kennedy Krieger Institute
707 North Broadway
Baltimore, Maryland 21205

Larry W. Desch, M.D.
Associate Professor of Clinical Pediatrics
University of Illinois–Chicago
Director of Developmental Pediatrics
Advocate Hope Children's Hospital
4440 West 95th Street
Oak Lawn, Illinois 60453

Julie Gosselin, O.T., Ph.D.
Associate Professor, School of Rehabilitation
University of Montreal
C.P. 6128, Succ. Centre-Ville
Montréal (Québec)
Canada H3C 3J7

Hilary Gwynn, M.D.
Instructor
The Johns Hopkins University School of
    Medicine
Faculty
Neurology and Developmental Medicine
Kennedy Krieger Institute
707 North Broadway
Baltimore, Maryland 21205

Alexander H. Hoon, Jr., M.D., M.P.H.
Associate Professor of Pediatrics
The Johns Hopkins University School of
    Medicine
Director
Phelps Center for Cerebral Palsy and
    Neurodevelopmental Medicine
707 North Broadway
Baltimore, Maryland 21205

Chris Plauché Johnson, M.Ed., M.D.
Clinical Professor of Pediatrics
University of Texas of Health Science Center at
    San Antonio
1014 Bay Horse Drive
San Antonio, Texas 78245

Daniel C. Johnson, M.D.
Associate Chair, Department of Pediatrics
University of Chicago
5841 South Maryland Avenue, MC6082
Chicago, Illinois 60637

Sonja Johnson-Brooks, Ph.D.
Research Associate
Kennedy Krieger Institute Family Center
2901 East Biddle Street
Baltimore, Maryland 21213

Michael V. Johnston, M.D.
Professor of Neurology, Pediatrics and Physical
    Medicine and Rehabilitation
The Johns Hopkins University School of
    Medicine
Chief Medical Officer
Kennedy Krieger Institute
707 North Broadway
Baltimore, Maryland 21205

SungWoo Kahng, Ph.D.
Assistant Professor of Psychiatry and Behavioral
    Sciences
The Johns Hopkins University School of
    Medicine
Director of Training, Department of Behavioral
    Psychology
Kennedy Krieger Institute
707 North Broadway
Baltimore, Maryland 21205

Walter E. Kaufmann, M.D.
Professor of Pathology, Neurology, Pediatrics,
    Psychiatry, and Radiology
The Johns Hopkins University School of
    Medicine
Director, Center for Genetic Disorders of
    Cognition and Behavior
Kennedy Krieger Institute
3901 Greenspring Avenue
Baltimore, Maryland 21211

Richard I. Kelley, M.D., Ph.D.
Professor of Pediatrics
The Johns Hopkins University School of
    Medicine
Director, Division of Metabolism
Kennedy Krieger Institute
707 North Broadway
Baltimore, Maryland 21205

Shelly J. Lane, Ph.D., OTR/L, FAOTA
Professor and Chair, Department of
    Occupational Therapy
Assistant Dean of Research, School of Allied
    Health Professions
Virginia Commonwealth University
1000 East Marshall Street
Post Office Box 980008
Richmond, Virginia 23298

Christopher T. Leffler, M.D., M.P.H.
Assistant Professor of Ophthalmology
Virginia Commonwealth University
403 North 11th Street, Fourth Floor
Richmond, Virginia 23298

Mary L. O'Connor Leppert, M.D.
Assistant Professor of Pediatrics
The Johns Hopkins University School of
    Medicine
Kennedy Krieger Institute
707 North Broadway
Baltimore, Maryland 21205

David N. Lieberman, M.D., Ph.D.
Instructor in Neurology
The Johns Hopkins University School of
    Medicine
200 North Wolfe Street, Suite 2158
Baltimore, Maryland 21287

Doris D.M. Lin, M.D., Ph.D.
Assistant Professor of Radiology, Division of
    Neuroradiology
Department of Radiology and Radiological
    Sciences
The Johns Hopkins University School of
    Medicine
600 North Wolfe Street, Phipps B-100
Baltimore, Maryland 21287

Paul H. Lipkin, M.D.
Assistant Professor of Pediatrics
The Johns Hopkins University School of
    Medicine
Director, Center for Development and Learning
Kennedy Krieger Institute
707 North Broadway
Baltimore, Maryland 21205

Thomas R. Montgomery, M.D.
Director, Neurodevelopmental Pediatrics
Children's Hospital of the King's Daughters
733 Volvo Parkway, Suite 300
Chesapeake, Virginia 23320

Olga Morozova, M.D.
Assistant Professor of Pediatrics
The George Washington University
Pediatric Physiatrist
Children's National Medical Center
111 Michigan Avenue, N.W.
Washington, D.C. 20010

Emily R. Msall
Teaching Fellow, Citizen Schools of Boston
Mildred Avenue Middle School
5 Mildred Avenue
Mattapan, Massachusetts 02126

Michael E. Msall, M.D.
Professor of Pediatrics
The University of Chicago
Chief, Neurodevelopmental and Behavioral
  Pediatrics
Comer Children's and LaRabida Children's
  Hospitals
Kennedy Center on Neurodevelopmental
  Disabilities
Research Scientist
Institute of Molecular Pediatric Sciences
Section of Community Health, Ethics and Policy
950 East 61st Street, Suite 207
Chicago, Illinois 60637

Scott M. Myers, M.D.
Assistant Professor of Pediatrics
Jefferson Medical College
Neurodevelopmental Pediatrician
Geisinger Health System
100 North Academy Avenue
Danville, Pennsylvania 17822

Frederick B. Palmer, M.D.
Shainberg Professor of Pediatrics
Director, Boling Center for Developmental
  Disabilities
University of Tennessee Health Science Center
711 Jefferson Avenue
Memphis, Tennessee 38105

Sandra A. Palomo-Gonzalez, Ph.D.
Senior Program Coordinator
The University of Texas at San Antonio
Center for Policy Studies
501 West Durango Boulevard
San Antonio, Texas 78205

Joan E. Pellegrino, M.D.
Associate Professor of Pediatrics
State University of New York Upstate Medical
  University
750 East Adams Street
Syracuse, New York 13210

Louis Pellegrino, M.D.
Assistant Professor of Pediatrics
State University of New York Upstate Medical
  University
750 East Adams Street
Syracuse, New York 13210

Frank S. Pidcock, M.D.
Associate Professor of Pediatrics and Physical
  Medicine and Rehabilitation
The Johns Hopkins University School of
  Medicine
Associate Director, Rehabilitation
Kennedy Krieger Institute
707 North Broadway
Baltimore, Maryland 21205

Nancy J. Roizen, M.D.
Professor of Pediatrics
Case Western Reserve University School of
  Medicine
Director of Behavioral/Developmental Pediatrics
Rainbow Babies and Children's Hospital
11100 Euclid Avenue
Cleveland, Ohio 44106

Erin M. Rosier, B.A.
Research Assistant
Kennedy Krieger Institute
707 North Broadway
Baltimore, Maryland 21205

Cristina Sadowsky, M.D.
Assistant Professor of Physical Medicine and
  Rehabilitation
The Johns Hopkins University School of
  Medicine
Director of Restoration Paralysis Clinic
International Center for Spinal Cord Injury
Kennedy Krieger Institute
707 North Broadway, Suite 518
Baltimore, Maryland 21205

Cynthia Salorio, Ph.D.
Assistant Professor of Physical Medicine and
  Rehabilitation
The Johns Hopkins University School of
  Medicine
Pediatric Neuropsychologist
Kennedy Krieger Institute
707 North Broadway
Baltimore, Maryland 21205

Mitchell Schertz, M.D.
Director
Institute for Child Development
Kupat Holim Meuhedet, Central Region
6 Lancet Avenue
Herzeliya 46782 Israel

Bruce K. Shapiro, M.D.
The Arnold J. Capute, M.D., M.P.H. Chair in
    Neurodevelopmental Disabilities
Associate Professor of Pediatrics
The Johns Hopkins University School of
    Medicine
Vice President of Training
Kennedy Krieger Institute
707 North Broadway
Baltimore, Maryland 21205

Peter J. Smith, M.D., M.A.
Assistant Professor of Pediatrics
University of Chicago
Chief of the Medical Staff
La Rabida Children's Hospital
East 65th Street at Lake Michigan
Chicago, Illinois 60649

Usha T. Sundaram, M.D.
Assistant Professor of Human Genetics
Virginia Commonwealth University
Campus Box 980033
1101 East Marshall Street
Richmond, Virginia 23298

Edwin Trevathan, M.D., M.P.H.
Director, National Center on Birth Defects and
    Developmental Disabilities
Centers for Disease Control and Prevention
Mail Stop E-87
1600 Clifton Road
Atlanta, Georgia 30333

Melissa K. Trovato, M.D.
Assistant Professor of Physical Medicine and
    Rehabilitation
The Johns Hopkins University School of
    Medicine
Kennedy Krieger Institute
707 North Broadway
Baltimore, Maryland 21205

Kim Van Naarden Braun, Ph.D.
Epidemiologist
National Center on Birth Defects and
    Developmental Disabilities
Centers for Disease Control and Prevention
Mail Stop E-86
1600 Clifton Road
Atlanta, Georgia 30333

Robert G. Voigt, M.D.
Assistant Professor of Pediatrics
Mayo Clinic
200 First Street, S.W.
Rochester, Minnesota 55905

Toni M. Whitaker, M.D.
Assistant Professor of Pediatrics
Neurodevelopmental Disabilities
University of Tennessee Health Science Center
Boling Center for Developmental Disabilities
711 Jefferson Avenue
Memphis, Tennessee 38105

Barbara Y. Whitman, Ph.D.
Associate Professor
St. Louis University School of Social Services
Director of Family Services and Family Studies
The Knights of Columbus Medical Center
Cardinal Glennon Children's Hospital
1465 South Grand Boulevard
St. Louis, Missouri 63104

Marshalyn Yeargin-Allsopp, M.D.
Medical Epidemiologist
National Center on Birth Defects and
    Developmental Disabilities
Centers for Disease Control and Prevention
Mail Stop E-86
1600 Clifton Road
Atlanta, Georgia 30333

Introduction

When the American Academy of Pediatrics established the Arnold J. Capute Award in Developmental Pediatrics and presented the first award to Dr. Capute, I proposed to Dr. Capute to collect the acceptance speeches from the future honorees as a historical document from leaders in the field. Dr. Capute sent me several fragmentary versions of his comments that I have smoothed out below. A more formal biographical sketch can be found in Accardo, P.J. (2004). The Father of Developmental Pediatrics: Arnold J. Capute, MD, MPH (1923–2003). Journal of Child Neurology, 19(12), 978–981.

Pasquale J. Accardo, M.D.

Upon completion of my developmental disability fellowship in the 1960s (the era of "inborn errors of metabolism"), it was already apparent that the training program was weak in addressing the neurological basis of the spectrum of developmental disorders. The existing 4-month inpatient and outpatient neurology rotation was insufficient. Despite rapid progress in other areas of pediatric medicine, the static encephalopathies of developmental disabilities had remained static. I felt that increased input from neurology was urgently needed if the field was ever to achieve academic respectability.

In order to meet neurology on more equal terms, subspecialty recognition was in order, and this was vigorously pursued from 1972 on, even though the majority of developmentalists were hesitant to endorse the idea wholeheartedly. The first application to the American Board of Medical Specialties was denied in 1978. John Griffiths, M.D., of the American Board of Pediatrics had the foresight and wisdom to recommend that developmental pediatrics should dialogue with pediatric neurology about the possibility of developing a joint program. Based on perceived weaknesses in the state of the art, a number of long-term measures were initiated to provide greater academic respectability to the field of neurodevelopmental disabilities:

- The Kennedy Fellows Association (KFA), with more than 100 graduates of the Developmental Pediatrics Program from the Kennedy Krieger Institute at The Johns Hopkins University, was established in 1975 and held an annual fall academic and business meeting in Williamsburg, Virginia.

- A "Spectrum of Developmental Disabilities" spring continuing medical education course was inaugurated in 1978 at The Johns Hopkins University/Kennedy Krieger Institute in Baltimore. The attendees included both physicians and nonmedical professionals who evaluated and managed children with handicapping conditions. It was a successful enough adventure to support other endeavors that were paramount in obtaining board recognition such as meeting with chairs of pediatrics throughout the nation (Boston, New York, Philadelphia, Chicago, Seattle, and Los Angeles) to tell them what developmental disabilities represented, to differentiate the field from *behavioral pediatrics,* and to educate them about the subspecialty endeavor. Pasquale J. Accardo, M.D., Bruce K. Shapiro, M.D., Renee C. Wachtel, M.D., Frederick B. Palmer, M.D., and Lawrence Taft, M.D., were most helpful in this activity.

- The Society for Developmental Pediatrics (SDP) was established in 1978 as a professional association of pediatricians either formally trained in or with in-depth exposure to the entire spectrum of developmental disabilities.

- Textbooks were written, and pediatric test instruments (the Cognitive Adaptive Test/ Clinical Linguistic and Auditory Milestone Scale) were developed.

- After finding that the educational input on neurodevelopmental disabilities at their annual meetings had been inadequate, the American Academy of Pediatrics (AAP) founded a Section on Children with Disabilities at the urging of the SDP.

My most cherished endeavor was setting up an "academic orchestra" in the late 1970s at The Johns Hopkins University: this included KFA developmental pediatricians with expertise and interest in clinical research. This consortium made "academic music" by carrying out several large research projects, one on the evolution of primitive reflexes, and one on the effect of physical therapy on diplegia. This clinical research unit was composed of Pasquale J. Accardo, Bruce K. Shapiro, Frederick B. Palmer, and Renee C. Wachtel, all of whom went on the direct training programs. I have always considered the graduates of the Hopkins/Kennedy Neurodevelopmental Training Program as my "academic" children, and my greatest pleasure is in keeping in touch with them to keep abreast of their academic and social undertakings.

Through 2000, negotiations were held to finalize the development of a new specialty. This conjoint endeavor was finally approved, and the first subboard examination was held in April 2001. The next generation of developmentalists will be better trained to respond to their high legacy.

Arnold J. Capute, M.D., M.P.H.
(1923–2003)

for

Arnold
vidi il maestro di color che sanno

and Patricia
chè non pur nei miei occhi è Paradiso

Introduction

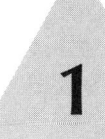

A Neurodevelopmental Perspective on the Continuum of Developmental Disabilities

PASQUALE J. ACCARDO,
JENNIFER A. ACCARDO, AND ARNOLD J. CAPUTE

Implicit in the term *developmental* is the effect of time. Development is a rate phenomenon. Even though a child's developmental rate may appear stable, the component behaviors exhibit a complex evolution over time. The resulting interweaving of continuity and change can appear confusing and may complicate both diagnosis and prognosis. An example of a child with attention-deficit/hyperactivity disorder (ADHD) and a specific learning disability will help clarify the difficulties (Figure 1.1).

Whereas severe neurodevelopmental disorders are easy to diagnose, with appropriate intervention and support typically initiated in early infancy, milder central nervous system (CNS) impairment is frequently misinterpreted by both professionals and parents as inadequate parenting. Regardless of how challenging the irritability of an infant is to parents, the subsequent clumsiness, disarticulation, and hyperactivity of the toddler tend to be viewed as an entirely new set of problems—and one that reconfirms the perception of parental inadequacy. Preschool behavior problems can set the stage for misinterpreting the academic underachievement that follows. By the time an accurate, comprehensive diagnosis is made, secondary emotional complications such as learned helplessness and possibly depression may render late intervention more difficult.

Underlying any ostensible change in the condition of a child with a neurodevelopmental disability is the permanent CNS impairment. The more severe the degree of intellectual disability, the more stable the intelligence quotient (IQ) over time. Disorders of attention and learning (disorders of higher cortical functioning) also exhibit continuity over time; for example, fairly constant rates of reading acquisition are reported for specific learning disorder in reading. The persistence of the neurodevelopmental disability into adulthood contributes to the impact of secondary emotional diagnoses. Although the underlying CNS pathology remains constant, both the manner in which a neurodevelopmental disability presents clinically and the priorities on the child's problem list will change over time. Helping families and involved professionals comprehend this evolving temporal expression represents a major goal of neurodevelopmental pediatrics.

Before breaking up the process of neurodevelopment into its phenomenological components, it is necessary to stress the importance of the forest over the trees. There is effectively no practical limit to the potential number of gene defects and organic brain syndromes that could contribute to neurodevelopmental disabilities, nor is there any anticipated ceiling on the number of odd and atypical behaviors, splinter skills, and unique stereotypies that may at first defy explanation. However, understanding and interpretation of the global pattern and what influences it represent the fundamental goals of neurodevelopmental pediatrics. The number of basic patterns is quite limited, but variety and novelty

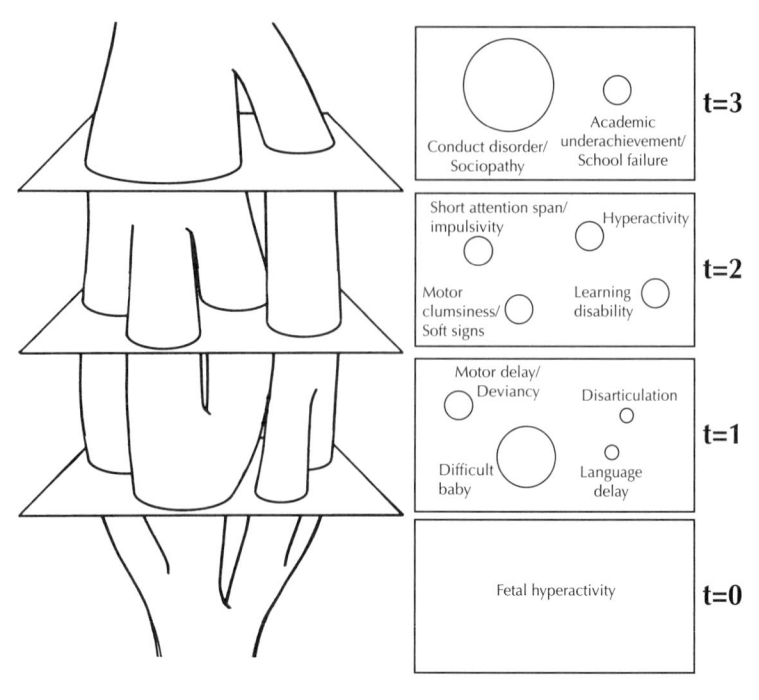

Figure 1.1. Temporal evolution of symptoms in a child with attention-deficit/hyperactivity disorder and a specific learning disability. The disarticulation noted in *t* = 1 is more strongly associated with language delay than any oral-motor pathology. At *t* = 2, conduct disorder criteria may not yet be fulfilled, but behavior problems may include lying, stealing, cheating, arson, and cruelty to animals.

are not absent from their presentations. Unexpected curves have been described, and the diversity hidden within many rare genetic syndromes is only beginning to be explored (Figure 1.2). The roots of this diversity lie in the interaction among four levels or paradigms of the developmental process: 1) the three developmental phenomena of delay, dissociation, and deviance; 2) the streams of development; 3) the spectrum and continuum of developmental disorders; and 4) patternological diagnosis.

DELAY, DISSOCIATION, AND DEVIANCE

What mothers worry most about in young children are a perceived lateness in achieving certain developmental milestones and an unevenness or peculiarity in the way their children achieve these milestones. These parental concerns appropriately presume the normative, orderly, and sequential process of child development within well-recognized age cutoffs. In addressing such parental concerns in a clini-

cally responsible manner, the neurodevelopmental pediatrician attempts to understand and interpret both individual milestones and milestone sequences in terms of delay, dissociation, and deviance.

Developmental quotient (DQ) is used to quantify lags in development. This consists simply of a ratio: the child's functional age equivalent in one or more areas of development divided by the child's chronological age. DQ may be perceived to imply rate—a child with a DQ of 50 in expressive language could easily be assumed to have acquired milestones in speech at half the rate of his or her typically developing peers. This is a potentially misleading interpretation as the rate may have been stable over time, accelerated, or altered by regression (see Figure 1.2). Detailed developmental history and multiple assessments separated in time are required to determine a clinically predictive developmental rate.

Delay refers to a significant lag in one or more areas of development, and sometimes a global delay across all areas of development. When using a DQ to quantitate the degree of

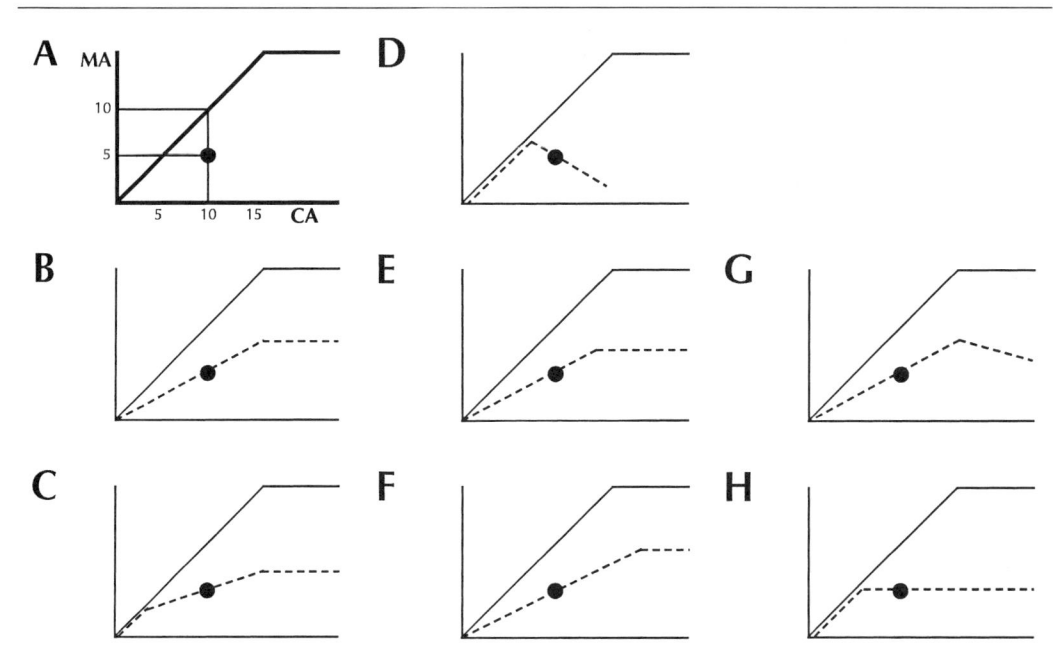

Figure 1.2. A child whose development is significantly delayed (A) may represent a case of intellectual disabilities from birth (B) or postnatal insult (C), or the delay may be secondary to a degenerative disorder (D). The pattern or time course is of much greater significance than the simple fact of delay. Some children with specific genetic syndromes may plateau in their development, either before or after mid-adolescence, giving rise to a decrease (E) or an increase (F) in their intelligence quotient (IQ) scores. Finally, some genetic syndromes appear to include a mild degenerative component as part of their long-term prognosis (G). The child who simply plateaus in development (leading to a progressive decline in DQ/IQ until adolescence) is a rare outcome of the loss of long-term memory storage ability (H). (*Key:* CA, chronological age; MA, mental age.)

delay, cutoff points for concern, further evaluation, and intervention will depend on any concurrent medical diagnoses, the age of the child, previous therapeutic response, and the specific areas of delay. If an infant is progressing at or below a DQ of 80 and this degree of delay is confirmed on two consecutive examinations, serious consideration should be given to a comprehensive neurodevelopmental assessment. If the DQ is 60 or below in any single area of development, then a full assessment is indicated. Global retardation refers to a DQ of 70 or less in all of the streams of development; in infancy, it presents with a DQ below 70 in both the language and problem-solving components of assessments such as The Capute Scales (see Chapter 19, this volume).

The degree of delay has biological implications. For children with DQs below 50 in a given area, it is often easy to find a cause through evaluation for organic etiology, even if it is "presumed genetic syndrome." However, this can contribute to a misunderstanding of the role of organic CNS damage in developmental delay by presuming the precedence of emotional, sociocultural, or environmental factors alone for children with DQs in the 50–75 range. Logic and common sense would suggest that mild but real brain damage leading to less severe neurodevelopmental disabilities should occur much more frequently than severe brain damage and severe disabilities. Recent research in twins has indeed described a much higher percentage of people with mild intellectual disabilities and slow learners, or those with "borderline" intellectual disabilities, as having genetic-based etiologies. Thus, although severity of delay appears to be directly correlated with the ease of identifying a specific organic etiology, the absence of an identified specific etiology in cases of milder delays does not necessarily imply nonorganic etiologies (Table 1.1).

Dissociation is manifested by a difference between the developmental rates of two streams of development, with one stream significantly more delayed. If severe intellectual disability is present, language is often more delayed than motor-dependent skills. In communication disorders and pervasive develop-

Table 1.1.   The three-group classification of developmental disabilities

I: Severe intellectual disability	II: Mild intellectual disability	III: Learning and language disabilities
High incidence of chromosomal abnormalities, genetic syndromes, and organic brain syndrome	Increasing incidence of chromosomal abnormalities, genetic syndromes, and organic brain syndrome	Increasingly higher identified incidence of familial/genetic patterns of learning and language disorders, academic underachievement, and adult psychopathology
Major organ system malformations and classic neurological findings, including cerebral palsy	Mild dysmorphic features and mild motor clumsiness	Mild dysmorphic features and soft neurological signs
Seizure disorders	Abnormal EEG findings	Abnormal EEG findings
Familial IQ/learning pattern: normal/achiever	Familial IQ/learning pattern: borderline/underachiever	Familial IQ/learning pattern: normal/underachiever

Key: EEG, electroencephalogram; IQ, intelligence quotient.

mental disorders, language abilities typically lag behind visual-motor problem solving. The dissociation phenomenon is most often observed in older children with learning disabilities. In these children, school underachievement reflects an underlying dissociation between academic achievement and general intellectual potential (Table 1.2). Significant dissociation is probably more common among people with various degrees of intellectual disability than are learning disabilities among the general population, but education tends to downplay the importance of this phenomenon by its insistence that learning disability and intellectual disability are mutually exclusive educational classifications. They are in fact neurologically quite compatible.

In a more individual context, the term *dissociation* is sometimes used to refer to the breaking of an expected linkage or coupling between given milestones. This type of dissociation is typically indicative of inadequacies in parental reporting or professional elicitation of the milestones. For example, in 2-year-olds, a 50-word vocabulary is linked to the use of 2-word phrases. When a parent reports either a 100-word vocabulary with no 2-word phrases or a 25-word vocabulary with several 2-word phrases, the linked milestones have been dissociated, or uncoupled. On further investigation, parental recollection of one or both milestones will usually be found to be incorrect; however, in some children with neurodevelopmental disabilities, this uncoupling may represent deviancy or isolated splinter skills, such as inflated rote auditory memory. In children with disabilities and spuriously large vocabularies, an unusually high proportion of their spoken words tend to be personal names.

Deviancy is manifested by nonsequential unevenness in the achievement of milestones within one or more streams of development. The phenomena of delay and dissociation present nothing intrinsically abnormal in their se-

Table 1.2.   Dissociation between the streams of development with different developmental diagnoses

Stream of development	Intellectual disability	Cerebral palsy	Blindness	Deafness	Autism	Communication disorders	Learning disability
Motor							
Gross	V	D	D	N	N	N	N
Fine	V	D	D	N	N	N	V
Problem solving	D	V	D	N	V	N	V
Language							
Expressive	D	V	N	D	D	D	V
Receptive	D	V	N	D	D	V	V
Social/adaptive	D	D	D	V	V	N	V

Key: N, normal; D, delayed; V, variable.

quences: the delayed milestones are attained in a fashion indistinguishable from what would be expected in a typically developing younger child. But the nonsequential deviant pattern is not typical for any age. The more common examples of deviancy involve failing simple items in a given developmental sequence while passing more difficult items. In formal psychometrics, this presents as the phenomenon of "double basals" or "double ceilings." Alternatively, a child may appear to perform well in one area of development that depends on another area of development in which he or she performs poorly. This latter form of deviancy is usually illusory. For example, expressive language skills cannot be more mature than receptive language skills: neither children nor adults can say more than they can understand. Whenever this contradictory situation is reported, alternative explanations should be sought. Artificially inflated rote expressive language skills are typical of communication disorders, pervasive developmental disorders, certain genetic syndromes such as Williams syndrome, and hydrocephalus.

In school-age children with learning disabilities, intelligence tests can reveal verbal performance or inter-subtest score scatter, or dissociation. It is not uncommon also to find intra-subtest score scatter or deviancy. One of the factors that contribute to such deviancy is the presence of rote sequencing abilities at a functional level that is superior to discrimination or comprehension skills. This kind of disproportion can be observed at a fairly early age. For example, an 18-month-old infant may demonstrate a vocabulary of 30 words (above age level) coupled with immature use of jargon (a 15-month skill). This pattern suggests a good auditory rote memory accompanied by a weakness in connected language and possibly verbal comprehension. Attentional deficits can contribute to extreme irregularities (and unreliability) in formal psychometric testing of older children.

In the motor arena, deviancy may also be exemplified by the infant who rolls or flips over by 1 month of age. Rather than representing advanced motor ability, this premature milestone may reflect an abnormal tonic labyrinthine reflex that places the child at risk for a later motor diagnosis, such as cerebral palsy. Alternatively, it could be the result of opisthotonus, an ominous neurological sign. Premature standing when a child is unable to sit up alone may similarly indicate increased risk of motor disability resulting from lower extremity hypertonia.

In addition to deviancy, which implies a lack of sequencing or an inversion of the typical expected pattern, there are certain signs and symptoms that suggest the presence of a neurodevelopmental disability (Table 1.3). The presence or history of any of these findings should be considered a risk marker for these disorders and should raise the possibility of formal neurodevelopmental assessment.

Although the term *deviancy* frequently has psychiatric implications to the layperson, no such connotations apply in neurodevelopmental disabilities. Even in autism, many characteristic behaviors represent deviancy in the neuromaturational sense. Still, some continue to misperceive autism as a psychoemotional disorder rather than an organic brain syndrome—a neurodevelopmental disability.

In infants and young children, the neurodevelopmental assessment attempts to interpret both historical milestones and current developmental performance in light of the three fundamental processes of delay, dissociation, and deviance. The mapping of these three processes onto the six streams of development will generate the spectrum and the continuum of developmental disabilities.

Table 1.3. Risk markers for neurodevelopmental disorders

Fetal hyperactivity
Fetal hypoactivity
Prematurity
Failure to thrive
Arching
Standoffishness
Acting as if deaf
Acting as if blind
Quietness
Central nervous system infection (meningitis, encephalitis)
Neurosurgical procedure
Toe walking
Echolalia

STREAMS OF DEVELOPMENT: PROCESS VERSUS PRODUCT

In the early decades of the 20th century, Gesell identified and highlighted various areas of infant and child development by relating functional activities or milestones achieved to chronological age. To be clinically useful, a developmental milestone should occur during a narrow normative time frame and should be easily observable to the clinician, useful to the child, and predictive of whether and when future milestones are attained. The concept of the DQ was easy to understand but all too open to misuse. Failure to achieve developmental milestones reflects the complex interactions among neuromaturational processes, environmental stimulation, educational history, temperament, intercurrent illnesses (with their impact on strength and physical growth), and genetic factors. Overreliance on a single milestone (e.g., age of walking) or on a handful of milestones averaged to yield a single developmental age or quotient is risky. The assessment of developmental milestones in infancy and childhood should be a comprehensive overview of the pattern or profile that the complex process of development is following in a particular child.

The analogy implied in the phrase "streams of development" is accurate in its suggestion of ongoing constant progress and of the child perpetually being in some kind of forward movement. Neuronal structures continue to grow, differentiate, and develop new connections and circuits throughout childhood so that forward momentum is always maintained.

The main streams of development derived from Gesell's work are gross motor, fine motor, visual-motor problem solving, expressive language, receptive language, and social and self-help (adaptive) skills. Variations in the relationships among these different streams will describe patterns that at different ages will suggest or confirm the presence of specific developmental diagnoses. The individual developmental milestones achieve importance only as part of a larger picture, one that accurately describes the developmental process and is only roughly indicated by a DQ. The following sections explore each of these streams of development.

Gross Motor Skills

Gross motor milestones (Table 1.4) describe posture and locomotion—how a child gets from one place to another. Although they have the weakest correlation with general functional ability (intelligence or global developmental level), they comprise the common substrate for any evaluation of the preverbal child. Factors that interfere with motor performance in turn interfere with the assessment of skills that depend on intact motor skills for their expression. This limits the use and complicates the interpretation of most infant scales, which tend to be highly motor dependent. Such limitations, however, are not binding: The clinician skilled in working with children with motor impairments can usually accommodate test administration and interpretation, just as the child with a physical disability can accommodate test performance.

The ordered, sequential appearance of motor milestone behaviors comes closest to the maturational ideal of the clockwork unfolding of a preprogrammed, myelinization-dependent, environment-independent evolution. Race, sex, and sociocultural influences are minimal. It is striking how little impact specific deficits, such as blindness, have on motor development; however, the principal way in which chronic debilitating diseases that are not caused by CNS damage affect general development is by means of weakening the motor substrate.

Table 1.4. Age of attainment of gross motor milestones

Milestone	Mean age of attainment (months)
Roll (prone to supine)	3.6
Roll (supine to prone)	4.8
Sit (supported)	5.3
Sit (unsupported)	6.3
Creep (locomotion in prone)	6.7
Come to sit	7.5
Crawl (locomotion in quadruped)	7.8
Pull to stand	8.1
Cruise	8.8
Walk	11.7
Walk backward	14.3
Run	14.8

Table 1.5. Milestone sequence for walking

No head lag when pulled to sit
Head control in supported sitting
Anterior propping
Lateral propping
Absent plantar grasp
Cruising
Anterior parachute
Posterior propping
Wide-based gait with short stride and high guard
Narrow-based gait with long stride and low guard

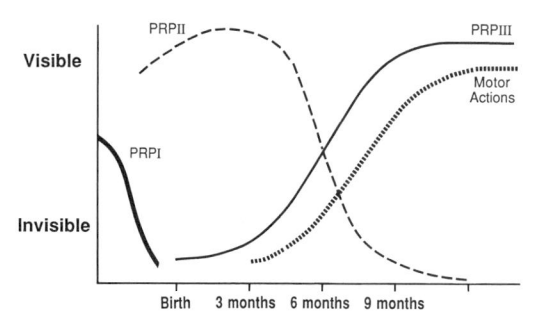

Figure 1.3. Interactions among primitive and postural reflexes and motor milestones. Although the correlations between reflex appearance (primitive reflex profile [PRP] III) and disappearance (PRP II) and the emergence of various motor milestones remain weak, these interrelations can still be clinically useful. For the child who is not yet walking and whose neurological examination is normal, the key indices for readiness to walk are the disappearance of the plantar grasp (PRP II) and the appearance of the anterior parachute (PRP III).

Gross motor milestones have little association with general intelligence: Children with profound intellectual disabilities may walk on time. Milder motor delays also do not correlate to any significant degree with milder cognitive delays. Achievement of gross motor milestones is the most accurate measure of gross motor development—and little else. Before attributing other delays to impaired motor functioning, it is important to assess carefully both the age level and the quality of motor functioning. The motor quotient must be derived from the child's progress in attaining an ordered sequence of milestones rather than from the attainment of a single milestone. Clinically, this involves not only observing whether a child walks but also noting how close the child is to walking (Table 1.5). In infants and young children, many milder neuromotor abnormalities (e.g., hypotonia) are transient. The interpretation of such findings must be subordinated to the child's functional level. A profile

of primitive reflexes (Table 1.6) can provide further supportive data in discriminating degrees of motor disability. Interactions among primitive and postural reactions and motor milestones are shown in Figure 1.3.

The cutoff for serious disability is lower for gross motor development than for other streams of development. Quotients consistently in the 50–75 range in language and problem solving typically indicate significant developmental problems, such as language disorders and intellectual disabilities. In the gross motor area, cerebral palsy usually presents with motor quotients below 50. Motor quotients in the 50–75 range are more consistent with hypotonia and developmental coordination disorder. Such mild motor disorders are

Table 1.6. Primitive and postural reflexes by age categories

PRP I (Intrauterine, suppressed before birth)	PRP II (Present at birth, suppressed during first 6 months)	PRP III (Postural reactions appearing during second 6 months)
Twitching	Moro	Head righting
Fetal startle	Neck righting	Landau response
	Galant	Derotative righting (DR)
	Tonic labyrinthine	Head on body (DRHB)
	Asymmetrical tonic neck	Body on body (DRBB)
	Positive support	Equilibrium responses
	Crossed extension	Anterior propping
	Stepping	Lateral propping
	Palmar grasp	Posterior propping
	Plantar grasp	Forward parachute
	Lower extremity placing	

Key: PRP, primitive reflex profile.

commonly associated with other neurodevel-opmental disabilities. Thus, a careful neuromo-tor assessment of both infants and children should be routinely included as part of the neu-rodevelopmental assessment. Motor delay is obligatory before a motor diagnosis can be made. Deviance in the absence of delay (the child who stands before he or she sits or who walks before he or she crawls) remains of ques-tionable significance.

Fine Motor Skills and Visual-Motor Problem-Solving Skills

Fine motor and visuomotor problem-solving skills refer to upper extremity and hand manip-ulative abilities and hand–eye coordination. In infants and young children, these skills are as-sessed by observing the child's interaction with test objects, such as blocks, formboards, and puzzles. In older children, they are usually tested via visual-motor or drawing and writing tasks. Although all of these test items depend to some degree on an intact motor substrate, they also require a given level of nonverbal cognitive ability.

The neurodevelopmental pediatrician at-tempts to distinguish between the motor and cognitive components when a child fails a par-ticular item. For example, the 10-month-old infant classically exhibits a neat pincer grasp. A 2-year-old child with intellectual disabilities may, with much encouragement and repeated refocusing of his or her short attention span, smoothly pluck a pellet with a pincer grasp, but, when distracted, he or she quickly loses interest and drops the pellet. Another 2-year-old child with cerebral palsy exhibits strong vis-ual interest in the same pellet, but all attempts at grasping it are frustrated by an overshoot in the child's reach as well as persistent fisting. The first child passes the fine motor item but fails the problem-solving item. The second child fails the fine motor item but passes the problem-solving item. The type of discrimina-tion represented by these examples is espe-cially important because problem-solving abili-ties represent the best measure of nonverbal intelligence in infants and young children. The difficulties in reliably and comfortably making this distinction are eased for the neurodevelop-

Table 1.7. Early visual-motor milestones

Age (months)	Milestone
1	Visually alerts, orients
	Visually fixates momentarily on face, red ring
	Moves eyes vertically
2	Coordinates eye movements with limited head movements
	Visually follows red ring horizontally and vertically through 90-degree arc
	Follows in prone, but not across midline
3	Coordinates eye movement with complete head turning
	Begins coupling eye-head coordination with hand–eye coordination/upper extremity function
	Follows red ring in a circle
	Follows past midline through 180-degree arc

mental pediatrician by familiarity with the range and impact of various motor diagnoses.

The earliest visual milestones that involve sequencing and discrimination may actually be fairly predictive of later cognitive function (Ta-bles 1.7 and 1.8). They represent the founda-tion for later nonverbal problem-solving abili-ties. The neurodevelopmental assessment for young children should routinely include non-verbal tasks involving blocks and formboards.

For school-age children, drawing tests provide a readily available, nonthreatening ap-proach to the assessment of graphomotor abili-ties (Table 1.9). Results on drawing tests corre-late with overall intellectual ability, learning disorders, and other psychological and psychi-atric disorders. Identifying the relative contri-butions of disability, experience, talent, and emotional factors is aided considerably by the use of more than one drawing test.

Expressive and Receptive Language Skills

In the absence of a communication disorder or significant hearing impairment, language de-velopment represents the best predictor of fu-ture intellectual performance. One of the major contributions of the neurodevelopmen-tal pediatrician has been to highlight the im-portance of the sequential appearance of pre-linguistic vocalizations to the early diagnosis of

Table 1.8. Age of attainment of CAT milestones

Milestone	Mean age of attainment (months)
Visually fixates momentarily on red ring Lifts chin off table in prone	1
Visually follows red ring horizontally and vertically Lifts chest off table in prone	2
Visually follows red ring in a circle Supports on forearm in prone Blinks in response to hand rapidly approaching eyes	3
Unclenches hands at rest more than half the time Manipulates fingers Supports on wrists in prone	4
Pulls down ring Transfers object from one hand to the other Regards pellet	5
Obtains cube Lifts cube Reaches for objects with the thumb and forefinger sliding across the table surface	6
Attempts pellet Pulls out peg Inspects ring	7
Pulls ring by string Secures pellet Inspects bell	8
Performs 3-finger scissor grasp Rings bell Looks for toy dropped over edge	9
Combines cube and cup Uncovers bell Fingers pegboard	10
Displays mature overhand pincer movement Looks for cube hidden under cup	11
Releases 1 cube in cup Marks with crayon	12
Reaches for toy around intervening glass pane Pushes peg in and out Solves pellet-bottle with demonstration	14
Solves pellet-bottle spontaneously Puts round block in formboard Scribbles in imitation	16
Puts 10 cubes in cup Solves round hole in reversed formboard Spontaneously scribbles with crayon Completes pegboard spontaneously	18
Obtains object with stick Solves square in formboard Builds tower of 3 cubes	21

(continued)

Table 1.8. *(continued)*

Milestone	Mean age of attainment (months)
Attempts to fold paper	24
Builds train of 4 cubes	
Imitates stroke with pencil	
Completes formboard	
Makes horizontal and vertical strokes with pencil	30
Solves 3-hole formboard rotated 180 degrees	
Folds paper with definite crease	
Builds train of 4 blocks with fifth block as smokestack in imitation	
Builds bridge of 3 cubes	36
Draws circle	
Names one color	
Draws a person with head plus one other body part	

Key: CAT, Clinical Adaptive Test (Accardo & Capute, 2005).

neurodevelopmental disability. The development of expressive language in the first few years of life is triphasic: prelinguistic vocalizations during the first year, verbalizations in the third year, and a transitional phase in the second year of life. This evolution is orderly and sequential and, therefore, susceptible to standardization (Table 1.10) and capable of yielding diagnostic predictability. Validity studies have correlated performance on the language component of the Capute Scales in infancy with later IQ score, language age, and development of communication disorders and learning disabilities. These associations strongly support the interpretation of prelinguistic vocalizations as neuromaturational markers for the entire neurodevelopmental disabilities spectrum.

Logically, expressive language cannot be more advanced than receptive language. Children should not be able to say more than they can understand. Thus, when receptive language is impaired, so is expressive language. This results in two common patterns of delayed language: 1) expressive language delay with mild to no receptive language impairment, and 2) combined expressive and receptive language delays. Pure receptive language disorders are found in adults with receptive aphasia, but their occurrence in the developing child is illogical. In a child with excellent rote memory and good auditory sequential skills, the illusion of expressive language that is superior to receptive language may result from memorized but inappropriately used language bits, or "scripted" speech. This pattern is most often observed in children with autism, severe communication disorders, and the "cocktail chatter" syndrome that can accompany hydrocephalus.

The neurodevelopmental assessment of language in infants and young children requires that both the parent and the examiner pay detailed attention to infant vocalizations. The one-way association between expressive and receptive skills can help in the assessment based on the coupling phenomenon. For example, not only is a vocabulary of 50 words associated with 2-word phrases (both expressive milestones), but a given age level for ex-

Table 1.9. Graphomotor milestones for ages 1–12

Age	Drawing skill
12 months	Marks with pencil
15 months	Imitates scribble
18 months	Scribbles spontaneously
26 months	Makes vertical/horizontal strokes
30 months	Imitates circle
36 months	Copies circle
40 months	Draws circle on command; draws cross
4 years	Draws square
5 years	Draws triangle
6 years	Draws horizontal diamond and Union Jack
7 years	Draws vertical diamond
8 years	Draws Greek cross
9 years	Draws cylinder
10 years	Draws transparent cube
12 years	Draws solid cube

Table 1.10. Expressive and receptive language milestones (CLAMS) for ages 2 weeks to 36 months

Expressive language milestones	Age (months)	Receptive language milestones
	0.5	Alert
Coo	1.5	Smiles
Ah-goo	4.0	Orients to voice
Razzing	4.5	
	5.0	Orients to bell I
Babbles	6.5	
	7.0	Orients to bell II
Dada/mama, nonspecific	7.5	
	9.0	Understands "no"
		Gestures
		Orients to bell III
Dada/mama, specific	11.0	Follows 1-step command with gesture
First word	11.5	
Immature jargon	12.0	
Second word	12.5	
Third word	13.0	
	14.0	Follows 1-step command without gesture
4–6 words	15.0	
Mature jargon	16.5	Recognizes five body parts
7–20 words	17.0	
	18.0	Points to one picture
		Recognizes eight body parts
2-word combinations	19.0	
2-word sentences	20.5	
50 words	21.0	Points to two pictures
Three pronouns, indiscriminately	24.0	
Three pronouns, discriminately	30.0	
250 words	36.0	
3-word sentences		
Gives age, sex, name		
Repeats three digits		

Key: CLAMS, Clinical Linguistic and Auditory Milestone Scale (Accardo & Capute, 2005).

pressive language requires receptive skills at or above that level.

Language must be clearly differentiated from articulation, and care must be taken not to penalize the assessment of a child's level of expressive language because of a significant disarticulation. A severe articulation disorder is sometimes associated with the early history or continued presence of an oral-motor problem evidenced by a feeding disorder, drooling, or occasionally a more generalized motor disorder, such as cerebral palsy. Language and ar-

ticulation are logically and clinically distinct in adults with aphasia but perhaps less so in children. It is certainly difficult to conceive how a child with delayed expressive language but age-appropriate articulation as well as receptive abilities can be suspected of having hearing loss as a major cause of the language delay.

The impact of hearing loss on language development varies with age and severity. Prelinguistic vocalizations are little affected by even severe hearing loss through about 9 months of age. After that time, vocalizations tend to decrease and the child with severe hearing impairment becomes quieter. Milder, intermittent hearing impairment has not been documented to slow language development significantly or to contribute to variable degrees of disarticulation. Recurrent otitis media in early childhood is probably unrelated to later learning disabilities. Some children with learning disabilities and a strong history of otitis media exhibit a perceptual-motor rather than a language-based learning disability pattern.

Expressive language delay is probably the most common developmental problem encountered in a general pediatric setting. When mild and accompanied by normal receptive language and problem-solving abilities, it represents either a mild communication disorder or an understimulating environment. When accompanied by a receptive delay, the level of problem-solving abilities becomes critical in distinguishing a mixed receptive-expressive language disorder from intellectual disability. When the differential diagnosis of a language delay in a 2-year-old is unclear, the most useful information to have available is a detailed history of prelinguistic vocalizations in the first year. It is not until the third year of life that the influence of the child's specific linguistic environment starts to become significant.

Somewhat more challenging than the differential diagnosis between communication disorders and intellectual disabilities is the discrimination of language disorders from emotional disorders. The two diagnoses frequently coincide. A psychiatric diagnosis is sometimes made when a language disorder is missed or improperly treated or when a psychiatric problem exists but is secondary to a language disorder and a result of the same underlying organic pathology. When a child is raised in a bilingual household, diagnosis of a language disorder becomes more difficult. The presence of bilingualism should not excuse the physician from attempting to identify the contribution of an underlying neurodevelopmental disability: Bilingual children are no less at risk for developmental disorders than other children and are entitled to accurate diagnosis and appropriate special services. Children of normal to superior intelligence have no difficulty acquiring a second language; children with cognitive, lan-

guage, and learning disorders exhibit problems with both languages.

Social-Adaptive Skills

Whereas motor milestones are almost entirely neuromaturationally determined and influenced only minimally by the environment, social behaviors and self-help skills depend heavily on environmental factors such as social expectations, parenting skills, education, and training. Patterns of social interaction and feeding and dressing behaviors are culturally diverse and largely do not reflect biological factors. In the face of wide diversity, the utility of social and adaptive milestones in the assessment of development is twofold. First, because they have cognitive and motor skill prerequisites and represent an amalgamation of certain problem-solving and language skills, social and adaptive milestones can be used for independent confirmation of the overall pattern yielded by the neurodevelopmental assessment. As useful as they may be in the detection and teasing out of significant discrepancies in a child's profile, however, such milestones should never provide the sole or main support for a developmental diagnosis. Second, in adults, a detailed description of social and adaptive behaviors is much more important to the developmental evaluation than any of the other streams of development or global IQ score in reflecting actual function and disability.

Social milestones are communicative in origin and represent the cumulative impact of language comprehension and problem-solving skills (Figure 1.4). Social behaviors might be considered the functional expression resulting

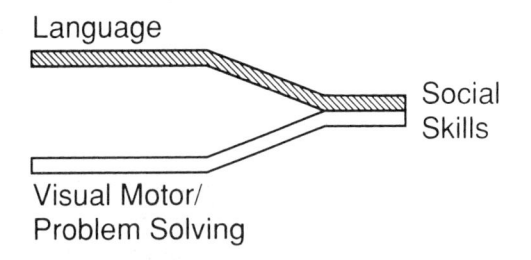

Figure 1.4. Social interactive and play skills represent a final common pathway for language and visual-motor/problem-solving skills, with an emphasis on the communicative aspect of the resultant adaptive behaviors.

from the interaction of these two streams of development. Some milestones that cross over from the language to the social arena include the social smile (4–6 weeks), parallel play (24 months), and group play (36 months). The development of interactive play obviously also requires visual-motor problem-solving skills and imitative behaviors. Moving from social milestones that are heavily loaded with communication prerequisites ("proper manners") toward milestones that are more concerned with self-help, one encounters purer "adaptive" skills or "activities of daily living" (Figure 1.5). These are represented by the typical feeding and dressing skills charted on many developmental checklists. A closer look at one important self-help skill, toilet training, helps clarify some of the difficulties in interpreting such behaviors.

The first hurdle in unraveling any given milestone is definition. Does toilet training refer to bowel control or bladder control, or both? To nocturnal control or diurnal control? To a certain frequency of accidents or none at all? The practitioner should note any discrepancy between maternal report and the presence or absence of diapers.

The range of ages reported for successful toilet training is wide. These ages tend to cluster around two means, 15 months and 33 months. One group of children tends to achieve toileting between 1 and $1\frac{1}{2}$ years; another tends to do so between $2\frac{1}{2}$ and 3 years. The rationale for this diphasic pattern becomes apparent through analysis of the prerequisites for toileting. The minimum requirements for toilet training are the ability to walk (gross motor), lower the pants (visual-motor), and follow one-step commands (receptive language). Typically developing children will have achieved all these milestones, along with sphincter control, by 18 months of age.

It would seem difficult to explain the almost 3-year cutoff for a large population of children, but the difference between the two groups reflects the children's learning environment. Those infants trained closer to 1 year need to be actively drilled by their caregivers; they are behaviorally reinforced to act out a functional pattern they do not understand. Those children who achieve toilet training closer to age 3 train themselves through a process of social imitation, with its requirement of a more advanced developmental level. Thus, the lower limit for toileting approaches a 1-year-old level; most older children with severe intellectual disabilities can be toilet trained even though their expressive language skills are preverbal. The upper age limit for toileting may be raised by deviant social expectations so that some children will arrive at kindergarten without having been toilet trained.

Parents may delay a child's achievement of self-help skills by "babying" the child. It should be noted that babying alone rarely accounts for severe developmental deficits, however. Parents may be reinforced in their inappropriate expectations by inadequate or incorrect child-rearing information. Parents of children with neurodevelopmental disabilities may offer dramatic overestimates or underestimates of their children's capabilities. In the presence of a disability, maternal denial and overprotection can severely restrict both the reliability and validity of parental reporting. Cross-cultural differences in areas such as weaning, toileting, and co-sleeping make the interpretation of self-help skills even more variable.

SPECTRUM AND CONTINUUM OF DEVELOPMENTAL DISABILITIES

In infants and young children, the neurodevelopmental assessment attempts to interpret both historic milestones and current developmental performance in light of the three fundamental processes of delay, dissociation, and deviance. The mapping of these three processes onto the six streams of development will generate the spectrum and the continuum of developmental disabilities. Neurodevelopmental

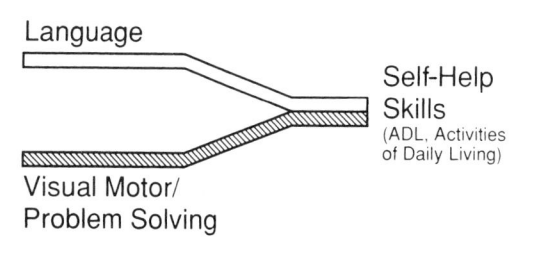

Figure 1.5. Self-help skills represent a final common pathway for language and visual-motor/problem-solving skills, with an emphasis on the motor aspects of the resultant activities of daily living.

pediatrics is concerned with applying the three phenomena of delay, dissociation, and deviance to the streams of development to generate a comprehensive developmental profile. Because, for an individual child, each of the streams of development are assessed by both observation and history, a temporal pattern emerges. In some cases, this pattern yields a specific diagnosis and prognosis. In other cases, the resulting profile markedly restricts the range of neurodevelopmental disabilities that must be considered and provides both clues and suggestions as to the follow-up and additional tests that will most likely complete the diagnostic evaluation. It cannot be stated too strongly that accurate neurodevelopmental assessment should precede other biomedical evaluations.

Most children presenting for developmental assessment have one specific stream of development highlighted. The *spectrum* of developmental disabilities (Table 1.11) includes the more common diagnostic categories that reflect the most prominent areas of functional delay. It is rare, however, for brain involvement severe enough to produce a significant delay in one area to affect only that single stream of development. The underlying *continuum* of cerebral dysfunction focuses on the wide range of associated dysfunctions that tend to occur in addition to the primary disorder. Even when a child with a disability fits the criteria for more than one neurodevelopmental disability, signs and symptoms relating to the other disorders listed in the continuum for which the child does not meet full diagnostic

criteria are often present. These remain unintelligible unless the contribution of the full continuum is taken into account.

One way to analyze this interaction might be to construct a grid in which primary developmental categories are cross-tabulated with their own milder manifestations and other neurodevelopmental symptoms (Figure 1.6). The primary neurodevelopmental diagnosis is often merely a marker for the much larger underlying continuum of CNS dysfunction. An alternative way to represent the interaction between the spectrum and the continuum is to generate other "iceberg" schemata for each specific neurodevelopmental disability (Figure 1.7).

The ability of the triangular pattern of the spectrum to be internally repeated for each of the major neurodevelopmental disabilities suggests that a simpler "inner continuum" or inner triangle can be used to categorize dissociation phenomena (Figure 1.8). These inner continua generate the dissociation and deviancy characteristic of each neurodevelopmental disability. In the same way that developmental delay is the target of primary care screening, assessment and interpretation of dissociation and deviance are properly the domain of neurodevelopmental pediatrics.

PATTERNOLOGICAL DIAGNOSIS

The application of the phenomena of delay and dissociation to the various streams of development allows a clear distinction of the patterns associated with each of the items on the neurodevelopmental disabilities spectrum (see Table 1.2). This represents patternological diagnosis at its broadest level; there are more subtle patternological differences among the disabilities on the spectrum. Although the pattern for each neurodevelopmental disability differs from the other patterns, it is interesting to note that, for each one that can be diagnosed in infancy, either gross motor or expressive language presents as delayed. Instead of attempting to screen all the major streams of development, the primary care pediatrician can more closely inspect these two areas, expanding to the others in the event

Table 1.11. The spectrum of developmental disabilities

Cerebral palsy

Intellectual disabilities

Communication disorders

  Central

    Language disorder

    Specific learning disability

    Autism

  Peripheral

    Hearing impairment

    Visual impairment

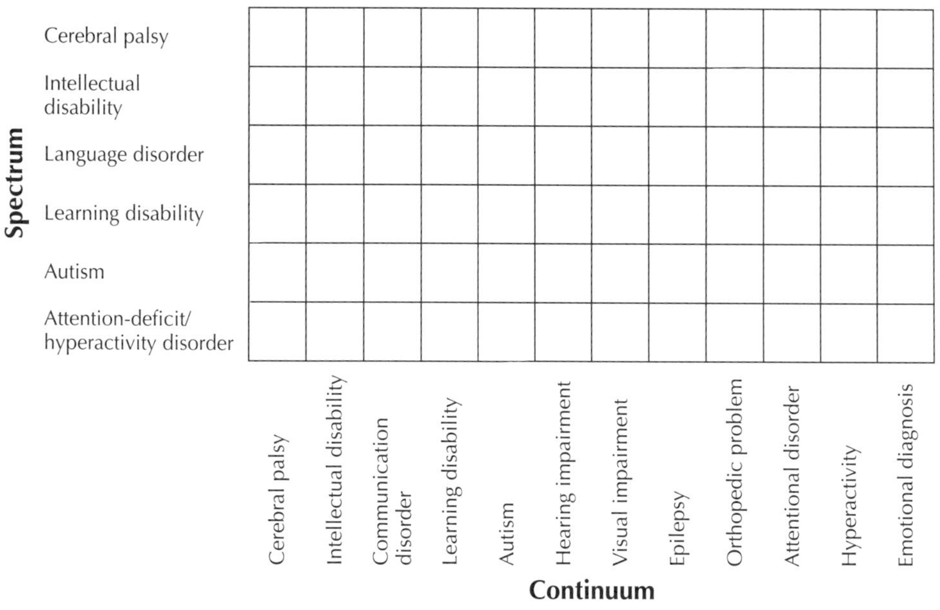

Spectrum

Cerebral palsy

Intellectual disability

Language disorder

Learning disability

Autism

Attention-deficit/ hyperactivity disorder

Cerebral palsy

Intellectual disability

Communication disorder

Learning disability

Autism

Hearing impairment

Visual impairment

Epilepsy

Orthopedic problem

Attentional disorder

Hyperactivity

Emotional diagnosis

Continuum

Figure 1.6. Interaction between the spectrum and the continuum of developmental disabilities.

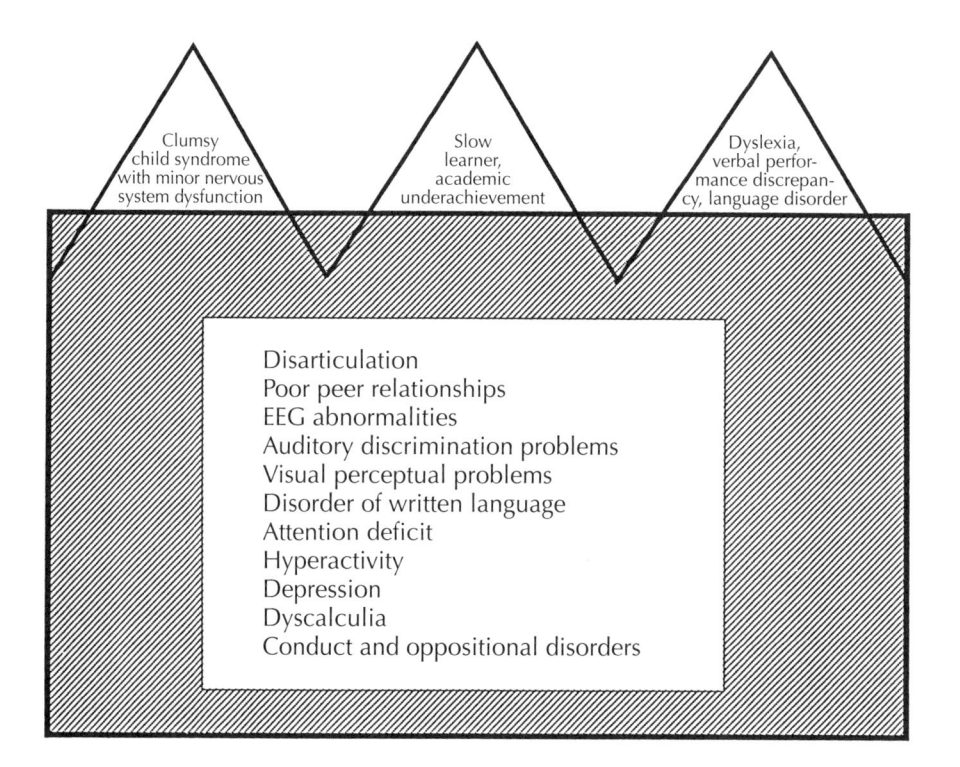

Clumsy child syndrome with minor nervous system dysfunction

Slow learner, academic underachievement

Dyslexia, verbal performance discrepancy, language disorder

Disarticulation
Poor peer relationships
EEG abnormalities
Auditory discrimination problems
Visual perceptual problems
Disorder of written language
Attention deficit
Hyperactivity
Depression
Dyscalculia
Conduct and oppositional disorders

Figure 1.7. Continuum of dysfunction applied to neurologically based specific learning disability. (*Key:* EEG, electroencephalographic.)

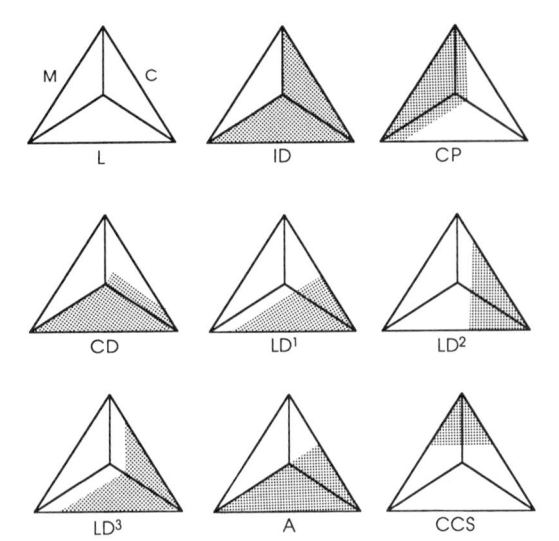

Figure 1.8. The inner continuum of developmental disabilities. Each diagram shows the impact of disability (shading) in the three primary areas of function: motor (M), cognitive (nonlanguage) (C), and language (L). (*Key:* A, autism; CCS, clumsy child syndrome; CD, communication disorder; CP, cerebral palsy; ID, intellectual disabilities; LD[1], language-based learning disability; LD[2], non–language-based learning disability; LD[3], language- and non–language-based learning disability.)

that a significant delay is noted in one of these two. By ignoring the "whole child" and focusing quite narrowly on these two developmental streams, a rapid and efficient screening for specific developmental diagnoses can be performed. Investigating all the streams in detail is of more use to confirm a diagnosis as well as provide information about the continuum of problems associated with a specific disability.

PEDIATRIC NEURODEVELOPMENTAL ASSESSMENT

The pediatric neurodevelopmental assessment is intended to identify markers for risk of later developmental problems, describe associated deficits and the range of neurodevelopmental behaviors, and formally diagnose the neurodevelopmental disabilities spectrum. Components of the assessment include a detailed developmental history, a review of previous testing, and physical examination with added focus on syndrome identification via both major and minor dysmorphic features, as well as an expanded neurological examination that

concentrates on subtle neurological signs (sometimes referred to as "soft signs") and quality of fine motor skills and gait. Direct observation and formal and informal testing of problem-solving behavior, graphomotor abilities, language usage, reading and mathematics abilities, and general cognitive processing are critical to allow the practitioner to reach a diagnosis and interact effectively with other professionals participating in patient assessment and management.

As in all medical diagnosis, a meticulous history usually provides the greatest contribution to the final neurodevelopmental diagnosis. Especially when details about milestone achievement in infancy are required, mothers remain a more accurate source of information on development than fathers. When there is any concern about maternal reliability, the history can be supplemented by interviewing grandparents and other relatives as well as alternative caregivers, such as baby sitters and teachers. Baby books, home movies and videos, and dated photographs can provide additional documentation. A number of historical factors are commonly associated with neurodevelopmental disability diagnosis. It is imperative to interpret them as relating to the entire range of disability rather than to any single specific diagnosis or an artificial quantitative cutoff, such as IQ score.

Prematurity and its associated complications represent one of the most important historical contributors to the incidence of developmental disabilities. As the degree of prematurity increases, birth weight declines, and the duration of ventilatory support lengthens, the risks for both an increased incidence and greater severity of neurodevelopmental disability rise proportionally. Although even at the lower limits of viability many premature infants escape major disability, this population exhibits a sharp increase in the prevalence of learning and language disorders—the new morbidity of minor neurological dysfunction or disorders of higher cortical function.

Overall, modern neonatal intensive care technology does not appear to be increasing the prevalence of disabilities. Rather, the incidence curve appears to be shifting: Some infants who decades ago would have died in the newborn period with severe disabilities are now being helped to survive with moderate disability, and other infants who decades ago would have survived with moderate disability are now being allowed by the same technology to achieve developmental normality. Thus, the overall incidence of neurodevelopmental disabilities appears relatively unchanged to the practicing clinician. The major fluctuations that have been noted would seem to result more from redefinition and refined diagnostic sensibility.

The surge in diagnoses of pervasive developmental disorders, including autism, is the most prominent example of such fluctuation. Previously, reclassification by the American Association on Mental Deficiency in 1973 of those individuals with IQ scores in the 70–85 range as having borderline intelligence rather than borderline mental retardation reduced the prevalence of mental retardation from 16% to 3%. Currently, there is little agreement on the incidence of learning disorders and attentional problems, with estimates for each of these disorders ranging from 2% to 15%. Neither of these conditions would have been diagnosed 50 years ago. It is not unreasonable to suggest that their observed incidence may continue to increase but that their true incidence will probably remain stable.

Another factor associated with increased risk for neurodevelopmental disability is a history of meningitis, severe head trauma, or brain surgery. It is troubling to encounter a child with a history of shunt revisions whose family has been led to believe that, as long as the latest shunt is working, their child's brain is not at risk. Pediatric neurosurgical procedures represent a significant risk for neurodevelopmental disability.

Failure to thrive (FTT) in infancy and early childhood is a complex syndrome with symptoms of disordered growth, development, and behavior. Regardless of specific etiology, the mere occurrence of FTT in infancy places the child at higher risk of exhibiting a neurodevelopmental disability. FTT often reflects one end of the spectrum of child abuse, and in general all the diagnoses in this category (sexual abuse, physical abuse, deprivation, neglect, malnutrition, emotional abuse, and parenting by adults with intellectual disabilities) are associated with an increased incidence of neurodevelopmental disabilities, especially in language, in both the children and the adults involved. The widely accepted correlation between socioeconomic variables (including homelessness and foster care) and the occurrence of the various types of child abuse often merely reflects the impact of underlying parental neurodevelopmental disabilities that have been misdiagnosed, mistreated, or simply never identified.

The major contribution of the spectrum–continuum concept is the idea that all of the characteristic variables associated with a specific neurodevelopmental disability are in varying degrees also correlated with all of the other disabilities on the entire spectrum–continuum. For example, although different levels of lead exposure in childhood can be causally associated with later intellectual disabilities, ADHD, and learning disabilities, plumbism has also been implicated in the development of autism. Toe walking, long recognized as a puzzling behavioral phenomenon common in early infantile autism, has been suggested as a nonspecific marker for language disorders. Microcephaly (a head circumference greater than 1.5 standard deviations below the mean for a given age), especially when severe, has been related to intellectual disabilities; however, it is also associated with learning disabilities and language disorders.

Microcephaly is also included in a standardized group of minor malformations (hypertelorism, low-set/rotated pinnae, high-arched palate, geographic tongue, electric hair, unusual hair whorl pattern, abnormal palmar creases, short curved fifth fingers, syndactyly, and sandal gap deformity of the toes) that have been related specifically to the early identification of hyperactive children but that also seem to relate more generally to the entire spectrum of disabilities. Minor malformation patterns combine with major organ system malformations to help identify genetic and congenital disorders; however, it must be remembered that the developmental implications of most genetic disorders remain inadequately worked out. For example, fragile X syndrome is associated not only with varying degrees of intellectual disabilities but also with autistic behaviors. Neurofibromatosis is associated with a low incidence of intellectual disabilities (approximately 10%) but a much higher incidence of learning disabilities and ADHD.

The model for chronic CNS impairment at the severe end of the spectrum also applies to the mild end of the spectrum. Professionals who work with children with learning disabilities often feel uncomfortable with the description of a delay in reading as "reading retardation"—intellectual disabilities isolated to the specific area of reading acquisition—yet, using this term might suggest that the two delay phenomena are not fundamentally and structurally different and could contribute to each other's understanding. Recognition of an underlying etiological unity between these two conditions as implied by the spectrum–continuum concept allows cross-fertilization of diagnostic perceptions and therapeutic research lessons, and facilitates the discovery of learning disabilities, language disorders, autistic features, and mild cerebral palsy syndromes in people with intellectual disabilities. Recalling the major categories of brain dysfunction will readily suggest the striking degree to which milder expressions of cerebral involvement are frequently associated with severe expressions

relating to other CNS functional areas (Table 1.12).

The details of the neurodevelopmental assessment have been alluded to in this chapter and are much expanded in later chapters. More than most other professionals, the neurodevelopmental pediatrician places a high value on a meticulous review of the earliest milestones (especially language), regardless of the child's age. As the child gets older, the assessment moves toward incorporating psychological instruments, either directly or indirectly. The reading of these test results by the neurodevelopmental pediatrician may differ from the psychologist's interpretation of the same data. The broader holistic neurodevelopmental pediatrics perspective allows a more comprehensive integration of relevant information than that afforded by other disciplines.

ASSOCIATED DEFICITS: CEREBRAL PALSY AS THE PARADIGM FOR THE SPECTRUM OF DEVELOPMENTAL DISABILITIES

Both therapeutically and prognostically, the continuum of neurodevelopmental disabilities dominates the spectrum of disabilities. In other words, the associated deficits often reveal more about the severity of the disability and the likelihood of various outcomes than does the pri-

Table 1.12. Functional expression of different degrees of central nervous system dysfunction

Affected area	Severe expression	Mild expression
Cognition	Intellectual disabilities	Borderline intelligence Slow learner
Motor abilities	Cerebral palsy	Clumsy child syndrome Benign cerebral hypotonia Soft neurological signs
Language	Aphasia Autism	Developmental disorders of language (expressive/receptive) and articulation
Perception	Developmental dyslexia Reading retardation Deafness Blindness	Learning disability Hearing impairment Vision impairment
Electrical activity	Epilepsy	EEG abnormalities without clinical seizures
Morphology	Major organ system malformation Chromosomal disorder Genetic syndrome Malformation syndrome	Dysmorphic features Microcephaly

Key: EEG, electroencephalographic.

mary diagnosis. Thus, in cerebral palsy, motor impairment is rarely the most disabling aspect of the disorder. Other effects of diffuse brain damage—intellectual disabilities, cognitive impairment, learning and language disorders, attentional problems, central visual and auditory processing problems, and seizure disorders—often outweigh the impact of the motor disorder.

In the same way, the most limiting aspect of intellectual disabilities is not the cognitive aspect but the societal aspect. There is nothing inherently disabling about being a 10-year-old who has the intellectual abilities of a 5-year-old. It is the unmet expectations of the significant adults in the life of the child with intellectual disabilities—parents, teachers, and the larger society, which demand a given level of production and consumption on the part of each social unit—that create the disability status.

With neurologically based learning disabilities, the focus is almost exclusively on academic difficulties and the need to determine and obtain the most appropriate classroom supports and interventions; yet, the most significant disabilities these children face as adults include social maladjustment, personality disorders, and other deficits in human interrelationships, which tend not to be addressed by current intervention strategies.

The tendency to focus inappropriately on spectrum diagnosis to the exclusion of the underlying continuum limits creation of a truly comprehensive habilitation program. The most practical way of resisting this trend is to consider the paradigm for neurodevelopmental disabilities, the disorder with the greatest potential to exhibit all aspects of chronic brain damage: cerebral palsy. Cerebral palsy, the most common severe motor disability in children, is frequently associated with the entire range of CNS dysfunctions. Neurobehaviorally, cerebral palsy can serve as a guide through, for example, the labyrinth of learning disabilities. It is difficult, if not impossible, to go as far starting with any disability other than cerebral palsy. If the six streams of development are collapsed into two—motor and central processing (Figure 1.9)—and the spectrum of disabilities that can be generated from these streams of development (Figures 1.10 and 1.11) is exam-

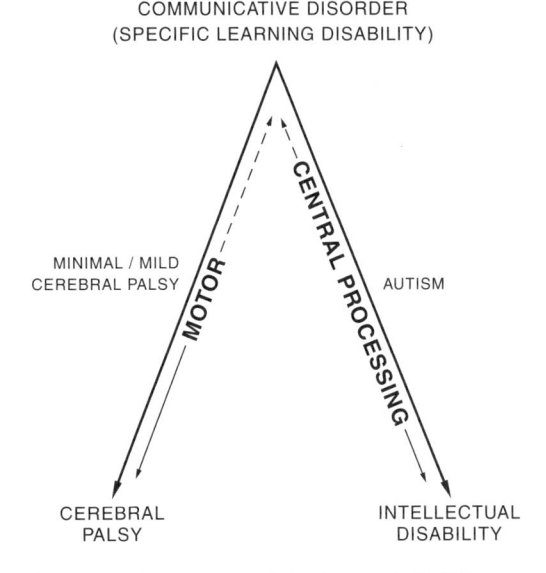

Figure 1.9. The spectrum of developmental disabilities expressed by two streams of development: motor and central processing.

ined, the result is the full spectrum (Figure 1.12).

FUNDAMENTAL TENETS OF NEURODEVELOPMENTAL PEDIATRICS

1. The etiology for neurodevelopmental disabilities is some form of central neurological damage, brain pathology, or organic cerebral deficit; however, behavioral symptomatology can identify these as neurological disorders even in the absence of classic neurological findings. In other words, behavioral and cognitive as well as subtle motor signs can confirm their CNS origin.

2. A neurodevelopmental disability reflects an underlying static encephalopathy, a lesion that is permanent and chronic. Thus, children with neurodevelopmental disabilities rarely arise de novo but evolve from infants with neurodevelopmental disabilities. Similarly, although some degree of adaptation is not unusual (and is the desired and expected goal of educational and other interventions), for the most part children with neurodevelopmental disabilities grow up to be adults

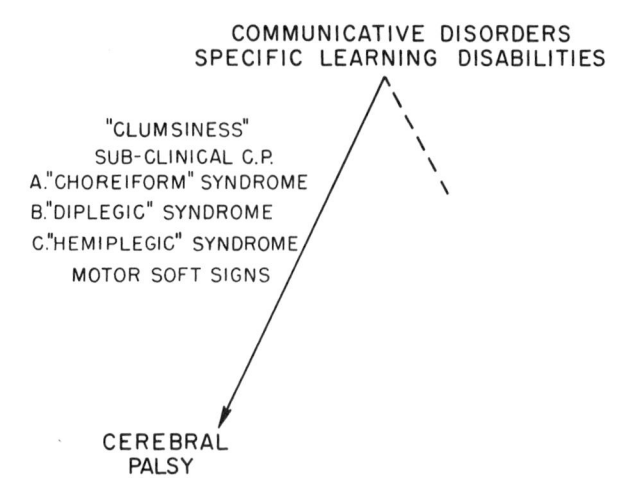

Figure 1.10.   The motor development portion of the spectrum of developmental disabilities. (*Key:* C.P., cerebral palsy.)

with neurodevelopmental disabilities. Neurodevelopmental disabilities represent lifelong differences, although not necessarily lifelong handicaps.

3. The screening and assessment of neurodevelopmental disabilities in infants and young children is the proper domain of pediatrics. The fundamental limitation inherent in any screening program is the lack of appreciation by professionals of the natural history of the disabilities for which they are screening.

4. Any strict segregation between high-severity, low-incidence neurodevelopmental disabilities (cerebral palsy, intellectual disabilities) and low-severity, high-incidence disabilities (learning disabilities, ADHD) is potentially misleading. Neurodevelopmental pediatrics interprets learning disability and ADHD as

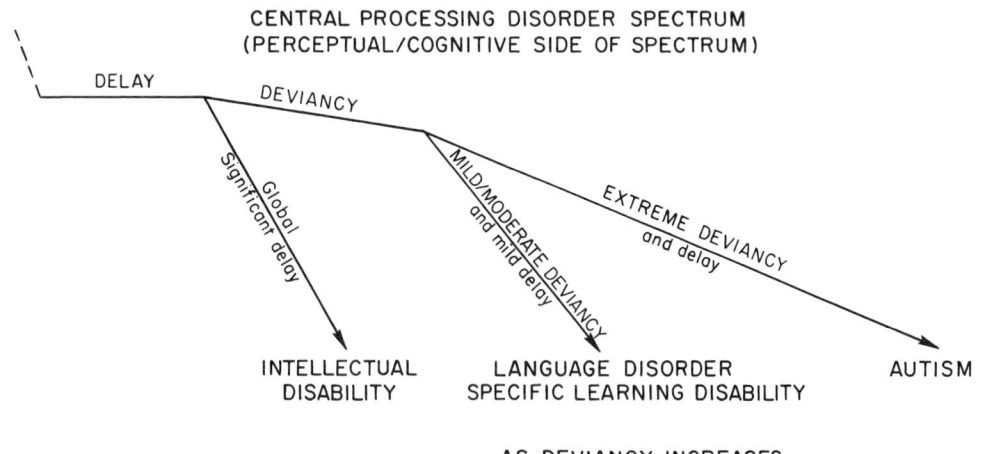

Figure 1.11.   The central processing development portion of the spectrum of developmental disabilities.

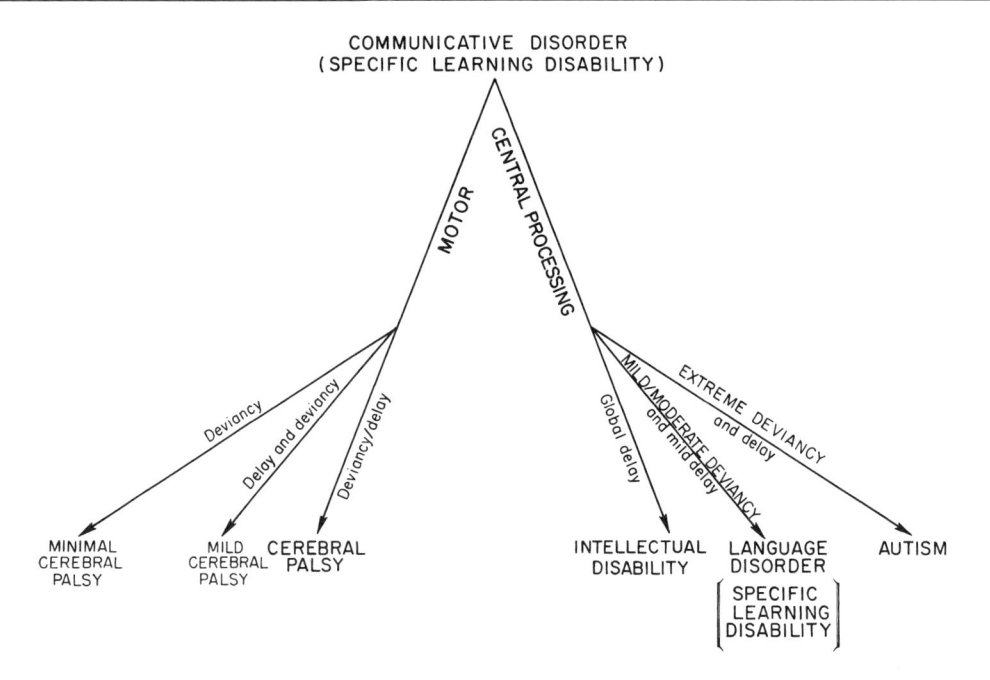

Figure 1.12. The full spectrum of developmental disabilities.

milder variants of intellectual disabilities and cerebral palsy. To conclude that, because learning disability and ADHD appear to be more amenable to environmental and behavioral modifications, they are therefore somehow less organic is inaccurate.

5. As with all pathology, the milder forms of neurodevelopmental disabilities are much more common than the most severe cases. Epidemiologically, the prevalence of the more common milder forms is thus also much more likely to overlap the prevalence of confounding variables that contribute to, result from, or are associated with the primary CNS insult.

6. A child's assessment cannot be reduced to or summarized by a single number, such as an IQ or DQ score. The developmental pattern is better described by a series of quantifiers reflecting the major streams of development: gross motor, fine motor, problem solving, expressive language, receptive language, and social-adaptive skills. In the older child, strengths and weaknesses in these quantifiers may be reflected in psychometric subtest scatter and unevenness in the profile of the child's learning skills.

7. Neurodevelopmental disabilities in children are best interpreted as occupying varying positions on both a spectrum and a continuum of chronic neurological handicaps.

8. An analysis of the three fundamental developmental pediatric processes of delay, dissociation, and deviance best explains the nature of and relationships among the various diagnostic entities subsumed under the neurodevelopmental disabilities continuum and spectrum. It is crucial to attempt to clarify the relative contribution of each of these processes to the presenting neurobehavioral symptomatology of each child.

9. Current research supports the primacy of genetic etiologies rather than perinatal and obstetric factors. Although improvements in the quality and quantity of obstetric and perinatal care continue to receive high priority, it is unlikely that the incidence of neurodevelopmental disabil-

ities will change significantly as a result of developments in these areas.

10. By failing to focus on the fixed organic nature of neurodevelopmental disabilities, professionals involved in the care of children with disabilities and the counseling of their families contribute to the parental perception that, if only they had employed different child-rearing techniques, the child's diagnosis or eventual outcome would have been radically different. Failure to emphasize the organic component tends to leave parents in a heightened and prolonged state of anxiety because the professional declines to venture a diagnosis or prognosis until multiple interventions have been tried. Such a delay in diagnosis is rarely appreciated by families, particularly in the case of a genetic syndrome in an infant whose family is left unaware of the possibility of recurrence.

11. There are no medically effective therapies to cure neurodevelopmental disabilities. The major effective therapeutic modalities for these conditions lie in the realm of education, along with modification of family and social expectations. There are, however, medical interventions that can be classified as preventive, ancillary, or peripheral and that can have significant impact on the comprehensive management of the child.

12. Neurodevelopmental pediatrics does not seek to in any way downplay the importance of emotional, familial, sociocultural, economic, and cross-cultural influences on normal and abnormal child development. The neurodevelopmental practitioner must heed, follow, and contribute to research on the influence of such factors. Such factors, however, remain a secondary responsibility, just as organic factors remain of secondary importance to the nonmedical professional working with children with neurodevelopmental disabilities.

CONCLUSION

Adult brain models do not apply to infancy in any clinically meaningful manner, yet it is in this earliest period that parents begin to note delays and become concerned about what to do about them. Screening tests corroborate the parental perception of delay but do not include any organized approach for interpreting or investigating such delays. Even in older children, the neuropsychology and localization studies of learning disabilities remain at a fairly primitive level, with much conflicting evidence and no generally accepted model.

Screening for the early diagnosis of milder and more subtle patterns of neurodevelopmental disabilities is further hampered by a lack of both information on their natural history and even cross-disciplinary agreement on diagnostic criteria. Refinement of diagnostic techniques and increased sensitivity to the multiple presentations and problems that neurodevelopmental disabilities can exhibit require novel epidemiological studies.

Therapy issues remain even less clear than diagnostic ones. There are no effective cures for neurodevelopmental disabilities. There are several preventive techniques whereby conditions such as cretinism (hypothyroidism), phenylketonuria, and certain hyperammonemia syndromes can be treated by hormone supplementation or dietary manipulation. Neurosurgical procedures for hydrocephalus, optimal medical management of bacterial meningitis, and rigorous environmental control of lead exposure are other examples of ways in which the impact of disease on the developing CNS can be minimized, with later and less effective intervention being associated with increasing degrees of irreversible brain damage. There is no medication, surgery, or physical or educational training that can restore damaged brain tissue to normal function. There do exist, however, medical and nonmedical interventions that can lessen the impact of this damage, treat associated deficits, and facilitate learning response to normal experiences. The limitations of treatment contribute to parental frustration and make unorthodox therapies, such as dietary manipulations, appear valid. Scientific illiteracy and the will to believe contribute to parental projection onto even standard treatments of curative powers that they do not have. The long-term ineffectiveness or even negative impact of a number of widely accepted interventions is only beginning to be appreciated.

The diagnosis of brain damage on the basis of deviations from a normal pattern of milestone behavior, whether quantitative or qualitative deviance and however broad the range of normal, represents a radical departure from the philosophical underpinnings of 20th-century behavioral science. Human nature is viewed as limited and definable (if not defined), and organic damage to its neurological substrate is interpreted as restricting in a predictable fashion the expression of human nature.

REFERENCE

Accardo, P.J., & Capute, A.J. (2005). *The Capute Scales: Cognitive adaptive test/clinical linguistic and auditory milestone scale (CAT/CLAMS).* Baltimore: Paul H. Brookes Publishing Co.

2

Human Brain Development

GEORGE T. CAPONE AND WALTER E. KAUFMANN

The brain is unquestionably the most complex organ in the human body. Its proper development and maturation are necessary for the acquisition of the full repertoire of integrated functions and behaviors that make us human. More than any other organ, the brain demonstrates enormous cellular and biochemical heterogeneity, which is necessary to support the full range of highly specialized functions it performs. Changes in gross morphology associated with brain development have been documented for well over a century. Much less, however, is known about the biochemical and molecular events that result in these changes. The biological processes contributing to brain development are enormously complex, and the underlying mechanisms that regulate these events are rather stringently controlled. Despite this complexity, the basic strategy utilized in constructing the brain is remarkably well conserved among higher organisms and mammalian species in particular. Studies of human autopsy material have contributed substantially to our understanding of the morphological and cellular changes that occur during development. They also provide a unique opportunity to correlate neuropathological changes with clinical descriptions of the acquisition and development of function and behavior. In contrast, most of our understanding of dynamic biochemical and molecular mechanisms has been derived largely through the use of animal models.

A detailed understanding of brain development has emerged largely during the past four decades. Many of the central questions of developmental neurobiology were originally formulated toward the end of the 19th century.

These questions, which focus on "major developmental events," were set forth by Cowan (1979) and are outlined as follows:

1. How are the various cellular components of the nervous system generated?

2. How do these cells come to occupy their definitive location within the brain?

3. How do separate neuronal and glial cell lines become established?

4. How do neurons in different regions of the brain establish their connections?

5. How do neurons acquire their distinctive morphological, physiological, and biochemical properties?

It would be impossible to give an account of developmental processes throughout the entire brain without becoming overwhelmed by details; therefore, this chapter focuses on one region, the cerebral cortex, and its connections. Unarguably, it is this structure more than any other region that endows us with our uniquely human capacities and frailties. A great deal is already known about the fine structure and development of the cerebral cortex in humans and related species. It is hoped that, by focusing on a single region, it will be possible to integrate information derived from numerous sources to construct a more comprehensive picture of brain development. Equally important is the recognition that cerebrocortical system dysfunction probably accounts for many of the clinical signs and symptoms seen in children with chronic neurodevelopmental disability. Contemporary neuroscience is now well positioned to address complex questions of cognitive-genetics, -evolution and -dysfunction, including causes of individual variation, as major research themes in coming decades. Undoubtedly, the regulatory mechanisms subserving higher cognitive function and conserved across the millenia of primate evolution are waiting to be discovered through the careful study of cerebrocortical development.

BRAIN DEVELOPMENT: A CONCEPTUAL FRAMEWORK

Our conceptual understanding of brain development has been greatly enhanced by the introduction of terminology that denotes discrete time periods that are critical for the continued progression of normal development. Conceptually based terminology, when misused, often contributes to confusion, which results in ambiguity or oversimplification of ideas rather than clarification. The concepts of *critical periods* and *sensitive periods* grew out of work in experimental embryology, teratology, and later behavioral neurobiology. Erzurumlu and Killackay (1983) defined a critical period as "the time during which the action of a specific external or internal condition or stimulus is required for the normal progress of development" (p. 208). In contrast, a sensitive period is defined as "the time period in development during which the nervous system is highly susceptible to the effects of harmful internal or external conditions" (p. 208).

Major Developmental Events

The developmental organization of the brain is the result of a multitude of heterogeneous yet remarkably well-orchestrated processes involving complex molecular biochemical and cellular mechanisms, each operative over a distinct time period in various regions of the brain. These organizational events occur in a highly ordered sequence for which proper timing is critical, each process being dependent to some degree on the outcome of related preceding events. The mechanisms that control these processes are highly regulated during ontogenesis and are under stringent genetic control. Throughout the development of the mammalian brain and the cerebral cortex in particular,

critical periods do not necessarily occur as discrete events, separable from one another by distinct beginning and end points. Rather, there is considerable overlap between successive critical periods, with the outcome of later events being significantly influenced by each of the preceding events.

Much of the information regarding the major events in human brain development was first summarized and presented with exceptional clarity by Volpe (2001). These events are summarized in Table 2.1. Cowan (1992) has further subdivided the period of neuronal organization in the mammalian brain to include morphological, physiological, and molecular differentiation; acquisition of positional information; axonal pathfinding; target recognition; synaptogenesis; synapse turnover and elimination; and cell death. Clearly, organizational events are immensely complex and may be best conceptualized as consisting of numerous interdependent critical periods occurring either concomitantly or in rapid succession. The details of the organization period, however, remain to be defined in humans.

Disturbances of Brain Development

Malformation of the developing brain remains a significant cause of severe intellectual disabilities (defined as an intelligence quotient [IQ] score < 50), cerebral palsy, and developmental disability worldwide. Epidemiological studies have indicated that prenatal factors are of

Table 2.1. Major events in human brain development

Major developmental event	Peak occurrence
Dorsal induction	3rd–4th wk prenatal
Ventral induction	5th–6th wk prenatal
Neuronal proliferation and programmed cell death	2nd–4th mo prenatal
Neuronal migration	3rd–5th mo prenatal
Neuronal differentiation and organization	
Synaptogenesis	6th mo–3 yr
Initial pruning	3–5 yr
Secondary reorganization	Adolescence
Myelination	6th mo–3 yr . . . 30 yr

This article was published in Neurology of the Newborn, Fourth Edition, J.J. Volpe, Copyright Elsevier 2001.

major etiological significance in a large percentage of cases of severe intellectual disabilities (McLaren & Bryson, 1987). Pathological studies indicate that a large percentage of cases of severe intellectual disabilities are associated with structural-anatomical malformation of the brain (Warkany, Lemire, & Cohen, 1981d). In their review of the topic, Warkany et al. stated,

> Understandably, medical research tends to emphasize combating mental retardation by prevention of the immediate causes, with reliance on perinatal and neonatal measures. Although such an expedient approach is commendable, it must be realized that the hardcore of severe mental retardation will persist even after solution of perinatal and neonatal problems. . . . The bulk of the problem is teratologic, and the causes of severe mental retardation are similar to those of congenital malformation in general: mutant genes, chromosomal anomalies and prenatal environmental teratologic factors. (1981d, p. 3–4)

A *primary malformation* refers to an anomaly resulting from a perturbation of developmental events resulting in failure of an anatomical structure to be formed and is distinguished from a *secondary malformation,* which results from the breakdown of a previously formed structure as a result of a destructive event (e.g., vascular insult, infection). Although many cases of primary brain malformation are causally related to specific genetic and chromosomal disorders, major congenital anomaly/intellectual disability (MCA/ID) syndromes, or exposure to a known teratogen, in a large number of instances a specific etiology cannot be determined despite recent progress.

This chapter cannot review disturbances of brain development and malformation in a comprehensive fashion, so the interested reader is referred to the excellent monographs by Warkany et al. (1981d), Volpe (2001), and Barkovich (2005) for further details regarding the prevalence, pathogenesis, and associated clinical aspects of malformation.

Neuroembryological Classification: All Things Reconsidered

Rapid scientific progress during the past two decades is revolutionizing our understanding of the molecular mechanisms controlling major developmental events, and the etiological mechanisms responsible for disorders of neurodevelopment (Sarnat, 2005). As the molecular genetic basis for these disturbances becomes more firmly established, the existing morphologically based terminology and classification scheme is challenged to remain functionally meaningful. The development of a new, more comprehensive nomenclature seems inevitable. Sarnat and Flore-Sarnat (2004) have proposed an etiological classification of central nervous system (CNS) malformation, based on *patterns of gene expression,* that incorporates both morphological and genetic criteria yet retains the flexibility necessary to account for acquired (nongenetic) causes as well. An expanded classification system based on *genetics and magnetic resonance imaging (MRI) morphometry* has also been advanced (Barkovich, Kuzniecky, Jackson, Guerrini, & Dobyns, 2005). The molecular genetic basis of malformation is discussed in several reviews, which are recommended reading (Clark, 2004; Sarnat, 2005; Tanaka & Gleeson, 2000).

EMBRYONIC BRAIN DEVELOPMENT

During the embryonic period (4–8 weeks' gestation), the flat trilaminar embryonic disc is transformed into a nearly cylindrical embryo as the general body plan begins to emerge (Moore & Persaud, 1993). By the end of this period, known as *organogenesis,* each of the major organ systems, including the brain and spinal cord, has been established.

Dorsal Induction (Third to Fourth Week of Gestation)

The process of *neurulation,* during which the primordial nervous system begins to form along the dorsal aspect of the embryo, is nearly complete by the end of the fourth week postconception. At about 18 days' gestation, the *neural plate* develops from a thickened area of embryonic *ectoderm.* The neural epithelium of the neural plate forms in response to the inductive influence of the underlying *mesoderm.* Both the *notochord* and the *paraxial mesoderm* exert an irreversible inductive influence on the overlying ectoderm. Under the continuing influence of the notochord and paraxial mesoderm, the lateral margins of the neural plate begin to elevate to form the *neural folds.* The forces necessary to create the appearance and deformation of the neural folds are generated by microtubules and microfilaments arranged within the neural epithelium itself (Karfunkel, 1974). The fusion of the neural folds begins toward the end of the third week of gestation. Fusion begins initially at what corresponds to the cervical region of the spinal cord and then proceeds "zipper-like" in both caudal and rostral directions until the *neural tube* is completely closed (Figure 2.1). The opening at cephalic end of the neural tube, or *anterior neuropore,* remains patent until approximately 24 days, whereas the caudal-most *posterior neuropore* closes at approximately 26 days (Volpe, 2001).

Initially, the neural tube resembles a straight pipe with its solid cylindrical wall and hollow lumen. The lumen of the tube eventually becomes the brain ventricles and central canal of the spinal cord. The wall of the neural tube can be thought of as having three dimensions: length, radius, and circumference. Changes in the longitudinal and circumferential dimensions result in regional subdivision of the CNS. Continued development along the radial dimension results in the distinctive laminar pattern specific to each region of the brain (Nowakowski, 1987).

Central Nervous System Segmentation

Segmentation of the neural tube along its longitudinal axis is fundamentally the most important stage in the early transformation of the developing brain. The position of each cell within the longitudinal and radial axes of the neural tube will determine to which one of the five embryonic vesicles it will belong. Specific subclasses of genes, many responsible for transcriptional regulation, are critical in determining the pattern and regional boundaries between adjacent vesicles (Kammermeier & Reichert, 2001) (Table 2.2).

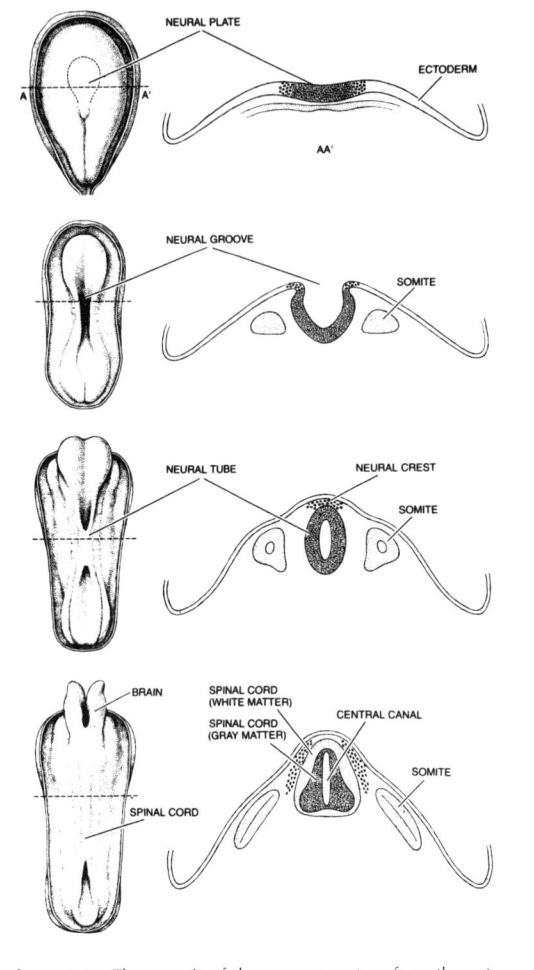

Figure 2.1. The genesis of the nervous system from the ectoderm, or outer cell layer, of a human embryo during the third and fourth weeks after conception is represented in these four pairs of drawings, which show an external view of the developing embryo (*left*) with a corresponding cross-sectional view at the level of the future spinal cord (*right*). The central nervous system begins as the neural plate, a flat sheet of ectodermal cells on the dorsal surface of the embryo. The plate subsequently folds into a hollow structure called the neural tube. The cephalic end of the central canal widens to form the ventricles of the brain. The peripheral nervous system is derived largely from the cells of the neural crest and spinal cord. (From Cowan, W.M. [1979]. The development of the brain. *Scientific American, 241,* 114, 1979; reprinted by permission.)

Embryonic Brain Vesicles

The brain is derived from the anterior-most portion of the neural tube, and the middle and posterior portions form the spinal cord. Even before the closure of the anterior neuropore on day 24, the cephalic region of the neural tube begins to expand rapidly. By Day 25, the three *primary embryonic brain vesicles,* each separated by a groove, have formed. These three brain vesicles are referred to as the *prosencephalon* (forebrain

Table 2.2. Regional specification and segmentation of the embryonic brain

Spatial gradient	Brain region	Gene(s)	Function
Anterior-posterior neuraxis	Hindbrain and spinal cord: HOXB	Homeotic (HOX) genes: HOXA, HOXB, HOXC, HOXD	Transcription factor
Anterior-posterior neuraxis	Forebrain and midbrain: all	Cephalic head (GAP) genes: OTX1, OTX2, EMX1, EMX2	Transcription factor
Entire neuraxis	Forebrain and midbrain: PAX6	Paired-box homeotic (PAX) genes: PAX2, PAX3, PAX5, PAX6, PAX7, PAX8	Transcription factor
	Midbrain and hindbrain: PAX3, PAX7		
	Hindbrain: all others		
Dorsal-ventral neuraxis	Cortex and basal ganglia	Fibroblast growth factor 8 (FGF8)	Diffusible morphogens
		Wingless-type MMTV integration site family (WNT)	
		Bone morphogenetic protein (BMP)	
		Sonic hedgehog (SHH)	

Sources: Gotz and Sommer (2005); Kammermeier and Reichert (2001); Shimogori, Banuchi, Ng, Strauss, and Grove (2004); and Urbach and Technau (2004).

vesicle), the *mesencephalon* (midbrain vesicle), and the *rhombencephalon* (hindbrain vesicle) (Moore & Persaud, 1993). By Day 32, the prosencephalon and the rhombencephalon begin to divide in two while the mesencephalon remains a single cavity. This results in five *secondary embryonic vesicles* (Figure 2.2). The prosencephalon divides into the *telencephalon* and the *diencephalon* while the rhombencephalon divides into the *metencephalon* and the *myelencephalon*.

Ventral Induction (Fifth to Sixth Week of Gestation)

Induction along the anterior-most ventral aspect of the embryo influences formation of both the face and forebrain structures. The *pre-*

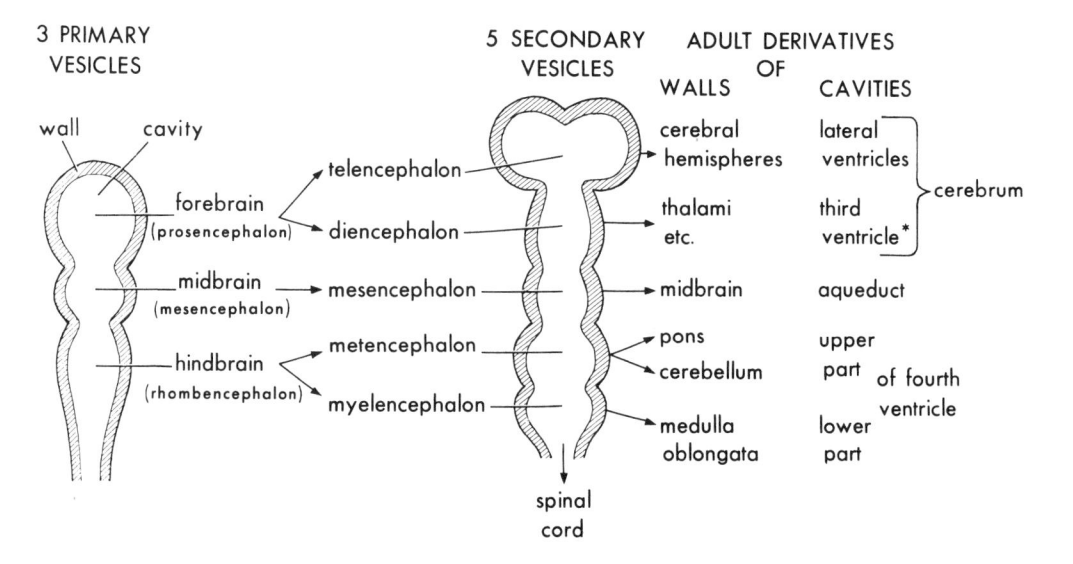

Figure 2.2. Diagramatic sketch of the brain vesicles indicating the adult derivatives of their walls and cavities. (This article was published in The Developing Human, Fifth Edition, K. Moore & T.V. Persaud, p. 401, Copyright Elsevier 1993.)

chordal mesoderm interacts with the developing forebrain vesicle to initiate cleavage through the prosencephalon. Cleavage along the horizontal plane results in paired optic vesicles, olfactory bulbs, and tracts. Separation between telencephalic and diencephalic structures results from cleavage in the transverse plane. Finally, the paired cerebral vesicles, basal ganglia, and lateral ventricles form as a result of cleavage along the sagittal plane. This process occurs during the fifth and sixth weeks of gestation. Thus, the basic structural subdivisions of the adult brain are formed by the end of the first 6 weeks of gestation.

Neurodevelopmental Disorders of Induction and Segmentation

Primary disturbances of dorsal induction result in errors of neural tube closure. The morphological appearance and clinical severity of these conditions depend on the timing and specific location of the resulting lesion. The two most common errors of dorsal induction, which affect the brain primarily, are *anencephaly* and *encephalocele* (Table 2.3).

Anencephaly results from the failure of the anterior portion of the neural tube to close by 24 days' gestation (Lemire, Beckwith, & Warkany, 1978). Prosencephalic structures are more severely affected than diencephalic, midbrain, or hindbrain regions. This defect is incompatible with life.

Encephalocele is a more restricted disorder resulting from failure of the anterior portion of the neural tube to close by 26 days' gestation. Typically, this occurs in the occipital region and less often in the frontal regions of the brain (Warkany, Lemire, & Cohen, 1981a). Many cases are complicated by hydrocephalus or other congenital abnormalities. Intellectual disabilities, motor deficits, or both are common.

Primary disturbances of ventral induction are the result of impairments in the interaction between the prechordal mesoderm, the face, and the developing prosencephalic vesicle. Typically, these disturbances are characterized by involvement of the eyes, nose, and mouth, which often result in a rather striking facial appearance (DeMeyer, Zeman, & Palmer, 1964). The disorders most characteristic of disturbances of ventral induction are the *holoprosencephalies* (see Table 2.3). This heterogeneous group of disorders results from failure of one or more of the cleavage planes to develop within the prosencephalon by the sixth week of gestation. The hallmark of the holoprosencephalies is severe midline dysgenesis and failure to form distinct telencephalic, dience-

Table 2.3. Disorders of segmentation and dorsal and ventral induction

Disorder	Termination period	Gene(s)	Function
Telencephalic segmentation			
Schizencephaly	2 months of gestation	Empty spiracles-like protein (*EMX2*)	Transcription factor
Dorsal induction			
Anencephaly	24 days of gestation		
Encephalocele	26 days of gestation	Collagen XVIII alpha-1 polypeptide (endostatin) (*COL18A1*)	Heparan sulfate proteoglycan
Ventral induction			
Holoprosencephalies	5th–6th weeks of gestation	Sonic hedgehog (*SHH*)	Diffusible morphogen
		Zinc finger cerebellar expressed-2 (*ZIC2*)	Transcription factor
		Sine oculis transcription factor-x3 (*SIX3*)	Transcription factor
		Transforming growth factor-β interacting factor (*TGIF*)	Transcription factor
		Also trisomies 13 and 18	

Sources: Clark (2004); Dubourg, Lazaro, Blayau, Pasquier, and Duron (2003); Kinsman, Plawer, and Hahn (2000); and Tanaka and Gleeson (2000).

phalic, and olfactory structures. The morphological appearance depends on the stage of maturation reached prior to the developmental arrest (Leech & Shuman, 1986). In the most severe form, there is a single cerebral vesicle with a common ventricle. The thalamus and basal ganglia are fused at the midline, and the corpus callosum and septum are usually absent. MRI is useful in determining the extent of prosencephalic dysgenesis and further classification into anatomical subtypes. Neurological symptoms are readily apparent during the neonatal period in those individuals who survive to birth. Infants may exhibit seizures, apneic episodes, and failure to regulate body temperature. Cognitive and motor development is usually profoundly impaired (Hahn & Pinter, 2002; Kinsman, Plawer, & Hahn, 2000).

A group of related disorders also representing midline prosencephalic dysgenesis includes *septo-optic dysplasia, agenesis of the corpus callosum,* and *agenesis of the septum pellucidum* (Leech & Shuman, 1986) (Table 2.4). Leech and Schuman proposed that these disorders constitute a spectrum of anomalies resulting from dysgenic alteration within the midline structures of the prosencephalon. They conceived of the midline as composed of a series of independent but closely related segments that interact during development. MRI is particularly helpful in diagnosing this related group of disorders and has provided important infor-

mation regarding their association with other congenital malformations of the brain (Barkovich, 2005).

Schizencephaly had previously been considered a disorder of migration but is now considered a result of disordered segmentation whereby primordial cells destined to become part of the cortex fail to form. It is characterized by complete agenesis of a part of the cerebral wall, resulting in a thickened cortical mantle with deep seams or clefts (Granata, Freri, Caccia, & Setola, 2005). The cortex surrounding the clefts is frequently associated with large neuronal heterotopia and microgyria. The deficit may be unilateral or, more often, bilateral. MRI is helpful in determining the extent of schizencephaly (Barkovich, 2005) (see Table 2.3).

ENCEPHALIZATION AND FORMATION OF THE CEREBRAL CORTEX

After about the fourth or fifth week, the brain begins to grow quite rapidly. In higher mammals and especially humans, the growth of the telencephalic structures is particularly striking and is often referred to as *encephalization.* As the paired telencephalic structures expand to form the cerebral hemispheres, growth is in a rostral-to-caudal direction, eventually covering the deeper structures of the brain.

Table 2.4. Disorders of related midline structures

Disorder	Termination period	Gene(s)	Function
Agenesis of septum pellucidum	6th weeks of gestation		
Septo-optic dysplasia	6th–7th weeks of gestation	Homeobox-containing, embryonic stem cell t-conscription factor-X (*HESX1*)	Transcription factor
Agenesis of corpus callosum	4th–5th months of gestation	Solute carrier family 12 member 6 (*SLC12A6*)	Ion transport K⁺/Cl⁻ protein
		GLI-Krumppel family member 3 (*GLI3*)	Transcription regulator
		Aristaless-related homeobox (*ARX*)	Transcription factor
		Paired-box homeotic gene 6 (*PAX6*)	Transcription factor
		Zinc finger homeobox-1B (*ZFHX1B*)	Transcription factor

Sources: Dattani, Martinez-Barbera, Thomas, Brickman, and Gupta (2000); Elson, Perveen, Donnai, Wall, & Black (2002); Free et al. (2003); Howard, Mount, Rochefort, Byun, and Dupre (2002); Kato, Das, Petras, Kitamura, and Morahashi (2004); Sarnat (2005); and Sztriha, Esponosa-Parrilla, Gururaj, and Amiel (2003).

Throughout gestation, the size of the hemispheres and width of the cerebral wall continue to expand. The cortex forms its characteristic pattern of *sulci* and *gyri* as it continues to acquire an increasing complement of neurons and glia (Figure 2.3).

By the end of the embryonic period, the basic outline and form of the CNS is complete. As the fetal period begins, dramatic growth is occurring in the radial dimension of the brain vesicles. Most of the discussion here now focuses on the events occurring in the wall of the telencephalic vesicle from which the cerebral cortex arises. The cerebral cortex is one of the most remarkable products of our evolutionary history. The framework for this highly laminated structure emerges early in development. It is remarkable that, in spite of the astounding number of neurons and glia residing in the cortex, these cells are actually generated outside the cortex itself, often at considerable distance from their final location in the mature brain.

The cerebral cortex is not a homogeneous structure. Most classification schemes attempt to subdivide the mature cortex into distinct regions based on differences in cell size, shape, and arrangement that, although functionally important, are of little use in trying to understand its developmental history. A more suitable classification scheme based on develop-

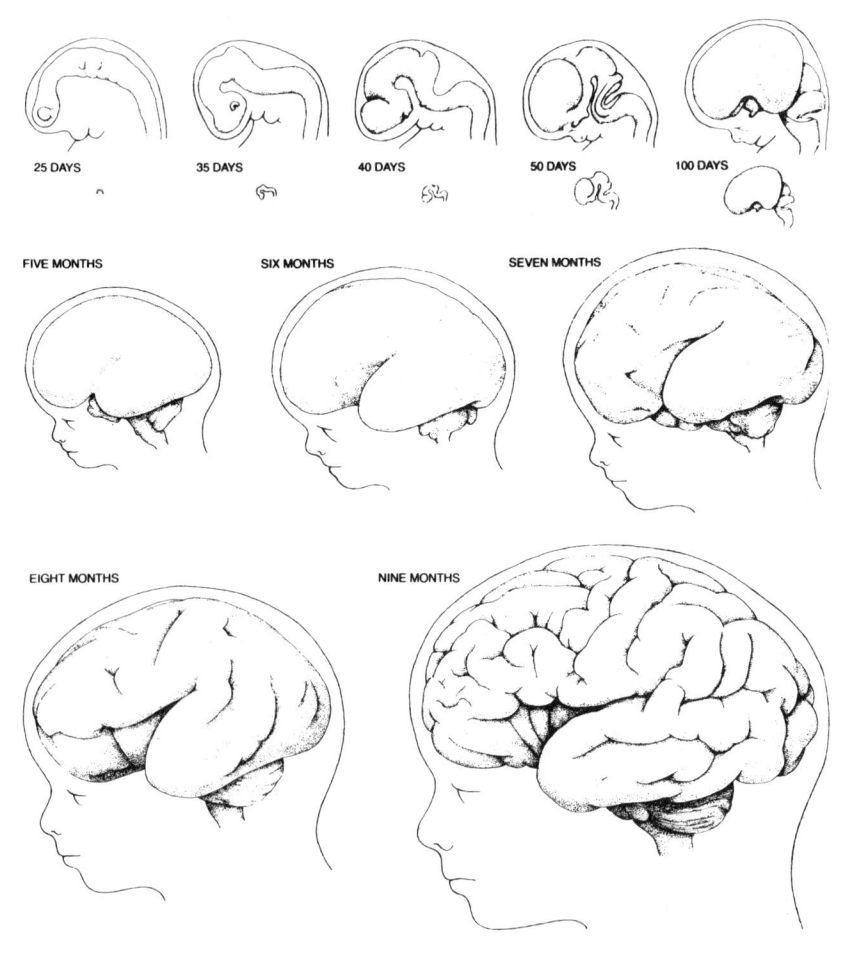

Figure 2.3.   The developing human brain is shown from the side in this sequence of drawings, which show a succession of embryonic and fetal stages. The first five embryonic stages are shown enlarged to clarify their structural details (*top*). The three main parts of the brain (forebrain, midbrain, and hindbrain) originate as prominent swellings at the cephalic end of the neural tube. In human beings, the cerebral hemispheres eventually overgrow the midbrain and the hindbrain and also partly obscure the cerebellum. The characteristic pattern of gyri and sulci on the brain surface do not begin to appear until about mid-gestation. (From Cowan, W.M. [1979]. The development of the brain. *Scientific American, 241,* 116; reprinted by permission.)

mental criteria was established by Filimonoff (1947). According to this scheme, *neocortex* comprises the cortical territory having all four fundamental embryonic zones and in addition a cortical plate. *Allocortex* refers to regions where the fundamental embryonic zones are incomplete and the structure and appearance of the cortical plate are quite variable. The *periallocortex* is characterized by a special type of transitional structure that forms the boundary between neocortex and allocortex. Accordingly, the cerebral cortex of the adult human brain is 95.5% neocortex and 4.5% allocortex (Rakic & Goldman-Rakic, 1982).

NEURONAL PROLIFERATION (SECOND TO FOURTH MONTH OF GESTATION)

Estimates of actual neuron number in the adult human cortex are technically difficult to establish. Investigators had previously estimated the total number of neurons in both cerebral hemispheres to be between 10 and 18 billion (Blinkov & Glezer, 1968). The total number of glial cells is estimated to be nearly 10 times greater. Regulatory mechanisms that determine the total number of neurons generated include the number of stem cell precursors, the length of the cell cycle, and the duration of neuron generation (Cowan, 1979). Stereological techniques have allowed for revised estimates of cell number and distribution in various gray matter structures as a function of development and aging. Thus, the total number of cells in the telencephalic wall of the human newborn is estimated at 32.6 billion, and the total number of neurons within the cortical plate is estimated to be 19.8 billion (Larsen, Larsen, Bogdanovic, & Laursen, 2006).

Early Proliferation (Second Month of Gestation)

Until about 6 weeks' gestation, the neural tube consists of a single layer of pseudostratified columnar neuroepithelium. These cells occupy the *ventricular zone* (VZ), immediately adjacent to the lumen of the neural tube, and are referred to as *ventricular cells*. Prior to neurogene-

sis, the pool of neural progenitor cells rapidly expands through successive rounds of symmetrical (proliferative) division that gives rise to two daughter progenitor cells (Haydar, Ang, & Rakic, 2003). Virtually 100% of the ventricular cells are actively proliferating, which results in a geometric increase in cell number during this period. Differential rates of cell proliferation within the dorsal and ventral compartments provide the forces necessary to transform the neural tube from a linear structure of uniform diameter into the primary and secondary vesicles, with their characteristic flexures and curvatures.

Later Proliferation (Second to Fourth Month of Gestation)

The peak period of neuronal proliferation in the cerebral cortex occurs between the second and fourth months of gestation. Quantitative studies of cell proliferation in the human forebrain show that the rate of proliferation increases exponentially through the first half of gestation (20 weeks) and continues into the second and third years postnatally before leveling off (Dobbing & Sands, 1970, 1973). Most neurons are produced by asymmetrical (neuronogenic) cell division, which yields two daughter cells of different fates, one neuron and one neural progenitor (Haydar et al., 2003; Noctor, Martinez-Cerdeno, Ivic, & Kriegstein, 2004). There are two distinct phases of proliferative activity in the forebrain. The first occurs between 10 and 20 weeks and is thought to represent the major period of *neuroblast* production. Most *pyramidal neurons* in the cerebral cortex are generated during this time. A second proliferative phase begins at 4–5 months postnatally and is associated with glial genesis. Certain glial subtypes can continue to multiply for several years postnatally. Smaller *interneurons* follow their own distinct time course compared with pyramidal neurons because they originate in a different proliferative compartment, the ganglionic eminence, located in the ventral telencephalon (Molnar, Metin, Stoykova, & Tarabykin, 2006).

The Fundamental Embryonic Zones

Both neuronal and glial stem cell precursors are actively dividing within the VZ at the earliest stages; however, these cells eventually become committed exclusively to either neuronal or glial lineage (Levitt, Cooper, & Rakic, 1981). As newly created postmitotic neuroblasts begin their journey out of the VZ, they come to occupy a new position in the *intermediate zone* (IZ), which is located just below the *marginal zone* (MZ). In this way, the telencephalic wall is transformed into four embryonic cell layers. These layers are classified according to their own special terminology because they lack a direct counterpart in the adult brain (Angevine et al., 1969). Beginning from the inner-most lumenal surface and moving radially outward toward the pial surface (which does not reflect the sequence of their appearance in development), they are the VZ, the *subventricular zone* (SVZ), the IZ, the *subplate* (SP), and the MZ (Figure 2.4).

Nearly all cell proliferation takes place in the VZ and SVZ, which constitute the primary sites of neuroblast production. Early-generated postmitotic neuroblasts begin to differentiate as they pass through the intermediate zone to form the SP, and later generated neuroblasts migrate through the SP to form the *cortical plate* (CP). The cells of the CP give rise to the familiar six-layered structure of the adult cerebral cortex. Neurons within the SP continue to differentiate, mature, and maintain their position

because they are destined to influence the future connectivity of the cerebral cortex. The MZ, which is largely devoid of cell bodies, will eventually accommodate the axonal and dendritic terminals of developing neurons and serve as a "synaptic field" within the most superficial cortical layer.

Neurodevelopmental Disorders of Neuronal Proliferation

Primary disturbances of neuronal proliferation result in too few or too many neurons being produced. The disorders that best represent the two extremes of dysfunctional cell proliferation are *micrencephaly* and *megalencephaly*. The molecular pathogenesis of these disorders is discussed in recent reviews (Crino, 2005; Woods, Bond, & Enard, 2005) (Table 2.5).

Micrencephaly refers to a heterogeneous group of disorders characterized by reduced brain size and weight (Warkany, Lemire, & Cohen, 1981e). Typically, individuals with micrencephaly manifest *microcephaly* (small head circumference), defined as greater than 2 or 3 standard deviations below the mean for age and sex; however, these terms are not synonymous, and not all cases of micrencephaly represent a true primary disturbance of neuronal proliferation. It is far more common to have

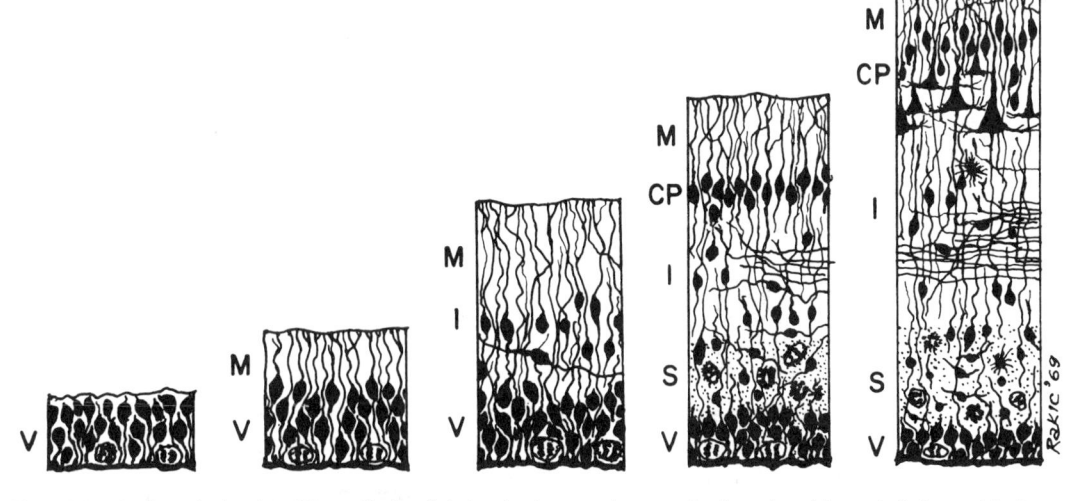

Figure 2.4. A schematic drawing of the cerebral wall during development demonstrating formation of the cortical plate and the four fundamental embryonic zones. (From Anatomical Record, Vol. 166, No. 2, 1970, page 258. Copyright © 1970 John Wiley & Sons, Inc. Reprinted with permission of John Wiley & Sons, Inc.) (*Key:* CP, cortical plate; I, intermediate zone; M, marginal zone; S, subventricular zone; V, ventricular zone.)

Table 2.5. Disorders of proliferation

Disorder	Termination period	Gene(s)	Function
Micrencephaly (primary) or autosomal recessive	4 months of gestation	Microcephalin (*MCPH1*)	Cell cycle control and telomorase regulation
		Cyclin-dependent kinase 5 regulatory subunit–associated protein 2 (*CDK5RAP2, MCPH3*)	Centrosomal microtubule production
		Abnormal spindle-like microcephaly-associated (*ASPM, MCPH5*)	Microtubule and spindle organization
		Centromeric protein J (*CENPJ, MCPH6*)	Regulation of microtubule nucleation and depolymerization
Megalencephaly	4–5 months of gestation	Nuclear receptor SET domain containing gene 1 (*NSD1*)	Chromatin-mediated transcriptional regulation

Sources: Bond and Woods (2006); Sarnat (2005); and Woods, Bond, and Enard (2005).

micrencephaly in association with other primary disturbances of brain development or secondary to an intrauterine or postnatal destructive lesion. Such cases are best considered secondary micrencephaly. Primary micrencephaly, or micrencephaly vera, is usually associated with genetic or chromosome abnormalities, MCA/MR syndromes, maternal toxic-metabolic disorders, or intrauterine exposure to a known CNS teratogen. This condition may be caused by decreased neuronal proliferation or increased cell death during the peak period of neurogenesis, resulting in cellular depletion and a smaller brain. Genetic forms of micrencephaly appear to result from mutation in genes controlling cell cycle and mitotic spindle organization (Bond & Woods, 2006).

In cases of isolated micrencephaly, without other associated malformations, neurological deficits may not be present during infancy, although minor abnormalities of the eyes, ears, nose, and scalp are common. Nonfocal, minor motor impairments are common, although severe motor impairment or seizures are usually not observed. There is considerable variation in the level of cognitive function attained by people with micrencephaly. Caution should be exercised when issuing a developmental prognosis early in life (Rossi et al., 1987).

Megalencephaly refers to a widely heterogeneous group of disorders characterized by increased brain size and weight (Warkany, Lemire, & Cohen, 1981c). Individuals with megalencephaly always manifest *macrocephaly* (large head circumference), defined as 2 or 3 standard deviations above the mean for age and sex. Megalencephaly is known to occur in a variety of forms and is associated with several genetic, chromosomal, endocrine, and overgrowth syndromes. Attempts to classify megalencephaly are anything but straightforward. Most classification schemes have attempted to distinguish between *hypertrophy* of the brain resulting from increased size of neural and glial elements and *hyperplasia* resulting from an increased number of neurons or glia. Megalencephaly occurring within the context of a more generalized endocrine or metabolic disorder is sometimes distinguished as a distinct category. Generally megalencephaly involves both hemispheres, but cases of hemimegalencephaly, in which only one hemisphere is overdeveloped, are seen.

DeMeyer (1986) proposed an etiological-pathogenic classification scheme that recognizes two basic forms of megalencephaly: metabolic and anatomic. Metabolic megalencephaly includes those brains enlarged because of an accumulation of normal or abnormal metabolic product within the cell. Anatomic megalencephaly includes those brains enlarged because of an increase in cell number or size and most closely represents primary megalencephaly. In bilateral megalencephaly, the brain may be increased one and one half to two times normal in the newborn period. MRI is useful in determining the extent of hemispheric involvement and the presence of associated neuromigrational disturbances (Barkovich, 2005).

In severe cases of megalencephaly, intellectual disabilities, motor impairment, and seizures may be present (Dekaban & Sakuragawa, 1977). In less severe cases, specific learning disabilities, language impairments, and minor neuromotor problems may be the only indication of neurological dysfunction. There are also familial forms of anatomical megalencephaly that are not associated with frank neurodevelopmental impairment (Day & Schutt, 1979). Such benign forms are a diagnosis of exclusion, and the term *benign megalencephaly* should be reserved for those individuals who meet very specific criteria (DeMyer, 1986).

NEURONAL MIGRATION (THIRD TO FIFTH MONTH OF GESTATION)

Migration refers to those events related to the mass movement of neurons from their birthplace in the germinal zone to their ultimate destination, where they will reside permanently. The peak period of neuronal migration in the cerebral cortex occurs between the third and fifth months of gestation (Sidman & Rakic, 1973). These events transform the four fundamental embryonic layers of the telencephalic wall into the familiar six-layer structure of the adult cerebral cortex. Neuronal migration occurs in several distinct trajectories within the telencephalic wall: radially (straight-out), tangentially (across-then-out), or diagonally (across-and-out) (Figure 2.5). The cellular and molecular mechanisms of neuronal migration are discussed in several reviews (Gressens, 2006; Kanatani, Tabata, & Nakajima, 2005; McManus & Golden, 2005).

The Subplate

Early-generated neuroblasts will differentiate as they migrate radially through the IZ and come to reside in the SP. Neurons within the SP undergo morphological maturation as they

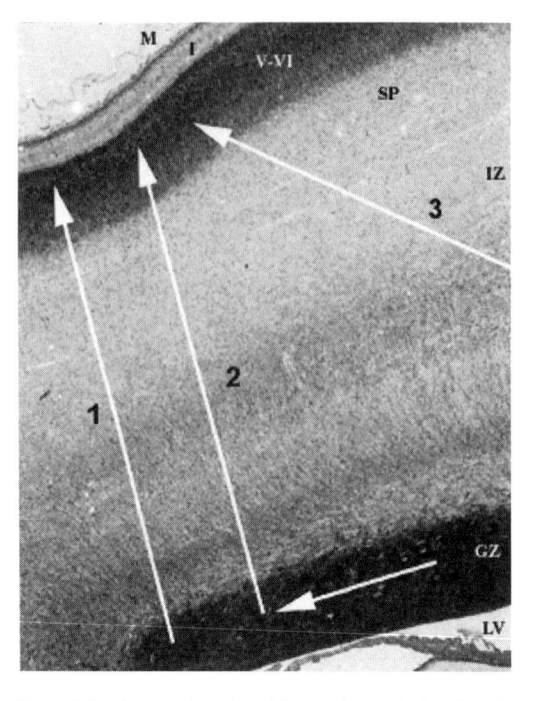

Figure 2.5. A coronal section of the cerebrocortical wall at the 15th prenatal week showing a schematic representation of the different migratory pathways adopted by neuroblasts. *1,* Radial migration along radial glial cells of neuroblasts originating in the GZ (germinal zones). *2,* Tangential migration of neuroblasts within the GZ followed by radial migration along glial guides. *3,* Tangential migration in the IZ (intermediate zone) of neuroblasts originating in the ganglionic eminence (From Gressens, P. [2000]. Mechanisms and disturbances of neuronal migration. *Pediatric Research, 48*(6), 726; reprinted by permission.)

begin to express several biochemical markers (neuropeptides, neurotrophins, and γ-aminobutyric acid [GABA]) characteristic of this cell population. These SP neurons are thus poised to orchestrate the directionality and positioning of ingrowing afferent fibers originating from the thalamus and striatum.

The Cortical Plate

The CP begins to appear between the seventh and tenth weeks of gestation as the result of neuroblasts migrating radially outward from the VZ and SVZ, through the IZ and SP, and then condensing within the CP. The SP, the CP, and remnants of the MZ are transformed into the adult cerebral cortex. Although some neurons continue to migrate into the CP during the third trimester, essentially the cerebral cortex acquires its full complement of neurons by the end of the fifth month. Two predominant "waves" of neuronal migration to the CP occur at 8–10 weeks' and 11–15 weeks' gestation (Sidman & Rakic, 1973). The earliest generated neurons occupy the deep cortical layers, and those generated later in gestation come to reside in more superficial layers. Thus, the cerebral cortex is constructed in an "inside-out" sequence.

Cellular Mechanisms of Neuronal Migration

Early in the formation of the CP, when the distance from the VZ is relatively short (100 microns), neurons appear to migrate by an ameboid mechanism whereby the neuron is propelled forward in a radial direction. The ability of the neuron to selectively attach, detach, and contract its cytoplasmic processes is dependent on the integrity of various components of the cytoskeletal matrix, composed of microtubules and microfilaments, and the signaling molecules regulating cytoskeletal dynamics.

Later in gestation, as the cortical plate thickens, the telencephalic wall measures up to 6,000 microns in width, a distance 10 times the length of the fully extended leading process (Sidman & Rakic, 1973). The presence of *radial-glial* cells provides a preferred substrate for larger neurons and facilitates migration by serving as a "guidewire" that establishes a direct radial trajectory to the outermost layer of the CP (Figure 2.6). It has been observed that multiple neurons generated in the same region of the VZ will most often choose the same radial glia fiber along which to migrate. Such *cell–cell interactions* demonstrate the selective binding affinities exhibited by migrating neurons for glial fibers as well as the extracellular matrix (Lambert de Rouvroit & Goffinet, 2001). The distinct migrational trajectory of smaller neurons originating from within the ganglionic eminence may employ novel cellular and molecular mechanisms versus those used by the pyramidal neurons (Metin, Baudoin, Rakic, & Parnavelas, 2006). Interneurons appear to use the corticofugal axonal system of the developing cortex as a scaffold for their migration into the cortex (Parnavelas, 2000).

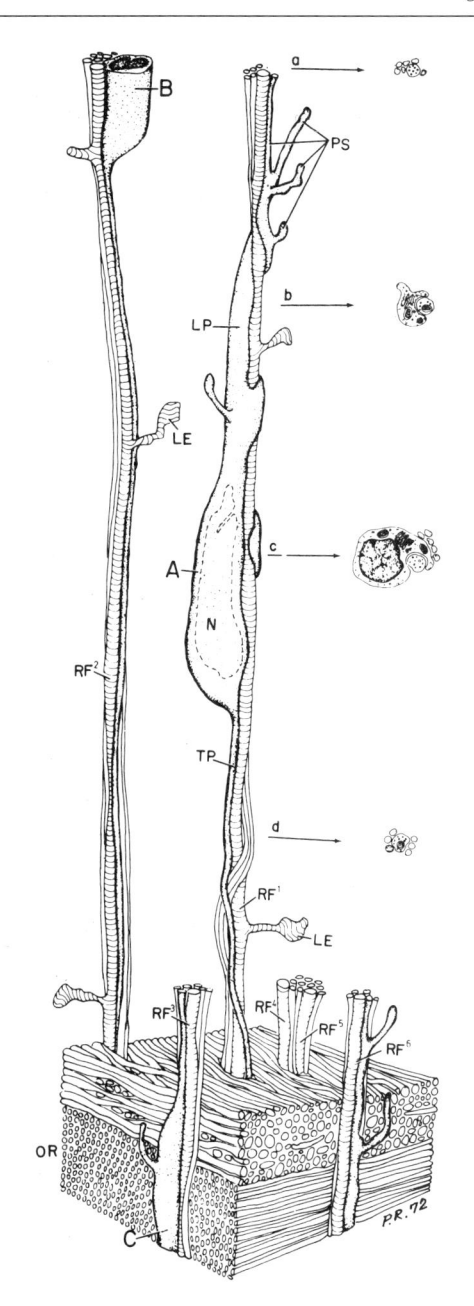

Figure 2.6. A three-dimensional recontruction of migrating neurons, based on electron micrographs from semiserial sections. Note the close apposition between the migrating neuron (A), its radial glial fiber (RF), the voluminous leading process (LP), and the attenuated trailing process (TP) of the migrating neuron. Cross sections of neuron A in relation to the several vertical fibers in the fascicle are drawn at levels a–d to the right of the figure. (This article was published in Brain Research, 62, R.L. Sidman & P. Rakic, Neuronal migration, with special reference to the developing human brain: A review, p. 10, Copyright Elsevier 1973.)

Functional Specificity within the Cerebral Cortex

Functionally distinct regions of the neocortex are often distinguishable based on differences in cytoarchitecture; there is a rather long and distinguished history of research into this aspect of cortical function. Most cartographers of the human neocortex have produced extensively detailed parcellations of cortical regions based on variations in cell number and packing density, as well as variation in cell type and cortical laminae (Kemper & Galabruda, 1984). Mountcastle (1979) has advanced the view that the *intrinsic* organization of the neocortex is more similar than different and that cytoarchitectonic differences between different regions reflects differences in their pattern of *extrinsic* connections. He postulated that cytoarchitectural differences in particular areas reflect the grouping together of vertically oriented *cortical columns* that are linked together by specific sets of input–output connections. These columns, then, make up the basic functional or *physiological unit* of information processing and distribution within the cortex. Rakic's radial-unit hypothesis attempts to explain the grouping of cortical (ontogenetic) columns to form functionally distinct regions, as arising from neighboring proliferative units that produce cohorts of related neurons (Rakic, 1988). These cohorts are thought to contain a certain amount of area-specific competence prior to their arrival in the CP. The identity of neurons within an ontogenetic column is then modified further by afferent connections arriving from ipsilateral and contralateral cortex as well as from the thalamus (Figure 2.7).

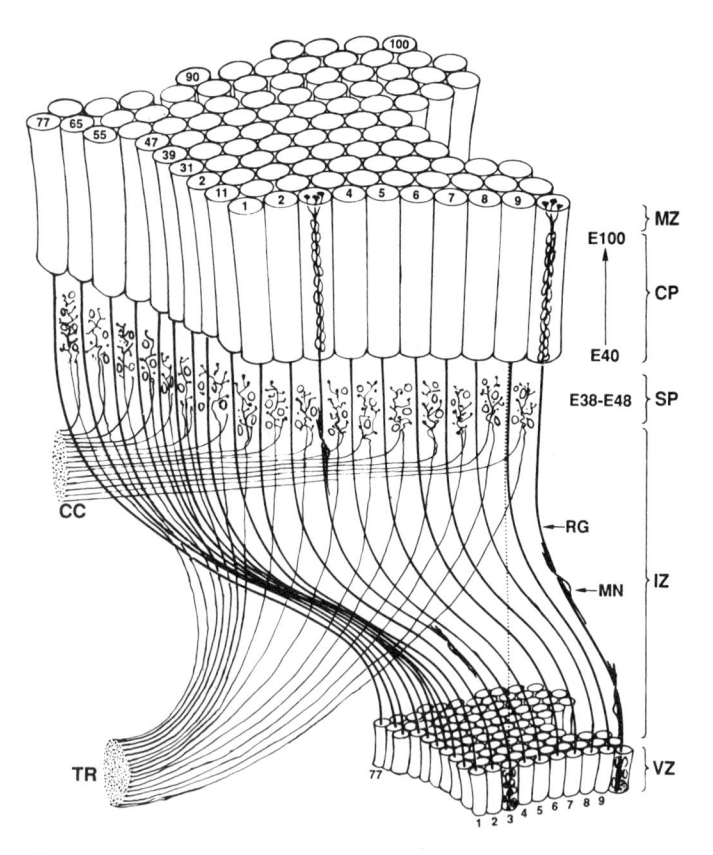

Figure 2.7. The relation between a small patch of the proliferative ventricular zone (VZ) and its corresponding area in the cortical plate (CP) in the developing cerebrum. Proliferative units 1–100 produce ontogenetic columns 1–100 in the same relative position without lateral mismatch. The specification of cytoarchitectonic and functional areas, then, depends on the spatial distribution of stem cells within the proliferative units, whereas the laminar position and neuronal phenotype within ontogenetic columns depend on the time of their origin. Note the subplate (SP), which contains "waiting" afferents from the thalamic radiation (TR) and ipsilateral and contralateral corticocortical connections (CC). (From Rakic, P. [1988]. Specification of cerebral cortical areas. *Science, 241,* 171. Reprinted with permission from AAAS.)

Formation of Gyri and Sulci

During the fifth month of gestation, the cerebral convolutions first appear and begin to transform the topography of the cortical surface. The *primary and secondary convolutions* appear rather predictably relative to specific cortical cytoarchitectonic fields. That is, their location, configuration, and appearance during gestation are fairly constant among individuals. In contrast, *tertiary convolutions* begin to develop during the final months of gestation. They are more random in both their morphological appearance and relationship to specific cortical regions. Tertiary convolutions may continue to develop well into the first year of postnatal life (Chi, Dooling, & Gilles, 1977; Richman, Stewart, Hutchinson, & Caviness, 1975). Initial expansion and folding of the cortical surface can be explained by the rapid influx of the migrating neurons to the CP. After the fifth month of gestation, other factors such as the growth, differentiation, and pattern of connections established by cortical neurons are critical to this process.

Neurodevelopmental Disorders of Neuronal Migration

In most disorders of neuronal migration, abnormality of cell proliferation is a concomitant finding. Neuronal migration disorders (NMDs) are a morphologically related group of disorders that result from either a focal or a generalized disruption in the migration process. Primary disturbances in neuronal migration result in anomalous formation of the cortical plate and cortical laminae. A spectrum of defects involving a few or all laminae of the cerebral cortex is produced. The most salient morphological feature of NMDs is aberration in the normal pattern of gyri and sulci. The molecular pathogenesis of these disorders is discussed in several reviews (Guerrini & Filippi, 2005; Kanatani et al., 2005; Kato & Dobyns, 2003).

Early Neuronal Migration Disorders

Early disturbance in neuronal migration (2–4 months' gestation) results in severe, often diffuse defects in cortical lamination. Large numbers of neurons are either absent or malpositioned, resulting in a reduced number of functional neuronal connections. *Agryyia (lissencephaly), pachygyria,* and *microgyria* constitute the spectrum of early NMD (Table 2.6). Generally, the early forms of NMD will coexist with one another, and it is far less often that one of the "pure varieties" exists in isolation. Each of the early forms of NMD discussed is causally related to specific genetic and chromosomal disorders, MCA/MR syndromes, or teratogenic agents (Barth, 1987; Warkany, Lemire, & Cohen, 1981b). Because of the distinctive morphological appearance of these conditions on MRI, a clinical diagnosis of NMD can be made early in life and may be helpful in determining etiology or prognosis (Barkovich, 2005).

Agyria (lissencephaly) is a severe form of NMD with onset probably no later than the third month of gestation. Agyria, as the name implies, is characterized by the near or complete absence of secondary and tertiary gyri so that the cortical surface appears smooth (Aicardi, 1991; Warkany et al., 1981b). MRI has proven especially useful in defining the spectrum of lissencephaly and its associated clinical manifestations (Barkovich, 2005). In classic type I lissencephaly, the cerebral wall consists of the four embryonic cortical laminae and a layer of vertically oriented columns of nonmigrated heterotopic neurons. A thin layer of underlying white matter may be present (Barth, 1987).

Pachygyria is closely related to agyria, and these two conditions often coexist in the same brain. The onset of pachygyria is probably no later than the fourth month of gestation. It is characterized by relatively few, unusually broad, gyri and few sulci. The cortical mantle is thickened, and the same embryonic cortical architecture seen in agyria is present (Crome, 1956; Hanaway, Lee, & Netsky, 1968).

Microgyria (polymicrogyria) has an onset probably no later than the fourth to fifth month of gestation. The cortex is composed of an increased number of very small gyri and shallow or absent sulci, which gives the cortical surface a remarkably wrinkled appearance (Crome, 1952). What distinguishes the cerebral wall in microgyria is that the molecular layers (layer I) of adjacent gyri are fused to-

Table 2.6. Disorders of migration

Disorder	Termination period	Gene(s)	Function
Lissencephaly type I ("classic")	3 months of gestation	Platelet-activating factor acetylhydrolase isoform 1B (*LIS1*)	Microtubule-associated protein
		Doublecortin (*DCX*)	Microtubule polymerization and stabilization
Lissencephaly type II	3 months of gestation	Reelin (*RELN*)	Cell signaling, synaptic remodeling, and memory
Polymicrogyria	4–5 months of gestation	G protein–coupled receptor (*GPR56*)	Intracellular signaling
		Protein O-mannose α-1,4-*N*-acetylglucosaminyltransferase (*POMGNT1*)	Glycosyltransferase
		Mitochondrial tRNA-leucine 1 (*MTTL1*)	Mitochondrial tRNA-leucine
Subcortical band heterotopia	5–6 months of gestation	Doublecortin (*DCX*) Platelet-activating factor acetylhydrolase isoform 1B (*LIS1*)	
Periventricular nodular heterotopia	5–6 months of gestation	Filamin 1 (*FLN1*)	Nonmuscle actin-binding protein
		ADP-ribosylation factor guanine nucleotide–exchange factor-2 (*ARFGEF2*)	Intracellular vesicular trafficking

Sources: Fox, Lamperti, Eksioglu, Hong, and Feng (1998); Guerrini and Filippi (2005); Kanatani, Tabata, and Nakajima (2005); Lambert de Rouvroit and Goffinet (2001); Piao, Hill, Bodell, Chang, and Basel-Vanagaite (2004); Sarnat (2005); Sheen, Ganesh, Topcu, Sebire, and Bodell (2004); and Vervoort, Holden, Ukadike, Collins, and Saul (2004).

gether, thus obliterating the intervening sulcus. The histological features of microgyria are not uniform and have led to the distinction between layered and unlayered types, unlayered microgyria being the more common (Barth, 1987).

Neurodevelopmental outcome in individuals with an early NMD is often quite poor as manifested by hypoactivity, hypotonia, motor dysfunction, intellectual disabilities (often severe), and seizures.

Late Neuronal Migration Disorders
Disturbances that affect the later stages of neuronal migration (5–6 months' gestation) often result in less severe or focal defects in cortical lamination. Unlike the early disorders, some of these neurons survive and appear capable of forming limited numbers of connections. The relationship between late NMD and specific pre- and perinatal pathogenic factors has been reviewed (Sarnat, 1987). *Neuronal heterotopias* and *verrucose dysplasia* (brain warts) are two forms of late NMD (see Table 2.6).

Neuronal heterotopias are clusters of ectopically positioned neurons that may be distributed anywhere along the migratory trajectory. Frequently, these nodular masses are located adjacent to the lateral ventricles in the subcortical white matter (Barth, 1987). Heterotopias are often found in association with the severe forms of NMD, and onset is probably no later than the end of the fifth or early sixth month of gestation. Detection of neuronal heterotopias using MRI is often difficult, but they may be visualized if the nodules are large, particularly if they are surrounded by white matter, or bulge into the wall of the ventricle (Barkovich, 2005; Osborn, Sharon, Naidich, Bohan, & Friedman, 1988). There is an association between intractable partial epilepsy and infantile spasms with neuronal heterotopia as well as other focal cortical dysplasias (Palm, Blennow, & Brun, 1986; Palmini et al., 1991).

Verrucose dysplasia or "brain warts" are tiny herniations of neurons from layer II that protrude into layer I and spill over onto the cortical surface. Viewed with the naked eye, brain warts appear as round, flat disks of tissue poised atop the gyrus (Barth, 1987). Verrucous dysplasia is not within the resolution capabilities of MRI scanners and is often only an incidental finding at autopsy. Several studies have noted an association between neuronal ectopias, verrucose dysplasia, and developmental language disability (Galaburda, Sherman, Rosen, Aboitiz, & Geschwind, 1985; Humphreys, Kaufmann, & Galaburda, 1990); however, subsequent studies have demonstrated these same microscopic lesions in up to 26% of brains from neurologically normal individuals (Kaufmann & Galaburda, 1989). Perhaps the nature and severity of neurological symptoms are dependent on the size, number, and distribution of these lesions within the cortex, or other associated ultrastructural deficits.

NEURONAL DIFFERENTIATION AND ORGANIZATION (SIXTH MONTH OF GESTATION TO THIRD YEAR)

Differentiation and organization refer to the processes by which the newly migrated sheet of neurons of the cortical plate express their distinctive morphological and biochemical phenotype (differentiation) and arrange themselves into large-scale networks of functional circuits (organization), which subserve the higher-order processing capabilities of the brain. It is difficult to determine a peak period for neuronal organization because it represents a cascade of highly synchronized cellular and molecular events occurring in rapid succession. The most rapid period of neuronal organization in the cerebral cortex begins around 6 months of gestation and extends through the second and third years of postnatal life. The cellular events that determine neuronal organization, in the approximate sequence of their occurrence, are

1. Axonal and dendritic outgrowth (morphological differentiation)

2. Axonal pathfinding and target recognition (connectivity)

3. Dendritic arborization and spine formation (connectivity)

4. Synapse formation, pruning, and stabilization (synaptogenesis)

5. Expression of neurotransmitter phenotype (biochemical differentiation)

Axonal and Dendritic Outgrowth

Morphological differentiation of neurons begins soon after final cell division. Among the many neurites that a neuron projects, it is not known which one is destined to become the *axon* and which the *dendrites*.

The axonal compartment consists of a longitudinally oriented cytoskeletal network and contains a variety of membranous organelles such as mitochondria, lysosomal bodies, synaptic vesicles, and axoplasmic reticulum that are arranged within the cytoskeletal matrix in a three-dimensional array (Bunge, 1986). Because axons lack the capability for local protein synthesis, they depend on intact transport mechanisms to support and maintain normal function. Proteins synthesized in the neuronal cell body are carried by *axoplasmic transport,* which occurs both anterograde and retrograde. Axoplasmic transport is regulated by ''molecular motors'' that slide along microtubles and microfilament tracks as they bind, transport, and release specific protein cargoes (Hirokawa & Takemura, 2004, 2005). Axons elongate by continuously incorporating newly synthesized neurofilaments and microtubules into the advancing *growth cone*; thus, the primary axon is extended while collateral branches remain short.

The dendritic compartment is rich in ribosomes, the organelle responsible for translation of protein from messenger RNA (mRNA). It is known that a select group of mRNAs are transported from the cytoplasm into the dendritic compartment proper, where they may become associated with polyribosomal aggregates that are associated with *dendritic spines*. These spines, which are distributed along the main dendritic shaft and its branches, represent the major postsynaptic targets of excitatory synaptic input and are critical for the normal coding, storage, and retrieval of information (Carlisle & Kennedy, 2005; Koch, Zador, & Brown, 1992). Local protein synthesis, regulated within the dendrite in response to synaptic activity, allows the dendrite to alter its shape, branching pattern, and spine morphology in response to neurally coded, environmentally regulated stimuli (Martin, 2004; Sutton & Schuman, 2005). Trafficking of mRNA into the dendrite is an important mechanism regulating translation in response to patterned synaptic activity.

Axonal Pathfinding and Target Recognition

There is a remarkable degree of consistency in the pathway that axons from the same cell group travel to reach their respective target field. The total number of axonal connections that must be made would appear to warrant an almost infinite number of genetically coded instructions to assure proper connectivity. It is well beyond the capacity of the human genome to supply this many specific instructions a priori. Thus, epigenetic strategies have been developed to account for the guidance and pathfinding capabilities exhibited by growing axons. *Chemotrophic signals* originating from target neurons and components of the *extracellular matrix* serve as guidance cues within the microenvironment, steering axonal growth. A network of signaling pathways that link cell surface receptors to the production and organization of cytoskeletal proteins orchestrates these complex events (Dickson, 2003; Kalil & Dent, 2005; Martin, 2004).

Dendritic Arborization and Spine Formation

The dendritic tree provides a major proportion of the membrane surface area utilized by individual neurons to integrate information from a multitude of individual synaptic inputs. Dendritic spines serve as the postsynaptic targets of corticocortical and cortical afferent fibers. Some of the most elaborate descriptions of dendritic branching and arborization in the developing human cortex resulted from research conducted by Conel (1939–1963) using the Golgi staining method. He described progressive enrichment of the *neurophil* from birth to 8 years of age (Figure 2.8). Observations made from different cortical regions suggest a "gra-

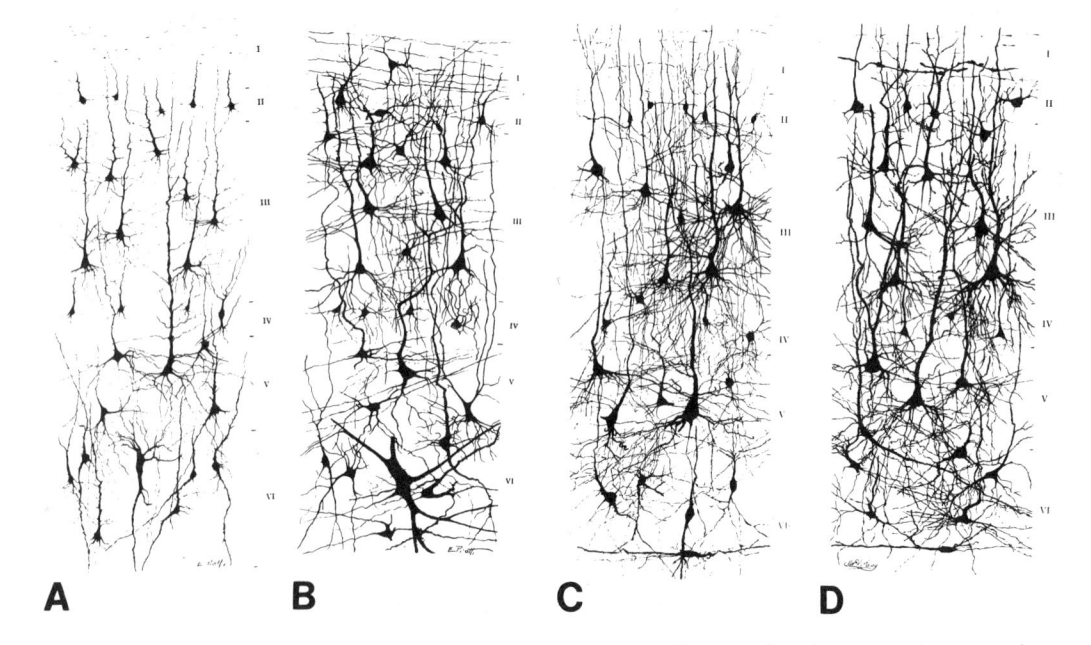

A   **B**   **C**   **D**

Figure 2.8.   Camera lucida composite drawings made from Golgi preparations of human prefrontal cortex at various postnatal ages. The six layers of Brodman and Economo are indicated by roman numerals. *A,* One month. Neurons are immature in appearance. The uppermost apical dendrites on the pyramidal neurons are easily distinguished, although the length, number, and branching pattern of dendrites are still relatively simple. *B,* Six months. Neuronal cell bodies are increased in size. The apical and basal dendrites appear longer, larger, and more numerous. *C,* Twenty-four months. All dendrites show a greater degree of bifurcation and collateral branching. The number of spines is dramatically increased on all cell types compared to 6 months. *D,* Forty-eight months. Dendrites are longer and larger, but not more numerous at this age. The number of spines is increased compared to 24 months. (Reprinted by permission of the publisher from THE POSTNATAL DEVELOPMENT OF THE HUMAN CEREBRAL CORTEX, VOLUMES I–VIII by Jesse LeRoy Conel, Cambridge, Mass.: Harvard University Press, Copyright © 1939; 1975 by the President and Fellows of Harvard College.)

dient of maturation" both within and between functional areas.

The Synapse

The synapse is composed of presynaptic and postsynaptic elements that allow neurons to rapidly communicate with one another using chemical signals. Presynaptic terminals are enriched in mitochondria, neurotransmitter synthesizing enzymes, and specialized vesicles for neurotransmitter storage and release. The postsynaptic terminals contain specialized receptors and enzymes for neurotransmitter inactivation or degradation (Cooper, Bloom, & Roth, 1991). Specific receptor families are also linked via G proteins to intracellular signal transduction pathways and are refered to as metabotropic-linked receptors (Chen & Bazan, 2005; Heuss & Gerber, 2000). Metabotropic signaling pathways are capable of regulating a variety of biochemical and metabolic processes within the cytoplasm and nucleus (Maise & Chong, 2005; Worley, Baraban, & Snyder, 1987). In this way, neurotransmitters act not only as mediators of electrochemical signaling but also as regulators of gene expression and differentiation during synaptic development (Lauder, 1993; Mattson, 1988).

Early Synaptogenesis The earliest synapses to appear in the developing cortex are found by 15 weeks' gestation. These pioneer synapses are found immediately above the CP in the MZ and below the CP within the SP, but not within the CP itself (Molliver, Kostovic, & Loos, 1973). Subplate neurons express a rich variety of neuropeptides and neurotrophin receptors in conjunction with the developmental appearance of dendrites and spines. Transient synaptic connections are made between these SP neurons and incoming cortical afferent fibers (Kostovic & Judas, 2002, 2006). Thus, the SP functions as both a "waiting compartment" and "traffic cop" for afferent fibers, ultimately directing them toward specific cortical laminae, thereby influencing the columnar organization and functional specification of the cortex itself (Kanold, 2004).

Later Synaptogenesis It appears to be a basic strategy of neuronal development that synapses are overproduced early in development and selectively eliminated at a later time. Studies of the human neocortex reveal that the first 2 years of postnatal life constitute a period of rapid cortical expansion. Cell packing density decreases as expansion of the neuropil results in separation of neuronal cell bodies from one another during this period. Total synaptic number and density continue to increase dramatically until about 2 or 3 years of age, when they reach a maximum. After about 5 years of age, when cortical expansion has ceased, cell packing density continues to decrease. During this period, synaptic density also begins to decrease markedly. By adolescence, synaptic density is about 60% of the maximum seen at 2 years of age (Huttenlocher, 1979, 1984) (Figure 2.9). Synaptic reorganization and diminution in gray matter volume occur throughout adolescence and the early adult years, which may account for increased susceptibility to neuropsychiatric disorders during this period (Andersen, 2003; Gogtay, Giedd, Lusk, & Hayashi, 2004).

In phylogenetically older regions of the brain, genetically determined *hardwiring* of neural structures is the rule, whereas in primates much of the neocortex is *softwired,* and synaptic survival may in part be dependent on functional stimulation of neuron activity. The strategy of redundancy during the initial for-

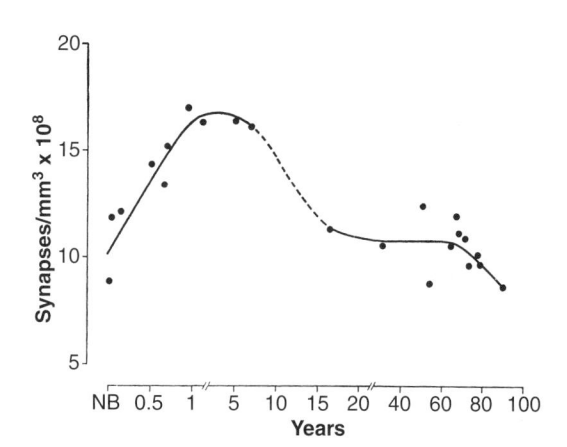

Figure 2.9. Density of synapses in layer III of the middle frontal gyrus as a function of age. Note the sharp decline in synaptic density beginning around 4 years of age. (This article was published in Brain Research, 163, P. Huttenlocher, Synaptic density in human frontal cortex—developmental changes and effects of aging, p. 199, Copyright Elsevier 1979.)

mation of neural connections is probably designed to ensure prompt and complete innervation of all available targets. Selective pruning of synapses could then occur later in development to assure greater specificity in the pattern of connections and shaping of specific functional areas within the cortex.

Neurodevelopmental Disorders of Neuronal Differentiation, Synaptogenesis, and Organization

Disturbances in neuronal differentiation and synaptic organization result in aberrant cortical microcircuitry that alters the integrity of electrochemical signaling in the brain. Synaptic disorganization may occur secondarily, as a consequence of the disorders discussed previously. These disturbances may also be an associated feature in a variety of genetic, chromosomal, and toxic-metabolic disturbances (Huttenlocher, 1991; Marin-Padilla, 1972) (Figure 2.10). In the absence of other patholog-

ical findings, disorders of synaptic organization appear to be the primary neurobiological disturbance in several well-recognized genetic syndromes (Kaufmann & Moser, 2000). Genetic defects in cell signaling pathways and transcriptional regulation appear to be common mechanisms leading to structural and functional synaptic impairment in certain genetic and acquired conditions (Johnston, 2004).

Several investigators have examined cortical neurons in individuals with intellectual disabilities of undetermined etiology for evidence of organizational disturbance. The ultrastructural findings reported most consistently are *impaired dendritic arborization* and *dendritic spine dysgenesis* (Table 2.7). It is difficult to know if these entities represent etiologically distinct findings or they are a manifestation of some common underlying disturbance. Dendritic spine dysgenesis, exemplified by spine loss or a preponderance of very long, thin, immature spines on apical dendrites has also been demonstrated on pyramidal neurons from the frontal cortex (Purpura, 1974). Additional studies revealed the formation of distinct varicosities along the length of apical and basilar dendrities on both pyramidal and nonpyramidal neurons (Purpura, Bodick, Suzuki, Rapin, & Wurzelmann, 1982) (Figure 2.11).

SYNAPTIC NEUROCHEMISTRY OF THE CEREBRAL CORTEX

Biochemical differentiation of young neurons occurs in conjunction with their morphological differentiation. As cortical neurons differentiate, they begin to express the specific molecules necessary for neurotransmitter synthesis, storage, inactivation, or degradation. Specific receptors are also expressed on the cell body and along the dendritic tree of postsynaptic neurons. Receptors bind the neurotransmitter to induce an electrochemical response (depolarization or hyperpolarization) via linkage to sodium, potassium, or chloride ion channels. The appearance of specialized biochemical pathways responsible for neurotransmitter synthesis generally occurs after migration is completed and the differentiating neuron has

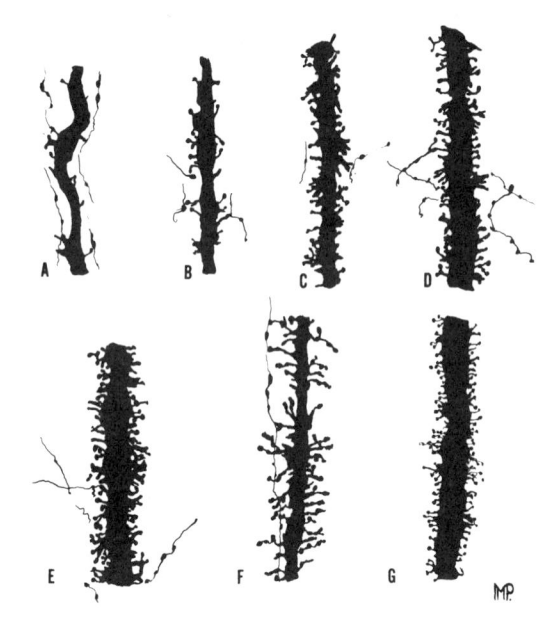

Figure 2.10. Camera lucida drawings made from Golgi preparations of the apical dendrites of layer V pyramidal neurons from the human cerebral cortex. They illustrate the morphological characterisics of dendritic spines during normal prenatal and postnatal development, and in two cases of trisomy. The dendritic segments illustrated are from the following: (A) a 5-month fetus, (B) a 7-month fetus, (C) a newborn, (D) a 2-month-old infant, (E) an 8-month-old infant, (F) a newborn with D1 (13–15) trisomy, and (G) an 18-month-old with trisomy 21. (This article was published in Brain Research, 44, M. Marin-Padilla, Structural abnormalities of the cerebral cortex in human chromosomal aberrations: A Golgi study, p. 627, Copyright Elsevier 1972.)

Table 2.7. Disorders associated with synaptic dysorganization

Disorder	Gene(s)	Function
Defective dendritic arborization or spine dysgenesis	Methyl-CpG–binding protein-2 (*MECP2*) (Rett syndrome)	Transcriptional regulator
	Fragile X mental retardation-1 (*FMR1*) (fragile X syndrome)	Activity-dependent protein translation regulator
	Cyclic AMP response element binding protein (*CREBBP*) (Rubinstein-Taybi syndrome)	Transcription factor
	Ribosomal protein S6 kinase 2 (*RSK2*) (Coffin-Lowry syndrome)	Protein kinase
	Tuberin (*TSC2*) (tuberous sclerosis)	Receptor signaling
	X-linked mental retardation (numerous)	
	Cromosomal aneuploidy syndromes (trisomies 13 and 21)	

Sources: Gardiner (2003); Inlow and Restifo (2004); Johnston (2004); Kaufmann and Moser (2000); Newey, Velamoor, Govek, and Van Aelst (2005); Ramakers (2002); and Renieri, Pescucci, Longo, Ariani, and Mari (2005).

arrived at its final position in the cortex. Neuronal expression of neurotransmitter phenotype is under the control of both the genetic and epigenetic influences.

Neurotransmitters are commonly divided into different classes based on their mode of synthesis or chemical composition, including catecholamines, monoamines, acetylcholine (Ach), amino acids, and the neuropeptides. The catecholamines, monoamines, Ach, and amino acid neurotransmitters are synthesized directly within the nerve terminal by the synthesizing enzymes contained therein. Their production is ideally suited to respond to rapidly occurring changes in the electrical activity in the brain. Neuroactive peptides, which constitute the largest class of neurotransmitters in the brain, are synthesized within the neuronal cytoplasm, and their production is dependent on RNA and protein synthesis (Hokfelt, 1991; Krieger, 1983).

Traditionally, the synaptic neurochemical composition of the neocortex can be thought of as consisting of three tiers: 1) *afferent,* 2) *efferent,* and 3) *intrinsic* systems. This designation reflects patterns of connectivity among (intrinsic) and between (afferent and efferent) cortical neurons and other regions of the brain (Coyle, 1982). The developmental appearance of neurotransmitters and neuromodulators, and their role in shaping cortical development, are discussed in several reviews (Herlenius & Lagercrantz, 2001; Lauder, 1993, 1995; Mattson, 1988).

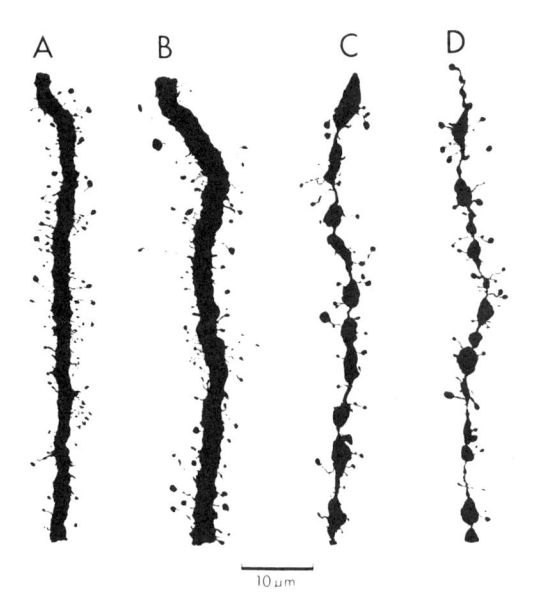

Figure 2.11. Camera lucida drawings of proximal (*A* and *B*) and distal (*C* and *D*) dendritic segments from a 5-month-old boy with seizures and profound developmental delays. In proximal segments, thin spines with long necks and beaded terminations predominate. In distal segments, irregular varicosities are connected by thinner strands. Abnormal spines extend from both swollen and constricted regions. (This article was published in Developmental Brain Research, 5, D.P. Purpura, N. Bodick, K. Suzuki, I. Rapin, & S. Wurzelmann, Microtuble disarray in cortical dendrites and neurobehavioral failure: I. Golgi and electron microscopic studies, p. 290, Copyright Elsevier 1982.)

Afferent System

Much of what is known about neocortical transmission is derived from knowledge of the extrathalamic afferent systems. Four of the classic neurotransmitter substances found in the neocortex—norepinephrine (NE), serotonin (or 5-hydroxytryptamine [5-HT]), dopamine (DA), and Ach—arise from cell bodies located within specific nuclei in the brain stem, midbrain, and basal forebrain regions, respectively (Figure 2.12). Overall, these classic neurotransmitters are probably responsible for no more than 10% of the total synaptic complement of the neocortex (Krieger, 1983).

Norepinephrine Norepinephrine-synthesizing neurons are located in the *nucleus locus coeruleus* in the rostral portion of the pons. These noradrenergic neurons send out axons that innervate nearly all of the neurons in the cerebral cortex and limbic system (Coyle & Molliver, 1977). Initially, the NE innervation to cortex is quite dense, but it diminishes as cortical volume increases. The distribution of NE fibers is most dense in primary motor and sensory cortices, sparsest in temporal cortex,

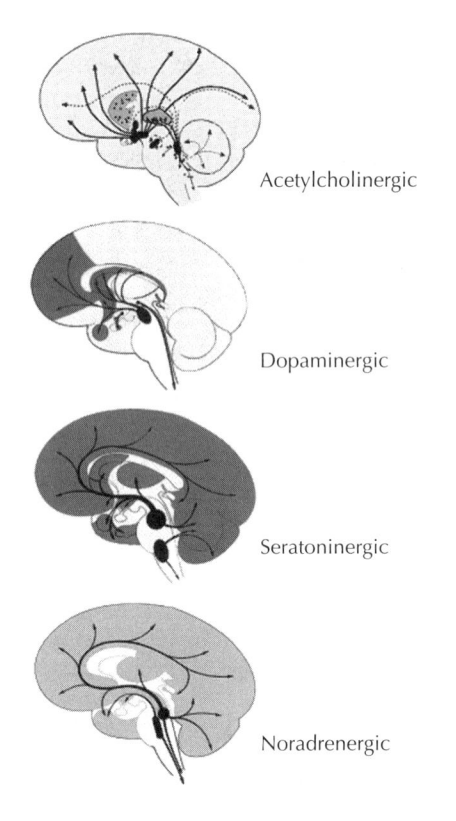

Acetylcholinergic

Dopaminergic

Seratoninergic

Noradrenergic

Figure 2.12. Schematic illustrations of neuronal cell bodies and cortically projecting (afferent) transmitter systems. Acetylcholinergic, dopaminergic, serotoninergic, and noradrenergic pathways in the human brain. (This article was published in Early Human Development, 65, E. Herlenius & H. Loger Crantz, Neurotransmitter and neuromodulators during early human development, p. 21, Copyright Elsevier 2001.)

and intermediate in the occipital cortex (Foote & Morrison, 1987). Norepinephrine appears to increase the "signal-to-noise" characteristics of cortical neurons, thereby enhancing the selectivity and vigor of the cortical response to incoming sensory stimuli from the thalamus. Norepinephrine helps to regulate the sleep–wake cycle and has been implicated in the modulation of mood and affective states, as well as learning and memory (Slaby & Tancredi, 2001).

Serotonin Serotonin-synthesizing neurons arise from the *dorsal and median raphe nuclei* in the midbrain and rostral brain stem. Like the noradrenergic neurons, the serotonergic neurons provide a very diffuse innervation to the cerebral cortex and limbic system. In primate cortex, 5-HT innervation is very dense (Foote & Morrison, 1987). Compared with the pattern of NE axon terminals in the same cortical laminae, it appears that the 5-HT axons terminate on different cell types, on different portions of the same neuron, or both. It has been proposed that these two systems play a distinct yet complementary role in cortical information processing. Serotonin has been implicated in the modulation of internal behavioral states such as mood, appetite, sexual behavior and aggression, sensory perception, temperature regulation, and regulation of the sleep–wake cycle (Slaby & Tancredi, 2001).

Dopamine Dopamine-synthesizing neurons are located in the ventral tegmental area of the midbrain, giving rise to the mesolimbic and mesocortical DA systems that innervate the limbic system and frontal cortex, respectively. There is a heterogeneous rostrocaudal gradient of DA innervation throughout the cortex (Foote & Morrison, 1987). In addition to the prefrontal cortex, which receives a dense innervation of DA fibers, primary motor areas and sensory association areas also receive a particularly dense input. Both regional and laminar patterns of innervation suggest that DA exerts an influence on corticocortical rather than thalamocortical circuitry. Dopamine is implicated in a variety of frontal lobe functions, including motivation, drive, motor function, and mood-aggression and memory-attentional mechanisms (Slaby & Tancredi, 2001).

Acetylcholine   Acetylcholine-synthesizing neurons are located in the *basal forebrain complex,* which is scattered throughout the base of the midbrain and telencephalon. This system provides diffuse innervation to the cortex, hippocampus, and limbic system. In primates, most of the cortically projecting Ach fibers arise from the *nucleus basalis of Meynert* and to a lesser extent from the *diagonal band of Broca* (Foote & Morrison, 1987). Like the monoamine fibers, Ach fibers show considerable regional heterogeneity in both density and laminar distribution. There is compelling evidence implicating the cholinergic system in memory, attention, and vigilance (Perry, Walker, Grace, & Perry, 1999; Richardson & DeLong, 1988).

Intrinsic System

Neurotransmitters classified as intrinsic are localized within neurons whose connections, by definition, originate and terminate within the cerebral cortex itself. The two principal and best-studied classes of intrinsic neurotransmitters are GABA and the neuropeptides: somatostatin, vasoactive intestinal polypeptide, cholecystokinin, and neuropeptide Y.

Gamma-Aminobutyric Acid   GABA is the primary inhibitory neurotransmitter in the cerebral cortex. Some estimates indicate that GABA may be utilized by up to 30%–40% of cortical synapses (Krieger, 1983). GABA localizes to the small interneurons, which are widely distributed throughout all cortical layers, especially laminae II and IV. GABAergic interneurons play a critical role in cortical excitability and local information processing and thus are implicated in neurodevelopmental and psychiatric disorders (Levitt, Eagleson, & Powell, 2004; Woo & Lu, 2006). GABAergic neurons provide inhibitory input to pyramidal neurons, the primary source of excitatory output from the cortex, and are primarily involved in cognition, anxiety, and seizure susceptibility (Ben-Ari, Khalilov, Represa, & Gozlan, 2004; Lydiard, 2003; Markram et al., 2004).

Neuropeptides   The brain is a rich and abundant source of neuroactive peptides. The hypothalamic-releasing hormones, neurohypophyseal hormones, and pituitary hormones are perhaps the most well-studied brain peptides. Peptides originally demonstrated to occur in the gastrointestinal tract and endocrine system are also found in the brain (Hokfelt, 1991; Krieger, 1983). Several of these "brain–gut" peptides are found throughout the cerebral cortex. Somatostatin, vasoactive intestinal polypeptide, cholecystokinin, and neuropeptide Y are found in each of the cortical layers, where they localize to the small interneurons (Parnavelas, 1986). In primates, these peptide-producing neurons probably comprise no more than 3%–4% of the total neocortical neuron population and are most heavily concentrated in cortical laminae II and III and between layer VI and the adjacent subcortical white matter. In primates, up to 90%–95% of neuropeptide-producing cortical neurons also contain the inhibitory neurotransmitter GABA (Hendry et al., 1984).

Efferent System

The efferent system is composed of neurons whose cell bodies are located within the cortex and send axonal projections to a more distant region outside the cortex. Although less is known about the neurochemical anatomy of the efferent system, it appears that the excitatory amino acid (EAA) neurotransmitters glutamate and aspartate are utilized to a large degree. Other endogenous amino acid compounds may be utilized to a lesser degree.

Glutamate and Aspartate   Glutamate and aspartate, in addition to being common amino acids, double as neurotransmitters in the brain. It is estimated that up to 50% of all cortical synapses utilize EAA transmitters (McDonald & Johnston, 1990). Most neurons are capable of excitation with glutamate. Glutamate is found in the pyramidal neurons, which constitute the primary output neurons from the cortex. Pyramidal neurons project to a number of subcortical regions, including the striatum, thalamus, lateral geniculate nucleus, superior colliculus, red nucleus, pontine nuclei, and spinal cord (Fagg & Foster, 1983). There is also evidence that glutamate and aspartate are used extensively by the commissural and association fibers of the hippocampus (Cotman, Monaghan, Ottersen, & Storm-Mathisen, 1987).

During development, an optimal amount of EAA activity is necessary to mediate certain critical events such as dendritic outgrowth and synaptogenesis (Kleinschmidt, Bear, & Singer, 1988; Mattson, 1988). Too little activity may result in delayed maturation or disruption of neural differentiation, whereas overactivity can produce neural damage (Choi, 1988; Hattori & Wasterlain, 1990; McDonald et al., 1991).

Neurodevelopmental Disorders

Knowledge of disturbances in synaptic neurochemistry as a component of the underlying pathology in diverse types of neurodevelopmental disorder is limited but expanding. Several of the idiopathic developmental epilepsies are caused by genes coding for components of membrane-associated ion channels (channelopathies), resulting in physiological imbalance of excitation–inhibition in the developing brain (Wong, 2005) (Table 2.8). A group of inherited neurometabolic conditions caused by a primary disturbance of neurotransmitter metabolism or transport has been described that encompasses disorders of biopterine, catecholamines, serotonin, tetrahydrobiopterin, folate, glycine, pyridoxine, and GABA (Pearl, Capp, Novotny, & Gibson, 2005). Current understanding regarding the neurochemical substrate of neurobehavioral conditions associated with intellectual disabilities is quite limited; however, complex interactions between neurotransmitter systems and their signaling systems appear to be involved in the pathogenesis of several neurobehavioral disorders such as attention-deficit/hyperactivity disorder, autism, and obsessive-compulsive disorder. In the absence of direct evidence, involvement of specific neurotransmitter systems are often inferred due to the nature of the observed neurobehavioral symptom complex or by the response to selective psychotrophic medication intervention (Slaby & Tancredi, 2001).

Table 2.8. Disorders associated with altered synaptic neurochemistry

Disorder	Transmitter interaction(s)
Autism[a]	Serotonin and glutamate
	Acetylcholine
ADHD[a]	Dopamine and noradrenaline
	Glutamate and dopamine
Lesch-Nyhan syndrome[a]	Dopamine
Obsessive-compulsive disorder[a]	Glutamate, serotonin, and acetylcholine
	Serotonin and dopamine
Tourette syndrome[a]	Dopamine, noradrenaline
Idiopathic epilepsies[b]	Glutamate and GABA
Neurometabolic-neurotransmitter disorders[c]	Biopterine, catecholamines, and serotonin
	Tetrahydrobiopterin, folate, glycine
	Pyridoxine, GABA

[a]*References:* Carlsson (1998, 2000); Castellanos and Tannock (2002); Chappell, Leckman, Pauls, and Cohen (1990); Chugani (2002); Chugani et al. (1999); Leckman, Walkup, and Riddle (1987); Loyd, Hornykiewicz, and Davidson (1981); Page and Nyhan (1990); Perry, Lee, Martin-Ruiz, Court, and Volsen (2001); Rosenberg and Keshavan (1998); and Solanto (2000)

[b]*Reference:* Wong (2005)

[c]*Reference:* Pearl, Capp, Novotny, and Gibson (2005)

Key: ADHD, attention-deficit/hyperactivity disorder; GABA, γ-aminobutyric acid.

MYELINATION (SIXTH MONTH OF GESTATION TO ADULTHOOD)

Initial myelin formation in the brain takes place over a prolonged period of time. In some regions, myelination begins as early as the sixth month of gestation, whereas in others it may start as late as several months postnatally and proceed well into the third and fourth decades of life.

The myelin membrane consists of a lipid bilayer sandwiched between monolayers of protein. The process of synthesizing and laying down the myelin membrane in the CNS is carried out by oligodendroglial cells. These cells, like neurons, originate from within the VZ and SVZ of the embryonic neural tube. Glial proliferation appears to peak during early the first 2 postnatal years (Dobbing & Sands, 1973).

Cellular Interactions During Myelination

The process of CNS myelination has been well studied using light and electron microscopy

(Bunge, 1968). A single oligodendroglia can myelinate multiple axons in the CNS. Initially, the oligodendroglial cell extends a portion of its cytoplasm to enfold the axon; it then proceeds to wrap itself around the axonal cylinder many times, like a "scroll around a wooden rod." The cellular and molecular mechanisms of oligodendrocytic-axonal signaling involve cellular adhesion molecules and activity-induced promyelinating factors (Coman, Barbin, Charles, & Zalc, 2005; Sherman & Brophy, 2005).

Myelination in the Cerebral Cortex

Ever since the pioneering work of Flechsig (1901), it has been recognized that there exist regional cycles of myelination throughout the developing brain. He proposed that the timing of myelination reflects the hierarchical position of a fiber system within the functional organization of the brain. In this schema, functionally related systems would myelinate together. A lifetime of studies led Flechsig to propose a number of rules governing myelination: 1) proximal pathways myelinate before distal pathways, 2) sensory pathways myelinate before motor pathways, and 3) projection pathways myelinate before association pathways. In his meticulously detailed studies of the cerebral cortex, Flechsig was able to subdivide the white matter core of the cerebral convolutions into 36 *myelogenetic fields*. Extending Flechsig's original observations, Yakovlev and Lecours (1967) introduced the concept of the *myelogenetic cycle*. This refers to the time period of myelination within a given fiber system from beginning to end.

The detailed studies of Brody and Kinney have further refined the understanding of the topography and sequence of myelination during the first 2 years of postnatal life (Brody, Kinney, Kloman, & Gilles, 1987; Kinney, Brody, Kloman, & Gilles, 1988). They introduced the concept that myelination, in general, progresses from the central sulcus outward toward the occipital, frontal, and temporal poles (Figure 2.13), and that the frontal pole completes its myelination before the temporal pole, the last of the higher order association areas to mature.

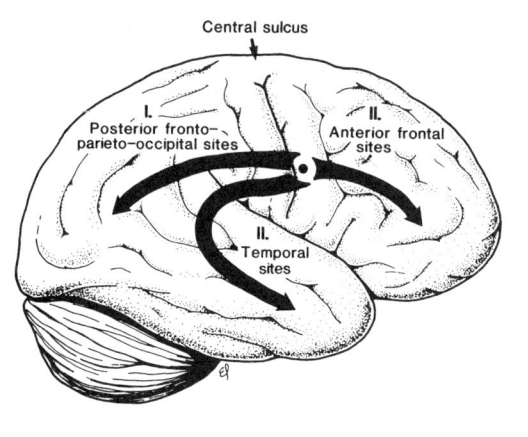

Figure 2.13. Drawing of the cerebrum depicting the progression of myelination in telencephalic sites from the central sulcus outward toward the poles, with the posterior sites preceding anterior frontotemporal sites. The occipital pole myelinates slightly earlier than the posterior parietal white matter. The frontal and temporal poles are the last regions to myelinate. (From Kinney, H.C., Brody, B.A., Kloman, A.S., & Gilles, F.H. [1988]. Sequence of central nervous system myelination in human infancy: II. Patterns of myelination in autopsied infants. *Journal of Neuropathology and Experimental Neurology, 47*(3), 224; reprinted by permission.)

MRI has been used to document the sequential pattern of white matter formation throughout childhood (Paus, Collins, Evans, & Leonard, 2001). Several excellent studies have been performed that establish normative standards for typically developing children and have proven helpful in the evaluation of children with neurodevelopmental disorders that affect myelination (Dietrich et al., 1988; Holland, Haas, Morman, Brant-Zawadzki, & Newton, 1985). The development of quantitative diffusion tensor imaging and three-dimensional fiber tractography is advancing knowledge of myelination and axonal connectivity in the developing brain (Mukherjee & McKinstry, 2006; Schneider, Il'yasov, Hennig, & Martin, 2004).

Neurodevelopmental Disorders

Primary disturbances refers to those conditions in which deficient myelin production is the most salient pathological finding in the absence of other anatomical or histological anomalies. These conditions are further classified as failure of myelination to occur and delay or diminution in myelin production (dysmyelination). Loss of preexisting myelin (demyelination) as a result of genetic (leukodystrophies) or acquired disorders is considered secondary. Mal-

Table 2.9. Disorders of dysmyelination

Dysmyelination
Pelizaeus-Merzbacher disease

Delay or diminution
Phenylketonuria
Homocystinuria
Maple syrup urine disease
Galactosemia
Glutaric aciduria 1
Nonketotic hyperglycinemia

Source: Kolodny (1993).

formation syndromes may also be associated with secondary dysmyelination (Kolodny, 1993). The conditions associated with primary deficits in myelination include *Pelizaeus-Merzbacher disease, amino acid defects,* and *organic acid defects* (Table 2.9).

CONCLUSION

If neuroscience in the 20th century was engaged in answering fundamental questions about cellular development, diversity, and organization, neuroscience in the 21st century will be about complex genetic traits, functional organization, and cognitive and disease mechanisms. Genotype-phenotype studies of genetically based cognitive-behavioral syndromes have provided an extraordinary opportunity to integrate information across multiple levels of neuroinquiry, and neuroinformatics promises to catalogue and demonstrate exactly how genetic variation influences developmental events to produce individual variation in human cognitive traits. What is to be done with all of this information? The revelation is exhilarating and, at the same time, a bit frightening.

REFERENCES

Aicardi, J. (1991). The agyria-pachygyria complex: A spectrum of cortical malformations. *Brain and Development, 13,* 1–8.

Andersen, S.L. (2003). Trajectories of brain development: Point of vulnerability or window of opportunity? *Neuroscience and Biobehavioral Reviews, 27,* 3–18.

Angevine, J.B., Bodian, D., Coulombre, A., Edds, J.M., Hamburger, V., Jacobson, M., et al. (1969). Embryonic vertebrate central nervous system. *Anatomical Record, 166,* 257–262.

Barkovich, A.J. (2005). *Congenital malformations of the brain and skull: Pediatric neuroimaging.* Philadelphia: Lippincott, Williams & Wilkins.

Barkovich, A.J., Kuzniecky, R.I., Jackson, G.D., Guerrini, R., & Dobyns, W.B. (2005). A developmental and genetic classification for malformations of cortical development. *Neurology, 65,* 1873–1887.

Barth, P.G. (1987). Disorders of neuronal migration. *Canadian Journal of Neurological Sciences, 14,* 1–16.

Ben-Ari, Y., Khalilov, I., Represa, A., & Gozlan, H. (2004). Interneurons set the tune of developing networks. *Trends in Neurosciences, 27,* 422–427.

Blinkov, S.M., & Glezer, I.I. (1968). *The human brain in figures and tables* (B. Haigh, Trans.). New York: Basic Books.

Bond, J., & Woods, C.G. (2006). Cytoskeletal genes regulating brain size. *Current Opinion in Cell Biology, 18,* 95–101.

Brody, B.A., Kinney, H.C., Kloman, A.S., & Gilles, F.H. (1987). Sequence of central nervous system myelination in human infancy: I. An autopsy study of myelination. *Journal of Neuropathology and Experimental Neurology, 46,* 283–301.

Bunge, M.B. (1986). The axonal cytoskeleton: Its role in generating and maintaining cell form. *Trends in Neurosciences, 9,* 477–482.

Bunge, R.P. (1968). Glial cells and the central myelin sheath. *Physiological Review, 48,* 197–251.

Carlisle, H.J., & Kennedy, M.B. (2005). Spine architecture and synaptic plasticity. *Trends in Neurosciences, 28,* 182–187.

Carlsson, M.L. (1998). Is infantile autism a hypoglutamatergic disorder? Relevance of glutamate-serotonin interactions for pharmacotherapy. *Journal of Neural Transmission, 105,* 525–535.

Carlsson, M.L. (2000). On the role of cortical glutamate in obsessive-compulsive disorder and attention-deficit hyperactivity disorder, two phenomenologically antithetical conditions. *Acta Psychiatrica Scandinavica, 102,* 401–413.

Castellanos, F.X., & Tannock, R. (2002). Neuroscience of attention-deficit/hyperactivity disorder: The search for endophenotypes. *Nature Reviews: Neuroscience, 3,* 617–628.

Chappell, P.B., Leckman, J.F., Pauls, D., & Cohen, D.J. (1990). Biochemical and genetic studies of Tourette's syndrome. In S.I. Deutch, A. Weizman, & R. Weizman (Eds.), *Application of basic neuroscience to child psychiatry* (pp. 241–260). New York: Plenum.

Chen, C., & Bazan, N.G. (2005). Lipid signaling: Sleep, synaptic plasticity, and neuroprotection. *Prostaglandins and Other Lipid Mediators, 77,* 65–76.

Chi, J., Dooling, E., & Gilles, F. (1977). Gyral development of the human brain. *Annals of Neurology, 1,* 86–93.

Choi, D.W. (1988). Glutamate neurotoxicity and diseases of the nervous system. *Neuron, 1,* 623–634.

Chugani, D.C. (2002). Anatomy and neurobiology of autism: Role of altered brain serotonin mechanisms in autism. *Molecular Psychiatry, 7,* s16–s17.

Chugani, D.C., Muzik, O., Behen, M., Rothemel, R., Janisse, J. J., Lee, J., et al. (1999). Developmental changes in brain serotonin synthesis capacity in autistic and nonautistic children. *Annals of Neurology, 45,* 287–295.

Clark, G.D. (2004). The classification of cortical dysplasias through molecular genetics. *Brain and Development, 26,* 351–362.

Coman, I., Barbin, G., Charles, P., & Zalc, B. (2005). Axonal signals in central nervous system myelination, demyelination and remyelination. *Journal of Neurological Sciences, 233,* 67–71.

Conel, J.L. (1939–1963). *The postnatal development of the human cerebral cortex* (Vols. 1–7). Cambridge, MA: Harvard University Press.

Cooper, J.R., Bloom, F.E., & Roth, R.H. (1991). *The biochemical basis of neuropharmacology* (6th ed.). New York: Oxford University Press.

Cotman, C.W., Monaghan, D.T., Ottersen, O.P., & Storm-Mathisen, J. (1987). Anatomical organization of excitatory amino-acid receptors and their pathways. *Trends in Neuroscience, 10,* 273–279.

Cowan, W.M. (1979). The development of the brain. *Scientific American, 241,* 113–133.

Cowan, W.M. (1992). Development of the nervous system. In A.K. Asbury, G.M. McKhann, & W.I. McDonald (Eds.), *Diseases of the nervous system: Clinical neurobiology* (2nd ed., pp. 5–24). Philadelphia: W.B. Saunders.

Coyle, J. (1982). Development of neurotransmitters in the neocortex. *Neurosciences Research Program Bulletin, 20,* 479–491.

Coyle, J.T., & Molliver, M.E. (1977). Major innervation of newborn rat cortex by monoaminergic neurons. *Science, 196,* 444–447.

Crino, P.B. (2005). Molecular pathogenesis of focal cortical dysplasia and hemimegalencephaly. *Journal of Child Neurology, 20,* 330–336.

Crome, L. (1952). Microgyria. *Journal of Pathology and Bacteriology, 64,* 479–494.

Crome, L. (1956). Pachygyria. *Journal of Pathology and Bacteriology, 71,* 335–352.

Dattani, M.L., Martinez-Barbera, J., Thomas, P.Q., Brickman, J.M., & Gupta, R. (2000). Molecular genetics of septo-optic dysplasia. *Hormone Research, 53,* 26–33.

Day, R.E., & Schutt, W.H. (1979). Normal children with large heads—benign familial megalencephaly. *Archives of Disease in Childhood, 54,* 512–517.

Dekaban, A.S., & Sakuragawa, N. (Eds.). (1977). *Handbook of clinical neurology: Vol. 30. Megalencephaly.* Amsterdam: North Holland.

DeMeyer, W., Zeman, W., & Palmer, C. (1964). The face predicts the brain: Diagnostic significance of median facial anomalies for holoprosencephaly. *Pediatrics, 34,* 256.

DeMyer, W. (1986). Megalencephaly: Types, clinical syndromes, and management. *Pediatric Neurology, 2,* 321–328.

Dickson, B.J. (2003). Molecular mechanisms of axon guidance. *Science, 298,* 1959–1964.

Dietrich, R.B., Bradley, W.G., Zaragoza, E.J., Otto, R.J., Taira, R.K., Wilson, G.H., et al. (1988). MR evaluation of early myelination patterns in normal and developmentally delayed infants. *AJNR: American Journal of Neuroradiology, 9,* 69–76.

Dobbing, J., & Sands, J. (1970). Timing of neuroblast multiplication in developing human brain. *Nature, 226,* 639–640.

Dobbing, J., & Sands, J. (1973). Quantitative growth and development of human brain. *Archives of Disease in Childhood, 48,* 757–767.

Dubourg, C., Lazaro, L., Blayau, M., Pasquier, L., & Duron, M.R. (2003). Genetic study of holoprosencephaly. *Annales de Biologie Clinique, 61,* 679–687.

Elson, E., Perveen, R., Donnai, D., Wall, S., & Black, G. (2002). De novo *GLI3* mutation in acrocallosal syndrome: Broadening the phenotypic spectrum of *GLI3* defects and overlap with murine models. *Journal of Medical Genetics, 39,* 804–806.

Erzurumlu, R.S., & Killackey, H.P. (1983). Critical and sensitive periods in neurobiology. *Current Topics in Developmental Biology, 17,* 207–240.

Fagg, G.E., & Foster, A.C. (1983). Amino acid neurotransmitters and their pathways in the mammalian central nervous system. *Neuroscience, 9,* 701–719.

Filimonoff, I. (1947). A rational subdivision of the cerebral cortex. *Archives of Neurology and Psychiatry, 58,* 296–311.

Flechsig, P. (1901). Developmental (myelogenetic) localization of the cerebral cortex in the human subject. *Lancet, 2,* 1027–1029.

Foote, S.L., & Morrison, J.H. (1987). Extrathalamic modulation of cortical function. *Annual Review of Neuroscience, 10,* 67–95.

Fox, J.W., Lamperti, E.D., Eksioglu, Y.Z., Hong, S.E., & Feng, Y. (1998). Mutations in filamin 1 prevent migration of cerebral cortical neurons in human periventricular heterotopia. *Neuron, 6,* 1315–1325.

Free, S., Mitchell, T., Williamson, K., Churchill, A., Shorvorrn, S., Moore, A., et al. (2003). Quantitative MR image analysis in subjects with defects in *PAX6* gene. *Neuroimage, 20,* 2281–2290.

Galaburda, A., Sherman, G.F., Rosen, G.D., Aboitiz, F., & Geschwind, N. (1985). Developmental dyslexia: Four consecutive patients with cortical anomalies. *Annals of Neurology, 18,* 222–233.

Gardiner, K. (2003). Predicting pathway perturbations in Down syndrome. *Journal of Neural Transmission: Supplement, 67,* 21–37.

Gogtay, N., Giedd, J.N., Lusk, L., & Hayashi, K.M. (2004). Dynamic mapping of human cortical development during childhood through early adulthood. *Proceedings of the National Academy of Sciences of the United States of America, 101,* 8174–8179.

Gotz, M., & Sommer, L. (2005). Cortical development: The art of generating cell diversity. *Development, 132,* 3327–3332.

Granata, T., Freri, E., Caccia, C., & Setola, V. (2005). Schizencephaly: Clinical spectrum, epilepsy, and pathogenesis. *Journal of Child Neurology, 20,* 313–318.

Gressens, P. (2000). Mechanisms and disturbances of neuronal migration. *Pediatric Research, 48,* 726.

Gressens, P. (2006). Pathogenesis of migration disorders. *Current Opinion in Neurology, 19,* 135–140.

Guerrini, R., & Filippi, T. (2005). Neuronal migration disorders, genetics, and epileptogenesis. *Journal of Child Neurology, 20,* 287–299.

Hahn, J.S., & Pinter, J.D. (2002). Holoprosencephaly: Genetic, neuroradiological and clinical advances. *Seminars in Pediatric Neurology, 9,* 309–319.

Hanaway, J., Lee, S.I., & Netsky, M.G. (1968). Pachygyria: Relation of findings to modern embryologic concepts. *Neurology, 18,* 791–799.

Hattori, H., & Wasterlain, C.G. (1990). Excitatory amino acids in the developing brain: Ontogeny, plasticity, and excitotoxicity. *Pediatric Neurology, 6,* 219–228.

Haydar, T.F., Ang, E., Jr., & Rakic, P. (2003). Mitotic spindle rotation and mode of cell division in the developing telencephalon. *Proceedings of the National Academy of Sciences of the United States of America, 100,* 2890–2895.

Hendry, S.H.C., Jones, E.G., DeFelipe, J., Schmechel, D., Brandon, C., & Emson, P.C. (1984). Neuropeptide-containing neurons of the cerebral cortex are also GABAergic. *Proceedings of the National Academy of Sciences of the United States of America, 81,* 6526–6530.

Herlenius, E., & Lagercrantz, H. (2001). Neurotransmitters and neuromodulators during early human development. *Early Human Development, 65,* 21–37.

Heuss, C., & Gerber, U. (2000). G-protein-independent signaling by G-protein-coupled receptors. *Trends in Neurosciences, 23,* 469–475.

Hirokawa, N., & Takemura, R. (2004). Molecular motors in neuronal development, intracellular transport and diseases. *Current Opinion in Neurobiology, 14,* 564–573.

Hirokawa, N., & Takemura, R. (2005). Molecular motors and mechanisms of directional transport in neurons. *Nature Reviews: Neuroscience, 6,* 201–214.

Hokfelt, T. (1991). Neuropeptides in perspective: The last ten years. *Neuron, 7,* 867–879.

Holland, B.A., Haas, D.K., Morman, D., Brant-Zawadzki, M., & Newton, T.H. (1985). MRI of normal brain maturation. *AJNR: American Journal of Neuroradiology, 7,* 201–208.

Howard, H.C., Mount, D.B., Rochefort, D., Byun, N., & Dupre, N. (2002). The K-Cl cotransporter KCC3 is mutant in a severe peripheral neuropathy associated with agenesis of the corpus callosum. *Nature Genetics, 32,* 384–392.

Humphreys, P., Kaufmann, W.E., & Galaburda, A.M. (1990). Developmental dyslexia in women: Neuropathological findings in three patients. *Annals of Neurology, 28,* 727–738.

Huttenlocher, P. (1979). Synaptic density in human frontal cortex—developmental changes and effects of aging. *Brain Research, 163,* 195–205.

Huttenlocher, P. (1984). Synapse elimination and plasticity in developing human cerebral cortex. *American Journal of Mental Deficiency, 88,* 488–496.

Huttenlocher, P.R. (1991). Dendritic and synaptic pathology in mental retardation. *Pediatric Neurology, 7,* 79–85.

Inlow, J.K., & Restifo, L.L. (2004). Molecular and comparative genetics of mental retardation. *Genetics, 166,* 835–881.

Johnston, M.V. (2004). Clinical disorders of brain plasticity. *Brain and Development, 26,* 73–80.

Kalil, K., & Dent, E.W. (2005). Touch and go: Guidance cues signal to the growth cone cytoskeleton. *Current Opinion in Neurobiology, 15,* 521–526.

Kammermeier, L., & Reichert, H. (2001). Evolution of the nervous system: Common developmental genetic mechanisms for patterning invertebrate and vertebrate brains. *Brain Research Bulletin, 55,* 675–682.

Kanatani, S., Tabata, H., & Nakajima, K. (2005). Neuronal migration in cortical development. *Journal of Child Neurology, 20,* 274–279.

Kanold, P.O. (2004). Transient microcircuits formed by subplate neurons and their role in functional development of thalamocortical connections. *NeuroReport, 15,* 2149–2153.

Karfunkel, P. (1974). The mechanisms of neural tube formation. *International Review of Cytology, 38,* 245.

Kato, M., Das, S., Petras, K., Kitamura, K., & Morahashi, K. (2004). Mutations of *ARX* are associated with striking pleiotropy and consistent genotype-phenotype correlation. *Human Mutation, 23,* 147–159.

Kato, M., & Dobyns, W.B. (2003). Lissencephaly and the molecular basis of neuronal migration. *Human Molecular Genetics, 12,* r89–r96.

Kaufmann, W.E., & Galaburda, A.M. (1989). Cerebrocortical microdysgenesis in neurologically normal subjects: A histopathologic study. *Neurology, 39,* 238–244.

Kaufmann, W.E., & Moser, H.W. (2000). Dendritic anomalies in disorders associated with mental retardation. *Cerebral Cortex, 10,* 981–991.

Kemper, T.L., & Galabruda, A.M. (1984). Principles of cytoarchitectonics. In A. Peters & E.G. Jones (Eds.), *Cerebral cortex: Vol. 1. Cellular components of the cerebral cortex* (pp. 35–57). New York: Plenum.

Kinney, H.C., Brody, B.A., Kloman, A.S., & Gilles, F.H. (1988). Sequence of central nervous system myelination in human infancy: II. Patterns of myelination in autopsied infants. *Journal of Neuropathology and Experimental Neurology, 47,* 217–234.

Kinsman, S.L., Plawer, L.L., & Hahn, J.S. (2000). Holoprosencephaly: Recent advances and new insights. *Current Opinion in Neurology, 13,* 127–132.

Kleinschmidt, A., Bear, M., & Singer, W. (1987). Blockade of NMDA receptors disrupts experience-dependent plasticity of kitten striate cortex. *Science, 238,* 355–358.

Koch, C., Zador, A., & Brown, T. (1992). Dendritic spines: Convergence of theory and experiment. *Science, 256,* 973–974.

Kolodny, E.H. (1993). Dysmyelinating and demyelinating conditions in infancy. *Current Opinion in Neurology and Neurosurgery, 6,* 379–386.

Kostovic, I., & Judas, M. (2002). Correlation between the sequential ingrowth of afferents and transient patterns of cortical lamination in preterm infants. *Anatomical Record, 1,* 1–6.

Kostovic, I., & Judas, M. (2006). Prolonged coexistence of transient and permanent circuitry elements in the developing cerebral cortex of fetuses and preterm infants. *Developmental Medicine and Child Neurology, 48,* 388–393.

Krieger, D.T. (1983). Brain peptides: What, where and why? *Science, 222,* 975–985.

Lambert de Rouvroit, C., & Goffinet, A.M. (2001). Neuronal migration. *Mechanisms of Development, 105,* 47–56.

Larsen, C.C., Larsen, K.B., Bogdanovic, N., & Laursen, H. (2006). Total number of cells in the human newborn telencephalic wall. *Neurosciences Research Program Bulletin, 139,* 999–1003.

Lauder, J. (1993). Neurotransmitters as growth regulatory signals: Role of receptors and second messengers. *Trends in Neurosciences, 16,* 233–240.

Lauder, J.M. (1995). Ontogeny of neurotransmitter systems: Substrates for developmental disabilities? *Mental Retardation and Developmental Disabilities Research Reviews, 1,* 151–168.

Leckman, J.F., Walkup, J.T., & Riddle, M.A. (1987). Tic disorders. In H.Y. Meltzer (Ed.), *Psychopharmacology: The third generation of progress* (pp. 1239–1246). New York: Raven.

Leech, R.W., & Shuman, R.M. (1986). Holoprosencephaly and related midline cerebral anomalies: A review. *Journal of Child Neurology, 1,* 3–17.

Lemire, R.J., Beckwith, J.B., & Warkany, J. (1978). *Anencephaly.* New York: Raven Press.

Levitt, P., Cooper, M., & Rakic, P. (1981). Coexistence of neuronal and glial precursor cells in the cerebral ventricular zone of the fetal monkey: An ultrastructural immunoperoxidase analysis. *Journal of Neuroscience, 1,* 27–39.

Levitt, P., Eagleson, K.L., & Powell, E.M. (2004). Regulation of neocortical interneuron development and the implications for neurodevelopmental disorders. *Trends in Neurosciences, 27,* 400–406.

Loyd, K.G., Hornykiewicz, O., & Davidson, L. (1981). Biochemical evidence of dysfunction of brain neurotransmitters in the Lesch-Nyhan syndrome. *New England Journal of Medicine, 305,* 1106–1111.

Lydiard, R.B. (2003). The role of GABA in anxiety disorders. *Journal of Clinical Psychiatry, 64*(3), 21–27.

Maise, K., & Chong, Z.Z. (2005). Driving cellular plasticity and survival through the signal transduction pathways of metabotropic glutamate receptors. *Current Neurovascular Research, 2,* 425–446.

Marin-Padilla, M. (1972). Structural abnormalities of the cerebral cortex in human chromosomal aberrations: A Golgi study. *Brain Research, 44,* 625–629.

Markram, H., Toledo-Rodriguez, M., Wang, Y., Gupta, A., Silberberg, G., & Wu, C. (2004). Interneurons of the neocortical inhibitory system. *Nature Reviews: Neuroscience, 5,* 793–807.

Martin, K.C. (2004). Local protein synthesis during axon guidance and synaptic plasticity. *Current Opinion in Neurobiology, 14,* 305–310.

Mattson, M.P. (1988). Neurotransmitters in the regulation of neuronal cytoarchitecture. *Brain Research Reviews, 13,* 179–212.

McDonald, J.W., Garofalo, E.A., Hood, T., Sackellares, J.C., Gilman, S., McKeever, P.E., et al. (1991). Altered excitatory and inhibitory amino acid receptor binding in hippocampus of patients with temporal lobe epilepsy. *Annals of Neurology, 29,* 529–541.

McDonald, J.W., & Johnston, M.V. (1990). Physiological and pathophysiological roles of excitory amino acids during central nervous system development. *Brain Research Reviews, 15,* 41–70.

McLaren, J., & Bryson, S. (1987). Review of recent epidemiological studies of mental retardation: Prevalence, associated disorders and etiology. *American Journal of Mental Retardation, 92,* 243–254.

McManus, M.F., & Golden, J.A. (2005). Neuronal migration in developmental disorders. *Journal of Child Neurology, 20,* 280–286.

Metin, C., Baudoin, J., Rakic, S., & Parnavelas, J.G. (2006). Cell and molecular mechanisms involved in the migration of cortical interneurons. *European Journal of Neuroscience, 23,* 894–900.

Molliver, M., Kostovic, I., & Loos, H. (1973). The development of synapses in cerebral cortex of the human fetus. *Brain Research, 50,* 403–407.

Molnar, Z., Metin, C., Stoykova, A., & Tarabykin, V. (2006). Comparative aspects of cerebral cortical development. *European Journal of Neuroscience, 4,* 921–934.

Moore, K.L., & Persaud, T.V. (1993). *The developing human: Clinically oriented embryology* (5th ed.). Philadelphia: W.B. Saunders.

Mountcastle, V.B. (1979). An organizing principle for cerebral function: The unit module and the distributed system. In F.O. Schmitt & F.G. Worden (Eds.), *The neurosciences: Fourth study program* (pp. 21–42). Cambridge, MA: M.I.T. Press.

Mukherjee, P., & McKinstry, R.C. (2006). Diffusion tensor imaging and tractography of human brain development. *Neuroimaging Clinics of North America, 16,* 19–43.

Newey, S.E., Velamoor, V., Govek, E., & Van Aelst, L. (2005). Rho GTPases, dendritic structure, and mental retardation. *Journal of Neurobiology, 64,* 58–74.

Noctor, S.C., Martinez-Cerdeno, V., Ivic, L., & Kriegstein, A.R. (2004). Cortical neurons arise in symmetric and asymmetric division zones and migrate through specific phases. *Nature Neuroscience, 7,* 136–144.

Nowakowski, R. (1987). Basic concepts of CNS development. *Child Development, 58,* 568–595.

Osborn, R.E., Sharon, E.B., Naidich, T.P., Bohan, T.P., & Friedman, H. (1988). MR imaging of neuronal migrational disorders. *AJNR: American Journal of Neuroradiology, 9,* 1101–1106.

Page, T., & Nyhan, W. (1990). Biochemical correlates of auto aggressive behavior. In S. Deutsch, A. Weizman, & R. Weizman (Eds.), *Application of basic neuroscience to child psychiatry* (pp. 297–312). New York: Plenum.

Palm, L., Blennow, G., & Brun, A. (1986). Infantile spasms and neuronal heterotopias. *Acta Paediatrica Scandinavica, 75,* 855–859.

Palmini, A., Andermann, F., Olivier, A., Tampieri, D., Robitaille, Y., Andermann, E., et al. (1991). Focal neuronal migration disorders and intractable partial epilepsy: A study of 30 patients. *Annals of Neurology, 30,* 741–749.

Parnavelas, J.G. (1986). Morphology and distribution of peptide-containing neurones in the cerebral cortex. *Progress in Brain Research, 66,* 119–134.

Parnavelas, J.G. (2000). The origin and migration of cortical neurones: New vistas. *Trends in Neurosciences, 23,* 126–131.

Paus, T., Collins, D.L., Evans, C., & Leonard, B. (2001). Maturation of white matter in the human brain: A review of magnetic resonance studies. *Brain Research Bulletin, 54,* 255–266.

Pearl, P.L., Capp, P.K., Novotny, E.J., & Gibson, K.M. (2005). Inherited disorders of neurotransmitters in children and adults. *Clinical Biochemistry, 38,* 1051–1058.

Perry, E.K., Lee, M., Martin-Ruiz, C.M., Court, J.A., & Volsen, S.G. (2001). Cholinergic activity in autism: Abnormalities in the cerebral cortex and basal forebrain. *American Journal of Psychiatry, 158,* 1058–1066.

Perry, E.K., Walker, M., Grace, J., & Perry, R. (1999). Acetylcholine in mind: A neurotransmitter correlate of consciousness? *Trends in Neurosciences, 22,* 273–280.

Piao, X., Hill, R.S., Bodell, A., Chang, B.S., & Basel-Vanagaite, L. (2004). G protein-coupled receptor-dependent development of human frontal cortex. *Science, 303,* 2033–2036.

Purpura, D.P. (1974). Dendritic spine "dysgenesis" and mental retardation. *Science, 186,* 1126–1128.

Purpura, D.P., Bodick, N., Suzuki, K., Rapin, I., & Wurzelmann, S. (1982). Microtubule disarray in cortical dendrites and neurobehavioral failure: I. Golgi and electron microscopic studies. *Developmental Brain Research, 5,* 287–297.

Rakic, P. (1988). Specification of cerebral cortical areas. *Science, 241,* 170–176.

Rakic, P., & Goldman-Rakic, P.S. (1982). Development and modifiability of the cerebral cortex: Overview. *Neurosciences Research Program Bulletin, 20,* 433–438.

Ramakers, G. (2002). Rho proteins, mental retardation and the cellular basis of cognition. *Trends in Neurosciences, 25,* 191–199.

Renieri, A., Pescucci, C., Longo, I., Ariani, F., & Mari, F. (2005). Non-syndromic X-linked mental retardation: From a molecular to a clinical point of view. *Journal of Cellular Physiology, 204,* 8–20.

Richardson, R.T., & DeLong, M.R. (1988). A reappraisal of the functions of the nucleus basalis of Meynert. *Trends in Neuroscience, 11,* 264–267.

Richman, D., Stewart, M., Hutchinson, J., & Caviness, V. (1975). Mechanical model of brain convolutional development. *Science, 189,* 18–21.

Rosenberg, D.R., & Keshavan, M.S. (1998). Toward a neurodevelopmental model of obsessive-compulsive disorder. *Biological Psychiatry, 43,* 623–640.

Rossi, L.N., Candini, G., Scarlatti, G., Rossi, G., Prina, E., & Alberti, S. (1987). Autosomal dominant microcephaly without mental retardation. *Archives of Disease in Childhood, 141,* 655–659.

Sarnat, H.B. (1987). Disturbances of late neuronal migrations in the perinatal period. *Archives of Diseases of Childhood, 141,* 969–979.

Sarnat, H.B. (2005). CNS malformations: Gene locations of known human mutations. *European Journal of Paediatric Neurology, 9,* 427–431.

Sarnat, H.B., & Flore-Sarnat, L. (2004). Integrative classification of morphology and molecular genetics in central nervous system malformations. *American Journal of Medical Genetics, 126A,* 386–392.

Schneider, J.F., Il'yasov, K.A., Hennig, J., & Martin, E. (2004). Fast quantitative diffusion-tensor imaging of cerebral white matter from the neonatal period to adolescence. *Neuroradiology, 46,* 258–266.

Sheen, V.L., Ganesh, V.S., Topcu, M., Sebire, G., & Bodell, A. (2004). Mutations in *ARFGEF2* implicate vesicle trafficking in neural progenitor proliferation and migration in the human cerebral cortex. *Nature Genetics, 36,* 69–76.

Sherman, D.L., & Brophy, P.J. (2005). Mechanisms of axon ensheathment and myelin growth. *Nature Reviews: Neuroscience, 6,* 683–690.

Shimogori, T., Banuchi, V., Ng, H.Y., Strauss, J.B., & Grove, E.A. (2004). Embryonic signaling centers expressing BMP, WNT, and FGF proteins interact to pattern the cerebral cortex. *Development, 131,* 5639–5647.

Sidman, R., & Rakic, P. (1973). Neural migration, with special reference to developing human brain: A review. *Brain Research, 62,* 1–35.

Slaby, A.E., & Tancredi, L.R. (2001). Micropharmacology: Treating disturbances of mood, thought, and behavior as specific neurotransmitter dysregulations rather than as clinical syndromes. *Primary Psychiatry, 8*(4), 28–32.

Solanto, M.V. (2000). Dopamine dysfunctionin AD/HD: Integrating clinical and basic neuroscience research. *Behavioural Brain Research, 130*, 65–71.

Sutton, M.A., & Schuman, E.M. (2005). Local translational control of dendrites and its role in long-term synaptic plasticity. *Journal of Neurobiology, 64*, 116–131.

Sztriha, L., Espinosa-Parrilla, Y., Gururaj, A., & Amiel, J. (2003). Frameshift mutation of the zinc finger homeobox 1B gene in syndromic corpus callosum agenesis (Mowat-Wilson syndrome). *Neuropediatrics, 34*, 322–325.

Tanaka, T., & Gleeson, J.G. (2000). Genetics of brain development and malformation syndromes. *Current Opinion in Pediatrics, 15*, 523–528.

Urbach, R., & Technau, G.M. (2004). Neuroblast formation and patterning during early brain development in Drosophila. *BioEssays, 26*, 739–751.

Vervoort, V.S., Holden, K.R., Ukadike, K.C., Collins, J.S., & Saul, R.A. (2004). *POMGnT1* gene alterations in a family with neurological abnormalities. *Annals of Neurology, 56*, 143–148.

Volpe, J.J. (2001). *Neurology of the newborn* (4th ed.). Philadelphia: W.B. Saunders.

Warkany, J., Lemire, R.J., & Cohen, M.M., Jr. (1981a). Encephaloceles. In *Mental retardation and congenital malformations of the central nervous system* (pp. 158–175). Chicago: Year Book Medical Publishers.

Warkany, J., Lemire, R.J., & Cohen, M.M., Jr. (1981b). Lissencephaly: Agyria and pachygyria. In *Mental retardation and congenital malformations of the central nervous system* (pp. 200–210). Chicago: Year Book Medical Publishers.

Warkany, J., Lemire, R., & Cohen, M.M., Jr. (1981c). Megalencephaly. In *Mental retardation and congenital malformations of the central nervous system* (pp. 101–121). Chicago: Year Book Medical Publishers.

Warkany, J., Lemire, R. J., & Cohen, M.M., Jr. (1981d). *Mental retardation and congenital malformations of the central nervous system* Chicago: Year Book Medical Publishers.

Warkany, J., Lemire, R., & Cohen, M.M., Jr. (1981e). Microcephaly. In *Mental retardation and congenital malformations of the central nervous system* (pp. 13–39). Chicago: Year Book Medical Publishers.

Wong, M. (2005). Advances in the pathophysiology of developmental epilepsies. *Seminars in Pediatric Neurology, 12*, 72–87.

Woo, N.H., & Lu, B. (2006). Regulation of cortical interneurons by neurotrophins: From development to cognitive disorders. *Neuroscientist, 1*, 43–56.

Woods, C.G., Bond, J., & Enard, W. (2005). Autosomal recessive primary microcephaly (MCPH): A review of clinical, molecular, and evolutionary findings. *American Journal of Human Genetics, 76*, 717–728.

Worley, P.F., Baraban, J.M., & Snyder, S.H. (1987). Beyond receptors: Multiple second-messenger systems in brain. *Annals of Neurology, 21*, 217–229.

Yakovlev, P.I., & Lecours, A.R. (1967). The myelogenetic cycles of regional maturation of the brain. In A. Minkowski (Ed.), *Regional development of the brain in early life* (pp. 3–70). Oxford: Blackwell.

Scientific Basis

▽ II

3

The Epidemiology of Developmental Disabilities

MARSHALYN YEARGIN-ALLSOPP, COLLEEN BOYLE,
KIM VAN NAARDEN BRAUN, AND EDWIN TREVATHAN

Epidemiology is defined as the study of the distribution and determinants of disease frequency (MacMahon & Pugh, 1970). It has been widely applied in the study of developmental disabilities to understand how the prevalence of these disorders varies in populations (*descriptive epidemiology*), to monitor trends in disease over time (*epidemiological surveillance*), and to conduct special investigations to try to understand risk and protective factors associated with disease occurrence (*analytical epidemiology*).

ANALYTICAL TOOLS

The basic observations in epidemiology are of disease occurrence (Rothman, 2002). Two primary measures of disease occurrence are used in epidemiological studies: disease incidence and disease prevalence. *Disease incidence* refers to the rate of new cases in a defined population expressed as a function of time and can be defined as 1) an incidence proportion or disease risk

$$\frac{\text{Number of new cases in the population during time } x}{\text{Number of people at risk of the disease in the population during time } x} \times 1{,}000$$

or 2) an incidence rate

$$\frac{\text{Number of new cases in population during time } x}{\text{Person-time (in years) contributed by the population at risk during time } x} \times 1{,}000$$

The incidence rate calculation can accommodate issues such as loss to follow-up or competing risks because individuals only contribute person-time for the period that they are known to be at risk for the disease.

Disease prevalence refers to the burden or status of a disease in a defined population at a specified time and includes all cases of disease in the population whether they are newly diagnosed or previously recognized (Rothman, 2002). It is defined as

$$\frac{\text{Number of people in a defined population with disease during time } x}{\text{Number of people in the population during time } x} \times 1{,}000$$

Prevalence is affected by the incidence of the disease in the population and the duration of the disease. Prevalence has been used for health- and policy planning–related activities in an attempt to anticipate the type and quantity of health services that will be needed.

Incidence rates or disease risks are commonly used in etiological studies; however, in developmental disabilities research, calculation of incidence rates is challenging, if not impossible. Because the majority of developmental disabilities have a prenatal origin, the population at risk is theoretically all pregnancies. Any pregnancy, even if lost or terminated prior to birth, could have resulted in a child with a developmental disability. For most epidemiological studies, it is not feasible to include such pregnancies in calculating disease occurrence for developmental disabilities.

Another characteristic of developmental disabilities that impinges on the calculation of incidence is that the variable clinical manifestation of disease is difficult to define in time and is generally identified when developmental milestones are delayed or missed in early childhood (Rogers & DiLalla, 1990; Stanley, Blair, & Alberman, 2000). As a result of these challenges, most epidemiological studies of developmental disabilities have used disease prevalence (with fewer using an incidence proportion based on a cohort of neonatal or infant survivors) as a measure of occurrence. Each measure and its complementary study design have limitations that need to be recognized when interpreting the study's findings.

STUDY DESIGNS

The major epidemiological study designs are the cohort and case–control designs. Table 3.1 highlights the major strengths and limitations of these two study designs. A *cohort* is defined as any "designated group of individuals who are followed or traced over a period of time" (MacMahon & Pugh, 1970). A birth cohort would include all live-born children in a specified geographic region during a defined period of time. A *cohort study* design involves measur-

ing disease occurrence among individuals by whether or not they are exposed to a factor of interest. A clinical trial is a special type of cohort study, generally used to evaluate treatments, that uses a randomized protocol to "assign" exposure (treatment interventions) and then follows study participants for the onset of illness or changes in the severity of the illness.

Cohort studies can be either prospective or retrospective in nature. *Prospective* means defining the population at risk of disease and following it concurrently in time. *Retrospective* refers to going back in time to historically assemble the cohort and ascertain exposure status and disease occurrence. A retrospective study requires the use of historical records that are relatively complete (e.g., hospital labor and delivery records, vital birth records) to establish the cohort and assign exposure. Retrospective studies are considerably less costly than prospective studies and usually, depending on the nature of the research question, take much less time to conduct.

In contrast to the cohort study, which begins with the population at risk, the *case–control study* begins with identifying individuals with a disorder in a defined population and then looking retrospectively among those with the disorder and a comparison group of those with-

Table 3.1.   Methodologic strengths and limitations of epidemiological cohort and case–control studies

Strengths	Limitations
Cohort	
An unexposed comparison group may be naturally defined in the cohort.	It may incur high study cost because of the need for large sample sizes and the examination of exposure and disease status in many individuals.
Exposure is obtained sequentially prior to disease onset (or determined retrospectively with the establishment of the cohort).	Studies may take many years to conduct depending on the prevalence of outcome and sample size.
Retrospective cohort studies are more timely, if exposure can be accurately measured from existing records (or interviews).	It is not always clear if exposure preceded disease onset.
Incidence rates or risk and their differences and ratios can be calculated.	
Multiple disease/conditions can be examined in the same study.	
Case–control	
Studies allow for a more rapid assessment of the problem.	Researchers need to retrospectively determine exposure from existing records or interviews.
Studies are often less resource intensive and more efficient; that is, fewer study subjects are needed to evaluate in terms of exposure and disease outcome.	It is challenging to identify the control (people without the disease) group; participants need to come from the same population at risk as the case group.
Researchers can study many exposures for the same disease/condition.	Researchers can only calculate the ratio of incidence rates or risks.

out the disorder to determine prior exposure. A case–control study is generally considered the design of choice when the disease of interest is uncommon. For many developmental disabilities, a cohort study would be cost prohibitive, particularly if the study involved multiple exposures. To illustrate, of the developmental disabilities listed in Table 3.2 with prevalence in the range of 2–7 per 1,000 (cerebral palsy, epilepsy, and autism), following 10,000 live-born children to 5 years of age (or the equivalent age to ensure that most of these developmental disabilities would be accurately identified) would identify approximately 20–60 children with each of these disorders. Such small numbers of children would provide little insight for exposure–disease associations of moderate magnitude (risk ratio < 3) or for uncommon exposures (prevalence < 5%), or both.

Cohort and case–control studies are both considered *longitudinal* studies in that the exposure is clearly separated in time from the onset of disease. In contrast, *cross-sectional* studies examine a snapshot of exposure and disease at a particular point in time. Population surveys, such as the National Health Interview Survey (NHIS) of the Centers for Disease Control and Prevention's (CDC) National Center for Health Statistics (NCHS), include questions about developmental disabilities in children and adults and a range of other topics, such as sociodemographic factors (e.g., household income, employment of head of household, and education) (Woodruff et al., 2004). Cross-sectional studies yield prevalence data describing the burden or status of disease for various subgroups of the population.

MEASURES OF DISEASE ASSOCIATION

Measures of association are used to quantify the relationship between a risk (protective) factor and disease outcome. (Rothman, 2002). A *risk ratio* is used to compare the probability of developing the disease among those exposed with the probability of developing the disease among those unexposed. The *rate ratio* takes into account the person-years of observation and describes the ratio of the incidence rate of

Table 3.2. Prevalence of major neurodevelopmental disorders in the United States

Disorders	Average prevalence per 1,000 children	References
Cerebral palsy	2–4	Karapurkar Bhasin, Brocksen, Avchen, and Van Naarden Braun (2006); Stanley, Blair, and Alberman (2000)
Intellectual disabilities	10 (all levels)	Karapurkar Bhasin et al. (2006); Kiely (1987); Leonard and Wen (2002); Murphy, Boyle, Schendel, Decouflé, and Yeargin-Allsopp (1998); Murphy, Yeargin-Allsopp, Decouflé, and Drews (1995); Roeleveld, Zielhuis, and Gabreels (1997)
Autism	2–7	ADDM (2007a, 2007b), Fombonne (1999); Gillberg and Wing (1999); Yeargin-Allsopp et al. (2003)
Epilepsy	4–9	Cowan, Bodensteiner, and Leviton (1989); Murphy, Trevathan, and Yeargin-Allsopp (1995); Waaler, Blom, Skeidsvoll, and Mykletun (2000)
Speech and language disorders	20–60	Shamas, Wiig, and Secord (1998); Tomblin, Smith, and Zhang (1997)
Behavior disorders	3–15	Cohen, Cohen, Kasen, and Velex (1993); Shaffer, Fisher, and Dulcan (1996)
Hearing loss	1–2	Darin, Hanner, and Thiringer (1997); Davis and Wood (1992); Fortnum, Summerfield, Marshall, Davis, and Bamford (2001); Karapurkar Bhasin et al. (2006); Van Naarden and Decouflé (1999)
Vision impairment	0.4–0.8	Gilbert, Anderton, Dandona, and Foster (1999); Karapurkar Bhasin et al. (2006); Mervis, Boyle, and Yeargin-Allsopp (2002); Steinkuller et al. (1993)

Key: ADDM, Autism and Developmental Disabilities Monitoring Network Surveillance Year 2000 Principal Investigators.

disease in the exposed group relative to that in the unexposed group. These two measures of effect are calculated as follows:

$$\text{Risk ratio} = \frac{\text{Probability of disease in the exposed group}}{\text{Probability of disease in the unexposed group}}$$

$$\text{Rate ratio} = \frac{\text{Incidence rate of disease in the exposed group}}{\text{Incidence rate of disease in the unexposed group}}$$

The *prevalence odds ratio* is used to describe the ratio of people with disease to those without disease, comparing subgroups of various risk or protective factors of interest. It is defined as the odds of having a disease relative to the odds of not having the disease. The prevalence odds ratio is calculated as follows:

$$\frac{\dfrac{\text{Prevalence}^1 \text{ of disease in the population}}{1 - \text{Prevalence}^1 \text{ of disease in the population}}}{\dfrac{\text{Prevalence}^2 \text{ of disease in the population}}{1 - \text{Prevalence}^2 \text{ of disease in the population}}}$$

Prevalence[1] is the prevalence of disease among individuals with characteristic A, and Prevalence[2] is the prevalence of disease among individuals with characteristic B.

EPIDEMIOLOGICAL SURVEILLANCE

Surveillance refers to the ongoing monitoring of disease in the population. Surveillance data are used to detect new outbreaks, provide information on the natural history of disease, describe the size and scope of health problems, and evaluate the effect of health interventions (Stroup, Brookmeyer, & Kalsbeek, 2004). Cases identified from surveillance activities can be used as the basis of analytical epidemiological studies to investigate risk factors for and causes of developmental disabilities. Surveillance of developmental disabilities has been an ongoing activity in the United States and in several other countries (Surman, Newdick, & Johnson, 2003; Yeargin-Allsopp, Murphy, Oakley, & Sikes, 1992).

CASE ASCERTAINMENT

Epidemiological studies (including surveillance studies) have used primarily three methods to identify children with developmental disabilities: 1) ongoing questionnaire surveys that ask a parent or primary caregiver information on children's functioning, 2) reviews of administrative medical and school records for children with developmental problems, and 3) screening of population samples (either total population or high-risk subgroups). Questionnaire surveys are dependent on the understanding of the parent or primary caregiver about the specific aspects of the child's diagnosis, as well as the ability of the survey questions to elicit such information correctly. Misclassification undoubtedly occurs, and the level of misclassification is directly related to the specificity of the information being ascertained. The validity of using administrative records (medical and education) to identify case children is dependent on children coming to the attention of a provider, appropriate testing being performed, recording of that information in the medical record, and obtaining appropriate access to such records. This method is assumed to yield reasonably complete ascertainment of children with moderate to severe disabilities, but will miss children with milder disabilities; however, issues of accurate diagnosis, particularly for conditions that have evolving case definitions or those that are based exclusively on behavioral signs and symptoms, such as autism and attention-deficit/hyperactivity disorder (ADHD), can be particularly challenging. Finally, population screening followed by clinical assessment of the child, while the "gold standard" from the standpoint of the validity of the diagnostic assessment, has challenges in terms of getting good participation (and thereby avoiding a biased sample) and the prohibitive cost of individualized assessments (particularly for large samples).

PREVALENCE OF DEVELOPMENTAL DISABILITIES IN U.S. CHILDREN

In epidemiological research, developmental disabilities are commonly defined as a group of severe chronic conditions that are attributable to an impairment in physical, cognitive, speech or language, psychological, or self-care areas and that are manifested during the developmental period (younger than 18 [or 21] years of age) (Crocker, 1989; Yeargin-Allsopp et al., 1992). Epidemiological research often uses administrative data such as medical and special education school records to ascertain children with developmental disabilities. Therefore, in such studies service provision is implicitly incorporated into the definition.

The average prevalence of major developmental disabilities ranges from 1 per 1,000 for sensory disorders to 20–60 per 1,000 for speech and language disorders (see Table 3.2). The majority of studies that have examined the prevalence of developmental disabilities have focused specifically on one disability. Therefore, comprehensive data on the frequency and range of developmental disabilities in children in the United States are available from a limited number of sources. Three commonly referenced data sources that report prevalence of a range of developmental disabilities are the National Health Interview Survey, the Office of Special Education Programs (OSEP) of the U.S. Department of Education, and the Metropolitan Atlanta Developmental Disabilities Surveillance Program (MADDSP).

The National Health Interview Survey on Disability (NHIS-D), which relies on parental or legal guardian interview, revealed that approximately 3%–4% of children 6–17 years of age were reported to have ever been diagnosed with intellectual disabilities (ID) or other developmental delays (ODD) (Larson, Lakin, Anderson, Kwak, & Lee, 2000; NCHS, 1999–2000). It was also found that approximately 9% of children ages 6–17 years had ever had a diagnosis of a learning disability, and slightly more than 7% had been diagnosed with ADHD.

By identifying children through their receipt of special education services, OSEP found that, based on the 2000–2001 school year, 8.8% of children 6–21 years of age were receiving services for a disability (U.S. Department of Education, 2001). The frequencies for the specific type of primary special education exceptionality (special service) were 4.3% for specific learning delay, 1.7% for speech and language impairment, 0.9% for ID, 0.51% for other health impairment, 0.15% for autism, 0.11% for hearing impairment, 0.11% for orthopedic impairment, and 0.04% for vision impairment.

One of the few ongoing sources of data on children with severe developmental disabilities is MADDSP, an active, population-based surveillance system for ID, cerebral palsy, autism spectrum disorders (ASDs), hearing loss, and vision impairment in 8-year-old children in metropolitan Atlanta (Boyle et al., 1996). MADDSP identifies children with developmental disabilities through comprehensive review of individual children's records from school, and medical and service provider data sources. In 2000, MADDSP found the prevalence of having at least one of the five serious developmental disabilities to be 1.9%. More specifically, the prevalence for ID among 8-year-old children was 1.2%, for ASDs, 0.7%; for cerebral palsy, 0.3%; for hearing loss, 0.1%; and for vision impairment, 0.1% (Karapurkar Bhasin, Brocksen, Avchen, & Van Naarden Braun, 2006).

The percentage of multiple developmental disabilities in MADDSP was 23.1%, with decreasing percentages (19.1% for one coexisting developmental disability; 3.8% for two developmental disabilities; and 0.2% for three developmental disabilities) as the number of coexisting developmental disabilities increased. Of the group of children with more than one developmental disability, children with ID were most likely to have another developmental disability (22.4%), followed by children with ASDs (13.8%) and then children with cerebral palsy (10.0%). The majority of children with ID and a coexisting developmental disability are those who also have an ASD. The definitions of and methods for identifying children with developmental disabilities differ considerably across these three data sources, which may account for some of the variability between estimates and highlights the challenges in understanding the epidemiology of developmental disabilities.

Examination of the variability of the prevalence of developmental disabilities by race or ethnicity and sex characteristics has provided descriptive insight into developmental disabilities and clues for further etiological research. Data from NHIS 1999–2000 and MADDSP both suggest that the prevalence of most developmental disabilities is higher in boys than girls. With the exception of ASDs, in both the OSEP and the MADDSP data, the prevalence of all disabilities was notably higher among black children. The prevalence of ASDs among white non-Hispanic children from the MADDSP data was slightly elevated, whereas the OSEP data showed no racial or ethnic disparity among children with ASDs. Although OSEP data also showed a slightly increased prevalence of learning disability among black children, the distributions for the developmental disabilities of vision impairment and hearing loss in the MADDSP and the OSEP data did not differ by race or ethnicity. The prevalence of ID in black children was approximately 2.5-fold that among white children in both the OSEP and the MADDSP data. There were, however, no differences for the categories of Other Health Impaired, Orthopedically Impaired, and Speech and Language Impaired. Data from the NHIS reported higher prevalence estimates for ID/ODD and learning disability for both white and black children compared with Hispanic children. These data also showed that the prevalence of ADHD is considerably higher among white children. Further epidemiological research needs to be conducted to examine these racial or ethnic and sex disparities.

Over time, there has been an evolution toward a greater understanding of how to incorporate functioning into defining an individual's disability. Although both the American Psychiatric Association (APA) and American Association on Intellectual and Developmental Disabilities (AAIDD) definitions use functioning as a component of the definition of mental retardation, the World Health Organization (WHO) *International Classification of Functioning, Disability and Health* (ICF) provides a new conceptual framework and classification scheme for capturing disability (WHO, 2001). The components of functioning and disability within the ICF are described from the perspective of the body, the individual, and society as 1) Body Functions and Structures and 2) Activities and Participation. Formerly referred to as *impairment, disability,* and *handicap,* the ICF terminol-

ogy measures both positive and negative experiences.

Using functioning as the measure of disability, the Survey of Income and Program Participation data for 1991–1992 for children 17 years of age or younger captured conditions most frequently reported as a cause of functional limitations among children (Table 3.3).

Table 3.3. Relationship between functional limitations and developmental disabilities

Condition	%
Learning disability	29.5
Speech problems	13.1
Intellectual disabilities	6.8
Asthma	6.4
Mental or emotional problems or disorders	6.3
Blindness or vision problems	3.0
Cerebral palsy	2.7
Epilepsy or seizure disorder	2.6
Impairment or deformity of back, side, foot, or leg	2.5
Deafness or serious hearing impairment	2.4
Tonsillitis or repeated ear infections	1.6
Hay fever or other respiratory allergies	1.6
Paralysis of any kind	1.5
Missing legs, feet, toes, arms, hands, or fingers	1.4
Autism	1.0
Drug or alcohol problems	1.0
Head or spinal cord injury	0.9
Heart disease	0.9
Impairment or deformity of hands, fingers, or arms	0.6
Cancer	0.5
Diabetes	0.3
Other	13.4

From Centers for Disease Control and Prevention. (1995). Disabilities among children aged less than or equal to 17 years—United States 1991–1992. *MMWR: Morbidity and Mortality Weekly Report, 44,* 609–613.

Note: The definition of functional limitation(s) varied by age group. For children ages birth to 5 years, the definition was: 1) limitation in the usual kinds of activities done by most children the same age or 2) receipt of therapy or diagnostic services by the child for developmental needs. For children 6 years of age or older, the definition was any limitation in the ability to do regular schoolwork. For children ages 3–14 years, additional indications included a long-lasting condition that limited the ability to walk, run, or use stairs. For children ages 15–17 years, additional indicators included problems in personal care, problems in personal management, and the use of assistive aids.

Condition was most frequently reported as a cause of functional limitations among children 17 years of age or younger (*n* = 4,858).

Data from the Survey of Income and Program Participation for 1991–1992 for children 17 years of age or younger. Parents or legal guardians were asked about disabilities among their children 14 years or younger and adolescents ages 15–17 years were asked directly.

"Learning disability" was the condition most commonly reported as responsible for a functional limitation (29.5%), with speech problems representing the next highest percentage (13.1%). ID, asthma, and mental or emotional problems each had a frequency of about 6% (CDC, 1995). Although this information was reported by a parent or legal guardian for children 14 years of age or younger and was self-reported by children 15–17 years of age, because there was no verification of disability status from examination or records, the data likely reflect an overall representation of health and developmental conditions of concern among the general population of parents.

As the pediatric population with developmental disabilities ages, questions of transition to adulthood arise. There are very few epidemiological data on how these children function in adulthood (Halpern, 1993). The National Longitudinal Transition Study (NLTS), a study of more than 8,000 special education students, provided data on educational experiences, social activities, postsecondary employment, and residential independence in youth 13–21 years of age who were receiving special education services in secondary school in 1985 (Blackorby & Wagner, 1996). The sample was weighted so as to provide comparisons with a national sample of youth. Experiences were captured from completion of secondary school until 2 years later, and again 3–5 years later. Findings from the NLTS indicated that there were many gains between these two time periods in numbers employed, wages, postsecondary school enrollment, and residential independence; however, there was a significant gap between the numbers of youth with disabilities who were enrolled in postsecondary education programs compared with youth in general (27% vs. 47%), even after adjusting for a number of sociodemographic factors. As more is learned about the functioning of children with disabilities as they move through adulthood, a better understanding of not only the negative long-term consequences of impairment but also the positive attributes and abilities of these individuals will be possible.

INTELLECTUAL DISABILITIES

There is an extensive and rich history of terminology and definition of ID (or mental retarda-

tion). Although more than one definition continues in current use, there is general agreement that the core feature of ID is significantly subaverage general intellectual functioning accompanied by significant limitations in adaptive functioning. The three most common definitions represent those of the *Diagnostic and Statistical Manual of Mental Disorders* (DSM) of the APA, those of the AAIDD, and those of the family of WHO definitions known as the *International Classification of Diseases and Related Health Problems* (ICD), *International Classification of Impairments, Disabilities, and Handicaps* (ICIDH) and the ICF (Table 3.4). The DSM and AAIDD definitions are similar in that they both stress significant limitations in adaptive functioning as well as intellectual functioning; however, the AAIDD definition uses a multidimensional approach comprising the following four dimensions: 1) intellectual functioning and adaptive skills; 2) psychological or emotional considerations; 3) physical, health, or etiology considerations; and 4) environmental considerations. The AAIDD paradigm reflects *the interaction of the individual with the environment* and *the outcomes of the interaction* with regard to independence, relationships, societal contributions, participation in school and community, and personal well-being (Luckasson et al., 2002). The WHO classification schemes (the ICD Tenth Revision [ICD-10], ICIDH, or ICF) do not specify an age cutoff for defining ID, in contrast to the AAP and AAIDD definitions, which require the diagnosis of ID before 18 years of age.

Levels of Intellectual Disabililties

ID have traditionally been divided into levels of severity based on the statistical distribution of intelligence quotient (IQ) scores as measured by standardized psychometric testing. The cutoff points for these levels are based on the number of standard deviations (1 standard deviation = 15 points) below the accepted statistical population mean IQ score of 100 and take into consideration the concept of standard error, which is approximately 5 points on either side of the cutoff score and varies according to the particular test used.

The APA has retained the conventional severity levels of intellectual impairment based

Table 3.4. Definitions of mental retardation/intellectual disabilities

Source	Definition
Diagnostic and Statistical Manual of Mental Disorders, Fourth Edition (American Psychiatric Association, 1994)	Significantly subaverage general intellectual functioning (Criterion A) that is accompanied by significant limitations in adaptive functioning in at least two of the following skill areas: communication, self-care, home living, social/interpersonal skills, use of community resources, self-direction, functional academic skills, work, leisure, health, and safety (Criterion B). The onset must occur before 18 years (Criterion C).
American Association on Intellectual and Developmental Disabilities (Luckasson et al., 2002)	A disability characterized by significant limitations in both intellectual functioning and adaptive behavior as expressed in conceptual, social, and practical adaptive skills. The disability originates before age 18.
International Classification of Diseases, Ninth Revision, Clinical Modification (ICD-9-CM; U.S. Department of Health and Human Services, 1988)	Subnormal intellectual functioning that originates during the developmental period.
International Classification of Diseases, Tenth Revision (ICD-10; World Health Organization, 1992)	A condition of arrested or incomplete development of the mind, which is especially characterized by impairment of skills manifested during the developmental period that contribute to the overall level of intelligence (i.e., cognitive, language, motor, and social abilities).
International Classification of Impairments, Disabilities and Handicaps (ICIDH; World Health Organization, 1980)	Intellectual impairments include those of intelligence, memory, and thought. Includes disturbances of the rate and degree of development of cognitive functions, such as perception, attention, memory, and thinking, and their deterioration as a result of the pathological process.
International Classification of Functioning, Disability and Health (ICF; World Health Organization, 2001)	Classified with intellectual growth, intellectual retardation, and dementia under Intellectual Functions: "General mental functions, required to understand and constructively integrate the various mental functions, including all cognitive functions and their development over the life span."

on IQ scores and maintained an IQ score cutoff point at 70 or below (APA, 1994). In contrast, the AAIDD uses a three-step approach to definition, classification, and "intensity of needed levels of support" that replaced the previous classification of severity (Luckasson et al., 1992; Luckasson et al., 2002). This change is believed to be more relevant to the provision of services and desired outcomes (Leonard & Wen, 2002). Whereas the subclassifications for the *ICD, Ninth Revision, Clinical Modification* (ICD-9-CM), ICD-10, and ICIDH are very similar to each other and have levels of mild, moderate, severe, and profound based on IQ cutoff scores, the ICF represents a departure in that IQ is not a construct in the ICF. Three components—Body Functions and Structures, Activities and Participation, and Environmental Factors—are quantified using the same generic scale, from "no problem" to "complete problem" (Table 3.5).

Incorporating additional aspects of the environment in the definition of ID has implica-tions for epidemiological research. Because adaptive functioning, which has been generally accepted as a necessary component of the ID case definition for clinical and service provision purposes, has not been considered in the case definition for most epidemiological studies to date, it may be difficult to operationalize the new AAIDD definition of mental retardation that uses intensity of supports for epidemiological research that relies on previously collected data. Likewise, the new ICF paradigm, although useful from a consumer and services perspective, will likely be challenging to use for most epidemiological research.

Prevalence

Estimates of ID prevalence from epidemiological studies have varied considerably for a number of reasons, including the differences in case definitions applied within a community or across studies, or both; variations in methods of ascertainment; and relationship of preva-

Table 3.5. Subclassifications of mental retardation/intellectual disabilities by intelligence quotient (IQ) score

Level of intellectual disability	DSM-IV IQ range	AAIDD intensity of support	ICD-9CM IQ range	ICD-10 IQ range	ICIDH impairments of intelligence	ICF
Mild	50–55 to 70	Intermittent	50–70	50–69	Mild: IQ score 50–70 Individuals who can acquire practical skills and functional reading and arithmetic abilities with special education, and can be guided toward social conformity	Mild problem (slight, low: 5%–24%)
Moderate	35–40 to 50–55	Limited	35–49	35–49	Moderate: IQ score 35–49 Individuals who can learn simple communication, elementary health and safety habits, and simple manual skills, but do not progress in functional reading or arithmetic	Moderate problem (medium, fair: 25%–49%)
Severe	20–25 to 35–40	Extensive	20–34	20–34	Severe: IQ score 20–34 Individuals who can profit from systematic habit training	Severe problem (high, extreme: 50%–95%)
Profound	Below 20–25	Pervasive	0–20	0–20	Profound: IQ score under 20 Individuals who might respond to skills training in the use of legs, hands, and jaws	Complete problem (total: 96%–100%)

Note: IQ is not a construct in the ICF. All three components classified in the ICF—Body Functions and Structures, Activities and Participation, and Environmental Factors—are quantified using the same generic scale, from "no problem" to "complete problem."

Key: AAIDD, American Association on Intellectual and Developmental Disabilities (Luckasson et al., 2002); DSM, *Diagnostic and Statistical Manual of Mental Disorders, Fourth Edition* (American Psychiatric Association, 1994); ICD-9CM, *International Classification of Diseases, Ninth Revision, Clinical Modification* (U.S. Department of Health and Human Services, 1988); ICD-10, *International Classification of Diseases, Tenth Revision* (World Health Organization, 1992); ICIDH, *International Classification of Impairments, Disabilities, and Handicaps* (World Health Organization, 1980); ICF, *International Classification of Functioning, Disability and Health* (World Health Organization, 2001).

lence to the sociodemographic characteristics (age, sex, race or ethnicity, and socioeconomic status) of the population studied. Revisions and variations in definitions and classification systems could have a direct influence on differences in reported prevalence rates of ID through their influence on data collection. For example, incorporating adaptive functioning into case definitions for epidemiological studies has been difficult because of the lack of standardization of adaptive functioning until recently; however, when adaptive functioning has been used, the prevalence of ID is lower (Hansen, Belmont, & Stein, 1980). An "administrative" prevalence is often used as a surrogate for "true" prevalence because it is difficult

to obtain a "true" prevalence of ID and other developmental disabilities in some countries, most notably in the United States.

Most epidemiological studies conducted to determine the prevalence of ID use a case definition that relies exclusively on the results of IQ testing. Using an assumed normal distribution for intelligence, with a mean of 100, about 2.3% of children are *expected* to score approximately 2 standard deviations below the mean on a standardized intelligence test (Larson et al., 2001); however, it has been shown that the "true" prevalence as ascertained from community studies of ID is closer to 10 per 1,000 than to 23 per 1,000 (Jacobson & Janicki, 1983; Karapurkar et al., 2006; Larson et al., 2001;

Munro, 1986; Murphy, Yeargin-Allsopp, De-couflé, & Drews, 1995). For epidemiological study purposes, the prevalence of ID is usually examined using two IQ levels, with an IQ ranging from 50–55 to 70–75 being considered mild ID and an IQ less than 50 being considered severe ID (Kiely, 1987; Roeleveld, Zielhuis, & Gabreels, 1997). Most studies have shown that approximately 75%–80% of individuals with ID have mild ID. A recent review by Roeleveld et al. (1997) concluded that 3.8 per 1,000 is a reliable estimate of the prevalence of severe ID and 29.8 per 1,000 is a reasonable estimate for the prevalence of mild ID. These authors also found the prevalence of severe ID for a school-aged population to be fairly stable across studies. The prevalence of mild ID was much more variable, and it was not known whether this represented true differences or differences in methodologies.

The prevalence of ID has been reported to vary with a number of characteristics of the population, such as age, sex, and socioeconomic status. In most studies, the prevalence peaks at 10–14 years of age, with a few studies showing the highest prevalence at 14 years of age (Kiely, 1987; McLaren & Bryson, 1987). In a recent review, variation in the prevalence of ID was found to be from 1 per 1,000 in children 4 years of age or younger to 97 per 1,000 in children 10–14 years of age, emphasizing the importance of considering age when examining the prevalence of ID (Murphy, Boyle, Schendel, Decoufle, & Yeargin-Allsopp, 1998).

Most studies have reported a slightly higher prevalence of ID among boys compared with girls, with the boy-girl ratio overall being approximately 1.5:1 (Leonard & Wen, 2002); this difference is even more pronounced for mild ID than for severe ID (Kiely, 1987; Murphy, Yeargin-Allsopp, et al., 1995; Roeleveld et al., 1997). Reasons for the male preponderance in mild ID are thought to be related to social factors. Certain behaviors might cause boys to receive greater attention (and hence get tested) than girls. Also, biological reasons, such as X-linked conditions, could result in greater identification of boys (Chelly & Mandel, 2001; Partington, Mowat, Einfeld, Tonge, & Turner, 2000; Tariverdian & Vogel, 2000).

Racial and ethnic differences in the prevalence of ID have also been reported with a pre-ponderance of black children having ID (Croen, Grether, & Selvin, 2001; Leonard & Wen, 2002; Murphy, Yeargin-Allsopp, et al., 1995). Confounding by socioeconomic factors is assumed to contribute to these racial and ethnic differences; however, there was an excess prevalence of ID among black children compared with white children in metropolitan Atlanta after controlling for the sociodemographic factors of sex, maternal age, birth order, maternal education, and economic status (Yeargin-Allsopp, Drews, Decouflé, & Murphy, 1995). More studies are needed in order to better elucidate the impact of race and ethnicity on ID.

The inverse relationship between socioeconomic status and prevalence of ID has been well documented (Broman, Nichols, Shaughnessy, & Kennedy 1987; Decouflé & Boyle, 1995; Yeargin-Allsopp, Drews, et al., 1995) and has been shown to be related to severity of ID (Drews, Yeargin-Allsopp, Decouflé, & Murphy, 1995; Munro, 1986; Kiely, 1987). Many studies have consistently shown that mild ID is largely of unknown etiology and is highly correlated with lower socioeconomic status, and that a greater proportion of cases of severe ID have been reported to have a biological basis (Leonard & Wen, 2002; McLaren & Bryson, 1987). It has even been suggested that mild ID is rarely found in the highest socioeconomic groups, unless accompanied by evidence of organic damage. This dichotomy in terms of biological causation associated with level of functioning has led to the notion that ID can be subclassified into two different types: the "two-group theory" of ID, with a smaller IQ curve shifted to the left for "organic damage" superimposed on the normal gaussian curve for overall intelligence (Zigler, Balla, & Hodapp, 1984).

This theory has been supported by several epidemiological studies showing a strong inverse association with socioeconomic factors across the ID spectrum for children with ID without neurological conditions but not for those with ID and concomitant impairment (Drews et al., 1995; Decouflé & Boyle, 1995; Croen, Grether, & Selvin, 2001).

Maternal age at delivery is another risk factor for ID but has not been shown to be as pronounced as that for maternal education (Broman et al., 1987; Drews et al., 1995). In one study, this relationship was found to be correlated with the level of ID in that women who delivered at 15–19 years of age demonstrated a slightly increased risk for *mild* ID, whereas women who delivered at 40–44 years of age demonstrated a greater risk for *moderate to severe* ID (Chapman, Scott, & Mason, 2002). This may be due in part to the increased risk of various chromosomal disorders with increased maternal age.

Etiology and Risk Factors

Prenatal Risk Factors Although more than 500 genetic diseases are known to cause ID, most are of low frequency and individually do not contribute substantially to the overall prevalence of ID (Flint & Wilkie, 1996; Murphy et al., 1998). Down syndrome has been shown to consistently account for about two thirds or more of all genetic causes of ID (Cans et al., 1999; Fernell, 1998; Hou, Wang, & Chuang, 1998; Stromme & Hagberg, 2000; Yeargin-Allsopp, Murphy, Cordero, Decouflé, & Hollowell, 1997). A review by Leonard and Wen (2002) that updates previous epidemiological studies of ID found that the proportion of cases of ID with a known etiology varied from 22% in metropolitan Atlanta to 77% in Sweden. Down syndrome accounted for roughly 10%–15% of all cases, with a range of approximately 5% in metropolitan Atlanta to about 20% in Sweden. Other prominent causes of ID included fragile X syndrome, fetal alcohol syndrome (FAS), and Prader-Willi syndrome. Overall, the most common causes of ID in the United States continue to be Down syndrome, with a prevalence of about 1 per 800 live births (National Center on Birth Defects and Developmental Disabilities, 2004); FAS, with a prevalence of 0.2–1.5 per 1,000 live births (Abel, 1995; Abel & Sokol, 1986); and fragile X syndrome, with a prevalence of 1 per 4,000 boys and 1 per 8,000 girls (Turner, Webb, Wake, & Robinson, 1996). These three conditions account for approximately 30% of all identifiable cases of severe ID (Moser, 1995).

Causes of ID have been reported to differ by level of severity of ID. The proportion of children with severe ID *with* an identified cause is roughly 75%–80% (Leonard & Wen, 2002; Yeargin-Allsopp et al., 1997). Earlier studies reported that roughly 25%–40% of cases of mild ID did not have a recognized etiology (McLaren & Bryson, 1987); however, with improved diagnostic capabilities, such as fluorescence in situ hybridization, DNA testing using methylation studies or gene sequencing, and testing to identify submicroscopic deletions in the subtelomeric chromosomal regions, there are challenges to this assumption (Shevell et al., 2003). In addition, an effort to look more closely for environmental factors, such as lead and mercury, is being encouraged (Mendola, Selevan, Gutter, & Rice, 2002).

The prevalence of idiopathic ID was increased by 50% in children whose mothers smoked during pregnancy, and the prevalence of ID increased with the amount of smoking (Drews, Murphy, Yeargin-Allsopp, & Decouflé, 1996). The mechanism by which smoking increases the risk of ID is not clear. One meta-analysis found a twofold increase in the risk of low birth weight (LBW) infants to smoking mothers (English et al., 1995); however, Drews et al. (1996) suggested that maternal smoking might increase the occurrence of ID by mechanisms other than LBW. Alcohol exposure resulting from maternal alcohol ingestion is also a risk factor for ID (Abel, 1995; Streissguth, Barr, & Sampson, 1990; Streissguth et al., 1991). The prevalence of FAS remains uncertain because of challenges in getting accurate information on the exposure (maternal alcohol ingestion) and the lack of a consistent epidemiological case definition. Maternal medications that have been shown to be teratogenic and associated with ID include antiepileptics (hydantoins, trimethadione, and valproate), warfarin, and retinoic acid (Adams, Voorhees, & Middaugh, 1990; Hanson, 1986; Holmes, Coull, Dorfman, & Rosenberger, 2005; Jones, 1997; Scolnik et al., 1994). Maternal medical conditions have also been shown to incur risk for ID in offspring. A report using data from the Collaborative Perinatal Project (McDermott, Daguise, Mann, Szwejbka, & Callaghan, 2001) found an increased relative risk of 1.4 for ID or developmental delay in the children of mothers who had a urinary tract infection in the third trimester. A thyroid deficiency state (whether a maternal untreated, often unrecognized, deficiency state during pregnancy or congenital hypothyroidism, a recognized risk factor for ID) remains an important contributor to lowered IQ scores and ID in children (Haddow et al., 1999, Qian, Wang, & Chen, 2000; Van Naarden Braun, Yeargin-Allsopp, Schendel, & Fernhoff, 2003).

Another important risk factor for ID is maternal phenylketonuria (PKU). Children born to women with PKU whose metabolic status was not under control were found to have serious congenital malformations, including cardiac defects, microcephaly, and ID (Lenke & Levy, 1980; Waisbren et al., 1997). Fortunately, a maternal PKU study found that women with PKU who kept their blood phenylalanine levels within the recommended range of 2–6 mg/dL during pregnancy had the same probability of having a typically developing infant as women without PKU (Koch, 2000).

Since the 1970s, when 3%–8% of children had ID as a result of an intrauterine infection, the percentage continues to decrease because of immunizations and better recognition and practice of prevention measures (Hagberg & Kyllerman, 1983; Yeargin-Allsopp et al., 1997). Neonatal cytomegalovirus (CMV) infection is the most common congenital cause of ID (Fowler et al., 1992; National Center for Infectious Diseases, 2002). Although neonatal CMV occurs in only 0.3%–1% of all live births and 90%–95% of these infections are not apparent, 15%–25% of those infants will have neurological sequelae, including ID (Naessens, Casteels, Decatte, & Foulon, 2005). The greatest risk of congenital CMV infection is for infants born to women who previously have not been infected with CMV and have their first infection during pregnancy (1%–3%). In a follow-up study of children 5 years of age or younger, 13% of children born to mothers who seroconverted during pregnancy developed ID.

Congenital toxoplasmosis occurs in 1 per 1,000 live births (Buyse, 1990). A follow-up study of children who were born to mothers with toxoplasmosis showed a 30% increase in the prevalence of ID (Sever et al., 1988). There are protocols for treating women who are infected during pregnancy and treating both the mother and infant if the infant is shown to be infected; however, there have been no randomized controlled trials to evaluate the effectiveness of treatment in preventing the long-term developmental sequelae of congenital toxoplasmosis in children (Gilbert et al., 2001).

Congenital rubella, with a prevalence of less than 1 per 100,000 live births in the United States, is no longer a major contributor to ID during childhood (CDC, 2000, 2005). From 2001 through 2004, only four cases of congenital rubella syndrome were reported to the CDC, and three of the four mothers were born outside the United States.

Sexually transmitted infections are also decreasing in their importance as causes of ID. The rate of congenital syphilis declined to about 13.4 per 10,000 live births in 2000 (CDC, 2001). ID occurs in about one third of children with congenital syphilis (Rozien & Johnson, 1996). Neonatal herpes simplex virus (HSV) infection occurs in 1 in 3,000–20,000 live births; however, congenital HSV infection is often severe, with high mortality rates (AAP, 2003b). In 2-year survivors of HSV encephalitis, up to 50% have permanent neurological impairment, including ID. Children who are perinatally infected with the human immunodeficiency virus (HIV) have been reported to have involvement of the central nervous system, with 20%–50% showing evidence of neurological signs (Chadwick & Yogev, 1995; Wachtel & Conlon, 1996).

A study by Pearson et al. (2000) found that neuropsychological and neurological (cortical atrophy on magnetic resonance imaging or computed tomography scans and abnormal motor functioning) tests were predictive of disease progression in HIV-infected children. A more recent study by Foster et al. (2006) found that 22% of HIV-1–infected children had significant motor impairment that persisted in spite of highly active antiretroviral treatment. These results are important because antiretroviral treatment has prolonged life expectancy in these children, yet long-term developmental functioning, as well as the effect of antiretroviral treatment on the developing nervous system, still warrant further study.

Another important risk factor for ID is birth defects. Analysis of data from two metropolitan Atlanta surveillance systems found that 7.2% of children with a major birth defect had a developmental disability and that approximately 18% of children with a developmental disability (ID, cerebral palsy, hearing loss, or vision impairment) had a major birth defect (Decouflé, Boyle, Paulozzi, & Lary, 2001).

Perinatal Risk Factors Perinatal risk factors for ID include LBW, perinatal asphyxia, infection (group B streptococcus), newborn endocrine and metabolic disorders, and multiple births. Both LBW (< 2,500 g) and preterm delivery (< 37 weeks' gestation) have been shown to be risk factors for ID (Cooke, 1994; Hack et al., 1994; Mervis, Decouflé, Murphy, & Yeargin-Allsopp, 1995). Developmental outcomes for premature infants have been reported primarily in terms of birth weight because of difficulties with reliability of data on gestational age (Allen, 1993). Mervis et al. (1995) found that LBW children had nearly three times the risk of ID as compared with normal birth weight children. The risk varied inversely by birth weight and was greater for severe ID than for mild ID. Children with normal birth weight who were born preterm were also at increased risk of ID. Camp, Borman, and Nichols (1998) found that up to 16.5% of infants with a birth weight of less than 2,000 g had ID at 7 years of age.

Perinatal asphyxia, once thought to be a major contributor to ID/ODD, was found to account for about 5% of all ID in one study in which asphyxia was defined as having been recorded in medical records (Yeargin-Allsopp et al., 1997). There are definitional problems with the use of this term, however. Infants who do experience ID as a result of "perinatal asphyxia" are likely to have had prolonged and severe asphyxia, and they are more likely to have had clinical evidence of moderate to severe neonatal encephalopathy; also, the ID is more likely to be associated with clinical evidence of cerebral palsy (Murphy et al., 1998; Nelson & Emery, 1993; Paneth & Stark, 1983; Robertson & Finer, 1985).

At present, the attributable fraction of ID that is due to perinatal infections, including group B streptococcus (GBS) and HSV (discussed previously), is very small (CDC, 1997). In the 1970s, GBS was the leading cause of sepsis in the newborn. Because of changes in the identification and treatment of GBS, by 2003, the rate of GBS infection had declined to 0.5 cases per 1,000 live births compared with 1.3 per 1,000 live births during the period 1993–1995 (AAP, 2003c). HSV remains a low-incidence condition and, therefore, is not a major contributor to the prevalence of ID.

Most metabolic and endocrine disorders that are screened for in the newborn period are genetic disorders that, if untreated in the early neonatal period, result in ID. In a study of children born from 1981 to 1991, newborn screening was found effective in preventing ID associated with PKU, homocystinuria, maple syrup urine disease, tyrosinemia, hypothyroidism, and classic galactosemia, with only 2 of 148 potential cases of ID identified as being due to a metabolic disorder (CDC, 1999). In a population-based follow-up study of children born during the same time period, however, there were at least 12 children with a developmental disability that could be attributed to a metabolic or endocrine disorder (Van Naarden Braun et al., 2003). These data indicate that, although newborn screening for these disorders is effective, long-term follow-up of the neurodevelopmental status of children who screen positive and are diagnosed with one of these disorders is needed.

It is recognized that children of multiple births are at increased risk for ID (Boyle, Keddie, & Holmgreen, 1997; Croen, Grether, & Selvin, 2001; Rydhstroem, 1995). Twins have twice the risk of singleton births, but this increased risk appears to be due to the increased prevalence of LBW infants of twin gestation.

Postnatal Risk Factors Postnatal causes are estimated to account for ID in 3%–15% of children (McLaren & Bryson, 1987; Murphy et al., 1998; Yeargin-Allsopp et al., 1997). Although the percentages appear small in comparison with those for prenatal and perinatal causes, postnatal cases are often preventable; hence, they deserve attention. Postnatal factors shown to be associated with ID include environmental exposures such as lead and mercury, injuries, and postnatally acquired infections.

Although ID is recognized as one of the most devastating long-term outcomes of high lead levels (60 mcg/dL and higher), studies have shown that lead exposure produces a continuum of developmental effects, from death at very high doses to subtle deficits in cognition, memory, and behavior at low levels (Mendola et al., 2002; Needleman, 1992a, 1992b). Increased lead levels in children remain a public health problem because, although blood lead levels have declined significantly since the 1950s, the proportion of children 1–5 years of age with blood levels greater than the current cutoff for defining lead toxicity (10 mcg/dL) was 2.2% during the 1999–2000 period (CDC, 2003a).

Methylmercury is a recognized powerful neurotoxin that has caused ID when associated with very high levels of *prenatal* exposure resulting from acute poisonings; the range of neurodevelopmental effects from lower levels of exposure are not as clear (Davidson, Myers, & Weiss, 2004; Marsh et al., 1987; Mendola et al., 2002). Likewise, the relationship of polychlorinated biphenyls (PCBs) to *prenatal* exposure and later neurodevelopmental outcomes has been studied extensively. When pregnant women were exposed to very high levels of PCBs, ID and other deficits did occur in their offspring (Chen, Guo, & Hsu, 1992; Jacobson & Jacobson, 1996, 1997; Yu, Hsu, Gladen, & Rogan, 1991); however, *postnatal* exposure at usual environmental levels has not been shown to be associated with ID.

Infectious organisms, specifically *Haemophilus influenzae* type b (Hib), *Streptococcus pneumoniae*, and *Neisseria meningitidis* are known to cause ID in children who have had meningitis associated with one of these organisms. Baraff, Lee, and Schriger (1993) examined studies of outcomes from bacterial meningitis in children 2 months of age or older caused by one of these organisms and found that 2.1% of children with *Neisseria*, 6.1% of children with Hib, and 17% of children infected with *S. pneumoniae* had ID. In a study examining postnatally acquired causes of developmental disabilities in children 3–10 years of age in 1991, infectious diseases (primarily Hib) were found to have

contributed to 35% of such cases (CDC, 1996); however, since the introduction of Hib vaccine in 1988, the incidence of invasive Hib disease in infants and young children has decreased by 99% to less than 1 case (0.3) per 100,000 children younger than 5 years of age (AAP, 2003a; CDC, 2002). The incidence of *S. pneumoniae* infections in young children is decreasing; however, there have been outbreaks in child care settings (CDC, 2003b).

Another major postnatal cause of ID is head injury. In children in metropolitan Atlanta, 52% of postnatally acquired ID was due to injuries (CDC, 1996). Of these injuries, child battering was the most frequent cause (18%), followed by being hit by a motor vehicle (9%) and by falls (7.8%). Near drownings, stroke (primarily related to sickle cell disease), and brain tumors accounted for 4%, 7%, and 1%, respectively. There is a statistically significant association between sickle cell disease and ID, with sickle cell disease contributing to 0.4% of ID in black children (Ashley-Koch, Murphy, Khoury, & Boyle, 2001). The association between sickle cell disease and developmental disabilities overall was due almost entirely to the presence of stroke.

CEREBRAL PALSY

Cerebral palsy is an "umbrella term covering a group of nonprogressive, but often changing, motor impairment syndromes secondary to lesions or anomalies of the brain arising in the early stages of development" (Mutch, Alberman, Hagberg, Kodama, & Perat, 1992, p. 549). This definition recognizes the clinical and etiological heterogeneity of the cerebral palsy diagnosis, which is based exclusively on the clinical signs and symptoms of motor impairment. Cerebral palsy is analogous to ID in that both are the overt signs of central nervous system dysfunction (Nelson & Grether, 1999). Clinical classification of cerebral palsy is generally by the type of motor disability, the extent of involvement of the limbs, and the severity of the motor disability (Table 3.6). The most prominent type of motor impairment is spasticity, which represents about 80% of all cerebral palsy cases. Individuals with spastic cerebral palsy are evenly divided among the

Table 3.6. Classification of cerebral palsy by type of movement disorder and location of impairment

Type of cerebral palsy	Percentage of cases
Spastic	76–86
Hemiplegia	27–37
Diplegia	18–45
Quadriplegia	8–32
Dyskinesia	4–10
Hypotonia	0.2–2.0
Ataxia	5–7
Mixed	5–11
Other	4–21

From Stanley, F., Blair, E., and Alberman, E. (2000). *Cerebral palsies: Epidemiology and causal pathways.* London: Mac Keith Press; adapted by permission.

subtypes of hemiplegia, diplegia, and quadriplegia, although some population-based registries have found lower proportions of children with quadriplegic cerebral palsy (Stanley et al., 2000).

Because the classification of cerebral palsy is based on clinical findings, the reliability of clinical subtype might be less certain, especially for less common subtypes (Blair & Stanley, 1985). This could explain some of the variation in subtypes of cerebral palsy across prevalence studies; however, this variation in diagnosis does not appear to greatly affect the overall prevalence of cerebral palsy. Attempts to examine the severity of cerebral palsy have used more objective indices, such as use of assistive devices, receipt of physical therapy, and use of motor scores from standardized developmental tests (Pinto-Martin et al., 1995).

A diagnosis of cerebral palsy is generally not given until a child reaches at least 2 years of age. Many registry programs for cerebral palsy use a later age (3–5 years) for reporting because clinical findings of motor disability may be transient in young children. As Nelson and Ellenberg (1982) showed in their analysis of the Collaborative Perinatal Project data, 52% of children who had clinical findings of motor impairment at 1 year of age no longer had signs of such impairment at 7 years of age.

Descriptive Epidemiology

Because cerebral palsy represents a heterogeneous condition, it is important in descriptive studies to examine the overall prevalence of not only cerebral palsy but also specific subgroups, particularly those defined by type and gestational age at birth (or birth weight as a proxy measure). Case finding methods in epidemiological studies of cerebral palsy (as with other developmental disabilities) have primarily used records of specialists who diagnose or provide services to children with cerebral palsy and other developmental disorders. Some studies have used clinical examinations of children to confirm diagnosis and to determine the specific type of cerebral palsy (Cummings, Nelson, Grether, & Velie, 1993), whereas others have relied exclusively on medical records, including physical and occupational therapy reports (Murphy, Yeargin-Allsopp, Decouflé, & Drews, 1993). Age-specific prevalence rates are important to report for comparison across studies, especially when examining the type of cerebral palsy, because the type may continue to evolve as the child grows older.

Prevalence

The prevalence of cerebral palsy from recent studies is remarkably similar—ranging from 1.2 to 3.6 per 1,000 live births, with the majority of studies at about 2.0 to 3.0 per 1,000 live births, despite any methodological differences (Clark & Hankins, 2003; Stanley et al., 2000). The majority of the studies are from northern European countries (e.g., Hagberg, Hagberg, Olow, & von Wendt, 1996; Pharoah, Cooke, Johnson, King, & Mutch, 1998; Topp, Uldall, & Langhoff-Roos, 1997), although there is a long-standing surveillance program for cerebral palsy in Western Australia (Stanley et al., 2000) and in the United States, where the CDC has an ongoing monitoring program for cerebral palsy in Atlanta, Georgia (Karapurkar et al., 2006).

The prevalence of cerebral palsy tends to increase up to early elementary school age. This, as with autism and ID, reflects undiagnosed children who do not come to medical attention or do not have a definitive diagnosis prior to the need for special education services at school entry (Boyle et al., 1996). In addition, a small fraction of this increase is due to postnatal cerebral palsy, that is, motor disability resulting from brain damage from such causes as postnatal infections and trauma (Cans et al., 2004; CDC, 1996).

Among children, boys are more likely to have cerebral palsy than are girls. The sex ratios range from 1.1:1 to 1.5:1, although there might be some variation by birth weight (Stanley et al., 2000). In metropolitan Atlanta, black children had lower rates of cerebral palsy than white children if their birth weight was less than 2,500 g, but higher rates if their birth weight was 2,500 g or greater (Winter, Autry, Boyle, & Yeargin-Allsopp, 2002).

Prematurity (or birth weight as a proxy) is the most prominent risk factor for cerebral palsy (O'Shea, 2002; Stanley et al., 2000). There is a bimodal distribution of birth weights among children with cerebral palsy—one peaking at about 1,000 g and the second paralleling the distribution of birth weights for all 3-year-old survivors (Figure 3.1). About one fourth of children with cerebral palsy were born weighing less than 1,500 g and about one half were born weighing less than 2,500 g, compared with about 1% and 5%, respectively, in the general population (A. Autry, unpublished data, 2005).

In studies of cerebral palsy in preterm infant survivors, it has generally been assumed that the risk and protective factors are similar among survivors with serious neurological disability and their counterparts who die in the first year of life. Brain imaging techniques are currently being used to try to identify early markers of motor impairment (Leviton & Gilles, 1999). Periventricular echolucency as measured by ultrasound is evidence of white matter damage and is strongly linked to later motor disability (Pinto-Martin et al., 1995; Serdaroglu, Tekgul, Kitis, Serdaroglu, & Gokben, 2004). Comparison of epidemiological characteristics of children with early signs of brain damage and those who survive and develop cerebral palsy will determine if there are differences in risk or protective factors between these groups.

Children from multiple births have a higher risk of cerebral palsy, which for the most part seems to be attributable to being born premature. Death of a co-twin in utero is a risk factor for cerebral palsy in the surviving twin, and it is thought that at least some cases of cerebral palsy in singletons could be attributable to the early in utero death of an unrecognized co-twin (Grether, Nelson, & Cummins, 1993; Petterson, Nelson, Watson, & Stanley, 1993; Pharoah, 2001; Scher et al., 2002).

Examining trends from 1958 to 1989 from five different registry systems, Blair and Stanley (1997) did not find consistent trends in the overall birth prevalence of cerebral palsy, even though there have been remarkable improvements in obstetric and neonatal care during that time period. Trends over time in neonatal survivors with birth weights less than 1,500 g,

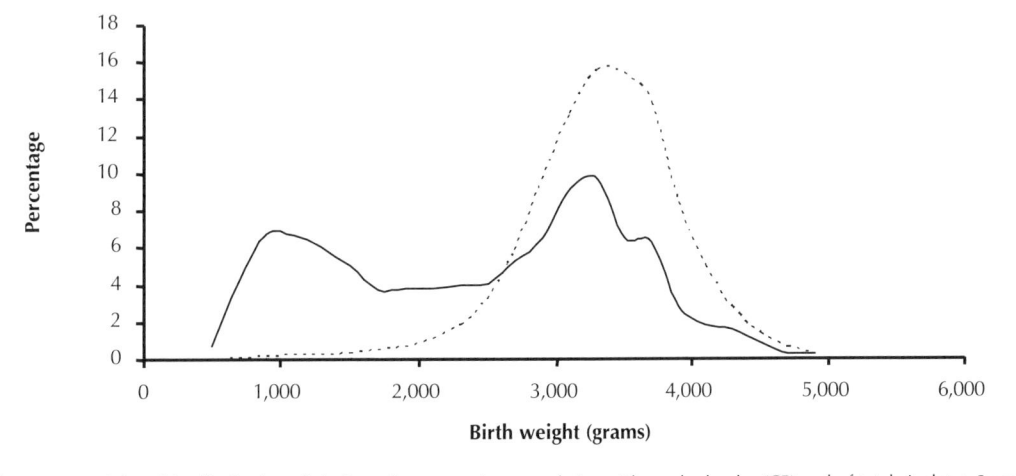

Figure 3.1. Birth weight distribution of singleton 3-year survivor population with cerebral palsy (CP) and of total singleton 3-year survivor population, Atlanta, 1981–1991. (*Source*: Unpublished data from the Metropolitan Atlanta Developmental Disabilities Surveillance Program [MADDSP], 2005.) (*Key*: ···· total population; — individuals with cerebral palsy.)

however, suggest an increase in the rate of cerebral palsy from the mid-1960s to the late 1980s (Stanley et al., 2000; Winter et al., 2002). In contrast, several studies of children born in the mid-1990s suggest a possible downward trend in the rate of cerebral palsy in very low birth weight (VLBW) neonatal survivors (Grether & Nelson, 2000; O'Shea, Preisser, Klinepeter, & Dillard, 1998; Surman et al., 2003).

There is some familial aggregation in cerebral palsy, but it tends to occur in association with unusual circumstances, such as populations with high rates of consanguineous marriages (Bundey, 1997). One interesting observation is that women who have given birth to a child with cerebral palsy are at increased risk for other adverse reproductive outcomes in subsequent pregnancies, such as prematurity or intrauterine growth retardation; however, this might be a result of maternal rather than genetic factors (Palmer, Petterson, Blair, & Burton, 1994). Several studies have shown a higher proportion of birth defects in children with cerebral palsy relative to that in the general population, suggesting a common prenatal, and perhaps genetic, etiology (Croen, Grether, Curry, & Nelson, 2001; Nelson & Ellenberg, 1986).

Analytical Epidemiology

Among VLBW infants, preeclampsia is associated with a reduced risk of cerebral palsy; however, there is a modest increase in risk of cerebral palsy associated with preeclampsia in normal birth weight infants (Collins & Paneth, 1998). It is unclear why preeclampsia would be a protective factor in preterm infants, given that preeclampsia results in infants who have lower birth weight for gestational age, a risk factor for cerebral palsy. One suggestion is that this is an artifact of selection resulting from higher mortality in infants born very preterm to preeclamptic mothers (Murphy, Squier, Hope, Sellers, & Johnson, 1996). Congenital infections, primarily rubella and CMV, are known to cause various neurological impairments, including cerebral palsy, primarily in term infants (Gilbert, 1996). A number of markers of maternal infection in pregnancy, such as clinical chorioamnionitis, maternal fever and antibiotic use, uterine tenderness, and neonatal sepsis, have been linked to cerebral palsy in preterm infants in some (Murphy, Sellers, MacKenzie, Yudkin, & Johnson, 1995; O'Shea, 2002) but not all (Grether & Nelson, 1996; Grether, Nelson, Walsh, Willoughby, & Redline, 2003) studies. Although it is unclear whether the link between maternal infection and cerebral palsy is independent of factors associated with preterm birth, these same markers of maternal infection, including biomarkers of neonatal inflammatory response, have been associated with cerebral palsy in term infants (Nelson, Dambrosia, Grether, & Phillips, 1998; Schendel, 2001). A variety of abnormalities in coagulation, both hereditary and acquired (e.g., antiphospholipid antibodies and factor V Leiden), have been linked to neonatal strokes and cerebral palsy in term infants (Harum et al., 1999; Nelson, 2002).

Obstetric complications and birth asphyxia, long thought to be the main causes of cerebral palsy, in fact account for at most a small proportion (Nelson, 2002). In preterm infants, intrapartum indications of fetal distress and factors that might reflect a compromised oxygen supply were not found to be associated with cerebral palsy (Grether & Nelson, 1996; Murphy, Sellers, et al., 1995). In term infants, a study that examined obstetric complications that might have resulted in birth asphyxia found only one factor—tight nuchal cord—to be associated with cerebral palsy. From this study, it was estimated that approximately 6% of spastic cerebral palsy is associated with potentially asphyxiating obstetric events (Nelson & Grether, 1998).

Studies have found that between 10% and 16% of cerebral palsy is due to postnatal causes (Cans et al., 2004; CDC, 1996; Stanley et al., 2000). There is a variable upper age limit for what is included as cerebral palsy, which could account for some of the variability in the proportion resulting from a postnatal cause. The major causes of postnatal cerebral palsy include infection, cerebrovascular events, and head injuries.

AUTISM SPECTRUM DISORDERS

ASDs—specifically autism, Asperger syndrome, and pervasive developmental disorder not otherwise specified (PDD-NOS)—are a group of neurodevelopmental disorders that are characterized by impairments in three areas: 1) communication and language, 2) reciprocal social interaction, and 3) behavior and interests (APA, 1994). Children with autism have the classic abnormalities of communication and language, impairment of reciprocal social behavior, and restricted behavior and interests. Asperger syndrome is characterized by significant impairment of social behavior and by restriction of interests and behavior with relative preservation of cognitive, language, and communication skills (Szatmari, Archer, Fisman, Streiner, & Wilson, 1995; Szatmari, Bartolucci, & Bremmer, 1989; Szatmari, Tuff, Finlayson, & Bartolucci, 1990; Volkmar et al., 1996).

Children with ASDs have a developmental pattern that is distinctly different from that of children with many other developmental disorders in that their development is characterized by unusual rather than delayed development: idiosyncratic speech, toe walking, twirling, showing affection on their own terms, "selective hearing," and unusual preoccupations (Baird, Cass, & Slonims, 2003; Tidmarsh & Volkmar, 2003; Volkmar, Lord, Bailey, Schultz, & Klin, 2004). In order to help clinicians identify the behavioral features of ASDs, there are a number of standardized screening and diagnostic instruments (Tidmarsh & Volkmar, 2003). According to the DSM, Fourth Edition (DSM-IV; APA, 1994), the features of the disorder must be clinically apparent prior to 3 years of age; however, population studies have reported that the mean age of diagnosis of the disorder is anywhere from 4 to 10 years of age (Charman, 2003; Howlin & Moore, 1997; Wiggins, Baio, & Rice, 2006; Yeargin-Allsopp et al., 2003). By the time the diagnosis is apparent from most population-based studies, etiological studies are quite difficult to perform because the exposure(s) occurred several years prior to data collection and surveillance.

Prevalence

The methods used to study the prevalence of ASDs have generally involved a two-phase process of case finding followed by case confirmation (Boyle, Bertrand, & Yeargin-Allsopp, 1999; Fombonne, 1999). The most comprehensive method of case finding involves total population screening using schools or pediatric well-child visits as the venue for screening. The advantage of this method is that it allows previously undiagnosed children to be identified. This is especially important for children who are high functioning and are not receiving special services for ASDs; however, the process is labor intensive and has been done only in relatively small populations, which has limited the number of children identified with ASDs (Gillberg & Wing, 1999). Other methods used in case finding have targeted at-risk populations by focusing on programs and clinics specifically for children with ASDs, including special education programs, specialty diagnostic clinics, and other service programs. Methods used to identify children at such sources have varied from asking providers to identify children with behaviors associated with ASDs to a comprehensive review of all service provider records. An advantage of the at-risk approach is that large populations can be targeted, but its success is dependent on the quality and comprehensiveness of diagnostic and treatment services in the community, as well as the extent of detail that is recorded in the individual records.

Methods used in the second phase—case confirmation—have also been variable (Fombonne, 1999; Wing & Potter, 2002). The most comprehensive method has been the clinical evaluation with the Autism Diagnostic Observation Scales–Generic (ADOS-G; Lord et al., 2000) or Autism Diagnostic Interview- Revised (ADI-R; Lord, Rutter & Le Couteur, 1994) or both; however, this approach is cost prohibitive for large studies. Another approach has been to use expert review based on available diagnostic record information on the child (Yeargin-Allsopp et al., 2003). Although this approach has resource advantages and potentially allows for a developmental perspective of the child's behavior, it is dependent on the quality of the records and the experience of the reviewers. Finally, some investigators have relied solely on a diagnosis as provided by a service provider (Barbaresi, Katusic, Colligan, Weaver, & Jacobsen, 2005; Lauritsen, Pedersen, & Mortensen, 2004; Williams et al.,

2005); however, because the diagnosis of autism varies widely within communities, this approach needs to be used with caution.

Debate exists about the prevalence of autism (also referred to as classic autism or autistic disorder) and ASDs and whether the prevalence has increased over time. The first epidemiological studies examining the prevalence of autism did not appear in the scientific literature until the late 1960s and early 1970s. Since these earlier investigations, there have been an increasing number of population-based prevalence studies; however, these vary in terms of their methods, case definitions, and population size. Therefore, comparisons of temporal trends in rates of autism must be viewed with caution.

Early population-based studies of autism using the Kanner criteria (published in 1956) reported a prevalence of approximately 4–5 per 10,000 (Brask, 1972; Hoshino, Kumashiro, Yashima, Tachibana, & Watanabe, 1982; Lotter, 1966; McCarthy, Fitzgerald, & Smith, 1984; Wing & Gould, 1979). DSM-IV and ICD-10 criteria are consistent; however, recent studies using either criteria have yielded disparate rates, ranging from 0.4 per 1,000 in Norway (Sponheim & Skjeldae, 1998) to 8.3 per 1,000 in the United Kingdom (Trebruegge, Nandini, & Ritchie, 2004). Most recent studies have reported rates of 2–7 per 1,000 (Arvidsson et al., 1997; Autism and Developmental Disabilities Monitoring Network, 2007a, 2007b; Baird et al., 2000; Bertrand et al., 2001; Chakrabarti & Fombonne, 2001; Croen, Grether, Hoogstrate & Selvin, 2002; Fombonne & du Mazaubrun, 1992; Fombonne, du Mazaubrun, Cans, & Grandjean, 1997; Fombonne, Simmons, Ford, Meltzer, & Goodman, 2001; Honda, Shimizu, Misumi, Niimi, & Ohashi, 1996; Kadesjö, Gillberg & Hagberg, 1999; Kielinen, Linna, & Moilanen, 2000; Mágnússon & Saemundsen, 2001; Powell et al., 2000; Sponheim & Skjeldal, 1998; Webb, Lobo, Hervas, Scourfield, & Fraser, 1997; Yeargin-Allsopp et al., 2003).

There have been only a few studies of trends in autism prevalence in the same population. The prevalence was determined for two French birth cohorts (children born in 1972 and 1976); no change in prevalence (5.1 and 4.9 per 10,000 children, respectively) occurred over that short period of time (Fombonne & du Mazaubrun, 1992). In Sweden, the prevalence of autism was determined for two time periods, 1962–1976 and 1975–1984, and was reported to have increased from 4.0 to 11.6 per 10,000 children (Gillberg, 1984; Gillberg, Steffenburg, & Schaumann, 1991). The rates of autism in children with mild ID remained relatively stable, whereas the rates increased in children with severe ID (IQ score < 50) and in children with normal intelligence (IQ score > 70). The Swedish investigators suggested that changes in the overall prevalence were influenced by the improved ability to identify children with autism who had very low as well as normal to high functioning.

Another study reported the incidence from 1991 through 1996 in preschool children in two areas of the United Kingdom and found that, although the rates for classic autism increased by 18% per year, there was a much larger increase for the other ASDs (Powell et al., 2000). The investigators attributed this increase in incidence to better awareness among clinicians rather than to true changes in the occurrence of autism. A more recent study of autism in Olmsted County, Minnesota, found that the incidence of research-identified autism, defined as indications in records of DSM-IV criteria for autism, increased from 5.5 per 100,000 children during the period 1980–1983 to 44.9 per 100,000 during the period 1995–1997 (Barbaresi et al., 2005). Because the increased rates were confined to a subgroup of children who were younger than 10 years of age and born after 1987, the authors concluded that the increase was due to changes in diagnostic criteria, service availability, and increased awareness.

Because of the lack of prevalence data for the United States, considerable attention has been paid to trends in service provider data, which have shown an increase in the number of children receiving services for autism (California Department of Developmental Services, 1999, 2003; U.S. Department of Education, 2004). A study by Newschaffer, Falb, and Gurney (2005) using data on special education utilization during the period from 1992 through 2001 found that the autism prevalence increase was higher in younger cohorts, with a suggestion of a recent slowing of the rate of increase. Under the category of "other health impairment," which is often the category used to provide services for many children with ADHD, there was a pattern of increased prevalence very similar to that for autism.

Beginning in the 1990s, the CDC initiated a number of prevalence studies to address this lack of prevalence data for ASDs in the United States. In response to a concern about a suspected large number of ASD cases, a study was conducted in Brick Township, New Jersey (Bertrand et al., 2001). It included an intensive case identification phase using schools and service providers, followed by case verification (clinical examinations, psychological examinations, and administration of the Autism Diagnostic Observation Scales–Generic). The prevalence of autism was found to be 40 per 10,000 children (95% confidence interval [CI], 28–56), and the prevalence for ASDs was 67 per 10,000 children (95% CI, 51–87). The prevalence of autism in Brick Township was higher than most previously published rates for ASDs.

In a second effort, the CDC conducted a population-based study to determine the prevalence of autism in five counties of metropolitan Atlanta (Yeargin-Allsopp et al., 2003). Children with autism were identified through screening and abstraction of records at multiple medical and educational sources, with expert review to determine autism case status. A total of 987 children who displayed behaviors consistent with the DSM-IV criteria for autistic disorder, PDD-NOS, or Asperger syndrome were identified. The prevalence for autism was 3.4 per 1,000 children, with boys more affected than girls and with no differences in prevalence by race.

Building on the experience in metropolitan Atlanta, the CDC developed the Autism and Developmental Disabilities Monitoring (ADDM) Network, a multisite, multiple source records-based surveillance system to determine the prevalence of autism and other developmental disabilities (ADDM, 2007a, 2007b). A report for study years 2000 and 2002 for 6 and 14 sites, respectively, found that the average ASD prevalence was 6.7 per 1,000 for 8-year-olds in 2000 and 6.6 per 1,000 8-year-olds in 2002 in the study areas across the United States. The range of ASD prevalence in these areas of the United States in 2002 was between 3.3 and 10.6 per 1,000 with most sites between 5.0–7.6 per 1,000 8-year-olds, but 12 of the 14 sites had a closer range of 5.2–7.6 per 1,000 children. The ADDM Network is based on access to multiple (clinical and educational) sources of previously recorded information; in 2002, four sites (Alabama, Missouri, Pennsylvania, and Wisconsin) relied on information from health sources only, and, on average, the prevalence was lower in those sites than in the other 10 sites that combined information from health and education sources.

The ADDM Network data found differences in ASD prevalence by sex and race/ethnicity. ASD prevalence was higher among boys than among girls, ranging from more than 3 to more than 6 boys for every girl with ASD. Five of the 14 sites identified more white non-Hispanic children with autism than black non-Hispanic children. Females with ASD were more likely to have cognitive impairment than males in most sites.

The prevalence was stable from 2000 to 2002 in four of the six sites that had data for both years with a statistically significant increase in only one area. In addition, the median age of earliest ASD diagnosis ranged from 4 years, 1 month to 5 years, 6 months, but for 51%–91% of children with an ASD, developmental concerns had been recorded before 3 years of age. The prevalence of autism found across the United States in the ADDM sites was consistent with recent studies outside the United States that reported estimates of about 6 per 1,000 children and higher than rates from studies conducted in the United States during the 1980s and early 1990s.

It remains uncertain what role factors such as greater awareness of the conditions or better availability of services have played in the higher rates of autism. Methodological issues related to the conduct of the studies could also have played a role, or the increased prevalence might reflect a true increase in occurrence of the disorder. Nevertheless, there appear to be more children with autism today than in the past, and continued monitoring of the prevalence of autism might shed some light on the contribution of each of these factors. Although attempting to apply criteria in use today to individuals identified in the past is fraught with many assumptions, Wing and Potter (2002) have estimated that only about 30%–50% of children meeting ICD-10 diagnostic criteria for autism would satisfy Kanner's (1943) original requirements for the diagnosis.

Sociodemographic Factors

All studies have found more boys than girls with autism, with sex ratios ranging from 2:1 to 4:1, with a few exceptions (Fombonne 1999; Gillberg & Wing, 1999). Although it is likely that sex difference is due to a genetic susceptibility, it might also be that diagnostic criteria differentially identify autistic behaviors in boys compared with girls. Of note, when considering the sex ratio by IQ level, there is a decreasing male–female ratio with decreasing IQ score; the sex ratio is close to 1:1 for children with IQ scores less than 50, whereas for higher functioning children with IQ scores greater than 50 the sex ratio is 3:1 to 4:1 (Lord & Schopler, 1985; Nordin & Gillberg, 1996; Yeargin-Allsopp et al., 2003).

Little is known about variations in the prevalence of autism among various racial or ethnic groups because most studies have been conducted in northern European countries or Japan. A study in metropolitan Atlanta found that the rates were the same in black and white children (3.4 per 1,000 in children 3–10 years of age); however, when examined by the presence or absence of associated disabilities (primarily ID), black children had a much higher prevalence of nonisolated autism than white children (Yeargin-Allsopp et al., 2003). Although the ASD prevalence data from metropolitan Atlanta did not show a difference by race, CDC ADDM Network data found that ASD was more prevalent in non-Hispanic white children in 5 of 14 U.S. communities, and Hispanic children had a lower prevalence in some communities (ADDM, 2007a, 2007b). There are a small number of studies of ethnic differences in autism prevalence; however, in a few studies, there is a suggestion of higher rates in immigrant populations (Gillberg & Gillberg, 1996).

Early studies of autism reported an association with higher social class, but there have been questions as to whether this is an artifact of biased ascertainment. In a study by Schopler, Andrews, and Strupp (1979), it was found that families of higher social class were more able to travel longer distances for services and gave more detailed responses to questions about their children's development. Wing (1980) also supported the idea of a possible social class bias in autism because of differences in referral and diagnosis. Another factor that might affect reports of race and social class in children with autism and other developmental disabilities relates to the perception and experience of diagnosticians. A study by Cuccaro (1996) found that diagnoses made by clinicians differed for children of different racial backgrounds, and the diagnosis of autism was more reliant on the experience of the clinician examining the child, with psychiatrists (assumed to be more experienced with autism) recognizing the behaviors associated with autism more often than school psychologists.

A few epidemiological studies have shown an increased risk for autism among families with higher socioeconomic status and in mothers with higher levels of education (Croen et al., 2002). Some studies have also shown increased maternal age to be associated with autism (Gillberg, 1980; Hoshino et al., 1982), whereas others have shown no such effect (Lotter, 1967; Steinhausen, Gobel, Breinlinger, & Wohllenben, 1986). Croen et al. (2002) found that there was a fourfold increased risk for autism in children born to mothers 35 years of age or older when compared with mothers 20 years of age; data from metropolitan Atlanta for 1996 also showed a 70% increased risk for autism associated with other disabilities in children born to older mothers (Bhasin & Schendel, 2007).

Genetic Risk Factors and Etiologies

Twin studies provided compelling evidence of a strong genetic component to the etiology of autism. They showed a significant difference in the concordance of autism between monozygotic (MZ) and dizygotic (DZ) twins, ranging from 36% to 96% for MZ twins and from 0% to 24% among DZ twins (Bailey et al., 1995; Ritvo, Freeman, Mason-Brothers, Mo, & Ritvo, 1985; Steffenburg et al., 1989). Although these works provide strong evidence of genetic factors in autism, the fact that MZ twins do not have 100% concordance indicates the presence of environmental factors (Piven & Folstein, 1997).

Although the role of nongenetic factors due to a shared intrauterine physical environment cannot be ruled out, the finding of no increase in the prevalence of twins among those with autism has been supported by studies from Western Australia, California, and Sweden (Hallmayer et al., 2002). Family studies have consistently shown that the rate of autism in siblings ranges from 2% to 6%; the recurrence risk estimates range from 10 to 30 times greater than the population prevalence (Newschaffer, Fallin, & Lee, 2002; Smalley, Asarnow, & Spence, 1988).

Associated Conditions

Autism has been shown to be associated with several genetic disorders; the most common are fragile X syndrome and tuberous sclerosis, with 4% and 1% of such individuals having autism (Cohen et al., 1991; Oberle et al., 1991; Smalley, Tanguay, Smith, & Gutierrez, 1992). Prader-Willi and Angelman syndromes, untreated PKU, Down syndrome, and neurofibromatosis type 1 are examples of additional disorders with known genetic etiologies that have been shown to be associated with autism (Folstein & Rutter, 1988; Kent, Evans, Paul, & Sharp, 1999; Page, 2000; Rasmussen, Borjesson, Wentz, & Gillberg, 2001; Steffenburg, Gillberg, & Steffenburg, 1996; Williams & Hersh, 1998). Given the low prevalence of these comorbid genetic disorders, it is unlikely that their co-occurrence with autism is coincidence. Although the association between autism and various known genetic disorders is present, all of these conditions do not account for a significant fraction of autism in the population.

Identification of the genes that cause autism might help in understanding the underlying neurological pathways and mechanisms, assist in identification of environmental risks, and enable the development of pharmaceutical treatments and other protective interventions. Since 2002, genome-wide scans and candidate gene studies have been conducted in efforts to identify the responsible genes. These genetic studies have produced promising findings supporting the notion that multiple genes are involved in the etiology of autism, with several genes potentially interacting with weak or moderate effects. Investigators have suggested that as many as 15 distinct loci could be involved in autism, operating in such a manner that the expression of one gene is altered or suppressed by other loci with the interaction of three genes being the best model (Pickles et al., 1995; Risch et al., 1999), although suggestions that up to 100 different genes might be involved likely reflect clinically heterogeneous study populations that were assumed to be homogeneous. A recent finding that tiny gene mutations, each individually rare, pose more risk for autism than had been previously thought supports this idea (Sebat et al., 2007).

Nongenetic Risk Factors

One of the few well-documented prenatal risk factors is in utero exposure to thalidomide. In a group of 15 adults prenatally exposed to thalidomide at 20–24 weeks' gestation, 4 were found to have autism (Stromland, Nordin, Miller, Akerstrom, & Gillberg, 1994). The importance of this association is that it documents the timing of the exposure when the brain abnormality responsible for this manifestation of autism occurred and also supports the search for other early exposures in pregnancy that might be responsible for autism (Rodier, Ingram, Tisdale, Nelson, & Romano, 1996).

The earliest evidence for the role of viruses in ASDs comes from a report in which 12 of 243 preschool children with congenital rubella were found to have ASDs (Chess, 1971). There have been a few other reports implicating herpes simplex, rubella, mumps, and varicella (Karapurkar, Lee, Curran, Newschaffer, & Yeargin-Allsopp, 2004). Another report examined the possible role of maternal autoimmune disease, asthma, and allergies and found no association except with maternal psoriasis; therefore, the authors concluded that these maternal conditions are not likely to contribute significantly to the development of ASDs in offspring (Croen, Grether, Yoshida, Obouli, & Van de Water, 2005).

The early literature suggested that parents of children with autism have a history of more reproductive problems than parents of children who do not have autism. These include infertility, spontaneous abortions, and maternal menstrual irregularities (Campbell, Hardesty, & Burdock, 1978). Perinatal risk factors have also been examined as possible causes for ASDs, singly and in combination, to produce an "optimality score" for pregnancy and delivery; however, although some researchers have found that children with ASDs have lower optimality scores that controls (Bolton, 1997; Bryson, Clark, & Smith, 1988; Gillberg & Gillberg, 1983), others have found no difference in optimality scores between children with ASDs and typically developing controls (Cryan, Byrne, O'Donovan, & O'Callaghan, 1996; Lord, Mulloy, Wendelboe, & Schopler, 1991; Piven et al., 1993).

The possible increase in prevalence of ASDs has prompted parents and investigators alike to search for an explanation. The question of whether the measles, mumps, and rubella (MMR) vaccine is causally associated with autism was initially raised by a case series of children with autistic regression and colitis with the onset of autistic behavior occurring shortly after receipt of the MMR vaccination (Wakefield et al., 1998); however, the Institute of Medicine (Stratton, Gable, Shetty, & McCormick, 2001; IOM, 2004), the American Academy of Pediatrics (Halsey & Hyman, 2001), and the Medical Research Council (2001) have reviewed the available scientific information on the proposed relationship between the MMR vaccine and ASDs and have concluded that there is no evidence of a causal association at the population level. Questions have also been raised about the safety of mercury-containing vaccines and whether these vaccines are related to the increased prevalence of ASDs. Using large data sets from the United States, Sweden, and Denmark, to date no consistent association has been found between mercury-containing vaccines and neurodevelopmental outcomes (Stehr-Green, Tull, Stellfeld, Mortenson, & Simpson, 2003; IOM, 2004). Also, none of the studies from these countries has supported a causal relationship between mercury-containing vaccine exposure in the general population and the prevalence of ASDs specifically.

SEIZURES AND EPILEPSY

An *epileptic seizure,* according to the International League Against Epilepsy (ILAE), is the transient occurrence of signs, symptoms, or both resulting from abnormal excessive or synchronous neuronal activity in the brain (Fisher et al., 2005). The manifestations of seizures are determined by whether the seizure begins simultaneously over the entire cortex ("generalized" seizure) or the onset is localized within a single cortical region ("partial" seizure). Single seizures provoked by specific insults to the cortex are considered *symptomatic seizures* and may occur only once, caused, for example, by a closed head injury, hyponatremia, or viral meningitis. *Epilepsy,* as defined by the ILAE, is a disorder of the brain characterized by an enduring predisposition to generated epileptic seizures and by the neurobiological, cognitive, psychological, and social consequences of this condition. Although the new definition of epilepsy proposed by the ILAE requires the occurrence of at least one seizure, most epidemiological studies of epilepsy have used an operational definition of epilepsy of two or more seizures, as up to 50% of children who have a single seizure do not have a second, whereas the vast majority of those with two or more seizures have recurrences (Commission on Epilepsy and Prognosis, 1993; Shinnar et al., 1996).

Epilepsy is not a single condition, but rather a very diverse family of disorders. Furthermore, many epilepsy syndromes have genetic and electroencephalographic (EEG) markers; epidemiologists have only recently started to consider these factors in the study of epilepsy. The diagnostic technologies as well as the classification of individual seizures and that of epilepsy syndromes have changed over the years, making accurate determination of trends from population-based data difficult (Commission on Classification and Terminology, 1981, 1989). Furthermore, several investigators have noted that a significant number of children ascertained in population-based studies cannot be adequately classified based on currently used classification schemes (Eriksson & Koivikko, 1997; Waaler, Blom, Skeidsvoll, & Mykletun, 2000).

The diagnosis of epilepsy and of specific epilepsy syndromes is often a complex clinical process that relies on an experienced clinician combining historical variables with EEG data. Analysis of the accuracy of epilepsy diagnosis among general practitioners (GPs) in the United Kingdom has documented significant problems of overdiagnosis when their evaluations were compared with those of neurologists. Therefore, epidemiological surveys that rely on the diagnosis of GPs may be of questionable accuracy (Cockerell, Eckle, Goodridge, Sander, & Shorvon, 1995; Wallace, Shorvon, & Tallis, 1998), prompting some recent studies to "verify" the diagnosis of epilepsy by GPs with record reviews by expert neurologists (Kurtz, Tookey, & Ross, 1998).

Prevalence of Childhood Epilepsy

The prevalence of epilepsy among children in developed countries has been reported to be 4 to 9 per 1,000, with almost 1% of children having experienced active epilepsy by the age of 20 years (Table 3.7). The prevalence of childhood epilepsy is significantly higher (up to 23 per 1,000) in certain areas of the developing world, especially in rural regions of Central America (Medina et al., 2005) and South America (Del Brutto et al., 2005; Nicoletti et al., 1999) and regions of sub-Saharan Africa (Preux & Druet-Cabanac, 2005). Although the increased prevalence of childhood epilepsy in developing countries has not been adequately explained, neurocysticercosis may be responsible for up to one third of the excess burden of epilepsy, particularly in rural areas of Latin American and East Africa (Andriantsimahavandy et al., 1997; Del Brutto et al., 2005; Nsengiyumva et al., 2003).

In developed countries, the prevalence of epilepsy increases with age (Kurtz et al., 1998; Wallace et al., 1998). A slightly higher prevalence is typically reported among boys than among girls. In the United States, a slightly higher prevalence of epilepsy has been reported among African American children compared with white children.

Trends over Time in Incidence of Childhood Epilepsy

The overall incidence of childhood epilepsy in developed countries is about 50 per 100,000 person-years (Bell & Sander, 2002); however, the incidence rates reported vary and have ranged from 43 to 82.3 per 100,000 person-years (Camfield, Camfield, Gordon, Wirrell, & Dooley, 1996; Sidenvall, Forsgren, Blomquist, & Heijbel, 1993) (Table 3.8). Higher rates have also been reported among studies that included single seizures or acute symptomatic seizures (Jallon, Goumaz, Haenggeli, & Morabia, 1997). The incidence of epilepsy seems to be higher among lower socioeconomic status groups, both in rural and in urban areas (Heaney et al., 2002).

The incidence of childhood epilepsy from early childhood to 14 years of age was reported to have decreased by 26% from 1935 to 1984 (Annegers, Hauser, & Lee, 1995; Annegers, Hauser, Lee, & Rocca, 1995). Epilepsy definitions and diagnostic methods changed dramatically between 1935 and 1984, and therefore the significance of these reported changes is unclear. The disorders that "look like" epilepsy in children (e.g., breathholding spells, syncope) are likely diagnosed with more accuracy now than in the 1930s to 1970s, probably accounting for some of the reported decrease in childhood epilepsy incidence; however, the decrease may have been clear as early as the mid-1960s, which predates the use of diagnostic EEG-video monitoring, but not the recognition of breathholding and syncope as being disorders separate and distinct from epileptic seizures. Early aggressive treatment of a first seizure and prevention of a second seizure (and the diagnosis of epilepsy) is not a likely explanation of the reported decrease in epilepsy incidence, as treatment of the first seizure is less common now than in the 1980s and earlier.

Part of the reported decrease in childhood epilepsy incidence might be due to prevention of some of the known preventable causes of childhood epilepsy. For example, prevention of childhood bacterial meningitis and serious head trauma (e.g., as a result of use of seat belts) could theoretically have reduced epilepsy incidence (Annegers, Hauser, Lee, et al.,

Table 3.7. Prevalence studies of childhood epilepsy

Study years	Prevalence (per 1,000)	Age range	Comments	References
1985–1988	6	10 years	Multiple-source population-based surveillance in Atlanta	Murphy, Trevathan, and Yeargin-Allsopp (1995)
1980s	4.7	Birth to 19 years	Multiple-source population-based surveillance in Oklahoma City	Cowan, Bodensteiner, and Leviton (1989)
1940–1980	6.8		Mayo Clinic (Rochester, MN) record linkage system	Hauser, Annegers, and Kurland (1993)
1985	4.2	Birth to 16 years	Identification via pediatrician reporting of suspected epilepsy cases in northern Sweden, followed by questionnaires to families	Sidenvall, Forsgren, and Heijbel (1996)
1995	5.1	6–12 years	Multiple source surveillance in western Norway, including study area's only electroencephalography (EEG) laboratory	Waaler, Blom, Skeidsvoll, and Mykletun (2000)
1992	3.94	Birth to 15 years	Multiple source ascertainment in Finland using physician records and EEG laboratories	Eriksson and Koivikko (1997)
1993	2.2 3.7 4.4 4.2	0–4 years 5–9 years 10–14 years 15–24 years	Multiple source ascertainment in Iceland using records from primary care physicians, neurologists, and EEG laboratories	Olafsson and Hauser (1999)
1995	3.16 4.05	5–9 years 10–14 years	General practitioner (GP) database in England and Wales. Accuracy of epilepsy diagnosis reported by GPs is a concern.	Wallace, Shorvon, and Tallis (1998)
1987–1988	3.89 4.28 4.91 6.28	7 years 11 years 16 years 23 years	National Child Development Study cohort in England, Scotland, and Wales	Kurtz, Tookey, and Ross (1998)
1997	23.3	Birth to adults	Door-to-door survey in rural Honduras; 15.4 per 1,000 with active epilepsy	Medina et al. (2005)
1994	20.4	15–24 years	Door-to-door survey in rural Bolivia	Nicoletti et al. (1999)
2003	9.9	Birth to adults	Door-to-door survey in rural Ecuador.	Del Brutto et al. (2005)
1987	9.3 (Pakistan) 10.7 (Turkey) 9.9 (Pakistan) 7.3 (Turkey)	< 10 years 11–19 years	Simultaneous studies in rural and urban Pakistan and Turkey using same methods and door-to-door survey. Rural areas had about twice the epilepsy prevalence of urban areas.	Aziz, Guvener, Akhtar, and Hasan (1997)
1993–1995	8.8	Birth to adults	Higher epilepsy prevalence in rural areas in India, but details not reported	Gourie-Devi, Gururaj, Satishchandra, and Subbakrishna (2004)

(continued)

Table 3.7.   *(continued)*

Study years	Prevalence (per 1,000)	Age range	Comments	References
1996	8.0	Birth to 16 years	Stratified two-stage cluster probability sample design among children ages birth to 16 years living in Turkey	Serdaroglu, Tekgul, Kitis, Serdaroglu, and Gokben (2004)
1999	8.9	Birth to 13 years	Multiple source ascertainment in Okayama, Japan	Oka (2002)

Table 3.8.   Incidence studies of childhood epilepsy

Study years	Annual incidence (per 100,000 person-year)	Age range	Comments	References
1974–1983 1984–1993	152.4 60.9	Birth to 20 years	Study in England. Includes some single seizures.	Cockerell, Eckle, Goodridge, Sander, and Shorvon (1995)
1958–1999	41.4	Birth to 14 years	General practitioner (GP) database in England, Scotland, and Wales. Recurrent unprovoked seizures. Data reviewed by neurologist and diagnosis of epilepsy "validated."	Kurtz, Tookey, and Ross (1998)
1995	72.3	5–19 years	GP database in England and Wales. Includes some single seizures.	Wallace, Shorvon, and Tallis (1998)
1977–1985	41	28 days to 15 years	Study in Nova Scotia. Recurrent unprovoked seizures.	Camfield, Camfield, Gordon, Wirrell, and Dooley (1996)
1985–1987	88.8 72.6	Birth to 15 years 28 days to 15 years	Study in northern Sweden. Excludes neonatal seizures.	Sidenvall, Forsgren, Blomquist, and Heijbel (1993)
1961–1964	35	Birth to 15 years	Study in Turku, Finland. Recurrent unprovoked seizures.	Sillanpaa (2000)
1990–1991	72	Birth to 19 years	Study in Geneva. Includes some single seizures.	Jallon, Goumaz, Haenggeli, and Morabia (1997)
1995–1997	190 75.4	Birth to 4 years 5–14 years	GP database in southeast England. Higher incidence of epilepsy in lower socioeconomic status groups.	Heaney et al. (2002)
1935–1974 1975–1984	71 52	All ages	Study in Rochester, MN. Recurrent unprovoked seizures.	Hauser, Annegers, and Kurland (1993)
1990	94 74	Birth to 9 years 10–19 years	Door-to-door survey in rural Ethiopia. Recurrent unprovoked seizures.	Tekle-Haimanot, Forsgren, and Ekstedt (1997)
1993	256.5 77.5 53 37 34	< 1 year 1–4 years 5–9 years 10–14 years 15–24 years	Multiple source surveillance system, including primary care physicians, neurologists, and electroencephalography laboratories, in Iceland.	Olafsson, Hauser, Ludvigsson, and Gudmundsson (1996)

1995). The reported reduction in seizures and epilepsy occurred after the introduction of widespread antibiotic use, but prior to the use of seat belts and prior to the introduction of vaccines such as the Hib vaccine. The reported decrease in childhood epilepsy incidence is likely due to a combination of improved diagnostic methods and prevention of some preventable causes (e.g., sequelae of infections).

Prevalence and Incidence Studies of Seizure Types and Epilepsy Syndromes

Several studies have reported the prevalence of specific seizure types (Eriksson & Koivikko, 1997; Murphy, Trevathan, & Yeargin-Allsopp, 1995; Waaler et al., 2000), but few have reported the relative distribution of seizure types and epilepsy syndromes among newly diagnosed children or incidence rates of specific seizure types (Berg, Levy, Testa, & Shinnar, 1999; Camfield et al., 1996; Hauser, Annegers, & Kurland, 1993; Jallon et al., 1997; Sidenvall et al., 1993; Zarrelli, Beghi, Rocca, & Hauser, 1999). Although generalized seizures are relatively more common among children than among adults, most prevalence studies have reported that partial seizures are more common among children than are generalized seizures (Cowan, Bodensteiner, & Leviton, 1989; Murphy, Trevathan, & Yeargin-Allsopp, 1995; Waaler et al., 2000).

The incidence rates for specific seizure types and epilepsy syndromes vary by age (Sidenvall et al., 1993; Zarrelli et al., 1999). For example, absence seizures have a peak incidence between 5 and 10 years of age, whereas the peak incidence of primary generalized tonic-clonic seizures occur between ages 11 and 15 years. Many primarily generalized epilepsies are genetically determined (e.g., childhood absence epilepsy, juvenile myoclonic epilepsy), with age of onset part of the epilepsy syndrome.

Infantile Spasms Infantile spasms are rare, with incidence rates ranging from 2 to 5 per 10,000 live births per year, with slightly higher incidence among boys (Cowan & Hudson, 1991; Lee & Ong, 2001; Ludvigsson, Olafsson, Sigurthardottir, & Hauser, 1994; Riiko-

nen & Donner, 1979; Sidenvall & Eeg-Olofsson, 1995). The lower incidence rates are from studies that tend to use the more rigid diagnostic criteria for infantile spasms, typically those studies that required hypsarrhythmia on EEG for the diagnosis of infantile spasms (Trevathan, Murphy, & Yeargin-Allsopp, 1999). Infantile spasms are known to be etiologically heterogeneous and are thought to represent an age-related response by the developing brain to a wide variety of exposures. The most common reported etiologies include tuberous sclerosis, cerebral malformations, intrauterine infections, chromosomal abnormalities, and inherited metabolic disorders (Wong & Trevathan, 2001).

The developmental prognosis of infantile spasms is poor. Although those children with normal development at the onset of spasms and no identified etiology have the best neurodevelopmental outcome, those children in the lowest risk groups have 30% or greater odds of ID (Riikonen, 1982; Trevathan et al., 1999; Wong & Trevathan, 2001). In studies that require the presence of hypsarrhythmia for the diagnosis of infantile spasms, about 70%–90% of children with known etiologies have ID, and most of these children have severe to profound ID. About 50%–60% of children with infantile spasms go on to develop long-term epilepsy, and many of these children develop Lennox-Gastaut syndrome (Trevathan, Murphy, & Yeargin-Allsopp, 1997).

Lennox-Gastaut Syndrome Lennox-Gastaut syndrome (LGS) is a relatively rare, yet devastating, epilepsy syndrome with multiple types of seizures (all of which tend to be refractory to aggressive medical treatment), slow spike-wave discharge on EEG, and significant intellectual impairment (Trevathan, 2002). The seizure types include generalized tonic-clonic seizures, atypical absence seizures, partial seizures, and generalized tonic seizures in sleep, as well as "drop attacks" that may be due to atonic seizures, tonic seizures, or massive myoclonic spasms.

Determining the incidence of LGS is methodologically difficult because children may have onset of seizures during the first year of life, but the insidious clinical transition until an individual child meets diagnostic criteria for LGS may take a decade. Even when carefully following a patient in the clinic, it is often difficult to determine when the patient first meets diagnostic criteria for LGS; timing the onset from surveillance records is virtually impossible. Therefore, most epidemiological studies have chosen to study the prevalence of LGS.

The prevalence is about 1.3–2.6 per 10,000 children and is slightly higher in boys (Cowan et al., 1989; Sidenvall et al., 1993; Trevathan et al., 1997). The estimated incidence of LGS is 1–2 per 100,000 children per year (Heiskala, 1997). Among children with LGS, 20%–60% have a history of infantile spasms. More than 90% of individuals with LGS have ID, in most cases severe to profound, whereas among children with multiple seizure types but without the slow spike-wave on EEG characteristic of LGS, only about half have ID. Although rare, LGS is an important contributor to childhood morbidity. For example, among children with profound ID ascertained in the MADDSP, 17% had LGS.

Benign Rolandic Epilepsy Benign rolandic epilepsy (BRE; also known as benign epilepsy with centrotemporal spikes) is a relatively common epilepsy syndrome with onset of partial seizures involving the face, tongue, and larynx during childhood (Lundberg & Eeg-Olofsson, 2003). The EEGs of children with BRE show rolandic (centrotemporal) spikes with unique morphology (Commission on Classification and Terminology, 1989), and these typical EEG findings are also reported in the siblings of children with BRE, raising questions about whether the EEG findings are a genetic marker of susceptibility. The genetics of BRE, however, are not simple and continue to be debated, and the role of gene–environment interactions has not been defined (Vadlamudi et al., 2004).

The incidence of benign rolandic seizures in Iceland was 6.2 per 100,000 children per year (Astradsson, Olafsson, Ludvigsson, Bjorgvinsson, & Hauser, 1998). An analysis of children with BRE from Nova Scotia demonstrated that all individuals achieved remission from their seizures regardless of treatment (Peters, Camfield, & Camfield, 2001); however, a rela-

tionship between BRE and impairment of language development has been reported, and the authors suggested a relationship between "epileptic activity" and impaired language development and educational difficulties that may persist into adulthood (Monjauze, Tuller, Hommet, Barthez, & Khomsi, 2005). Whether there is a cause-and-effect relationship between seizure frequency, duration, and intensity and language problems is uncertain (Papavasiliou, Mattheou, Bazigou, Kotsalis, & Paraskevoulakos, 2005).

Childhood Absence Epilepsy Childhood absence epilepsy (CAE) is an idiopathic, primarily generalized epilepsy of apparent multifactorial genetic etiology, with onset typically between 4 and 12 years of age, that is associated with 3-per-second spike-wave complexes on EEG that are time-locked with the clinical absence seizures, each of which usually lasts for 1–10 seconds and which occur up to 100 times per day in untreated children (Commission on Classification and Terminology, 1989; Crunelli & Leresche, 2002). The incidence of CAE is about 6–12 per 100,000 children per year (Camfield et al., 1996; Sidenvall et al., 1993), and the prevalence among school-age children is about 2 per 10,000 children (Cowan et al., 1989). CAE may be more common among girls. The risk of accidental injury associated with absence seizures is significant at 9% per person-year (Wirrell, Camfield, Camfield, Dooley, & Gordon, 1996). Although the prognosis in terms of seizure control is fairly good, with up to 90% of children with CAE achieving spontaneous remission, psychosocial functioning (school performance, behavior, and social relationships) is impaired in one third of children with CAE (Wirrell et al., 1997). Although a majority of children with CAE will undergo a spontaneous remission of their epilepsy by some time in adolescence, up to 44% of children with CAE progress to juvenile myoclonic epilepsy, which is a lifelong autosomal dominant generalized epilepsy with absence, myoclonic, and generalized tonic-clonic seizures (Wirrell, Camfield, Camfield, Gordon, & Dooley, 1996).

Seizures and Epilepsy Among Children with Developmental Disabilities

About 25%–45% of children with epilepsy have another coexisting developmental disability. Approximately 20% of children with cerebral palsy have epilepsy, and about one third of children with ID have epilepsy. About 16% of children with epilepsy have both ID and cerebral palsy (Cowan et al., 1989; Murphy, Sellers, et al., 1995).

Among children with developmental disabilities, epilepsy is a major cause of additional morbidity and contributes to an increased risk of death. The Standardized Mortality Ratio among children with epilepsy only was 1.5, whereas that among children with both epilepsy and another developmental disability was 13.2 (Decouflé & Autry, 2002). Among children and young adults with ID, partial seizures were associated with a Standardized Mortality Ratio of 3.7, whereas generalized seizures were associated with a ratio of 8.1 (Forsgren, Edvinsson, Nystrom, & Blomquist, 1996). Lack of seizure control significantly increased the risk of death among those with ID (Standardized Mortality Ratio of 2.0 among those with controlled epilepsy vs. 16.8 among those with 51 or more seizures per year). Furthermore, children with epilepsy and ID had a much higher risk of death (Standardized Mortality Ratio of 39.7; 95% CI = 23.5–67.1) compared with adults ages 20–59 years (5.0; 95% CI = 2.9–8.7). The reasons for the increased risk of death among children with developmental disabilities plus epilepsy are not well established, and whether the risk of death can be reduced by early effective treatment is not known

ATTENTION-DEFICIT/ HYPERACTIVITY DISORDER

ADHD is a common developmental disorder that is characterized by impulsivity, hyperactivity, and inattention to a degree that leads to impairment in functioning. Although there are case reports in the literature dating back to the early 1900s, the evolution of the understanding of clinical features of the disorder is relatively recent (Barkley, 1998). With the publication of the DSM-III-R (APA, 1987), the variability in the ADHD phenotype was first acknowledged with diagnostic criteria distinguishing between those individuals with and without hyperactivity. In the DSM-IV, this distinction between phenotypes further evolved with separate subtypes of ADHD for children who are primarily inattentive, those who are primarily hyperactive, and those who have a combined presentation (APA, 1994). The DSM-IV also requires that symptoms be present in at least two settings, manifest before 7 years of age, be present for at least 6 months, and result in significant clinical impairment. Also important, the diagnosis should be made in the context of an everyday setting, such as home or school. The DSM-IV subclassification is important from an epidemiological perspective, allowing for more meaningful groupings to examine the etiology of and risk factors for the disorder.

Current diagnosis of ADHD relies on interviews with or ratings of the child's behavior by key informants, including teachers and parents. The challenge in epidemiological studies has been to take the clinical case definitions and adapt them to large-scale studies. When limiting studies to those from school-based settings using DSM-IV criteria, the prevalence rates are generally high, between 11%–16% (Wolraich, Hannah, Baumgaertel, & Feurer, 1998; Wolraich, Hannah, Pinnock, Baumgaertel, & Brown, 1996). With the exception of a higher ratio of boys to girls (about 4:1), other demographic characteristics of ADHD have not been well described (Cantwell, 1996). It is unclear if there is a socioeconomic gradient or differences in prevalence rates by race, although a recent school-based epidemiological study suggested little difference in the rate of ADHD by race. There was variability, however, in ADHD-related medication use, being highest in whites and lowest in Hispanics (Rowland et al., 2001; Rowland, Umbach, et al., 2002). A number of explanations have been advanced for the excess of boys with ADHD, including referral bias because of greater impulsive behaviors in boys and potentially an underdiagnosis of inattentive subtypes in girls.

Many conditions appear to occur more often in children with ADHD than in unaffected children. Conditions that have been described most often to co-occur with ADHD include other emotional and behavioral disorders—oppositional defiant disorder, obsessive-compulsive disorder, anxiety disorder, and depression (Biederman, Newcorn, & Sprich, 1991; Cantwell, 1996). Some of these conditions have symptoms similar to ADHD, which makes it challenging to distinguish between a diagnosis of ADHD and a co-occurring disorder in epidemiological studies. The challenges in accurate assessment of comorbidities might result in spuriously high ADHD prevalence estimates (Rowland, Lesesne, & Abramowitz, 2002).

ADHD has been described as a complex genetic condition. Evidence to support a genetic etiology includes a higher prevalence of a positive family history of ADHD and a higher concordance among MZ compared with DZ twin pairs (Acosta, Arcos-Burgos, & Muenke, 2004). Although epidemiology has not played a role yet in evaluating candidate genes (e.g., dopamine transporter and receptor genes), epidemiological case–control studies (and other epidemiological methods) can play an important role in investigating potential gene–environment interactions.

A few non-genetic risk factors have been identified for ADHD. The most convincing of these are LBW (as a proxy measure for preterm delivery) and environmental lead exposure (Bellinger, Leviton, Allred, & Rabinowitz, 1994; Botting, Powls, & Cooke, 1997; Fergusson, Lynsdey, Horwood, & Kinzett, 1988). Additional epidemiological studies are needed to examine, in a systematic manner, candidate preconceptional, prenatal, and early childhood environmental exposures.

COMMUNICATION DISORDERS

Speech-language disorders are problems in communication and related areas such as oral-motor function. The disorders range from sound substitutions to an inability to understand or use language or use the oral-motor mechanism for functional speech and feeding. Causes include hearing loss, neurological disorders, brain injury, ID, drug abuse, and physical impairments such as cleft lip or palate.

Often the cause is unknown (National Information Center, 2000). Some communication disorders of childhood are developmental in nature; hence, they might be transient, whereas others are more serious, with lifelong consequences that affect learning, socialization, and employment.

Sixteen in every 1,000 children younger than 18 years of age are reported to have a chronic speech disorder, defined as difficulty producing speech sounds or problems with voice quality (American Speech-Language-Hearing Association, 2004). In the 2000–2001 school year, 18.9% of children 6–21 years of age served under Part B of the Individuals with Disabilities Education Act (IDEA) of 1990 (PL 101-476) received services for speech or language disorders. This number did not include children who had speech or language problems that were secondary to another condition (U.S. Department of Education, 2002).

Specific language impairment is a significant deficit in linguistic functioning that does not appear to be accompanied by deficits in hearing, intelligence, or motor functioning (Shamas, Wiig, & Secord, 1998). The estimated prevalence of specific language impairment during preschool and early years is 2%–8%, with an overall median prevalence of 5.9% (8% for boys and 6% for girls) (Tomblin, Smith, & Zhang, 1997). There was a 9.5% increase in services for children with speech or language impairment from the 1991–1992 to the 2000–2001 school years (U.S. Department of Education, 2002). In 2003, more than 1.1 million children were receiving special services under IDEA Part B for speech or language impairments, making it the second most common disability classification after specific learning disabilities (U.S. Department of Education, 2003).

HEARING LOSS

The prevalence of bilateral permanent childhood hearing loss is reported to be roughly 0.6–2.6 per 1,000 children in population-based studies in which the criterion for hearing loss (decibel threshold level) ranged from 20 to 55 dB (Darin, Hanner, & Thiringer, 1997; Davis & Wood, 1992; Drews, Yeargin-Allsopp, Murphy, & Decouflé, 1994; Fortnum, Summerfield, Marshall, Davis, & Bamford, 2001; Kankkunen & Lidén, 1982; Karapurkar et al., 2006; Martin, 1982; Parving, 1993; Sehlin, Holmgren, & Zakrisson, 1990; Sorri & Rantakallio, 1985; Van Naarden & Decouflé, 1999; Vartiainen, Kemppinen, & Karjalainen, 1997). Differences in methods of clinical assessment as well as ascertainment for studies might be responsible for much of these differences. Data from MADDSP showed that the rate of hearing loss increased steadily with age, a trend that was seen for all levels of severity, and that more boys than girls were found to have a hearing loss and there were more black children with a hearing loss than white children (K. Van Naarden Braun, unpublished data, 2005). When the types of hearing loss were examined, sensorineural hearing loss was much more prevalent (79%) than conductive (6%); in approximately 12% of children the type of hearing loss could not be determined using the MADDSP surveillance method of record review. Approximately 30% of children in metropolitan Atlanta with a hearing loss were found to have another developmental disability, most often ID (Van Naarden & Decouflé, 1999).

Of note, children with congenital hearing loss are being identified earlier in the United States through universal newborn hearing screening; however, it is important to screen children for a hearing loss at later ages also. Fortnum et al. (2001) reported that it is likely that late-onset and progressive hearing impairment (e.g., that resulting from disorders such as CMV infection, postnatally acquired loss, and genetic disorders that present clinically after the newborn period) are more prevalent than previously thought. They found that the prevalence of permanent childhood hearing loss of 40 dB or greater in children in the United Kingdom born from 1980 through 1995 has risen with age to at least 1.65 per 1,000 live births and may be as high as 2.05 per 1,000 live births among children 9 years of age or older. This increase in prevalence has implications for service needs for children with hearing loss.

Genetic causes of hearing loss account for up to 50% of cases (Kenneson, Van Naarden Braun, & Boyle, 2002). In about 30% of cases, a specific syndrome can be identified, with more than 400 syndromes having an associated hearing loss; the other 70% are nonsyndromic, either familial or sporadic. Of the familial nonsyndromic cases, 75%–80% are autosomal recessive, 20%–25% are autosomal dominant, and 1%–1.5% are X-linked. Variants in one locus, gap junction beta-2 or *GJB2* (connexin 26), account for up to 50% of cases of nonsyndromic sensorineural hearing loss in some populations, most notably in the Ashkenazic Jewish population, whites of northern European descent, the Japanese population, and individuals from Ghana.

VISION IMPAIRMENT

Impaired vision can significantly affect a child's neurological, cognitive, physical, and emotional development. Recent prevalence rates of childhood vision impairment in the United States range from 0.2 to 0.9 per 1,000 children in population-based studies in which the criterion for vision impairment (visual acuity in the better eye) ranged from blindness in one or both eyes to visual acuity of 3/30 to 20/70 (Boyle, Decouflé, & Yeargin-Allsopp, 1994; Karapurkar Bhasin et al., 2006; Gilbert et al., 1999; Mervis et al., 2002; Riise et al., 1992; Steinkuller et al., 1993; Stewart-Brown & Haslum, 1988; Thylefors, Negrel, Pararajasegaram, & Dadzie, 1995; Wilson et al., 1996). This range of rates is likely due to the different methods of ascertaining cases of childhood blindness, different survival rates of very preterm infants, and different case definitions (low vision vs. legal blindness). Children 3–10 years of age in metropolitan Atlanta identified in 1991 were found to have a prevalence of vision impairment of 0.8 per 1,000 children. Vision impairment was defined as a measured visual acuity of 20/70 or worse, with correction, in the better eye. This prevalence was similar to the prevalence of legal blindness in 10-year-old children in the same population ascertained during the period 1985 through 1987. As with hearing loss, the prevalence of vision impairment in 1991 increased with age (up to 7 years); however, unlike hearing loss, the prevalence of vision impairment was similar for all race- and sex-specific subgroups (K. Van Naarden Braun, unpublished data, 2005).

When the underlying causes of vision impairment were examined in this same population, prenatal causes accounted for 43%, whereas 27% of the etiologies were found to be perinatal in origin. Postnatal etiologies were very uncommon. Of the prenatal etiologies, 38% were genetic, with the largest percentage being due to ocular or oculocutaneous albinism. The distribution of timing of insult associated with the vision impairment differed significantly by birth weight categories, with children of normal birth weight (> 2,500 g) having a larger percentage of prenatal etiologies, and children with LBW (< 2,500 g) having a larger percentage of perinatal etiologies.

CONCLUSION

The epidemiology of developmental disabilities and disorders is a rapidly evolving field that is an important complement to clinical investigation and practice. The public health model uses the determination of prevalence and description of the conditions, followed by epidemiological research into risk and protective factors and causes, to inform prevention programs and public policy. More and more, pediatricians and other health practitioners are called on to understand clinical conditions in the context of populations, not merely individual patients. Epidemiology is the science that provides the information on which decisions can be responsibly made for the benefit of children and families affected by developmental disabilities. Knowledge and understanding of epidemiological principles is important in order to best serve the large and increasing number of children with developmental disabilities and their families.

REFERENCES

Abel, E.L. (1995). An update on incidence of FAS: FAS is not an equal opportunity birth defect. *Neurotoxicology and Teratology, 17,* 437–443.

Abel, E.L., & Sokol, R.J. (1986). Fetal alcohol syndrome is now leading cause of mental retardation. *Lancet 2,* 1222.

Acosta, M.T., Arcos-Burgos, M., & Muenke, M. (2004). Attention deficit/hyperactivity disorder (ADHD): Complex phenotype, simple genotype? *Genetics in Medicine, 6,* 1–15.

Adams, J., Voorhees, C.V., & Middaugh, L.D. (1990). Developmental neurotoxicity of anticonvulsants: Human and animal evidence on phenytoin. *Neurotoxicology and Teratology, 12,* 203–214.

Allen, M. (1993). The high risk infant. *Pediatric Clinics of North America, 40,* 479–490.

American Academy of Pediatrics. (2003a). *Haemophilus influenzae* infections. In L.K. Pickering, C.J. Baker, S.S. Long, et al. (Eds.), *2003 Red book: Report of the Committee on Infectious Diseases* (26th ed.). Elk Grove Village, IL: Author.

American Academy of Pediatrics. (2003b). Herpes simplex. In L.K. Pickering, C.J. Baker, S.S. Long, et al. (Eds.), *2003 Red book: Report of the Committee on Infectious Diseases* (26th ed., pp. 344–345). Elk Grove Village, IL: Author.

American Academy of Pediatrics. (2003c). Group B streptococcal infections. In L.K. Pickering, C.J. Baker, S.S. Long, et al. (Eds.), *2003 Red book: Report of the Committee on Infectious Diseases* (26th ed., p. 584). Elk Grove Village, IL: Author.

American Psychiatric Association. (1987). *Diagnostic and statistical manual of mental disorders* (3rd ed., rev). Washington, DC: Author.

American Psychiatric Association. (1994). *Diagnostic and statistical manual of mental disorders* (4th ed.). Washington, DC: Author.

American Speech-Language-Hearing Association. (2004). *Communication facts: Incidence and prevalence of communication disorders and hearing loss in children.* Retrieved November 11, 2004, from http://www.asha.org

Andriantsimahavandy, A., Lesbordes, J.L. Rasoaharimalala, B., Peghini, M., Rabarijaona, L., & Boiser, P. (1997). Neurocysticercosis: A major aetiological factor of late-onset epilepsy in Madagascar. *Tropical Medicine and International Health, 2,* 741–746.

Annegers, J.F., Hauser, W.A., & Lee, J.R. (1995). Incidence of acute symptomatic seizures in Rochester, Minnesota 1935–1984. *Epilepsia, 36,* 327–333.

Annegers, J.F., Hauser, W.A., Lee, J.R., & Rocca, W.A. (1995). Secular trends and birth cohort effects in unprovoked seizures: Rochester, Minnesota 1935–1984. *Epilepsia, 36,* 575–579.

Arvidsson, T., Danielsson, B., Forsberg, P., Gillberg, C., Johansson, M., & Kjellgren, G. (1997). Autism in 3–6 year-old children in a suburb of Goteborg, Sweden. *Autism, 1,* 163–171.

Ashley-Koch, A., Murphy, C.C., Khoury, M.J., & Boyle, C.A. (2001). Contribution of sickle cell disease to the occurrence of developmental disabilities: A population-based study. *Genetics in Medicine, 3,* 181–186.

Astradsson, A., Olafsson, E., Ludvigsson, P., Bjorgvinsson, H., & Hauser, W.A. (1998). Rolandic epilepsy: An incidence study in Iceland. *Epilepsia, 39,* 884–886.

Autism and Developmental Disabilities Monitoring Network Surveillance Year 2000 Principal Investigators (ADDM). (2007a). Prevalence of autism spectrum disorders—Autism and Developmetnal Disabilities Monitoring Network, six sites, United States, 2000. *Morbidity and Mortality Weekly Report: CDC Surveillance Summaries, 56*(SS01), 1–11.

Autism and Developmental Disabilities Monitoring Network Surveillance Year 2000 Principal Investigators (ADDM). (2007b). Prevalence of autism spectrum disorders—Autism and Developmental Disabilities Monitoring Network, 14 sites, United States, 2002. *Morbidity and Mortality Weekly Report: CDC Surveillance Summaries, 56*(SS01), 12–27.

Aziz, H., Guvener, A., Akhtar, S.W., & Hasan, K.Z. (1997). Comparative epidemiology of epilepsy in Pakistan and Turkey: Population-based studies using identical protocols. *Epilepsia, 38*, 716–722.

Bailey, A., Le Couteur, A., Gottesman, I., Bolton, P., Simonoff, E., & Rutter, M. (1995). Autism is a strongly genetic disorder: Evidence from a British twin study. *Psychological Medicine, 25*, 63–77.

Baird, G., Cass, H., & Slonims, V. (2003). Diagnosis of autism. *BMJ, 327*, 488–493.

Baird, G., Charman, T., Baron-Cohen, S., Swettenham, J., Whellwright, S., & Drew, A. (2000). A screening instrument for autism at 18 months of age: A 6-year follow-up study. *Journal of the American Academy of Child and Adolescent Psychiatry, 39*, 694–702.

Baraff, L.J., Lee, S.I., & Schriger, D.L. (1993). Outcomes of bacterial meningitis in children: A meta-analysis. *Pediatric Infectious Disease Journal, 12*, 389–394.

Barbaresi, W.J., Katusic, S.K., Colligan, R.C., Weaver, A.L., & Jacobsen, S.J. (2005). The incidence of autism in Olmsted County, Minnesota, 1976–1997: Results from a population-based study. *Archives of Pediatrics and Adolescent Medicine, 159*, 37–44.

Barkley, R.A. (1998). *Attention-deficit hyperactivity disorder: A handbook for diagnosis and treatment* (2nd ed.). New York: The Guilford Press.

Bell, G.S., & Sander, J.W. (2002). The epidemiology of epilepsy: The size of the problem. *Seizure, 11*(Suppl. A), 306–314.

Bellinger, D., Leviton, A., Allred, E., & Rabinowitz, M. (1994). Pre- and postnatal lead exposure and behavior problems in school-aged children. *Environmental Research, 66*(1), 12–30.

Berg, A.T., Levy, S.R., Testa, F. M., & Shinnar, S. (1999). Classification of childhood epilepsy syndromes in newly diagnosed epilepsy: Interrater agreement and reasons for disagreement. *Epilepsia, 40*, 439–444.

Bertrand, J., Mars, A., Boyle, C., Bove, F., Yeargin-Allsopp, M., & Decouflé, P. (2001). Prevalence of autism in a United States population: The Brick Township, New Jersey, investigation. *Pediatrics, 108*, 1155–1161.

Bhasin, T.K., & Schendel, D. (2007). Sociodemographic risk factors for autism in a U.S. metropolitan area. *Journal of Autism Developmental Disorders, 37*(4), 667–677.

Biederman, J., Newcorn, J., & Sprich, S. (1991). Comorbidity of attention deficit hyperactivity disorder with conduct, depressive, anxiety, and other disorders. *American Journal of Psychiatry, 148*, 564–577.

Blackorby, J., & Wagner, M. (1996). Longitudinal postschool outcomes of youth with disabilities: Findings from the National Longitudinal Transition Study. *Exceptional Children, 62*, 399–413.

Blair, E., & Stanley, F. (1985). Interobserver agreement in the classification of cerebral palsy. *Developmental Medicine and Child Neurology, 27*, 615–622.

Blair, E., & Stanley, F.J. (1997). Issues in the classification and epidemiology of cerebral palsy. *Mental Retardation and Developmental Disabilities Research Reviews, 3*, 184–193.

Bolton, P.F. (1997). Obstetric complication in autism: Consequences or causes of the condition? *Journal American Academy of Child Adolescent Psychiatry, 36*, 272–281.

Botting, N., Powls, A., & Cooke, R.W.I. (1997). Attention deficit hyperactivity disorder and other psychiatric outcomes in very low birthweight children at 12 years. *Journal of Child Psychology and Psychiatry and Allied Disciplines, 38*, 931–941.

Boyle, C.A., Bertrand, J., & Yeargin-Allsopp, M. (1999). Surveillance of autism. *Infants and Young Children, 12*, 75–78.

Boyle, C.A., Decouflé, P., & Yeargin-Allsopp, M. (1994). Prevalence and health impact of developmental disabilities in U.S. children. *Pediatrics, 33*, 399–403.

Boyle, C.A., Keddie, A., & Holmgreen, P. (1997). The risk of mental retardation in twins. *Paediatric and Perinatal Epidemiology, 11*, A10.

Boyle, C.A., Yeargin-Allsopp, M., Doernberg, N., Holmgreen, P., Murphy, C.C., & Schendel, D. (1996). Prevalence of selected developmental disabilities in children aged 3–10 years: The Metropolitan Atlanta Developmental Disabilities Surveillance Program, 1991. *Morbidity and Mortality Weekly Report: CDC Surveillance Summaries, 45*(SS02), 1–14.

Brask, B. (1972). *Barnepsykiatrisk.* Presentation at the Nordic Symposium of the Comprehensive Care of Psychotic Children, Oslo, Norway.

Broman, S., Nichols, P.L., Shaughnessy, P., & Kennedy, W. (1987). *Retardation in young children: A developmental study of cognitive development.* Hillsdale, NJ: Lawrence Erlbaum Associates.

Bryson, S., Clark, B., & Smith, I.M. (1988). First report of a Canadian epidemiological study of autistic syndromes. *Journal of Child Psychology and Psychiatry and Allied Disciplines, 29*, 433–446.

Bundey, S. (1997). Prevalence and type of cerebral palsy. *Developmental Medicine and Child Neurology, 39*, 568.

Buyse, M.L. (1990). *Birth defects encyclopedia.* Cambridge, UK: Blackwell Scientific Publications.

California Department of Developmental Services. (1999). *Changes in the population of persons with autism and pervasive developmental disorders in California's developmental services system: 1987–1998. A report of the Legislature.* Sacramento: California Department of Developmental Services.

California Department of Developmental Services. (2003). *Autistic spectrum disorders changes in the California caseload an update: 1999 through 2002. A report of the Legislature.* Sacramento: Author.

Camfield, C.S., Camfield, P.R., Gordon, K., Wirrell, E., & Dooley, J.M. (1996). Incidence of epilepsy in childhood and adolescence: A population-based study in Nova Scotia from 1977 to 1985. *Epilepsia, 37,* 19–23.

Camp, B.W., Borman, S.H., & Nichols, P.L. (1998). Maternal and neonatal risk factors for mental retardation: Defining the "at risk" child. *Early Human Development, 50,* 159–173.

Campbell, M., Hardesty, A.S., & Burdock, E.I. (1978). Demographic and perinatal profile of 105 autistic children: A preliminary report. *Psychopharmacology Bulletin, 14,* 36–39.

Cans, C., McManus, V., Crowley, M., Guillem, P., Platt, M.J., Johnson, A., et al. (2004). Surveillance of Cerebral Palsy in Europe Collaborative Group. Cerebral palsy of post-neonatal origin: Characteristics and risk factors. *Paediatric and Perinatal Epidemiology, 18,* 214–220.

Cans, C., Wilhelm, L., Baille, M.F., du Mazaubrun, C., Grandjean, H., & Rumeau-Rouquette, C. (1999). Aetiological findings and associated factors in children with severe mental retardation. *Developmental Medicine and Child Neurology, 41,* 233–239.

Cantwell, D.P. (1996). Attention deficit disorder: A review of the past 10 years. *Journal American Academy Child Adolescent Psychiatry, 35,* 978–987.

Centers for Disease Control and Prevention. (1995). Disabilities among children aged less than or equal to 17 years—United States 1991–1992. *MMWR: Morbidity and Mortality Weekly Report, 44,* 609–613.

Centers for Disease Control and Prevention. (1996). Postnatal causes of developmental disabilities in children aged 3–10 years—Atlanta, Georgia, 1991. *MMWR: Morbidity and Mortality Weekly Report, 45,* 130–134.

Centers for Disease Control and Prevention. (1997). Decreasing incidence of perinatal group B streptococcal disease—United States, 1993–1995. *MMWR: Morbidity and Mortality Weekly Report, 46,* 473–477.

Centers for Disease Control and Prevention. (1999). Mental retardation following diagnosis of a metabolic disorder in children aged 3–10 years—metropolitan Atlanta, Georgia, 1991–1994. *MMWR: Morbidity and Mortality Weekly Report, 48,* 353–356.

Centers for Disease Control and Prevention. (2000). Measles, rubella, and congenital rubella syndrome—United States and Mexico, 1997–1999. *MMWR: Morbidity and Mortality Weekly Report, 49,* 1048–1050.

Centers for Disease Control and Prevention. (2001). Congenital syphilis—United States, 2000. *MMWR: Morbidity and Mortality Weekly Report, 50,* 573–577.

Centers for Disease Control and Prevention. (2002). Progress toward elimination of *Haemophilus influenzae* type B invasive disease among infants and children—United States, 1998–2000. *MMWR: Morbidity and Mortality Weekly Report, 51,* 234–237.

Centers for Disease Control and Prevention. (2003a). Surveillance for elevated blood lead levels among children—United States, 1997–2001. *Morbidity and Mortality Weekly Report: CDC Surveillance Summaries, 52* (SS10).

Centers for Disease Control and Prevention. (2003b). *Streptococcus pneumoniae disease.* Retrieved March 5, 2005, from http://www.cdc.gov/ncidod/dbmd/diseaseinfo/streppneum_t.htm.

Centers for Disease Control and Prevention. (2005). Achievements in public health: Elimination of rubella and congenital rubella syndrome—United States, 1969–2004. *MMWR: Morbidity and Mortality Weekly Report, 54,* 279–282.

Chadwick, E.G., & Yogev, R. (1995). Pediatric AIDS. *Pediatric Clinics of North America, 42,* 969–992.

Chakrabarti, S., & Fombonne, E. (2001). Pervasive developmental disorders in preschool children. *JAMA, 285,* 3093–3099.

Chapman, D.A., Scott, K., & Mason, C. (2002). Early risk factors for mental retardation: Role of maternal age and maternal education. *American Journal on Mental Retardation, 107,* 46–59.

Charman, T. (2003). Epidemiology and early identification of autism: Research challenges and opportunities. *Novartis Foundation Symposium, 251,* 10–19; discussion 19–25, 109–111, 281–297.

Chelly, J., & Mandel, J.L. (2001). Monogenic causes of X-linked mental retardation. *Nature Reviews: Genetics, 2,* 669–680.

Chen, Y-C.J., Guo, Y-L., & Hsu, C-C. (1992). Cognitive development of Yu-Cheng ("oil disease") in children prenatally exposed to heat-degraded PCBs. *JAMA, 268,* 3213–3218.

Chess, S. (1971). Autism in children with congenital rubella. *Journal of Autism and Childhood Schizophrenia, 1,* 33–47.

Clark, S.L., & Hankins, G.D. (2003). Temporal and demographic trends in cerebral palsy—fact and fiction. *American Journal of Obstetrics and Gynecology, 188,* 628–633.

Cockerell, O.C., Eckle, I., Goodridge, D.M., Sander, J.W., & Shorvon, S. (1995). Epilepsy in a population of 6000 re-examined: Secular trends in first attendance rates, prevalence, and prognosis. *Journal of Neurology, Neurosurgery and Psychiatry, 60,* 247. [Published erratum in *Journal of Neurology, Neurosurgery and Psychiatry, 60,* 247 (1996).]

Cohen, I.L., Sudhalter, V., Pfadt, A., Jewnkins, E.C., Brown, W.T., & Vietze, P.M. (1991). Why are autism and the fragile X syndrome associated? Conceptual and methodological issues. *American Journal of Human Genetics, 48,* 195–202.

Cohen, P., Cohen, J., Kasen, S., & Velex, C.N. (1993). An epidemiological study of disorders in late childhood and adolescence I: Age and gender-specific prevalence. *Journal of Child Psychology and Psychiatry and Allied Disciplines, 34,* 851–867.

Collins, M., & Paneth, N. (1998). Pre-eclampsia and cerebral palsy: Are they related? *Developmental Medicine and Child Neurology, 40,* 207–211.

Commission on Classification and Terminology of the International League Against Epilepsy. (1981). Proposal for revised clinical and electroencephalographic classification of epileptic seizures. *Epilepsia, 22,* 489–501.

Commission on Classification and Terminology of the International League Against Epilepsy. (1989). Proposal for revised classification of epilepsies and epileptic syndromes. *Epilepsia, 30,* 389–399.

Commission on Epilepsy and Prognosis of the International League Against Epilepsy. (1993). Guidelines for epidemiologic studies on epilepsy. *Epilepsia, 34,* 592–596.

Cooke, R.W.I. (1994). Factors affecting survival and outcome at 3 years in extremely preterm infants. *Archives of Disease in Childhood: Fetal and Neonatal Edition, 71,* F28–F31.

Cowan, L.D., Bodensteiner, J.B., & Leviton, A. (1989). Prevalence of the epilepsies in children and adolescents. *Epilepsia, 30,* 94–106.

Cowan, L.D., & Hudson, L.S. (1991). The epidemiology and natural history of infantile spasms. *Journal of Child Neurology, 6,* 355–364.

Crocker, A.C. (1989). The spectrum of medical care for developmental disabilities. In I.L. Rubin & A.C. Crocker (Eds.), *Developmental disabilities: Delivery of medical care for children and adults.* Philadelphia: Lea & Febiger.

Croen, L.A., Grether, J.K., Curry, C.J., & Nelson, K.B. (2001). Congenital abnormalities among children with cerebral palsy: More evidence for prenatal antecedents. *Journal of Pediatrics, 138,* 804–810.

Croen, L.A., Grether, J., Hoogstrate, J., & Selvin, S. (2002). The changing prevalence of autism in California. *Journal of Autism and Developmental Disorders, 32,* 207–215.

Croen, L.A., Grether, J.K., & Selvin, S. (2001). The epidemiology of mental retardation of unknown cause. *Pediatrics, 107,* e86.

Croen, L.A., Grether, J.K., Yoshida, C.K., Odouli, R., & Van de Water, J. (2005). Maternal autoimmune diseases, asthma and allergies, and childhood autism spectrum disorders: A case control study. *Archives of Pediatrics and Adolescent Medicine, 159,* 151–157.

Crunelli, V., & Leresche, N. (2002). Childhood absence epilepsy: Genes, channels, neurons and networks. *Nature Reviews: Neuroscience, 3,* 371–382.

Cryan, E., Byrne, M., O'Donovan, A., & O'Callaghan, E. (1996). Brief report: A case-control study of obstetric complications and later autistic disorder. *Journal of Autism and Developmental Disorders, 26,* 453–460.

Cuccaro, M.L. (1996). Professional perceptions of children with developmental difficulties: The influence of race and socioeconomic status. *Journal of Autism and Developmental Disorders, 26,* 461–469.

Cummings, S.K., Nelson, K.B., Grether, J.K., & Velie, E.M. (1993). Cerebral palsy in four northern California counties, births 1983 through 1985. *Journal of Pediatrics, 123,* 230–237.

Darin, N., Hanner, P., & Thiringer, K. (1997). Changes in prevalence, etiology, age at detection, and associated disabilities in preschool children with hearing impairment born in Göteborg. *Developmental Medicine and Child Neurology, 39,* 797–802.

Davidson, P.W., Myers, J., & Weiss, B. (2004). Mercury exposure and child development outcomes. *Pediatrics, 113,* 1023–1027.

Davis, A., & Wood, S. (1992). The epidemiology of childhood hearing impairment: Factors relevant to planning of services. *British Journal of Audiology, 26,* 77–90.

Decouflé, P., & Autry, A. (2002). Increased mortality in children and adolescents with developmental disabilities. *Paediatric and Perinatal Epidemiology, 16,* 375–382.

Decouflé, P., & Boyle, C.A. (1995). The relationship between maternal education and mental retardation in 10-year old children. *Annals of Epidemiology, 5,* 347–353.

Decouflé, P., Boyle, C.A., Paulozzi, L., & Lary, J. (2001). Increased risk for developmental disabilities in children who have major birth defects: A population-based study. *Pediatrics, 108,* 728–734.

Del Brutto, O.H., Santibanez, R., Idrovo, L., Rodriguez, S., Diaz-Calderon, E., Navas, C., et al. (2005). Epilepsy and neurocysticercosis in Atahualpa: A door-to-door survey in rural coastal Ecuador. *Epilepsia, 46,* 583–587.

Drews, C.D., Murphy, C.C., Yeargin-Allsopp, M., & Decouflé, P. (1996). The relationship between idiopathic mental retardation and maternal smoking during pregnancy. *Pediatrics, 97,* 547–553.

Drews, C.D., Yeargin-Allsopp, M., Decouflé, P., & Murphy, C.C. (1995). Variation in the influence of selected sociodemographic risk factors for mental retardation. *American Journal of Public Health, 85,* 329–334.

Drews, C.D., Yeargin-Allsopp, M., Murphy, C.C., & Decouflé, P. (1994). Hearing impairment among 10-year-old children: Metropolitan Atlanta, 1985 through 1987. *American Journal of Public Health, 84,* 1164–1166.

English, D.R., Holman, C.D.J., Milne, E., Winter, M.G., Hulse, G.K., Codde, J.P., et al. (1995). *The quantification of drug caused morbidity and mortality in Australia, 1995 edition.* Canberra, Australia: Commonwealth Department of Human Services and Health.

Eriksson, K.J., & Koivikko, M.J. (1997). Prevalence, classification, and severity of epilepsy and epileptic syndromes in children. *Epilepsia, 38,* 1275–1282.

Fergusson, D.M., Lynsdey, M.T., Horwood, L.J., & Kinzett, N.G. (1988). A longitudinal study of dentine lead levels, intelligence, school performance and behavior: Part III. Dentine lead levels and attention/activity. *Journal of Child Psychology and Psychiatry and Allied Disciplines, 29,* 811–824.

Fernell, E. (1998). Aetiological factors and prevalence of severe mental retardation in children in a Swedish municipality: The possible role of consanguinity. *Developmental Medicine and Child Neurology, 40,* 608–611.

Fisher, R.S., van Emde Boas, W., Blume, W., Elger, C., Genton, P., Lee, P., et al. (2005). Epileptic seizures and epilepsy: Definitions proposed by the International League Against Epilepsy (ILAE) and the International Bureau for Epilepsy (IBE). *Epilepsia, 46,* 470–472.

Flint, J., & Wilkie, A.O.M. (1996). The genetics of mental retardation. *British Medical Bulletin, 52,* 453–464.

Folstein, S.E., & Rutter, M.L. (1988). Autism: Familial aggregation and genetic implications. *Journal of Autism and Developmental Disorders, 18,* 3–20.

Fombonne, E. (1999). The epidemiology of autism: A review. *Psychological Medicine, 29,* 769–786.

Fombonne, E., & du Mazaubrun, C. (1992). Prevalence of infantile autism in four French regions. *Social Psychiatry and Psychiatric Epidemiology, 27,* 203–210.

Fombonne, E., du Mazaubrun, C., Cans, C., & Grandjean, H. (1997). Autism and associated medical disorders in a French epidemiological survey. *Journal of the American Academy of Child and Adolescent Psychiatry, 36,* 1561–1569.

Fombonne, E., Simmons, H., Ford, T., Meltzer, H., & Goodman, R. (2001). Prevalence of pervasive developmental disorders in the British nationwide survey of child mental health. *Journal of the American Academy of Child and Adolescent Psychiatry, 40,* 820–827.

Forsgren, L., Edvinsson, S.O., Nystrom, L., & Blomquist, H.K. (1996). Influence of epilepsy on mortality in mental retardation: An epidemiologic study. *Epilepsia, 37,* 956–963.

Fortnum, H.M., Summerfield, A.Q., Marshall, D.H., Davis, A.C., & Bamford, J.M. (2001). Prevalence of permanent childhood hearing impairment in the United Kingdom and implications for universal neonatal hearing screening: Questionnaire based ascertainment study. *BMJ, 323,* 536–540.

Fowler, K.B., Stagnos, S., Paas, R.F., Britt, W.J., Boll, T.J., & Alsord, C.A. (1992). The outcome of congenital cytomegalovirus infection in relation to maternal antibody status. *New England Journal of Medicine, 326,* 663–667.

Foster, C.J., Biggs, R.J., Melvin, D., Walters, M.D.S., Tudor-Williams, G., & Lyall, E.G.H. (2006). Neurodevelopmental outcomes in children with HIV infection under 3 years of age. *Developmental Medicine & Child Neurology, 48,* 677–682.

Gilbert, C.E., Anderton, L., Dandona, L., & Foster, A. (1999). Prevalence of visual impairment in children: a review of available data. *Ophthalmic Epidemiology, 6,* 73–82.

Gilbert, G.L. (1996). Congenital fetal infections. *Seminars in Neonatology, 1,* 91–105.

Gilbert, R., Dunn, D., Wallon, M., Hayde, M., Prusa, A., Lebech, M., et al. (2001). Ecological comparison of the risks of mother-to-child transmission and clinical manifestations of congenital toxoplasmosis according to prenatal treatment period. *Epidemiology and Infection, 127,* 113–120.

Gillberg, C. (1980). Maternal age and infantile autism. *Journal of Autism and Developmental Disorders, 10,* 293–297.

Gillberg, C. (1984). Infantile autism and other childhood psychoses in a Swedish urban region: Epidemiological aspects. *Journal of Child Psychology and Psychiatry and Allied Disciplines, 25,* 35–43.

Gillberg, C., & Gillberg, I.C. (1983). Infantile autism: A total population study of reduced optimality in the pre-, peri-, and neonatal period. *Journal of Autism and Developmental Disorders, 13,* 153–166.

Gillberg, C., Steffenburg, S., & Schaumann, H. (1991). Is autism more common now than ten years ago? *British Journal of Psychiatry, 158,* 403–409.

Gillberg, C., & Wing, L. (1999). Autism: Not an extremely rare disorder. *Acta Neurologica Scandinavica, 99,* 399–406.

Gillberg, I., & Gillberg, C. (1996). Autism in immigrants: A population-based study from Swedish rural and urban areas. *Journal of Intellectual Disability Research, 40*(Pt. 1), 24–31.

Gourie-Devi, M., Satishchandra, P., & Subbakrishna, D.K. (2004). Prevalence of neurological disorders in Bangalore, India: A community-based study with a comparison between urban and rural areas. *Neuroepidemiology, 23,* 261–268.

Grether, J.K., & Nelson, K.B. (1996). Prenatal and perinatal factors and cerebral palsy in very low birth weight infants. *Journal of Pediatrics, 128,* 407–414.

Grether, J.K., & Nelson, K.B. (2000). Possible decrease in prevalence of cerebral palsy in premature infants. *Journal of Pediatrics, 136,* 133.

Grether, J.K., Nelson, K.B., & Cummins, S.K. (1993). Twinning and cerebral palsy: Experience in four northern California counties, births 1983 through 1985. *Pediatrics, 92,* 854–858.

Grether, J.K., Nelson, K.B., Walsh, E., Willoughby, R.E., & Redline, R.W. (2003). Intrauterine exposure to infection and risk of cerebral palsy in very preterm infants. *Archives of Pediatrics and Adolescent Medicine, 157,* 26–32.

Hack, M., Taylor, H.G., Klein, N., Eiben, R., Schatschneider, C., & Mercuri-Minich, N. (1994). School-age outcomes in children with birth weights under 750 g. *New England Journal of Medicine, 331,* 753–759.

Haddow, J.E., Palomaki, G.E., Allan, W.C., Williams, J.R., Knight, G.J., Gagnon, J., et al. (1999). Maternal thyroid deficiency during pregnancy and subsequent neuropsychological development of the child. *New England Journal of Medicine, 341,* 549–555.

Hagberg, B., Hagberg, G., Olow, I., & von Wendt, L. (1996). The changing panorama of cerebral palsy in Sweden VII. Prevalence and origin in the birth year period 1987–90. *Acta Pediatrica, 85,* 954–960.

Hagberg, B., & Kyllerman, M. (1983). Epidemiology of mental retardation—a Swedish survey. *Brain and Development, 5,* 441–449.

Hallmayer, J., Glasson, E. J., Bower, C., Petterson, B., Croen L., Grether, J., et al. (2002). On the twin risk in autism. *American Journal of Human Genetics, 71,* 941–946.

Halpern, A.S. (1993). Quality of life as a conceptual framework for evaluating transition outcomes. *Exceptional Children, 59,* 486–498.

Halsey, N.A., & Hyman, S.L. (2001). Measles-mumps-rubella vaccine and autistic spectrum disorder: Report from the New Challenges in Childhood Immunizations Conference convened in Oak Brook, Illinois, June 12–13, 2000. *Pediatrics, 107*(5), e84.

Hansen, H., Belmont, L., & Stein, Z. (1980). Epidemiology. *Mental Retardation, 11,* 21–54.

Hanson, J.W. (1986). Teratogen update: Fetal hydantoin effects. *Teratology, 33,* 349–353.

Harum, K.H., Hoon, A.H., Kato, G.J., Casella, J.F., Breiter, S.N., & Johnston, M.V. (1999). Homozygous factor-V mutation as a genetic cause of perinatal thrombosis and cerebral palsy. *Developmental Medicine and Child Neurology, 41,* 777–780.

Hauser, W.A., Annegers, J.F., & Kurland, L.T. (1993). Incidence of epilepsy and unprovoked seizures in Rochester, Minnesota: 1935–1984. *Epilepsia, 34,* 453–468.

Heaney, D.C., MacDonald, B.K., Everitt, A., Stevenson, S., Leonardi, G.S., Wilkinson, P., et al. (2002). Socioeconomic variation in incidence of epilepsy: Prospective community based study in south east England. *BMJ, 325,* 1013–1016.

Heiskala, H. (1997). Community-based study of Lennox-Gastaut syndrome. *Epilepsia, 38,* 526–531.

Holmes, L.B., Coull, B.A., Dorfman, J., & Rosenberger, P. (2005). The correlation of deficits in IQ with midface and digit hypoplasia in children exposed in utero to anticonvulsant drugs. *Journal of Pediatrics, 146,* 118–122.

Honda, H., Shimizu, Y., Misumi, K., Niimi, M., & Ohashi, Y. (1996). Cumulative incidence and prevalence of childhood autism in children in Japan. *British Journal of Psychiatry, 169,* 228–235.

Hoshino, Y., Kumashiro, H., Yashima, Y., Tachibana, R., & Watanabe, M. (1982). The epidemiological study of autism in Fukushima-ken. *Folia Psychiatric et Neurologica Japonica, 36,* 115–124.

Hou, J.W., Wang, T.R., & Chuang, S.M. (1998). An epidemiological and aetiological study of children with intellectual disability in Taiwan. *Journal of Intellectual Disability Research, 42,* 137–143.

Howlin, P., & Moore, A. (1997). Diagnosis of autism: A survey of over 1200 patients in the UK. *Autism, 1,* 135–162.

Individuals with Disabilities Education Act (IDEA) of 1990, PL 101-476, 20 U.S.C. §§ 1400 *et seq.*

Institute of Medicine, Board on Health Promotion and Disease Prevention, Immunization Safety Review Committee. (2001). *Immunization safety review: Measles-mumps-rubella vaccine and autism.* Washington, DC: National Academies Press.

Institute of Medicine, Board of Health Promotion and Disease Prevention, Immunization Safety Review Committee. (2004). *Immunization safety review: Thimerosal-containing vaccines and neurodevlopmental disorders.* Washington, DC: National Academies Press.

Jacobson, J.L., & Jacobson, S.W. (1996). Intellectual impairment in children exposed to polychlorinated biphenyls in utero. *New England Journal of Medicine, 333,* 783–789.

Jacobson, J.L., & Jacobson, S.W. (1997). Teratogen update: Polychlorinated biphenyls. *Teratology, 55,* 338–347.

Jacobson, J.W., & Janicki, M.P. (1983). Observed prevalence of multiple developmental disabilities. *Mental Retardation, 21*(3), 87–94.

Jallon, P., Goumaz, M., Haenggeli, C., & Morabia, A. (1997). Incidence of first epileptic seizures in the canton of Geneva, Switzerland. *Epilepsia, 38,* 547–552.

Jones, K.I. (1997). *Smith's recognizable patterns of human malformation* (5th ed.). Philadelphia: W.B. Saunders.

Kadesjö, B., Gillberg, C., & Hagberg, B. (1999). Brief report. Autism and Asperger syndrome in seven-year-old children: A total population study. *Journal of Autism and Developmental Disorders, 29,* 327–332.

Kankkunen, A., & Lidén, G. (1982). Early identification of hearing handicapped children. *Acta Otolaryngologica: Supplement, 386,* 31–35.

Kanner, L. (1943). Autistic disturbances of affective contact. *Nervous Child, 2,* 217–250.

Karapurkar, T., Lee, N.L., Curran L.K., Newschaffer, C.J., & Yeargin-Allsopp, M. (2004). The epidemiology of autism and autism spectrum disorders. In V.B. Gupta (Ed.), *Autistic spectrum disorders in children* (pp. 17–42). New York: Marcel Dekker.

Karapurkar Bhasin, T., Brocksen, S., Avchen, R.N., & Van Naarden Braun, K. (2006). Prevalence of four developmental disabilities among children age 8 years—Metropolitan Atlanta Developmental Disabilities Surveillance Program: 1996 and 2000. *Morbidity and Mortality Weekly Report: CDC Surveillance Summaries, 55*(SS01), 1–9.

Kenneson, A., Van Naarden Braun, K., & Boyle, C. (2002). GJB2 (connexin 26) variants and nonsyndromic sensorineural hearing loss. *Genetics in Medicine, 4,* 258–274.

Kent, L., Evans, J., Paul, M., & Sharp, M. (1999). Comorbidity of autistic spectrum disorders in children with Down syndrome. *Developmental Medicine and Child Neurology, 41,* 153–158.

Kielinen, M., Linna, S., & Moilanen, I. (2000). Autism in northern Finland. *European Child and Adolescent Psychiatry, 9,* 162–167.

Kiely, M. (1987). The prevalence of mental retardation. *Epidemiologic Reviews, 9,* 194–218.

Koch, R. (2000). *Maternal PKU.* Retrieved June 18, 2005, from http://www.pku-allieddisorders.org/maternalpku.htm

Kurtz, Z., Tookey, P., & Ross, E. (1998). Epilepsy in young people: Twenty-three year follow-up of the British National Child Development Study. *BMJ, 316,* 339–342.

Larson, S.A., Lakin, K.C., Anderson, L., Kwak, N., & Lee J.H. (2000). Prevalence of mental retardation and/or developmental disabilities: Analysis of the 1994–1995 NHIS-DS. *MR/DD Data Brief, 2*(1). Retrieved January 18, 2005, from http://rtc.umn.edu/nhis/pubs.asp

Larson, S.A., Lakin, K.C., Anderson, L., Kwak, N., Lee J.H., & Anderson, D. (2001). Prevalence of mental retardation and developmental disabilities: Estimates from the 1994/1995 National Health Interview Survey Disability Supplements. *American Journal of Mental Retardation, 106,* 231–252.

Lauritsen, M.B., Pedersen, C.B., & Mortensen, P.B. (2004). The incidence and prevalence of pervasive developmental disorders: A Danish population-based study. *Psychological Medicine, 34,* 1339–1346.

Lee, W.L., & Ong, H.T. (2001). Epidemiology of West syndrome in Singapore. *Brain and Development, 23,* 584–585.

Lenke, R.R., & Levy, H.L. (1980). Maternal phenylketonuria and hyperphenylalaninemia: An internation survey of the outcome of untreated and treated pregnancies. *New England Journal of Medicine, 303,* 1202–1208.

Leonard, H., & Wen, X. (2002). The epidemiology of mental retardation: Challenges and opportunities in the new millennium. *Mental Retardation and Developmental Disabilities Research Reviews, 8,* 117–134.

Leviton, A., & Gilles, F. (1999). Ventriculomegaly, delayed myelination, white matter hypoplasia, and "periventricular" leukomalacia: How are they related? *Pediatric Neurology, 15,* 127–136.

Lord, C., Mulloy, C., Wendelboe, M., & Schopler, E. (1991). Pre- and perinatal factors in high-functioning females and males with autism. *Journal of Autism and Developmental Disorders, 21,* 197–209.

Lord, C., Rutter, M., & Le Couteur, A. (1994). Autism Diagnostic Interview–Revised: A revised version of a diagnostic interview for caregivers of individuals with possible pervasive developmental disorders. *Journal of Autism and Developmental Disorders, 24,* 659–685.

Lord, C., Risi, S., Lambrecht, L., Cook, E.H., Jr., Leventhal, B.J., DiLavore, P.C., et al. (2000). The Autism Diagnostic Observation Schedule–Genetic: A standard measurement of social and communication defects associated with the spectrum of autism. *Journal of Autism and Developmental Disorders, 30,* 205–223.

Lord, C., & Schopler, E. (1985). Difference in sex ratios in autism as a function of measured intelligence. *Journal of Autism and Developmental Disorders, 15,* 185–193.

Lotter, V. (1967). Epidemiology of autistic conditions in young children. II: Some characteristics of the parent and children. *Social Psychiatry, 1,* 163–173.

Luckasson, R., Coulter, D.L., Polloway, E.A., Reiss, S., Schalock, R.L., Snell, M.E., et al. (1992). *Mental retardation: Definition, classification, and systems of supports* (9th ed.). Washington, DC: American Association on Mental Retardation.

Luckasson, R., Coulter, D.L., Polloway, E.A., Reiss, S., Schalock, R.L., Snell, M.E., et al. (2002). *Mental retardation: Definition, classification, and systems of supports* (10th ed.). Washington, DC: American Association on Mental Retardation.

Ludvigsson, P., Olafsson, E., Sigurthardottir, S., & Hauser, W.A. (1994). Epidemiologic features of infantile spasms in Iceland. *Epilepsia, 35,* 802–805.

Lundberg, S., & Eeg-Olofsson, O. (2003). Rolandic epilepsy: A challenge in terminology and classification. *European Journal of Pediatric Neurology, 7,* 239–241.

MacMahon, B., & Pugh, T.F. (1970). *Epidemiology: Principles and methods.* Boston: Little, Brown.

Mágnússon, P., & Saemundsen, E. (2001). Prevalence of autism in Iceland. *Journal of Autism and Developmental Disorders, 31,* 153–163.

Marsh, D.O., Clarkson, T.W., Cox, C., Myers, G.J., Amin-Zaki, L., & Al-Tikriti, S. (1987). Fetal methylmercury poisoning: Relationship between concentration in single strands of maternal hair and child effects. *Archives of Neurology, 44,* 1017–1022.

Martin, J.A.M. (1982). Aetiological factors relating to childhood deafness in the European Community. *Audiology, 21,* 149–158.

McCarthy, P., Fitzgerald, M., & Smith, M. (1984). Prevalence of childhood autism in Ireland. *Irish Medical Journal, 77,* 129–130.

McDermott, S., Daguise, V., Mann, H., Szwejbka, L., & Callaghan, W. (2001). Perinatal risk for mortality and mental retardation associated with maternal urinary tract infections. *Journal of Family Practice, 50,* 433–437.

McLaren, J., & Bryson, S.E. (1987). Review of recent epidemiological studies of mental retardation: Prevalence, associated disorders, and etiology. *American Journal of Mental Retardation, 92,* 243–254.

Medical Research Council. (2001). *MRC review of autism research: Epidemiology and causes.* London: Author.

Medina, M.T., Duron, R.M., Martinez, L., Osorio, J.R., Estrada, A.L., Zuniga, C., et al. (2005). Prevalence, incidence, and etiology of epilepsies in rural Honduras: The Salama Study. *Epilepsia, 46,* 124–131.

Mendola, P., Selevan, S., Gutter, S., & Rice, D. (2002). Environmental factors associated with a spectrum of neurodevelopmental deficits. *Mental*

Retardation and Developmental Disabilities Research Reviews, 8, 188–197.

Mervis, C.A., Boyle, C.A., & Yeargin-Allsopp, M. (2002). Prevalence and selected characteristics of childhood vision impairment. *Developmental Medicine and Child Neurology, 44,* 538–541.

Mervis, C.A., Decouflé, P., Murphy, C.C., & Yeargin-Allsopp, M. (1995). Low birthweight and the risk for mental retardation later in childhood. *Paediatric and Perinatal Epidemiology, 9,* 455–468.

Monjauze, C., Tuller, L., Hommet, C., Barthez, M.A., & Khomsi, A. (2005). Language in benign childhood epilepsy with centro-temporal spikes. *Brain and Language, 92,* 300–308.

Moser, H.W. (1995). A role for gene therapy in mental retardation. *Mental Retardation and Developmental Disabilities Research Reviews, 1,* 4–6.

Munro, J.D. (1986). Epidemiology and the extent of mental retardation. *Psychiatric Perspectives on Mental Retardation, 9,* 591–624.

Murphy, C.C., Boyle, C., Schendel, D., Decouflé, P., & Yeargin-Allsopp, M. (1998). Epidemiology of mental retardation in children. *Mental Retardation and Developmental Disabilities Research Reviews, 4,* 6–13.

Murphy, C.C., Trevathan, E., & Yeargin-Allsopp, M. (1995). Prevalence of epilepsy and epileptic seizures in 10-year-old children: Results from the metropolitan Atlanta developmental disabilities study. *Epilepsy, 6,* 866–872.

Murphy, C.C., Yeargin-Allsopp, M., Decouflé, P., & Drews, C.D. (1993). Prevalence of cerebral palsy among ten-year-old children in metropolitan Atlanta, 1985 through 1987. *Journal of Pediatrics, 123,* S13–S19.

Murphy, C.C., Yeargin-Allsopp, M., Decouflé, P., & Drews, C. (1995). The administrative prevalence of mental retardation in 10-year-old children in metropolitan Atlanta, 1985 through 1987. *American Journal Public of Health, 85,* 319–323.

Murphy, D.J., Sellers, S., MacKenzie, I.A., Yudkin, P.L., & Johnson, A.M. (1995). Case-control study of antenatal and intrapartum risk factors for cerebral palsy in preterm singleton babies. *Lancet, 346,* 1449–1454.

Murphy, D.J., Squier, M.V., Hope, P.L., Sellers, S., & Johnson, A. (1996). Clinical associations and term of onset of cerebral white matter damage in very preterm babies. *Archives of Disease in Childhood: Fetal and Neonatal Edition, 75,* F27–F32.

Mutch, L.W., Alberman, E., Hagberg, B., Kodama, K., & Perat, M.V. (1992). Cerebral palsy epidemiology: Where are we now and where are we going? *Developmental Medicine and Child Neurology, 34,* 547–555.

Naessens, A., Casteels, A., Decatte, L., & Foulon, W. (2005). A serologic strategy for detecting neonates at risk for congenital cytomegalovirus infection. *Journal of Pediatrics, 146,* 194–203.

National Center for Health Statistics. (1999–2000). *National Health Interview Survey.* Retrieved from http://www.cdc.gov/nchs/data/factsheets/DevDisabilities.pdf

National Center for Infectious Diseases. (2002). *Cytomegalovirus (CMV) infection.* Retrieved June 18, 2005, from website http://www.cdc.gov/ncidod/diseases/cmv.htm

National Center on Birth Defects and Developmental Disabilities. (2004). *How common is fetal alcohol syndrome?* Retrieved January 18, 2005, from http://www.cdc.gov/ncbddd/fas/fasask.htm#how

National Information Center for Children and Youth with Disabilities. (2000). *NICHCY—Info about speech & language disorders: Fact sheet number 11 (FS11).* Retrieved February 28, 2005, from http://www.kidsource.com/NICHCY/speech.html

Needleman, H. (1992a). *Human lead exposure.* Boca Raton, FL: CRC Press.

Needleman, H. (Ed). (1992b). *Low level lead exposure: The clinical implications of current research.* New York: Raven Press.

Nelson, K.B. (2002). The epidemiology of cerebral palsy in term infants. *Mental Retardation and Developmental Disabilities Research Reviews, 8,* 146–150.

Nelson, K.B., Dambrosia, J.M., Grether, J.K., & Phillips, T.M. (1998). Neonatal cytokines and coagulation factors in children with cerebral palsy. *Annals of Neurology, 44,* 665–675.

Nelson, K.B., & Ellenberg, J.H. (1982). Children who "outgrew" cerebral palsy. *Pediatrics, 69,* 529–536.

Nelson, K.B., & Ellenberg, J.H. (1986). Antecedents of cerebral palsy: Multivariate analysis of risk. *New England Journal Medicine, 315,* 81–86.

Nelson, K.B., & Emery, E.S. (1993). Birth asphyxia and the neonatal brain: What do we know and when do we know it? *Clinics in Perinatology, 20,* 327–344.

Nelson, K.B., & Grether, J.K. (1998). Potentially asphyxiating conditions and spastic cerebral palsy in infants of normal birthweight. *American Journal of Obstetrics and Gynecology, 179,* 507–513.

Nelson, K.B., & Grether, J.K. (1999). Causes of cerebral palsy. *Current Opinion in Pediatrics, 11,* 487–491.

Newschaffer, C., Falb, D., & Gurney, J.G. (2005). National autism prevalence trends from United States special education data. *Pediatrics, 115,* 277–282.

Newschaffer, C.J., Fallin, D., & Lee, N.L. (2002). Heritable and nonheritable risk factors for autism spectrum disorders. *Epidemiologic Reviews, 24,* 137–153.

Nicoletti, A., Reggio, A., Bartoloni, A., Fallia, G., Sofia, V., Bartalesi, F., et al. (1999). Prevalence of epilepsy in rural Bolivia: A door-to-door survey. *Neurology, 53,* 2064–2069.

Nordin, V., & Gillberg, C. (1996). Autism spectrum disorders in children with physical or mental disability or both 1: Clinical and epidemiological aspects. *Developmental Medicine and Child Neurology, 38,* 297–313.

Nsengiyumva, G., Druet-Cabanac, M., Ramanan-kandrasana, B., Bouteille, B., Nasizabira, L., & Preux, P.M. (2003). Cysticercosis as a major risk factor for epilepsy in Burundi, east Africa. *Epilepsia, 44,* 950–955.

Oberle, I., Rousseau, F., Heitz, D., Kretz, C., Devys, D., Hanauer, A., et al. (1991). Instability of a 550-base pair DNA segment and abnormal methylation in fragile X syndrome. *Science, 252,* 1087–1102.

Oka, E. (2002). Childhood epilepsy in Okayama Prefecture, Japan—a neuroepidemiological study. *No to Hattatsu, 35,* 95–102.

Olafsson, E., & Hauser, W.A. (1999). Prevalence of epilepsy in rural Iceland: A population based study. *Epilepsia, 40,* 1529–1534.

Olafsson, E., Hauser, W.A., Ludvigsson, P., & Gudmundsson, G. (1996). Incidence of epilepsy in rural Iceland: A population-based study. *Epilepsia, 37,* 951–955.

O'Shea, T.M. (2002). Cerebral palsy in very preterm infants: New epidemiologic insights. *Mental Retardation and Developmental Disabilities Research Reviews, 8,* 135–145.

O'Shea, T.M., Preisser, J.S., Klinepeter, K.L., & Dillard, R.G. (1998). Trends in mortality and cerebral palsy in a geographically based cohort of very low birth weight neonates born between 1982 to 1994. *Pediatrics, 101*(4 Pt. 1), 642–647.

Page, T. (2000). Metabolic approaches to the treatment of autism spectrum disorders. *Journal of Autism and Developmental Disorders, 30,* 463–469.

Palmer, L., Petterson, B., Blair, E., & Burton, P. (1994). Family patterns of gestational age at delivery and growth in utero in moderate and severe cerebral palsy. *Developmental Medicine and Child Neurology, 36,* 1108–1119.

Paneth, N., & Stark, R.I. (1983). Cerebral palsy and mental retardation in relation to the indicators of perinatal asphyxia. *American Journal of Obstetrics and Gynecology, 147,* 960–966.

Papavasiliou, A., Mattheou, D., Bazigou, H., Kotsalis, C., & Paraskevoulakos, E. (2005). Written language skills in children with benign childhood epilepsy with centrotemporal spikes. *Epilepsy and Behavior, 6,* 50–58.

Partington, M., Mowat, D., Einfeld, S., Tonge, B., & Turner G. (2000). Genes on the X chromosome are important in undiagnosed mental retardation. *American Journal of Medical Genetics, 92,* 57–61.

Parving, A. (1993). Congenital hearing disability—epidemiology and identification: A comparison between two health authority districts. *International Journal of Pediatric Otorhinolaryngology, 27,* 29–46.

Pearson, D., Mcgrath, N., Nozyce, M., Nichols, S., Raskino, C., Brouwers, P., et al. (2000). Predicting HIV disease progression in children using measures of neuropsychological and neurological functioning. *Pediatrics, 106*(6), e76.

Peters, J.M., Camfield, C.S., & Camfield, P.R. (2001). Population study of benign rolandic epilepsy: Is treatment needed? *Neurology, 57,* 537–539.

Petterson, B., Nelson, K.B., Watson, L., & Stanley, F. (1993). Twins, triplets, and cerebral palsy in births in Western Australia in the 1980s. *BMJ, 307,* 1239–1243.

Pharoah, P.O. (2001). Cerebral palsy in the surviving twin associated with infant death of the co-twin. *Archives of Disease in Childhood. Fetal and Neonatal Edition, 84*(2), F111-F116.

Pharoah, P.O.D., Cooke, T., Johnson, M.A., King, R., & Mutch, L. (1998). Epidemiology of cerebral palsy in England and Scotland 1984–9. *Archives of Disease in Childhood: Fetal and Neonatal Edition, 79,* F21–F25.

Pickles, A., Bolton, P., Macdonald, H., Bailey, A., LeCouteur, A., Sim, C.H., et al. (1995). Latent class analysis of recurrence risk for phenotypes with selection and measurement error: A twin and family history study of autism. *American Journal of Human Genetics, 57,* 717–726.

Pinto-Martin, J.A., Riolo, S., Cnaan, A., Holzman, C., Susser, M.W., & Paneth, N. (1995). Cranial ultrasound prediction of disabling and nondisabling cerebral palsy at age two in a low birth weight population. *Pediatrics, 95,* 249–254.

Piven, J., & Folstein, S. (1997). *The genetics of autism: The neurobiology of autism.* Baltimore: The Johns Hopkins University Press.

Piven, J., Simon, J., Chase, G.A., Wzorek, M., Landa, R., Gayle, J., et al. (1993). The etiology of autism: Pre-, peri-, and neonatal factors. *Journal of the American Academy of Child and Adolescent Psychiatry, 32,* 1256–1263.

Powell, J.E., Edwards, A., Edwards, M., Pandit, B.S., Sungum-Paliwal, S.R., & Whitehouse, W. (2000). Changes in the incidence of childhood autism and other autistic spectrum disorders in preschool children from two areas of the West Midlands, U.K. *Developmental Medicine and Child Neurology, 42,* 624–628.

Preux, P.M., & Druet-Cabanac, M. (2005). Epidemiology and aetiology of epilepsy in sub-Saharan Africa. *Lancet Neurology, 4,* 21–31.

Qian, M., Wang, D., & Chen, Z. (2000). A preliminary meta-analysis of 36 studies on impairment of intelligence development induced by iodine deficiency. *Journal of Preventive Medicine, 24,* 75–77.

Rasmussen, P., Borjesson, O., Wentz, E., & Gillberg, C. (2001). Autistic disorders in Down syndrome: Background factors and clinical correlates. *Developmental Medicine and Child Neurology, 43,* 750–753.

Riikonen, R. (1982). A long-term follow-up study of 214 children with the syndrome of infantile spasms. *Neuropediatrics, 13,* 14–23.

Riikonen, R., & Donner, M. (1979). Incidence and aetiology of infantile spasms from 1960 to 1976: A population study in Finland. *Developmental Medicine and Child Neurology, 21,* 333–343.

Riise, R., Flage, T., Hansen, E., Rosenberg, T., Rudanko, S.L., Viggosson, G., et al. (1992). Visual impairment in Nordic children. *Acta Ophthalmologica, 70,* 145–154.

Risch, N., Spiker, D., Lotspeich, L., Nouri, N., Hinds, D., Hallmayer, J., et al. (1999). A genomic screen of autism: Evidence for a multilocus etiology. *American Journal of Human Genetics, 65*, 493–507.

Ritvo, E.R., Freeman, B.J., Mason-Brothers, A., Mo, A., & Ritvo, A.M. (1985). Concordance for the syndrome of autism in 40 pairs of afflicted twins. *American Journal of Psychiatry, 142*, 74–77.

Robertson, C., & Finer, N. (1985). Term infants with hypoxic-ischemic encephalopathy: Outcome at 3.5 years. *Developmental Medicine and Child Neurology, 27*, 473–484.

Rodier, P.M., Ingram, J.L., Tisdale, B., Nelson, S., & Romano, J. (1996). Embryological origin for autism: Developmental anomalies of the cranial nerve motor nuclei. *Journal of Comparative Neurology, 370*, 247–261.

Roeleveld, N., Zielhuis, G.A., & Gabreels, F. (1997). The prevalence of mental retardation: A critical review of recent literature. *Developmental Medicine and Child Neurology, 39*, 125–132.

Rogers, S.J., & DiLalla, D.L. (1990). Age of symptom onset in young children with pervasive developmental disorders. *Journal of the American Academy of Child and Adolescent Psychiatry, 29*, 863–872.

Rothman, K.J. (2002). *Epidemiology: An introduction.* Philadelphia: Lippincott–Raven.

Rowland, A.S., Lesesne, C.A., & Abramowitz, A.J. (2002). The epidemiology of attention-deficit/hyperactivity disorder (ADHD): A public health view. *Mental Retardation and Developmental Disabilities Research Reviews, 8*, 162–170.

Rowland, A.S., Umbach, D.M., Catoe, K.E., Stallone, L., Long, S., Rabiner, D., et al. (2001). Studying the epidemiology of attention deficit hyperactivity disorder: Screening method and pilot results. *Canadian Journal of Psychiatry, 46*, 931–940.

Rowland, A.S., Umbach, D.M., Stallone, L., Naftel, A.J., Bohlig, E.M., & Sandler, D.P. (2002). Prevalence of medication treatment for attention deficit hyperactivity disorder among elementary school children, Johnston County, NC. *American Journal of Public Health, 92*, 231–234.

Rozien, N.J., & Johnson, D. (1996). Congenital infections. In A.J. Capute & P.J. Accardo (Eds.), *Developmental disabilities in infancy and childhood: Vol. I. Neurodevelopmental diagnosis and treatment* (2nd ed., pp. 175–193). Baltimore: Paul H. Brookes Publishing Co.

Rydhstroem, H. (1995). The relationship of birth weight and birth weight discordance to cerebral palsy or mental retardation later in life for twins weighing less than 2500 grams. *American Journal of Obstetrics and Gynecology, 173*, 680–686.

Schendel, D.E. (2001). Infection in pregnancy and cerebral palsy. *Journal of the American Medical Women's Association, 56*, 105–108.

Scher, A.L., Petterson, B., Blair, E., Ellenberg, J.H., Grether, J.K., Haan, E., et al. (2002). The risk of mortality or cerebral palsy in twins: A collaborative population-based study. *Pediatric Research, 52*, 671–681.

Schopler, E., Andrews, C., & Strupp, K. (1979). Do autistic children come from upper-middle-class parents? *Journal of Autism and Developmental Disorders, 9*, 139–152.

Scolnik, D., Nulman, I., Rovet, J., Gladstone, D., Czuchat, D., Gardner, H.A., et al. (1994). Neurodevelopment of children exposed in utero to phenytoin and carbamazepine monotherapy. *Journal of the American Medical Association, 271*, 767–770.

Sebat, J., et al. (2007). *Strong Association of de novo copy number mutations with autism.* Retrieved March 15, 2007, from Sciencexpress web site, http://www.sciencexpress.org.

Sehlin, P., Holmgren, G., & Zakrisson J. (1990). Incidence, prevalence, and etiology of hearing impairment in children in the county of Vasterbotten, Sweden. *Scandinavian Audiology, 19*, 193–200.

Serdaroglu, G., Tekgul, H., Kitis, O., Serdaroglu, E., & Gokben, S. (2004). Correlative value of magnetic resonance imaging for neurodevelopmental outcome in periventricular leukomalacia. *Developmental Medicine and Child Neurology, 46*, 733–739.

Sever, J.L., Ellenberg, J.H., Ley, A.C., Madden, D.L., Fuccillo, D.A., Tzan, N.R., et al. (1988). Toxoplasmosis: Maternal and pediatric findings in 23,000 pregnancies. *Pediatrics, 82*, 181–192.

Shaffer, D., Fisher, P., & Dulcan, M.K. (1996). The NIMH Diagnostic Interview Schedule for Children Version 2.3 (DISC-2.3): Description, acceptability, prevalence rates, and performance in the MECA Study. Methods for the Epidemiology of Child and Adolescent Mental Disorders Study. *Journal of the American Academy of Child and Adolescent Psychiatry, 35*, 865–877.

Shamas, G.H., Wiig, E.H., & Secord, W.A. (1998). *Human communication disorders: An introduction* (5th ed). Boston: Allyn & Bacon.

Shevell, M., Ashwal, S., Donley, D., Flint, J., Gingold, M., Hirtz, D., et al. (2003). Practice parameter: Evaluation of the child with global developmental delay. *Neurology, 60*, 367–380.

Shinnar, S., Berg, A., Moshe, S., O'Dell, C., Alemany, M., Newstein, D., et al. (1996). The risk of seizure recurrence after a first unprovoked afebrile seizure in childhood: An extended follow-up. *Pediatrics, 98*, 216–225.

Sidenvall, R., & Eeg-Olofsson, O. (1995). Epidemiology of infantile spasms in Sweden. *Epilepsia, 36*, 572–574.

Sidenvall, R., Forsgren, L., Blomquist, J.K., & Heijbel, J. (1993). A community-based prospective incidence study of epileptic seizures in children. *Acta Paediatrica, 82*, 60–65.

Sidenvall, R., Forsgren, L., & Heijbel, J. (1996). Prevalence and characteristics of epilepsy in children in northern Sweden. *Seizure, 5*, 139–146.

Sillanpaa, M. (2000). Long-term outcome of epilepsy. *Epileptic Disorder, 2*, 79–88.

Smalley, S.L., Asarnow, R.F., & Spence, M.A. (1988). Autism and genetics: A decade of research. *Archives of General Psychiatry, 45*, 953–961.

Smalley, S.L., Tanguay, P.E., Smith, M., & Gutierrez, G. (1992). Autism and tuberous sclerosis. *Journal of Autism and Developmental Disorders, 22*, 339–355.

Sorri, M., & Rantakallio, P. (1985). Prevalence of hearing loss at the age of 15 in a birth cohort of 12,000 children from Northern Finland. *Scandinavian Audiology, 14,* 203–207.

Sponheim, E., & Skjeldal, O. (1998). Autism and related disorders: Epidemiological findings in a Norwegian study using IDC-10 diagnostic criteria. *Journal of Autism and Developmental Disorders, 28,* 217–228.

Stanley, F., Blair, E., & Alberman, E. (2000). *Cerebral palsies: Epidemiology and causal pathways.* London: Mac Keith Press.

Steffenburg, S., Gillberg, C., Hellgren, L., Andersson, L., Gillberg, I.C., Jakobsson, G., et al. (1989). A twin study of autism in Denmark, Finland, Iceland, Norway, and Sweden. *Journal of Child Psychology and Psychiatry and Allied Disciplines, 30,* 305–316.

Steffenburg, S., Gillberg, C.L., & Steffenburg, U. (1996). Autism in Angelman syndrome: A population based study. *Pediatric Neurology, 28,* 131–136.

Stehr-Green, P., Tull, P., Stellfeld, M., Mortenson, P.B., & Simpson, D. (2003). Autism and thimerosal-containing vaccines: Lack of consistent evidence for an association. *American Journal of Preventive Medicine, 25,* 101–106.

Steinhausen, H.C., Gobel, D., Breinlinger, M., & Wohllenben, B. (1986). A community survey of infantile autism. *Journal of the American Academy of Child and Adolescent Psychiatry, 25,* 189.

Steinkuller, P.G., Du, L., Gilbert, C., Foster, A., Collins, M.L., & Coats, D.K. (1993). Childhood blindness. *Journal of Pediatric Ophthalmology and Strabismus, 3,* 26–32.

Stewart-Brown, S.L., & Haslum, M.N. (1988). Partial sight and blindness in children of the 1970 birth cohort at 10 years of age. *Journal of Epidemiology and Community Health, 42,* 17–23.

Stratton, K., Gable, A., Shetty, P., & McCormick, M. (Eds.). (2001). *Immunization safety review: Measles-mumps-rubella vaccine and autism.* Washington, DC: National Academies Press.

Streissguth, A.P., Aase, J.M., Clarren, S.K., Randels, S.P., LaDue, R.A., & Smith, D.F. (1991). Fetal alcohol syndrome in adolescents and adults. *JAMA, 265,* 1961–1967.

Streissguth, A.P., Barr, H.M., & Sampson, P.D. (1990). Moderate prenatal alcohol exposure: Effects on child IQ and learning problems at age 7 1/2 years. *Alcoholism: Clinical and Experimental Research, 14,* 662–669.

Strömberg, B., Dahlquist, G., Ericson, A., Finnström, O., Köster, M., & Stjernqvist, K. (2002). Neurological sequelae in children born after in vitro fertilization: A population based study. *Lancet, 359,* 461–465.

Stromland, K., Nordin, V., Miller, M., Akerstrom, B., & Gillberg, C. (1994). Autism in thalidomide embryopathy: A population study. *Developmental Medicine and Child Neurology, 36,* 351–356.

Stromme, P., & Hagberg, G. (2000). Aetiology in severe and mild mental retardation: A population-based study of Norwegian children. *Developmental Medicine and Child Neurology, 42,* 76–86.

Stroup, D.F., Brookmeyer, R., & Kalsbeek, D. (2004). Public health surveillance in action: A framework. In R. Brookmeyer & D.F. Stroup (Eds.), *Monitoring the health of populations: Statistical principles and methods for public health surveillance.* Oxford, UK: Oxford University Press.

Surman, G., Newdick, H., & Johnson, A. (2003). Cerebral palsy rates among low-birthweight infants in the 1990s. *Developmental Medicine and Child Neurology, 45,* 456–462.

Szatmari, P., Archer, L., Fisman, S., Streiner, D.L., & Wilson, F. (1995). Asperger's syndrome and autism: Differences in behavior, cognition, and adaptive functioning. *Journal of the American Academy of Child and Adolescent Psychiatry, 34,* 1662–1671.

Szatmari, P., Bartolucci, G., & Bremner, R. (1989). Asperger's syndrome and autism: Comparison of early history and outcome. *Developmental Medicine and Child Neurology, 31,* 709–720.

Szatmari, P., Tuff, L., Finlayson, M.A., & Bartolucci, G. (1990). Asperger's syndrome and autism: Neurocognitive aspects. *Journal of the American Academy of Child and Adolescent Psychiatry, 29,* 130–136.

Tariverdian, G., & Vogel, F. (2000). Some problems in the genetics of X-linked mental retardation. *Cytogenetics and Cell Genetics, 91,* 278–284.

Tebruegge, M., Nandini, V., & Ritchie, J. (2004). Does routine child health surveillance contribute to the early detection of children with pervasive developmental disorders? An epidemiologic study in Kent, U.K. *BMC Pediatrics, 4*(4), 1–7.

Tekle-Haimanot, R., Forsgren, L., & Ekstedt, J. (1997). Incidence of epilepsy in rural central Ethiopia. *Epilepsia, 38,* 541–546.

Thylefors, B., Negrel, A.D., Pararajasegaram, R., & Dadzie, K.Y. (1995). Global data on blindness. *Bulletin of the World Health Organization, 73,* 115–121.

Tidmarsh, L., & Volkmar, F.R. (2003). Diagnosis and epidemiology of autism spectrum disorders. *Canadian Journal of Psychiatry, 48,* 517–525.

Tomblin, J.B., Smith, E., & Zhang, X. (1997). Epidemiology of specific language impairment: Prenatal and perinatal risk factors. *Journal of Communication Disorders, 30,* 325–344.

Topp, M., Uldall, P., & Langhoff-Roos, J. (1997). Trend in cerebral palsy birth prevalence in eastern Denmark: Birthyear period 1979–86. *Paediatric and Perinatal Epidemiology, 11,* 451–460.

Trevathan, E. (2002). Infantile spasms and Lennox-Gastaut syndrome. *Journal of Child Neurology, 17*(Suppl. 2), 2S9–2S22.

Trevathan, E., Murphy, C.C., & Yeargin-Allsopp, M. (1997). Prevalence and descriptive epidemiology of Lennox-Gastaut syndrome among Atlanta children. *Epilepsia, 38,* 1283–1288.

Trevathan, E., Murphy, C.C., & Yeargin-Allsopp, M. (1999). The descriptive epidemiology of infantile spasms among Atlanta children. *Epilepsia, 40,* 748–751.

Turner, G., Webb, T., Wake, S., & Robinson, H. (1996). Prevalence of fragile X syndrome. *American Journal of Medical Genetics, 64,* 196–197.

U.S. Department of Education. (2001). *Office of Special Education Programs, Data Analysis System: December 2001 count updated as of August 30, 2002.* Retrieved January 18, 2005, from http://www.ideadata.org/tables25th/ar.aa11htm

U.S. Department of Education. (2002). *24th Annual report to Congress on the implementation of the Individuals with Disabilities Education Act, Section 618.* Jessup, MD: Education Publication Center.

U.S. Department of Education. (2003). *25th Annual report to Congress on the implementation of the Individuals with Disabilities Education Act, Section 618.* Jessup, MD: Education Publication Center.

U.S. Department of Education. (2004). *Individual with Disabilities Education Act (IDEA) data: Number of children served under IDEA by disability and age group, 1994–2003.* Retrieved January 21, 2005, from http://www.ideadata.org/tables27th/ar_aa9.xls

U.S. Department of Health and Human Services. (1988). *International classification of diseases, ninth revision, clinical modification.* Washington, DC: Author

Vadlamudi, L., Harvey, A.S., Connellan, M.M., Milne, R.L., Hopper, J.L., Scheffer, I.E., et al. (2004). Is benign rolandic epilepsy genetically determined? *Annals of Neurology, 56,* 129–132.

Van Naarden, K., & Decouflé, P. (1999). Relative and attributable risks for moderate to profound bilateral sensorineural hearing impairment associated with lower birth weight in children 3 to 10 years old. *Pediatrics, 104,* 905–910.

Van Naarden Braun, K., Yeargin-Allsopp, M., Schendel, D., & Fernhoff, P. (2003). Long-term developmental outcomes of children identified through a newborn screening program with a metabolic or endocrine disorder: A population-based approach. *Journal of Pediatrics, 143,* 236–242.

Vartiainen, E., Kemppinen, P., & Karjalainen, S. (1997). Prevalence and etiology of bilateral sensorineural hearing impairment in a Finnish childhood population. *International Journal of Pediatric Otorhinolaryngology, 41,* 175–185.

Volkmar, F.R., Klin, A., Schultz, R., Bronen, R., Marans, W.D., Sparrow, S., et al. (1996). Asperger's syndrome. *Journal of the American Academy of Child and Adolescent Psychiatry, 35,* 118–123.

Volkmar, F.R., Lord, C., Bailey, A., Schultz, R.T., & Klin, A. (2004). Autism and pervasive developmental disorders. *Journal of Child Psychology and Psychiatry and Allied Disciplines, 45,* 135–170.

Waaler, P.E., Blom, B.H., Skeidsvoll, H., & Mykletun, A. (2000). Prevalence, classification, and severity of epilepsy in children in western Norway. *Epilepsia, 41,* 802–810.

Wachtel, R.C., & Conlon, C.J. (1996). Pediatric neuro-AIDS. In A.J. Capute & P.J. Accardo (Eds.), *Developmental disabilities in infancy and childhood: Vol. I. Neurodevelopmental diagnosis and treatment* (2nd ed., pp. 195–213). Baltimore: Paul H. Brookes Publishing Co.

Waisbren, S.E., Rokni, H., Bailey, I., Rohr, F., Brown, T., & Warner-Rogers, J. (1997). Social factors and the meaning of food in adherence to medical diets: Results of a maternal phenylketonuria summer camp. *Journal of Inherited Metabolic Disease, 20,* 21–27.

Wakefield, A.J., Murch, S.H., Anthona, A., Linnell, J., Casson, D.D., Malik, M., et al. (1998). Ileal-lymphoid-nodular hyperplasia, non-specific colitis, and pervasive developmental disorder in children. *Lancet, 351,* 637–641.

Wallace, H., Shorvon, S., & Tallis, R. (1998). Age-specific incidence and prevalence rates of treated epilepsy in an unselected population of 2,052,922 and age-specific fertility rates of women with epilepsy. *Lancet, 352,* 1970–1973.

Webb, E.V., Lobo, S., Hervas, A., Scourfield, J. & Fraser, W.I. (1997). The changing prevalence of autistic disorder in a Welsh health district. *Developmental Medicine and Child Neurology, 39,* 150–152.

Wiggins, L.D., Baio, J., & Rice, C. (2006). Examination of the time between first evaluation and first autism spectrum diagnosis in a population-based sample. *Journal of Developmental Behavior Pediatrics, 27*(2 Suppl.), S79–S87.

Williams, K., Glasson, E., Wray, J., Tuck, M., Helmer, M., Bower, C.I., et al. (2005). Incidence of autism spectrum spectrum disorders in children in two Australian states. *Medical Journal of Australia, 182,* 108–111.

Williams, P.G., & Hersh, J.H. (1998). Brief report: The association of neurofibromatosis type 1 and autism. *Journal of Autism and Developmental Disorders, 28,* 567–571.

Wilson, M.R., Mansour, M., Ross-Degnan, D., Moukouri, E., Fobi, G., Alemayehu, W., et al. (1996). Prevalence and causes of low vision and blindness in the Extreme North Province of Cameroon, West Africa. *Opthalmic Epidemiology, 3,* 23–33.

Wing, L. (1980). Childhood autism and social class: A question of selection? *British Journal of Psychiatry, 137,* 410–417.

Wing, L., & Gould, J. (1979). Severe impairments of social interaction and associated abnormalities in children: Epidemiology and classification. *Journal of Autism and Developmental Disorders, 9,* 11–29.

Wing, L., & Potter, D. (2002). The epidemiology of autistic spectrum disorders: Is the prevalence rising? *Mental Retardation and Developmental Disabilities Research Reviews, 8,* 151–161.

Winter, S., Autry, A., Boyle, C., & Yeargin-Allsopp, M. (2002). Trends in the prevalence of congenital cerebral palsy in Atlanta, Georgia. *Pediatrics, 10,* 1220–1225.

Wirrell, E.C., Camfield, P.R., Camfield, C.S., Dooley, J.M., & Gordon, K.E. (1996). Accidental injury is a serious risk in children with typical absence epilepsy. *Archives of Neurology, 53,* 929–932.

Wirrell, E.C., Camfield, P.R., Camfield, C.S., Gordon, K.E., & Dooley, J.M. (1996). Long-term prognosis of typical childhood absence epilepsy: Remission or progression to juvenile myoclonic epilepsy. *Neurology, 47,* 912–918.

Wirrell, E.C., Camfield, P.R., Camfield, C.S., Dooley, J.M., Gordon, K.E., & Smith, B. (1997). Long-term psychosocial outcome in typical absence epilepsy: Sometimes a wolf in sheeps' clothing. *Archives of Pediatrics and Adolescent Medicine, 151,* 152–158.

Wolraich, M.L., Hannah, J.N., Baumgaertel, A., & Feurer, I.D. (1998). Examination of DSM-IV criteria for attention deficit/hyperactivity disorder in a county-wide sample. *Journal of Developmental and Behavioral Pediatrics, 19,* 162–168.

Wolraich, M.L., Hannah, J.N., Pinnock, T.Y., Baumgaertel, A., & Brown, J. (1996). Comparison of diagnostic criteria for attention deficit hyperactivity disorder in a county-wide sample. *Journal of the American Academy of Child and Adolescent Psychiatry, 35,* 319–323.

Wong, M., & Trevathan, E. (2001). Infantile spasms. *Pediatric Neurology, 24,* 89–98.

Woodruff, T.J., Axelrod, D.A., Kyle, A.M., Nweke, O., Miller, G.G., & Hurley, B.J. (2004). Trends in environmentally related childhood illnesses. *Pediatrics, 113,* 1133–1140.

World Health Organization. (1980). *International classification of impairments, disabilities, and handicaps.* Geneva: World Health Organization.

World Health Organization. (1992). *International classification of diseases, tenth revision.* Geneva: World Health Organization.

World Health Organization. (2001). *International classification of functioning, disability and health.* Geneva: Author.

Yeargin-Allsopp, M., Drews, C.D., Decouflé, P., & Murphy, C.C. (1995). Mild mental retardation in black and white children in metropolitan Atlanta: A case-control study. *American Journal of Public Health, 85,* 324–328.

Yeargin-Allsopp, M., Murphy, C.C., Cordero, J.F., Decouflé, P., & Hollowell, J. (1997). Reported biomedical causes and associated medical conditions for mental retardation among 10-year-old children, metropolitan Atlanta, 1985 to 1987. *Developmental Medicine and Child Neurology, 39,* 142–149.

Yeargin-Allsopp, M., Murphy, C.C., Oakley, G.P., & Sikes, K. (1992). A multiple-source method for studying the prevalence of developmental disabilities in children: The Metropolitan Atlanta Developmental Disabilities Study. *Pediatrics, 89,* 624–630.

Yeargin-Allsopp, M., Rice, C., Karpurkar, T., Doernberg, N., Boyle, C., & Murphy, C. (2003). Prevalence of autism in a U.S. metropolitan area. *JAMA, 289,* 49–55.

Yu, M-L., Hsu, C-C., Gladen, B., & Rogan, W.J. (1991). In-utero PCB/PCDF exposure: Relation of developmental delay and dysmorphology and dose. *Neurotoxicology and Teratology, 13,* 195–202.

Zarrelli, M.M., Beghi, E., Rocca, W.A., & Hauser, W.A. (1999). Incidence of epileptic syndromes in Rochester, Minnesota: 1980–1984. *Epilepsia, 40,* 1708–1714.

Zigler, E., Balla, D., & Hodapp, R. (1984). On the definition and classification of mental retardation. *American Journal of Mental Deficiency, 89,* 215–230.

Genetics

USHA T. SUNDARAM AND JOANN N. BODURTHA

The developmental pediatrician who evaluates children with the broad spectrum of developmental disorders needs to incorporate a genetic perspective in the assessment. Assessing the child within the family history context and in light of the increasing array of available genetic tests can lead to diagnostic clarity, tailored health monitoring, supports and services, and the most accurate genetic counseling. No chapter or book can provide an algorithm for testing for all of the expanding number of identified syndromes and gene changes. Resources on the Internet that build on the advances of the Human Genome Project (e.g., Online Mendelian Inheritance in Man [OMIM], GeneTests, POSSUM, Genetics Home Reference, London Dysmorphology Database, Genetic Alliance) are important tools for specialist physicians to use in exploring and understanding the links between genetic variation and developmental disorders. This chapter provides a brief review of genetic mechanisms of developmental disorders, basic genetic differentials for each of the major types of developmental disorders, and criteria and suggestions for testing and referral. This information will continue to evolve in clarity and complexity.

MODES OF INHERITANCE

The different inheritance patterns of genetic conditions are autosomal recessive or dominant, X-linked recessive or dominant, and mitochondrial (Table 4.1). In *autosomal recessive* inheritance, the genetic condition is the result of mutation in genes located on autosomes, and the altered allele is manifested only in the homozygous state. An individual with one mu-

tated allele for a recessive condition is called a *carrier* and is usually asymptomatic. In disorders inherited in an autosomal recessive manner, males and females are affected, usually multiple siblings in one generation are affected, the parents are obligate heterozygotes for the disorder, and the parents can be consanguineous. Good examples of autosomal recessive genetic conditions are metabolic disorders such as phenylketonuria.

When both parents are carriers for a recessive condition, there is a 25% chance of having a homozygous affected child, a 25% chance of having a nonaffected and noncarrier child, and a 50% chance of having a nonaffected but carrier child. An individual with an autosomal recessive condition produces only gametes with the disease allele. If such a person marries a noncarrier individual, who will always contribute a normal allele, all of their children will be unaffected carriers. If an individual with an autosomal recessive condition marries a carrier, then the partner can pass on the normal or altered allele (50/50). Thus, there is a 50% chance they will have an affected child and a 50% chance they will have a carrier child.

In *autosomal dominant* inheritance, the genetic condition is the result of mutation in genes located on autosomes, and the altered allele is dominant to the wild-type allele and is manifested in the heterozygous state. Some autosomal dominant conditions are the result of new mutations, and, hence, family history may be negative. For example, two thirds of cases of tuberous sclerosis, 25% of Marfan syndrome cases, and 50% of neurofibromatosis type 1 (NF1) cases are the result of new mutations. Another factor to remember is the vari-

Table 4.1. Inheritance patterns of genetic conditions

Condition	Features	Examples
Autosomal recessive	Affected males and females Multiple affected members in one generation History of consanguinity	Phenylketonuria, methylmalonic acidemia, propionic acidemia, homocystinuria, cystic fibrosis, mucopolysaccharidosis, mucolipidosis, Tay-Sachs disease, Niemann-Pick disease, metachromatic leukodystrophy, Pendred syndrome
Autosomal dominant	Affected males and females At least one male-to-male transmission Successive or multiple generations affected Some are the result of new mutations, with only one affected individual in the family	Tuberous sclerosis, neurofibromatosis, Noonan syndrome, Sotos syndrome, Huntington disease, 22q11 deletion, achondroplasia
X-linked recessive	No male-to-male transmission Affected males are related through carrier females Males are affected almost exclusively Affected males are at risk of transmitting the disease to their grandsons through their daughters Mild expression in females	Fragile X syndrome
X-linked dominant	No male-to-male transmission Twice as many females with the disorder as males Males with the disorder transmit to all daughters and to no sons Females have variable expression due to X inactivation	Incontinentia pigmenti, hypophosphatemic rickets, Rett syndrome
Mitochondrial	Affected males and females Affected males do not have affected offspring	Nonsyndromic sensorineural deafness, MELAS, MERRF, Leber's hereditary optic neuropathy

Key: MELAS, mitochondrial encephaly with lactic acidosis and stroke-like episodes; MERRF, myoclonic epilepsy with ragged red fibers.

ability in severity of many autosomal dominant genetic conditions. Careful examination is needed to diagnose a mildly affected parent when it appears that the family history is negative for the condition. In each pregnancy, an individual with an autosomal dominant genetic condition has a 50% chance of passing on the mutated allele, resulting in an affected child.

X-linked inheritance is the result of mutation in genes located on the X chromosome. Males, having one X chromosome, are hemizygous for most genes on the X chromosome, and, if they have a mutant allele, they will manifest the condition. Females, having two X chromosomes, will usually manifest an X-linked recessive condition only if homozygous for the mutant allele. Because it is rare for females to be homozygous for an X-linked

recessive disorder, *X-linked recessive disorders* are usually manifested only in males.

A male with an X-linked recessive condition will pass on his Y chromosome to his sons and will never have an affected son; he will pass on his X chromosome with the mutant allele to all his daughters, so all of his daughters will be carriers. A female carrier of an X-linked recessive condition has a 50% chance of passing on the X chromosome with the mutant allele or the normal X chromosome; thus her sons have a 50% chance of being affected, and her daughters have a 50% chance of being carriers.

X-linked dominant disorders are the result of mutation of genes on X chromosomes that are lethal in males. Examples include incontinentia pigmenti and Rett syndrome. Most of these disorders are thought to arise as new mutations, though there can be gonadal mosaicism in females for these X-linked dominant disorders.

Mitochondrial DNA is inherited only from the mother, and mutations in mitochondrial DNA are passed down the maternal line. Mitochondrial DNA codes for proteins/enzymes involved in oxidative phosphorylation. Diseases resulting from mutation in the mitochondrial DNA can affect both males and females; affected males do not have affected offspring. Examples of conditions resulting from mutations in mitochondrial DNA include nonsyndromic sensorineural deafness, MELAS (mitochondrial encephalopathy with lactic acidosis and stroke-like episodes), MERRF (myoclonic epilepsy with ragged red fibers), and Leber's hereditary optic neuropathy.

Genetic and medical conditions may underlie the symptom complex for which a patient is referred to a developmental pediatrician. Some of the reasons for referral to a developmental pediatrician include autism, pervasive developmental disorder (PDD), intellectual disability/developmental delay (ID/DD), speech delay, and learning disability. Some of the genetic conditions in which these symptoms are prominent include tuberous sclerosis complex (TSC), Rett syndrome, fragile X syndrome, chromosomopathies, Prader-Willi syndrome (PWS), Angelman syndrome (AS), and NF1.

INTELLECTUAL DISABILITIES AND GENETIC CONDITIONS

Intellectual disabilities (ID) are seen in 1%–10% of the population (McLaren & Bryson, 1987; Stevenson, 1996; Xu & Chen, 2003). Both genetics and environmental factors play a role in the etiology of ID. A search of OMIM reveals 1,180 conditions with associated ID, showing the diversity of the genetic factors that influence brain development. The diagnostic yield is greater in individuals with more severe ID (Barton & Volkmar, 1998). A consensus conference of the American College of Medical Genetics produced guidelines regarding the evaluation of individuals with ID/DD (Curry et al., 1997). Battaglia and Carey (2003) also provided an excellent overview of the evaluation of individuals with ID/DD. Table 4.2 gives the frequency of various causes of ID. The ad-

Table 4.2. Causes of intellectual disabilities in literature surveys

	%
Chromosomal abnormalities	4–28
Recognizable syndromes	3–7
Known monogenic conditions	3–9
Structural central nervous system abnormalities	7–17
Complications of prematurity	2–10
Environmental/teratogenic causes	5–13
"Cultural-familial" mental retardation	3–12
Provisionally unique, monogenic syndromes	1–5
Metabolic/endocrine causes	1–5
Unknown	3–50

From American Journal of Medical Genetics, Vol. 72, No. 4, 1997, pp. 468–477; Copyright © 1997 Wiley-Liss. Reprinted with permission of Wiley-Liss, a subsidiary of John Wiley & Sons, Inc.

vantages to finding a cause include a sense of closure for the parents, direction to planning care, specific treatments where indicated, and discussion of prognosis and recurrence risk.

Chromosomal abnormalities are seen in 4%–34.1% of individuals with ID/DD (Battaglia, Bianchini, & Carey, 1999). Down syndrome is a common genetic cause of mild to moderate ID. Down syndrome does not usually present a diagnostic challenge and usually should not be referred to a developmental pediatrician as ID of unknown etiology. Besides Down syndrome, other chromosomal anomalies underlying some cases of ID/DD include interstitial duplication in the Prader-Willi/Angelman syndrome, inverted duplication of 15q, UPD14mat, 16p deletion, 22q11 duplication, 22q13.3 deletion, marker chromosomes, and unbalanced translocations. These patients may or may not have dysmorphic features, hypotonia, seizures, speech delay, and autism spectrum disorder. Hence, referral to a geneticist for consideration and workup for these conditions is useful in patients with unexplained ID/DD.

Subtelomeric regions, just below the ends of chromosomes, are rich in genes. A deletion or rearrangements of subtelomeric regions is seen in 6.5%–7.4% of people with ID/DD (de Vries et al., 2001; Knight & Flint, 2003). De Vries et al. (2001) developed a checklist of characteristics to look for in patients with ID/DD that will increase the yield of finding deletions in the subtelomeric region. According to these authors, family history of ID, prenatal-onset growth retardation, postnatal poor growth/overgrowth, two or more facial dysmorphic features, and one or more nonfacial dysmorphic features with or without congenital anomalies are good predictors of the presence of deletion of the subtelomeric regions of chromosomes.

Inverted duplicated chromosome 15 results from duplication of the PWS/AS critical region. The clinical features of this condition include ID ranging from mild to severe, facial dysmorphism, language delay, and neurological signs such as hypotonia, ataxia, and epilepsy. The psychological impairment seen in these individuals includes autism and PDD (Borgatti et al., 2001).

AUTISM AND GENETIC CONDITIONS

Autism is etiologically and genetically heterogeneous. There are data to support the genetic influence in autism (Folstein & Piven, 1991; Rutter, Bailey, Bolten, & Le Couteur, 1994; Smalley, 1997). The likelihood of finding an underlying medical condition is dependent on criteria used to diagnose autism as well as a definition of *medical condition* (Barton & Volkmar, 1998). The prevalence of medical conditions in patients with autism is 10%–15% (Rutter et al., 1994). In a retrospective study, Barton and Volkmar (1998) found the prevalence of medical conditions in patients with autism to be 10%–15%. The patient with more severe ID and autism is more likely to have a medical condition (Barton &Volkmar, 1998; Ritvo et al., 1990; Steffenburg, 1991). Examples of medical conditions that may be found in patients with autism include TSC, fragile X syndrome, untreated phenylketonuria, fetal alcohol syndrome, and fetal rubella syndrome. An excellent review of the genetic basis of autism is available in the article by Muhle, Trentacoste, and Rapin (2004).

Tuberous Sclerosis Complex

TSC involves abnormalities of the skin, brain, kidney, and heart (Northrup & Au, 2004). There is variability in clinical findings both between families and within families. The skin is affected in 100% of patients; findings include hypomelanotic macules, facial angiofibromatosis, shagreen patches, fibrous facial plaques, and ungual and periungual fibromata. None of the skin lesions causes serious medical problems. Central nervous system (CNS) involvement leads to the most serious morbidity and mortality. CNS findings include subependymal glial nodules, cortical or subcortical tubers, and subependymal giant cell astrocytomas. Clinical features of CNS involvement are seizures, ID, PDD, autism, attention-deficit/hyperactivity disorder, and aggression. Kidney involvement includes benign angiomyolipoma, epithelial cysts, malignant angiomyolipoma, and renal cell carcinoma. Heart involvement is characterized by cardiac rhabdomyomas. These tumors regress with time and eventually disappear. Retinal lesions of TSC are hamartomas and achromic patches.

Diagnostic criteria for TSC were revised at the TSC consensus conference (Roach, Gomez, & Northrup, 1998). Diagnosis of TSC is made in an individual with either two major features or one major plus two minor features (Table 4.3). A probable diagnosis of TSC is made when an individual has one major plus one minor feature, and a diagnosis of possible TSC is made when an individual has one major feature or two or more minor features.

TSC1 (chromosome 9q34) and *TSC2* (chromosome 16p13) are two causative genes. Two thirds of affected individuals with TSC have the condition as a result of a new mutation. TSC is inherited in an autosomal dominant manner. The offspring of an individual with TSC have a 50% risk of inheriting the altered TSC gene.

The association between autism and TSC is well documented (Gillberg, Gillberg, & Ahlsen, 1994; Hunt & Shepherd, 1993; Smalley, Tanguay, Smith, & Gutierrez, 1992). The frequency of autism in TSC patients ranges from 17% to 58%. In a study by Gutierrez, Smalley, and Tanguay (1998), the frequency of autism was 28.6%, and the frequency of autism/PDD was 43%. The study by Baker, Piven, and Sato (1998) found an association between hypsarrhythmia and autism. In their study, electroencephalographic hypsarrhythmia in a patient with TSC was more often observed if the patient also had autism. They did not find an association between number, type, or location of CNS tumors and the presence of autism. The frequency of TSC in patients with autism is 0.4%–4% (Smalley et al., 1992).

Table 4.3. Major and minor features of tuberous sclerosis complex (TSC)

Major features

Facial angiofibromas or forehead plaque
Nontraumatic ungual or periungual fibromas
Hypomelanotic macules (three or more)
Shagreen patch (connective tissue nevus)
Multiple retinal nodular hamartomas
Cortical tuber[a]
Subependymal nodule
Subependymal giant cell astrocytoma
Cardiac rhabdomyoma (single or multiple)
Lymphangiomyomatosis[b]
Renal angiomyolipomas[b]

Minor features

Multiple randomly distributed pits in dental enamel
Hamartomatous rectal polyps
Bone cysts
Cerebral white matter radial migration lines
Gingival fibromas
Nonrenal hamartoma
Retinal achromic patch
"Confetti" skin lesions
Multiple renal cysts

From Roach, E.S., Gomez, M.R., and Northrup, H. (1998). Tuberous Sclerosis Consensus Conference: Revised clinical diagnostic criteria. *Journal of Child Neurology, 13,* 625; adapted by permission.

[a]When cerebral cortical dysplasia and cerebral white matter migration tracts occur together, they are counted as one rather than two features of TSC.

[b]When both lymphangiomyomatosis and renal angiomyolipomas are present, other features of tuberous sclerosis must be present before TSC is diagnosed.

Imprinting Disorders

AS and PWS are examples of disorders of imprinting. The genes in the region of chromosome 15 are expressed differently depending on the sex of the parent from whom they are inherited (Table 4.4). Genes that are critical in AS are normally expressed on the maternally inherited chromosome 15, and those critical in PWS on the paternally inherited chromosome 15. AS is due to the loss of maternal 15q 11–13, and PWS is due to loss of paternally inherited 15q 11–13.

AS is characterized by severe ID, jerky ataxic gait, absent speech, microcephaly, inappropriate laughter, protruding tongue, prognathism, skin hypopigmentation, seizures, wide mouth, fascination with water, and flexed arms during walking (Williams et al., 1995). PWS is characterized by severe hypotonia, feeding difficulties in infancy followed later by excessive eating and gradual development of morbid obesity, some degree of cognitive impairment, short stature, and hypogonadism (Table 4.5).

Fragile X Syndrome

Fragile X syndrome is the most common cause of inherited ID. It is seen in 1 in 1,200 males and 1 in 2,500 females (American College of Medical Genetics, 1994). Fragile X syndrome is due to mutation in the *FMR1* gene (Xq27.3), which was identified in 1991. The mutation consists of expansion of the CGG trinucleotide repeat. Normal alleles range from approximately 5 to 44 repeats. These are stably transmitted without increase or decrease of repeat number. Intermediate alleles, also known as gray zone alleles, range from approximately 45 to 58 CGG repeats. Alleles in this range are transmitted by females with minor increase or decrease in repeat number. Thus far, transmission of alleles with 58 or fewer repeats has not been reported to result in an affected individual with full mutation.

Table 4.4. Genetic abnormalities in Prader-Willi syndrome (PWS) and Angelman syndrome (AS)

| | Frequency of genetic abnormalities | |
	PWS (%)	AS (%)
Deletion 15q11–13	70	70
Uniparental disomy	25–28 (maternal)	3–5 (paternal)
Imprinting center defect	2–5	2–5
Translocation within PWS/AS critical region	< 1	< 1
Single-gene mutation	0?	10–15 (*UBE3A*)
Unknown	0?	~10

From American Journal of Medical Genetics, Part C (Seminars in Medical Genetics), Vol. 97, No. 2, pp. 136–146; Copyright © 2000 Wiley-Liss. Reprinted with permission of Wiley-Liss, Inc., a subsidiary of John Wiley & Sons, Inc.

Table 4.5.   Characteristics of Prader-Willi syndrome and Angelman syndrome

Clinical features	Prader-Willi syndrome	Angelman syndrome
Cognitive function	Mild to moderate ID	Severe ID
Feeding problems	In infancy, FTT; obesity when older	May have feeding difficulty in infancy
Neurological function	Hypotonia	Ataxia, seizures, microcephaly
Behavior	Temper tantrum, obsessive-compulsive behavior, stealing, skin picking, high pain threshold	Unprovoked laughter, fascination with water, severe speech delay
Facial features	Almond-shaped eyes; bifrontal narrowing; downturned mouth	Wide mouth; prognathism; protruding tongue
Endocrine features	Hypogonadotrophic hypogonadism; short stature	None
Genital features	Scrotal hypoplasia, cryptorchidism, hypoplasia of labia	None

Key: FTT, failure to thrive; ID, intellectual disabilities.

Premutation alleles range from approximately 59 to 200 CGG repeats. Alleles in this range are unstable and can expand to full mutation range during ovum formation. Thus, women with alleles in this range are considered to be at risk for having affected children. Full-mutation alleles have more than 200 CGG repeats, with several hundred to several thousand repeats being typical. Males with full mutation have moderate to severe ID and may or may not have a distinctive appearance. About 50% of females with full mutation experience ID, and about 50% have normal intellect (Saul & Tarleton, 2004).

The clinical features in males with fragile X syndrome include developmental delay, large head, long face, prominent forehead, large ears, prominent jaw, and macro-orchidism. The clinical features vary with age and are more prominent in postpubertal children and adults. Females with the full mutation have the physical and behavioral features seen in males but with lower frequency and milder involvement. Females with premutation alleles have premature ovarian failure (Schwartz et al., 1994). Males and females with premutation alleles have normal intellect and appearance. A recently described feature is tremor/ataxia syndrome in older males with premutation alleles (Hagerman et al., 2004).

Behavior abnormalities in fragile X syndrome include hyperactivity, hand flapping, hand biting, temper tantrum, and autism. Autism spectrum behavior is seen in 25% of patients with fragile X syndrome (Bailey et al., 1998), and fragile X syndrome is seen in 2.1%

of patients with autism (Kielinen, Rantala, Timonen, Linna, & Moilanen, 2004). Although fragile X syndrome is common, many patients are being missed. Using a checklist such as that in Table 4.6 might help identify patients likely to have fragile X syndrome (Hagerman, Amiri, & Cronister, 1991).

Rett Syndrome

Rett syndrome is another genetic condition to consider in the differential diagnosis of patients referred for ID/DD. It is classically seen in girls and is characterized by a progressive neurological disorder that starts after a period of 6–18 months of normal development. The neurological disorder starts as a period of develop-

Table 4.6.   Clinical characteristics of males with fragile X syndrome

Mental retardation
Family history of mental retardation
Large, prominent ears
Simian crease
Hyperextensible finger joints
Large testicles
Short attention span
Hyperactivity
Perseverative speech
Hand flapping
Hand biting
Tactile defensiveness
Poor eye contact

From *American Journal of Medical Genetics*, Vol. 38, No. 2–3, pp. 283–287; Copyright © 1991 Wiley-Liss. Reprinted with permission of Wiley-Liss, Inc., a subsidiary of John Wiley & Sons, Inc.

mental arrest followed by regression of language and motor skills. Loss of purposeful hand use and replacement by repetitive stereotypic hand movement is a characteristic finding. Additional clinical features include ataxia, autistic features, bruxism, seizures, and acquired microcephaly.

There is variability in the clinical features, with more mildly and more severely affected individuals. The mildly affected girls have less dramatic regression and milder ID. The more severely affected girls do not have a period of normal development. Clinical features that are clues to a diagnosis of Rett syndrome are acquired microcephaly, stereotypic hand movements, and family history of multiple pregnancy loss (loss of male fetus). Rett syndrome is to be considered in the differential diagnosis of ID and autism.

Rett syndrome is inherited as a X-linked dominant disorder. About 99.5% of cases are single occurrences in a family, resulting from a de novo mutation in the child with Rett syndrome (Zoghbi, 2004). The gene for Rett syndrome is on Xq28 and is called the *MECP2* (methyl-CpG–binding protein 2) gene.

Even though classic Rett syndrome is described in females, males with the *MECP2* mutation have been reported in the literature (Schanen, 2001). There are three ways in which a male presents: 1) with neonatal encephalopathy and early death (diagnosed when there is an affected female in the family) (Hoffbuhr et al., 2001); 2) with classic Rett syndrome (males with 47,XXY and mosaicism for the *MECP2* mutation) (Leonard et al., 2001); and 3) with nonspecific ID (Couvert et al., 2001).

APPROACH TO THE PATIENT WITH ID/DD, AUTISM, OR PDD

History

A comprehensive history is necessary in the patient who may have ID/DD, autism, or PDD. The history should include the following elements:

- *Family history*—recurrent miscarriage, ID, infant death

- *Pregnancy history*—alcohol, infections (cytomegalovirus), drugs (anticonvulsants), in vitro fertilization

- *Birth history*—head circumference, prematurity, postmaturity, birth asphyxia

- *Developmental history*—period of normal development (Rett syndrome) followed by regression

Examination

Clinical features of genetic conditions associated with developmental disabilities include

- Seizures, autism (AS, Rett syndrome, fragile X syndrome)

- Fascination with water, toe walking, inappropriate laughter (AS)

- Failure to thrive followed by obesity; obsessive-compulsive disorder (PWS)

- Dysmorphic features, ID, microcephaly, multiple congenital anomalies (chromosomal condition), long face with large ears (fragile X syndrome)

Laboratory Investigations

At a minimum, all patients with ID/DD must have chromosome analysis. Fluorescent in situ hybridization testing should be conducted for AS and PWS, and subtelomeric probes should be considered if additional features as described previously are present. Molecular genetic testing for mutations in single genes (Rett and fragile X syndromes) should be considered if there are features to suggest these. Also, any male with ID should be tested for fragile X syndrome because the classic clinical features may not always be present; as well, early diagnosis helps with recurrence risk counseling. Comparative genome hybridization, multicolor karyotyping, and microarray analysis are newer cytogenetic techniques that will aid in the evaluation of patients with ID/DD and autism.

CONCLUSION

Genetic conditions are an important consideration in the evaluation of patients referred to developmental pediatricians. Making a genetic diagnosis for these children helps tremendously the families of these patients. Though rare individually, collectively genetic conditions contribute significantly to the symptom complex that is seen by developmental pediatricians. With advances in genetic technologies, we hope to make a specific diagnosis in patients with ID and autism. Remaining informed of these advances and using a team approach in taking care of this patient population should be a goal of every developmental pediatrician.

RESOURCES

- *Gene tests* (http://www.genetests.org)— web site that provides comprehensive and current review articles about genetic conditions, including availability of tests and the laboratories that offer these

- *Online Mendelian Inheritance in Man* (http://www.ncbi.nih.gov/omim)—on-line database of genes and genetic conditions authored by Dr. Victor A. McKusick and colleagues at The Johns Hopkins University

- *Prader-Willi Syndrome Association* (http://www.pwsausa.org)—support group providing education and information to families and professionals

- *National Angelman Syndrome Foundation* (http://www.angelman.org)—national organization providing information, education, and services to patients, families, and professionals about Angelman syndrome

- *National Fragile X Foundation* (http://www.nfxf.org)—national organization providing information and services and promoting research into fragile X syndrome

REFERENCES

American College of Medical Genetics. (1994). Policy statement. Fragile X syndrome: Diagnostic and carrier testing. *American Journal of Medical Genetics, 53,* 380–381.

Bailey, D.B., Mesibov, G.B., Hatton, D.D., Clark, R.D., Roberts, J.E., & Mayhew, L. (1998). Autistic behavior in young boys with fragile X syndrome. *Journal of Autism and Developmental Disorders, 28,* 499–508.

Baker, P., Piven, J., & Sato, Y. (1998). Autism and tuberous sclerosis complex: Prevalence and clinical features. *Journal of Autism and Developmental Disorders, 28,* 279–285.

Barton, M., & Volkmar, F. (1998). How many commonly known medical conditions are associated with autism? *Journal of Autism and Developmental Disorders, 28,* 273–278.

Battaglia, A., Bianchini, E., & Carey, J.C. (1999). Diagnostic yield of the comprehensive assessment of developmental delay/mental retardation in an institute of child neuropsychiatry. *American Journal of Medical Genetics, 82,* 60–66.

Battaglia, A., & Carey, J.C. (2003). Diagnostic evaluation of developmental delay/mental retardation: An overview. *American Journal of Medical Genetics, Part C (Seminars in Medical Genetics), 117C,* 3–14.

Borgatti, R., Piccinelli, P., Passoni, D., Dalpra, L., Miozzo, M., Micheli, R., et al. (2001). Clinical and genetic features in inverted dup (15). *Pediatric Neurology, 24,* 111–116.

Cassidy, S.B., Dykens, E., & Williams, C.A. (2000). Prader-Willi and Angelman syndrome: Sister imprinted disorders. *American Journal of Medical Genetics, Part C (Seminars in Medical Genetics), 97,* 136–146.

Couvert, P., Bienvenu, T., Aquaviva, C., Poirier, K., Moraine, C., Gendrot, C., et al. (2001). *MECP2* is highly mutated in X-linked mental retardation. *Human Molecular Genetics, 10,* 941–946.

Curry, C.J., Stevenson, R.E., Aughton, D., Byrne, J., Carey, J.C., Cassidy, S., et al. (1997). Evaluation of mental retardation: Recommendations of a consensus conference. *American Journal of Medical Genetics, 72,* 468–477.

De Vries, B.B.A., White, S.M., Knight, S.J.L., Regan, R., Homphray, T., et al. (2001). Clinical studies on submicroscopic subtelomeric rearrangements: A checklist. *Journal of Medical Genetics, 38,* 145–150.

Folstein, S.E., & Piven, J. (1991). Etiology of autism: Genetic influences. *Pediatrics, 87,* 767–771.

Gillberg, I.C., Gillberg, C., & Ahlsen, G. (1994). Autistic behavior and attention deficits in tuberous sclerosis: A population based study. *Developmental Medicine and Child Neurology, 36,* 50–56.

Gutierrez, G.C., Smalley, S.L., & Tanguay, P.E. (1998). Autism in tuberous sclerosis. *Journal of Autism and Developmental Disorders, 28,* 97–103.

Hagerman, R.J., Amiri, K., & Cronister, A. (1991). Fragile X checklist. *American Journal of Medical Genetics, 38,* 283–287.

Hagerman, R.J., Leavitt, B.R., Farzin, F., Jacquemont, S., Greco, C.M., Brunberg, J.A., et al. (2004). Fragile-X–associated tremor/ataxia syndrome (FXTAS) in females with the *FMR1* premutation. *American Journal of Human Genetics, 74,* 1051–1056.

Hoffbuhr, K., Devaney, J.M., LaFleur, B., Sirianni, N., Scaleri, C., Giron, J., et al. (2001). *MECP2* mutations in children with and without the phenotype of Rett syndrome. *Neurology, 56,* 1486–1495.

Hunt, A., & Shepherd, C. (1993). A prevalence study of autism in tuberous sclerosis. *Journal of Autism and Developmental Disorders, 23,* 323–340.

Kielinen, M., Rantala, H., Timonen, E., Linna, S.-L., & Moilanen, I. (2004). Associated medical disorders and disabilities in children with autistic disorder: A population based study. *Autism, 8,* 49–60.

Knight, S.J.L., & Flint, J. (2003). Perfect endings: A review of subtelomeric probes and their use in clinical diagnosis. *Journal of Medical Genetics, 37,* 401–409.

Leonard, H., Silberstein, J., Falk, R., Houwink-Manville, I., Ellaway, C., Raffaele, L.S., et al. (2001). Occurrence of Rett syndrome in boys. *Journal of Child Neurology, 16,* 333–338.

McLaren, J., & Bryson, S.E. (1987). Review of recent epidemiological studies of mental retardation: Prevalence, associated disorders, and etiology. *American Journal on Mental Retardation, 92,* 243–254.

Muhle, R., Trentacoste, S.V., & Rapin, I. (2004). The genetics of autism. *Pediatrics, 113*(5), e472–e486.

Northrup, H., & Au, K.-S. (2004, September 27). *Tuberous sclerosis complex.* Retrieved October 25, 2004, from http://www.genetests.org

Ritvo, E.R., Mason-Brothers, A., Freeman, B.J., Pingree, C., Jenson, W.R., McMahon, W.M., et al. (1990). The UCLA–University of Utah epidemiological survey of autism: The etiologic role of rare disease. *American Journal of Psychiatry, 147,* 1614–1621.

Roach, E.S., Gomez, M.R., & Northrup, H. (1998). Tuberous Sclerosis Consensus Conference: Revised clinical diagnostic criteria. *Journal of Child Neurology, 13,* 624–628.

Rutter, M., Bailey, A., Bolten, P., & Le Couteur, A. (1994). Autism and known medical conditions: Myth and substance. *Journal of Child Psychology and Psychiatry, 35,* 311–322.

Saul, R.A., & Tarleton, J.C. (2004, September 13). *Fragile X syndrome.* Retrieved October 25, 2004, from http://www.genetests.org

Schanen, C. (2001). Rethinking the fate of males with mutation in the gene that causes Rett syndrome. *Brain & Development, 23,* S144–S146.

Schwartz, C.E., Dean, J., Howard-Peebles, P.N., Bugge, M., Mikkelsen, M., Tommerup, N., et al. (1994). Obstetrical and gynecological complications in fragile X carriers: A multicenter study. *American Journal of Medical Genetics, 51,* 400–402.

Smalley, S.L. (1997). Genetic influences in childhood onset psychiatric disorders: Autism and attention deficit hyperactivity disorders. *American Journal of Human Genetics, 60,* 1276–1283.

Smalley, S.L., Tanguay, P.E., Smith, M., & Gutierrez, G.(1992). Autism and tuberous sclerosis. *Journal of Autism and Developmental Disorders, 22*(97), 339–355.

Steffenburg, S. (1991). Neuropsychiatric assessment of children with autism: A population based study. *Developmental Medicine and Child Neurology, 33,* 495–511.

Stevenson, R. (1996). Mental retardation: Overview and historical perspective. *Proceedings of the Greenwood Genetics Center, 15,* 19–25.

Williams, C.A., Angelman, H., Clayton-Smith, J., Driscoll, D.J., Hendrickson, J.E., Knoll, J.H., et al. (1995). Angelman syndrome: Consensus for diagnostic criteria. Angelman Syndrome Foundation. *American Journal of Medical Genetics, 56,* 237–238.

Xu, J., & Chen, Z. (2003). Advances in molecular cytogenetics for the evaluation of mental retardation. *American Journal of Medical Genetics, Part C (Seminars in Medical Genetics), 117C,* 15–24.

Zoghbi, H.Y. (2004, February 11). *Rett syndrome.* Retrieved October 25, 2004, from http://www.genetests.org

5

Metabolic Diseases and Developmental Disabilities

RICHARD I. KELLEY

Recognizing a metabolic disease is not difficult for the pediatrician confronted with a newborn who develops severe hyperammonemia on the third day of life or an older infant who startles easily and has a retinal cherry-red spot. More difficult is knowing when and how to look for an inborn error of metabolism in the 2-year-old who has little understanding of language, the 4-year-old with hypotonia and delays, or a child with extrapyramidal cerebral palsy. Almost every day pediatricians see children with developmental problems, but only a few of these children will prove to have a recognizable inborn error of metabolism. In addition, although many physicians do not think of children with static encephalopathies as victims of metabolic disease, the advances in biochemical and molecular genetics have blurred, if not erased, the etiological distinction between progressive and nonprogressive genetic encephalopathies.

We now know that, for almost every inborn error of metabolism that presents as a neonatal catastrophe, there exist milder forms of the disease that present in later infancy, in childhood, or even during the adult years with behavior disturbances, seizures, or other neurological disabilities. The challenge to the nonspecialist is to know 1) when to suspect a metabolic disease, 2) how to gather additional historical and clinical information to guide a metabolic workup, 3) what tests to order for a comprehensive yet cost-effective evaluation, and 4) when to call for help. This chapter should provide both the developmental specialist and the general pediatrician with a basic

understanding of the many faces of metabolic disease and the tools to organize a simple and sensible approach to diagnosing an inborn error of metabolism in the child with a developmental disability.

SCOPE OF GENETIC METABOLIC DISEASES

The rapidly growing number of recognizable metabolic diseases not only limits the nonspecialist's ability to identify and diagnose more than a handful of better-known metabolic diseases, but also keeps diagnostic laboratories struggling to provide pediatricians and neurologists with a reasonably comprehensive testing menu. Whereas 30 years ago the majority of known metabolic diagnoses could be detected by a single laboratory with a combination of amino acid chromatography and a few simple urine tests, today's diagnostic evaluation of a child with a suspected metabolic disease often is a nightmare of sending specimens to a half dozen or more laboratories and then trying to make sense of an equal number of incomprehensible laboratory reports. The goal of this chapter, therefore, is not to present an exhaustive list of biochemical diseases and diagnostic tests, but instead to provide developmentalists and pediatricians with a guide through this increasingly complicated maze of metabolic diseases and their varied presentations in children.

CATEGORIES OF METABOLIC DISEASE

Even with the best molecular and biochemical diagnostic resources, a specific biochemical or

Table 5.1. Inborn errors of metabolism causing developmental disabilities (selected)

Category	Examples
Disorders of amino acid metabolism	Phenylketonuria Ornithine transcarbamylase deficiency
Disorders of organic acid metabolism	Glutaric aciduria type I Methylmalonic aciduria
Lactic acidoses and mitochondrial disorders	Leigh's disease; MELAS syndrome Cytochrome-c oxidase deficiency
Disorders of lipid metabolism	Sjögren-Larssen syndrome Multiple acyl–coenzyme A dehydrogenase deficiency
Lysosomal storage diseases	Sanfilippo syndrome (mucopolysaccharidosis type III) Tay-Sachs disease
Peroxisomal disorders	X-linked adrenoleukodystrophy Zellweger syndrome
Disorders of cholesterol biosynthesis	Smith-Lemli-Opitz syndrome Mevalonic aciduria
Disorders of neurotransmitter metabolism	Phenylketonuria–biopterin defects L-amino acid decarboxylase deficiency
Disorders of mineral metabolism	Molybdenum cofactor deficiency Menkes disease

Key: MELAS, mitochondrial myopathy, encephalopathy, lactic acidosis, and stroke-like episodes.

molecular genetic cause of a developmental disability, especially a less-severe one, can be found in only about half of children who come to testing, even under the guidance of an experienced geneticist or developmental pediatrician. Table 5.1 summarizes the basic categories of metabolic disease, many of which are considered in this chapter. Despite its length, this list does not include all metabolic diseases of infancy and childhood, but it encompasses all of the more common metabolic diseases as well as some of the rarer ones for which there are effective therapies.

GENERAL DIAGNOSTIC APPROACHES

Past Medical History

All children with unexplained motor or cognitive delays should be tested for a metabolic disease. Even children with apparent, but not proven, causes of their developmental disability, such as perinatal asphyxia or a damaging viral "encephalitis," should be considered for metabolic testing because past medical problems may have been the setting for acute neurological injury that would not have occurred in the absence of an underlying metabolic disease. For example, prematurity can be a sign of

a fetus compromised by intrinsic biochemical abnormalities, a traumatic delivery secondary to macrocephaly is a feature of glutaric aciduria, the congenital hypotonia associated with many neurometabolic disorders also can predispose to a traumatic birth, and an immunization or viral syndrome that occurs during the "window of vulnerability" of certain metabolic diseases may be the only damaging event in a child with no other outward signs of a metabolic disease.

Classic metabolic signs—hypoglycemia, metabolic acidosis, hyperammonemia, abnormal odors, and acute encephalopathy—often are characteristic only of the more severe forms of a metabolic disease, which usually are the first cases reported in the medical literature. However, once tools for definitive biochemical or molecular diagnosis are developed, the spectrum of most metabolic diseases that present as an acute infantile disease expands to include partial enzymatic deficiencies that present as mild systemic disease or isolated developmental delay. For example, infants with biotinidase deficiency may present with an idiopathic seizure disorder but lack any of the other elements of the textbook constellation of hair loss, skin rashes, hypotonia, seizures, meta-

Table 5.2. Signs and symptoms of metabolic disease

Episodic disease, especially neurological and precipitated by simple illnesses or fasting

Progressive neurological deterioration

Abnormal startle

Nystagmus and other oculomotor abnormalities

Loss of auditory or visual function

Chronic or intermittent extrapyramidal dysfunction: dystonia, chorea, choreoathetosis

Hypotonia—central, muscular, or both

Metabolic acidosis, renal tubular acidosis

Protein avoidance, persistent vomiting, pyloric stenosis

Growth retardation

Acquired skin and hair disorders, storage deposits in skin

Hepatosplenomegaly

Coarse facial features

---

bolic acidosis, and a diagnostic organic aciduria (Table 5.2). In such cases, there may be partial dietary compensation providing a serum level of a cofactor that is adequate for systemic functions of the enzyme but insufficient for supplying the needs of the nervous system.

Regardless of preexisting assumptions about the cause of a child's disabilities, the medical history for a child with developmental disability should document carefully all perinatal events and the early development of the child, with special attention to dietary changes and infectious diseases that could have initiated a metabolic injury. Subtle or more obvious changes in the trajectory of an infant's psychomotor development may follow a viral syndrome that caused unusual lethargy and irritability but no overt signs of metabolic compromise. Seeking such a metabolic history is especially important for evaluating children with "cerebral palsy" because most studies show that only 15%–25% of children with cerebral palsy have a history of perinatal injury that unquestionably explains the child's psychomotor disability (Nelson & Ellenberg, 1986) and because other studies document a substantial heritability of cerebral palsy. Other causes of disability among individuals with cerebral palsy but no perinatal injury include many metabolic disorders, a variety of other Mendelian syndromes, and submicroscopic chromosomal aneuploidies. A group deserving special attention are children with extrapyramidal ce-

rebral palsy and other movement disorders caused by dysfunction of the cerebellum or basal ganglia, which are sites of increased vulnerability in children with disorders of mitochondrial, organic acid, or energy metabolism, as discussed later. Important examples include type I glutaric aciduria, propionic acidemia, pyruvate dehydrogenase deficiency, and the primary disorders of mitochondrial energy metabolism.

The increasing understanding of the mechanisms of brain injury, such as glutamate excitotoxicity and the role of mitochondrial compromise in neuronal apoptosis, has shown that there are discrete windows of vulnerability during which certain types of brain injury occur. This phenomenon is typified by type I glutaric aciduria, in which the neostriatal injury that leads to extrapyramidal cerebral palsy rarely occurs in the first few weeks of life and never after age 3 years, even when there are recurrent episodes of metabolic decompensation. Patients with methylmalonic aciduria, propionic acidemia, and some forms of mitochondrial complex I deficiency have similar windows of vulnerability for basal ganglial injury and may have a transiently progressive encephalopathy in early childhood but no other clinical signs of metabolic disease in later years. Such a child examined at 5 or 10 years may be given a diagnosis of just idiopathic extrapyramidal cerebral palsy. Thus, careful chronicling and correlation of medical events and neurological changes during the first 2 or 3 years of life is especially important for the detection of metabolic disease among children with static encephalopathies. Even if the child is no longer at risk of injury, the benefit of a correct diagnosis to future children can be great.

Diet and nutrition have important roles in the evolution of many metabolic diseases, especially those involving amino acid, organic acid, and fatty acid metabolism. For example, a change from breast milk to formula will often double an infant's protein intake and lead to subacute neurological injury in a child with a protein-sensitive organic aciduria or urea cycle defect. Moreover, as an infant's intrinsic rate of protein accretion decreases over the first 2 years, the amount of protein amino acid that must be catabolized increases and often exceeds the capacity of a genetically limited pathway in children with partial inborn errors of metabolism. The result may be hyperammonemia, metabolic acidosis, or other metabolic intoxication that can have many different clinical manifestations, including just delayed development.

Children with amino acid–derived metabolic diseases may learn to refuse protein, but the signs of disease are often more subtle, and protein tolerance can be good until the time of an illness or fasting, which can increase protein catabolism three- or four-fold and thereby lead to metabolic autointoxication. The state of hydration during a gastrointestinal illness is another important factor in the evolution of neurological injury in many organic acidurias, especially glutaric aciduria and methylmalonic aciduria. Even relatively mild degrees of volume contraction caused by vomiting or a diarrheal illness can greatly limit renal excretion of a toxic metabolite and set the conditions for rising metabolite levels and acute cerebral injury.

Smith-Lemli-Opitz syndrome, an autosomal recessive multiple anomaly syndrome caused by a defect in the last step of cholesterol biosynthesis, illustrates best a metabolic disease with a natural history opposite to that of inborn errors of amino acid and organic acid metabolism. The inability of the fetus with Smith-Lemli-Opitz syndrome (SLOS) to synthesize cholesterol, compounded by limited placental transport of cholesterol, causes retarded fetal growth, microcephaly, and multiple malformations. A presumptive diagnosis is made by recognition of the characteristic dysmorphic appearance and a specific pattern of malformations, including cleft palate, polydactyly, and hypospadias. At the mild end of the clinical spectrum, however, the older child with SLOS may have mild to moderate intellectual disabilities, autism, and difficult-to-recognize dysmorphic facial features. Two other defects of cholesterol biosynthesis at earlier steps

in the pathway, desmosterolosis and lathosterolosis, cause similar static encephalopathies with multiple malformations. The phenomenon of postnatal amelioration of abnormal growth and behavior in SLOS when treated with cholesterol supplementation is the opposite of the classic paradigm of maternal correction of a metabolic disease before birth. The same phenomenon involving other essential lipids may underlie many undiagnosed static encephalopathies and explain the occasional infant with hypotonia and poor development who makes better-than-expected gains in subsequent years.

Family History

Most inborn errors of metabolism observe autosomal recessive inheritance wherein both parents are carriers (heterozygotes), and only infrequently will there be a similarly affected child in the family outside the primary sibship. The rarer a disorder, the more likely the parents will have a common relative or descend from a population for which a particular disease has an increased prevalence, such as Tay-Sachs disease (*Mendelian Inheritance in Man* [MIM] 272800)[1] in Ashkenazic Jews or Cohen syndrome (MIM 216550) in the Amish-Mennonites of northeastern Ohio. Thus, a careful but tactful exploration of the family background to look for consanguinity is always important. In some regions, such as the Middle East, cousin marriages are often favored, and in some relatively isolated religious sects, such as the Old Order Amish of Lancaster County, Pennsylvania, there is restricted gene diversity, and marriages of distant cousins are inevitably common.

In contrast to autosomal recessive disorders, both X-linked inheritance and maternal (mitochondrial) inheritance can present a substantial recurrence risk for other sibships and generations in a family. For possible X-linked recessive disorders, one must consider carefully diseases and disabilities in maternal uncles and other male relatives of a

---

[1]MIM numbers are provided for all disorders for which a listing in *Mendelian Inheritance in Man* (McKusick, 1992) is available. Readers interested in additional information and literature resources for these disorders can access a web-based version (Online Mendelian Inheritance in Man) at http://www.ncbi.nlm.nih.gov/entrez/query.fcgi?db = OMIM.

male proband. For "mitochondrial inheritance," all offspring, both males and females, of a mother carrying a mitochondrial DNA (mtDNA) mutation will inherit different proportions of normal and abnormal mitochondrial genomes. The threshold for disease typically is crossed when the fraction of abnormal mtDNA exceeds 70%–80%, which can vary substantially from person to person and from organ to organ. Those tissues with the highest demand for oxidative metabolism, such as brain and muscle, are more likely to cross the disease threshold at a lower percentage of abnormal mtDNA. Certain other mitochondrial diseases of childhood, such as Pearson marrow–pancreas syndrome, most often are sporadic and caused by de novo deletions of the mitochondrial genome.

Physicians should explore the family history in detail for disorders associated with abnormal energy metabolism: myopathy, myoclonus, myoclonic seizures, cardiomyopathy, ophthalmoplegia, retinitis pigmentosa, sensorineural deafness, and peripheral neuropathies. Young children with mitochondrial disorders may develop any of these problems or have only hypotonia, delayed development, or an uncomplicated seizure disorder for years before there is evidence of a progressive disease. However, in a substantial number of milder pediatric mitochondrial diseases, brain injury and neurodevelopmental decline may be restricted to a "window of vulnerability" in the early years. This phenomenon is seen in patients with regressive pervasive developmental disorder who often have biochemical evidence of a mitochondrial disease.

PHYSICAL EXAMINATION

Apart from the neurological examination and assessment for signs of metabolic acidosis and odors, there are relatively few physical signs that aid in the diagnosis of metabolic diseases. Nevertheless, some physical findings can be important diagnostic clues for a number of metabolic diseases for which routine metabolic "screening" is not available. Such physical findings may be the first to suggest a specific diagnosis, which must then be established by an enzymatic assay or other specific test.

General Features

The appreciation of coarse facial features in the mucopolysaccharidoses and oligosaccharidoses can be difficult in the early years, especially for children with Sanfilippo syndrome (mucopolysaccharidosis type III), whose somatic changes can be subtle. However, because facial coarsening is progressive in most mucopolysaccharidoses, comparing infant photographs with the later appearance of a child often is revealing and helps distinguish familial features from those of a storage disease. Facial coarsening also occurs in several mendelian syndromes and chromosome aneuploidies, most notably Williams syndrome (MIM 194050) and cardio-facio-cutaneous syndrome (MIM 115150). If caused by a lysosomal storage disease, facial coarsening almost always is accompanied by identifiable storage on biopsy. Those storage diseases with more visceral involvement, such as Hunter and Hurler syndromes, usually have clinically appreciable storage in the tongue, liver, spleen, or cornea.

Hair and Skin Abnormalities

Table 5.3 lists the diagnostically most important skin abnormalities in metabolic diseases. In some storage diseases, such as Hunter syndrome (mucopolysaccharidosis type II) and Niemann-Pick disease type A, relatively specific and diagnostic skin lesions occur. For these and several other diseases listed, the skin and hair abnormalities are not always present or may even be intermittent. Not listed in Table 5.3 are many genetic syndromes that combine relatively specific hair or skin abnormalities and psychomotor retardation but for which the suspected metabolic error is unknown.

Eye Abnormalities

The eye examination is important for identifying specific neuro-opthalmological abnormalities and for detecting diagnostically important structural or degenerative abnormalities. Corneal clouding is an important feature of many

Table 5.3. Skin and hair abnormalities in metabolic diseases

Metabolic disease	Skin and hair abnormalities
Amino acid disorders	
Tyrosinemia and phenylketonuria	Pale, reddish hair
Argininosuccinic aciduria	Friable hair (trichorrhexis nodosa)
Hartnup disease	Photosensitive dermatitis/pellagra
Organic acid disorders	
Biotinidase deficiency	Acquired hair loss; excoriating skin lesions
Lysosomal storage diseases	
Mucopolysaccharidosis disorders	Thick skin; coarse facies, coarse hair; mucopolysaccharide skin deposits
Niemann-Pick disease type A	Nodular skin lesions
Fabry disease	Angiokeratomata
Schindler disease	Angiokeratomata (older patients)
Other lipid disorders	
Smith-Lemli-Opitz syndrome	Sparse, reddish hair; cold mottled skin (distal extremities)
Carbohydrate-deficient glycoprotein syndromes	Abnormal skin fat pads; inverted nipples
Steroid sulfatase deficiency	Ichthyosis
Sjögren-Larssen syndrome	Ichthyosis
Other disorders	
Menkes disease	Wiry hair (pili torti)
Acrodermatitis enteropathica	Excoriative diaper and perioral rashes

of the mucopolysaccharidoses, oligosaccharidoses, sialidoses, gangliosidoses, and mucolipidoses, almost all of which today can be diagnosed by specific enzymatic assays. Congenital or acquired cataracts occur in galactosemia (MIM 230400), SLOS (MIM 270400), pseudohypoparathyroidism (Albright hereditary osteodystrophy; MIM 103580), and Senger syndrome (cataracts, cardiomyopathy, and lactic acidosis; MIM 212350), among others. Important retinal lesions for the differential diagnosis of metabolic disorders include cherry-red spots (GM_1 and GM_2 gangliosidoses, Niemann-Pick disease), optic hypoplasia or atrophy (pyruvate dehydrogenase deficiency and mitochondrial disorders), and pigmentary retinopathies (ceroid lipofuscinosis, mucopolysaccharidoses, mitochondrial diseases, Refsum disease, and generalized peroxisomal disorders). Although many of the disorders associated with ocular lesions are intrinsically degenerative diseases, they can also present as variant forms that appear to be nonprogressive for years or decades. Among these diseases, Niemann-Pick disease type C, peroxisomal diseases (e.g., "infantile Refsum disease"), and mitochondrial diseases are best known. Ceroid lipofuscinosis in a child with seizures yet with normal or near-normal development can also go unsuspected for many months or years if retinal lesions are not detected and a diagnostic electroretinogram is not performed.

Hepatomegaly and Splenomegaly

Hepatomegaly and splenomegaly, well-known features of lysosomal storage diseases, are variably severe but can be subclinical or absent in some of the better-known visceral storage diseases, such as neuronopathic Gaucher disease, GM_1 gangliosidosis, and Niemann-Pick disease, especially type C, recently shown to be caused by a defect in intracellular cholesterol transport. In such cases, tissue biopsies (e.g., rectal mucosa, bone marrow, conjunctiva, skin) can be crucial for establishing the true nature of the disease. Some metabolic diseases that cause only motor delay, such as several glycogen storage diseases, can have hepatomegaly alone. Among diseases with splenomegaly, the spleen sometimes is palpable only during or shortly after viral infections, when there is activation of the reticuloendothelial system and increased trapping of poorly degraded cellular elements. At the same time, thrombobycytopenia and petechiae resulting from hypersplenism may become the first sign of an underlying storage process.

Neurological Abnormalities

Hypotonia Mild hypotonia is common to many neurological syndromes, both metabolic and nonmetabolic, and, by itself, has little diagnostic specificity. However, profound hypotonia is less common and should suggest a generalized peroxisomal disorder (e.g., Zellweger syndrome, neonatal adrenoleukodystrophy), 4-hydroxybutyric aciduria (succinic semialdehyde dehydrogenase deficiency), propionic acidemia, Smith-Lemli-Opitz syndrome, fumarase deficiency, and mitochondrial diseases. Rapid metabolic diagnosis of the hypotonic infant with motor delay but normal cognitive development also is important because death or serious morbidity from several of these diseases, such as fasting-sensitive mitochondrial diseases, can be prevented with simple dietary interventions.

Cerebral Palsy, Spasticity, and Movement Disorders Children with cerebral palsy, especially those who lack a convincing history of perinatal injury, constitute a group of patients with a higher risk of a metabolic disease than those with otherwise unexplained developmental delays. Too often, a child with cerebral palsy due to an underlying metabolic disease is missed until a biochemical stress, such as an orthopedic operation, causes additional brain injury. In general, spastic or mixed spastic/dystonic cerebral palsy is more likely to be caused by mitochondrial diseases and disorders of amino acid metabolism than by other categories of metabolic disease. Although the classic forms of these disorders are not easily missed when they present as catastrophic neonatal illnesses, milder variants may present in the first few years as static encephalopathies. Neurological abnormalities in children with milder variants of a generalized peroxisomal disease (e.g., neonatal adrenoleukodystrophy, infantile Refsum disease) and various lysosomal storage diseases may be interpreted as only hypotonic or spastic cerebral palsy for many months or years before neurodegenerative changes become evident. Because of the substantial cortical involvement in most of these disorders, major cognitive impairment is a common associated finding.

When caused by a metabolic disease, choreoathetotic or mixed choreoathetotic/dystonic cerebral palsy is most often associated with disorders of organic acid metabolism, such as type I glutaric aciduria, propionic acidemia, and diseases of mitochondrial metabolism. Many of these diseases can be rapidly progressive or episodic in the first few months of life but also relatively or completely stable for years or decades after acute or chronic injury in early childhood. Lesch-Nyhan syndrome, the classic disorder of purine metabolism associated with self-mutilation and hyperuricemia, can present as only extrapyramidal cerebral palsy or hyperuricemia until the third or fourth year and be diagnosable biochemically only by measurement of the urinary uric acid–to–creatinine ratio or enzymatic assay of hypoxanthine guanine phosphoribosyltransferase (HGPRT) in red blood cells in that period. However, in contrast to metabolic diseases associated with spasticity, children with metabolic diseases that cause predominantly extrapyramidal injury often have no or minimal cortical injury. Some metabolic diseases of childhood with predominantly extrapyramidal neurological disease, most notably type I glutaric aciduria and methylmalonic aciduria, often have a history of normal or relatively normal psychomotor development until the metabolic stress of fasting or dehydration from gastroenteritis causes basal ganglial injury. The most important of these diseases are listed in Table 5.4.

Ataxia Disorders of pyruvate and energy metabolism form the largest group of metabolic diseases with ataxia: pyruvate dehydrogenase deficiency, Leigh's disease, specific mitochondrial respiratory chain defects, and mutations or deletions of the mitochondrial genome (Table 5.5). The diagnostic marker for most of these diseases, pyruvic or lactic acidemia or both, can be persistent or deceptively intermittent and often must be evaluated by carefully timed provocative tests or enzymatic assays. Certain organic acidemias, in particular biotinidase deficiency and those that involve 2-ketoacids, can present with chronic or intermittent

Table 5.4. Metabolic diseases with basal ganglial injury

Metabolic disease	Site of injury
Organic acid disorders	
Glutaric aciduria type I	Caudate/putamen
Glutaric aciduria type II	Caudate/putamen
Propionic acidemia	Putamen ± globus pallidus
Methylmalonic aciduria	Globus pallidus
Pyruvate dysmetabolism	
Pyruvate dehydrogenase deficiency	Globus pallidus; thalamus
Leigh's disease	Caudate/putamen; brain stem
Mitochondrial encephalomyopathies	Caudate/putamen
Lysosomal storage diseases	
Niemann-Pick disease type C	Putamen
Tay-Sachs disease and variants	Putamen
GM_1 gangliosidosis	Caudate/putamen
Other disorders	
Pantothenate kinase-associated neurodegeneration (Hallervorden-Spatz syndrome)	Globus pallidus
Wilson disease	Globus pallidus
Triose phosphate isomerase deficiency	Caudate/putamen
Lesch-Nyhan syndrome	None structural
Molybdenum cofactor deficiency and isolated sulfite oxidase deficiency	Caudate
Guanidinoacetate methyltransferase deficiency	Globus pallidus

ataxia. Mild variants of classic urea cycle defects, especially X-linked ornithine transcarbamylase deficiency heterozygosity, in which periodic elevations of blood ammonia and glutamine occur, also are important metabolic causes of intermittent ataxia. Fortunately, most metabolic diseases with intermittent ataxia are at least partially treatable. In many of these disorders, cerebellar atrophy is evident at diagnosis or later in the course of the disease.

Nystagmus and Other Oculomotor Abnormalities
Nystagmus and related oculomotor abnormalities occur most commonly in metabolic diseases associated with ataxia but also serve as important diagnostic clues in other neurometabolic diseases. These include leukodystrophies, lysosomal storage diseases such as Niemann-Pick disease type C (impaired upward gaze), neuronopathic Gaucher disease (horizontal and rotatory nystagmus), mitochondrial cytopathies (nystagmus, ptosis, and external ophthalmoplegia), the ceroid lipofuscinoses, generalized peroxisomal disorders, and other diseases with early or severe visual loss.

Seizures
Seizures are characteristic of many neurometabolic diseases; however, seizures in a child without other neurological problems usually are not the first sign of a metabolic disease because, as a rule, seizures reflect old cerebral injury, not acute metabolic disturbances. Notable diseases whose first sign can be seizures include mitochondrial encephalomyopathies, ceroid lipofuscinoses, and several of the oligosaccharidoses and gangliosidoses. For many of the mitochondropathies and lysosomal storage diseases, myoclonic seizures often predominate.

Seizures in the first few days of life are characteristic of nonketotic hyperglycinemia, "pyridoxine-responsive" seizures, and folinic acid–responsive seizures; however, treatable metabolic seizure disorders can be missed when seizures are attributed to perinatal difficulties that many congenitally hypotonic children have. Nonketotic hyperglycinemia typically is a fulminant neonatal disorder with rapid respiratory depression, seizures, a characteristic burst-suppression pattern on electroencephalography, and early death. Neonatal or even prenatal seizures are common in children with metabolic diseases that affect neuronal migration, such as Zellweger syndrome and multiple acyl-coenzyme A (CoA) dehydrogenase deficiency.

Table 5.5. Metabolic diseases associated with ataxia

Mitochondrial disorders
Kearns-Sayre syndrome
MERRF syndrome, MELAS syndrome, NARP
Leigh's disease (NARP mutation in some)
Respiratory chain subunit deficiency

Pyruvate dysmetabolism
Pyruvate dehydrogenase deficiency (e.g., E1α subunit)

Aminoacidopathies
Maple syrup urine disease
Hartnup disease
Argininosuccinate lyase deficiency
Ornithine transcarbamylase deficiency

Organic acid disorders
Mevalonate kinase deficiency
2-Hydroxyglutaric aciduria
3-Methylglutaconyl-CoA hydratase deficiency

Peroxisomal disorders
Neonatal adrenoleukodystrophy
Infantile Refsum disease
X-linked adrenoleukodystrophy

Storage diseases
GM$_1$ gangliosidosis
Juvenile GM$_2$ gangliosidosis (B1 variant and others)
Juvenile metachromatic leukodystrophy

Other lipid disorders
Abetalipoproteinemia (Bassen-Kornzweig disease)
Hypobetalipoproteinemia
Carnitine acetyltransferase deficiency
Cerebrotendinous xanthomatosis

Key: MERRF, myoclonic epilepsy associated with ragged-red fibers; MELAS, mitochondrial myopathy, encephalopathy, lactic acidosis, and stroke-like episodes; NARP, neuropathy, ataxia, and retinitis pigmentosa.

For most other metabolic diseases in which seizures are common, the seizures usually develop following an acute metabolic crisis or months of chronic milder cerebral toxicity. The development of seizures in a child with chronic neurological problems can be the first sign of a deteriorating condition, such as Leigh's disease and mtDNA transfer RNA mutations, that prior to seizures had been manifest as an apparently static condition. The onset of a metabolic regression, however, can be difficult to distinguish from seizure-induced regression in a child with a fixed brain injury.

Other Neurological Signs Other important neurological signs of metabolic disease include peripheral neuropathy in several leuko-dystrophies and Leigh's disease; macrocephaly in Canavan disease, mucopolysaccharidoses, and some sphingolipidoses; and bulbar dysfunction in neuronopathic Gaucher disease and other infantile sphingolipidoses. Congenital or postnatal macrocephaly caused by increased subarachnoid fluid or cysts also is characteristic of organic acidurias associated with increased blood and cerebrospinal fluid (CSF) levels of substituted and unsubstituted five-carbon dicarboxylic acids: glutaric acid and glutaconic acid (glutaric aciduria type I), 3-hydroxy-3-methylglutaric acid (hydroxymethylglutaryl-CoA lyase deficiency), 2-hydroxyglutaric acid (L-2-hydroxyglutaric aciduria), and 3-methylglutaconic acid (3-methylglutaconyl-CoA hydratase deficiency). Not uncommonly, macrocephaly-related delivery complications suffered by these children are blamed for subsequent delayed development before recognition of the underlying metabolic diagnosis.

Autism and Other Behavior Disorders

Although the cause of most cases of autism remains undetermined, an increasing number of metabolic diseases and other genetic disorders have been linked to infantile autism and other forms of pervasive developmental disorder. Metabolic and genetic disorders traditionally associated with autism include phenylketonuria (PKU), several disorders of purine biosynthesis, and Rett syndrome. In addition, with better appreciation of subtle forms of mitochondrial disease, an increasing number of studies show biochemical evidence of mitochondrial abnormalities in up to 25% of children with autism, largely those with regression. When studied by muscle biopsy, most of these patients have complex I deficiency and often respond to therapies designed to augment complex I activity. X-linked creatine transporter deficiency, which also impairs ATP metabolism, has been identified as a cause of autism, although children with classic creatine transporter deficiency characteristically have a seizure disorder and progressive worsening. Partial deficiencies of pyruvate dehydrogenase deficiency also often manifest an autism spectrum disorder. Especially interesting among the more recently identified metabolic causes of autism is Smith-Lemli-Opitz syndrome, a genetic deficiency of cholesterol biosynthesis, because cholesterol supplementation to correct the cholesterol deficiency often largely eliminates the autistic behaviors.

Episodic Disease Occasionally, a child with an apparently static developmental disability who has been followed for months or years will develop an acute encephalopathy, usually at the time of an otherwise simple childhood infection or a surgical procedure. Many of these children will be found to have an inborn error of amino acid, organic acid, or pyruvate metabolism caused by a partial enzymatic deficiency. For diagnosis of these children, it is important to obtain "acute" urine and blood specimens for metabolic testing because once a child with an organic aciduria or fatty acid oxidation defect is treated, diagnostic metabolites may largely clear from the urine. An order to "send urine for metabolic screening" that is not executed until the next morning can miss a critical opportunity for diagnosis, requiring additional provocative studies if a metabolic disorder is suspected.

A child who experiences substantial cerebral damage during infancy from an unrecognized, fasting-dependent episodic metabolic disease may become more stable once a gastrostomy and regular scheduled feedings are introduced, as often happens when brain damage is substantial. Such a child, however, may again become encephalopathic or die during the catabolic stress of a surgical procedure, or the same disease may appear suddenly in a sibling. Similarly, children with persistent vomiting who improve with more frequent or continuous feedings may have a protein-dependent (i.e., amino acid–dependent) metabolic disease that is then ameliorated by, in effect, reducing the amount of protein given at one feeding.

CATEGORIES OF METABOLIC DISEASE

Disorders of Amino Acid Metabolism

Although the list of known amino acid disorders has grown substantially since the first description of PKU more than 50 years ago, amino acid disorders now constitute a rela-

tively small proportion of identifiable metabolic diseases. At the same time, however, the variety of presentations for each amino acid disorder has grown, making clinical and laboratory diagnosis more difficult. Table 5.6 lists the most important amino acid disorders to consider today in the evaluation of developmental disabilities.

All 50 states in the United States as well as most other developed countries screen at birth for PKU, the most common inherited disorder of amino acid metabolism. As a result, the classic phenylketonuric syndrome of intellectual disabilities, microcephaly, spasticity, and a "musky" odor is now rarely seen. An increasing number of children with PKU, however, are being missed by newborn screening programs because of the more common practice of discharging newborns on the first or second day of life, often before amino acid levels have crossed the diagnostic threshold. Therefore, missed PKU must now more routinely be entertained as the cause of an undiagnosed

Table 5.6. Amino acid disorders causing developmental disability

Primary amino acid disorders
Phenylketonuria
    Phyenylalanine hydroxylase deficiency
    Biopterin synthesis deficiency
    Maternal phenylketonuria
Homocystinuria
    Cystathionine β-synthase deficiency
    Homocysteine remethylation defect (several forms)
Maple syrup urine disease
    Classic
    Intermittent, partial, and thiamine-responsive
Disorders of ureagenesis
    Ornithine transcarbamylase deficiency
    Carbamylphosphate synthase deficiency
    Citrullinemia (argininosuccinate synthase deficiency)
    Argininosuccinic aciduria (argininosuccinate lyase deficiency)
    Hyperargininemia (arginase deficiency)

Amino acid transport defects
Lysinuric protein intolerance (dibasic amino acid transport deficiency)
Hyperornithinemia with homocitrullinuria (ornithine transporter deficiency)

Secondary amino acid disorders
Secondary hyperalaninemia (pyruvate dysmetabolism and hyperammonemia syndromes)

static encephalopathy. Children with variants of PKU caused by defects in the synthesis of biopterin, a cofactor for both phenylalanine hydroxylase and tyrosine hydroxylase, develop intellectual disabilities despite careful dietary management of phenylalanine intake because of deficient synthesis of biogenic amines from tyrosine. Furthermore, as women with PKU reach childbearing age, there will be more cases of maternal PKU, a syndrome of phenylalanine-induced fetal abnormalities including microcephaly, intellectual disabilities, heart defects, and other malformations.

The term *homocystinuria* describes not one disease but a family of diseases having in common increased plasma levels of the sulfhydryl amino acid homocysteine in several different forms: free monomeric homocysteine, dimeric "homocystine," cysteine–homocysteine mixed disulfide, and complexes of homocysteine with cysteine in proteins. Classic homocystinuria, caused by a deficiency of cystathionine β-synthase (MIM 236200), has three major serum amino acid abnormalities: increased homocystine and methionine levels and a low cystine level. This is the form associated with "marfanoid" features, including arachnodactyly and dislocated lenses, but the dysmorphic physical characteristics may not be recognized until after developmental problems appear, and some biochemically affected patients lack the physical features entirely. More difficult to identify both clinically and biochemically are forms of homocystinuria associated with a failure of remethylation of homocysteine to methionine caused by a primary deficiency of methionine synthase or one of its vitamin cofactors, methylcobalamin and tetrahydrofolate (MIM 250940, 277410, 277380, 236270, 236250). These remethylation defects are characterized by mildly to moderately increased plasma homocystine levels, low or borderline-low plasma methionine levels, and no marfanoid features.

Because blood levels of free homocysteine may appear to be normal in patients with remethylation defects owing to rapid complexing of free homocysteine to blood proteins, a total blood homocysteine level should be measured. This test is now available as part of adult screening for cardiovascular disease risk. Several remethylation defects are easily treated with vitamin B_{12} or other cofactors. If untreated, homocystinuria caused by a remethylation defect can present as developmental delay, cerebral palsy, a leukodystrophy, or multisystem degeneration.

Patients with urea cycle defects who do not present with textbook neonatal hyperammonemic crisis are not rare. X-linked ornithine transcarbamylase deficiency, argininosuccinic aciduria (argininosuccinate lyase deficiency), lysinuric protein intolerance (MIM 222700), and hyperargininemia (arginase deficiency; MIM 207800) have well-recognized presentations with developmental delay and failure to thrive beyond early infancy. Although hyperammonemic encephalopathy typically occurs episodically with infections, fasting, or excessive protein intake, some affected children may be followed for years for an apparent static encephalopathy before a catabolic crisis leads to an acute encephalopathy. Self-imposed protein restriction is common and often extreme in affected children, who may first be evaluated for recurrent vomiting, a "behavioral" feeding disorder, and nutritional failure to thrive, occasionally without significant developmental delay. Because the encephalopathy of urea cycle defects is largely a gray matter disease, affected children can have any combination of mild to moderate intellectual disabilities, seizures, spasticity, cerebral atrophy, and microcephaly.

Nonketotic hyperglycinemia (NKH; MIM 238300, 238330, 238310), caused by defective conversion of glycine to serine via the glycine cleavage enzyme, is another amino acid disorder with both severe neonatal and milder later-onset presentations. In the neonatal period, children with classic NKH rapidly develop hypotonia, apnea, seizures, and burst-suppression patterns on electroencephalography. Those infants with NKH who are identified later in infancy or childhood typically have developmental delay, dystonia, and seizures and may regress during fevers or simple viral infections. The diagnostic hallmark of all forms of NKH is hyperglycinemia, with a glycine-to-serine ratio in plasma greater than 3:1. Cerebrospinal glycine also is disproportionately increased, and the CSF-to-plasma glycine ratio is greater than 0.12:1 (normal is < 0.06:1). Because CSF glycine levels in NKH can be pathologically increased at the same time that plasma glycine levels are only high-normal, a possible diagnosis of NKH is one of the important indications for measurement of CSF amino acid levels. Whereas treatment of classic NKH is all but futile, the more mildly affected patients with only developmental delay and seizures occasionally respond favorably to treatment with vitamin cofactors for the glycine cleavage enzyme (e.g., folate, pyridoxine) and sodium benzoate to trap excess glycine as hippurate. Dextromethorphan given to block glycine activation of the neuronal glutamate N-methyl-D-aspartate (NMDA) receptors also has had some success in controlling seizures.

3-Phosphoglycerate dehydrogenase (3PGD) deficiency (MIM 601815) is a recently delineated disorder of serine biosynthesis with principal manifestations of seizures, global developmental delay, microcephaly, and low plasma and CSF levels of serine. Unlike most other amino acid disorders, 3PGD deficiency is a disorder of amino synthesis and, therefore, is treatable by dietary supplementation with serine and glycine. Unfortunately, this diagnosis has been missed in several children because of the inclination of clinicians to think of metabolic disease diagnosis only in terms of abnormally high values in amino acid and organic acid testing and to ignore results flagged as low.

Secondary Abnormalities of Amino Acid Metabolism

Abnormal levels of amino acids often are important markers for metabolic diseases that are not primary defects of amino acid metabolism. The most important of these is an absolutely or relatively increased level of alanine, which may indicate either high levels of pyruvate or high levels of ammonia. Similarly, secondarily increased levels of glycine are found in all hyperammonemic syndromes and in the several organic acidurias originally described as the "ketotic hyperglycinemias": propionic acidemia (MIM 232000), methylmalonic acidemia (MIM 251000), and isovaleric acidemia (MIM 243500).

Disorders of Organic Acid and Fatty Acid Metabolism

The introduction of clinical urinary organic acid analysis by gas chromatography–mass spectrometry (GC-MS) in the 1970s almost doubled the number of known inborn errors of metabolism within a decade. Today, urinary organic acid quantification is an essential component of metabolic testing for any child with an unexplained developmental disability. Table 5.7 lists some of the better-known organic acid disorders associated with developmental disability.

The classic description of an organic aciduria is that of a neonatal or infantile catastrophe with encephalopathy and metabolic acidosis; however, at least as many children with an organic aciduria present with nonacute signs—hypotonia, a movement disorder, or leukodystrophy—without metabolic acidosis. Although there may also be evidence of episodic worsen-

Table 5.7. Common disorders of organic acid metabolism

Disorders of branched-chain organic acid catabolism
Branched-chain 2-ketoacid dehydrogenase deficiency (maple syrup urine disease)
Isovaleryl-CoA dehydrogenase deficiency (isovaleric acidemia)
3-Methylglutaconic aciduria
    3-Methylglutaconyl-CoA hydratase deficiency
    Idiopathic (normal 3-methylglutaconyl-CoA hydratase activity)
Methylmalonic aciduria (several genetic forms)
Propionic acidemia

Disorders of fatty acid β-oxidation
Short-, medium-, and long-chain acyl-CoA dehydrogenase deficiency
Very-long-chain acyl-CoA dehydrogenase deficiency
Mitochondrial trifunctional enzyme deficiency
β-Ketothiolase deficiency
Multiple acyl-CoA dehydrogenase deficiency (type II glutaric aciduria)
Carnitine plasmalemmal transporter deficiency
Acylcarnitine translocase deficiency

Other organic acidurias
Biotinidase and holocarboxylase synthase deficiencies
Glutaryl-CoA dehydrogenase deficiency (type I glutaric aciduria)
L-2-hydroxyglutaric aciduria

Key: CoA, coenzyme A.

ing with protein-enriched foods, fevers, or viral infections, all of which increase amino acid catabolism and overload the limited catabolic pathway, a clear history of protein avoidance is less common for an organic aciduria than for a urea cycle defect. Furthermore, because there appears to be a window of vulnerability for metabolic brain injury during early childhood in several organic acidurias, affected older children whose critical injury may have occurred subclinically as infants are sometimes found in cerebral palsy clinics, especially among patients with extrapyramidal cerebral palsy.

As discussed previously, this is particularly true for type I glutaric aciduria (glutaryl-CoA dehydrogenase deficiency; MIM 231670), in which acute or subacute injury to the caudate and putamen never occurs after the age of 3 years, even when there is severe metabolic decompensation. Surprisingly, intellect can be largely spared, even superior, in a child who has severe physical disability caused by glutaric aciduria or several similar organic acidurias. Nonprogressive, dystonic cerebral palsy also is common among injured children with methylmalonic aciduria (MIM 251000), which damages the globus pallidi, again usually sparing the intellect, but primary disorders of mitochondrial energy metabolism are more common causes of dystonic cerebral palsy. The mildest cases of these organic acidurias may be found among children with attention deficit disorder, poor fine motor skills, and mild extrapyramidal abnormalities.

Special attention should be paid to the collectively large group of patients with increased urinary excretion of 3-methylglutaconic acid. A few children with this abnormality have a primary deficiency of leucine catabolism (3-methylglutaconyl-CoA hydratase deficiency; MIM 250950) and usually present during childhood with mild to moderate speech delay and, less commonly, episodic metabolic illness. These patients are distinguished from those with other genetic forms of 3-methylglutaconic aciduria by the associated increased excretion of 3-hydroxyisovaleric acid.

A much larger number of patients have leucine-independent 3-methylglutaconic aciduria and one of several different phenotypes with, variably, hypotonia, neutropenia, optic atrophy, hypomyelination, myopathy, cardiomyopathy, growth failure, choreoathetosis, and moderate to severe developmental delays. On further investigation, most of these patients are found to have evidence of abnormal mitochondrial energy metabolism, although the specific genetic lesion often remains undetermined. As a result, 3-methylglutaconic aciduria without accompanying 3-hydroxyisovaleric aciduria should be viewed as a diagnostic marker for mitochondrial disease in the same way that increased blood or CSF lactate levels are. The two best characterized syndromes with leucine-independent 3-methylglutaconic aciduria are X-linked recessive Barth syndrome (dilated cardiomyopathy, skeletal myopathy, neutropenia, and growth retardation; MIM 302060), caused by a defect in mitochondrial phospholipid synthesis, and autosomal recessive Costeff syndrome (optic atrophy, ataxia, progressive spasticity, and Iraqi Jewish heritage; MIM 258501), resulting from mutations in OPA3, a small gene of unknown function.

Defects of mitochondrial fatty acid β-oxidation constitute another relatively common group of disorders that may come to medical attention because of hypotonia and motor delay rather than their better-known presentation as hypoketotic hypoglycemia, cardiomyopathy, and progressive liver disease. Whereas some of the disorders, such as very-long-chain acyl-CoA dehydrogenase (VLCAD) deficiency (MIM 201475) and long-chain 3-hydroxyacyl-CoA dehydrogenase (LCHAD) deficiency (MIM 609016), may manifest hypotonia and cardiomyopathy at birth, others—including the most common, medium-chain acyl-CoA dehydrogenase (MCAD) deficiency (MIM 201450)—may present in later childhood as hypotonia, motor delay, and "systemic carnitine deficiency." VLCAD and LCHAD deficiencies also commonly present as progressive hepatocellular disease. Classic multiple acyl-CoA dehydrogenase (MAD) deficiency (MIM 130410, 231675), also called "type II glutaric aciduria," is caused by a deficiency of one of two electron acceptors for all mitochondrial acyl-CoA dehydrogenases. MAD deficiency therefore combines blocks in several fatty acyl-CoA dehydrogenases with those of the branched-chain acyl-CoA dehydrogenase and is the only β-oxidation disorder with prenatal involvement of the central nervous system, including, in its more severe forms, cerebral dysgenesis not unlike Zellweger syndrome. Fortunately, almost all fatty acid oxidation disorders and most of the common organic acidurias can now be detected presymptomatically by acylcarnitine newborn screening using tandem mass spectrometry (TMS).

Although the addition of TMS to newborn screening in many states has prevented much injury through early detection and treatment of metabolic disease, TMS also detects metabolic defects of uncertain clinical significance and labels newborns who may have no increased risk for injury. The two most important diagnoses in this group are short-chain acyl-CoA dehydrogenase (SCAD) deficiency (MIM 201470), a fatty acid oxidation defect, and 3-methylcrotonyl-CoA carboxylase (3MCC) deficiency (MIM 210200), a defect in the leucine catabolic pathway. Many asymptomatic adults with normal physical and mental development and biochemically severe 3MCC deficiency have now been found, mostly mothers whose own abnormal metabolites were found in their infants' blood at the time of newborn screening. Also apparent is that most individuals with SCAD deficiency have a metabolic disorder but not a metabolic disease and that the attribution of the cause of pathology to the metabolic disorders in historically identified patients with SCAD deficiency or 3MCC deficiency was incorrect. As yet unresolved is whether or not there are special conditions under which these disorders will cause brain injury or otherwise impair development. Another disorder detected by TMS in this uncertain disease category is 3-methylglutaconyl-CoA hydratase deficiency.

Episodic symptoms—irritability, vomiting, and morning lethargy—caused by abnormal fatty acid metabolism after simple fasting or during illness-induced fasting are common to most fatty acid oxidation defects. Therefore, specific questions should be asked about morning symptoms and response to illnesses when considering a fatty acid oxidation disorder and most of the more common organic acidurias. A marked, unexplained medium-chain dicarboxylic aciduria also is common in infantile

spinal muscular atrophy and other neuromuscular disorders associated with profound muscle hypoplasia or muscle wasting. This same group of disorders and any chronic debilitating condition or nutritional disorder that leads to severe muscle wasting can manifest a syndrome of hyperketosis, hypoglycemia, and cyclic vomiting, a condition that is often mistaken for a primary metabolic disease or "ketotic hypoglycemia." The primary pathology in these children is suppression of insulin synthesis because of inadequate muscle mass for gluconeogenesis. Although muscle protein catabolism is a normal physiological adaptation for maintenance of blood glucose levels during normal overnight fasting, the same process leads to maladaptation to longer periods of fasting and lack of regulation of free fatty acid release if muscle mass is too limited to supply adequate amounts of amino acids for gluconeogenesis. Treatment is provision of an intravenous insulin infusion with glucose for acute attacks and bedtime cornstarch, a higher protein diet, and more exercise, if possible, for restoration of normal glucose-insulin homeostasis.

Biotinidase deficiency (MIM 253260) is a well-known organic acid disorder caused by defective recycling of biotin, resulting in deficiencies of four biotin-dependent mitochondrial carboxylases: propionyl-CoA carboxylase (MIM 232000), acetyl-CoA carboxylase (MIM 200350, 601557), methylcrotonyl-CoA carboxylase (MIM 210200), and pyruvate carboxylase (MIM 266150). Although some children with biotinidase deficiency present with the classic combination of developmental delay, dermatitis, alopecia, seizures, acidosis, and a characteristic organic aciduria, others will manifest only seizures or hypotonia and have normal urinary organic acid profiles. This is because the postnatally acquired deficiency of biotin is typically manifest first in the central nervous system. Treatment with 10 mg biotin daily is simple and effective.

Lactic Acidoses and Other Disorders of Mitochondrial Metabolism

Lactic acidemia and aciduria are important markers for a large number of diseases, most of which are caused by defects of mitochondrial energy metabolism or gluconeogenesis. Although many diseases of amino acid and organic acid metabolism are caused by the deficiency of a mitochondrial matrix enzyme, the term *mitochondrial disease* implies a fundamental defect of energy metabolism, the electron transport chain, or the citric acid cycle (Table 5.8). The clinical and metabolic manifestations of mitochondrial disorders are protean.

Although some children with mitochondrial disorders have lethal or life-threatening lactic acidosis in the newborn period, most affected children come to medical attention for nonspecific problems, such as developmental delay, failure to thrive, hypotonia, seizures, and developmental regression. Common clinical phenotypes include intermittent ataxia, Leigh's disease, MELAS (mitochondrial myopathy, encephalopathy, lactic acidosis, and stroke-like episodes) syndrome (MIM 540000), Pearson syndrome (MIM 557000), progressive myoclonus, Alpers cerebrohepatic syndrome (MIM 203700), and renal tubular acidosis. As in many organic acidurias and urea cycle defects, episodic crises may occur, especially with defects that impair gluconeo-

genesis, such as pyruvate carboxylase deficiency (MIM 266150) and fructose-1,6-bisphosphatase deficiency (MIM 229700). Seizures, progressive microccphaly, and developmental regression are common, but many children with lactic acidoses have intermittent, limited problems and can lead relatively normal lives throughout childhood. At institutions that specialize in the diagnosis and treatment of developmental delay, autism, and cerebral palsy, disorders of mitochondrial energy metabolism account for the largest fraction of diagnosable genetic causes of developmental disabilities.

Three major problems are associated with the diagnosis and treatment of mitochondrial diseases: 1) the primary genetic defect causing unmistakable mitochondrial disease often remains unknown despite exhaustive testing, 2) biochemical evidence for a mitochondrial disease may be missed because of intermittent abnormalities or a biochemical deficiency limited to the central nervous system, and 3) treatment of mitochondrial disease is often unsuccessful. Because mitochondrial function varies substantially with nutrition, biochemical testing for mitochondrial diseases requires careful timing of specimen collection—lactate, pyruvate, amino acids, and organic acids—to assure capturing a diagnostic abnormality. Fortunately, molecular testing is able to identify an increasing number of point mutations causing mitochondrial disorders, such as MELAS syndrome (mtDNA A3243G); MERRF (myoclonic epilepsy associated with ragged-red fibers) syndrome (mtDNA A8344G; MIM 545000); and NARP (neuropathy, ataxia, and retinitis pigmentosa) (mtDNA T8993G; MIM 551500), a common cause of Leigh's disease (subacute necrotizing encephalomyopathy).

Not infrequently, children with progressive mitochondrial syndromes such as Leigh's disease and MELAS syndrome will be followed for a number of years for ''cerebral palsy'' or other apparently static developmental disorders before signs of deterioration and brain lesions develop. Although treatment of mitochondrial diseases once was rarely successful, 30 years of treatment experimentation and new knowledge about the role of free radical damage in the progression of mitochondrial

Table 5.8. Mitochondrial diseases

Single enzyme deficiency syndromes
Pyruvate dehydrogenase deficiency
Pyruvate carboxylase deficiency
Fumarase deficiency
2-Ketoglutarate dehydrogenase deficiency
Dihydrolipoyl dehydrogenase deficiency (multiple 2-ketoacid dehydrogenase deficiency)

Electron transport chain defects
Succcinate dehydrogenase (complex II) deficiency
NADH-dehydrogenase/complex I deficiency
Complex III deficiency
Cytochrome-*c* oxidase (complex IV) deficiency
ATP synthase (complex V) deficiency

Mitochondrial deficiency syndromes
Leigh's disease
Kearns-Sayre syndrome
Pearson marrow–pancreas syndrome
MELAS syndrome (mitochondrial myopathy, encephalopathy, lactic acidosis, and stroke-like episodes)
MERRF syndrome (myoclonic epilepsy associated with ragged-red fibers)
NARP (neuropathy, ataxia, and retinitis pigmentosa)

diseases have substantially increased the chance of success, especially for children who develop normally for the first few years. Nevertheless, the management of a child with a mitochondrial disorder remains complex and usually requires the combined efforts of a pediatrician, neurologist, and metabolic specialist.

Peroxisomal Diseases

Peroxisomal diseases are characterized by the deficiency of one or more enzymes localized to the peroxisome, a small subcellular organelle. In the most severe peroxisomal diseases—Zellweger syndrome (MIM 214100), neonatal adrenoleukodystrophy (MIM 202370), and infantile Refsum disease (MIM 266510)—an apparent complete absence of intact peroxisomes is associated with a large number of diagnostically useful biochemical abnormalities. Although classic Zellweger syndrome is a multiple congenital anomaly syndrome diagnosable by physical examination alone, children with milder peroxisomal deficiency syndromes may have only nonspecific physical anomalies and must be identified by biochemical testing. Collectively, the peroxisomal diseases are not uncommon causes of severe congenital hypotonia, intractable neonatal seizures, progressive liver disease, pigmentary retinopathy, sensorineural deafness, and adrenal insufficiency. The combination of any two of these problems should prompt biochemical testing for a peroxisomal disease. In addition, X-linked adrenoleukodystrophy (XALD; MIM 300100) and its adult form, adrenomyeloneuropathy (AMN), also are caused by the deficiency of a peroxisomal protein, one that appears to be required for oxidation of very-long-chain fatty acids. In both XALD and AMN, there are variable combinations of adrenal insufficiency (Addison's disease), peripheral neuropathy, and leukodystrophy. New-onset behavior problems, gait problems, and auditory/visual problems in a previously normal male child, especially between the ages of 5 and 10 years, should suggest XALD.

Molecular studies in the 1990s delineated two separate peroxisomal enzyme import systems whose mutated protein products account for most of the known peroxisomal disorders. A deficiency of any component of peroxisomal targeting system 1 (PTS1), which is responsible for the uptake of most peroxisomal enzymes, causes Zellweger syndrome or other generalized peroxisomal diseases, whereas a deficiency of a component of peroxisomal targeting system 2 (PTS2), which transports a much smaller ensemble of enzymes, causes rhizomelic chondrodysplasia punctata (RCDP; MIM 215100) and its milder variants. The spectrum of peroxisomal disorders has now expanded to include many diseases caused by a deficiency of a single peroxisomal enzyme with phenotypes overlapping with peroxisomal disorders caused by a deficiency of the PTS1 or PTS2 enzyme import systems.

In the early years of peroxisomal diagnosis, almost all peroxisomal diseases identified were progressive, but variants with long survival and partially treatable deficiencies are now more commonly recognized. Whereas the primary biochemical defects in most peroxisomal disorders are not treatable, treatment of specific deficiencies that may occur, such as adrenal insufficiency and deficiency of essential fatty acids, can be beneficial.

Lysosomal Storage Diseases and Nonlysosomal Leukodystrophies

Lysosomal Storage Diseases Lysosomal storage diseases (Table 5.9) constitute a large group of disorders related by the lysosomal localization of their deficient enzymes. Because most lysosomal enzymes serve a degradative function in the cell, most lysosomal diseases are characterized by the intralysosomal storage of cellular by-products, such as complex membrane lipids and mucopolysaccharides. Whereas in some disorders the pathogenesis of the disease is the mechanical effect of stored lysosomal material on the involved tissue, in others the disease process reflects a discrete toxicity of the accumulated metabolites. For example, some of the severe neurological effects of Tay-Sachs disease (MIM 272800) and other gangliosidoses have been attributed to the effect of abnormal gangliosides on neurotransmitter receptors, for which gangliosides have important structural roles.

Table 5.9. Lysosomal storage diseases

Disease class	Examples
Mucopolysaccharidoses	Sanfilippo syndrome (MPS III), Hurler syndrome (MPS I H), Hunter syndrome (MPS II)
Oligosaccharidoses	Mannosidosis Fucosidosis
Sphingolipidoses	Tay-Sachs disease; Gaucher disease Niemann-Pick disease GM_1 gangliosidosis
Leukodystrophies	Metachromatic leukodystrophy Krabbe disease (globoid cell leukodystrophy)
Sialidoses	Neuraminidase deficiency Combined neuraminidase/β-galactosidase deficiency
Glycogen storage diseases	Acid maltase deficiency (Pompe disease) Lysosomal glycogen storage with normal acid maltase level

Like most categories of metabolic diseases, lysosomal storage diseases are individually rare but collectively common as genetic causes of severe motor and mental disability with developmental regression at some stage of the disease; however, steady developmental progress can be achieved for many years before developmental stagnation or loss of skills ensues. In retrospect, most of these children will have had some physical signs of storage from an earlier age. Although not every child with unexplained developmental delay need have exhaustive testing for storage diseases, careful consideration of storage diseases should be incorporated into the physical examination.

Several storage diseases commonly present with apparently isolated developmental delay, behavior problems, or gait disturbances. Sanfilippo syndrome (mucopolysaccharidosis [MPS] III; MIM 252900, 252920, 252930, 252940) is a group of mucopolysaccharidoses that often have minimal visceral storage and facial coarsening, which can be difficult to appreciate in the first several years. Motor development can be normal, but language acquisition usually is very delayed and behavior hyperactive. Other MPS disorders, such as Hunter syndrome (MPS II; MIM 309900) and Hurler syndrome (MPS I H; MIM 252800), are more readily recognized because of visceromegaly and more obvious coarsened facial features. Some children with neuronopathic Gaucher disease (MIM 230800) may lack the characteristic hepatosplenomegaly yet present in the first year with delayed development, hypotonia, oculomotor abnormalities, and dys-

phagia and other signs of bulbar dysfunction. Similarly, some children with Niemann-Pick disease type C (MIM 257220), a disorder of intracellular cholesterol trafficking, may lack hepatosplenomegaly and present instead with dystonia, seizures, and failure of upward gaze, the most characteristic neurological sign. With effective screening of Ashkenazic Jewish and at-risk populations, classic Tay-Sachs disease (GM_2 gangliosidosis; MIM 272800) of the young infant is now much less common than it once was. As a result, a higher proportion of cases of GM_2 gangliosidosis now present in other ethnic groups, later in the first decade with developmental stagnation, and in the early adult years as a form of motor neuron disease. The biochemically related disease GM_1 gangliosidosis (MIM 230500), caused by lysosomal β-galactosidase deficiency, combines neurological features of Tay-Sachs disease with visceral storage and erosive skeletal disease; however, GM_1 gangliosidosis also is one of the most variable storage diseases and may have no findings outside the central nervous system.

Another important group of lysosomal storage diseases are the oligosaccharidoses, principally α-mannosidosis (MIM 248500), β-mannosidosis (MIM 248510), and α-fucosidosis (MIM 230000). These diseases have many features in common with the mucopolysaccharidoses—psychomotor retardation, coarse facial features, organomegaly, and dysostosis multiplex—but have negative mucopolysaccharide spot tests and a wide range of clinical expression. Patients with α- or β-mannosidosis may not develop significant disabilities until the second or third decade, nor do affected patients always have a neurodegenerative phase.

Neuraminidase deficiency (mucolipidosis type I [ML I]; MIM 256550) is one of a group of diseases, the sialidoses, that resemble the mucopolysaccharidoses. As in mucopolysaccharide disorders, sialidoses feature psychomotor retardation, coarse facies, and hepatosplenomegaly but also have cherry-red maculae and myoclonic seizures, not typically found in mucopolysaccharidoses. Because myoclonic seizures can be the only clinical sign, testing for the sialidoses is integral to the evaluation of children with myoclonic seizures and complicated or refractory seizure disorders. An important related disease is a deficiency of the sialic acid transporter SLC17A5, which combines intralysosomal storage of sialic acid with increased urinary excretion of sialic acid, the most useful marker for laboratory diagnosis. The severe form, infantile sialic acid storage disease (MIM 269920), features marked visceral storage or even fetal hydrops in addition to seizures and other signs of major central nervous system maldevelopment and damage. The milder variants, collectively called Salla disease (MIM 604369), extend to a phenotype of simple developmental delay with minimal facial coarsening or visceral storage. A distinctive feature that can develop in all forms of sialic acid storage disease is marked hypointensity of white matter, including the U fibers, which are spared in most leukodystrophies.

Two other lipidoses, ML II and ML III (MIM 252500), are caused by, respectively, severe and mild deficiencies of an enzyme that glycosylates many different lysosomal enzymes with mannose 6-phosphate, which serves as a targeting signal for lysosomal uptake of the tagged enzyme. ML II and ML III, therefore, are characterized by deficiencies of multiple lysosomal enzymes and the expected clinical sequelae. The clinical presentation is similar to that of a mucopolysaccharidosis except that tight skin, "clawhand," and progressive joint contractures often dominate. ML II, also known as "I-cell disease," is an infantile disease, whereas ML III usually has an onset beyond infancy. Like the oligosaccharidoses, the mucolipidoses have characteristic excretion patterns of oligosaccharides or sialylated oligosaccharides that can be identified by thin-layer chromatography or by their characteristic appearance as storage material on rectal or conjunctival tissue biopsy. The diagnoses are confirmed by enzymatic assay in plasma or cultured fibroblasts.

Leukodystrophies Leukodystrophies have often been grouped with the lysosomal storage diseases because two of the first leukodystrophies to be delineated biochemically, metachromatic leukodystrophy (MIM 250100) and globoid cell leukodystrophy (Krabbe disease; MIM 245200), are caused by lysosomal storage of complex lipids. Most of the more recently biochemically defined leukodystrophies, however, such as Canavan disease (MIM 271900), L-2-hydroxyglutaric aciduria (MIM 236792), and Salla disease, are abnormalities of small, soluble metabolites (Table 5.10). As disorders that affect primarily white matter, leukodystrophies often present first with long tract signs and other motor disabilities rather than the early cognitive failure and seizures common to many other metabolic diseases that affect the brain.

Metachromatic leukodystrophy and globoid cell leukodystrophy (Krabbe disease), two well-known white matter storage diseases, usually present in the first or second year as rapidly progressive diseases with loss of motor milestones, irritability, intermittent fevers, and blindness. Later onset forms of both diseases, however, sometimes come to medical attention because of school problems, changes in personality, and gait disturbances, followed only later by losses of motor and cognitive abilities. Such a period of "soft" neurological signs may last for several years in cases that present in later childhood or the teenage years. Adult cases have been found among patients with psychosis or dementia. Although tissue sampling will show storage material characteristic of the disorder, most cases now are identified by enzymatic analysis of peripheral white cells. Krabbe disease is also distinguished by very high levels of CSF protein, pleocytosis, and, occasionally, calcification of the basal ganglia.

XALD, although not a lysosomal storage disease, involves the storage of complex lipids, including very-long-chain fatty acids, in the

Table 5.10. Principal childhood leukodystrophies

Disorder	Protein deficiency	Metabolite excess
Metachromatic leukodystrophy	Arylsulfatase A	Cerebroside sulfate
Krabbe disease	Galactocerebrosidase	Galactosylceramides
X-linked adrenoleukodystrophy (ALD)	ALD protein	Very-long-chain fatty acids
Pelizeaus-Merzbacher disease	Proteolipid protein	None
Canavan disease	Aspartoacylase	N-acetyl-L-aspartate
Sialic acid storage disease (Salla disease, sialuria)	Lysosomal sialic acid transporter (*SLC17A5*)	Sialic acid
Vanishing white matter disease and childhood ataxia with central hypomyelination	Translation initiation factor eIF2B subunits α, β, γ, δ, and ε	None
L-2-hydroxyglutaric aciduria	L-2-hydroxyglutaric acid dehydrogenase	L-2-hydroxyglutaric acid
Polyol leukoencephalopathy	Ribose-5-phosphate isomerase	Arabitol, ribitol, and other polyols and pentoses

cytoplasm of many cell types, including neurons and macrophages. Unlike most other leukodystrophies, however, central nervous system damage in the most severe "cerebral" form of the disease is mediated by an inflammatory process with white matter lesions reminiscent of multiple sclerosis. XALD typically has onset of gait disturbance, behavior problems, and hearing loss between 5 and 10 years but also presents as AMN, an adult-onset syndrome of peripheral neuropathy, spasticity, and variable adrenal insufficiency. Childhood XALD and adult AMN may also present as apparently isolated Addison's disease without neurological signs. Another X-linked recessive leukodystrophy, Pelizeaus-Merzbacher disease (MIM 312080), once thought to be a possible metabolic disorder, has now been shown to be caused by mutations of the proteolipid protein, an essential structural protein of central myelin. Other leukodystrophies doubtless will be assigned to defects in several other structural proteins, but there also remain many myelin-specific structural lipids for which metabolic defects have not been found. Among other important nonmetabolic leukodystrophies not considered in this chapter is vanishing white matter disease (MIM 603896), caused by mutations in one of five genes encoding the eIF2B transcription initiation complex.

Canavan disease, an unusual leukodystrophy most commonly found in children of Ashkenazic Jewish heritage, is characterized by developmental delay, hypotonia, optic atrophy, and macrocephaly. Canavan disease is one of a small number of leukodystrophies in which all of the white matter, including the subcortical U fibers, is abnormal on cranial magnetic resonance imaging (MRI). Involvement of the globus pallidus and thalamus also is seen in more advanced disease. Although most patients present with developmental delay and accelerated head growth shortly after birth or in early infancy, onset of the neurodegenerative phase of Canavan disease in later years in a child with mild developmental delays and no microcephaly also occurs. Canavan disease is caused by deficiency of the neuronal enzyme aspartoacylase, which deacetylates N-acetyl-L-aspartate. This leads to increased levels of N-acetyl-L-aspartate in all body fluids, which also allows simple definitive diagnosis by urinary organic acid analysis. Although the mechanism by which aspartoacylase deficiency leads to white matter disease is unknown, N-acetyl-L-aspartate may be a primary cerebral osmolyte, and the inability to regulate its levels may lead to increased brain water and the white matter changes on MRI.

L-2-hydroxyglutaric aciduria is a rare but distinctive metabolic disorder that presents as ataxia and mild to moderate developmental delay. Although the diagnostic metabolite, L-2-hydroxyglutaric acid, is indistinguishable by routine urinary organic acid GC-MS from D-2-hydroxyglutaric acid (MIM 600721), another cause of childhood encephalopathy, the finding on MRI of diffuse white matter hyperintensity out of proportion to the mildness of the neurological findings in effect establishes the diagnosis without need for chemical differentiation of the two stereoisomers of 2-hydroxyglutaric acid. Whereas some patients with L-2-hydroxyglutaric acid follow a slowly degenerative course of progressively severe ataxia, seizures, and cerebral and cerebellar atrophy, others have no seizures, show little progression, and develop steadily throughout childhood at a rate between 50% and 75% of normal. The biochemical origin of L-2-hydroxyglutaric acid is presumed to be 2-ketoglutaric acid, but both the primary enzymatic defect and the specific cause of the white matter abnormalities are unknown, and no effective therapy has been found.

Ribose-5-phosphate isomerase deficiency (MIM 608611), a recently identified metabolic leukodystrophy, is a defect in the pentose phosphate shunt that blocks the interconversion of ribose 5-phosphate and ribulose 5-phosphate and shunts five-carbon aldoses into the synthesis of ribitol and D-arabitol. The single known patient had global developmental delay, seizures at age 4, regression by age 7, and a physical examination notable for spasticity, cerebellar ataxia, optic atrophy, and a sensorimotor peripheral neuropathy. By MRI there was extensive T2 hyperintensity of all white matter, including the U fibers, and, by magnetic resonance spectroscopy (MRS), large peaks of the two pentitols were identified. The very high total level of ribitols in brain suggests that the white matter abnormalities are osmotic in nature, although a toxic disruption of myoinositol regulatory pathways by the pentitols also is possible. This is the first of potentially many disorders of ribose and polyol metabolism, some of which could have similar effects on white matter.

In addition to what may be called the primary metabolic leukodystrophies listed in Table 5.10, both peroxisomal disorders and mitochondrial diseases should be remembered as causes of a leukodystrophy that dominates both the clinical and MRI findings. This is particularly true of mitochondrial diseases, in which the MRI abnormalities can vary from multiple lesions of different sizes and ages in the subcortical white matter, to extensive changes in the centrum semiovale, and to diffuse hyperintensity of most of the central white matter reminiscent of adrenoleukodystrophy or metachromatic leukodystrophy. The finding of basal ganglial involvement or, in more recent years, increased lactate levels by brain MRS, points out the true nature of the disease, although abnormal MRS lactate peaks can also appear in active areas of white matter damage in nonmitochondrial leukodystrophies. The combination of white matter disease of both cerebral and cerebellar white matter, especially when accompanied by cerebellar atrophy, should suggest a mitochondrial disease. Maternally inherited mtDNA mutations such as mtDNA A3243G (MELAS syndrome) and mtDNA G11778A (Leber hereditary optic neuropathy [LHON]; MIM 535000), de novo mtDNA deletions (Kearns-Sayre syndrome; MIM 530000), and mutations of nuclear-encoded mitochondrial enzymes have been found in cases of white matter–predominant mitochondrial disease. In addition to peroxisomal X-linked ALD or neonatal adrenoleukodystrophy (NALD), a number of patients with generalized peroxisomal diseases somewhat less severe than Zellweger syndrome carried the diagnosis of NALD in the years before the recognition that such patients all had mutations allelic with Zellweger syndrome PTS1 mutations.

Disorders of Sterol Biosynthesis

Although SLOS (MIM 270400) was known for the first 30 years as an autosomal recessive, multiple malformation syndrome with principal findings of cleft palate, polydactyly, ambiguous genitalia, and characteristic facies, the discovery in 1993 that SLOS is caused by a primary defect of cholesterol biosynthesis allowed the biochemical identification of mildly affected SLOS patients with no malformations and minimally dysmorphic facies. The recognized spectrum of SLOS is now continuous, from a lethal prenatal malformation syndrome to a few normal-appearing individuals with mild developmental delays and a behavior disorder. Also important has been the recognition that the behavioral and personal-social deficits in children with SLOS fulfill criteria for autism and that cholesterol supplementation of affected children often eliminates their autistic behaviors. As a result, developmental pediatricians are now including testing for SLOS in the evaluation of minimally dysmorphic patients with developmental delays and autistic spectrum behaviors.

Important diagnostic findings in many of the mildly affected children with SLOS are congenital microcephaly, 2/3 toe syndactyly, oral and tactile hypersensitivities, feeding disorders, short tempers, and sleep disturbances. With rare exceptions, even the most mildly affected children will have diagnostic abnormalities by GC-MS analysis of plasma sterols, which shows increased levels of 7-dehydrocholesterol and 8-dehydrocholesterol resulting from a deficiency of 7-dehydrocholesterol reductase, the last step in cholesterol biosynthesis. With an incidence of 1 in 40,000 births, SLOS is one of the more common genetic developmental disorders, although only about 20% of patients are not easily recognized by their typical facial appearance and characteristic malformations.

In contrast to most metabolic diseases, which are manifest only after metabolic compensation afforded by the maternal circulation is lost at birth, SLOS is one of few metabolic diseases wherein pathology is caused by the inability of the fetus to make adequate amounts of an essential metabolite, cholesterol, that cannot be supplied in sufficient amounts by the mother. Both clinical and experimental studies indicate that almost all of the physical and functional abnormalities of SLOS are caused by the deficiency of cholesterol and not toxicity of 7-dehydrocholesterol and 8-dehydrocholesterol. Because genetic deficiencies of other steps in cholesterol biosythesis also should cause a prenatal cholesterol deficiency syndrome, perhaps resembling SLOS, other SLOS-like conditions were tested for defects of cholesterol biosynthesis and three other disorders were identified. These are desmosterolosis, caused by desmosterol reductase (DHCR24; MIM 602398) deficiency; lathosterolosis, caused by sterol C5-desaturase (SC5DL; MIM 607330) deficiency; and males with hypomorphic mutations of the gene encoding X-linked sterol isomerase (EBP; MIM 302960). Females with sterol isomerase deficiency have a very different, asymmetrically expressed disorder known as Conradi-Hünermann syndrome, or X-linked dominant chondrodysplasia punctata. Although each of these four disorders has anomalies that overlap with those of SLOS, each also has distinctive abnormalities that would not usually be recognized as part of a sterol malformation syndrome, as listed in Table 5.11. All of these disorders can be diagnosed by GC-MS analysis of plasma sterols.

Disorders of Vitamin and Mineral Metabolism with Developmental Disabilities

Most vitamins serve as prosthetic groups for enzyme proteins that have no enzymatic function in the absence of the vitamin. Vitamin-dependent metabolic diseases can be divided as those wherein pharmacological amounts of the natural vitamin can stabilize or otherwise increase the residual activity of a mutant enzyme and those caused by a primary defect in vitamin transport or the conversion of a vitamin into its active form. The best known example of the former is pyridoxine (vitamin B_6)–responsive homocystinuria, and of the latter, biotinidase deficiency (MIM 253260). Although most vitamins have been known as essential nutrients having many effects on brain metabolism for more than 50 years, still relatively few genetic disorders of vitamin metabolism are known. In addition to biotinidase deficiency, described previously under disorders of organic acid metabolism, two recently delineated disorders of vitamin metabolism include a biotin-responsive form of basal ganglial disease (MIM 607483) and the syndrome of deafness, diabetes, and thiamine-responsive megaloblastic anemia (MIM 249270) caused by a defect of thiamine transport (SLC 19A2).

Other Neurometabolic Diseases

Defects of Neurotransmitter Metabolism

Abnormalities of neurotransmitter metabolism are an emerging group of diseases associated with developmental disabilities, neurologic dysfunction, and seizures. In addition to abnormalities of biogenic amine synthesis caused by defects of biopterin metabolism

Table 5.11. Disorders of cholesterol biosynthesis

Disorder	Enzyme deficiency	Principal abnormalities
Mevalonic aciduria	Mevalonate kinase	Hepatosplenomegaly, fevers, facial dysmorphism
Hyperimmunoglobulinemia D syndrome	Mevalonate kinase (mild)	Recurrent fevers and adenopathy, normal cognition, autism
Smith-Lemli-Opitz syndrome	7-Dehydrocholesterol reductase	Characteristic facial dysmorphism, microcephaly, cleft palate, polydactyly, hypospadias, short stature, 2/3 toe syndactyly
Desmosterolosis	Sterol Δ^{24}-reductase	Severe microcephaly, agenesis corpus callosum, severe intellectual disabilities
Greenberg dysplasia	Sterol Δ^{14}-reductase (severe)	Severe short-limbed dwarfism, "moth-eaten" skeletal dysplasia
Pelger-Huët anomaly	Sterol Δ^{14}-reductase (mild)	Undersegmented neutrophils, mild skeletal dysplasia, hand anomalies, short stature
Conradi-Hünermann syndrome (CDPX2)	Sterol Δ^8-isomerase	Ichthyosiform erythroderma, chondrodysplasia punctata, X-linked dominant inheritance
CHILD syndrome (NSDHL)	Sterol 4-demethylase (β-hydroxysteroid dehydrogenase subunit)	Asymmetric skeletal defects, psoriasiform skin lesions, X-linked dominant inheritance
Antley-Bixler syndrome	Lanosterol 14α-methyl oxidase (caused by p450 oxidoreductase deficiency)	Multiple craniosynostoses, bowed femora, femoral fractures, ambiguous genitalia

and manifest as variant PKU, three other defects of biogenic amine metabolism have been described. A deficiency of aromatic pyridoxine–dependent L-amino acid decarboxylase is associated with hypotonia, psychomotor retardation, and oculogyric spells in infancy. A deficiency of dopamine β-hydroxylase (MIM 223360) limits norepinephrine synthesis, causing orthostatic hypotension in adults and ptosis, hypotonia, and hypoglycemia in infancy and childhood. Cognitive function is normal. The third disorder is a deficiency of X-linked monoamine oxidase-A (MIM 309850), which is required for catabolism of serotonin and catecholamines. Affected young boys have mild psychomotor retardation, whereas adolescent boys and adult men manifest stereotypical hand movements and aggressive and violent behaviors. All three disorders can be diagnosed by measuring CSF levels of biogenic amines and related metabolites.

Congenital Disorders of Glycosylation: Carbohydrate-Deficient Glycoprotein Syndromes
Congenital disorders of glycosylation (CDG) constitute a relatively new group of diseases associated with hypotonia, psychomotor retardation, and diagnostically important abnormalities of plasma protein glycosylation. Among the originally identified patients, most of whom are now classified as CDG-Ia, affected children are noted for having hypotonia, growth retardation, developmental delays, and a number of unusual physical findings, including nipple inversion, cardiomyopathy, and a distinctive pattern of enlarged fat pads in the nuchal, perineal, and upper ischial areas. Among the first patients identified, the disease was progressive and sometimes fatal; however, as in most metabolic disorders, definitive biochemical diagnosis and mutation analysis have allowed the identification of milder CDG-Ia variants with nonprogressive disease as well as at least a dozen other clinically overlapping genetic disorders of both O-glycosylation and N-glycosylation.

With the extraordinary variety of glycolsylated proteins affecting essentially all systems in the body, the clinical and physiological signs of CGDs are protean. More than 95% of patients with well-defined disorders of glycosylation, however, are classed as either CDG-Ia (phosphomannomutase 2 deficiency; MIM 212065) or the similar but milder CDG-Ic (glucosyltransferase I deficiency; MIM 603147). In its classic form, CDG-Ia is readily diagnosed clinically, with most of the important diagnostic signs appearing at birth. In addition to the abnormal fat pads, the phenotype of CDG-Ia includes global psychomotor retardation, axial hypotonia, seizures, esotropia, feeding problems, and failure to thrive. By the end of the first year, deep tendon reflexes are lost due to a peripheral neuropathy, and ataxia due to cerebellar atrophy has developed. Abnormal brain stem auditory evoked potentials also are common. Few children with CDG-Ia learn to walk or speak, and joint contractures, scoliosis, and marked osteopenia are common. Other abnormalities reported in a smaller number of CDG-Ia patients include congenital hydrops, hypertrophic cardiomyopathy, pericardial effusion, and microcystic kidneys. Mortality has been 20% in the first year, but relative clinical stabilization occurs thereafter. CDG-Ic is similar to CDG-Ia but is a milder disorder with hypotonia, seizures, and strabismus and lacks the characteristic physical and neurophysiological stigmata of CDG-Ia. In addition, unlike CDG-Ia, most CDG-Ic patients lean to walk and speak. Although only one tenth as many CDG-Ic cases as CDG-Ia cases have been reported, because of the milder and mostly nonspecific abnormalities of CDG-Ic, it is likely that a large proportion of CDG-Ic patients go unrecognized.

CDG-Ib, caused by phosphomannose isomerase deficiency (MIM 602579), is distinguished from CDG-Ia and CDG-Ic by having normal psychomotor development and a principally gastrointestinal presentation, including failure to thrive, chronic diarrhea, cyclic vomiting, protein-losing enteropathy, and intestinal villus atrophy resembling celiac disease. Other common abnormalities include hypoglycemia, hypoalbuminemia, and persistently elevated serum transaminases. Children with CDG-Ib have abnormalities of serum clotting proteins causing hypercoagulability, and they may first come to the attention of a developmental pediatrician for rehabilitation after suffering thrombotic strokes. Unlike other CDG syndromes, CDG-Ib can be treated with oral mannose. Diagnostic screening for all CDG syndromes is by serum transferrin isoelectrofocusing, which detects incompletely glycosylated transferrin isoforms.

Disorders of Creatine Synthesis and Transport Creatine is a small molecule that functions—in the form of creatine phosphate—as a carrier and reservoir for high-energy phosphates for ATP synthesis. Creatine is synthesized in the liver and pancreas from the guanidino group of arginine by a two-step enzymatic process via the intermediate, guanidinoacetate (GUAA). Creatine is then transported in high concentrations into tissues, principally the brain and muscle, that have high rates of ATP synthesis and utilization. The first disorder of creatine synthesis described was a deficiency of the second enzyme, guanidinoacetate methyltransferase (GAMT; MIM 601240), in a boy with early developmental arrest, severe choreoathetosis, intractable seizures, and lesions of the globus pallidus. He was found to have absent creatine and creatine phosphate by MRS, which led to testing for GUAA and GAMT deficiency. A milder phenotype of GAMT deficiency has since been described in several patients with only autism and speech delay.

The second described disorder of creatine metabolism, a deficiency of the X-linked creatine transporter (caused by mutations in *SLC6A8*), also results in absent brain creatine by MRS and a clinical disorder characterized by mild mental retardation, severe speech delay, and seizures. The mother and grandmother of the first reported patient both had a history of learning disability, a possible expression of heterozygous deficiency of the creatine transporter. More recently, a mutation analysis of 288 individuals with X-linked intellectual disabilities (XLID) found disabling mutations of *SLC6A8* in 6 patients (2.1%), which is a proportion among XLID similar to that of fragile X syndrome. The third creatine disorder, a deficiency of the first enzyme of the pathway, L-arginine:glycine amidinotransferase (AGAT; MIM 602360), and the rarest of the three disorders of creatine metabolism, is characterized by moderately severe psychomotor retardation, hypotonia, and autistic features including severe language delay, poor social interaction, and sterotypies. Fewer than 10 patients are known.

The essential characteristics of disorders of creatine metabolism include global psychomotor retardation, hypotonia, disproportionately severe language delay, autism spectrum disorder, and essential absence of brain creatine and creatine phosphate by MRS. GAMT deficiency stands apart from the other two defects by the frequent occurrence of difficult-to-control seizures, which are believed to be a toxic effect of the high level of GUAA. Patients at the mild end of the spectrum may not be distinguishable from those with nonmetabolic autism, although several unpublished surveys show that creatine deficiency is not a common cause of autism. Nevertheless, because both GAMT deficiency and AGAT deficiency can be treated with creatine supplements, the threshold for testing should be relatively low, and the increasing use of MRS for metabolic testing will doubtless aid in the detection of other clinical forms of these diseases. Screening for all three disorders of creatine metabolism requires measurement of plasma and urine levels of creatine, GUAA, and creatinine.

The Neuronal Ceroid Lipofuscinoses: Batten Disease   The neuronal ceroid lipofuscinoses (NCLs) are a group of neurodegenerative disorders originally defined by the intralysosomal storage of an autofluorescent, lipofuscin-like material in patients with the clinical constellation of seizures, blindness, and dementia. Often collected under the term *Batten disease*, these are largely late infantile and childhood diseases that begin with seizures before cognitive or visual changes are apparent, although most patients will have abnormal electroretinograms before the earliest sign of the disease. The three most common forms of NCL—infantile (CLN1; MIM 256730), late infantile (CLN2; MIM 204500), and juvenile (CLN3; MIM 204200)—are caused by defects in the lysosomal system for protein degradation. At least five other, rarer genetic forms of NCL have been defined. Whereas formerly the definitive diagnosis of a form of NCL required biopsy identification of the characteristic storage material, mutation analysis is now available for the most common forms. Mutation analysis has also revealed that the age of presentation does not necessarily correlate with mutations in the gene originally identified with a particular form of NCL.

Glucose Transporter Deficiency   Hypoglycorrhachia caused by heterozygous disabling mutations in the gene encoding the GLUT1 protein (*SLC2A1*), which transports glucose into the central nervous system, is a treatable but often missed cause of seizures, language delay, microcephaly, extrapyramidal abnormalities, and ataxia in children (MIM 606777). Patients have 50%–75% of the normal GLUT1 activity, depending on the residual activity of the mutant GLUT1 protein, and CSF glucose levels between 23 and 40 mg/dL. The average CSF glucose level in one series was 37% of the simultaneous blood glucose level, or about half the expected CSF glucose level. Although all GLUT1-deficient patients in the original series reported in 1991 had seizures, several more recently identified patients have had language disability, dystonia, and intermittent ataxia, but no seizures. Treatment is by the ketogenic diet, which allows the brain to derive most of its energy from fat-derived acetoacetate rather than glucose.

LABORATORY DIAGNOSIS OF INBORN ERRORS OF METABOLISM
General Principles

Although developmental pediatricians, primary care physicians, and others not trained in metabolic diseases cannot be expected to coordinate exhaustive testing for inborn errors of metabolism without the assistance of a biochemical geneticist, basic screening for inborn errors of metabolism should be incorporated into the initial laboratory evaluation of most patients with a developmental disability and an abnormal neurological examination. Fortunately for the general practitioner, most metabolic screening tests are now readily available from national reference laboratories. Because most of the more routine tests, such as amino acid quantification and blood acylcarnitine analysis, are standardized, the results from different laboratories usually are comparable. The national centralization of testing in the United States to a handful of large commercial laboratories, however, has come at the expense of the well-informed interpretation of the results once offered by many smaller laboratories at academic centers. Therefore, to make timely diagnoses and avoid wasteful testing, pediatricians and developmental specialists must develop access to specialists in metabolic diseases. Another important consideration is that the range and complexity of metabolic testing increases substantially every decade, along with the discovery of many new metabolic disorders. Therefore, a child with a developmental disability who had metabolic testing 5 or 10 years ago may need to be retested. For example, metabolic testing for congenital disorders of glycosylation and many of the more recently defined leukodystrophies was not available 10 years ago. Adding to the complexity of the metabolic evaluation is the need in some cases to test for a disorder by mutation analysis, which for most metabolic disorders has only limited availability in clinically certified laboratories.

Before embarking on the evaluation of a child for a metabolic disease, the physician should also consider two general principles of metabolic testing. The first is that a laboratory test designed to detect all cases of a disease usually will identify as abnormal a number of patients who are ultimately determined to have normal metabolism. Although the ideal laboratory test should have absolute sensitivity (no false negatives) and specificity (no false positives), in reality, most metabolic tests must allow a percentage of false positives to minimize the number of false negatives. If the normal range is defined as the 95% of test values surrounding the mean, then 2.5% of test results will fall above and 2.5% below the normal range. The majority of these ''abnormal'' results will reflect the extremes of normal physiology, not a pathological process. For a test that measures 20 or more compounds, such as amino acid chromatography, there is a substantial probability that at least one value will fall outside the 2.5%–97.5% range. Not all of these tests must be repeated if the abnormal result seems trivial and, often, changes relative to other values will help determine if an abnor-

mal result truly indicates disease. Repeat testing or consultation with a biochemical geneticist for interpretation is sometimes necessary, though.

The second principle of diagnostic testing for inborn errors of metabolism is that the diagnosis ideally should be established by two independent methods, one that reflects the abnormal physiology and a second that directly measures the genetic defect, such as an abnormal enzymatic assay or DNA mutation. The biochemical abnormality alone can be essentially diagnostic, such as combined glutaric and 3-hydroxyglutaric aciduria in type I glutaric aciduria, or diagnostic only of a group of diseases, such as lactic acidemia in many mitochondrial diseases. Despite recent impressive advances in genetic analysis, DNA testing will not soon, if ever, supplant physiological and enzymatic testing for biochemical diseases, largely because there often exists an unmanageable multiplicity of DNA mutations for a single disease, all of which lead to the same enzymatic or physiological abnormality, for which a diagnostic result can be available in 24 hours. For example, although many dozens of hexosaminidase mutations have been found, each of which can be useful for diagnosis and prenatal diagnosis in a particular family, a simple hexosaminidase assay remains the most reliable single test for Tay-Sachs disease in a new patient with an undiagnosed neurodegenerative process. The same is true for diagnosis and prenatal diagnosis of Smith-Lemli-Opitz syndrome, for which mutation analysis usually is needed only for counseling the extended family.

Conversely, there are occasional, but collectively many, patients whose metabolic diagnoses can be established unequivocally by a physiological or histological test, but in whom the corresponding enzymatic assay was normal or equivocal. For some of the false-negative enzymatic assays, the artificial substrate used for the assay is metabolized by a specific mutant enzyme but the slightly different natural substrate is not. In other cases, the growth conditions used for culturing cells prior to assay correct the defect. Thus, independent methods of diagnosis should be available to confirm diagnosis or to help interpret a confusing or inconsistent result.

Basic Tests and Methods of Specimen Collection

To allow optimal interpretation of test results, patient information to be submitted with urine, plasma, and other specimens for metabolic testing should include the following:

- Age, clinical diagnosis, and major clinical findings

- Time of collection, relationship to last meal (plasma), and whether a random or timed collection was made (urine)

- Acute or recovery specimen, if applicable

- Special diets: medium-chain triglyceride oil; elemental or protein hydrolysate formulas

- Any unusual diet or dietary supplements

- Intravenous glucose or hyperalimentation

- Concurrent or recent intravenous contrast study

- Medications, especially anticonvulsants

Basic metabolic testing for a child with otherwise nonspecific developmental disabilities should include both first-tier and second-tier tests (Table 5.12). The first-tier tests are broad screening studies that should diagnose more than 75% of patients with an identifiable metabolic disease and also provide useful information about a patient's physiological status, which may help guide further diagnostic testing. The first-tier tests also identify most potentially treatable metabolic diseases. The second-tier tests each screen for several rare disorders that may have relatively nonspecific physical findings. Only a few of these disorders are treatable.

In general, a preprandial specimen (at least 3 hours fasting) can be drawn for quantification of plasma amino acids, blood ammonia, blood lactate and pyruvate, plasma very-long-chain fatty acids, and sterol analysis. Urinary

Table 5.12.   Basic metabolic testing

First-tier tests

Plasma amino acid quantification

Urinary organic acid quantification by GC-MS

Blood acylcarnitine analysis by tandem mass spectrometry

Blood lactate and pyruvate levels

Blood ammonia quantification

Comprehensive metabolic profile with creatine kinase

Second-tier tests

CSF lactate, protein, and amino acid quantification

Urinary amino acid quantification

Urinary orotic acid quantification (as test for urea cycle defects)

Urinary urate-creatinine ratio (Lesch-Nyhan syndrome)

Plasma very-long-chain fatty acid quantification

Plasma 7-dehydrocholesterol and other sterol intermediate quantification

Urinary mucopolysaccharide quantification or electrophoresis

Urinary oligosaccharide and sialylated oligosaccharide chromatography

Urinary free sialic acid level

Combined urinary and plasma creatine and guanidinoacetate levels

Serum transferrin electrophoresis (glycosylation disorders)

Urinary sulfite

Key: GC-MS, gas chromatography with mass spectrophotometry detection; CSF, cerebrospinal fluid.

amino acid quantification has limited value unless an amino acid transport defect not detectable in plasma, such as lysinuric protein intolerance, is suspected. The finding of a severe generalized aminoaciduria, a marker for partial or complete renal Fanconi syndrome, can be diagnostically useful, however. A urine collection for measuring orotic acid and uric acid levels also can be useful for diagnosis of, respectively, urea cycle defects and Lesch-Nyhan syndrome. Quantification of the special amino acid pipecolic acid, in both plasma and urine, is an important confirmatory test for a generalized peroxisomal disorder and pyridoxine-dependent seizures but is available in only a few laboratories. Quantification of amino acids in CSF is most useful for diagnosis of nonketotic hyperglycinemia, defects of serine biosynthesis, and disorders of pyruvate dysmetabolism (high alanine level). Spinal fluid is also the specimen of choice for diagnosis of disorders of biogenic amine metabolism.

Diagnosis of Amino Acid and Organic Acid Disorders

Partial enzymatic deficiencies often require careful timing of specimen collection to obtain diagnostic metabolite levels—for example, drawing a 60- to 90-minute postprandial blood sample for ammonia and lactate, which may return to normal by 4 hours after a meal in patients with, respectively, partial ornithine transcarbamylase deficiency and a mild mitochondrial disorder. In addition, care should be taken to separate, freeze, and deliver plasma specimens for amino acid analysis as quickly as possible to avoid processing artifacts and missed diagnoses. Low, but nonetheless diagnostic, levels of free homocysteine can complex completely with protein sulfhydryls in blood within a few hours and essentially disappear from the free amino acid pool. The loss of homocysteine, deamidation of glutamine to glutamate, and other postcollection artifacts are among problems associated with sending plasma samples to central reference laboratories, which often adds 2 or 3 days to sample processing time.

If an amino acid–dependent organic aciduria is suspected and the baseline organic acid analysis is normal or equivocal, a 6-hour urine collection following a meal containing 1 g protein/kg should be submitted for organic acid gas chromatography. Conversely, some organic acid disorders, especially fatty acid oxidation defects, may not be evident in the urine until after 18–24 hours of fasting, when fluxes through amino acid oxidation, fatty acid oxidation, and gluconeogenic pathways increase substantially. Fasting a child for diagnostic purposes more than a few hours beyond the usual overnight fast is not always safe and, in general, should not be done outside the hospital or unsupervised by a metabolic specialist. Fortunately, even a 12-hour overnight fasting urine specimen often demonstrates sufficient changes to be diagnostic. A morning fasting urine specimen also reduces contamination of the urine with drug metabolites and dietary and intestinal bacterial by-products. All urinary organic acid studies should be performed quantitatively with mass spectrometry for definitive compound identification.

For both organic acid and amino acid quantification, the amounts of specific analytes relative to other metabolites often are more important than absolute levels. Low as well as high values can be diagnostically significant. For example, a child with arginase deficiency may have only a high-normal plasma arginine level, but the arginine-ornithine ratio may be diagnostically increased. The plasma glycine level in nonketotic hyperglycinemia may fall within the high-normal range, but the glycine-serine ratio may exceed 4:1 (normal < 3:1). Also, low metabolite levels, such as a low methionine level in several genetic forms of homocystinuria or low citrulline levels in females heterozygous for ornithine transcarbamylase deficiency, can be diagnostically very important.

Diagnosis of Peroxisomal Diseases

The measurement of increased plasma levels of very-long-chain fatty acids (VLCFAs) is the most convenient screening test for most peroxisomal diseases. Other tests of peroxisomal function, such as levels of pipecolic acid and phytanic acid in plasma, levels of plasmalogens in red blood cells, and several assays in cultured fibroblasts, can be obtained for diagnosis of several less-common forms of peroxisomal disease in which the levels of VLCFAs are normal. For example, patients with classic rhizomelic chondrodysplasia punctata, caused by mutations in the PEX7 gene, which encodes the PTS2 receptor, and those with milder variants who might be evaluated for mild dysmorphism and idiopathic developmental delay, require measurement of red blood cell plasmalogen levels for diagnosis because VLCFA metabolism is normal.

Diagnosis of Lysosomal Storage Diseases

For analysis of neutral oligosaccharides, sialylated oligosaccharides, and mucopolysaccharides, a 24-hour urine collection is preferred. Separate screening tests are required for oligosaccharidoses (thin-layer chromatography), mucopolysaccharidoses (electrophoresis), and the sialidoses and related defects of sialic acid metabolism (thin-layer chromatography). In experienced hands, these urinary chromatographic studies are excellent screening tests for their particular disease groups; however, as with most tests, false negatives and false positives occasionally occur. For one of the more common mucopolysaccharidoses, Sanfilippo syndrome (MPS III), MPS electrophoresis can be normal because of the generally low level of excretion of the sulfated polysaccharides in that diagnosis. Ultimately, enzymatic assays in plasma, peripheral leukocytes, or skin fibroblasts are required for definitive diagnosis of most of the lysosomal storage diseases, but not all biochemical genetics laboratories offer a comprehensive panel of lysosomal enzyme assays. For many of the sphingolipidoses and gangliosidoses, for which urinary screening tests are not available or are less reliable, the diagnosis must be suspected clinically or histologically (see Tissue Biopsies later) and then be confirmed or excluded by assay of the particular lysosomal hydrolase. For example, there are four different enzyme deficiencies that cause Sanfilippo syndrome (MPS IIIA, B, C, and D), but many laboratories assay only for MPS IIIA and MPS IIIB, the two most common forms. Consultation with a biochemical geneticist usually is required at this point. A skeletal survey for signs of dysostosis muliplex is a useful adjunct to biochemical testing for many of the MPS and oligosaccharide storage diseases.

Diagnosis of Mitochondrial Diseases

The diagnosis of a mitochondrial disease is especially complicated and difficult. Usually, the diagnosis is suggested by the finding of a lactic acidosis or a specific neurological syndrome, such as Leigh's disease or MELAS syndrome (see Table 5.8); however, urinary organic acid analysis often is overlooked as a screening tool of equal sensitivity and specificity for the diagnosis of mitochondrial disease. Increased excretion of citric acid cycle intermediates and 3-methylglutaconic acid is characteristic of not only many mitochondrial disorders with lactic acidosis but also a subset of mitochondrial diseases with impaired energy metabolism but no lactic acidosis. A muscle biopsy for histology (e.g., for "ragged-red" fibers) and for assay of

respiratory chain enzyme complexes often is used as the first diagnostic study when a mitochondrial disorder is suspected. In most situations, the clinical and biochemical evaluation should be pursued as far as possible before a muscle biopsy is performed since, contrary to common belief, an abnormal muscle biopsy is not the "gold standard" for mitochondrial disease diagnosis, especially when clinical pathology is limited to the nervous system. Furthermore, it is not necessary in most cases to have a molecular or enzymatic diagnosis before initiating therapy for a mitochondrial disease. There are relatively few therapies that are clinically beneficial, and these can usually be selected on the basis of the initial biochemical studies alone. Occasionally, an unmistakable clinical response to an empirical therapy, such as treatment of lactic acidosis with pharmacological doses of thiamine in pyruvate dehydrogenase deficiency, points to one or a few possible diagnoses, which can be further evaluated enzymatically.

If a lactic acidemia is found, then whether the acidemia worsens with fasting or with feeding should be established. This result then dictates specific enzyme assays, such as pyruvate dehydrogenase or pyruvate carboxylase, that can be performed in white cells or cultured skin fibroblasts. A lactic acidosis secondary to an organic acid disorder, such as methylmalonic aciduria, also should be excluded by urinary organic acid analysis, blood acylcarnitine analysis, and, in the case of biotinidase deficiency, a Guthrie card enzymatic assay. Next, blood, urinary sediment, or tissue samples should be submitted to a mitochondrial genetics laboratory for DNA analysis for the more common mitochondrial DNA mutations. These include several different mutations commonly associated with classic MERRF and MELAS syndromes, which can cause a wide variety of clinical syndromes in children and adults because of variable tissue distribution of the abnormal mitochondrial DNA. Mitochondrial DNA mutation T8993G, causing a deficiency of subunit 6 of mitochondrial ATP synthase, is one of the more common causes of Leigh's disease but also causes other neuromuscular or neurodegenerative diseases in children. When other avenues of diagnosis prove fruitless or when a sample of muscle mtDNA is needed, a muscle biopsy can then be performed; however, for mtDNA analysis alone, some laboratories specify fresh urinary sediment, which contains renal tubular cells with a high abundance of mitochondria.

Additional Laboratory Tests

A number of radiological studies, neurophysiological tests, and other supplementary examinations can be helpful in narrowing the differential diagnosis or marshaling evidence for a specific metabolic diagnosis (Table 5.13). For example, the finding of a subtle dysostosis multiplex in a child with unexplained language or global delay would be a sign to pursue a diagnosis of mucopolysaccharidosis or oligosaccharidosis. A pigmentary retinopathy in a young child with hypotonia and a seizure disorder might be the first suggestion of an underlying mitochondrial or peroxisomal disorder. Judicious early use of these tests, although they are sometimes expensive, often can reduce a lengthy differential diagnosis to a short list of possibilities.

Tissue Biopsies

Histological examination of biopsied tissue, once the principal method for diagnosing a storage disease, is used less frequently today but is nonetheless useful in some settings, especially when a neurodegenerative process cannot be diagnosed by biochemical, enzymatic, or mutation analysis. Bone marrow biopsy still has usefulness either for a quick confirmation of a suspected storage process or when enzymatic assays are equivocal. For many metabolic diseases, there are rare cases wherein the in vitro enzymatic assay does not fall within the diagnostic range, but the disease nonetheless exists by pathological criteria. Although tissue biopsies are necessarily invasive, their use can abruptly focus the remaining evaluation down to one or just a few diagnoses when a distinct abnormality is found (Table 5.14). If a child has an apparent neurodegenerative process and the initial biochemical tests have been nondiagnostic, a conjunctival or rectal mucosal biopsy for histology often is useful because of the diversity of cellular elements captured: stromal cells, macrophages, glandular cells, neurons, and axons. Most lysosomal storage diseases will be detected by these biopsies, although the greatest factor limiting the diagnostic sensitivity and specificity of a tissue biopsy is the experience of the pathologist and the time spent searching the specimen for a diagnostic abnormality. A bone marrow aspi-

Table 5.13. Supplementary nonbiochemical tests for metabolic diseases

Test	Diseases with abnormal results
Magnetic resonance imaging	Leukodystrophies
	Organic acidurias
	Leigh's disease
Skeletal radiology	Mucopolysaccharidoses
	Oligosaccharidoses
	Gaucher disease
	Other lysosomal storage diseases
Chest radiography	Niemann-Pick disease (pulmonary lipidosis)
Electroretinography	Mitochondrial disorders
	Generalized peroxisomal diseases
	Mucopolysaccharidoses
	Ceroid lipofuscinosis
Nerve conduction velocity	Leukodystrophies
	Leigh's disease
	Mitochondrial diseases
	Long-chain fatty acid oxidation defects
Echocardiography	Pompe disease
	Senger syndrome (cataracts/cardiomyopathy)
	Mitochondrial diseases

Table 5.14. Metabolic diseases diagnosed by tissue biopsies

Tissue	Metabolic disease	Biopsy results
Skin	Ceroid lipofuscinosis	"Thumbprint" lipid deposits
Conjunctiva	Ceroid lipofuscinosis	"Thumbprint" lipid deposits
Rectal mucosa	Mucopolysaccharidoses Oligosaccharidoses Gangliosidoses I-cell disease	Lysosomal storage material
Sural nerve	Metachromatic leukodystrophy Neuroaxonal dystrophies Nonspecific leukodystrophies	Segmental demyelination
Liver	Peroxisomal disorders	Diminished number of peroxisomes
	Long-chain fatty acid oxidation disorders	Neutral lipid storage $\pm$ cirrhosis
	Lysosomal storage diseases	Lysosomal inclusions
Muscle	Mitochondrial diseases	Ragged-red fibers
	Histologically defined myopathies and neuropathies	Nemaline rod, central nuclei, group atrophy, and so forth
Bone marrow	Niemann-Pick disease	Lipid storage in macrophages
	Gaucher disease	Lipid storage in macrophages
	GM_2 gangliosidoses	Sea-blue histiocytes

rate may give more specific results when Gaucher disease or Niemann-Pick disease type C is strongly suspected. A full-thickness skin biopsy can also be diagnostic of ceroid lipofuscinosis and is always useful for establishing a fibroblast culture.

Abnormal Test Results

The most common causes of missed metabolic diagnoses are improper sample collection and inadequate history accompanying the sample. This is especially true for partial enzyme defects characterized by only intermittent or relatively subtle biochemical changes. An equally common cause of a missed metabolic diagnosis is inadequate interpretation of test results. Unfortunately, some commercial laboratories that perform metabolic testing do not offer adequate interpretation of abnormal results. A well-cultivated telephone relationship with a metabolic specialist or use of a laboratory that provides an informed medical interpretation of results is the best protection against a missed diagnosis.

CONCLUSION

Although recent advances in molecular diagnostic techniques have largely replaced enzymatic analysis and some other biochemical assays for confirming the diagnosis of an inborn error of metabolism, metabolic screening remains the primary diagnostic method for most groups of metabolic disease and will not be supplanted in the foreseeable future. This is because most genes have hundreds, if not thousands, of possible mutations, not all of which are recognizable as benign or disease causing. Moreover, in most enzymatic disorders for which molecular testing is available, at least 5% of patients with a proven enzymatic deficiency will have very difficult-to-identify mutations, such as those affecting upstream promoter regions. With few exceptions, biochemical profiling and specific biochemical tests will yield a diagnosis and dictate a therapy much more rapidly than DNA mutation analysis. Although not without their own pitfalls, most metabolic tests are, in effect, bioassays that establish a disease diagnosis regardless of the type of mutation or gene involved. Therefore, the prudent developmental pediatrician who must seek etiological diagnoses almost every day should develop a working understanding of basic metabolic testing, which this chapter has endeavored to provide. Although these are, for the most part, rare disorders, the student of inborn errors of metabolism will also gain a better understanding of nonmetabolic diseases, almost all of which are influenced by metabolic and genetic factors.

RESOURCES

A small library of reference works and articles is essential for the clinician undertaking a metabolic evaluation. Standard texts for metabolic diseases, such as *The Metabolic and Molecular Basis of Inherited Diseases,* are biochemically comprehensive but sometimes lack useful clinical details. An important print and on-line resource of metabolic information is *Mendelian Inheritance in Man,* which abstracts historically and diagnostically important medical literature concerning both recognized clinical disorders and individual genes and mutations. One of the more useful works for deciding on needed tests and the interpretation of abnormal test results is the *Physician's Guide to the Laboratory Diagnosis of Metabolic Diseases,* which is written at the level of the practicing pediatrician and developmental specialist. These and other resources are listed in the Selected Bibliography.

SELECTED BIBLIOGRAPHY

Batshaw, M.L. (1984). Hyperammonemia. *Current Problems in Pediatrics, 11,* 1–70.

Blau, N., Duran, M., Blaskovics, M.E., & Gibson, K.M. (Eds.). (2003). *Physician's guide to the laboratory diagnosis of metabolic diseases* (2nd ed.). Berlin: Springer-Verlag.

Burton[2], B.K. (1987). Inborn errors of metabolism: The clinical diagnosis in early infancy. *Pediatrics, 79,* 359–369.

Cohn[3], R.M., & Roth, K.S. (1983). *Metabolic disease: A guide to early recognition.* Philadelphia: W.B. Saunders.

Hyland, K. (1993). Abnormalities of biogenic amine metabolism. *Journal of Inherited Metabolic Disease, 16,* 676–690.

Kelley, R.I., Watkins, P.W., & Raymond, G. (1990). Peroxisomal disorders. In W.A. Walker, P.R. Durie, J.R. Hamilton, J.A. Walker-Smith, & J.B. White (Eds.), *Pediatric gastrointestinal disease* (pp. 1032–1054). Toronto: BC Decker.

McKusick, V.A. (1992). *Mendelian inheritance in man* (10th ed.). Baltimore: The Johns Hopkins University Press.

Nelson, K.B., & Ellenberg, J.H. (1986). Antecedents of cerebral palsy: Multivariate analysis of risk. *New England Journal of Medicine, 315,* 81–86.

Nyhan, W.L. (1984). *Abnormalities in amino acid metabolism in clinical disease.* East Norwalk, CT: Appleton-Century-Crofts.

Robinson, B.H. (1993). Lacticacidemia. *Biochimica Biophysica Acta, 1182,* 231–244.

Schutgens, R.B., Heymans, H.S., Wanders, R.J., van den Bosch, H., & Tager, J.M. (1986). Peroxisomal disorders: A newly recognized group of genetic disorders. *European Journal of Pediatrics, 144,* 30–44.

Scriver[4], C.R., Beaudet, A.L., Sly, W.S., & Valle, D. (Eds.). (1998). *The metabolic basis of inherited disease* (8th ed.). New York: McGraw-Hill.

---

[2]This reference offers practical differential gamuts; much of the information is applicable to older children as well.

[3]The reference has more discussion of systemic abnormalities (e.g., acidosis, hyperammonemia, hepatomegaly) than most texts.

[4]This reference offers a very comprehensive biochemical review of each diagnosis, although some chapters lack adequate clinical information.

6

Neonatal Encephalopathy

MICHAEL V. JOHNSTON

Encephalopathy in the newborn period is often a sign of a serious neurological disorder requiring urgent evaluation and treatment. The differential diagnosis is large, including sepsis, meningitis, encephalitis, hypoglycemia, genetic metabolic disorders, and malformations, as well as brain injuries from asphyxia and stroke (Table 6.1). The clinical syndrome of encephalopathy usually includes seizures, impaired consciousness, abnormal electroencephalogram (EEG), diminished muscle tone, poor oral feeding, depressed reflexes, abnormal central breathing, and diminished reaction to noxious stimuli. These signs can also be an early manifestation of a more chronic genetic disorder such as Rett or Angelman syndrome. Modern imaging technology and genetic diagnosis have been combined with epidemiological study of infants with neonatal encephalopathy to understand the differential diagnosis of neonatal encephalopathies. This information is relevant to care of infants in the neonatal period as well as to evaluation of older children with motor and other developmental disabilities.

INCIDENCE AND RISK FACTORS FOR ENCEPHALOPATHY

Population-based studies of term infants with all kinds of encephalopathy indicate that the condition occurs in about 1.9–3.8 per 1,000 infants, with a death rate of 9.1% (Badawi et al., 1997). The incidence was 3.8 per 1,000 in a case–control study of all term infants greater than 37 weeks' gestation with encephalopathy born in Perth, Western Australia, as well as in a similar study of infants born in Nepal (Badawi et al., 1998a, 1998b; Ellis, Manandhar, Manan-

dhar, & Costello, 2000). The Western Australian study, which compared 164 cases of encephalopathy and 400 control infants, showed that the risk of encephalopathy was increased by intrauterine growth restriction and gestation longer than 39 weeks (Table 6.2). Other prenatal risk factors associated with increased risk in this study included maternal thyroid disorders; preeclampsia; maternal bleeding; and family history of a neurological disorder, including maternal seizures. Low socioeconomic status of the mother was also associated with increased risk.

It is noteworthy that the vast majority (69%) of the infants in the Western Australian study had antenatal, but no intrapartum, factors that correlated with encephalopathy. Twenty-five percent had a combination of antenatal and intrapartum factors, including occipitoposterior presentation, maternal fever, an acute intrapartum event, or emergency cesarean delivery, whereas only 4% had evidence of intrapartum hypoxia alone. These data are consistent with the predominance of antepartum risk factors in children with cerebral palsy in the National Perinatal Collaborative Project (Nelson & Ellenberg, 1986); however, data from Nepal showing that 60% of infants with encephalopathy had intrapartum risk factors suggest that this distribution of causation may be different in developing countries (Ellis et al., 2000).

HYPOXIC-ISCHEMIC ENCEPHALOPATHY

Asphyxia leading to hypoxic-ischemic brain insult remains an important cause of encephalopathy in term newborns (Johnston, Trescher,

Table 6.1. Differential diagnosis of neonatal encephalopathy

Infection
  Meningitis
  Encephalitis
  Sepsis in infant or mother
  Chorioamnionitis
  Congenital infection
Hypoglycemia
Hypoxic-ischemic encephalopathy
Stroke and thrombophilic disorders
Venous sinus thrombosis
Intracranial hemorrhage
Electrolyte disturbances
Maternal drugs
Brain trauma
Brain malformations
Genetic metabolic disorders
Kernicterus

Ishida, & Nakajima, 2001). Signs of hypoxic-ischemic encephalopathy (HIE) usually appear after a latent period of 8–36 hours following the initial insult, during which time the infant may appear normal. Signs typically worsen and then improve over about a week. This pattern is probably related to the delayed evolution of energy failure and other biochemical events triggered by accumulation of glutamate and excessive stimulation of glutamate receptors in the brain. Delayed changes in gene expression also mediate a mixture of apoptosis or necrosis in selectively vulnerable regions of the brain.

Table 6.2. Risk factors for neonatal encephalopathy in the Western Australia study

	Odds ratio
Antenatal conditions	
Maternal thyroid disease	5.9
Late or no prenatal care	5.4
Severe preeclampsia	3.9
Maternal bleeding	2.3
Viral illness	2.1
Gestation of 42 weeks	3.9
Family history of seizures	2.6
Intrapartum conditions	
Acute intrapartum event	4.4
Occipitoposterior presentation	4.3
Maternal fever	3.8

Sources: Badawi et al. (1998a, 1998b).

Sarnat and Sarnat (1976) published an early clinical scale for encephalopathy related to asphyxia that included the EEG and distinguished mild, moderate, and severe categories. According to the Sarnat scale, infants with mild or stage 1 encephalopathy are hyperalert, with increased reflexes and normal muscle tone, but do not have seizures or an abnormal EEG. Infants with moderate encephalopathy are lethargic or obtunded, with mild hypotonia; weak or absent suck and Moro reflexes; seizures; and a moderately abnormal, slow EEG. Infants in the severe category or stage 3 have more severe reduction in consciousness and flaccid hypotonia, with very severe EEG slowing or a burst-suppression pattern. Levene, Grindulis, Sands, and Moore (1986) reported that infants with mild encephalopathy are likely to be normal on follow-up, whereas infants with moderate or severe encephalopathy have a significant risk of motor disability and developmental delay.

The clinical signs of HIE and the appearance of the EEG in the neonatal period are usually not specific enough to make a diagnosis of hypoxia-ischemia as the cause of encephalopathy; however, brain imaging, especially magnetic resonance imaging (MRI), often reveals specific signs of hemorrhage, asphyxial injury, arterial stroke, venous sinus thrombosis, or trauma (Johnston, 2003). Head ultrasound is sensitive to bleeding, ventricular size, edema, and white matter injury but is not as sensitive to injury in gray matter areas, especially the cerebral cortex, which may be outside the view of ultrasound. Computed tomographic imaging provides a more complete view of the brain, especially the cortex, where the gray matter–white matter contrast may be reduced by edema. This modality, however, is not much better than ultrasound for detecting tissue injury associated with HIE.

MRI is considerably more sensitive and specific than other modalities, and, in the study by Cowan et al. (2003), 77% of infants referred to tertiary care centers in the United Kingdom and the Netherlands had evidence of hypoxic-ischemic lesions, focal infarctions, or hemorrhages. They also found that 69% of a subgroup of 90 infants who had seizures without other signs of encephalopathy had focal infarctions or hemorrhages. In the first few weeks after a hypoxic-ischemic injury, MRI generally shows enhanced signal on T1-weighted images in the basal ganglia and perirolandic cortex or in extensive areas of cerebral cortex (Maller, Hankins, Yeakley, & Butler, 1998). The pattern of injury in the basal ganglia is generally confined to the putamen and thalamus and reflects very severe and relatively brief near-total asphyxial insults such as cord compression (Figure 6.1). The second, more diffuse cerebral cortical pattern of injury generally reflects less severe but more prolonged asphyxial episodes. After several weeks, the increased signal seen on T1-weighted imaging of near-total asphyxial lesions disappears, and smaller areas of T2 enhancement emerge in more restricted areas of the basal ganglia and thalamus. Areas of high T1 signal seen after partial prolonged asphyxia in the cerebral cortex are generally replaced by multicystic encephalomalacia. Watershed infarctions caused by asphyxia accompanied by severe hypotension are less common than the other two patterns but are easily seen on MRI. MRI is quite sensitive to acute brain injuries from hypoxia-ischemia in term infants. A normal MRI in the newborn period, especially when accompanied by a normal EEG, is strong evidence that there

has been no injury from asphyxia (Biagoni et al., 2001).

ENCEPHALOPATHY AND CEREBRAL PALSY

When older children are evaluated for motor disorders such as cerebral palsy, it is common for parents to ask if the child's problems had any relationship to the birth process. This relationship has been examined critically in considerable detail by several professional groups, in part related to the high number of lawsuits claiming that obstetric care contributed to brain injuries linked to cerebral palsy. A report entitled "Neonatal Encephalopathy and Cerebral Palsy" was prepared by an American College of Obstetricians and Gynecologists (ACOG) Task Force (2003) and endorsed by the ACOG, the American Academy of Pediatrics, and other groups. Based on a review of the literature, the report concluded that absence of moderate or severe encephalopathy in the newborn period rules out asphyxia as an intrapartum cause of cerebral palsy. When encephalopathy is present, the report concluded that asphyxia is probably not causally linked to cerebral palsy unless there was a severe metabolic acidosis at birth (cord arterial blood gas

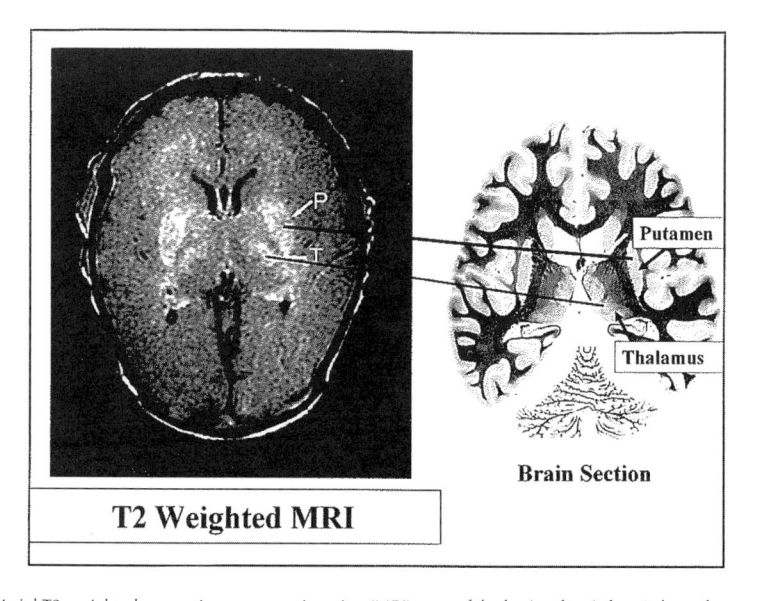

Figure 6.1. *Left,* Axial T2-weighted magnetic resonance imaging (MRI) scan of the brain of an infant 6 days after an episode of severe, near-total intrapartum asphyxia secondary to cord compression. Note increased signal in the putamen of the basal ganglia and thalamus on both sides. *Right,* Section through a stained postmortem brain specimen with lines connecting homologous areas of the putamen and thalamus to the same areas in the MRI scan.

with a pH < 7 and a base deficit of > 12 mEq/ L). In addition, the report concluded that cerebral palsy is probably not related to intrapartum asphyxia unless it is of the spastic quadriplegic or dyskinetic (extrapyramidal) type and other etiologies such as infectious or genetic disorders have been ruled out. Evidence suggests that other markers for intrapartum events, such as an episode of sudden bradycardia on a fetal heart rate monitor, an Apgar score of 3 or less beyond 5 minutes, and early onset of multiorgan dysfunction, are suggestive of but not specific for asphyxia.

INFECTION AND ENCEPHALOPATHY

Infections are an important cause of neonatal encephalopathy, which can result from direct invasion by viruses or bacteria or from systemic sepsis in the infant's bloodstream, or indirectly through exposure to maternal infection or chorioamnionitis (see Table 6.1). In a case–control study of term infants, Grether and Nelson (1997) found that maternal fever exceeding 38° C and a clinical diagnosis of chorioamnionitis were associated with an increased risk of cerebral palsy (odds ratio, 9.3) as well as encephalopathy. Exposure to maternal infection was associated with a higher incidence of low Apgar scores, neonatal seizures, intubation in the delivery room, need for medications to support blood pressure, acidosis, and a diagnosis of HIE in these infants. Most of these children did not have evidence of infection in the neonatal period. Previous studies, including the Western Australian study, have also shown an association between fever in labor and increased risk of cerebral palsy and neonatal encephalopathy (Adamson et al., 1995; Badawi et al., 1998b; Eastman & deLeon, 1955; Nelson & Ellenberg, 1984). The increased risk from exposure to infection as opposed to direct invasion by the infectious agent suggests that a systemic inflammatory response or sepsis-like syndrome, rather than direct exposure to an organism, may damage the infant's brain.

GENETIC METABOLIC DISORDERS, SYNDROMES, AND MALFORMATIONS

A diverse group of genetic metabolic disorders, syndromes, and malformations can also cause encephalopathy in neonates, sometimes mimicking more commonly recognized disorders such as HIE and infection. In the Western Australian study, 28% of infants with encephalopathy had birth defects, compared with 4% of controls, and these contributed to encephalopathy in 37% of cases (Felix et al., 2000).

Genetic metabolic disorders associated with neonatal encephalopathy include those that disrupt energy metabolism as well as the processing of amino acids, organic acids, ammonia, and fatty acids (Table 6.3). Many of these disorders appear to have an impact on the function of neuronal synapses. Nonketotic hyperglycinemia, which raises the level of glycine in the blood and the brain's extracellular space, causes seizures, coma, myoclonus, and hiccups in the first few days of life in association with an abnormally slow EEG with a burst-suppression pattern (Hamosh, Maher, Bellus, Rasmussen, & Johnston, 1998). The EEG resembles the pattern seen in HIE, probably because glycine is a co-agonist at the N-methyl-D-aspartate (NMDA)-type glutamate receptor that is a major trigger for brain injury in HIE. Urea cycle disorders and other diseases that raise brain ammonia, such as propionic and methylmalonic acidemia, can also raise brain glutamate levels by impairing the reuptake of glutamate from the synapses by glial

Table 6.3. Genetic metabolic disorders associated with neonatal encephalopathy

Nonketotic hyperglycinemia
Hyperammonemia and urea cycle disorders
Pyridoxine dependency
Maple syrup urine disease
Phenylketonuria
Medium-chain acyl-CoA dehydrogenase deficiency
Multiple carboxylase deficiency
Congenital lactic acidosis
Mitochondrial disorders
Glucose transporter disorders
Smith-Lemli-Opitz syndrome
Methylmalonic acidemia
L-Amino acid decarboxylase deficiency
Folinic acid–responsive seizures
Fumaric aciduria
Glutaric aciduria types I and II
Other organic acidurias
Sulfite oxidase (molybdenum cofactor) deficiency

pumps (Chan & Butterworth, 2003). This is similar to the effect of hypoglycemia, which impairs the delivery of glucose needed to supply reuptake pumps for glutamate in the brain (Ichord, Johnston, & Traystman, 2001). Pyridoxine dependency, a vitamin cofactor for conversion of glutamate to γ-aminobutyric acid (GABA) in the brain, also causes seizures by raising brain levels of glutamate and lowering levels of GABA (Baumeister, Gsell, Shin, & Egger, 1994). Mechanisms for encephalopathy in some of the other metabolic disorders are less well understood.

Whereas the potential role of metabolic disorders in neonatal encephalopathy is widely known, some of the other genetic disorders that can cause neonatal brain dysfunction are less well appreciated (Table 6.4). Angelman and Prader-Willi syndromes, resulting from deletions at similar loci on chromosome 15 inherited from the mother or father, respectively, can cause encephalopathy in the neonatal period. Infants with Prader-Willi syndrome are often very hypotonic with very poor sucking and feeding in the neonatal period, and those with Angelman syndrome also frequently have

hypotonia and feeding problems, as well as seizures (Richer, Shevell, & Miller, 2001). Seizures in Angelman syndrome may be related to the deletion of a subunit of the inhibitory GABA receptor, which is coded for by DNA on chromosome 15 (Sinnett et al., 1993). The abnormalities in both syndromes usually improve with age, although deceleration of head growth from a normal size at birth has been reported in Angelman syndrome (Smith et al., 1996).

Mutations in the *MECP2* transcription factor gene that cause Rett syndrome can cause behavioral abnormalities or encephalopathy in both male and female neonates (Geerdink et al., 2002; Hammer, Dorrani, Dragich, Kudo, & Shanen, 2002). Joubert syndrome is another intellectual disabilities syndrome that can present in the nursery (Maria, Boltshauser, Palmer, & Tran, 1999). These infants often present in the neonatal period with hypotonia, irregular breathing characterized by hyperpnea and apnea, and oculomotor apraxia. Joubert syndrome is caused by recessive inheritance of mutations in the *AHI1* gene coding for the protein jouberin and is usually diagnosed by visualizing the typical "molar tooth sign" associated with hypoplasia of the cerebellar vermis on brain imaging (Dixon-Salazar et al., 2004). A variety of early-onset degenerative disorders such as Canavan's disease can rarely present in the neonatal period. Neuromuscular disorders such as the Werdnig-Hoffman form of motor neuron disease and myotonic dystrophy should also be considered in the differential diagnosis of neonatal encephalopathy because they present with severe central hypotonia in the neonatal period (Richer et al., 2001).

CONCLUSION

Neonatal encephalopathy is a potentially serious neurological disorder with implications for acute diagnosis and management in the neonatal period as well as prognostic implications for future motor and cognitive disorders in older children. A diverse group of disorders should be considered in the differential diagnosis of neonatal encephalopathy. When older children are evaluated for motor dysfunction or other disabilities, it is useful to determine

Table 6.4. Genetic syndromes and malformations associated with neonatal encephalopathy

Angelman syndrome
Prader-Willi syndrome
Rett syndrome
Joubert syndrome
Ohtahara syndrome
Benign neonatal seizures
Trisomy 13 or 18
Fetal alcohol syndrome
Cortical dysplasias (e.g., Miller-Dieker syndrome, 1p36 deletion)
Hemimegalencephaly
Zellweger syndrome, other peroxisomal disorders
Menkes' syndrome
Infantile ceroid lipofuscinosis
Alpers disease
Sialic acid storage disease
Infantile neuroaxonal dystrophy
Leukodystrophies (Canavan's disease, Alexander's disease, metachromatic)
Gangliosidoses (GM$_1$ and GM$_2$)
Storage diseases (Gaucher, Niemann-Pick)
Myotonic dystrophy, other nerve and muscle disorders
Werdnig-Hoffmann disease

the presence and severity of any neonatal encephalopathy as well as any diagnostic testing done at that time. If the newborn course was entirely normal in a child who has cerebral palsy, it is very unlikely that the disability was caused by a hypoxic-ischemic or other injury at birth. If encephalopathy was present in the neonatal period in a child with cerebral palsy, additional criteria, including the type of cerebral palsy and brain imaging, are useful for determining if it was caused by HIE or some other disorder. Evidence suggests that infants exposed passively to a mother's infection are at increased risk for both encephalopathy and cerebral palsy. Genetic disorders, including Rett, Joubert, Prader-Willi, and Angelman syndromes, can also present first in neonates as encephalopathy, causing potential confusion with other more common causes.

REFERENCES

Adamson, J., Alessandri, L.M., Badawi, N., Burton, P.R., Pemberton, P.J., & Stanley, F. (1995). Predictors of neonatal encephalopathy in full term infants. *British Medical Journal, 311,* 598–602.

American College of Obstetrics and Gynecology (ACOG) Task Force on Neonatal Encephalopathy and Cerebral Palsy. (2003). *Neonatal encephalopathy and cerebral palsy.* Washington, DC: American College of Obstetricians and Gynecologists.

Badawi, N., Kurinczuk, J.J., Hall, D., Field, D., Pemberton, P.J., & Stanley, F.J. (1997). Newborn encephalopathy in term infants: Three approaches to population-based investigation. *Seminars in Neonatology, 2,* 181–188.

Badawi, N., Kurinczuk, J.J., Keogh, J.M., Alessandri, L.M., O'Sullivan, F., Burton, P.R., et al. (1998a). Antepartum risk factors for newborn encephalopathy: The Western Australian case-control study. *British Medical Journal, 317,* 1549–1553.

Badawi, N., Kurinczuk, J.J., Keogh, J.M., Alessandri, L.M., O'Sullivan, F., Burton, P.R., et al. (1998b). Intrapartum risk factors for newborn encephalopathy: The Western Australian case-control study. *British Medical Journal, 317,* 1554–1558.

Baumeister, F.A., Gsell, W., Shin, Y.S., & Egger, J. (1994). Glutamate in pyridoxine-dependent epilepsy: Neurotoxic glutamate concentration in the cerebrospinal fluid and its normalization by pyridoxine. *Pediatrics, 94,* 318–321.

Biagoni, E., Mercuri, E., Rutherford, M., Cowan, F., Azzopardi, D., Frisone, M.F., et al. (2001). Combined use of electroencephalogram and magnetic resonance imaging in full-term neonates with acute encephalopathy. *Pediatrics, 107,* 461–468.

Chan, H., & Butterworth, R.F. (2003). Cell-selective effects of ammonia on glutamate transporter and receptor function in mammalian brain. *Neurochemistry International, 43,* 525–532.

Cowan, F., Rutherford, M., Groenendaal, F., Eken, P., Mercuri, E., Bydder, G.M., et al. (2003). Origin and timing of brain lesions in term infants with neonatal encephalopathy. *Lancet, 361,* 736–742.

Dixon-Salazar, T., Silhavy, J.L., Marsh, S.E., Louie, C.M., Scott, L.C., Gururaj, A., et al. (2004). Mutations in the *AHI1* gene, encoding jouberin, cause Joubert syndrome with cortical polymicrogyria. *American Journal of Human Genetics, 75,* 979–987.

Eastman, N.J., & DeLeon, M. (1955). The etiology of cerebral palsy. *American Journal of Obstetrics and Gynecology, 69,* 950–961.

Ellis, M., Manandhar, N., Manandhar, D.S., & Costello, A.M.L. (2000). Risk factors for neonatal encephalopathy in Kathmandu, Nepal, a developing country: Unmatched case-control study. *British Medical Journal, 320,* 1229–1236.

Felix, J.F., Badawi, N., Kurinczuk, J.J., Bower, C., Keogh, J.M., & Pemberton, P.J. (2000). Birth defects in children with newborn encephalopathy. *Developmental Medicine and Child Neurology, 42,* 803–808.

Geerdink, N., Rotteveel, J.J., Lammens, M., Sistermans, E.A., Heikens, G.T., Gabreels, F.J., et al. (2002). *MECP2* mutation in a boy with severe neonatal encephalopathy: Clinical, neuropathological and molecular findings. *Neuropediatrics, 33,* 33–36.

Grether, J.K., & Nelson, K.B. (1997). Maternal infection and cerebral palsy in infants of normal birth weight. *JAMA, 278,* 207–211.

Hammer, S., Dorrani, N., Dragich, J., Kudo, S., & Shanen, C. (2002). The phenotypic consequences of *MECP2* mutations extend beyond Rett syndrome. *Mental Retardation and Developmental Disability Research Reviews, 8,* 94–98.

Hamosh, A., Maher, J.F., Bellus, G.A., Rasmussen, S.A., & Johnston, M.V. (1998). Long-term use of high dose benzoate and dextromethorphan for the treatment of nonketotic hyperglycinemia. *Journal of Pediatrics, 132,* 709–713.

Ichord, R.N., Johnston, M.V., & Traystman, R.J. (2001). MK801 decreases glutamate release and oxidative metabolism during hypoglycemic coma in piglets. *Brain Research: Developmental Brain Research, 128,* 139–148.

Johnston, M.V. (2003). MRI for neonatal encephalopathy in full-term infants. *Lancet, 361,* 713–714.

Johnston, M.V., Trescher, W.H., Ishida, A., & Nakajima, W. (2001). Neurobiology of hypoxic-ischemic injury in the developing brain. *Pediatric Research, 49,* 735–741.

Levene, M.I., Grindulis, H., Sands, C., & Moore, J.R. (1986). Comparison of two methods of predicting outcome in perinatal asphyxia. *Lancet, 1,* 67–69.

Maller, A.I., Hankins, L.L., Yeakley, J.W., & Butler, I.J. (1998). Rolandic type cerebral palsy in children as a pattern of hypoxic-ischemic injury in the full-term infant. *Journal of Child Neurology, 13,* 313–321.

Maria, B.L., Boltshauser, E., Palmer, S.C., & Tran, T.X. (1999). Clinical features and revised diagnostic criteria in Joubert syndrome. *Journal of Child Neurology, 14,* 583–590.

Nelson, K.B., & Ellenberg, J.H. (1984). Obstetric complications as risk factors for cerebral palsy or seizure disorders. *JAMA, 251,* 1843–1848.

Nelson, K.B., & Ellenberg, J.H. (1986). Antecedents of cerebral palsy: Multivariate analysis of risk. *New England Journal of Medicine, 315,* 81–86.

Richer, L.P., Shevell, M.I., & Miller, S.P. (2001). Diagnostic profile of neonatal hypotonia: An 11-year study. *Pediatric Research, 25,* 33–36.

Sarnat, H.B., & Sarnat, M.S. (1976). Neonatal encephalopathy following fetal distress. *Archives of Neurology, 33,* 696–705.

Sinnett, D., Wagstaff, J., Glatt, K., Woolf, E., Kirkness, E.J., & Lalande, M. (1993). High resolution mapping of the gamma-aminobutyric acid receptor subunit beta 3 and alpha 5 gene cluster on chromosome 15q11–q13, and localization of breakpoints in two Angelman syndrome patients. *American Journal of Human Genetics, 52,* 1216–1229.

Smith, A., Wiles, C., Haan, E., McGill, J., Wallace, G., Dixon, J., et al. (1996). Clinical features in 27 patients with Angelman syndrome resulting from DNA deletions. *Journal of Medical Genetics, 33,* 107–112.

7

Genetic Intellectual Disability

Neurobiological and Clinical Aspects

WALTER E. KAUFMANN, GEORGE T. CAPONE,
JOHN C. CARTER, AND DAVID N. LIEBERMAN

Intellectual disability (ID) is one of the most common and severe developmental neurological syndromes, affecting 1%–3% of individuals in the general population. ID is typically described as a nonprogressive primary impairment of cognitive function and adaptive behavior. The definition of ID depends on whether medical, educational, legal, or other aspects are emphasized; however, there is widespread agreement on classifying individuals with an intelligence quotient (IQ) lower than 70 at age 5 years or older (when delineation of cognitive performance is more stable) as having ID. Younger children with predominant or exclusive cognitive delay are typically labeled as having global developmental delay (GDD). Severe ID, corresponding to an IQ below 40–50, is frequently associated with genetic abnormalities, comprising 25%–50% of all forms of ID (Chiurazzi & Oostra, 2000; McLaren & Bryson, 1987). Although environmental factors appear to play an important role in the etiology of GDD/ID in mildly affected individuals (Chiurazzi & Oostra, 2000), it is unquestionable that even these exogenous agents act through disturbances in genetic developmental programs (Kaufmann, 1996; Kaufmann & Moser, 2000).

Because of space limitations, this chapter does not discuss metabolic and degenerative disorders of childhood, which may resemble ID during the course of their progressive evolution but usually evolve in the setting of a normally developed brain. Among the known "primary" genetic abnormalities associated with ID, a disproportionately high percentage involve genes on the X chromosome (6–8 times more frequent than expected for the proportion of X chromosome genes in the human genome) (Inlow & Restifo, 2004). Altogether, these observations suggest that important clues about the pathogenesis of ID will emerge from the study of key genes involved in brain development, particularly those located on the X chromosome.

Although the focus of this chapter is the neurobiology of ID, clinical and neurobiological evidence has suggested a considerable overlap between the presentations of ID and autism spectrum disorder (ASD). Some of the literature on neuroanatomic changes in ID is based on cases that, under current diagnostic standards that emphasize behavioral features, could also be labeled as autism or ASD (Kaufmann & Moser, 2000). Consequently, some of the principles and features described in the following sections could also be applicable to individuals with ASD. For these reasons, we propose that the study of GDD/ID should occur in the context of a new disease category en-

We are grateful to the families who have participated in research projects at our Center; their partnership is critical for advancing the field. We also thank Dr. Michael Johnston for his continuous support of our research and the Center and Irena Bukelis for assistance in the preparation of this manuscript.

compassing ID, ASD, and related clinical syndromes that we have termed *severe developmental neurobehavioral disorders.*

KEY ISSUES IN THE CLINICAL ASSESSMENT OF INDIVIDUALS WITH INTELLECTUAL DISABILITIES

Taking into consideration the prominent role of genetic factors in the etiology of GDD/ID (Chiurazzi & Oostra, 2000), and the close relationship between ID and behavior disorders, the clinical assessment of patients with GDD

Table 7.1. Overview of the Center for Genetic Disorders of Cognition & Behavior approach to clinical evaluation of children with global developmental delay/intellectual disabilities

1. Personal clinical history
   a. Present illness
   b. Developmental history
   c. Educational history
2. Family/social history
3. General physical examination
   a. Dysmorphology
   b. Non-neurological systems review
4. Neurological examination
   a. Standard examination
   b. Overall cognitive function
   c. Fine motor function
5. Behavioral/psychiatric assessment
   a. Mental status examination
   b. Adaptive functioning
   c. Aberrant behaviors
   d. Autistic behavior (preferably ADI-R)
   e. Psychopharmacology
6. Psychological evaluation
   a. Behavioral observation
   b. Intelligence/developmental tests
   c. Complementary cognitive tests[a]
   d. Language and speech assessment
   e. Academic tests
   f. Adaptive behavior scales
   g. Aberrant behavior scales
   h. Autistic behavior assessment (preferably ADOS-G)
7. Sensory deficit screening[b]
   a. Auditory
   b. Ophthalmological

[a]Perceptual, memory, attention, executive function, sensorimotor, socioemotional.

[b]If indicated by history.

Key: ADI-R, Autism Diagnostic Interview-Revised (Rutter, Le-Couteur, & Lord, 2003); ADOS-G, Autism Diagnostic Observation Schedule-Generic (Lord et al., 2000).

or ID should include, in addition to a detailed clinical and family history, the following four components: medical (i.e., search for dysmorphic features, non-neurological systems review), neurological (emphasis on motor and cognitive aspects), behavioral (emphasis on cognitive profiling, aberrant behaviors, and socialization), and laboratory (emphasis on genetic testing) (Tables 7.1 and 7.2). This approach is likely to yield information for individual patient-targeted management strategies, in addition to specific etiologies with obvious implications for genetic counseling and prognosis.

Several approaches that include most of the aforementioned components have been proposed for the diagnostic assessment of individuals with GDD/ID. A widely accepted strategy was published by a task force of the American Academy of Neurology and the Child Neurology Society (Shevell et al., 2003); as with other peer-reviewed guidelines, the Practice Parameter for the Evaluation of the Child with Global Developmental Delay emphasizes the quality of the supporting evidence for each diagnostic element (Shevell et al., 2003) (Figure 7.1). Figure 7.2 depicts a flow chart for the diagnostic evaluation of children with GDD/ID, with emphasis on genetic testing, published by the American Academy of Pediatrics' Committee on Genetics (Moeschler & Shevell, 2006). This approach is complementary to the one described in Figure 7.1, highlighting the salient features of the genetics component of the assessment. Srour, Mazer,

Table 7.2. Overview of the Center for Genetic Disorders of Cognition & Behavior approach to laboratory evaluation of children with global developmental delay/intellectual disabilities

1. Genetic
   a. Karyotype/cytogenetic evaluation
   b. FISH for subtelomere abnormalities
   c. Molecular genetic testing[a]
2. Targeted brain imaging (MRI)[b]
3. Targeted metabolic testing, including T$_4$[b]
4. Lead screen[b]
5. EEG[b]

[a]Highest yield: *FMR1, MECP2.*

[b]If indicated by history.

Key: EEG, electroencephalography; FISH, fluorescent in situ hybridization; MRI, magnetic resonance imaging; T$_4$, thyroxine.

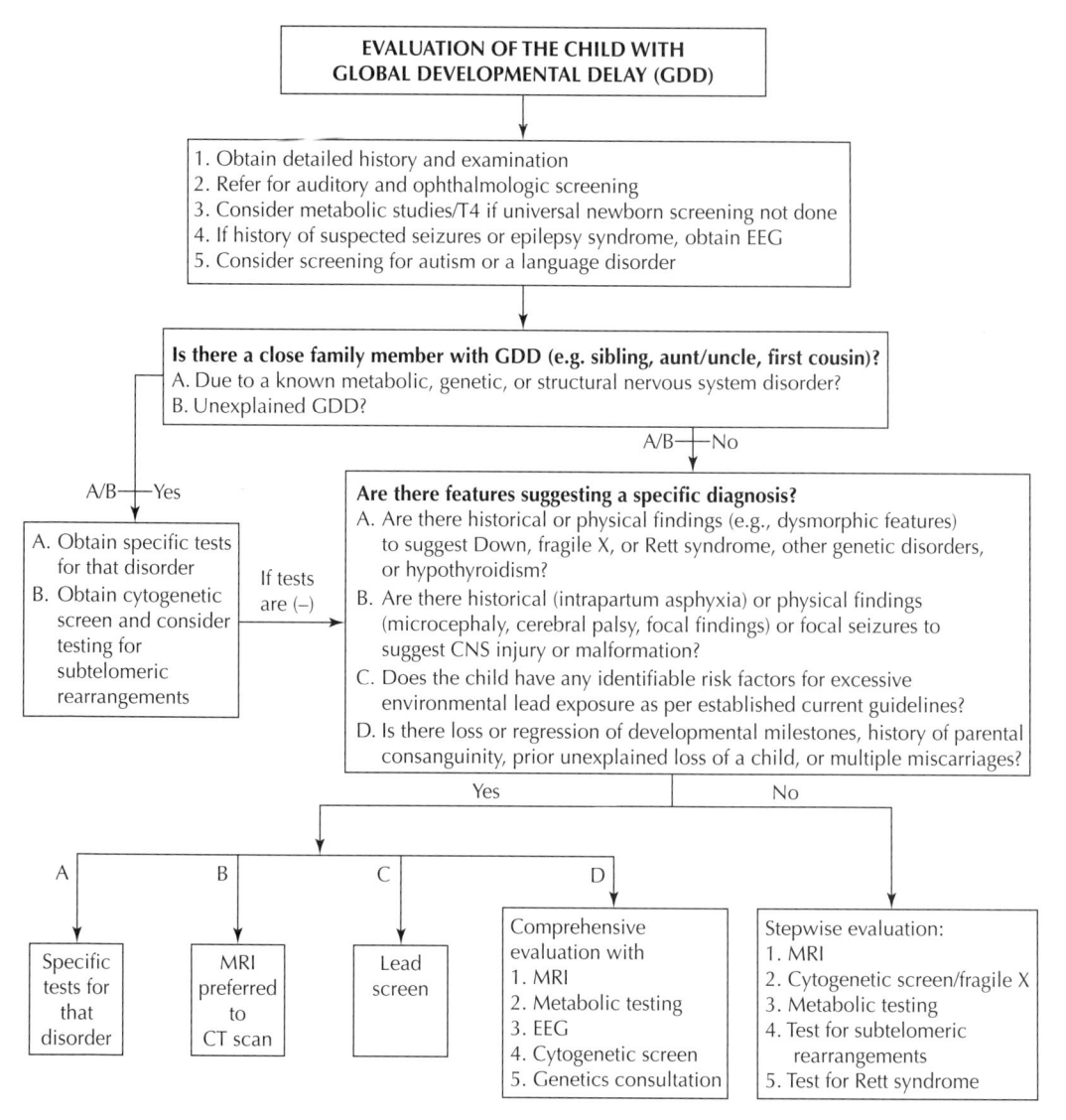

EVALUATION OF THE CHILD WITH GLOBAL DEVELOPMENTAL DELAY (GDD)

1. Obtain detailed history and examination
2. Refer for auditory and ophthalmologic screening
3. Consider metabolic studies/T4 if universal newborn screening not done
4. If history of suspected seizures or epilepsy syndrome, obtain EEG
5. Consider screening for autism or a language disorder

Is there a close family member with GDD (e.g. sibling, aunt/uncle, first cousin)?
A. Due to a known metabolic, genetic, or structural nervous system disorder?
B. Unexplained GDD?

A/B —— No

A/B —— Yes

A. Obtain specific tests for that disorder
B. Obtain cytogenetic screen and consider testing for subtelomeric rearrangements

If tests are (–)

Are there features suggesting a specific diagnosis?
A. Are there historical or physical findings (e.g., dysmorphic features) to suggest Down, fragile X, or Rett syndrome, other genetic disorders, or hypothyroidism?
B. Are there historical (intrapartum asphyxia) or physical findings (microcephaly, cerebral palsy, focal findings) or focal seizures to suggest CNS injury or malformation?
C. Does the child have any identifiable risk factors for excessive environmental lead exposure as per established current guidelines?
D. Is there loss or regression of developmental milestones, history of parental consanguinity, prior unexplained loss of a child, or multiple miscarriages?

Yes   No

A   B   C   D

A. Specific tests for that disorder

B. MRI preferred to CT scan

C. Lead screen

D. Comprehensive evaluation with
1. MRI
2. Metabolic testing
3. EEG
4. Cytogenetic screen
5. Genetics consultation

Stepwise evaluation:
1. MRI
2. Cytogenetic screen/fragile X
3. Metabolic testing
4. Test for subtelomeric rearrangements
5. Test for Rett syndrome

Figure 7.1. Algorithm for the evaluation of the child with global developmental delay/intellectual disability (American Academy of Neurology/Child Neurology Society). (From Shevell, M., Ashwal, S., Donley, D., Flint, J., Gingold, M., Hirtz, D., et al. [2003]. Practice Parameter. Evaluation of the child with global developmental delay: Report of the Quality Standards Subcommittee of the American Academy of Neurology and the Practice Committee of the Child Neurology Society. *Neurology, 60*(3), 367–380; reprinted by permission.) (*Key:* T4, thyroxine; EEG, electroencephalogram; CNS, central nervous system; MRI, magnetic resonance imaging; CT, computed tomography.)

and Shevell (2006) have reported that the etiological yield in unselected patients with GDD is 40% overall and up to 55% in the absence of autistic features. The discrepancy in the latter figures probably reflects the predominance of genetic disorders without available standardized testing in the severe GDD/ID group, the frequent association of autism and severe GDD/ID, and the lack of informative history and physical features (i.e., dysmorphia, multisystem syndromes) in a large proportion of

children with severe GDD/ID. Advances in several areas, in particular in the characterization of nonsyndromic X-linked ID, may lead in the near future to improved diagnostic yield for children with severe GDD/ID.

An in-depth discussion about diagnosis and management of children with GDD/ID is beyond the scope of this chapter (for details, see Tables 7.1 and 7.2 and Figures 7.1 and 7.2, as well as their source references). Nevertheless, a few points about the rationale of each

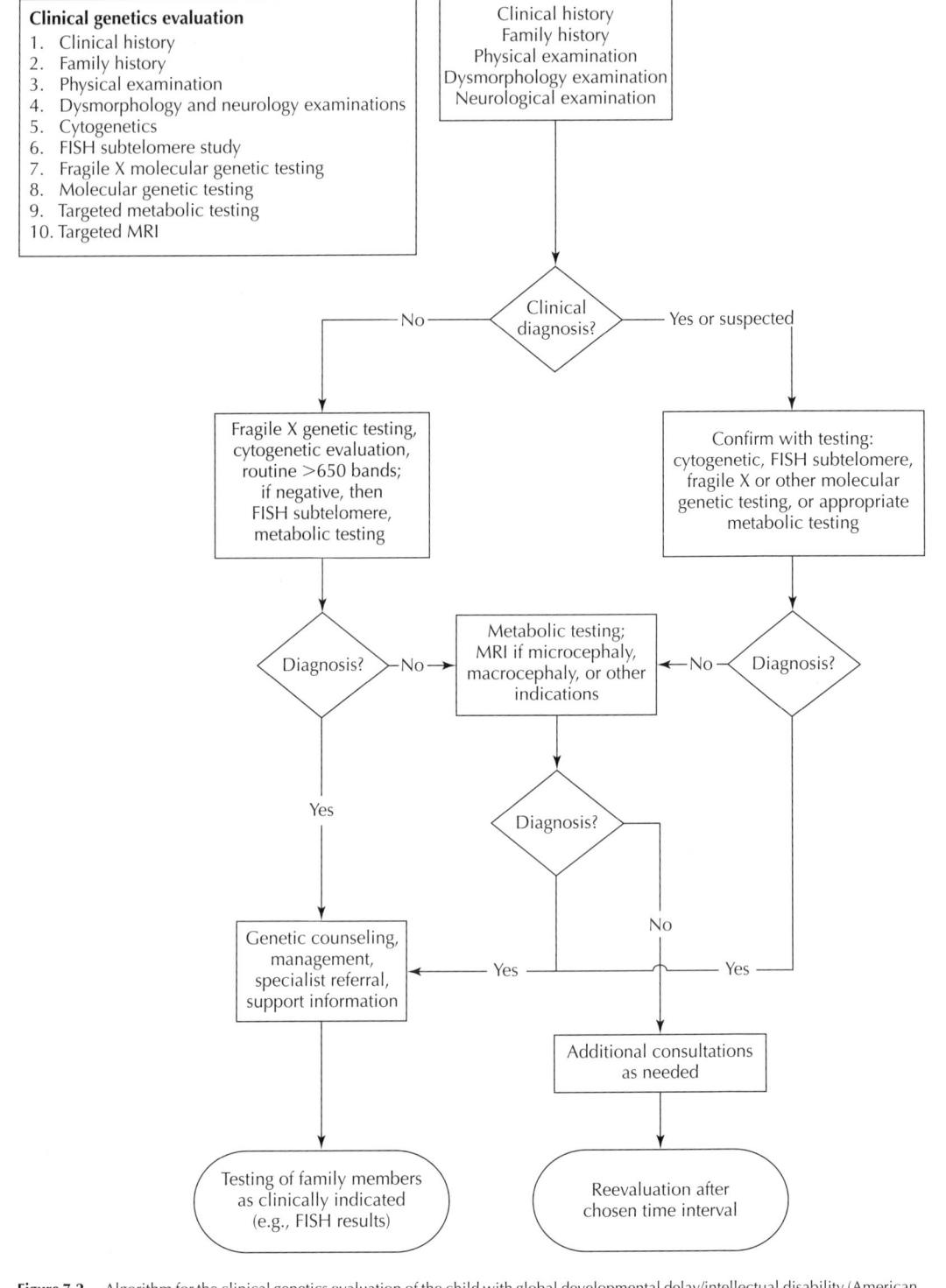

Figure 7.2. Algorithm for the clinical genetics evaluation of the child with global developmental delay/intellectual disability (American Academy of Pediatrics). (Reproduced with permission from *Pediatrics,* Vol. 117, Pages 2304–2316, Copyright © 2006 by the AAP.) (*Key:* FISH, fluorescent in situ hybridization; MRI, magnetic resonance imaging.)

component of the diagnostic assessment deserve consideration. In addition to its role in establishing etiology, by identifying features characteristic of a particular disorder (e.g., facial dysmorphia in fragile X syndrome [FXS]), physical examination of the child with GDD/ID is of great importance for the assessment and management of extraneurological abnormalities seen in syndromic ID (e.g., cardiac malformations in Down syndrome [DS]). Neuromotor assessments are also an essential component of the evaluation because they can assist in determining etiology (e.g., spastic diplegia characteristic of perinatal hypoxia-ischemia) and therapeutic management (e.g., occupational therapy in patients with fine motor impairment).

Cognitive and behavioral evaluations are required for establishing with certainty the diagnosis of ID and its level of severity (Fisch, 2000); however, often overlooked is their role in delineating the patient's individual neurobehavioral profile. For instance, severe behavior disorder is a relatively uncommon but challenging phenotype in DS (Capone, Goyal, Ares, & Lannigan, 2006; Capone, Grados, Kaufmann, Bernad-Ripoll, & Jewell, 2005; Carter, Capone, Gray, Cox, & Kaufmann, 2007). Neurobehavioral profiling is also critical for adequate management of single-gene disorders, such as FXS and Rett syndrome (RTT), because they show substantial phenotypic variability and limited genotype–phenotype correlation (Colvin et al., 2004; Kaufmann et al., 2004). Furthermore, some ID-associated disorders have a dynamic evolution that requires periodic assessments of neurological and behavioral features (e.g., four clinical stages in RTT; Hagberg, 2002). These diagnostic efforts are supported by a small but increasing body of literature emphasizing that the success of pharmacological and nonpharmacological therapies in ID depends on identifying the unique neurobehavioral profile of each patient (Berry-Kravis & Potanos, 2004). For example, special education programs aimed at improving functional communication will differ if the patient presents only with cognitive delay or if ID is associated with severe autistic features.

In addition to the laboratory tests outlined in Table 7.2 and Figures 7.1 and 7.2, specialized molecular genetic approaches are becoming available for a variety of less well-characterized disorders (e.g., nonsyndromic X-linked ID; Chiurazzi, Tabolacci, & Neri, 2004) as well as for atypical mutations in common conditions (e.g., mutations affecting exon 1 of *MECP2* in RTT; Philippe et al., 2006). As evident for more traditional diagnostic approaches (Shevell et al., 2003; Srour et al., 2006), the yield of new genetic tests will to a large extent depend on the information provided by focused clinical assessment as delineated earlier and in Table 7.1.

DENDRITIC AND SYNAPTIC ABNORMALITIES: A FUNDAMENTAL FEATURE OF GENETIC INTELLECTUAL DISABILITY

Since the application in the early 1970s of dendritic labeling techniques (e.g., Golgi impregnations) to postmortem brain samples, it has become evident that reductions in dendritic branching and abnormalities of dendritic spine morphology are the most consistent anatomic features in genetic and environmental conditions associated with ID (Marin-Padilla, 1972) (Table 7.3, Figure 7.3). More extensive anatomic derangements, such as cortical malformations secondary to disturbed neuronal proliferation and/or migration, are commonly associated with "stagnated" cognitive and motor development and, therefore, may resemble early GDD but not the slow acquisition of skills seen in patients with more typical ID disorders. The frequently reduced life expectancy in subjects with severe brain abnormalities and associated non–central nervous system (non-CNS) malformations complicates their inclusion in diagnostic and management strategies designed for common genetic ID syndromes (Kaufmann, 2003; Kaufmann & Moser, 2000). Although genetically identified causes of ID are more prevalent in syndromic than nonsyndromic forms of ID, there has been considerable progress in identifying single-gene causes of X-linked nonsyndromic forms of ID (Chiurazzi et al., 2004). The relevance of dendritic and other synaptic abnormalities to ID has been underscored by their reproduction in animal models of these genetic disorders and by the demonstration that many genes mu-

Table 7.3. Neocortical cytoarchitectonic and dendritic abnormalities in genetic disorders associated with intellectual disabilities[a]

Disorder	Laminar disturbance	Increased packing density	Reduced dendritic length	Spine dysgenesis
Down syndrome	Yes	No	Yes	Yes
Fragile X syndrome	No	No	No	Yes
Neurofibromatosis-1	Yes (focal)	No	?	?
Tuberous sclerosis	Yes (focal)	Yes (focal)	Yes (focal)	Yes (focal)
Williams syndrome	Yes	Yes	?	?
Rett syndrome	No	Yes	Yes	Yes
Phenylketonuria	No	Yes	Yes	Yes
Patau syndrome	Yes	No	Yes	Yes
Rubinstein-Taybi syndrome	No	Yes	?	?

Adapted from Kaufmann and Moser, Dendritic anomalies in disorders associated with mental retardation, Cerebral Cortex, 2000, 10(10), 981–991, by permission of Oxford University Press.

[a]The conditions have been listed according to estimated incidence.

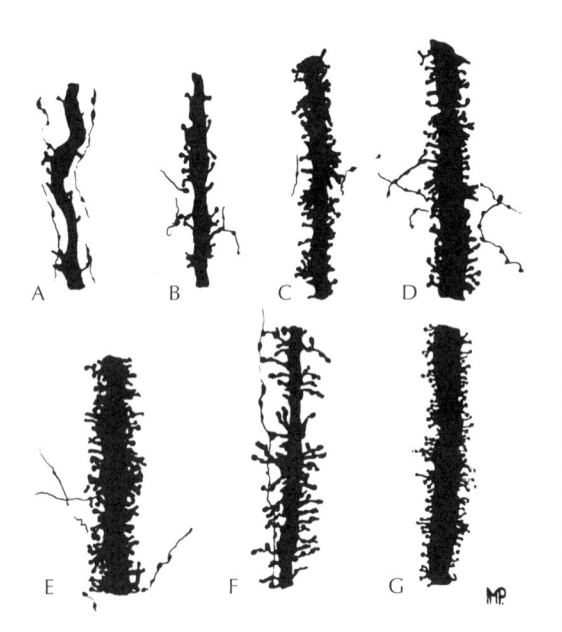

Figure 7.3. Dendritic spine abnormalities in Patau syndrome and Down syndrome (DS). Drawings are from Golgi preparations depicting comparable segments of apical dendrites from layer V pyramidal neurons (motor cortex). *A–E*, Different developmental stages in normal subjects (5th gestational month, 7th gestational month, neonatal period, 2nd postnatal month, and 8th postnatal month, respectively). *F*, A newborn with 13–15 trisomy. *G*, An 18-month-old infant with DS (trisomy 21). Note the progressive increase in spine density, associated with a reduction in spine length, during normal development. Spines in Patau syndrome are not only sparse, but also longer than expected for a neonate. Conversely, the infant with DS had shorter and thinner rather than longer spines. (Reprinted from Brain Research, 44, Marin-Padilla, M., Structural abnormalities of the cerebral cortex in human chromosomal aberrations: A Golgi study, 625–629, Copyright 1972, with permission from Elsevier.)

tated in ID are involved directly or indirectly in synaptic function (Inlow & Restifo, 2004). Comparative analyses of dendritic profiles of patients affected by genetic ID (e.g., FXS) and their related animal models (e.g., *Fmr1* knockout mouse) have also provided valuable insights into the nature and evolution of synaptic anomalies in these disorders.

DOWN SYNDROME

Down syndrome is the most common genetic cause of ID, occurring in an estimated 1 in 1,000 live births (Kaufmann, 1996; Roizen & Patterson, 2003). The DS phenotype is linked in most cases to chromosome 21 trisomy and involves characteristic aberrations of physical and neurological growth. Physical abnormalities include cardiac and gastrointestinal malformations. Neurological abnormalities include decreased brain size, immature gyral patterns, volumetric reductions in selective brain regions (e.g., frontal cortex), delayed myelination of cortical fibers, and abnormal neocortical lamination (Kates, Folley, Lanham, Capone, & Kaufmann, 2002; Kaufmann, 2003; Kaufmann & Moser, 2000; Roizen & Patterson, 2003). Table 7.4 presents a list of phenotypic features of DS. As in other ID disorders, and in correspondence with changes in dendritic length, there are also abnormalities in cortical cytoarchitecture (e.g., decrease in neuronal density in granular layers of the neocortex) (Benavides-Piccione et al., 2004; Kaufmann &

Table 7.4. Phenotypic features of Down syndrome

Physical features	Neurobehavioral features
Epicanthal folds	Mental retardation
Flat nasal bridge	Alzheimer-type dementia
Open mouth	
Short stature	Autistic-like features
Broad hands	Depression
Brachycephaly	Attention-deficit/ hyperactivity disorder
Brachydactyly	
Fifth finger clinodactyly	Obsessive-compulsive disorder
Cataracts	
Wide first-second toe gap	Anxiety
Lax ligaments	Aggressive-disruptive behaviors
Mitral valve prolapse	
Duodenal atresia	Hypotonia
Hypo/hyperthyroidism	Seizures
Cervical myelopathy	

Reprinted from The Lancet, 361, Roizon and Patterson, Down's Syndrome, 1281–1289, Copyright 2003, with permission from Elsevier.

Moser, 2000). In addition, poor laminar distinction in the superior temporal gyrus and aberrations of neuronal morphology and orientation have been noted (Benavides-Piccione et al., 2004; Kaufmann, 2003).

The profile of cortical dendritic abnormalities in DS suggests a postnatal process, characterized by initial normal development followed by progressive neurodegeneration. Several studies have reported normal numbers of dendrites and normal dendritic morphology in newborns with DS, with some reports of greater than normal dendritic arborization in infants with DS who are younger than 6 months, in contrast to marked reductions in length, branching, and spine density in early childhood (see Figure 7.3) (Benavides-Piccione et al., 2004; Kaufmann & Moser, 2000). Cross-sectional studies of adults with DS have revealed degenerative neuronal abnormalities of dendritic length and morphology (Benavides-Piccione et al., 2004). The course and nature of these dendritic abnormalities appear unique to DS and, in some reports, are related to the cognitive profile of DS (Benavides-Piccione et al., 2004; Kaufmann & Moser, 2000).

The study of the molecular bases of neuronal pathology in DS has been aided by the recent sequencing of the human genome and the application of data derived from animal models. Because DS involves triplication of an entire chromosome, estimated to contain upward of 200 genes (Benavides-Piccione et al., 2004), the number of related gene products is immense, and thus dendritic/synaptic abnormalities in this condition may be the result of altered expression levels of a variety of proteins coded for by genes on chromosome 21 (Table 7.5) (Capone, 2001). Dendritic development is a dynamic process involving changing expression profiles of dendritic proteins across the course of development, often in a time-dependent manner. In the case of DS, molecular analyses indicate that there is an accumulation of several cytoskeletal proteins in cortical neurons, most likely as a result of dendritic involution (Kaufmann, MacDonald, & Altamura, 2000). Recent genetic and molecular studies have implicated a number of chromosome 21 gene products in DS neuronal pathology.

DYRK1A, a serine-threonine kinase, controls dendrite growth and differentiation and is a modulator for cyclic AMP response element–binding protein (CREB), which is involved in neuronal differentiation and plasticity. In mouse models haploinsufficient for DYRK1A, cortical layer III pyramidal neurons show decreased soma size, dendritic arborization, and spine distribution compared to wild-type mice (Benavides-Piccione et al., 2004). In addition, Down syndrome cell adhesion molecule (DSCAM), an inhibitor of synaptogenesis and outgrowth of neurites, is elevated in brains of people with DS (Galdzicki, Siarey, Pearce, Stoll, & Rapoport, 2001). Drebrin, an actin-binding protein co-localized with actin in dendrites and filopodia in cortex, has been shown to be decreased in fetal DS brains during the second trimester of prenatal life. Similarly, levels of α-SNAP and SNAP-25, two synaptosomal proteins associated with drebrin, have also been reported to be lower in prenatal DS cortex during the second trimester (Galdzicki et al., 2001). Initial studies of channel and receptor function in the (partial trisomic) Ts65Dn mouse model have demonstrated abnormalities in action potential duration; rates of depolarization and repolarization; and sodium, potassium, and calcium channel kinetics, as well

Table 7.5. Genes in chromosome 21 that are possibly involved in brain development and degeneration in Down Syndrome

Symbol	MIM	Name	Possible effect in Down syndrome
SIM2	600892	Single-minded homologue 2 (*Drosophila*)	*Brain development:* required for synchronized cell division and establishment of proper cell lineage
DYRK1A	600855	Dual-specificity tyrosine-(Y)-phosphorylation–regulated kinase 1A	*Brain development:* expressed during neuroblast proliferation and believed an important homologue in regulation of cell cycle kinetics during cell division
GART	138440	Phosphoribosylglycinamide formyltransferase Phosphoribosylglycinamide synthetase Phosphoribosylaminoimidazole synthetase	*Brain development:* expressed during prenatal development of the cerebellum
PCP4	601629	Purkinje cell protein 4	*Brain development:* function unknown but found exclusively in the brain and most abundantly in the cerebellum
DSCAM	602523	Down syndrome cell adhesion molecule	*Brain development and possible candidate gene for congenital heart disease:* expressed in all regions of the brain and believed to have a role in axonal outgrowth during development of the nervous system
GRIK1	138245	Glutamate receptor, ionotropic, kainate 1	*Neuronal loss:* function unknown; found in the cortex in fetal and early postnatal life and in adult primates; most concentrated in pyramidal cells in the cortex
APP	104760	Amyloid beta A4 precursor protein (protease nexin-II, Alzheimer's disease)	*Alzheimer's-type neuropathy:* seems to be involved in plasticity, neurite outgrowth, and neuroprotection
S100B	176990	S100 calcium-binding protein, beta (neural)	*Alzheimer's-type neuropathy:* stimulates glial proliferation
SOD1	147450	Superoxide dismutase 1, soluble (amyotrophic lateral sclerosis 1, adult)	*Accelerated aging:* scavenges free superoxide molecules in the cell and might accelerate aging by producing hydrogen peroxide and oxygen

From Capone, G.T. (2001). Down syndrome: Advances in molecular biology and the neurosciences. *Journal of Developmental and Behavioral Pediatrics, 22*(1), 40–59, adapted by permission.

Key: MIM, Mendelian Inheritance in Man.

as unusual distribution patterns of those channels (Galdzicki et al., 2001). Further evidence from the Ts65Dn mouse suggests that hippocampal electrophysiology involving protein kinases A and C and the phosphoinositide pathway may be aberrant in DS, such that long-term potentiation and long-term depression and related learning and memory paradigms are affected (Galdzicki et al., 2001).

Taken together, the molecular, electrophysiological, and genetic data from DS and its animal models point to a predominantly functional (as opposed to structural) underlying neural abnormality. Although this information has not yet been applied toward improving the diagnostic classification of this relatively het-

erogeneous disorder, treatments aimed at remedying the neurological pathobiology in DS are beginning to emerge. Operating under the premise that homeostatic and metabolic processes are disrupted in DS (Roizen & Patterson, 2003), many dietary supplements, including vitamins and minerals, have been proposed to increase cognitive function, though such treatments have to date been largely ineffective (Roizen & Patterson, 2003; Salman, 2002). Pharmacological treatments have focused primarily on improving cognition in DS, mainly by targeting cholinergic and glutamatergic neurotransmission, although none of the currently available pharmacological interventions has consistently proven effective in this regard (note that there is still controversy about the type and magnitude of cholinergic abnormalities in children with DS). Nootropic drugs such as the cyclic γ-aminobutyric acid derivative piracetam, though initially promising in animal studies, have since shown poor results in patients with DS (Benavides-Piccione et al., 2004; Roizen & Patterson, 2003).

The association between DS and Alzheimer disease, including the accumulation of beta-amyloid (Aβ) plaques, the subsequent presynaptic cholinergic deficit, the development of dementia in both conditions, and the efficacy of cholinesterase inhibitors in targeting Alzheimer-related symptoms, has spurred research focusing on the effects of these drugs in DS. Nonetheless, drugs targeting the cholinergic system, including muscarinic agonists, acetylcholine analogues, and acetylcholinesterase inhibitors—specifically the cholinesterase inhibitor donepezil—have shown mixed results, with some studies reporting no significant clinical benefit and others reporting increases in socialization, expressive language, and adaptive behavior domains in subjects with and without dementia (Benavides-Piccione et al., 2004). Hormone therapies, including steroid, thyroid, and growth hormone treatments, have shown little promise, although new research on estrogen administration in the Ts65Dn mouse suggests that women with DS and dementia may benefit from such therapeutic regimens with respect to cognitive function and cholinergic phenotype (Benavides-Piccione et al., 2004). Lastly, in response to cognitive deficits and related long-term potentiation and long-term depression, drugs designed to target the glutamatergic system are emerging as a promising area of new research.

Alternative, nonpharmacological therapies, such as environmental/social enrichment, have shown mixed results, both in humans and in Ts65Dn mice (Kaufmann & Moser, 2000). Environmental enrichment and related interventions in the trisomic mouse have produced measurable improvements in cognitive function (e.g., performance in a Morris water maze), as well as increases in dendritic complexity and number of spines in female mice, though these results were strongly gender specific because environmental enrichment actu-

ally worsened Morris water maze performance in male Ts65Dn mice (Benavides-Piccione et al., 2004). In children with DS, educational interventions have demonstrated efficacy in improving performance on measures of cognitive function, though these effects appear minor and transient (Benavides-Piccione et al., 2004; Roizen & Patterson, 2003).

X-LINKED INTELLECTUAL DISABILITY DISORDERS

Among genetic disorders associated with ID, the group in which the primary defect involves genes on the X chromosome, termed X-linked ID (XLID), deserves special consideration because it comprises 20%–25% of cases of ID with a high proportion of inheritance. XLID includes a relatively large number of conditions in which the only clinical manifestations are ID-related cognitive and behavioral abnormalities (nonsyndromic XLID), as well as a few disorders in which there are physical or metabolic features (syndromic XLID) (Chiurazzi et al., 2004; Inlow & Restifo, 2004). Although at present mutated genes have been identified in only approximately 10% of families with XLID, this represents a comparatively high percentage in the context of ID in general. Of particular interest is the group of genes linked to nonsyndromic XLID because many of them are involved in the Rho-GTPase signaling pathway. Examples of these are oligophrenin-1, a RhoA-GAP (GTPase-activating protein) that interacts with several postsynaptic density proteins; α-PIX, a guanine nucleotide exchange factor (GEF) for Rac and Cdc42; and PAK 3, a RhoA effector protein.

Because the Rho signaling system is involved in key processes leading to dendritic and axonal formation, such as neuronal and spine morphogenesis polarity, neurite outgrowth, and synapse formation (Table 7.6) (Ramakers, 2002), it is reasonable to speculate that these XLID conditions are primary synaptic disorders. Because different components of the Rho system have opposite effects on dendritic development (e.g., Rac and Cdc42 promote, activated RhoA inhibits), these XLID disorders appear to represent imbalances in synaptic formation and plasticity. Novel therapeutic approaches targeting GTPase-related

Table 7.6. Genes involved in nonsyndromic and syndromic X-linked intellectual disabilities (ID), with emphasis on Rho signaling[a,b]

Gene	Locus	Protein name(s)	Function(s)	Effects of mutation(s)	MRX family[c]	MIM[d]
Nonsyndromic ID (MRX) genes						
ARHGEF6	Xq26	α-PIX, Cool-2	GEF for Rac/Cdc42; activator of PAKs	Exon skipping, 28–amino acid deletion in CH domain, loss of function owing to translocation	MRX46	300267
FMR2	Xq28	FMR2	Transcriptional activator? (AF-4 like)	Truncation, loss of expression		309548
GDI1	Xq28	α-GDI, RABGD1A	GDI for Rab3a, b; neurotransmitter release and vesicle trafficking	Decrease and loss of function, truncation, and loss of expression	MRX41, fam R MRX48	300104
IL1RAPL	Xp22	ILRAPL	IL signaling?	Deletions, truncation, and decreased expression	MRX34	300206
OPHN1	Xq12	Oligophrenin-1	Rho family GAP inhibitor of RhoA?	Frameshift and decreased expression, loss of function	MRX60	300127
PAK3	Xq22	PAK 3, β-PAK	Ser/Thr protein kinase; Cdc42/Rac1 effector	Truncation, loss of kinase activity, mutation in GTPase-binding domain	MRX30, MRX47	300142
TM4SF2	Xp11	Tetraspanin 2	Intergrin-mediated signaling?	Truncation, mutation in extracellular loop, translocation and decreased expression		300096
Syndromic ID genes involved in Rho signaling						
FGDY	Xp11	FGD1	GEF for Cdc42	Truncation, mutations in PH and GEF domain	Faciogenital dysplasia; Aarskog-Scott syndrome	305400
LIMK1	7q11	LIM kinase-1	Tyr kinase downstream of Rac/Cdc42 and PAK; phosphorylates and inactivates cofilin	Deletion of multiple genes, including elastin gene	Williams syndrome (probably involved)	601329

Reprinted from *Trends in Neurosciences, 25,* Ramakers, Rho proteins, mental retardation and the cellular basis of cognition, 191–199. Copyright 2002, with permission from Elsevier.

[a]It also includes a gene on chromosome 7, *LIMK1,* which is also implicated in Rho signaling.

[b]Only well-confirmed MRX genes (listed in the XLMR Update web site) are included. Genes involved in both nonsyndromic and syndromic MR are excluded. All genes are expressed in fetal and adult brain.

[c]As listed in the XLMR Update website (http://xlmr.interfree.it/home.htm).

[d]Entry numbers for Online Mendelian Inheritance in Man database; for further information and references, go to http://www.ncbi.nlm.nih.gov/entrez/query.fcgi?db = OMIM.

Key: MRX, nonspecific mental retardation/intellectual disability; ARHGEF, Rho guanine nucleotide exchange factor; PIX, PAK-interacting exchange factor; Cool-2, cloned out of library 2; GEF, guanine nucleotide exchange factor; PAK, p21-associated kinase; FMR, fragile site mental retardation; GDI, guanine dissociation inhibitor; RABGDIA, Rab GDP-dissociation inhibitor a; IL1RAPL, IL-1 receptor accessory protein like; IL, interleukin; TM4SF2, transmembrane-4 superfamily 2; FGD, faciogenital dysplasia; PH, pleckstrin homology; LIMK, LIM domain containing kinase.

disorders, including perturbations of the balance of the Rho system, may lead to specific treatments for this group of XLID conditions. Furthermore, recent approaches for the identification of mutations involving genes on the X chromosome (e.g., customary microarray technology), in conjunction with the characteristic pedigrees of families affected by X-linked disorders, hold the promise of increasing the number of identified XLID conditions (Chiurazzi et al., 2004). The following two sections review important neurobiological aspects of the two most common XLID syndromes: FXS and RTT.

Fragile X Syndrome

FXS is the most prevalent form of inherited ID, affecting 1 in 4,000 males and 1 in 6,000 females. The disorder is linked to the expansion of a CGG polymorphism in the 5'-untranslated regulatory region (5'UTR) of *FMR1*. When the normal approximately 30 CGG repeats increase to more than 200 (full mutation), *FMR1* promoter hypermethylation, *FMR1* transcriptional silencing, and the FXS phenotype occur. Intermediate-level expansions (60–200 CGG repeats), which are termed *premutation,* are not associated with FXS (Kaufmann & Reiss, 1999). In addition to mild to moderate ID, FXS is characterized by dysmorphic features, connective tissue abnormalities (e.g., lax joints), and other non-CNS phenotypic anomalies (e.g., macroorchidism after puberty); however, variable cognitive and language impairments and associated neurobehavioral problems, including attentional difficulties, hyperactivity, anxiety, and autistic disorder, constitute the major medical and educational concerns for patients with FXS (Table 7.7) (Kaufmann & Reiss, 1999). As in DS, the exact proportion of individuals with certain phenotypical features in FXS is unclear because the published range is quite wide (Hagerman, 2002). Ascertainment bias and variable diagnostic instruments and definitions are the main reasons for these discrepancies. As expected in an X-linked condition, the characteristic features of FXS are more prominent in affected males.

Neuroimaging studies have shown that in FXS the brain is in general larger (i.e., most cortical regions, caudate, hippocampus),

Table 7.7. Variable phenotypic features of Fragile X syndrome

Physical features	Neurobehavioral features
Large ears	Mild to moderate
Thick nasal bridge	intellectual disabilities
Prominent jaw	Language delay,
High-arched/narrow	predominantly expressive
palate	Rapid/burst-like speech
Pale blue irides	Attentional-organizational
Strabismus	dysfunction
Pectus excavatum	Visuospatial impairment
Kyphoscoliosis	Hyperactivity
Lax joints	Autistic-like features
Single palmar crease	Aggressive behavior
Flat feet	Hyperarousal
Cutis laxa	Anxiety, particularly social
Mitral valve prolapse	Stereotypic/perseverative
Macroorchidism	behavior
	Hypotonia
	Nystagmus
	Seizures

From Kaufmann W. E., and Reiss, A. L. (1999). Molecular and cellular genetics of fragile X syndrome. *American Journal of Medical Genetics, 88,* 11–24; adapted by permission.

though of normal configuration. Nonetheless, certain areas such as the temporal neocortex and the posterior cerebellar vermis are decreased in (absolute and relative) size (Kates et al., 2002). Postmortem analyses of the cerebral cortex in males with FXS demonstrate that the most consistent anatomic abnormality is an aberrant conformation of dendritic spines, which are longer and tortuous (Figure 7.4) (Irwin,

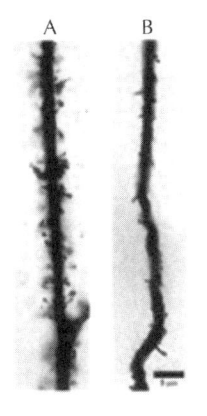

Figure 7.4. Examples of typical spine morphologies on Golgi-impregnated dendrites from a person with fragile X syndrome (*A*) and an unaffected control (*B*). Dendrites are at extremes of density differences and not intended to depict the norm. (From Irwin, S.A., Galvez, R., & Greenough, W.T., Dendritic spine structural anomalies in fragile-X mental retardation syndrome, *Cerebral Cortex, 2000, 10*(10), 1038–1044; by permission of Oxford University Press.)

Galvez, & Greenough, 2000; Kaufmann & Moser, 2000). Similar profiles have been observed in mice lacking the *Fmr1* product, the fragile X mental retardation protein (FMRP) (Kaufmann & Moser, 2000). This spine configuration resembles that of early stages of normal dendritic development (see Figure 7.3A–D), which suggests that in FXS there is a maturational arrest of dendritic spine formation.

The combination of studies on patient samples, animal models, and in vitro systems has led to an explosion of knowledge about the neurobiology of FXS, in particular on the dendritic and synaptic abnormalities in FXS (Bagni & Greenough, 2005; Bear, Huber, & Warren, 2004; Kaufmann & Moser, 2000). FMRP is an RNA-binding protein that associates with polyribosomes and is involved in the transport and translational regulation (i.e., mainly inhibition) of a selected subset of transcripts at synaptic sites (Bagni & Greenough, 2005). FMRP appears also to be linked to the microRNA pathway (Jin, Alisch, & Warren, 2004). Among the mRNAs regulated by FMRP are those coding for key cytoskeletal (e.g., MAP1-B) and synaptic (e.g., Arc) constituents. It is postulated that the role of FMRP is to regulate protein synthesis in response to synaptic activity, enabling in this way the adaptation of particularly the postsynaptic site to multiple influences during development and plasticity (Bagni & Greenough, 2005).

Of importance for understanding the mechanisms of action of FMRP deficiency is the consistent observation of long-term depression enhancement in the hippocampus of the *Fmr1* knockout mouse (other synaptic abnormalities are less well characterized). This group 1 metabotropic glutamate receptor (mGluR)– and protein synthesis–dependent type of long-term depression has been linked to a variety of neurobehavioral manifestations of FXS, as well as to the unique appearance of dendritic spines in the mouse model (Figure 7.5) (Bear et al., 2004). Exaggerated group 1 mGluR activity would lead to a reduction in the AMPA and NMDA subtypes of glutamate receptors on the postsynaptic surface that, in conjunction with an imbalance in key postsynaptic proteins, would result in a morphologically and functionally immature/deficient synapse unable to

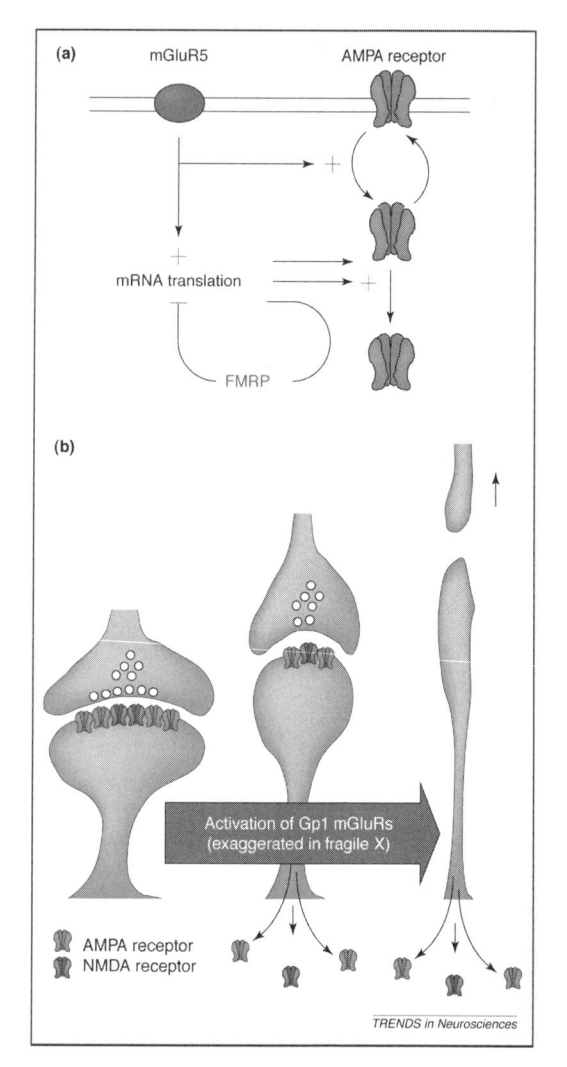

Figure 7.5. Models of protein synthesis–dependent, functional and structural consequences of group 1 (Gp1) metabotropic glutamate receptor (mGluR) activation at hippocampal synapses, and the role of FMRP. *A,* Model to account for exaggerated mGluR–long-term depression (mGluR-LTD) in the *Fmr1* knockout mouse, based on the assumption that FMRP is synthesized in response to mGluR activation and functions as a translational repressor. *B,* Model relating the net loss of synaptic AMPA and NMDA receptors and elongation of dendritic spines observed following Gp1 mGluR activation in cultured hippocampal neurons. (Reprinted from Trends in Neurosciences, 27, Bear, M.F., Huber, K.M., & Warren, S.T., The mGluR theory of fragile X mental retardation, 370–377, Copyright 2004, with permission from Elsevier.)

deal with subtle changes in synaptic activity. Another potential mechanism for dendritic changes in FXS is the interaction between FMRP and the cytoplasmic interacting proteins CYFIP1 and CYFIP2, which bind activated Rac1. This provides a pathogenetic link between FXS and the Rho system–dependent abnormalities (e.g., actin cytoskeleton remodeling) in the nonsyndromic XLID disorders described in the preceding section.

The knowledge of specific targets of FMRP in the CNS, as well as of defective synaptic processes, offers the opportunity to improve current diagnostic and therapeutic approaches to FXS. Despite the single-gene nature of FXS, at present it is not possible to anticipate which patients with *FMR1* full mutation will develop a severe neurobehavioral phenotype. Molecular profiling of patients with FXS, through the measurement in peripheral samples of relevant biomarkers, may help in diagnostic classification, prognosis, and subject selection for treatment. In addition, pharmacological interventions aimed at restoring a balance in glutamate receptor activity (some currently under development), such as decreasing group 1 mGluR activity and enhancing AMPA receptor function, would provide a neurobiologically based amelioration of FXS manifestations.

Rett Syndrome

RTT is an XLID condition that affects predominantly females, with an incidence of 1 in 10,000–15,000 births. RTT is a severe disorder, lethal in most male cases (Kankirawatana et al., 2006) and the second leading cause of GDD and severe ID in females (Akbarian, 2003; Hagberg, 2002). The majority of RTT cases are associated with mutations in the coding region of *MECP2,* a gene located on Xq28 that encodes the transcriptional repressor methyl-CpG–binding protein 2 (MeCP2) (Akbarian, 2003; Hagberg, 2002; Kaufmann, Johnston, & Blue, 2005). RTT is a dynamic condition; apparently normal development from birth until 6–18 months of age is followed by deceleration of head growth and failure to attain new milestones. During this "regressive" stage, progressive loss of language and motor skills characteristically develops. Additional manifestations include respiratory irregularities, impaired social interaction (i.e., "autistic-like" features), seizures, and the stereotypic hand-wringing movements that characterize the disorder (Tables 7.8 and 7.9) (Hagberg, 2002). Typically, after age 3–4 years, the neurological manifestations tend to stabilize or improve (e.g., language) for a period of years. By adolescence, a slow motor decline that lasts for decades becomes apparent and in most cases leads to wheelchair dependency (Hagberg, 2002). Other non-CNS clinical features, such as disturbed gastrointestinal motility and abnormal autonomic vascular regulation, appear to be related to peripheral neuronal dysfunction. The described "classic" RTT phenotype may not be fully developed in a variety of atypical forms of RTT, including rare male cases (Hagberg, 2002; Kaufmann et al., 2005). Mutations in *MECP2* and brain tissue changes in MeCP2 expression have been associated with other phenotypes, such as nonspecific ID, Angelman syndrome, and ASD (Hagberg, 2002; Kaufmann et al., 2005).

The neuroanatomic phenotype of RTT is characterized by a marked brain hypoplasia, with slightly greater involvement of the cerebral gray matter (Akbarian, 2003; Kaufmann et al., 2005; Naidu et al., 2001). At the microscopic level, there is a generalized increase in cell packing density and marked decrease in the size of the neuronal soma and dendritic tree. Abnormal dendritic spine profiles have also been described in postmortem cortical samples from people with RTT (Akbarian, 2003; Kaufmann &

Table 7.8. Diagnostic criteria for Rett syndrome

Manifestation/age	Comments
Infant apparently normal initially	Pre/perinatal period as well as first 6 months of life or longer
Head circumference stagnation at 3 months–4 years	Normal at birth, then a decelerating growth rate
Purposeful hand skill loss at 9 months–2.5 years	Communicative dysfunction, social withdrawal, mental deficiency, loss of speech/babbling
Classic stereotypic hand movements after 1–3 years	Hand washing/wringing or clapping/tapping
Gait/posture dyspraxia at 2–4 years	Gait "ataxia"/more or less jerky truncal "ataxia"

From Mental Retardation and Developmental Disabilities Research Reviews, Vol. 8, No. 2, 2002, pp. 61–65. Copyright © 2002 Wiley-Liss. Reprinted with permission of Wiley-Liss, Inc., a subsidiary of John Wiley & Sons, Inc.

Table 7.9. Clinical stages of classic Rett syndrome

Original staging system	Later additions
Stage I: Early-Onset Stagnation	
Onset age: 6 months to 1.5 years	Onset from 5 months of age
Developmental progress delayed	Early postural delay
Developmental pattern still not significantly abnormal	Dissociated development "Bottom-shufflers"
Duration: weeks to months	
Stage II: Developmental Regression	
Onset age: 1–3 or 4 years	
Loss of acquired skills/communication	Loss of acquired skills: fine finger, babble/words, active playing
Mental deficiency appears	Occasionally "in another world"
	Eye contact preserved
	Breathing problems still modest
	Seizures in only 15%
Duration: weeks to months, possibly 1 year	
Stage III: Pseudostationary Period	
Onset age: after passing Stage II	
Some communicative restitution	"Wake-up" period
Apparently preserved ambulant ability	Prominent hand apraxia/dyspraxia
Unapparent, slow neuromotor regression	
Duration: years to decades	
Stage IV: Late Motor Deterioration	
Onset age: when Stage III ambulation ceases	
Complete wheelchair dependency	Subgrouping introduced:
Severe disability: wasting and distal distortion	Stage IV A: previous walkers, now nonambulant
	Stage IV B: never ambulant
Duration: decades	

From Mental Retardation and Developmental Disabilities Research Reviews, Vol. 8, No. 2, 2002, pp. 61–65. Copyright © 2002 Wiley-Liss. Reprinted with permission of Wiley-Liss, Inc., a subsidiary of John Wiley & Sons, Inc.

Moser, 2000; Kaufmann et al., 2005). Although neuroimaging and postmortem anatomic studies indicate more severe changes in areas such as the frontal cortex, subcortical cholinergic neuronal groups, and the monoaminergic nuclei of the brainstem (e.g., substantia nigra hypopigmentation), severe neuronal pathology is a widespread finding in RTT (Akbarian, 2003; Kaufmann et al., 2005; Naidu et al., 2001). The previously mentioned neuronal structural features, as well as immunochemical data showing reductions in cytoskeletal proteins linked to neuronal differentiation (Figure 7.6) (Kaufmann et al., 2000), suggest that the fundamen-

tal cellular phenotype in RTT is a disturbance in neuronal maturation.

As in FXS, some of the key cellular and neurological features of the disorder have been reproduced in mouse models lacking MeCP2 expression (Akbarian, 2003; Kaufmann et al., 2005). This finding provides further evidence for the classification of RTT as a disorder of synaptic development. Neurotransmitter abnormalities associated with either the early stages (i.e., reduction in monoamines) or the period of regression (i.e., increase in glutamate levels and NMDA receptor binding) of RTT have not yet been reported in the recently developed an-

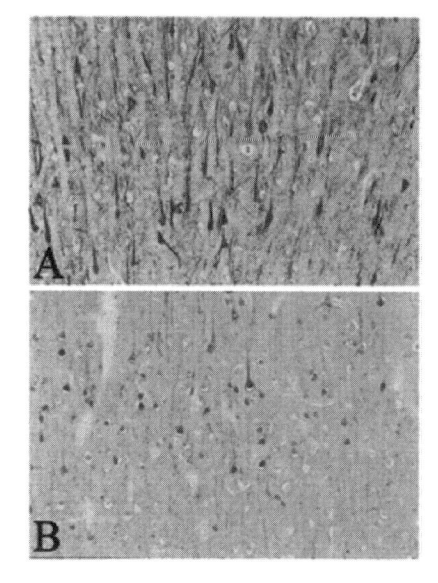

Figure 7.6. Immunohistochemical pattern of MAP-2 in motor cortex. *A,* In control subjects, perikaryal and, predominantly, dendritic staining is seen throughout layer V. *B,* In Rett syndrome, there is a marked reduction in MAP-2 staining involving both somas and dendrites in the same lamina. Note also the smaller cell bodies in Rett syndrome. (*A* and *B* both × 140.) (From Kaufmann, W.E., Mac-Donald, S.M., & Altamura, C., Dendritic cytoskeletal protein expression in mental retardation: An immunohistochemical study of the neocortex in Rett syndrome. *Cerebral Cortex, 2000, 10*(10), 992–1004, by permission of Oxford University Press.)

imal models of the disorder, which show cognitive and behavioral impairments (Moretti et al., 2006).

MeCP2 binds methylated DNA sequences through its methyl-binding domain and subsequently recruits histone deacetylases, via interactions between its transcriptional repressor domain and co-repressors (e.g., Sin3A). This process, which alters chromatin architecture from an active to an inactive state, may not be the only mechanism of action of MeCP2 (Akbarian, 2003; Young et al., 2005). Regardless, as expected from MeCP2 deficit, increases in levels of acetylated histones have been demonstrated in a mouse model of *MECP2* nonsense (i.e., protein truncation) mutation (Kaufmann et al., 2005). In contrast to FXS, the search for genes transcriptionally silenced by MeCP2 has been a frustrating endeavor. Brain-derived neurotrophic factor (BDNF) is one of the few recognized targets of MeCP2, which also supports a role for MeCP2 in synaptic plasticity (Chang, Khare, Dani, Nelson, & Jaenisch, 2006; Kaufmann et al., 2005).

The recent demonstration of two *MECP2* transcripts with differential tissue distribution,

and of MeCP2 immunoreactivities of different molecular weight and intracellular localization, suggests that MeCP2 regulation is a complex phenomenon with unique temporal and spatial dimensions (Kaufmann et al., 2005). Available data on the pattern of MeCP2 expression suggest that it plays a role in the maintenance of neuronal differentiation and in other synaptic activity–dependent processes. In the CNS, MeCP2 expression is almost exclusively neuronal and begins at the time in which the differentiated neuroblast phenotype is established and synaptogenesis begins (Figure 7.7) (Akbarian, 2003; Kaufmann et al., 2005; Mullaney, Johnston, & Blue, 2004).

In contrast with other transcriptional regulators, MeCP2 levels in several brain regions (e.g., cerebral cortex) increase steadily until the adult stage (Akbarian, 2003; Kaufmann et al., 2005). Neuronal activation and neural circuit manipulation lead to changes in MeCP2 levels and possibly in the protein's conformation, as suggested by the de-repression of the BDNF promoter secondary to MeCP2 phosphorylation in stimulated neurons. Altogether, these data support the hypothesis that MeCP2 plays a critical role in synaptic plasticity both during development and in the processes of learning and memory in the adult brain (Table 7.10) (Kaufmann et al., 2005). Consequently, MeCP2 deficit during synaptic formation and stabilization, after the establishment of the

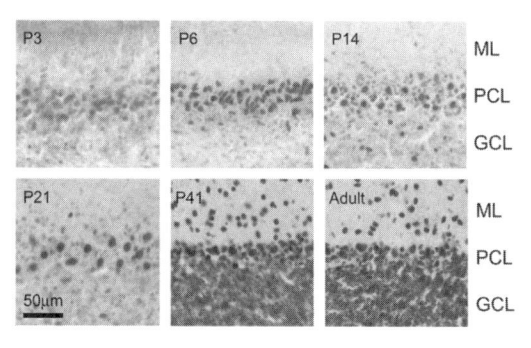

Figure 7.7. Ontogeny of MeCP2 staining in the rat cerebellum. MeCP2 expression patterns change dramatically with age; early postnatal ages exhibit significant staining only in Purkinje cells and Golgi cells within the granule cell layer (GCL). Granule cells exhibited minimal MeCP2 staining up through the first 3 postnatal weeks but were darkly stained by postnatal day (P) 41. (Reprinted from Neuroscience, 123, Mullaney B.C., Johnston, M.V., & Blue, M.E., Developmental expression of methyl-CpG binding protein 2 is dynamically regulated in the rodent brain, 939–949. Copyright 2004, with permission from Elsevier.) (*Key:* ML, molecular layer; PCL, Purkinje cell layer.)

Table 7.10. Evidence supporting role of MeCP2 in synaptic plasticity

Feature
ERK1-like N-terminal motif (MeCP2B)
Extranuclear localization (MeCP2A, MeCP2B)
Postsynaptic localization
Membrane depolarization–dependent BDNF silencing
100-kD MeCP2-like band in synaptic fractions
Neuronal group–specific pattern of expression
High-expressing neuronal subtype (postnatally)
Levels regulated by deafferentation (olfactory system)
Induction by hippocampal kindling

Reprinted from Brain and Development, 27, Kaufmann, W.E., Johnston, M.V., & Blue, M.E., MeCP2 expression and function during brain development: Implications for Rett syndrome's pathogenesis and clinical evolution, S77–S87, Copyright 2005, with permission from Elsevier.

neuronal phenotype, would lead to the marked reductions of dendritic arborization seen in RTT.

Although identification of MeCP2 targets is still in its early stages, preliminary work on histone acetylation and methylation profiles indicates that these and other indices of MeCP2 function in peripheral cells hold the promise of improving the limited predictive value of mutation patterns in RTT (Kaufmann et al., 2005). Alternative diagnostic classifications, or those complementary to the existing ones, which are based on type of mutation and clinical profile, could be of great importance in the near future because new treatments are emerging. As in DS, recently available modulators of cholinergic and glutamatergic activity are being considered as the first group of neurobiologically based pharmacological interventions for RTT. Insight into the genetic defect also offers the possibility of modifying defective DNA methylation binding and histone deacetylation; clinical trials with methyl group donors such as folate are currently in progress (Percy, 2002).

OTHER GENETIC INTELLECTUAL DISABILITY DISORDERS

There is indirect evidence that, in other genetic ID conditions, there are dendritic/synaptic abnormalities similar to those reported in DS and XLID (Kaufmann, 1996; Kaufmann & Moser, 2000). On the basis of studies of RTT and idiopathic autism, increased neuronal density by cytoarchitectonic analyses, which can be interpreted as a likely reduction in length and complexity of dendritic trees, has been demonstrated in Williams syndrome (WS) and Rubinstein-Taybi syndrome (RTS) (see Table 7.3) (Kaufmann & Moser, 2000).

WS is caused by a submicroscopic deletion on chromosome 7q11.23, which includes the elastin gene; the HPC-1/syntaxin 1A (*STX1A*) gene, which codes for a protein involved in the docking of synaptic vesicles; and the gene coding for LIM kinase-1 (*LIMK1*), which is linked to the Rho signaling system (see Table 7.6). Patients with WS show a distinctive cognitive and social phenotype; although they demonstrate relatively preserved language and face processing abilities, subjects with WS typically experience impairments in visuospatial domains. In addition, they are hypersociable, with engaging personalities and excessive sociability with strangers (Bellugi, Lichtenberger, Mills, Galaburda, & Korenberg, 1999).

In correspondence with their profile of strengths and weaknesses, morphometric neuroimaging studies have shown relative reductions in parieto-occipital regions and enlargement of frontal temporal structures involved in emotion and face processing (Reiss et al., 2004). Neuropathological data on WS are limited; however, generalized reductions in cortical columnar organization and increases in cell packing density, as well as abnormal neuronal orientation that is more severe in posterior regions, have been reported (Kaufmann & Moser, 2000). Despite the lack of direct evidence of postsynaptic abnormalities in WS, defective LIM kinase-1 function may lead to dendritic spine dysgenesis and enhanced long-term potentiation as shown in *Limk1* knockout mice (Meng et al., 2002). LIM kinase-1, which is downstream of Rac/Cdc42 and PAK, phosphorylates and inactivates cofilin, influencing in this way actin cytoskeletal dynamics (i.e., increasing turnover) and dendritic morphology (Meng et al., 2002; Ramakers, 2002). Interestingly, levels of phospho-cofilin are reduced in *Fmr1* knockout mice, suggesting that WS and FXS may share common dendritic spine abnormalities.

In addition to ID, RTS is characterized by selective deficits in expressive language and by maladaptive behavior. Initially described somatic/skeletal abnormalities include short stature, facial dysmorphia, and broad thumbs and first toes (Kaufmann & Moser, 2000). The genetic defect in RTS (16p13.3) has been reported to involve CREB-binding protein, a protein that is recruited by CREB to bind DNA and activates the basal transcription factor–enzyme complex (Kaufmann & Worley, 1999). Limited neuroimaging and neuropathological investigations have shown an association between RTS and several CNS malformations, such as agenesis of the corpus callosum. Nonetheless, the most comprehensive neuropathological evaluation of the brain of an adult with RTS reported mild reduction in brain weight, overall preserved cortical architecture, but decreased neuronal size and marked increase in cell packing density (Kaufmann & Moser, 2000). In correspondence to the critical role of CREB-binding protein in neuronal function both as a transcriptional activator and a histone acetyltransferase, mice modeling a haploinsufficiency form of RTS showed decreased chromatin acetylation and impairment in some forms of long-term memory and the late phase of hippocampal long-term potentiation (Alarcon et al., 2004). Of mechanistic and therapeutic importance, these memory and long-term potentiation deficits can be ameliorated by enhancing the expression of CREB-dependent genes and by inhibiting histone deacetylase activity (Alarcon et al., 2004).

CONCLUSION

There is considerable evidence that a disturbance of neuronal differentiation, and to a lesser extent of other CNS developmental processes, underlies most genetic forms of ID (Kaufmann, 2003; Kaufmann & Moser, 2000). Furthermore, morphological and molecular data indicate that impaired neuronal and synaptic formation in ID represents a defect in signaling pathways involved in synaptic plasticity (Johnston, 2004). The postsynaptic compartment, comprising neurotransmitter receptors (e.g., glutamate receptors), cytoskeletal elements (e.g., actin), signaling proteins (e.g., kinases), and anchoring molecules that "connect" the former constituents (e.g., Homer), seems to be particularly affected in ID. Therefore, the dendritic abnormalities in patients with ID appear to be the structural correlate of less "adaptable" postsynaptic sites.

Because there is an economy of genetic programs responsible for neuronal adaptation to environmental changes, most key molecules involved in the modeling of synapses during development are also implicated in cognition and complex behavior in the adult brain (Johnston, 2004; Kaufmann & Worley, 1999). This molecular "double jeopardy" in genetic ID results in an abnormally developed brain that also lacks the "machinery" for responding properly/optimally to environmental stimuli. Although this is an apparently negative situation, it also represents an opportunity because, as demonstrated in animal models (Alarcon et al., 2004; Bear et al., 2004), modifying the fundamental molecular or neurotransmitter disturbances in adulthood can lead to improvement of cognition and behavior. This means that there is a lifelong possibility of ameliorating the neurobehavioral phenotype in genetic ID, though the ultimate goal is to intervene before synaptic development is complete. Considering that environmental causes of ID (e.g., lead poisoning) could also affect signaling programs disturbed in genetic ID (Johnston, 2004), therapeutic approaches for genetic disorders may have a broader application.

Although neurobiologically based treatments for genetic ID are emerging, several major challenges remain in the field. First, there is a need for understanding how changes in dendritic morphology or in postsynaptic components translate into functional (e.g., neurotransmitter) alterations in synaptic transmission. The extent to which presynaptic abnormalities are also present in ID should be better characterized; the current emphasis on dendritic pathology is in part the consequence of methodological advantages for studying postsynaptic elements. Although knowledge of synaptic anomalies has led to novel pharmacological strategies, there is the possibility of using neurobiological information for planning more effective nonpharmacological interventions. For instance, the role of environmental stimulation in genetic ID treatment is still unclear. Neurobiologically supported pharmacological enhancement of different therapies is also a potential alternative. Despite all of these issues, the future of the clinical management of ID is quite promising because it will be able to take advantage of innovations in genetics, developmental neurobiology, neuroimaging, and other relevant fields.

REFERENCES

Akbarian, S. (2003). The neurobiology of Rett syndrome. *Neuroscientist, 9,* 57–63.

Alarcon, J.M., Malleret, G., Touzani, K., Vronskaya, S., Ishii, S., Kandel, E.R., et al. (2004). Chromatin acetylation, memory, and LTP are impaired in CBP + / – mice: A model for the cognitive deficit in Rubinstein-Taybi syndrome and its amelioration. *Neuron, 42,* 947–959.

Bagni, C., & Greenough, W.T. (2005). From mRNP trafficking to spine dysmorphogenesis: The roots of fragile X syndrome. *Nature Review: Neuroscience, 6,* 376–387.

Bear, M.F., Huber, K.M., & Warren, S.T. (2004). The mGluR theory of fragile X mental retardation. *Trends in Neurosciences, 27,* 370–377.

Bellugi, U., Lichtenberger, L., Mills, D., Galaburda, A., & Korenberg, J.R. (1999). Bridging cognition, the brain and molecular genetics: Evidence from Williams syndrome. *Trends in Neurosciences, 22,* 197–207.

Benavides-Piccione, R., Ballesteros-Yáñez, I., Martínez de Lagrán, M., Elston, G., Estivill, X., Fillat, C., et al. (2004). On dendrites in Down syndrome and DS murine models: A spiny way to learn. *Progress in Neurobiology, 74,* 111–126.

Berry-Kravis, E., & Potanos, K. (2004). Psychopharmacology in fragile X syndrome—present and future. *Mental Retardation and Developmental Disabilities Research Reviews, 10,* 42–48.

Capone, G.T. (2001). Down syndrome: Advances in molecular biology and the neurosciences. *Journal of Developmental and Behavioral Pediatrics, 22,* 40–59.

Capone, G., Goyal, P., Ares, W., & Lannigan, E. (2006). Neurobehavioral disorders in children, adolescents, and young adults with Down syndrome. *American Journal of Medical Genetics. Part C, Seminars in Medical Genetics, 142,* 158–172.

Capone, G.T., Grados, M.A., Kaufmann, W.E., Bernad-Ripoll, S., & Jewell, A. (2005). Down syndrome and comorbid autism-spectrum disorder: Characterization using the Aberrant Behavior Checklist. *American Journal of Medical Genetics. Part A, 134,* 373–380.

Carter, J.C., Capone, G.T., Gray, R.M., Cox, C.S., & Kaufmann, W.E. (2007). Autistic-spectrum disorders in Down syndrome: Further delineation and distinction from other behavioral abnormalities. *American Journal of Medical Genetics. Part B, Neuropsychiatric Genetics, 144,* 87–94.

Chang, Q., Khare, G., Dani, V., Nelson, S., & Jaenisch, R. (2006). The disease progression of Mecp2

mutant mice is affected by the level of BDNF expression. *Neuron, 49,* 341–348.

Chiurazzi, P., & Oostra, B.A. (2000). Genetics of mental retardation. *Current Opinion in Pediatrics, 12,* 529–535.

Chiurazzi, P., Tabolacci, E., & Neri, G. (2004). X-linked mental retardation (XLID): From clinical conditions to cloned genes. *Critical Reviews in Clinical and Laboratory Sciences, 41,* 117–158.

Colvin, L., Leonard, H., de Klerk, N., Davis, M., Weaving, L., Williamson, S., et al. (2004). Refining the phenotype of common mutations in Rett syndrome. *Journal of Medical Genetics, 41,* 25–30.

Fisch, G.S. (2000). Psychological assessment in XLID: A proposal for setting international standards. *Genetic Counseling, 11,* 85–101.

Galdzicki, Z., Siarey, R., Pearce, R., Stoll, J., & Rapoport, S.I. (2001). On the cause of mental retardation in Down syndrome: Extrapolation from full and segmental trisomy 16 mouse models. *Brain Research: Brain Research Reviews, 35,* 115–145.

Hagberg, B. (2002). Clinical manifestations and stages of Rett syndrome. *Mental Retardation and Developmental Disabilities Research Reviews, 8,* 61–65.

Hagerman, R.J. (2002). The physical and behavioral phenotype. In R.J. Hagerman & P.J. Hagerman (Eds.), *Fragile X syndrome: Diagnosis, treatment, and research* (3rd ed., pp. 3–110). Baltimore: The Johns Hopkins University Press.

Inlow, J.K., & Restifo, L.L. (2004). Molecular and comparative genetics of mental retardation. *Genetics, 166,* 835–881.

Irwin, S.A., Galvez, R., & Greenough, W.T. (2000). Dendritic spine structural anomalies in fragile-X mental retardation syndrome. *Cerebral Cortex, 10,* 1038–1044.

Jin, P., Alisch, R.S., & Warren, S.T. (2004). RNA and microRNAs in fragile X mental retardation. *Nature Cell Biology, 6,* 1048–1053.

Johnston, M.V. (2004). Clinical disorders of brain plasticity. *Brain and Development, 26,* 73–80.

Kankirawatana, P., Leonard, H., Ellaway, C., Scurlock, J., Mansour, A., Makris, C.M., et al. (2006). Early progressive encephalopathy in boys and *MECP2* mutations. *Neurology, 67,* 164–166.

Kates, W.R., Folley, B.S., Lanham, D.C., Capone, G.T., & Kaufmann, W.E. (2002). Cerebral growth in fragile X syndrome: Review and comparison with Down syndrome. *Microscopy Research and Technique, 57,* 159–167.

Kaufmann, W.E. (1996). Mental retardation and learning disabilities: A neuropathologic differentiation. In A.J. Capute & P.J. Accardo (Eds.), *Developmental disabilities in infancy and childhood* (Vol. 2, pp. 49–70). Baltimore: Paul H. Brookes Publishing Co.

Kaufmann, W.E. (2003). Cortical histogenesis. In M.J. Aminoff & R.B. Daroff (Eds.), *Encyclopedia of the neurological sciences* (Vol. 1, pp. 777–784). San Diego: Academic Press.

Kaufmann, W.E., Cortell, R., Kau, A.S., Bukelis, I., Tierney, E., Gray, R.M., et al. (2004). Autism spectrum disorder in fragile X syndrome: Communication, social interaction, and specific behaviors. *American Journal of Medical Genetics. Part A, 129,* 225–234.

Kaufmann, W.E., Johnston, M.V., & Blue, M.E. (2005). MeCP2 expression and function during brain development: Implications for Rett syndrome's pathogenesis and clinical evolution. *Brain and Development, 27,* S77–S87.

Kaufmann, W.E., MacDonald, S.M., & Altamura, C. (2000). Dendritic cytoskeletal protein expression in mental retardation: An immunohistochemical study of the neocortex in Rett syndrome. *Cerebral Cortex, 10,* 992–1004.

Kaufmann, W.E., & Moser, H.W. (2000). Dendritic anomalies in disorders associated with mental retardation. *Cerebral Cortex, 10,* 981–991.

Kaufmann, W.E., & Reiss, A.L. (1999). Molecular and cellular genetics of fragile X syndrome. *American Journal of Medical Genetics, 88,* 11–24.

Kaufmann, W.E., & Worley, P.F. (1999). The role of early neural activity in regulating immediate early gene expression in the cerebral cortex. *Mental Retardation and Developmental Disabilities Research Reviews, 5,* 41–50.

Lord, C., Risi, S., Lambrecht, L., Cook, E.H., Leventhal, B.L., DiLavore, P.C., et al. (2000). The Autism Diagnostic Observation Schedule-Generic: A standard measure of social and communication deficits associated with the spectrum of autism. *Journal of Autism and Developmental Disorders, 30*(3), 205–223.

Marin-Padilla, M. (1972). Structural abnormalities of the cerebral cortex in human chromosomal aberrations: A Golgi study. *Brain Research, 44,* 625–629.

McLaren, J., & Bryson, S.E. (1987). Review of recent epidemiological studies of mental retardation: Prevalence, associated disorders, and etiology. *American Journal of Mental Retardation, 92,* 243–254.

Meng, Y., Zhang, Y., Tregoubov, V., Janus, C., Cruz, L., Jackson, M., et al. (2002). Abnormal spine morphology and enhanced LTP in *Limk-1* knockout mice. *Neuron, 35,* 121–133.

Moeschler, J.B., & Shevell, M. (2006). Clinical genetic evaluation of the child with mental retardation or developmental delays. *Pediatrics, 117,* 2304–2316.

Moretti, P., Levenson, J.M., Battaglia, F., Atkinson, R., Teague, R., Antalffy, B., et al. (2006). Learning and memory and synaptic plasticity are impaired in a mouse model of Rett syndrome. *Journal of Neuroscience, 26,* 319–327.

Mullaney, B.C., Johnston, M.V., & Blue, M.E. (2004). Developmental expression of methyl-CpG binding protein 2 is dynamically regulated in the rodent brain. *Neuroscience, 123,* 939–949.

Naidu, S., Kaufmann, W.E., Abrams, M.T., Pearlson, G.D., Lanham, D.C., Fredericksen, K.A., et al. (2001). Neuroimaging studies in Rett syndrome. *Brain and Development, 23,* S62–S71.

Percy, A.K. (2002). Clinical trials and treatment prospects. *Mental Retardation and Developmental Disabilities Research Reviews, 8,* 106–111.

Philippe, C., Villard, L., De Roux, N., Raynaud, M., Bonnefond, J.P., Pasquier, L., et al. (2006). Spectrum and distribution of *MECP2* mutations in 424 Rett syndrome patients: A molecular update. *European Journal of Medical Genetics, 49,* 9–18.

Ramakers, G.J.A. (2002). Rho proteins, mental retardation and the cellular basis of cognition. *Trends in Neurosciences, 25,* 191–199.

Reiss, A.L., Eckert, M.A., Rose, F.E., Karchemskiy, A., Kesler, S., Chang, M., et al. (2004). An experiment of nature: Brain anatomy parallels cognition and behavior in Williams syndrome. *Journal of Neuroscience, 24,* 5009–5015.

Roizen, N.J., & Patterson, D. (2003). Down's syndrome. *Lancet, 361,* 1281–1289.

Rutter, M., LeCouteur, A., & Lord, C. (2003). *Autism Diagnostic Interview, Revised (ADI-R).* Los Angeles: Western Psychological Services.

Salman, M.S. (2002). Systematic review of the effect of therapeutic dietary supplements and drugs on cognitive function in subjects with Down syndrome. *European Journal of Paediatric Neurology, 6,* 213–219.

Shevell, M., Ashwal, S., Donley, D., Flint, J., Gingold, M., Hirtz, D., et al. (2003). Practice Parameter. Evaluation of the child with global developmental delay: Report of the Quality Standards Subcommittee of the American Academy of Neurology and the Practice Committee of the Child Neurology Society. *Neurology, 60,* 367–380.

Srour, M., Mazer, B., & Shevell, M.I. (2006). Analysis of clinical features predicting etiologic yield in the assessment of global developmental delay. *Pediatrics, 118,* 139–145.

Young, J.I., Hong, E.R., Castle, J.C., Crespo-Barreto, J., Bowman, A.B., Rose, M.F., et al. (2005). Regulation of RNA splicing by the methylation-dependent transcriptional repressor methyl-CpG binding protein 2. *Proceedings of the National Academy of Sciences of the United States of America, 102,* 17551–17558.

8

Human Behavior Genetics

Implications for Neurodevelopmental Disorders

BARBARA Y. WHITMAN

As recently as a few decades ago, psychological theorists believed that environmental influences determined most human behavior. Nevertheless, the roots of modern behavior genetic studies reach back to the end of the 19th century and Galton's investigations into the heritability of "talent and character" (Galton, 1869). Indeed, in a 1994 paper, Danish psychiatrist Eric Stromgren commented that, in the 1920s and 1930s, most European academic and "asylum" psychiatrists believed that schizophrenia and manic-depressive disorder were inherited. Unfortunately, Galton's early observations regarding the inheritance of behavioral traits became inextricably intertwined, even in his own thinking, with the eugenics movement.

Eugenics promulgated the notion that mental illness, feeble-mindedness, criminality, alcoholism, and sexual promiscuity were expressions of national or racial degeneracy whose remedy lay in legislating selective birth control and sterilization of those afflicted with these maladies because they were unfit to bear children. It is a historical tragedy that the eugenics movement served as the basis for the doctrine of racial hygiene in Nazi ideology used to justify the mass extermination of people with mental illness and those with disabilities, as well as people of Jewish faith (Eisenberg, 2001). This resulted in a scientific revulsion toward the study of a gene–behavior relationship in humans.

Animal researchers, however, were not constrained by an ideological misapplication of science. Using the fruit fly as a model system, Benzer isolated for study "behavior mutants," or animals that were incapable of performing specific behavioral tasks because of a specific genetic mutation (Benzer, 1967, 1971). His methodologies laid the foundation for modern human behavior genetic studies.

As medical researchers seeking to understand causation and improve treatment have utilized epidemiological methods to study such complex conditions as schizophrenia and bipolar disorder, the study of gene–behavior linkages has again emerged. As a result, multiple converging lines of evidence now make a strong case for biological (i.e., genetic) determinants of such diverse behavioral dimensions as overall intelligence, information processing, electroencephalographic evoked potentials, cerebral glucose metabolism, autism, depression, schizophrenia, anxiety and panic disorders, language disorders, antisocial personality, eating disorders, and Tourette syndrome (Plomin, Owen, & McGuffin, 1994).

Two research perspectives anchor opposite ends of a conceptual framework that seeks to link genetics with brain function, cognition, and ultimately behavior (Figure 8.1). Those in the behavioral sciences start with a defined neuropsychiatric disorder such as schizophrenia or attention-deficit/hyperactivity disorder (ADHD) and, within the framework of genetic epidemiology, utilize family, adoption, and twin studies complemented by molecular genetic methods to work "backward" toward the

175

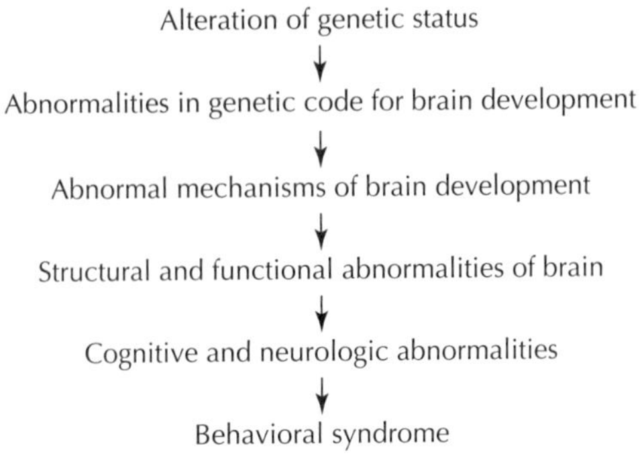

Alteration of genetic status

↓

Abnormalities in genetic code for brain development

↓

Abnormal mechanisms of brain development

↓

Structural and functional abnormalities of brain

↓

Cognitive and neurologic abnormalities

↓

Behavioral syndrome

Figure 8.1. A model of genetic impact on behavior. (*Source:* Bauman, 1998).

probable genetic origins (e.g., Brzustowicz, Chow, Honer, & Bassett, 2000; Karayiorgou & Gogos, 1997). By necessity, this approach focuses on complex, multivariate behavioral dimensions and multisymptom disorders with a spectrum of phenotypes that 1) are thought to be inherited because they tend to run in families but do not show the typical mendelian patterns of inheritance (Grigorenko, 2002), and 2) are presumed to reflect a *complex genetic* predisposition (i.e., result from the interplay of multiple genes of varying effect size, and possibly even multiple chromosomes). The majority of these disorders remain behaviorally defined with no clear biological diagnostic markers. In the absence of biological markers, research remains constrained by multiple and evolving diagnostic (phenotype) definitions as reflected in the polyphenotypic definitions of dyslexia and in the successive iterations of the American Psychiatric Association's *Diagnostic and Statistical Manual of Mental Disorders* (DSM) and the World Health Organization's *International Classification of Diseases* (ICD).

From the opposite end of the framework, and armed with the straightforward rationale that genes are required to produce the proteins that ultimately build neurons and that neuronal activity produces behavior, those working from the genetics and developmental perspective anchor their investigations in known disorders with a specific genetic etiology. By defining the associated behavior phenotype, these investigators attempt to trace the impact of the underlying genetic lesion from the level of DNA sequences through structural and func-

tional alterations of the central nervous system that ultimately result in a specific "behavior phenotype" (Asherson & Curran, 2001; McGuffin, Riley, & Plomin, 2001). Of particular interest are those genetic disorders in which the behavior phenotype appears to reflect strong potential susceptibility for psychiatric disorders. By necessity, the focus is on small numbers of subjects with rare (primarily single-gene) disorders and unusual behavior phenotypes (e.g., velocardiofacial syndrome, Smith-Magenis syndrome, Prader-Willi syndrome). This chapter briefly reviews the methods and findings of each of these research perspectives as they apply to neurodevelopmental disorders.

COMPLEX NEURODEVELOPMENTAL DISORDERS: QUANTITATIVE GENETIC EPIDEMIOLOGY STUDIES

Establishing a genetic diathesis for complex behavioral traits and disorders is neither simple nor direct. Nonetheless, several decades of genetic epidemiological studies document a genetic substrate for many neurodevelopmental disorders, including ADHD, autistic spectrum disorders, disorders of speech and language, and reading disorders. Epidemiological genetic research traditionally has relied on three approaches: family, twin, and adoption studies. Each has advantages and disadvantages that may be partially addressed by combining designs (Neiderhiser, 2001). These approaches are used primarily to establish that a trait or behavior *is* genetically influenced or heritable and to estimate the *strength* of heritability. Once heritability has been established, the molecular genetic techniques of linkage analysis and allelic association are used to establish "susceptibility" and "candidate" causal gene loci (Table 8.1).

With the completion of the full first draft of the human genome and the focus on molecularly derived interventions, new molecular techniques for genetic investigation are being developed at seemingly exponential speed. Furthermore, new quantitative genetic techniques are being developed that go beyond asking if and how much genetic factors influence

Table 8.1. Summary of designs employed in genetic epidemiology

Type of design	Sample	Best use
Quantitative genetic designs		
Family studies	Probands with psychiatric disorders (or complex neurodevelopmental disorders) and relatives	Determination of "familial aggregation" of disorder
Twin studies	Identical (MZ) and fraternal (DZ) twins	Disentangling of genetic and environmental contributions to disorder
Adoption studies	Adoptees and adoptive parents and/or birth parents	Disentangling of genetic and environmental contributions to disorder; especially useful for identifying "shared environmental" influences
Combination designs	*Twin/sibling:* MZ and DZ twins and siblings	Allows generalizability of results in twins to be assessed
	Sibling/adoption: adoptees and siblings and/or nonadoptive control siblings	Allows generalizability of results in adoptees to be assessed and increases power of adoption design
Molecular genetic designs		
Allelic association	Related or unrelated samples of individuals	When candidate gene strategy is employed, a powerful method of assessing associations between genes and disorders
Linkage analysis	Family members	Allows systematic examination of genome for associations between gene markers and disorder

From Neiderhiser, J. (2001). Understanding the roles of genome and environment: Methods in genetic epidemiology. *British Journal of Psychiatry, 178*(Suppl. 40), s12–s17; reprinted by permission.
Key: DZ, dizygotic; MZ, monozygotic.

behavior. With these newer techniques, it will soon be possible to investigate how genes and environment affect developmental change and continuity, heterogeneity and comorbidity, interactions and correlations between genetic and environmental influences, and the links between disorders and normal variation (Plomin, Defries, Craig, & McGuffin, 2002). Nonetheless, a review of these classic methods as they relate to multisymptom neurodevelopmental disorders is in order. The first step in establishing heritability is phenotype definition.

Defining the Phenotype

The validity of the heritability data hinges on how well the phenotype is defined. This remains a significant problem for the complex neurodevelopmental disorders, wherein phenotypes are often defined on the basis of reported symptoms and behaviors rather than on biological markers. For instance, the cognitive and behavioral spectrum referenced by the concept "dyslexia" ranges from spelling errors to difficulty reading single words. In part this definitional complexity reflects the multidimensional nature of the disorder; it may also reflect that dyslexia connotes a group of related phenotypes, rather than a single rigidly defined disorder (Schulte-Korne, 2001). Distinct from the issue of phenotypic complexity is whether dyslexia is the extreme of a behavioral dimension or a separate diagnostic category (quantitative vs. qualitative disruption).

Starting from the assumption that many of the conditions encountered in childhood, including dyslexia, appear to be extremes of normal trait variations, the question is posed whether dyslexia is the extreme lower end of a normal distribution of the behavioral dimension "reading skills," or is a distinct etiological condition (Snowling, Gallager, & Frith, 2003). Thus, a family study that employs a simple inquiry regarding family members who have difficulty reading may yield an overestimate of the heritability of the disorder because reading problems resulting from visual difficulties, intellectual disabilities, poor school attendance, and just plain disinterest may be included. Conversely, an inquiry regarding family members who were late in talking, had articulation difficulties when they started talking, and had trouble learning to read may yield a more restricted heritability estimate that may or may not encompass the full range of "dyslexia-related problems" present in the family.

Although the use of a broader-based clinical diagnostic system offers another approach to eliciting information, clinically acceptable definitions of disorders may not represent genetically valid phenotypes or may encompass several phenotypes of genetically diverse origins (Weissman, 2001). For example, earlier inheritance studies of attention disorders looked primarily at hyperactivity (Cantwell, 1972), whereas later studies were based on multidimensional clinical criteria that encompassed impaired attention, activity level, and impulsivity (e.g., Biederman et al., 1992, 1999). Furthermore, rapid evolution and multiple revisions of the two major clinical diagnostic systems (the DSM and the ICD) over the past two decades can mean that, by the time they are published, heritability studies are often out of sync with current definitions. With these constraints in mind, we review the process and outcomes of establishing heritability in the complex neurodevelopmental disorders.

Establishing Heritability

Classically, the first step in establishing a genetic predisposition for multidimensional behaviors or multisymptom behavior disorders is a test of familial aggregation; that is, is there an increased occurrence of the disorder among family members of affected individuals? To the extent that genetic mechanisms are at work, there should be an aggregation or increased occurrence of the disorder in the relatives of the index case compared with the occurrence noted in families of unaffected controls. Furthermore, that aggregation should proportionally decrease as familial biological closeness decreases (i.e., siblings vs. cousins). Thus, family pedigrees are examined for both an (excess) occurrence of the behavior complex and an aggregation pattern compatible with genetic transmission.

Family pedigree data are obtained in two ways: 1) a *family history* whereby information about noninterviewed family members is obtained from an index patient or close relative; or 2) a *family study* that includes direct interview of all family members regarding the presence or absence of the disorder(s) in question. There are inherent advantages and disadvantages in both methods. Family study methods are both labor intensive and extremely costly, and the data contain the usual biases associated with self-report measures. Family history methods depend on the index patient's knowledge and opinions of other family members. Although these studies are less expensive, it has been shown that the data frequently underestimate the true occurrence of a given disorder in a family and are biased toward the most severely affected.

Familial aggregation has clearly been established for a broad range of "dyslexia-related phenotypes," including reading and spelling disorders (Gayan et al., 1999; Pennington, 1990, 1994; Schulte-Korne, Diemel, Muller, Gutenbrunner, & Remschmidt, 1996); attention deficit disorders both with and without hyperactivity (Biederman & Faraone, 1990; Biederman et al., 1986, 1992; Faraone, Biederman, Keenan, & Tsuang, 1991a, 1991b; McGuffin, Owen, O'Donovan, Thapar, & Gottesman, 1994; Roizen et al., 1996); speech and language disorders (Bishop, 2001; Tomblin, 1989); and autism spectrum disorders (Belmonte et al., 2004; Pericak-Vance, 2002). Although family studies are a necessary first step for establishing familial aggregation, such studies are insufficient to assert genetic heritability. Many things that "run" in families are not genetic, such as bad manners (Pennington, 1994). Twin studies are used to disentangle genetic from environmental causes.

Twin Studies Twin studies rest on the assumption that, because monozygotic twins are genetically identical, differences between these two individuals must result from either subsequent genetic mutation or significantly different environmental influences (including but not limited to child rearing, infections, and trauma). Because postconception genetic mutation is extraordinarily rare, it is safe to assume that differences between identical twins result from environmental factors. It is also assumed that dizygotic twins share no more than 50% of their genetic material and are therefore no more similar than any two siblings born of the same parents. Thus, differences between dizygotic twins derive from both genetic and environmental influences. When dizygotic twins are more alike than serially born siblings, this increased alikeness is explained by their shared environment.

When examining rates of occurrence for a suspected genetic trait, it is assumed that, when raised in a common environment, monozygotic twins should be more alike than dizygotic twins, dizygotic twins more alike than serially born siblings, and siblings more alike than nonrelated people. To rule out the influence of common environment, this proportionally decreasing relationship should hold even when twins are separated early in life and raised in different environments. If a trait is due solely to genetic factors, then monozygotic twins reared apart should have the same disorder 100% of the time. If a trait is totally environmentally determined, then the twins should not have the same trait with any greater frequency than any two children raised in dissimilar environments. The role of gender differences in dizygotic twin pairs remains a methodological issue that is handled differently across studies.

Adoption Studies Studies of children adopted at birth are also used to investigate behavior heritability. Adoption studies rest on the assumption that, to the extent that a trait is genetic, affected children should resemble their biological relatives more closely than they do their adoptive relatives (assuming an absence of the trait in the adoptive family). Thus, a study of the biological families of adopted children should yield higher prevalence rates for a trait or disorder than are found in the family into which they were adopted. Similarly, unaffected adopted children should have lower prevalence rates in their biological families than affected adopted children. Although the preferred design of adoption studies utilizes

twins adopted at birth into separate families, non-twin studies are also utilized.

Combination Designs Starting from the logic of heritability estimates lodged in twin studies, several investigators have combined both twin and family studies or twin and adoption methodologies in a single design. Thus, when twins and their siblings are included in the same sample, genetic and environmental contributions to behavior can be dissected from those stemming solely from a special twin effect. Furthermore, when twins reside in families that have morphed through divorce and remarriage, the incorporation of siblings with increased genetic dilution (e.g., half siblings and stepsiblings) allows an extended statistical basis for heritability estimates.

Constraints and Limitations In addition to the genetic assumptions, both twin and adoption studies rest on a number of other assumptions, including random mating (people are equally likely to choose dissimilar as similar mates) and equal environments (fraternal and identical twins raised in the same home experience equally similar environments). Furthermore, twin studies assume that genes and environment separately influence behavior; recent evidence of a gene–environment interaction on behavior phenotype is not taken into account. Similarly, twin studies usually assume that multiple gene traits result from an additive effect of all involved genes; alternative genetic mechanisms such as dominant/recessive, interactive, and modifying mechanisms are outside the scope of most current models. In most instances, violation of these assumptions would lower heritability estimates.

Consider adoptive studies: prevalence in the biological family of an affected child will only be higher than prevalence in the adoptive family if the adoptive family is negative for the trait or disorder in question. Because adoption agencies frequently seek to match children with families along a number of dimensions, many of which are genetically determined (e.g., skin and eye color, temperament, family background), it is possible that such placement methods might also select for companion or correlated (if unintended) traits. Unless the research design is specifically controlled by sampling methodology, true genetic linkages could be masked by selective adoptive placement methods. Conversely, statistically significant differences may reflect a conservative, yet genetically true, estimate of heritability.

HERITABILITY OF COMPLEX NEURODEVELOPMENTAL DISORDERS: MOLECULAR GENETIC EPIDEMIOLOGICAL DESIGNS

Twin and adoptive study methodologies have been employed with virtually all of the complex neurodevelopmental disorders, using multiple phenotypic measures (Table 8.2), and, as with family aggregation studies, these studies yield strong evidence of heritability for a broad range of dyslexia-related phenotypes (Grigorenko, 2001; Schulte-Korne, 2001), attention deficit disorders both with and without hyperactivity (Thapar, Holmes, Poulton, & Harrington, 1999), speech and language disorders (Fisher, 2002), and autism spectrum disorders (Pericak-Vance, 2002), although the mode of inheritance for each remains an open question. Nonetheless, the strength of these heritability estimates has spawned molecular genetic studies in an effort to isolate candidate susceptibility genes.

Molecular Genetics: Searching for Susceptibility and Candidate Genes

Until recently, the primary methods for determining the genetic locus of a trait or disorder included linkage analysis and allelic association. Classically, genetic linkage maps are constructed by studying family histories and statistically measuring the frequency with which traits are linked or inherited together. If a trait can be shown to be linked to a known genetic marker locus, it is inferred that a major gene for that trait is located on the same chromosome as the marker. Linkage is statistically inferred using maximum likelihood methods to compute the likelihood of linkage, yielding a LOD score (log of the odds of linkage). A LOD score over 3 is generally accepted as evidence of linkage, whereas LOD scores less than -2 reject

linkage (Schulte-Korne, 2001). Linkage analysis has two attractive features: 1) it requires no knowledge of pathophysiological mechanisms of the disorder under investigation, and 2) its range extends over the entire genome.

In complex neurodevelopmental disorders, classic linkage methods have had less success than newer linkage models that focus on allele sharing in sibling pairs and small nuclear families. This model assumes that affected siblings share susceptibility genes inherited from the same parent; thus, affected sibling pairs are genotyped with markers spread evenly throughout the genome. A linkage between a susceptibility gene and the marker alleles is presumed when affected siblings are found to share parental alleles more often than by chance. The model is extended to small nuclear families by studying affected relatives in a pedigree to see how often a particular copy of a chromosomal region is shared, with the assumption that it is inherited from a common ancestor in the pedigree.

With completion of the first draft of the human genome map, the number and specificity of available markers for linkage studies continues to rapidly grow. A good random genomic screen uses markers evenly spaced across the entire genome. The goal of an initial screen is to quickly scan the genome to identify those regions most likely to harbor genes for the trait or disorder in question. Such an approach maximizes sensitivity, so many false-positive loci may be identified. This approach, however, lessens the likelihood of missing truly relevant regions (Pericak-Vance, 2002). Once a chromosomal region has been implicated, association studies and other methodologies can be used to target a particular gene.

Association Studies

Association studies follow a typical case–control methodology, testing whether a particular allele occurs at higher frequency among affected than unaffected individuals (Lander & Schork, 1994). Typically, genotyping for a genetic marker believed to be of etiological significance is conducted on DNA samples from both subjects with a trait of interest and controls without the trait. Statistical analysis compares

Table 8.2.   Representative twin studies of complex neurodevelopmental disorders

Author	Measure	MZ twins (N)	DZ twins (N)	Age	Concordance (%) or correlation		Heritability
					MZ	DZ	
Attention deficit disorders (with or without hyperactivity)							
Goodman and Stevenson (1989) and Stevenson (1992)	Hyperactivity, parent report	102	111[a]	13	51%	33%	.75
Edelbrock, Rende, Plomin, and Thompson (1995)	CBCL Attention Problems Scale	99	82	7–15	.68	.29	.66
Thapar and McGuffin (1995)	Rutter	113	85[a] + 83[b]	8–16	.61	−.10	.88
Gjone, Stevenson, and Sundet (1996)	CBCL (mother) Attention Problems Scale	327	389[a]	5–15	.72 .78	.21 .45	.73 .79 .87 (extreme scores)
Speech and language disorders							
Bishop, North, and Donlan (1995)	At least one twin and sibling met DSM-III criteria for Developmental Language Disorder	63	27[a]		70%	46%	
Tomblin and Buckwalter (1998)				4–16	.96	.69	

(continued)

Table 8.2. (continued)

Author	Measure	MZ twins (N)	DZ twins (N)	Age	Concordance (%) or correlation		Heritability
					MZ	DZ	
Dyslexia/reading and spelling disorders							
Hermann (1959)	Reading disability	10	33		100%	33%	
Olson, Forsberg, and Wise (1994)	Word recognition	183	126		.47		
	Phonological awareness	93	68		.60		
	Phonological coding	151	105				.59
Autism							
Bailey et al. (1995)					92%	10%	
Folstein (1996)							.90
Merikangas and Risch (2003)							

[a]Same sex pairs
[b]Opposite sex pairs
Key: CBCL, The Child Behavior Checklist (Achenbach, 1993); DSM-III, Diagnostic and Statistical Manual of Mental Disorders, Third Edition (American Psychiatric Association, 1980); DZ, dizygotic; MZ, monozygotic.

allele or genotype frequencies in cases versus controls (Sullivan, Eaves, Kendler, & Neale, 2001). An association approach is typically employed when there is evidence to suggest good candidate loci. As with any case–control study, care must be exercised to ensure that, to the extent possible, cases and controls are drawn from the same population, differing only on the trait or disorder under study. As a result of work over the past decade, molecular studies are making significant inroads into the genetic origins of dyslexia/reading disorders, ADHD, speech and language disorders, and autism.

Molecular Studies of Neurodevelopmental Disorders

Dyslexia/Reading Disorders Quantitative epidemiological studies have long documented familial transmission of dyslexia. Twin studies estimate a heritable component of between 50% and 79% (Cardon et al., 1994; Defries, Fulker, & LaBuda, 1987), although there is no consensus regarding the mode of transmission. Some researchers argue that dyslexia is likely to be polygenic and produce an increased risk of dyslexia in a continuous fashion, whereas others posit that dyslexia is transmitted in a mode consistent with a major gene, either additive or dominant. Molecular investigations have been based primarily on traditional linkage studies and date as early as 1983, when Smith et al. reported a linkage for dyslexia to chromosome 15 markers (Smith, Kimberling, Pennington, & Lubs, 1983; Smith, Pennington, Kimberling, & Ing, 1990).

Thus far, candidate regions of interest have been examined on chromosomes 1, 2, 6, and 15 (Table 8.3). Early follow-up studies failed to support a locus on chromosome 15, so subsequent linkage studies examined regions of the genome selected on the basis of a hypothesized link between dyslexia and immune system disorders (Galaburda et al., 1985). This has resulted in a number of studies that provided evidence for a linkage between reading disability and markers in the human leukocyte antigen region of chromosome 6 and the Rh locus on chromosome 1, and subsequently reconfirmed a possible locus near the β_2-microglobulin gene on chromosome 15. As-

sociation mapping has been used to screen the chromosome 6 and 15 regions, yielding a highly significant association with three markers on chromosome 15. To date, one genome-wide scan has been reported, resulting in the identification of a region on the short arm of chromosome 2 as a dyslexia susceptibility region (Fagerheim et al., 1999). No replication studies for this site have been reported at this time.

Attention-Deficit/Hyperactivity Disorder
Family, twin, and adoption studies document that ADHD is a highly heritable condition with heritability patterns that hold up whether using hyperactivity or more broadly based diagnostic criteria as the phenotypic index and regardless of whether categorical or continuous measures are applied. Heritability estimates range from 60% to 80% when rated by parents and from 39% to 72% when rated by teachers (Thapar et al., 1999). Molecular genetic studies have investigated genes in the dopaminergic, noradrenergic, and serotonergic systems as possible mediators of susceptibility to ADHD. Based on extensive neurochemical evidence supporting the involvement of the dopaminergic system, the bulk of molecular studies focus on the dopaminergic pathways, using principally family-based and case–control association strategies. To date, genes encoding the dopamine transporter *DAT1* and the dopamine receptors *DRD4* and *DRD5* have been implicated. Despite mixed results, the most robust of these findings is the association between ADHD and the *DRD4* gene, which encodes a protein receptor that mediates the postsynaptic action of dopamine. Positive associations are reported across a wide range of sampling procedures and across different diagnostic systems and measures of ADHD. More complete reviews of these studies can be found in the papers by Faraone et al. (Faraone & Doyle, 2001; Faraone, Doyle, Mick, & Biederman, 2002).

There are similar mixed findings regarding the *DAT1* gene. This gene is of particular interest because stimulant medications used to treat ADHD interact directly with the transporter protein (Cook et al., 1995). Although a number of subsequent studies support these findings, an almost equal number do not (summarized

Table 8.3. Identified susceptibility genes

Chromosome/gene	Measure of phenotype	Study
Attention		
DAT1 gene: loci on 17p11, 16p13, 6q12, 5p13, 5p13.3, 4p16.1	Multiple measures	For example, Cook et al. (1995) and Barr et al. (2001) (*Source*: OMIM)
DRD4 gene: locus on 11p15.5	Multiple measures	Reviewed by Faraone et al. (2002) and Thapar (2002) (*Source*: OMIM)
DRD5 gene: locus on 4p16.1–p15.3	Multiple measures	For example, Daly, Hawi, Fitzgerald, and Gill (1999) and Barr et al. (2000) (*Source*: OMIM)
NET1 gene: locus on 16q12.2	Multiple measures	Spencer et al. (1998); Barr et al. (2002) (*Source*: OMIM)
XP22.3	Multiple measures	Boycott et al. (2003)
Speech and language		
SPCH1 gene: locus on 7q31	One family with history of speech delay	Fisher et al. (1998)
Short arm of chromosome 6	Reading data	Fisher et al. (1999)
Chromosomes 16 and 19	−1.5 SD below mean for age on standard language tests	SLI Consortium (2002)
FOXP2 gene	Noted as severe impairment	Lai, Fisher, Hurst, Vargha-Khadem, and Monaco (2001)
Dyslexia/reading disorders		
1p34–36	Reading disability	Rabin et al. (1993); Mudad and Telen (1996); Huang (1997); Grigorenko et al. (1998)
2p15–16	Phonological decoding, phonological awareness, single-word reading, spelling	Fagerheim et al. (1999)
6p21	Reading disability	Smith, Kimberling, and Pennington (1991)
	Composite reading and spelling	Cardon et al. (1994)
6p21.1–p22.3	4 reading and coding measures	Fisher et al. (1999)
	Single-word reading, spelling, vocabulary	Grigorenko, Wood, Meyer, and Pauls (2000); Grigorenko et al. (1997)
15q15–q21	Reading disorder	Morris et al. (2000)
15q21	Spelling disorder	Schulte-Korne et al. (1998)
Autism		
6q16.3–21	Clinical diagnoses	Jamain et al. (2002)
7q13, 20–24, 32–35	Clinical diagnoses	Reviewed by Bespalova and Busbaum (2003)
15q11–13 (dup)	Clinical diagnoses	Cook et al. (1998); Bass et al. (2000)
17q11.2, 21.32	Clinical diagnoses	Mbarek et al. (1999); Plank et al. (2001)

Key: OMIM, Online Mendelian Inheritance in Man; SD, standard deviation.

by Curran et al., 2001). Future studies are needed to examine the impact of phenotypic heterogeneity for both the *DRD4* and *DAT1* genes. Additional dopamine system genes under study include the catechol-*O*-methyltransferase (COMT) gene, the A1 allele of the D_2 receptor gene, and the *DRD5* gene.

In addition to dopaminergic system abnormalities, adrenergic system dysregulation has been implicated as a factor in ADHD (see, e.g., Biederman & Spencer, 2000). A study of the norepinephrine transporter gene *NET1* found no evidence for linkage (Barr et al., 2002). The same group had previously examined the genes for the α_1C-, α_2A-, and α_2C-adrenergic receptors and found no evidence for linkage (Barr et al., 2001). Researchers are beginning to look at the impact of comorbidity (e.g., ADHD + conduct disorder, ADHD + reading disorder) as one explanation for previously mixed findings.

Speech and Language Disorders A genome-wide linkage scan was used to isolate a susceptibility region on chromosome 7 (q31) (Fisher et al., 1998); however, this single genetic locus (referred to as *SPCH1*) was specific to a single family; the significance of the findings for other families or milder forms of speech and language disorders is unclear. Two genome-wide scans, each using much larger samples, recently have been conducted. Using quantitative measures for a language disorder, 100 families from the United Kingdom have been examined. The scan implicated two loci on chromosomes 16 and 19. A second scan of 14 families, using both quantitative and qualitative measures of a specific language disorder, has yielded areas of interest on chromosomes 1, 6, and 15. These findings are of particular interest because these regions overlap with those implicated in dyslexia; it remains to be seen if this overlap reflects a common genetic origin for both specific language disorders and dyslexia. A further linkage with the *DRD4* locus at 11p15.5 has been reported, a finding that is strengthened by the known comorbidity of ADHD and language disorders (Hsiung, Kaplan, Petryshen, Lu, & Field, 2004).

Autism Epidemiological data compellingly implicate genetic factors in the etiology of autism, with heritability estimated to be greater than 90%. A number of genome-wide screens have been conducted in an effort to isolate candidate susceptibility genes. In addition to X-linked disorders such as fragile X syndrome, areas of interest have been identified on chromosomes 2, 3, 6, 7, 15, 17, and 19. Both linkage analysis and association studies implicate chromosome 2, particularly when the affected individuals demonstrate delayed onset of phrased speech until after 36 months of age (Pericak-Vance, 2002). Three sites on chromosome 7 have been implicated: 7q21,

7q31, and 7q32–35. An overlap with sites implicated in speech and language disorders is noted at 7q31, and a similar overlap is noted at 6q21; however, the full meaning of these overlaps has yet to be explored. Several studies have noted abnormalities of the 15q11–13 region, with duplications of the region the most common rearrangement associated with autism. Clearly, studies with larger sample sizes employing a more homogeneous phenotype are necessary to more definitively identify the autism susceptibility gene(s).

BEHAVIOR PHENOTYPE: SYNDROME-SPECIFIC BEHAVIOR COMPLEXES

Although both geneticists and developmental pediatricians have long recognized specific behaviors associated with a number of genetic disorders (e.g., hyperphagia associated with Prader-Willi syndrome, a specific pattern of self-injury unique to Lesch-Nyhan syndrome), the systematic study of syndrome-specific behavior complexes is relatively recent. Most authors attribute Nyhan's 1972 article describing the typical behavior profile of Lesch-Nyhan syndrome as the lynchpin for the study of syndrome-specific behavior phenotypes. Prior to the focus provided by Nyhan's article, most behavior studies in this population focused on IQ-based levels of impairment as the driving force behind (primarily maladaptive or aberrant) behavior (Borthwick-Duffy, 1994; Tager-Flusberg, 1999). Behavior comparisons were made between levels of cognitive functioning rather than between individuals affected with different genetic disorders; yet, two people with a developmental disability from different genetic origins might have the same global IQ but entirely different patterns of abilities and deficits on the subscales of an IQ test and widely differing patterns of ability and deficits on detailed neuropsychological testing (Levitas, 2000).

The search for behavior phenotypes depends on at least two assumptions: 1) individuals with the same genetic abnormality have a characteristic behavior pattern that is atypical for the nonaffected population and different from the characteristic behavior patterns associated with other genetic disorders, and 2) there is a causal relationship between the genetic abnormality and the characteristic behavior pattern via a specific effect of the genetic abnormality on brain development and functioning. Thus, many view studies of behavior phenotype as instrumental for understanding the pathways from genes to behavior via the brain, as well as clinically useful for detailing the range of variability between syndromes and among those individuals with the same syndrome and for improving clinical care by better defining the developmental, psychological, and academic needs of affected individuals.

Initially, studies of behavior phenotype concentrated on specific behavior dysmorphisms, including self-injury; sleep and circadian rhythm problems; eating behavior; motor concerns; and behavior, mood and psychiatric disorders. Subsequent work expanded the behavior profile to include cognitive and adaptive functioning, language and communication, social development, sensory issues, and behavior self-regulation. Early studies focused on such questions as

1. To what extent do we find different types of behavior (and behavior problems) in those individuals affected with different types of genetic disorders?

2. To what extent do we find commonalities and differences of behavior (and behavior problems) both between individuals affected by different types of disabilities and between those affected and those not affected?

3. Among those affected, how does the severity of the cognitive disability have an impact on behavior?

4. Are there associations between severity of cognitive disability and psychopathology?

As research has evolved, the complexity of the questions has similarly developed. For example, studies now focus on the question, "How do psychosocial influences affect both normal and abnormal behavioral development?" Research supports that children with genetic disorders and cognitive disabilities more often suffer social strain, have an increased risk of failure at school, frequently have poor lan-

guage and social skills, suffer increased peer rejection and ostracism, and are at higher risk of exploitation and abuse—all known risk factors for the development of mood and behavior disorders. Other studies ask, "Are apparent commonalities across genetic syndromes real?" Dykens and Rosner (1999) examined anxiety in two groups of children, one with Williams syndrome and the other with Prader-Willi syndrome. These authors indicated that, although both groups of children demonstrated high levels of anxiety, those with Williams syndrome tended to have more classic anxiety, fears, and occasionally phobias, whereas those with Prader-Willi syndrome expressed their anxiety as obsessions and compulsions.

Some syndromes have been extensively studied for the past two decades (e.g., Lesch-Nyhan, fragile X), whereas others have a short study history (e.g., Lowe's syndrome). Taken together, these studies document many behavioral commonalities across syndromes, as well as unique, syndrome-specific neurodevelopmental and neuropsychiatric profiles (Steinhausen et al., 2002). Recognizing significant within-syndrome variability, Tables 8.4 and 8.5 profile selected aspects of the behavior phenotype for a number of genetic syndromes. As the study of syndrome-specific behavior phenotypes has gained momentum over the past two decades, several conceptual, ethical, and methodological concerns have been raised, including the variable definition of behavior phenotype, imprecise definitions and measurement of specific behaviors and behavior disorders, and theoretical tunnel vision.

Definition of Phenotype

Although seemingly straightforward in concept, defining behavior phenotype has presented some difficulty. Early definitions specified a "characteristic pattern of motor, cognitive, linguistic and/or social abnormalities which is *consistently* associated with a biological disorder" (Flint & Yule, 1994; O'Brien & Yule, 1995, p.2). Although this definition recognizes potential variability between syndromes, it fails to recognize the wide variation in phenotype and severity among individuals with the same syndrome, even when the "core fea-

Table 8.4. Cognitive features of genetic syndromes

Syndrome and prevalence	Intelligence	Language Receptive	Language Expressive	Visuospatial abilities	Memory	Cognitive strengths	Learning disability
Down 1:650–1,000	ID (moderate to severe)	⇓	⇓⇓⇓	=	⇓ with age	Pragmatic language	Uneven profile
Fragile X (M) 1:4,000	ID (mild to severe)	⇓	⇓⇓⇓	⇓	ST ⇓, LT =		Uneven profile
Fragile X (F) 1:2,000	Borderline to ID (mild in 50%)		= (?)	=	=		Mild to moderate
Rett 1:10,000–15,000	ID (severe)	⇓⇓	⇓⇓	⇓⇓	⇓⇓		
Prader-Willi 1:10,000–12,000	Borderline to ID (mild to moderate)	⇓	⇓	⇑	ST ⇓, LT =	Exceptional abilities with jigsaw puzzles if deletion etiology	Uneven profile specific to etiology
Angelman 0.08:1,000	ID (severe)	⇓	none	⇓⇓	⇓⇓		
Williams 1:10,000	Borderline to ID (mild to moderate)	⇓	⇑	⇓⇓	=	Expressive language	
VCF 1:5,000	Normal to ID (mild)	=	=	=	=	Language skills	Moderate
Smith-Magenis 1:25,000	ID (moderate)	=	⇓	⇓	ST ⇓, LT =	Visual learning	Moderate
Turner 1:2,500 females	Usually normal	=	=	⇓	=		Variable but usually mild, particularly math

Adapted from Muldavsky, M., Lev, D., and Leeman-Sagie, T. (2001). Behavioral phenotypes of genetic syndromes: A reference guide for psychiatrists. *Journal of the American Academy of Child and Adolescent Psychiatry, 178* (Suppl. 40), S12–S17.

Key: F, female; ID, intellectual disability; LT, long-term; M, male; ST, short-term; VCF, velocardiofacial; ⇑, well-developed ability; =, not impaired; ⇓, impaired; ⇓⇓, very impaired.

Table 8.5. Psychopathology in genetic syndromes

Syndrome	Sleep disturbance	Anxiety	Depression	Hyperactivity	Aggression/psychoses	Autistic features	Other behaviors
Down	High incidence of both airway and CNS origin	Not inherent	In adulthood	+	+	Rarely	Early dementia
Fragile X (M)	Occasional obstructive airway problems	++	+	++	Rarely	++	Hypersensitive to external stimuli
Fragile X (F)	Occasional obstructive airway problems	++	+	+	Rarely	Asperger	Avoidant disorder
Rett	80% multiple day and night sleep problems—night problems can include behavioral oddities	–	–	–	–	+ mainly in infancy	Loss of purposeful movement, development of hand stereotypies
Prader-Willi	Central apnea, abnormal sleep architecture; can be worsened by weight-related hypoventilation syndrome or hypotonic airway	++	+	+	+	Can be + in infancy; Asperger from late childhood on	Lack of satiety, food foraging
Angelman	Reported to be prominent feature without further description	–	–	+	–	+	Frequent smiling, inappropriate outbursts of laughter
Williams	Reported to be prominent feature without further description	+	In adulthood	+	+	+	
VCF	Many evidence upper airway obstructions that can lead to cor pulmonale and sudden death	+	+	+	–	–	Increased prevalence of schizophrenia and bipolar disorders
Smith-Magenis	Reported to be prominent with abnormal nighttime behavior	–	–	+	+	–	Self-injury
Turner	Not reported as routinely present	+	+	+	Rarely	Rarely	Immature personality, social and self-esteem difficulties

Key: CNS, central nervous system; F, female; M, male; VCF, velocardiofacial; +, present; + +, marked; – , not characteristic.

tures" of a syndrome are readily accepted as such. For instance, few would deny that hyperphagia is a cardinal feature of Prader-Willi syndrome; however, population surveys indicate that skin picking occurs with a greater frequency than hyperphagia (i.e., Einfeld, Smith, Durvasula, Florio, & Tonge, 1999). For each behavior, a wide range of severity is observed among affected individuals.

Other authors place less emphasis on "consistently associated," suggesting that those individuals with a syndrome have a "predilection for a certain behavior" (Einfeld & Hall, 1994) or that there is "a heightened probability or greater likelihood that affected individuals will exhibit specific behavioral or developmental characteristics when compared to unaffected individuals" (Dykens, 1995). Although both definitions seek to accommodate within-syndrome variability, neither defines the implied statistical threshold for ruling a behavior in or out of the "phenotype." For example, if a behavior occurs in 51% of those affected, is it any more a "predilection" than a behavior that occurs in 49% of those affected—or 35%? Should some behaviors be more heavily weighted than others? For instance, clinically one would suspect that, if 20% of the affected population eventually develops psychoses, then developing psychoses should probably be considered a "predilection" despite the converse, that 80% of affected individuals do not develop psychoses. If only 20% of affected individuals develop psychoses, however, it must be questioned if psychosis is a direct genetic effect or an environmentally mediated genetic propensity. Pursuing the definition of "heightened probabilities" requires measurement against a comparison group; however, defining the appropriate comparison group also presents some difficulty, as is later discussed.

For clinical practice, the definition proposed by Carey and McMahon holds most promise:

A profile of behavior, cognition, or personality that represents a component of the overall pattern seen in many or most individuals with a particular condition or syndrome. Although the profile may not be specific, it is consistent in the syndromal pattern. (1999, p. 58)

Control/Comparison Groups

The assumption of a direct and specific genetic effect on behavior implies a comparison with a nonaffected population. Often such comparisons are made through the use of standardized testing, wherein the de facto comparison group is the normative population in which a test was standardized. Other studies make direct comparisons against either an age-matched or "mental age"–matched nonaffected group; however, as Finegan (1998) noted, comparing those individuals with a specific syndrome only to people in the general population is of little value because those with a syndrome will differ on other important and behaviorally determinant variables, such as overall intelligence when matched for age or specific cognitive abilities (e.g., memory, language), and environmental influences when matched by "mental age." Nonetheless, such comparisons do offer an opportunity for determining those abilities that may remain "relatively intact" even when most other abilities are depressed.

A third approach compares people with a specific syndrome either to those with another syndrome (e.g., Down syndrome) or to a heterogeneous group of people with intellectual disabilities for whom no etiology has been defined. Yet another approach compares those with a specific syndrome to other groups with discrete diagnosed conditions (e.g., comparing those with Sotos syndrome to those with other overgrowth conditions; comparing those with Prader-Willi syndrome to normal obese individuals). As with other methodological considerations, all approaches offer both merit and limitations depending on the nature of the underlying question (for a more complete review of this issue, see Hodapp & Dykens, 2001). It is likely that a variety of converging approaches will be necessary to fully determine the unique phenotypic characteristics associated with specific syndromes (Finegan, 1998).

Poor Measurement Tools and Reporting Bias

The search for behavior phenotype is hampered by imprecise measurement tools that 1) focus on only a small segment of behavior and qualities of the individual; 2) reduce complex, multidimensional cognitive or language abilities to a single score; and 3) are standardized on cognitively normal individuals and often do not provide norms that extend into the lower ranges of ability frequently found in those with genetic disorders. For instance, many IQ tests fail to detect or account for speech and language deficits. Although speech and language deficits can be separately measured, the interplay between speech and language deficits, uneven cognitive abilities, and behavior is more difficult to demonstrate.

Similar difficulties surround the measurement of psychiatric symptoms and diagnoses. Many question the applicability of traditional diagnostic schemas and formal psychiatric diagnoses (e.g., those listed in the DSM and the ICD), derived from cognitively normal populations, to people with intellectual disabilities (e.g., Sovner, 1986), arguing that traditional diagnostic categorizations overestimate the presence of psychiatric symptomatology and clinically lead to excessive use of chemical restraints. Independent of the validity of traditional diagnostic schemas, measurement problems can occur when intellectual and verbal impairments limit the affected individual's ability to reliably report fears, anxieties, and depressive and psychotic symptoms. Thus, a diagnosis of an anxiety disorder in a nonverbal individual may require an inferential leap based on interpreting behavior that appears fearful or anxious.

Similarly, an individual with a significant cognitive impairment may not be able to describe a delusion in the same way as another individual. In both instances, third-party reports frequently serve as data. Often these third-party reports originate from inadequately compensated, poorly prepared, often undersupervised caregiving staff who have high rates of turnover and often spotty or limited contact with the individual being assessed, possibly compromising the quality of observations on which behavioral descriptions are based. At the same time, these reports may not reveal that, as a result of the same lack of training and supervision, the caregiver interacts with the person in ways that provoke behaviors that, without provocation, would not be displayed—thus inflating reports of behavioral deviancies.

Inflated reporting may also occur when there is a failure to account for an individual's developmental level, leading to the erroneous labeling of developmentally age-appropriate behavior as a neuropsychiatric condition. A specific underreporting bias is also common. This occurs with "diagnostic overshadowing," or the uncritical attribution of behavioral characteristics to the behavior phenotype or the presence of intellectual disabilities when the behaviors in question actually signify a psychiatric difficulty. Finally, although many affected individuals may present with clear symptoms of standard emotional and psychiatric disorders, many of the most problematic behaviors associated with genetic disorders (e.g., specific self-injurious behaviors, hyperphagia) fall outside usual diagnostic schemas; for many of these behaviors, there are no validated measurement tools.

Theoretical Tunnel Vision

In many arenas, the data from syndrome-specific behavior studies have been invaluable for providing improved clinical care, for providing families with critical child-rearing information, for tailoring and executing more appropriate and more effective individual educational programs, and for more realistic, individually designed behavioral and psychopharmacological interventions. Even in the genomic disorders, however, the path from genes to behavior has not met expectations. Conceptually, many argue that assuming a direct causal effect is far too simplistic and ignores the crucial role of gene–gene interaction both in the development of behaviorally determinant neural networks and in the functional dynamics of gene expression (e.g., Inoue & Lupski, 2003; Seth & Edelman, 2003).

For example, fragile X syndrome results from the silencing of a single gene whose impact is to stop production of a specific RNA-binding protein; however, because of the critical role of this protein in multiple gene and neural networks, the overall disruptive impact mirrors that of a multiple-gene disorder (Belmonte et al., 2004). From this perspective, it is argued that the single-gene, direct-effect mode of expression is the rare exception rather than the rule. It is more likely that behavior results from the complex interactions of genetic, cellular, anatomical, and functional networks with environmental influences (Inoue & Lupski, 2003).

Furthermore, even for single-gene diseases, many allelic variants have been found. For instance, the *5-HTT* gene is involved in the transmission of serotonin. Two common alleles have been identified, one long and one short. Because pilot data indicated that those individuals with two long alleles handle stress better than those with two short alleles, Caspi and colleagues determined whether their subjects had two long, two short, or one of each allele. They then asked about the type and quantity of stressful events that had occurred between the ages of 21 and 26 years. Among those experiencing significant stress, those with two short alleles were twice as likely to become depressed as those with two long alleles (Caspi et al., 2003).

Finally, most studies fail to recognize the gene–environment interaction. There can be no more straightforward example of this than phenylketonuria. Moving to the behavioral arena, Caspi and colleagues examined the genetically mediated impact of monoamine oxidase type A (MAO-A) enzyme production on the relationship between child abuse and adult antisocial behavior (Caspi et al., 2002). The MAO-A enzyme is involved in the regulation of several neurotransmitters, including serotonin. The results indicated that boys who produced low levels of this enzyme and were abused as children were twice as likely to develop adult antisocial behavior as were those abused boys who produced high levels of this same enzyme. The need to study more complex models has led some authors to advocate alternative research models and strategies for investigating gene–behavior links.

Endophenotypes and Animal Models

An alternative approach to tracing gene–behavior relationships involves the use of endophenotypes, or measurable biological traits that are associated with target behavior phenotypes (Inoue & Lupski, 2003). For instance, local activity of the brain can be assessed by functional magnetic resonance imaging, an approach that has been successfully applied to identify the association between the *COMT* gene and frontal lobe function (a hallmark for schizophrenia). Event-related potentials have been utilized as endophenotypes in Down syndrome, in Prader-Willi syndrome, and in linkage studies of alcoholism and schizophrenia. The documented linkage between velocardiofacial syndrome and schizophrenia, possibly via the *COMT* gene, offers a starting point for gene–schizophrenia associations using endophenotypes as an intermediate step.

A second strategy employs animal models to study endophenotypes. For instance, one method employs single-gene mouse mutants for tracing endophenotype alterations, then applies these results to human studies. Both endpoints of the gene–behavior relationship are available using mouse models. One can start with a mouse mutant that displays characteristics that correspond to the physiological and behavior markers of a human behavior phenotype, search for candidate genes, then use targeted mutagenesis in known genes to test the gene–behavior relationship (for review, see Tarantino & Bucan, 2000). Conversely, one can utilize known single-gene knockout mouse models and track through to the resulting endotypes and phenotypes. Although mouse models are appealing because they can be easily genetically manipulated, they present clear limitations for studies of higher brain functions such as language, self-concept, or hallucinations.

Ethical Concerns

There is growing concern regarding the sociopolitical and ethical implications surrounding behavior genetics research. Many worry that the move toward genetic reductionism is simply the eugenics movement in new clothes. In the United States and elsewhere, the growing prospects of genetic screening for job selections (Gostin, 1991) and medical insurance (Wilke, 1998) have led some observers to conclude that the eugenics movement has not disappeared but has merely been privatized (Cooper, 2001).

The characterization of the completion of the first draft of the human genome as "The Book of Life" (Sulston, reported by McKie in the *London Observer,* October, 1999) has many critics concerned that human diseases may come to be regarded simply as typographical errors, with the implication that such errors are eminently erasable. Nowhere is this concern any more grave that among those who work with people affected by genetic disorders, developmental disabilities, and intellectual disabilities—for the evidence of history clearly relegates those so affected to lesser citizenship and, by extension, lesser rights and protections. The practice of moral equality in the light of clear (and by implication, undesirable) genetic differences is easily threatened by the unchecked desire for or inappropriate exercise of power and authority or by times of inadequate resources.

CONCLUSION

Several decades of quantitative genetic research recently supplemented with molecular studies suggest that the biological basis (i.e., genetic substrate) of complex human behaviors and individual behavioral differences, although both strong and pervasive, is rarely determinative (Rutter, 2002). From the perspective of the complex disorders, even when using several methods to triangulate on the same problem, most candidate loci and genes have failed to reproduce positive linkage or association, and no single gene has been conclusively identified (Inoue & Lupski, 2003). Although this may, in part, reflect phenotypic heterogeneity, it likely also reflects complex gene–gene and gene–environment interactions not fully accounted for in present models.

Research in this area has to grapple with the complexity of both environmental and confounding influences on behavioral and developmental outcomes. Whereas some behavioral and developmental outcomes are genetically determined, others are secondary phenomena resulting from variables unrelated to the syndrome, and yet others arise from genetic-environmental interactions (Finegan, 1998). In addition, the same behavioral outcome (e.g., depression) can result from these three disparate etiological sources, further complicating understanding and interpreting findings. Similar concerns apply even with single-gene disorders, whose influence on behavior is far more indirect and complex than originally envisioned. This has led some to suggest that biological parameters are best viewed as *delimiting factors constraining outcomes rather than causal agents determining a particular trait* (Kagan, 2002). Although major technological advances have been made, clearly bridging the gap between gene structure and function as related to behavioral outcomes remains a major challenge.

REFERENCES

Achenbach, T.M. (1993). *Manual for the Child Behavior Checklist and revised Child Behavior Profile.* Burlington, VT: University Associates in Psychiatry.

American Psychiatric Association. (1980). *Diagnostic and statistical manual of mental disorders.* (3rd ed.). Washington, DC: Author.

Asherson, P., & Curran, S. (2001). Approaches to gene mapping in complex disorders and their application in child psychiatry and psychology. *British Journal of Psychiatry, 179,* 122–128.

Bailey, A., LeCouteur, A., Gershon, I., Bolton, P., Simonoff, E., Yuzda, E., et al. (1995). Autism as a strongly genetic disorder: Evidence from a British twin study. *Psychological Medicine, 25,* 63–77.

Barr, C., Kroft, J., Feng, Y., Wigg, K., Roberts, W., Malone, M., et al. (2002). The norepinephrine transporter gene and attention-deficit hyperactivity disorder. *American Journal of Medical Genetics (Neuropsychiatric Genetics), 114,* 255–259.

Barr, C.W., Kroft, J., Feng, Y., Zai, G., Malone, M., Roberts, W., et al. (2000). Attention deficit hyperactivity disorder and the gene for the dopamine D5 receptor. *Molecular Psychiatry, 5,* 548–551.

Barr C., Xu, C., Kroft, J., Feng, Y., Wigg, K., Zai, G., et al. (2001). Haplotype study of three polymorphisms at the dopamine transporter locus confirm linkage to attention-deficit/hyperactivity disorder. *Biological Psychiatry, 49,* 333–339.

Bass, M.P., Menold, M.M., Wolpert, C.M., Donnelly, S.K., Ravan, S.A., & Hauser, E.R. (2000). Genetic studies in autistic disorder and chromosome 15. *Neurogenetics, 2,* 219–226.

Bauman, M. (1998). Neuroanatomy: Cerebellar dysfunction spectrum—cognition/motor. In *The spectrum of developmental disabilities XX: Autism—stretching the concept.* Baltimore: The Johns Hopkins University Press.

Belmonte, M.K., Cook, E.H. Jr., Anderson, G., Rubenstein, J.L., Greenough, W.T., Beckel-Mitchener, A., et al. (2004). Autism as a disorder of neural information processing: Directions for research and targets for therapy. *Molecular Psychiatry, 9,* 646–663.

Benzer, S. (1967). Behavioral mutants of *Drosophila* isolated by counter-current distribution. *Proceedings of the National Academy of Sciences of the United States of America, 58,* 1112–1119.

Benzer, S. (1971). From the gene to behavior. *Journal of the American Medical Association, 218,* 1015–1022.

Bespalova, I.N., & Busbaum, J. (2003). Disease susceptibility genes for autism. *Annals of Medicine, 35,* 274–281.

Biederman, J., & Faraone, S. (1990). Retrospective assessment of DSM-III attention deficit disorder in non-referred individuals. *Journal of Clinical Psychiatry, 51,*102–107.

Biederman, J., Faraone, S.V., Keenan, K., Benjamin, J., Krifcher, B., Moore, C., et al. (1992). Further evidence for family genetic risk factors in attention deficit hyperactivity disorder: Patterns of comorbidity in probands and relatives of psychiatrically and pediatrically referred samples. *Archives of General Psychiatry, 49,* 728–738.

Biederman, J., Faraone, S.V., Mick, E., Williamson, S., Wilens, T.E., Spencer, T.J., et al. (1999). Clinical correlates of attention deficit hyperactivity in females: Findings from a large group of pediatrically and psychiatrically referred girls. *Journal of the American Academy of Child and Adolescent Psychiatry, 38,* 966–975.

Biederman, J., Munir, K., Knee, D., Habelow, W., Armentano, M., Autor, S., et al. (1986). A family study of patients with attention deficit disorder and normal controls. *Journal of Psychiatric Research, 20,* 263–274.

Biederman, J., & Spencer, T.J. (2000). Genetics of childhood disorders: XIX. ADHD, Part 3: Is ADHD a noradrenergic disorder? *Journal of the American Academy of Child and Adolescent Psychiatry, 39,* 1330–1333.

Bishop, D.V.M. (2001). Genetic and environmental risks for specific language impairment in children. *Philosophical Transactions of the Royal Society of London, Series B, 356,* 369–380.

Bishop, D.V.M., North, T., & Donlan, C. (1995). Genetic basis for specific language impairment: Evidence from a twin study. *Developmental Medicine and Child Neurology, 37,* 56–71.

Borthwick-Duffy, S.A. (1994). Epidemiology and prevalence of psychopathology in people with mental retardation. *Journal of Consulting and Clinical Psychology, 62,* 17–27.

Boycott, K.M., Parslow, M., Ross, J.L., Miller, I.P., Bech-Hansen, N.T., & MacLeod, P.M. (2003). A familial contiguous gene deletion syndrome at $X_p22.3$ characterized by severe learning disabilities and ADHD. *American Journal of Medical Genetics, 122A,* 139–147.

Brzustowicz, L.M., Hodgkinson, K.A., Chow, E.W., Honer, W.G., & Bassett, A.S. (2000). Location of a major susceptibility locus for familial schizophrenia on chromosome 1q21–q22. *Science, 288,* 678–682.

Cantwell, D.P. (1972). Psychiatric illness in the families of hyperactive children. *Archives of General Psychiatry, 27,* 414–427.

Cardon, L.R., Smith, S., Fulker, D.W., Kimberling, W.J., Pennington, B.F., & Defries, J.C. (1994). Quantitative trait locus for reading disability on chromosome 6. *Science, 266,* 276–279.

Carey, J.C., & McMahon, W.M. (1999). Neurobehavioral disorders and medical genetics. In C. Reynolds & S. Goldstein (Eds.), *Handbook of neurodevelopmental and genetic disorders in children* (pp. 38–60). New York: The Guilford Press.

Caspi, A., McClay, J., Moffitt, T.E., Mill, J., Martin, J., Craig, I.W., et al. (2002). Role of genotype in the cycle of violence in maltreated children. *Science, 297,* 851–854.

Caspi, A., Sugden, K., Moffitt, T.E., Taylor, A., Craig, I.W., & Harrington, H., et al. (2003). Influence of life stress on depression: Moderation by a polymorphism in the 5-Htt gene. *Science, 301,* 386–389.

Cook, E.H., Courchesne, R., Cox, N.J., Lord, C., Gonen, D., Guter, S.H., et al. (1998). Linkage-disequilibrium mapping of autistic disorder with 15Q11–13 markers. *American Journal of Human Genetics, 62,* 1077–1083.

Cook, E., Stein, M., Krasowski, M., Cox, N., Olkon, D., Kieffer, J., et al. (1995). Association of attention deficit disorder and the dopamine transporter gene. *American Journal of Human Genetics, 56,* 993–998.

Cooper, B. (2001). Nature, nurture and mental disorder: Old concepts in the new millennium. *British Journal of Psychiatry, 178*(Suppl. 40), s91–s102.

Curran, S., Mill, J., Tahir, E., Kent, L., Richards, S., Gould, A., et al. (2001). Association study of a dopamine transporter polymorphism and attention deficit hyperactivity disorder in UK and Turkish samples. *Molecular Psychiatry, 6,* 425–428.

Daly, G., Hawi, Z., Fitzgerald, M., & Gill, M. (1999). Mapping susceptibility loci in attention deficit hyperactivity disorder: Preferential transmission of parental alleles at DAT1, DBH, and DRD5 to affected children. *Molecular Psychiatry, 4,* 192–196.

Defries, J.C., Fulker, D., & LaBuda, M.C. (1987). Evidence for a genetic aetiology in reading disability in twins. *Nature, 329,* 537–539.

Dykens, E. (1995). Measuring behavioral phenotypes: Provocations from the "new genetics." *American Journal on Mental Retardation, 99,* 522–532.

Dykens, E.M., & Rosner, B. (1999). Refining behavioral phenotypes: Personality-motivation in Williams and Prader-Willi syndromes. *American Journal on Mental Retardation, 104,* 158–169.

Edlebrock, C., Rende, R., Plomin, R., & Thompson, L.A. (1995). A twin study of competence of problem behavior in childhood and early adolescence. *Journal of Child Psychology and Psychiatry, 36,* 775–785.

Einfeld, S., & Hall, W. (1994). When is a behavioral phenotype not a phenotype. *Developmental Medicine and Child Neurology, 36*, 467–470.

Einfeld, S., Smith, A., Durvasula, S., Florio, T., & Tonge, B. (1999). Behavior and emotional disturbance in Prader-Willi syndrome. *American Journal of Medical Genetics, 82*, 123–127.

Eisenberg, L. (2001). Why has the relationship between psychiatry and genetics been so contentious? *Genetics in Medicine, 3*, 377–381.

Fagerheim, T., Raeymaekers, P., Tonnessen, F.E., Pedersen, M., Tranebjaerg, L., & Lubs, H.A. (1999). A new gene (*DYX3*) for dyslexia is located on chromosome 2. *Journal of Medical Genetics, 36*, 664–669.

Faraone, S., Biederman, J., Keenan, K., & Tsuang, M.T. (1991a). A family-genetic study of girls with DSM-III attention deficit disorder. *American Journal of Psychiatry, 148*, 112–115.

Faraone, S.V., Biederman, J., Keenan, K., & Tsuang, M.T. (1991b). Separation of DSM-III attention deficit disorder and conduct disorder: Evidence from a family-genetic study of American child psychiatric patients. *Psychological Medicine, 21*, 109–121.

Faraone, S.V., & Doyle, A. (2001). The nature and heritability of attention-deficit/hyperactivity disorder. *Child and Adolescent Psychiatry Clinics of North America, 10*, 299–317.

Faraone, S.V., Doyle, A.E., Mick, E., & Biederman, J. (2002). Meta-analysis of the association between the 7-repeat allele of the dopamine D(4) receptor gene and attention deficit hyperactivity disorder. *American Journal of Psychiatry, 159*, 496–497.

Finegan, J.A. (1998). Study of behavior phenotypes: Goals and methodological considerations. *American Journal of Medical Genetics (Neuropsychiatric Genetics), 81*, 148–155.

Fisher, S.E. (2002). Isolation of the genetic factors underlying speech and language disorders. In R. Plomin, J. Defries, I. Craig, & P. McGuffin (Eds.), *Behavioral genetics in the postgenomic era* (pp. 205–226). Washington, DC: American Psychological Association.

Fisher, S.E., Marlow, A.J., Lamb, J., Maestrini, E., Williams, D.F., Richardson, A.J., et al. (1999). A quantitative-trait locus on chromosome 6p influences aspects of developmental dyslexia. *American Journal of Human Genetics, 64*, 146–156.

Fisher, S.E., Vargha-Khadem, F., Watkins, K.E., Monaco, A.P., & Pembrey, M.E. (1998). Localisation of a gene implicated in a severe speech and language disorder. *Nature Genetics, 18*, 168–170.

Flint, J., & Yule, W. (1994). Behavioral phenotypes. In M. Rutter, E. Taylor, & L. Hersov (Eds.), *Child and adolescent psychiatry: Modern approaches* (3rd ed., pp. 666–687). Oxford, UK: Blackwell Scientific.

Folstein, S. (1996). Twin and adoption studies in child and adolescent psychiatric disorders. *Current Opinion in Pediatrics, 8*, 339–347.

Galaburda, A.M., Sherman, G., Rosen, G.D., Aboitiz, F., & Geschwind, N. (1985). Developmental dyslexia: Four consecutive patients with cortical anomalies. *Annals of Neurology, 18*, 222–233.

Galton, F. (1869). *Heredity talent and character.* London: Macmillan.

Gayan, J., Smith, S.D., Cherny, S.S., Cardon, L.R., Fulker, D.W., Brower, A.M., et al. (1999). Quantitative-trait for specific language and reading deficits on chromosome 6p. *American Journal of Human Genetics, 64*, 157–164.

Gjone, H., Stevenson, J., & Sundet, J. (1996). Genetic influence on parent-reported attention-related problems in a Norwegian general population twin sample. *Journal of the American Academy of Child and Adolescent Psychiatry, 35*, 588–598.

Goodman, R., & Stevenson, J. (1989). A twin study of hyperactivity: II. The aetiological role of genes, family relationship, and perinatal adversity. *Journal of Child Psychology and Psychiatry, 30*, 691–709.

Gostin, L. (1991). Genetic discrimination: The use of genetically based diagnostic and prognostic tests by employers and insurers. *American Journal of Law and Medicine, 17*, 109–144.

Grigorenko, E., Wood, F., Meyer, M.S., Pauls, J.E.D., Hart, L.A., & Pauls, D.L. (1998). Linkage studies suggest a possible locus for dyslexia near the Rh region on chromosome 1. *Behavior Genetics, 28*, 470.

Grigorenko, E., Wood, F.B., Meyer, M.S., & Pauls, D.L. (2000). Chromosome 6p influences on different dyslexia related cognitive processes: Further confirmation. *American Journal of Human Genetics, 66*, 715–723.

Grigorenko, E. (2001). Developmental dyslexia: An update on genes, brains, and environments. *Journal of Child Psychology and Psychiatry, 42*, 91–125.

Grigorenko, E. (2002). Epistasis and the genetics of complex traits. In R. Plomin, J. Defries, I. Craig, & P. McGuffin (Eds.), *Behavioral genetics in the postgenomic era*. Washington, DC: American Psychological Association.

Grigorenko, E.L., Wood, F.B., Meyer, M.S., Hart, L.A., Speed, W.C., & Schuster, A. (1997). Susceptibility loci for distinct components of developmental dyslexia on chromosomes 6 and 15. *American Journal of Human Genetics, 60*, 27–39.

Hermann, K. (1959). *Reading disability: A medical study of word blindness and related handicaps.* Springfield, IL: Charles C Thomas.

Hodapp, R., & Dykens, E. (2001). Strengthening behavioral research on genetic mental retardation syndromes. *American Journal on Mental Retardation, 106*, 4–15.

Hsiung, G.Y., Kaplan, B., Petryshen, T., Lu, S., & Field, L. (2004). A dyslexia susceptibility locus (DYX7) linked to dopamine D4 receptor (DRD4) region on chromosome 11p15.5. *American Journal of Medical Genetics, Part B, 125B*, 112–119.

Huang, C.H. (1997). Molecular insights into the Rh protein family and associated antigens. *Current Opinion in Hematology, 4*, 94–103.

Inoue, K., & Lupski, J. (2003). Genetics and genomics of behavioral and psychiatric disorders. *Current Opinion in Genetics and Development, 13,* 303–309.

Jamain, S., Betancur, C., Quach, H., Philippe, A., Fellpus, M., Giros, B., et al, (2002). Linkage and association of the glutamate receptor 6 gene with autism. *Molecular Psychiatry, 7,* 302–310.

Kagan, J. (2002). A behavioral science perspective. In R. Plomin, J.C. Defries, I.W. Craig, & P. McGuffin (Eds.), *Behavior genetics in the postgenomic era* (pp. xvii–xx). Washington, DC: American Psychological Association.

Karayiorgou, M., & Gogos, J.A. (1997). Dissecting the genetic complexity of schizophrenia. *Molecular Psychiatry, 2,* 211–223.

Lai, C.S.L., Fisher, S.E., Hurst, J.A., Vargha-Khadem, F., & Monaco, A.P. (2001). A forkhead-domain gene is mutated in a severe speech and language disorder. *Nature, 413,* 519–523.

Lander, E., & Schork, N. (1994). Genetic dissection of complex traits. *Science, 265,* 2037–2048.

Levitas A. (2000). Behavior and psychiatric phenotype of genetic syndromes: Part 1. *Healthy Times, 12*(1), 1–13.

Mbarek, O., Marouillat, S., Martineau, J., Barthelemy, C., Muh, J.P., & Andres, C. (1999). Association study of the NF1 gene and autistic disorder. *American Journal of Medical Genetics, 88,* 729–732.

McGuffin, P., Owen, M., O'Donovan, M.C., Thapar, A., & Gottesman, I.I. (Eds.). (1994). *Seminars in psychiatric genetics.* London: Gaskell.

McGuffin, P., Riley, B., & Plomin, R. (2001). Toward behavior genomics. *Science, 291,* 1232–1249.

McKie, R. (1999, October 3). Gene pioneers herald medical revolution. *London Observer,* p. 1.

Merikangas, K., & Risch, N. (2003). Will the genomics revolutions revolutionize psychiatry? *American Journal of Psychiatry, 160,* 625–635.

Morris, D.W., Robinson, K., Turic, D., Duke, M., Webb, V., Milham, C., et al. (2000). Family-based association mapping provides evidence for a gene for reading disability on chromosome 15q. *Human Molecular Genetics, 9,* 855–860.

Mudad, R., & Telen, M.J. (1996). Biological functions of blood group antigens. *Current Opinion in Hematology, 32,* 473–479.

Muldavsky, M., Lev, D., & Leeman-Sagie, T. (2001). Behavioral phenotypes of genetic syndromes: A reference guide for psychiatrists. *Journal of the American Academy of Child and Adolescent Psychiatry, 40*(7), 749–761.

Neiderhiser, J. (2001). Understanding the roles of genome and enviroment: Methods in genetic epidemiology. *British Journal of Psychiatry, 178*(Suppl. 40), s12–s17.

Nyhan, W.L. (1972). Clinical features of the Lesch-Nyhan syndrome. *Archives of Internal Medicine, 130,* 186–192.

O'Brien, G., & Yule, W. (1995). *Behavioral phenotypes.* London: Mac Keith Press.

Olson, R.K., Forsberg, H., & Wise, B. (1994). Genes, environment, and the development of orthographic skills. In V.W. Berninger (Ed.), *The varieties of orthographic knowledge 1: Theoretical and developmental issues* (pp. 27–71). Dordrecht, The Netherlands: Kluwer.

Pennington, B.F. (1990). Annotation: The genetics of dyslexia. *Journal of Child Psychology and Psychiatry and Allied Disciplines, 2,* 193–201.

Pennington, B.F. (1994). Genetics of learning disabilities. *Journal of Child Neurology, 10*(Suppl), S69–S76.

Pericak-Vance, M.A. (2002). The genetics of autistic disorder. In R. Plomin, J. Defries, I. Craig, & P. McGuffin (Eds.), *Behavioral genetics in the postgenomic era* (pp. 267–286). Washington, DC: American Psychological Association.

Plank, S.M., Coopeland-Yates, S., Sossey-Alaoui, K., Bell, J.M., Schroer, R.J., Skinner, C., et al. (2001). Lack of association of the (AAAT)6 allele of the GXAlu tetranucleotide repeat in intron 27b of the NF1 gene with autism. *American Journal of Medical Genetics, 105,* 404–405.

Plomin, R., Defries, J., Craig, I., & McGuffin, P. (2002). Behavior genomics. In R. Plomin, J. Defries, I. Craig, & P. McGuffin (Eds.), *Behavioral genetics in the postgenomic era* (pp. 529–540). Washington, DC: American Psychological Association.

Plomin, R., Owen, M., & McGuffin, P. (1994). The genetic basis of complex human behaviors. *Science, 264,* 1733–1739.

Rabin, M., Wen, X.L., Hepburn, M., Lubs, H.A., Feldman, E., & Duara, R. (1993). Suggestive linkage of developmental dyslexia to chromosome 1p34–p36. *Lancet, 342,* 178.

Roizen, N.J., Blondis, T.A., Irwin, M., Rubinoff, A., Kieffer, J., & Stein, M.A. (1996). Psychiatric and developmental disorders in families of children with attention-deficit hyperactivity disorder. *Archives of Pediatrics and Adolescent Medicine, 150,* 203–208.

Rutter, M. (2002). The interplay of nature, nurture and developmental influences: The challenge ahead for mental health. *Archives of General Psychiatry, 59,* 996–1000.

Schulte-Korne, G., Grimm, T., Nothen, M.M., Muller-Myhsok, B., Cichon, S., Vogt, I.R., et al. (1998). Evidence for linkage of spelling disability to chromosome 15. *American Journal of Human Genetics, 63,* 279–282.

Schulte-Korne, G. (2001). Annotation: Genetics of reading and spelling disorder. *Journal of Child Psychology and Psychiatry, 42,* 985–997.

Schulte-Korne, G., Diemel, W., Muller, K., Gutenbrunner, C., & Remschmidt, H. (1996). Familial aggregation of spelling disorder. *Journal of Child Psychology and Psychiatry, 37,* 817–822.

Seth, A., & Edelman, G. (2003). Environment and behavior influence the complexity of evolved neural networks. *Adaptive Behavior, 12,* 15–20.

SLI Consortium. (2002). A genome wide scan identifies two novel loci involved in specific language impairment. *American Journal of Human Genetics, 70,* 384–398.

Smith, S., Kimberling, W., Pennington, B., & Lubs, H. (1983). Specific reading disability: Identification of an inherited form through linkage analysis. *Science, 219,* 1345–1347.

Smith, S., Pennington, B.F., Kimberling, W.J., & Ing, P.S. (1990). Familial dyslexia: Use of genetic linkage data to define subtypes. *Journal of the American Academy of Child and Adolescent Psychiatry, 29,* 338–348.

Smith, S.D., Kimberling, W.J., & Pennington, B.F. (1991). Screen for multiple genes influencing dyslexia. *Reading and Writing: An Interdisciplinary Journal, 3,* 285–298.

Snowling, M., Gallager, A., & Frith, U. (2003). Family risk of dyslexia is continuous: Individual difference in the precursors of reading skill. *Child Development, 74,* 358–373.

Sovner, R. (1986). Limiting factors in the use of DSM-III criteria with mentally ill/mentally retarded persons. *Psychopharmacology Bulletin, 22,* 1055–1059.

Spencer, T, Biederman, J., Wilens, T.E., Prince, J., Hatch, M., Jones, J., et al. (1998). Effectiveness and tolerability of tomaxetine in adults with attention-deficit hyperactivity disorder. *American Journal of Psychiatry, 155,* 693–695.

Steinhausen, H.C., von Gontard, A., Spohr, H.L., Hauffa, B.P., Eiholzer, U., Backes, M., et al. (2002). Behavioral phenotypes in four mental retardation syndromes: Fetal alcohol syndrome, Prader-Willi syndrome, fragile X syndrome, and tuberosis sclerosis. *American Journal of Medical Genetics, 111,* 381–387.

Stevenson, J. (1992). Evidence for a genetic etiology in hyperctivity in children. *Behavior Genetics, 22,* 337–343.

Stromgren, E. (1994). Recent history of European psychiatry—ideas, developments and personalities: The Annual Eliot Slater Lecture. *American Journal of Human Genetics, 54,* 405–410.

Sullivan, P., Eaves, L., Kendler, K., & Neale, M. (2001). Genetic case-control association studies in neuropsychiatry. *Archives of General Psychiatry, 58,* 1015–1024.

Tager-Flusberg, H. (Ed.). (1999). *Neurodevelopmental disorders.* Cambridge, MA: The MIT Press.

Tarantino, L., & Bucan, M. (2000). Dissection of behavior and psychiatric disorders using the mouse as a model. *Human Molecular Genetics, 9,* 953–965.

Thapar, A. (2002). Attention deficit hyperactivity disorder: New genetic findings, new directions. In R. Plomin, I. Craig, & P. McGuffin (Eds.), *Behavioral genetics in the postgenomic era* (pp. 445–462). Washington, DC, American Psychological Association.

Thapar, A., Hervas, A., & McGuffin, P. (1995). Childhood hyperactivity scores are highly heritable and show sibling competition effects: Twin study evidence. *Behavior Genetics, 25,* 537–544.

Thapar, A., Holmes, J., Poulton, K., & Harrington, R. (1999). Genetic basis of attention deficit and hyperactivity. *British Journal of Psychiatry, 174,* 105–111.

Tomblin, J.B. (1989). Familial concentration of developmental language impairment. *Journal of Speech and Hearing Disorders, 54,* 287–295.

Tomblin, J.B., & Buckwalter, P.R. (1998). Heritability of poor language achievement among twins. *Journal of Speech, Language and Hearing Research, 41,* 188–199.

Weissman, M. (2001). Phenotype definitions: Some hidden issues in psychiatry. *American Journal of Medical Genetics, 105,* 45–47.

Wilke, T. (1998). Genetics and insurance in Britain: Why more than just the Atlantic divides the English-speaking nations. *Nature Genetics, 20,* 119–121.

III

Etiologies

Prematurity

MARILEE C. ALLEN

Prematurity implies relative immaturity for extrauterine life and therefore vulnerability to complications involving most of the major organ systems. Preterm infants are a heterogeneous population of infants born before 37 weeks' gestation. They differ as to degree of prematurity, etiology of preterm birth, environmental exposures, vulnerability to the complications of prematurity, and long-term health and neurodevelopmental outcomes. The major determinant of mortality and morbidity is maturity, but because it is difficult to directly measure it, gestational age and birth weight are often used as proxies for maturity. Although interrelated, maturity, gestational age (GA; i.e., duration of pregnancy) and birth weight (BW; i.e., a measure of infant size) are distinct entities, both conceptually and operationally (in that they vary as to how environmental factors influence them). The imprecise and interchangeable use of these terms has made it difficult to interpret much of the preterm outcomes literature.

Prematurity is not a disease for which a cure will be found. Preterm birth is a common, complex condition resulting from multiple interactions between the maternal and fetal genomes and conditions in the intrauterine environment, the mother's body, and her external environment (Institute of Medicine [IOM], 2006). It has multiple determinants, physiological pathways, and outcomes, and these vary among populations. Genetics, maternal illness, pregnancy conditions, infection and inflammation, psychosocial and behavioral factors, assistive reproductive technologies, and environmental exposures have all been implicated in preterm birth. Some directly influence fetal development.

The prevalence of preterm birth makes it a significant public health problem: 12.5% of infants born in the United States in 2004 were preterm (Alexander, 2006). Medical and technological advancements have dramatically reduced infant mortality rates for infants of all GA and BW categories, but the preterm birth rate has increased 30% since 1980 (Alexander, Tompkins, Allen, & Hulsey, 1999; Allen, Alexander, Tompkins, & Hulsey, 2000; IOM, 2006). Although the greatest increase has been in infants born at 32–36 weeks' gestation, sustained efforts to save smaller and more immature infants have lowered the limits of viability to now 22–23 weeks' gestation (with rare survival reported at 21 weeks' gestation) (Allen, 2002; Ho & Saigal, 2005). Preterm infants account for 75% of perinatal deaths (Slattery & Morrison, 2002). For the United States in 2005, an IOM report (2006) estimated the annual economic societal burden associated with preterm birth to be over $26.2 billion. Concerns about biological limits, higher rates of neurodevelopmental disability at the lowest gestational ages, increased risks of motor, cognitive, and behavior impairments associated with preterm birth, and rising health care costs have shifted society's attention toward preventing preterm births and improving health and neurodevelopmental outcomes (Green et al., 2005).

HISTORICAL PERSPECTIVE

A historical perspective provides insight into the emergence of high-risk obstetric and neonatal intensive care and subsequent dramatic improvements in preterm survival and outcomes (Allen, 2002). Although rare preterm infants occasionally survived, concerted efforts to save preterm infants began in Europe during the last quarter of the 19th century (Baker, 2000). French and German physicians, recognizing the detrimental effects of cold stress, devised various models of incubators for preterm infants. Starting with an adaptation of a chick embryo incubator from a science exhibition, obstetrician Stéphane Tarnier's efforts to provide warmth, good nursing care, and gavage feedings to French preterm infants reduced mortality by half. His student Adolph Pinard concentrated on preventing prematurity, while Pierre Budin continued his work, describing basic principles of caring for preterm infants in his book, *Le Nourisson* (Budin, 1907).

Alexandre Lion of Nice improved incubators by equipping them with thermostats and ventilation systems and supervised a display of preterm infants at the 1896 Berlin Exposition (a "child hatchery" funded by spectator admission fees) (Baker, 2000). As proof of the value of this work, a preterm survivor won the Croix de Guerre in World War I (Liebling, 1939). Martin Couney, a physician trained in Europe, set up preterm nurseries at a number of U.S. World's Fairs. Arnold Gesell observed and described the development of movement and behavior prior to term in preterm infants at the 1939 New York World's Fair (Gesell & Amatruda, 1945). At Coney Island, Dr. Couney established a permanent but seasonal preterm nursery, funded by admission fees (Baker, 2000; Liebling, 1939; Silverman, 1979).

The first successful hospital-based nursery for preterm infants in the United States was established in Chicago by Dr. Julian Hess and nurse Evelyn Lundeen (Baker, 2000; Hess, 1953). Preterm infants were transferred to their unit if they survived the first 7–10 days; no doubt many were small for their GA. Hess's 30-year follow-up study of 370 preterm survivors reported that most grew up to be functioning members of society, including their smallest survivor, who weighed 605 g (Hess, 1953). The work of these and other pioneers was so successful that, by the late 1940s, most tertiary care hospitals had established preterm nurseries.

The definition of prematurity changed from one based on BW (i.e., below 2,500 g) to one based on GA. When publishing a graph of growth percentiles as BW for each week of gestation, Battaglia and Lubchenco (1967) recognized the importance of identifying infants as small, appropriate, or large for gestational age. Lubchenco and colleagues went on to demonstrate that mortality and prevalence of neonatal complications and disabilities varied by BW for GA categories (Lubchenco, Delivoria-Papadopoulos, & Searls, 1972; Lubchenco, Searls, & Brazie, 1972). The World Health Organization currently defines prematurity as birth before 37 weeks' gestation. Nevertheless, many outcomes studies report outcomes in terms of BW categories: very low birth weight (BW < 1,500 g), extremely low birth weight (BW < 1,000 g), and more recently, infants with BW below 750 g, 600 g, and even 500 g.

Supplemental oxygen was routinely given to preterm infants in incubators because respiratory distress syndrome (RDS) is the most common complication of prematurity (Nelson, 2000; Silverman, 1980). In the early 1950s, recognition of an association of hyperoxia with retinopathy of prematurity (ROP, a cause of severe visual impairment) led to a curtailment of the liberal use of supplemental oxygen (with resulting hypoxia in some infants). Fluids and nourishment were difficult to provide to fragile, sick preterm infants during the first few days after birth, and many developed dehydration and hypoglycemia. Monitoring blood gases, electrolytes, and glucose levels was extremely difficult. Antibiotics used to treat infections had unfortunate side effects in preterm infants, including hearing impairment with streptomycin, hyperbilirubinemia with sulfonamides, and shock with chloramphenicol. Systematic follow-up studies of preterm survivors born in the 1950s and 1960s demonstrated high morbidity rates: more than half of infants with BW below 1,500 g had cerebral palsy, intellectual disabilities, and/or blindness (Drillien, 1961, 1967; Lubchenco, Horner, Reed, Hix, Metcalf, et al., 1963; Lubchenco, Delivoria-Papadopoulos, & Searls, 1972). These findings highlighted the importance of both carefully monitoring preterm infants and following health and neurodevelopmental outcomes to provide feedback regarding their medical care.

By the mid-1960s, basic science research had led to better understanding of the pathophysiology of asphyxia and RDS, which then led to better methods of resuscitating newborns (Allen, 2002; Hack, Fanaroff, & Merkatz, 1979). Respirators used in adults and children were adapted for neonates. Clinicians applied these technological and medical advances in their care of preterm and sick full-term infants, and this was the beginning of neonatal intensive care. They intubated and ventilated preterm infants or provided them with continuous positive airway pressure or both, and provided them with intravenous fluids and glucose. The widespread establishment of neonatal intensive care units (NICUs) in many tertiary care hospitals provided the stimulus for creation of NICU follow-up clinics. Preterm outcome studies have progressively increased in number since that time.

In the ensuing decades, technological advances in fetal and neonatal monitoring included electronic fetal heart rate monitoring; prenatal ultrasound to evaluate fetal anatomy and movements; electronic heart and respiratory rate monitors; blood pressure monitors; continuous monitors of transcutaneous oxygen, carbon dioxide, and oxygen saturations; and better isolettes and infant warmers with continuous feedback for maintaining a thermoneutral environment and minimizing energy expenditure. Meticulous attention to fluid, glucose, calcium, and electrolyte management, a focus on early nutrition that includes parenteral nutrition and gut stimulation, and efforts to reduce physiological instability have become hallmarks of neonatal intensive care. Infant ventilators are constantly being modified and improved, and high-frequency ventilation with oscillators and jet ventilators now augments conventional ventilation. Worrisome data from earlier preterm outcome studies raised the concern that dramatic improvements in survival of preterm infants would increase the number of children with major disabilities. Fortunately, follow-up studies from the 1970s and 1980s reported lower rates of major disability: 5%–16% for infants with BW below 1,500 g and 9%–24% for infants with BW below 1,000 g (Allen & Jones, 1986; Hack et al., 1979; Jones, Cum-

mins, & Davies, 1979; Saigal, Rosenbaum, Stoskopf, & Sinclair, 1984).

ROP, a neovascular disorder of the developing preterm retina that was recognized in the 1940s and associated with hyperoxia in the 1950s, continues to be a significant problem for the most immature and sick preterm infants (Repka, 2002; Silverman, 1980). It has become clear that its etiology is multifactorial. Uniform descriptions of ROP published in 1984 ("An international classification," 1984) facilitated large randomized controlled trials that demonstrated improved visual outcomes, first with cryotherapy, then with early laser treatment (Shalev, Farr, & Repka, 2001).

Survival of preterm infants continued to improve in the 1990s, and major advances included antenatal steroids, exogenous surfactant, and high-frequency ventilation (Allen, 2002). Widespread administration of betamethasone to mothers about to deliver preterm did not occur until a National Institutes of Health–sponsored Consensus Conference in 1994 reviewed 20 years of data, including multiple randomized controlled trials with follow-up into childhood, that demonstrated reductions in RDS, intraventricular hemorrhage (IVH), and neonatal mortality (Crowley, 2000; National Institute of Child Health and Human Development, 1994). When preterm delivery is successfully delayed, any benefit from giving multiple antenatal courses of steroids is controversial (Crowther & Harding, 2003). Similarly, multiple randomized controlled trials of exogenous surfactant have demonstrated benefits in terms of mortality, gas exchange, RDS, pulmonary air leak, and chronic lung disease/bronchopulmonary dysplasia (CLD/BPD), with no differences in neurodevelopmental outcomes (Soll, 2000).

"It is a pity that neonatologists who carefully and methodically evaluated surfactant treatment before its widespread use in clinical practice failed to do the same with postnatal steroids" (Halliday, 2001). After randomized controlled trials in the mid-1980s demonstrated that pharmacological doses of dexamethasone improved gas exchange, duration of mechanical ventilation, and incidence of CLD/BPD, steroids were widely used, despite multiple side effects (hyperglycemia, hypertension, and growth problems) (Halliday & Eh-renkranz, 2001a, 2001b; Halliday, Ehren-kranz, & Doyle, 2004; "Postnatal cortico-steroids," 2002). Fifteen years later, follow-up studies from several trials raised an alarm by reporting a higher incidence of cerebral palsy and cognitive deficits in children randomized to receive dexamethasone. Whether the short-term pulmonary benefits of dexamethasone outweigh concerns about an increased risk of motor or cognitive impairment or both re-mains controversial. This experience highlights both the difficulty of narrowly focusing on one organ system at the expense of another (i.e., respiratory vs. central nervous system [CNS]) as well as the importance of demonstrating safety with long-term neurodevelopmental and health follow-up in randomized controlled trials of NICU interventions.

The importance of demonstrating safety and efficacy before introducing obstetric and neonatal interventions has been increasingly recognized. The last decade has seen the publi-cation of multiple randomized controlled trials of antenatal medications (e.g., phenobarbital, magnesium sulfate), neonatal medications (e.g., indomethacin, caffeine, inhaled nitric oxide), new technologies (e.g., high-frequency ventilation), and treatment strategies (e.g., NICU developmental support) (Allen, 2002; Aucott, Donohue, Atkins, & Allen, 2002; Barrington & Finer, 2006; Crowther & Hender-son-Smart, 2003; Crowther, Hiller, Doyle, & Haslam, 2003; Fowlie & Davis, 2002; Hender-son-Smart, Bhuta, Cools, & Offringa, 2003; Henderson-Smart & Davis, 2000; Symington & Pinelli, 2006). Nonetheless, many of the medi-cations and treatment strategies commonly used in neonatal intensive care have not been evaluated for safety and efficacy (Brion & Soll, 2001; Clerihew & McGuire, 2004; Finer, Hig-gins, Kattwinkel, & Martin, 2006; Lawn, Weir, & McGuire, 2005; Walsh et al., 2006). Some of the greatest neonatal intensive care controversies revolve around the most basic is-sues, including what safe levels are for fragile preterm infants with respect to oxygen and carbon dioxide (Askie & Henderson-Smart, 2001; Saugstad, 2006; Van Marter, 2005).

Specific neuroprotective strategies for ex-tremely preterm infants are on the horizon, but results from many randomized controlled trials have been mixed (Allen, 2002; IOM, 2006). There is little doubt of the benefits of antenatal betamethasone in improving outcomes of ex-tremely preterm infants, but there is no clear evidence as yet as to benefits of antenatal vita-min K, phenobarbital, or magnesium sulfate (Crowley, 2000; Crowther & Henderson-Smart, 2001, 2003; Crowther, Hiller, & Doyle, 2002; Crowther et al., 2003; "Report," 1994). Prophylactic indomethacin does reduce symp-tomatic patent ductus arteriosus and severe IVH, but its effect on neurodevelopmental out-come is not as dramatic (it might benefit verbal abilities in boys) (Fowlie & Davis, 2002; Ment et al., 2000, 2004; Schmidt et al., 2001). Con-cerns about adverse effects were raised in stud-ies of intramuscular vitamin E (sepsis); post-natal phenobarbital for IVH (longer time on ventilator); and posthemorrhagic hy-drocephalus, diuretics (nephrocalcinosis, in-creased motor impairment), and streptokinase (secondary hemorrhage) (Brion, Bell, & Raghuveer, 2003; Whitelaw, 2001a, 2001b; Whitelaw, Kennedy, & Brion, 2001). Studies of naturally occurring neuroprotective sub-stances (i.e., thyroxin, hydrocortisone, and erythropoietin) have raised many questions re-garding whether supplementation will im-prove preterm neurodevelopmental outcomes (Osborn, 2001; O'Shea, 2002; Sola, Wen, Ham-rick, & Ferriero, 2005; Watterberg, Gerdes, & Cook, 2001; Watterberg et al., 2004).

Recognizing mistakes of the past and the need to evaluate new therapies has moved high-risk obstetrics and neonatal intensive care toward more evidence-based medicine. The focus has been shifting from all-out efforts to save smaller and more immature infants to rec-ognizing that "the ultimate goal of neonatal intensive care... [is]...to provide survival with-out impairment" (Hack & Fanaroff, 1999, p. 319). The importance of long-term follow-up is highlighted by recognition that adverse ef-fects of medications or treatment strategies are not limited to the targeted organ system and may not be detectable in the neonatal period.

The range of health and neurodevelopmental outcomes raises questions about possible undetected adverse effects of current obstetric and NICU medications and treatment strategies on the developing CNS of preterm infants.

SURVIVAL OF PRETERM INFANTS

Despite increases in preterm birth rates during the last few decades, advancements in obstetric and neonatal intensive care have dramatically reduced neonatal (within 28 days of birth) and infant (within 1 year of birth) mortality rates for infants of all GA and BW categories (Alexander, 2006; Alexander & Slay, 2002; Alexander, Thompkins, et al., 1999; Allen et al., 2000; Guyer, Freedman, Strobino, & Sondik, 2000; IOM, 2006; Martin, Kochanek, Strobino, Guyer, & MacDorman, 2005). Nonetheless, preterm infants account for the majority of infant deaths: in the United States in 2002, 64% of infant deaths occurred in the 12.1% of infants born before 37 weeks' gestation, and 53.7% of deaths occurred in the 2% of infants born before 32 weeks' gestation. Careful analysis reveals striking geographic, racial, and ethnic disparities in preterm birth rates and neonatal and infant mortality rates.

A rise in preterm births in the United States is attributed to increases in maternal age at delivery, multiple gestations, and indicated preterm births. Approximately half of twins and 90% of triplets are delivered preterm, and both advanced maternal age at delivery and assisted reproductive technologies have been implicated in the rising multiple birth rate (Gardner et al., 1995; Keith, Cervantes, Mazela, Oleszuk, & Papiernick, 1998; Kogan et al., 2002). Since GA- and BW-specific neonatal mortality rates and *fetal* mortality rates have decreased, the increase in preterm births may be partially due to an increased willingness of obstetricians to deliver infants preterm (Alexander, Tompkins, et al., 1999; Alexander, Kogan, Bader, Carlo, Allen, & Mor, 2003; Allen et al., 2000; Martin, Kochanek, et al., 2005; Martin et al., 2005). The most significant increase in preterm births has been in infants born at 32–36 weeks' gestation. The cesarean section rate has been increasing, especially for preterm twins. Concomitantly, late fetal deaths

(after 27 weeks' gestation) have decreased. Intensive prenatal care for multiple gestations, necessitated by increasing intrauterine growth restriction and fetal death rates as they approach term, increases the likelihood of preterm delivery (Kogan et al., 2000, 2002; Rydhstrom, 1990). This is sobering because mortality and morbidity rates remain higher for infants born just before term (33–36 weeks' gestation) than for full-term infants (Amiel-Tison, Allen, Lebrun, & Rogowski, 2002; Escobar et al., 2006; Huddy, Johnson, & Hope, 2001; Wang, Dorer, Fleming, & Catlin, 2004).

One reason for an increase in infant and neonatal mortality rates in the United States between 2001 and 2002 (from 6.8 to 7.0 and from 4.5 to 4.7 per 1,000 live births, respectively) was an increase in infants with BW below 750 g who were born alive and resuscitated (MacDorman, Martin, Mathews, Hoyert, & Ventura, 2005; Martin, Hamilton, et al., 2005). The fetal death rate during this time decreased, and there was no change in the *perinatal* mortality rate (6.9 per 1,000 live births and fetal deaths) between 2001 and 2002.

Infant mortality rates and preterm birth rates demonstrate considerable geographic variability, both within and between countries (Alexander, 2006; Alexander & Slay, 2002; IOM, 2006; Martin, Hamilton, et al., 2005; Martin, Kochanek, et al., 2005). Infant mortality rates vary from 4.3 to 11.3 per 1,000 live births among states, while preterm birth rates vary from 9.2 to 17.9 per 1,000 live births. These geographic variations have been attributed to major differences in methodology (e.g., how GA, live births, and fetal deaths are recorded), access to health care, and population differences.

Populations differ widely with respect to many biological, cultural, economic, social, and educational variables. Within the United States, racial and ethnic disparities have been well documented in BW distributions for GA, preterm birth rates, neonatal mortality, and GA-specific neonatal mortality (Alexander, 2006; Alexander & Slay, 2002; IOM, 2006; Martin, Hamilton, et al., 2005; Martin, Kochanek, et al., 2005). For lack of generally agreed upon definitions of race and ethnicity, these categories are socially defined (generally determined by the mother) and have social, economic, cultural, and educational dimensions. Population differences in socioeconomic status, maternal behaviors (including seeking prenatal care), stress, and infection rates do not fully explain observed racial and ethnic disparities. Within racial groups, geographic variations are observed in preterm birth rate. Although genetic differences have been invoked, the complex gene–environment interactions involved in fetal growth and development, preterm birth, and infant survival are poorly understood (Fiscella, 2005; IOM, 2006).

In preterm infants born in the United States, the greatest variation is between non-Hispanic whites and blacks (Alexander, 2006; Alexander, Kogan, Himes, Mor, & Goldenberg, 1999; Allen et al., 2000; Martin, Hamilton, et al., 2005; Martin, Kochanek, et al., 2005). Non-Hispanic blacks have the highest preterm birth rate, intrauterine growth restriction rate, low BW (below 2,500 g) rate, and very low BW (BW below 1,500 g) rate, as well as smaller BW for each GA category. The greatest increases in preterm birth rates have been in non-Hispanic white infants, however. Although they have the highest neonatal and infant mortality rates of all groups, *preterm* black infants have had a survival advantage over preterm white infants. This gap has been narrowing. The GA at which 50% of infants in South Carolina survived decreased from 26.8 to 24.5 weeks' gestation for whites and from 25.2 to 23.9 weeks' gestation for blacks (Allen et al., 2000).

While the upper limit of prematurity is defined as 36 weeks' gestation, the lower limit is determined by maturity of the infant's organs and the obstetric and neonatal intensive care provided. At the lower limit of viability, mortality and morbidity rates improve with an increase of only 1 or 2 weeks' gestation (Allen, 2002; Allen, Donohue, & Dusman, 1993; El Metwally, Vohr, & Tucker, 2000; Ho & Saigal, 2005; IOM, 2006; Wood, Marlow, Costeloe, Gibson, & Wilkinson, 2000). Survival has been reported in rare infants born at 21 and 22 weeks' gestation, 0%–55% of infants born at 23 weeks' gestation, and 9%–70% of infants born at 24 weeks' gestation. The majority of infants delivered with GA below 23 weeks' gestation or BW below 500 g are stillborn. Re-

ported survival rates that include data regarding stillbirths are as low as 0%–2% for infants born before 23 weeks' gestation, 0%–34% at 23 weeks' gestation, 9%–56% at 24 weeks' gestation, and 28%–79% at 25 weeks' gestation. Because infants born at the lower limit of viability do not survive without being resuscitated in the delivery room, geographic and temporal differences in survival at 21–26 weeks' gestation are in part related to a willingness to resuscitate these infants (Hakansson, Farooqi, Holmgren, Serenius, & Hogberg, 2004; Lorenz, Paneth, Jetton, den Ouden, & Tyson, 2001).

A number of concerns have been raised regarding the care of infants born at the limit of viability (Alexander, Petersen, & Allen, 2000; Allen et al., 1993; Hack & Fanaroff, 1999; Lorenz et al., 2001; Sanders, Donohue, Oberdorf, Rosenkrantz, & Allen, 1995; Vohr & Allen, 2005):

1. Does neonatal intensive care just prolong death for some infants?

2. Has a biological limit been reached in terms of the lowest GA at which an infant may survive?

3. Who should be involved in the medical decision making when outcome is so uncertain?

4. Should not our efforts be focused on preventing these preterm births?

5. If we continue our efforts to lower the limit of viability, should we not also be providing the health, educational, and societal support that survivors and their families need after hospital discharge?

Many believe that the focus needs to shift beyond providing neonatal intensive care to every infant born at the limit of viability toward providing support and resources for the long-term neurodevelopmental and health outcomes of the preterm infants that currently survive.

PRETERM OUTCOME STUDIES

Preterm outcome studies provide important information for parents of infants born preterm as well as feedback for the health care professionals who care for these high-risk infants. This feedback allows for modifications in neonatal intensive care to improve health and neurodevelopmental outcomes. Marked variations in health and neurodevelopmental outcomes reflect differences in etiologies and treatments of preterm birth, complications of prematurity, NICU management and treatments, and home environments (Allen, 2002; IOM, 2006; Vohr et al., 2004). Comparisons of outcomes of preterm infants from different NICUs and from one NICU over different time periods, with careful analysis of differences in population characteristics and obstetric/neonatal management strategies, can provide insight into factors or treatments that influence outcomes.

Judgment as to whether the results of a given study can be generalized to another preterm population requires careful assessment of details regarding study sample selection, study sample characteristics, obstetric and neonatal intensive care provided, rate and duration of follow-up, and how outcomes were assessed and reported (Allen, 2002; Aylward, 2002a, 2002b, 2005). Differences in referral patterns (inborns, outborns, and maternal transfers) and racial and ethnic group composition make generalizability and comparison of results difficult. Studies that include outcomes for all infants who meet study criteria who are born in a specific geographic region are preferred over studies of infants born at specific tertiary care centers. Preterm outcome studies generated from tertiary care centers are fraught with concerns regarding selection bias (i.e., what determines which babies or mothers are transferred to their center?). Survival data may be misleading if only infants who survive labor, delivery, and transition to extrauterine life are transported to tertiary care center NICUs. Studies that provide survival data limited to preterm infants admitted to a NICU are not useful for counseling parents anticipating a preterm delivery because many infants born at the limit of viability are stillborn or die in the delivery room.

Ideally, follow-up rates should be 100%. This is exceedingly difficult to achieve, and there is always concern about bias with respect to which children are brought back for follow-up (the ones doing well or the ones with major problems?). The length of follow-up is critical in determining the kind of problems the children experience. One to two years after birth may be enough to identify cerebral palsy or severe cognitive impairment, but it is too early to identify learning disability. The outcome measures used also determine what problems are reported. Not all studies perform intelligence, language, hearing, and visual assessments. There is considerable variability in intelligence tests chosen and in cutoffs used to report cognitive data. Some studies just determine and report the presence of a disability, with no detail as to severity or type of impairment (e.g., motor, cognitive). There are not well-accepted uniform definitions or criteria for many of the more subtle disorders of CNS function (e.g., language disorders, learning disability, attention deficit, executive dysfunction, and social and emotional problems).

Few studies provide a comparison group. Some studies present comparison data on full-term children, siblings, or classmates from similar home environments. The incidence of major disability is often compared with the general population, and performance on intelligence and language tests are compared with population norms. One study of 6-year-old children born before 26 weeks' gestation found that the rate of cognitive impairment increased from 21% to 41% when the definition of IQ score as 2 or more standard deviations below the norm for a sample of full-term control children was substituted for the test standardization population norm (Marlow, Wolke, Bracewell, & Samara, 2005). Most studies of school and behavior problems in preschool and school-age children born preterm generally provide full-term controls matched for demographic characteristics (e.g., socioeconomic status, gender).

The primary problem with preterm outcome studies is time lag: time required from the birth of the study sample to age at follow-up evaluation and then to study publication. Short-term follow-up studies only tell a small portion of the story in terms of neurodevelopmental outcomes, and how well early tests predict later cognitive abilities is controversial

(Doyle, 2001; Hack, Taylor, et al., 2005; Lefeb- vre, Mazurier, & Tessier, 2005; Ment et al., 2003). With appropriate testing of language, visual-motor abilities, visual-perceptual abili- ties, fine motor abilities, auditory and visual memory, sustained attention, vocabulary, ex- ecutive function, and academics, the full range of functioning can be evaluated in school-age children and adolescents. Several studies have begun to detail health, educational achieve- ment, and functional outcomes of young adults born preterm (Cooke, 2004; Hack et al., 2002, Saigal et al., 2006). Because high-risk obstetric and neonatal intensive care has changed sub- stantially, caution must be exercised when generalizing the outcomes of individuals born 10–20 years ago to infants born today.

NEURODEVELOPMENTAL DISABILITY

For preterm infants, advances in technology and obstetric and neonatal intensive care have yielded more dramatic improvements in sur- vival than in prevalence of neurodevelopmen- tal disabilities (Allen, 2002; IOM, 2006). As with survival, the prevalence of major neuro- developmental disability (e.g., disabling cere- bral palsy, cognitive scores below 2 standard deviations below the mean) or neurosensory impairment (e.g., disabling cerebral palsy, sig- nificant cognitive impairment, severe bilateral visual or hearing impairment) increases with decreasing GA and BW: 1% in full-term con- trols, 28% in infants born at 27–32 weeks' ges- tation, 13%–28% in infants with BW below 1,000 g, 27% in infants born with BW below 750 g, 45% in infants born before 27 weeks' gestation, 58% in infants born at 24 weeks' gestation, and 61% in infants born before 24 weeks' gestation (Hintz, Kendrick, Vohr, Poole, & Higgins, 2005; Saigal, Hoult, Streiner, Stoskopf, & Rosenbaum, 2000; Vohr, Wright, Poole, & McDonald, 2005; Wilson-Costello, Friedman, Minich, Fanaroff, & Hack, 2005). Studies of young adults find that 10% born with BW below 1,500 g and 27% with BW below 1,000 g had major neurodevelopmental disability (Hack et al., 2002; Saigal et al., 2006).

A small proportion of children born pre- term have multiple neurodevelopmental disa-

bilities. A study of kindergartners born before 28 weeks' gestation found that 5% had multi- ple neurodevelopmental disabilities (Msall, Buck, Rogers, & Catanzaro, 1992). In a study that surveyed parents and defined disability ac- cording to the Education for All Handicapped Children Act of 1975 (PL 94-142), the preva- lence of multiple disabilities varied with BW category: 2.5% with normal BW, 5% with BW 1,501–2,500 g, 12% with BW 1,001–1,500 g, and 14% with BW below 1,001 g (Klebanov, Brooks-Gunn, & McCormick, 1994).

The proportion of children born preterm who do not develop disability decreases with decreasing GA or BW category: as many as 56%–77% of survivors with BW below 1,000 g or BW below 750 g, but only 20% of survi- vors born before 26 weeks' gestation, develop *no* major neurodevelopmental disability or neurosensory impairment (Doyle & Anderson, 2005; Hack & Fanaroff, 1999; Hansen & Grei- sen, 2004; Hintz et al., 2005; Ho & Saigal, 2005; Marlow et al., 2005; Saigal, Szatmari, Rosen- baum, Campbell, & King, 1990; Wilson- Costello et al., 2005). For infants born at the limit of viability, reported "intact survival" (i.e., the number of survivors without major neurodevelopmental disability or neurosen- sory impairment divided by the number of live births) is 31%–56% of children born at 25 weeks' gestation, 13%–42% of children born at 24 weeks' gestation, 6%–35% of children born at 23 weeks' gestation, and 0%–0.7% of children born before 23 weeks' gestation (Doyle, 2001; Wood et al., 2000).

Cerebral Palsy

There is a wide range in prevalence rates of cerebral palsy for children born preterm in var- ious BW and GA categories, and this is due to methodological differences in addition to pop- ulation and management differences (Allen, 2002; Amiel-Tison et al., 2002; Bracewell & Marlow, 2002; Escobar, Littenberg, & Petitti, 1991; IOM, 2006). The greatest difficulty is in classifying the child with mild cerebral palsy, who may not walk until 1½–2½ years of age but has little functional motor impairment by school age. Many investigators focus more on disabling cerebral palsy, which seems to occur in 0.7%–1.6% of children with BW of 1,500–2,500 g, 5%–8% of children with BW below 1,500 g, and 10%–13% of children with BW below 1,000 g. Many longitudinal motor assessments show good stability in diagnosis of cerebral palsy over time (Hack et al., 2002; Marlow et al., 2005; Wood et al., 2000).

In a study of cerebral palsy in Sweden, Hagberg and colleagues noted a stepwise increase with decreasing GA category: 1.4 per 1,000 live births at term (i.e., at or after 37 weeks' gestation), 8 per 1,000 live births at 32–36 weeks' gestation, 54 per 1,000 live births at 28–31 weeks' gestation, and 80 per 1,000 live births before 28 weeks' gestation (Hagberg, Hagberg, Olow, & van Wendt, 1996). The prevalence of cerebral palsy is 10%–20% in children born before 26 weeks' gestation and as high as 46% in children with BW below 500 g (Marlow et al., 2005; Sauve, Robertson, Etches, Byrne, & Dayer-Zamora, 1998; Vohr et al., 2000). Any changes in prevalence of cerebral palsy over the years have been offset by much larger changes in survival of preterm infants (and therefore an increase in numbers of children with cerebral palsy born preterm) (Bhushan, Paneth, & Kiely, 1993; Bracewell & Marlow, 2002; Hagberg, Hagberg, Beckung, & Uvebrant, 2001; Hagberg et al., 1996; IOM, 2006; Stanley & Watson, 1992).

The most common type of cerebral palsy in children born preterm, spastic diplegia, has been attributed to the vulnerability of the periventricular white matter of the internal capsule to injury (Bracewell & Marlow, 2002; Dammann, Kuban, & Leviton, 2002; Hack, Wilson-Costello, et al., 2000; Hagberg et al., 1996; O'Shea, 2002). A complex interplay among a variety of factors has been implicated in the vulnerability of the preterm brain (this vulnerability is not limited to white matter). These factors include immature autoregulation of cerebral blood flow, poor regional blood flow as a result of hypotension or obstruction, hypoxia, vulnerability of supporting preoligodendrocytes, prominence of excitatory neurotransmitters (e.g., glutamate), toxicity from oxidative stress with free radicals, high levels of proinflammatory cytokines, and insufficient levels of naturally occurring developmentally regulated neuroprotective substances (e.g., cortisol, thyroxin).

Among children with cerebral palsy born preterm in Sweden, 66% had spastic diplegia, 22% had spastic hemiplegia, and 7% had spastic quadriplegia (Hagberg et al., 1996). The proportion of preterm children with cerebral palsy who had spastic diplegia increased with decreasing GA category (29% above 36 weeks, 58% at 32–35 weeks, 66% at 28–31 weeks, and 80% below 28 weeks). In contrast, the proportion of children with cerebral palsy with hemiplegia is highest at term and decreases with lower GA or BW (Stanley & Watson, 1992).

Degree of motor impairment varies widely in children with cerebral palsy who were born preterm, and associated deficits are common (Bracewell & Marlow, 2002; Hagberg et al., 1996; IOM, 2006). Associated deficits include cognitive impairments, learning disability, visual impairment, hydrocephalus, epilepsy, and sensorimotor integration problems. For children with mild cerebral palsy, these associated deficits often have a greater influence on function at school age and adolescence than does their motor impairment.

Cognitive Impairment

Children born preterm have a normal range of intelligence, but the data suggest that mean cognitive scores decrease with decreasing GA and BW categories (Aylward, 2002a, 2005; Aylward, Pfeiffer, Wright, & Verhulst, 1989; Bhutta, Cleves, Casey, Cradock, & Anand, 2002; IOM, 2006; Marlow et al., 2005; Ornstein, Ohlsson, Edmonds, & Asztalos, 1991). Mean differences in cognitive scores are reported to be 5–7 points for children born with BW below 2,500 g, 10.9 points for children born preterm, and 0.3–0.6 standard deviations for children with BW below 1,500 g or 1,000 g. Significant mean differences in cognitive scores remain even when children with severe neurological impairment are excluded from analysis. Studies suggest that children born before 26 weeks' gestation or with BW below 750 g have mean cognitive scores 1 or more standard deviations below the mean of full-term controls (Marlow et al., 2005; Taylor, Klein, Minich, & Hack, 2000).

The primary significance of these studies that show that children born preterm have lower mean cognitive scores than full-term controls is the higher prevalence of children born preterm who have intellectual disabilities (i.e., cognitive scores below 2 standard deviations below the general population mean) or borderline intelligence (i.e., cognitive scores 1–2 standard deviations below the general population mean). Children born at 32–36 weeks' gestation have a 1.4-fold increased risk of intellectual disabilities over children born full term, but this risk increases 7-fold for children born before 32 weeks' gestation (Stromme & Hagberg, 2000). Cognitive scores consistent with intellectual disabilities occurred in 10%–22% of children with BW below 1,000 g, 37% of children with BW below 750 g, 23%–30% of children born at 27–32 weeks' gestation, 21%–42% of children born before 26 weeks' gestation, 27%–44% of children born at 24 weeks' gestation, and 27%–52% of children born before 24 weeks' gestation (Aylward, 2002a, 2005; Bhutta et al., 2002; IOM, 2006; Ornstein et al., 1991). Borderline intelligence occurred in 16%–25% of children with BW below 1,000 g, 25%–34% of children born below 26 weeks' gestation, and 25%–40% of children born below 25 weeks' gestation. As many as 74% of children born with BW below 1,000 g had normal cognitive scores, but only 36%–54% of children born before 26 weeks' gestation and 28%–42% of children born before 25 weeks' gestation had normal cognitive scores.

Adolescents and young adults who were born preterm continue to demonstrate more cognitive impairments than those born full term, even when those with neurosensory impairments were excluded from analysis (Aylward, 2002a, 2005; Hack, 2006; IOM, 2006; Lefebvre et al., 2005; Saigal, 2000). In addition, children and adolescents born preterm demonstrate many more problems with specific cognitive processes than do full-term controls (Anderson & Doyle, 2003; Bhutta et al., 2002; Breslau, Chilcoat, DelDotto, Andreski, & Brown, 1996; Breslau et al., 1994; Caravale, Tozzi, Albino, & Vicari, 2005; Goyen, Lui, & Woods, 1998; Grunau, Whitfield, & Davis, 2002; Hack et al., 1994; Mikkola et al., 2005). These include tests of vocabulary, language, visual perception, visual-motor integration, memory, learning disability, sustained attention, and executive function.

Sensory Impairments

ROP is a neovascular retinal disorder that is a common complication of prematurity, especially in the most immature and sickest preterm infants. Early recognition of ROP is important, and guidelines for ophthalmologic screening of preterm infants have been revised ("Screening examination," 2006). Although it occurs in almost half of infants with BW below 1,000 g and most (90%) of infants with BW below 750 g, it generally resolves without significant visual loss, and only a small proportion (10%–20% with BW below 750 g or GA below 26 weeks) have severe ROP requiring laser surgery (IOM, 2006; Repka, 2002). Severe visual impairment occurs in 0.4% of children born at 27–32 weeks' gestation, 1%–3% of children born before 26–27 weeks' gestation or with BW below 1,000 g, 4% of children born at 24 weeks' gestation, and 8% of children born before 24 weeks' gestation. Although rare, late severe findings associated with severe ROP include cataracts, angle-closure glaucoma, and retinal detachments.

Myopia (nearsightedness) is a common visual sequela of preterm birth and ROP, and its prevalence increases with decreasing GA and BW categories (IOM, 2006; Repka, 2002). Myopia and other visual problems (e.g., hyperopia, astigmatism) require glasses in a significant proportion of children born preterm. In one study, 31% of adolescents with BW below 750 g required glasses, compared with 13% of children with BW 750–1,499 g and 11% of controls with normal BW (Hack, Taylor, Klein, & Mercuri-Minich, 2000). As many as 24% of 6-year-olds born before 26 weeks' gestation required glasses, whereas only 4% of full-term controls did (Marlow et al., 2005). Amblyopia and strabismus are also more frequent in children born preterm than in full-term controls.

Severe hearing impairment occurs in 2%–4% of children born before 25 or 26 weeks' gestation and in 1.5%–5% of children with BW below 1,000 g (Doyle & Anderson, 2005; Hansen & Greisen, 2004; Hintz et al., 2005; IOM, 2006; Marlow et al., 2005; Vohr et al., 2005). Although only 2% of full-term controls had hearing impairment (1% mild, 1% corrected with hearing aids), 4% of children born before 26 weeks' gestation had mild hearing impairment, 3% required hearing aids, and another 3% had profound sensorineural hearing impairment that could not be corrected (Marlow et al., 2005). All preterm children should have their hearing screened prior to hospital discharge, with follow-up hearing screens during the first few years if they had cytomegalovirus infection, frequent ear infections, or language delay.

Subtle Disorders of Central Nervous System Function

Before neonatal intensive care, a third of surviving children with BW below 1,500 g could not be educated in general education classrooms, and half of those with normal intelligence had school and behavior problems (Drillien, 1967; Lubchenco et al., 1963). By the 1970s, at least 95% of children with BW below 1,500 g attended general education classes (Drillien, Thomson, & Burgoyne, 1980; Kitchen et al., 1980). This dramatic improvement reflected, to some extent, changing attitudes and a movement toward including children with disabilities in general education classrooms.

More recent preterm outcome studies document school concerns for preterm children of all ages. In a study of kindergarten children born before 28 weeks' gestation, only half had the skills they needed, and many had difficulties with language, attention, or both (Msall et al., 1993). At 8–10 years, 13%–36% of preterm children with BW below 1,000 g repeated a grade, 15%–47% required some special education support, and 2%–16% were in special education classes (Anderson & Doyle, 2003; Buck, Msall, Schisterman, Lyon, & Rogers,

2000; Gross, Slagle, D'Eugenio, & Mettelman, 1992; Halsey, Collin, & Anderson, 1996; Klebanov et al., 1994; Saigal, Rosenbaum, Szatmari, & Campbell, 1991; Saigal et al., 2000; Whitfield, Grunau, & Holsti, 1997). A Dutch longitudinal study found that 9-year-olds born below 32 weeks' gestation or with BW below 1,500 g, compared with the general Dutch population, had significantly higher rates of requiring special education classes (19% vs. 1%), requiring special educational resources (38% vs. 6%), and functioning below grade level (32% vs. 14%) (Hille et al., 1994). By 14 years of age, 27% required special education services, compared with 7% of their peers (Walther, den Ouden, & Verloove-Vanhorick, 2000). In a region of Canada, significantly more 14-year-olds who were born between 1977 and 1982 with BW below 1,000 g received special education assistance and/or repeated a grade than did full-term controls (58% vs. 13%, odds ratio [OR] 9) (Saigal et al., 2000). Only 33%–50% of 8- to 10-year-olds with BW below 1,000 g were *in regular classes without grade failure or special education,* and this fell to 36% at 18 years of age (Klebanov et al., 1994; Lefebvre, Bard, Veilleux, & Martel, 1988; Lefebvre et al., 2005).

Even when children with neurosensory impairments are excluded from analysis, children born preterm have more difficulty with visual perception, visual-motor integration, visual-spatial skills, fine motor function, coordination, executive function, memory, language, attention, and behavior than do full-term controls (Aylward, 2002a, 2005; Bhutta et al., 2002; Grunau et al., 2002; IOM, 2006; Ornstein et al., 1991). School-age children with BW below 1,000 g who have normal intelligence have a 3- to 10-times increased risk of learning disabilities with respect to reading, writing, spelling, and/or arithmetic compared to full-term peers (Hall, McLeod, Counsell, Thomson, & Mutch, 1995; O'Callaghan et al., 1996; Saigal et al., 2000). Arithmetic and reading may be the most consistent learning disabilities associated with preterm birth, which Grunau et al. (2002) have suggested is due primarily to their difficulties with verbal intelligence, visual memory, and visual-motor integration abilities (Anderson & Doyle, 2003; Hack et al., 1994; Klebanov et al., 1994).

In preterm outcome studies, the lower the GA or BW category, the higher the risk of learning disabilities: 7%–18% in full-term controls; 30%–38% in children with BW 750–1,499 g; 50%–63% in children born with BW below 750 g, and 66% in children born before 28 weeks' gestation (Avchen, Scott, & Mason, 2001; Aylward, 2002a; Grunau et al., 2002; Hack et al., 1994; Halsey et al., 1996; Hille et al., 1994; Pinto-Martin et al., 2004; Taylor et al., 2000). Saigal et al. (2000) found that the proportion of children with test scores below 2 standard deviations below the mean increased with decreasing BW category (i.e., normal, BW 750–1,000 g, and BW below 750 g) for tests of arithmetic (5%, 32%, and 50%, respectively), reading (0, 12%, and 23%, respectively) and spelling (2%, 18%, and 38%, respectively). By parental report, even children born at 32–35 weeks' gestation have significant academic difficulties (29% with arithmetic, 21% with reading, 32% with writing, and 19% with speaking) (Huddy et al., 2001).

The proportion of children born preterm who have academic difficulties or require special education assistance increases with chronological age and grade (Aylward, 2002a; Dewey, Crawford, Creighton, & Sauve, 1999; Hille et al., 1994; O'Callaghan et al., 1996; Taylor et al., 2000; Walther et al., 2000). This may be due to an ability to compensate for mild cognitive deficits in the early grades, with failure of these compensatory mechanisms as the amount, complexity, and degree of difficulty of academic school work increases. It may be a matter of efficiency, with increasing difficulty keeping up when the demands on time and accuracy increase. Children who have subtle cognitive and executive function deficits can become increasingly frustrated, less likely to take advantage of learning opportunities, and less responsive to interventions and may lose their energy and motivation.

Children born preterm have an increased risk of mild motor impairment, called minor neuromotor dysfunction or developmental co-ordination disorder, which can affect their participation in preschool and playground activities, peer relationships, and self-esteem (Botting, Powls, Cooke, & Marlow, 1998; Hadders-Algra, 2002; Hall et al., 1995; Jongmans, Mercuri, de Vries, Dubowitz, & Henderson, 1997; Khadilkar, Tudehope, Burns, O'Callaghan, & Mohay, 1993; Mikkola et al., 2005; Pharoah, Stevenson, Cooke, & Stevenson, 1994a; Vohr & Garcia Coll, 1985; Weisglas-Kuperus et al., 1994; Whitfield et al., 1997). Common neuromotor abnormalities include asymmetries, generalized hypotonia, and tight heel cords. In a study of 5-year-olds with BW below 1,000 g, half (51%) had coordination problems, 18%–20% had abnormal reflexes or posture, and 17% had some problems with involuntary movements (Mikkola et al., 2005).

Fine motor dysfunction and visual-perceptual difficulties are common in children born preterm, especially in those born before 28 weeks' gestation (Aylward, 2002a; Bracewell & Marlow, 2002; Goyen et al., 1998). As many as 71% of 5-year-olds with BW below 1,500 g scored 1 or more standard deviations below the mean on tests of fine motor function, 17% had low scores on tests of visual-motor skills, and 11% had low scores on visual-perceptual tasks (Goyen et al., 1998). Children born before 28 weeks' gestation had the most difficulty with fine motor and visual-motor tasks. One third of parents of school-age children born at 32–36 weeks' gestation reported that their child had poor fine motor and writing skills (Huddy et al., 2001). Difficulty with fine motor, visual-motor, visual-perceptual, and visuospatial tasks can hamper efforts to write, copy figures, draw, dress, use scissors, tap one's fingers, and complete a pegboard. Children with neuromotor abnormalities and sensorimotor integration problems have difficulty tolerating certain foods (e.g., with lumps), clothes (e.g., tags on T-shirts), or movements (e.g., swinging), and may have great difficulty with following demonstrated directions (e.g., put on a jacket, tie their shoes).

The finding of neuromotor abnormalities on examinations during the first years of life increases the risk that a preterm infant will develop cognitive impairments, academic difficulties, and behavior problems (Bracewell & Marlow, 2002; Dammann et al., 1996; Drillien et al., 1980; Khadilkar et al., 1993; Marlow, Roberts, & Cooke, 1993; Stewart et al., 1989; Vohr & Garcia-Coll, 1985). These mild motor impairments may persist, and correlate with cognitive and academic difficulties (Botting et al., 1998; Dammann et al., 1996; Marlow et al., 1993; Powls, Botting, Cooke, & Marlow, 1995; Whitfield et al., 1997).

Symptoms of attention-deficit/hyperactivity disorder (ADHD) are more common in children and adolescents born preterm than children born at term. Children born preterm (with BW below 1,000 g, 1,500 g, or 2,000g) are 2–6 times more likely to have symptoms consistent with ADHD (Aylward, 2002a; Bhutta et al., 2002; Botting, Powls, Cooke, & Marlow, 1997; Breslau, 1995; Pharoah, Stevenson, Cooke, & Stevenson, 1994b; Szatmari, Saigal, Rosenbaum, Campbell, & King, 1990). Two thirds of 16 case–control studies of children born preterm compared with controls born at term found significantly more preterm children with attention deficit disorder, and 81% found significantly more behavior problems in children born preterm (Bhutta et al., 2002). Anderson and Doyle (2003) found that 8-year-olds born before 28 weeks' gestation or with BW below 1,000 g had significantly higher scores for hyperactivity and lower scores for freedom from distractibility, processing speed, and working memory than 8-year-olds with normal BW. Taylor et al. (2000) found a higher prevalence of difficulties with planning, problem solving, organizing, and abstracting in middle-school children with BW below 750 g than in children with higher BW (i.e., 750–1,500 g) or normal BW. These symptoms are suggestive of significant executive dysfunction, which can interfere with academic performance and behavior at school and at home.

Children with BW below 1,000 g or 1,500 g have more difficulties with social interactions, adaptability, leadership skills, and atypical behavior (Anderson & Doyle, 2003; Breslau, Klein, & Allen, 1988). More 14-year-olds with BW below 750 g went to a counselor, psychologist, or social worker than did 14-year-olds born at term (17% vs. 4%, $p < .05$) (Hack, Taylor, et al., 2000). Although conduct disorders are more common, children and adults born preterm are also more likely than controls born at term to be shy, withdrawn, and depressed and to lack social skills and assertiveness (Bhutta et al., 2002; Grunau, Whitfield, & Fay, 2004; Hack et al., 2002; Sommerfelt, Troland, Ellertsen, & Markestad, 1996). Adolescents who were born preterm (before 35 weeks' gestation or with BW below 800 or 1,500 g) vary as to whether they report more problems with self-esteem, self-confidence, or feeling themselves attractive than their peers (Cooke, 2004; Grunau et al., 2004; Tideman, Ley, Bjerre, & Forslund, 2001). School-age children born before 29 weeks' gestation are more likely to be bullied by their peers than are controls born at term, and this difference persists even when children with major disabilities are excluded from analysis (Nadeau, Tessier, Lefebvre, & Robaey, 2004).

FUNCTIONAL OUTCOMES

Although most preterm outcomes studies have described neurodevelopmental outcomes, a few have described how preterm survivors are able to function in their lives at home, at school, and in their communities. Many of these studies have been described in the previous section, but a few additional studies have added important data regarding functional outcomes.

Attainment of infant developmental milestones is one method of communicating how infants and toddlers function in their home environment. A study of developmental milestone data from the National Health and Nutrition Examination Survey found motor and social delays in children born preterm, even in those born at 33–36 weeks' gestation (Hediger, Overpeck, Ruan, & Troendle, 2002). When boys born preterm were compared with boys at term, developmental scores decreased by 0.1 point for each week of gestation. A study of toddlers with BW below 1,000 g who were 18 months from their due date revealed that 93% could sit, 83% could walk, and 86% could feed themselves (Vohr et al., 2000). At $2\frac{1}{2}$ years from term, 97% of children born before 26 weeks' gestation could sit, 90% could walk, 96% could feed themselves with their hands, and 6% could speak (Wood et al., 2000).

Of 149 children born before 28 weeks' gestation, 95% could walk, perform basic self-care skills, and stay continent during the day by kindergarten age (Msall et al., 1992). Even those with neurodevelopmental disabilities were relatively functional: 87% could walk one block, 84% talked in sentences, and 81% performed self-care tasks. At 6 years, most children born before 26 weeks' gestation had good function with respect to ambulation and hand use; only 6% could not walk and 6% walked independently with an abnormal gait (Marlow et al., 2005).

As expected, children born preterm who have neurodevelopmental disability have more functional limitations than those without disability. In a study of 5-year-olds with BW below 1,500 g, those with cerebral palsy had more functional limitations with respect to self-care (57% vs. 5%, respectively), mobility (89% vs. 21%, respectively), and social communication (32% vs. 8%, respectively) than those without cerebral palsy (Palta, Sadek-Badawi, Evans, Weinstein, & McGuinnes, 2000). In an ROP follow-up study, the proportion of 5-year-old children with severe functional limitations increased with increasing severity of ROP and visual impairment: 4% in those with no ROP, 11% in those with pre-threshold ROP, and 26% in those with severe ROP requiring laser surgery (Msall et al., 2000). As many as 77% of children with severe ROP and poor vision had severe limitations with self-care, 66% with social communication, 50% with continence, and 43% with mobility.

In a longitudinal study, only a few 14-year-olds with BW below 750 g had severe functional limitations, but the likelihood of functional limitations and need for special services was higher than for children with BW 750–1,499 g and children with normal BW (Hack, Taylor, et al., 2000). The OR for restrictions in activity was 5.1, with a confidence interval (CI) of 1.6–16.3. They had a greater need for special education (OR 5.0, CI 2.1–11.7), counseling (OR 4.8, CI 1.0–23.1), and special arrangements in school (OR 9.5, CI 2.1–43.6).

Although completing schooling and going on to higher education is sometimes more problematic, adolescents born preterm can make a successful transition to young adulthood. Several studies have documented that young adults born preterm (i.e., with BW below 1,000 or 1,500 g), when compared with controls born at term or with normal BW or both, continue to have more academic problems and a lower high school graduation rate (74% vs. 83%, respectively) or secondary school graduation rate (56% vs. 86%, respectively) and are older when they graduate from high school (18.2 vs. 17.9 years, respectively) (Bjerager, Steensberg, & Greisen, 1995; Ericson & Kallen, 1998; Hack, 2006; Hack et al., 2002; Lefebvre et al., 2005). One study found a significant difference in college attendance for men born preterm, but not for women (Hack et al., 2002). A more recent Canadian study found no differences between 23-year-olds born with BW below 1,000 g or with normal BW in completion of secondary school or going on to postsecondary or university education (Saigal et al., 2006).

Transition to adulthood for adolescents born preterm may be facilitated by their tendency to avoid risk-taking behaviors and by social supports provided by families and communities. Significantly decreased risk-taking behavior included fewer violations of the law and delinquent behaviors in men born preterm and fewer pregnancies and less experience with intercourse in women born preterm (Hack, 2006; Hack et al., 2002; Hack, Youngstrom, et al., 2005). Young adults born with BW below 1,500 g in Britain and the United States were less likely to drink alcohol or use illicit drugs than controls born at term (but there were no differences in smoking rates). Women with BW below 1,500 g were more likely than young women with normal BW to report anxiety or depression or both, withdrawn behaviors, fewer friends, and poorer family relationships. Once adults with disabilities were excluded, the Canadian study found no differences between 23-year-olds with BW below 1,000 g or normal BW as to whether they lived independently from their parents (42% vs. 53%), had children (11% vs. 14%), or were employed (48% vs. 57%) or married or cohabitating (23% vs. 25%) (Saigal et al., 2006). This cohort was from relatively advantaged homes and had access to universal health care.

HEALTH AND GROWTH

Infants born with BW below 1,500 g or 2,500 g have a 2- to 4-times increased risk of being rehospitalized during infancy, with a longer duration of hospital stay, than infants with normal BW (Cavalier, Escobar, Fernbach, Quesenberry, & Chellino, 1996; Escobar et al., 1999; Escobar et al., 2006; Martens, Derksen, & Gupta, 2004). Although all preterm infants are at increased risk for respiratory infections, especially with respiratory syncytial virus, those with CLD/BPD are at highest risk for respiratory illnesses and may require rehospitalization, intubation, and ventilation. Residual effects of CLD/BPD include an increased risk of asthma/reactive airways disease, exercise intolerance, persistent growth problems, and an increased vulnerability to secondhand smoke (Doyle, Ford, & Davis, 2003; Hack, Taylor, et al., 2000; Jacob et al., 1998).

Preterm birth can adversely influence health even into the school-age years and adolescence (Doyle, Ford, & Davis, 2003; Hack, Taylor, et al., 2000; McCormick, Brooks-Gunn, Workman-Daniels, Turner, & Peckham, 1992; Saigal, Stoskopf, Streiner, & Burrows, 2001). In addition to neurodevelopmental disabilities, adolescents born with BW below 1,000 g had more problems with vision (57% vs. 21%, respectively) and seizures (7% vs. 1%, respectively) than did controls born at term (Saigal et al., 2001). Adolescents born preterm with BW below 750 g are more likely than children with BW 750–1499 g to have chronic health conditions (41% vs. 30%), including constipation (22% vs. 2%) (Hack, Taylor, et al., 2000). Children born preterm often have poor growth compared to children born full term, but they can demonstrate "catch-up growth" into adolescence (Saigal et al., 2001). Longitudinal studies vary as to whether they find height or weight differences in young adults born with BW below 1,000 g or 1,500 g compared with controls with normal BW (Ericson & Kallen, 1998; Hack et al., 2002).

Concern about how preterm birth and neonatal intensive care influence adult health has been raised by a few studies that noted higher mean systolic blood pressures in adolescents with BW below 1,500 g compared with adolescents with normal BW (Doyle, Faber, Callanan, & Morley, 2003; Hack, Schluchter, Cartar, & Rahman, 2005). The "fetal origins of adult disease hypothesis" postulates that undernutrition during critical periods of development in utero (and perhaps infancy) has long-lasting metabolic and cardiovascular effects that increase vulnerability to high blood pressure, heart disease, stroke, and diabetes (Barker, Eriksson, Forsen, & Osmond, 2002; Huxley, Neil, & Collins, 2002). A few studies have documented metabolic differences (e.g., reduced insulin sensitivity, insulin and cholesterol levels) in children and young adults born preterm compared with those born full term (Hofman et al., 2004; Irving, Belton, Elton, & Walker, 2000). Far more research needs to be done to better understand these relationships.

PREDICTION OF NEURODEVELOPMENTAL DISABILITY

Preterm infants have a higher incidence of neurodevelopmental disability than the general population, but the majority are free of major disability. The wide variations in prevalence of neurodevelopmental disabilities results from variations in etiologies of preterm birth, intrauterine environments, maternal health, obstetric and neonatal management, complications of prematurity, and subsequent health and home environment. In a time of limited resources, it is helpful to focus comprehensive follow-up and early intervention services on infants with the highest risk for neurodevelopmental disability. Many preterm outcome studies have sought to identify those prenatal, perinatal, and neonatal factors that carry the highest risks of neurodevelopmental disability, especially cerebral palsy and cognitive impairments.

Demographic factors (e.g., socioeconomic status, parental education or occupations) have their strongest effects on cognition, behavior, and academic performance (Allen, 2002; Aylward, 2002a; Drillien et al., 1980; IOM, 2006; Ornstein et al., 1991). The effect of socioeconomic status on cognition is often not manifested until 2–2½ years. Poverty increases the likelihood of preterm delivery and has an adverse effect on outcomes for all children, not just those born preterm (Brooks-Gunn & Duncan, 1997; Hofman et al., 2004; Irving et al., 2000). It is no longer a question as to whether genes or environment determine who we are; they are continuously interacting and intertwined during development (Allen, 2005). Neuromaturation is a dynamic process that begins with patterns encoded in the genome and proceeds as scheduled with continual modification from the environment. Continuous gene–environment interactions determine neural network patterns, with reinforcement of circuits that are utilized and pruning of unused circuits. Demographic factors can be viewed as proxies for the enriched, child-oriented environment.

Many of the pathophysiological processes that lead to preterm delivery and its complications and subsequent treatments injure immature organ systems that are not ready for extrauterine life (IOM, 2006). Maternal chronic illness (e.g., hypertension, diabetes, heart disease), pregnancy-induced illness (e.g., preeclampsia), medications (e.g., phenytoin), and abused substances (e.g., narcotics, alcohol) can adversely influence fetal growth and development, and some can provide an indication for preterm delivery. Infection and inflammation have been implicated in the etiologies of preterm delivery, complications of prematurity (e.g., chronic lung disease, necrotizing enterocolitis, white matter injury), and neurodevelopmental disability (i.e., cerebral palsy and cognitive impairments) (Andrews, Hauth, & Goldenberg, 2000; Dammann & Leviton, 1999, 2000; Dammann, Leviton, Gappa, & Dammann, 2005; Dammann et al., 2001; Goldenberg, Culhane, & Johnson, 2005; Hagberg, Mallard, & Jacobsson, 2005; Hagberg, Wennerholm, & Savman, 2002; IOM, 2006). More research is needed to elucidate relationships among the maternal and fetal genomes and immune systems, factors that control inflamma-

tion, neuromaturation, development of fetal neurotransmitters, stress, and endogenous neuroprotective substances (e.g., cortisol, thyroxin).

Markers of severe neonatal illness (e.g., CLD/BPD, severe ROP, signs of severe brain injury) are good NICU predictors of neurodevelopmental outcome of preterm infants (Allen, 2002; Emsley, Wardle, Sims, Chiswick, & D'Souza, 1998; Hack, Wilson-Costello, et al., 2000; Hintz et al., 2005; Msall & Tremont, 2000; Msall et al., 2000; Schmidt et al., 2003; Vohr et al., 2005; Walsh et al., 2005). Inflammation and immaturity are implicated in the pathophysiology of each of these conditions. The adverse influence of CLD/BPD on cognitive impairment, cerebral palsy, and minor neuromotor dysfunction may be due to intermittent hypoxia, inflammation, treatments (e.g., ventilator strategies, oxygen supplementation, postnatal dexamethasone), and difficulty with nutrition and growth, or it may be because it is a marker of extreme immaturity (Halliday & Ehrenkranz, 2001b).

The strongest neonatal predictors of preterm neurodevelopmental outcome are the signs of severe brain injury on neuroimaging or clinical examination. On neuroimaging studies, severe (grade 3) IVH, posthemorrhagic hydrocephalus, intraparenchymal hemorrhage or infarction, porencephaly, and signs of white matter injury (e.g., periventricular leukomalacia; ventricular dilation, especially with irregular edges; large intraparenchymal cysts; punctuate white matter lesions) carry a significantly increased risk of neurodevelopmental disability, although most are not 100% predictive (de Vries & Groenendaal, 2002; Doyle, 2001; Hack, Wilson-Costello, et al., 2000; Ment et al., 2003; Pinto-Martin et al., 1995; Rogers et al., 1994). Cranial ultrasounds are routinely performed on preterm infants with BW below 1,500 g or who were acutely ill; however, research in the use of magnetic resonance imaging (MRI) with diffusion-weighted imaging, diffusion tensor imaging, or both and the use of nearinfrared spectroscopy and positron emission tomography may lead to future recommendations regarding clinical use in preterm infants (de Vries & Groenendaal, 2002; Huppi et al., 2001; Inder, Anderson, Spencer, Wells, & Volpe, 2003; Inder, Warfield, Wang, Huppi, & Volpe, 2005; Inder, Wells, Mogridge, Spencer, & Volpe, 2003; Murphy et al., 2001; Peterson et al., 2000, 2002). For example, if the significant reductions in gray and white matter volumes of the cortex (especially parietal and sensorimotor areas) and deep nuclear structures seen in some preterm infants at term correlate well with later neurodevelopmental outcomes, MRI scans with brain volume measurements may be recommended for preterm infants when they reach term (i.e., 40 weeks' postmenstrual age).

A comprehensive neurodevelopmental examination and careful observation of an infant's movements and responses can be used to evaluate brain function in the neonate, just as achievement of developmental milestones and careful neurodevelopmental examination are used to evaluate brain function in the older infant (see Chapter 18, this volume). A number of methods of assessing brain function in neonates and young infants help predict neurodevelopmental outcome, especially when used in conjunction with neuroimaging studies (Allen & Capute, 1989; Dubowitz, Bydder, & Mushin, 1985; Dubowitz, Ricciw, & Mercuri, 2005; Dubowitz et al., 1984; Einspieler & Prechtl, 2005; Gosselin, Gahagan, & Amiel-Tison, 2005; Mercuri, Ricci, Pane, & Baranello, 2005; Weisglas-Kuperus, Baerts, Fetter, & Sauer, 1992). Even if they do not develop cerebral palsy, preterm infants with neuromotor abnormalities during the first years after preterm birth are at increased risk for school and behavior problems (Bracewell & Marlow, 2002; Dammann et al., 1996; Drillien et al., 1980; Khadilkar et al., 1993; Marlow et al., 1993; Stewart et al., 1989; Vohr & Garcia-Coll, 1985).

Neuromaturation of the preterm infant in the NICU generally proceeds according to postmenstrual age, with only a few exceptions (e.g., mildly accelerated neuromaturation with intrauterine growth restriction or severe maternal illness) (Allen, 2005; Allen & Capute, 1986, 1990; Amiel-Tison, 2003; Amiel-Tison et al., 2004; Saint-Anne Dargassies, 1977). Despite some controversy over the years, most agree to fully correct for degree of prematurity for at least the first 2 years when evaluating the rate of a preterm infant's development (Allen, 2002, 2004; Aylward, 2002a, 2002b). Although it has less of an effect with age, correction for degree of prematurity can influence cognitive scores up to 8 years (Rickards, Kitchen, Doyle, & Kelly, 1989).

CONCLUSION

Progressive advances in obstetric and neonatal intensive care have led to marked improvement in survival for preterm infants and a lowering of the limit of viability to approximately 400–500 g BW and 22–23 weeks' gestation. Children born preterm demonstrate a wide range of health and neurodevelopmental outcomes. Although the incidence of major disability is higher than in the general population, the majority of children born preterm do not develop cerebral palsy or intellectual disabilities. Although infants born preterm may develop any type of cerebral palsy, more than half develop spastic diplegia, and it is frequently mild. Populations of children, adolescents, and young adults born preterm demonstrate a normal range of intelligence, but they tend to have lower mean cognitive scores and a greater incidence of intellectual disabilities or borderline intelligence than populations born at term. ROP is still a concern, but early recognition with appropriate treatment is effective in reducing visual impairment. Although cognitive, motor, hearing, and visual impairments are more common in the most immature and sickest preterm infants, all infants and children born preterm should have their development, vision, and hearing screened periodically during childhood.

Children and adolescents born preterm have an increased prevalence of minor neuromotor dysfunction/developmental coordination disorder, fine motor dysfunction, language disorder, visual-perceptual deficits, visuospatial difficulties, memory deficits, executive dysfunction, attention deficits, hyperactivity, specific learning disabilities, school failures, and behavior problems than do children and adolescents born full term. Although these problems are less severe than major disability, the cumulative effect can profoundly influence peer relationships, self-esteem, and ability to function at school and at home. Despite all this, the majority of adolescents with BW below 1,000 g or 1,500 g successfully make the transition to adulthood.

Many resources are required to provide the necessary medical, neurodevelopmental, and educational support for children born preterm and their families. Accurate and current data regarding health and neurodevelopmental outcomes are important for medical decision making and anticipating services needed following hospital discharge. Research on the relationships between brain structural and functional development, causes and mechanisms of brain injury, and how brain recovery and plasticity occur can develop better predictors of outcomes and can provide insight into treatment and prevention strategies that improve outcomes.

The most effective strategy for improving preterm outcomes would be to prevent prematurity. Preterm birth is not a single disorder but a complex cluster of problems with multiple overlapping factors that differ among populations. These include, but are not limited to, individual psychosocial and behavioral factors, neighborhood characteristics, environmental exposures, medical conditions, assisted reproductive technology, biological factors, and genetics. Multiple determinants across the life span need to be considered, including gene–environment interactions even before conception. No one magic bullet will prevent prematurity. Research that provides insight into the multiple interactions among the maternal and fetal genomes and conditions in the intrauterine environment, the mother's body, and her external environment may lead to more effective strategies for preventing delivery before the infant's organs are mature enough to support extrauterine life.

REFERENCES

Alexander, G.R. (2006). Prematurity at birth: Determinents, consequences and geographic variations. In Institute of Medicine Committee on Understanding Premature Birth and Assuring Healthy Outcomes (Ed.), *Preterm birth: Causes, consequences and prevention* (pp. 493–527). Washington, DC: National Academies Press.

Alexander, G.R., Kogan, M., Bader, D., Carlo, W., Allen, M., & Mor, J. (2003). U.S. birth weight-gestational age specific neonatal mortality: 1995–7 rates for Whites, Hispanics and African-Americans. *Pediatrics, 111*(1)e61–e66.

Alexander, G.R., Kogan, M.D., Himes, J.H., Mor, J.M., & Goldenberg, R. (1999). Racial differences in birthweight for gestational age and infant mortality in extremely-low-risk US populations. *Paediatric and Perinatal Epidemiology, 13,* 205–217.

Alexander, G.R., Petersen, D.J., & Allen, M.C. (2000). Life on the edge: Preterm births at the limit of viability—committed to their survival, are we equally committed to their prevention and long-term care? *Medicolegal OB/Gyn Newsletter, 8*(1), 18–21.

Alexander, G.R., & Slay, M. (2002). Prematurity at birth: Trends, racial disparities, and epidemiology. *Mental Retardation and Developmental Disabilities Research Reviews, 8,* 215–220.

Alexander, G.R., Tompkins, M.E., Allen, M.C., & Hulsey, T.C. (1999). Trends and racial differences in birth weight and related survival. *Maternal and Child Health Journal, 3,* 71–79.

Allen, M.C. (2002). Preterm outcomes research: A critical component of neonatal intensive care. *Mental Retardation and Developmental Disabilities Research Reviews, 8,* 221–233.

Allen, M.C. (2004). Risk assessment and neurodevelopmental outcomes. In Taeusch, H.W., Ballard, R., & Gleason, C.A. (Eds.), *Avery's diseases of the newborn* (8th ed.). Philadelphia: W.B. Saunders.

Allen, M.C. (2005). Assessment of gestational age and neuromaturation. *Mental Retardation and Developmental Disabilities Research Reviews, 11,* 21–33.

Allen, M.C., Alexander, G.R., Tompkins, M.E., & Hulsey, T.C. (2000). Racial differences in temporal changes in newborn viability and survival by gestational age. *Paediatric and Perinatal Epidemiology, 14,* 152–158.

Allen, M.C., & Capute, A.J. (1986). The evolution of primitive reflexes in extremely premature infants. *Pediatric Research, 20,* 1284–1289.

Allen, M.C., & Capute, A.J. (1989). Neonatal neurodevelopmental examination as a predictor of neuromotor outcome in premature infants. *Pediatrics, 83,* 498–506.

Allen, M.C., & Capute, A.J. (1990). Tone and reflex development before term. *Pediatrics, 85,* 393–399.

Allen, M.C., Donohue, P.K., & Dusman, A.E. (1993). The limit of viability—neonatal outcome of infants born at 22 to 25 weeks' gestation. *New England Journal of Medicine, 329,* 1597–1601.

Allen, M.C., & Jones, M.D., Jr. (1986). Medical complications of prematurity. *Obstetrics and Gynecology, 67,* 427–437.

Amiel-Tison, C. (2003). Neurologic maturation of the neonate. *NeoReviews, 4,* e199–e206.

Amiel-Tison, C., Allen, M.C., Lebrun, F., & Rogowski, J. (2002). Macropremies: Underprivileged newborns. *Mental Retardation and Developmental Disabilities Research Reviews, 8,* 281–292.

Amiel-Tison, C., Cabrol, D., Denver, R., Jarreau, P.H., Papicrnik, E., & Piazza, P.V. (2004). Fetal adaptation to stress. Part I: Acceleration of fetal maturation and earlier birth triggered by placental insufficiency in humans. *Early Human Development, 78,* 15–27.

Anderson, P., & Doyle, L.W. (2003). Neurobehavioral outcomes of school-age children born extremely low birth weight or very preterm in the 1990s. *JAMA, 289,* 3264–3272.

Andrews, W.W., Hauth, J.C., & Goldenberg, R.L. (2000). Infection and preterm birth. *American Journal of Perinatology, 17,* 357–365.

Askie, L.M., & Henderson-Smart, D.J. (2001). Restricted versus liberal oxygen exposure for preventing morbidity and mortality in preterm or low birth weight infants. *Cochrane Database of Systematic Reviews,* (4), CD001077.

Aucott, S., Donohue, P.K., Atkins, E., & Allen, M.C. (2002). Neurodevelopmental care in the NICU. *Mental Retardation and Developmental Disabilities Research Reviews, 8,* 298–308.

Avchen, R.N., Scott, K.G., & Mason, C.A. (2001). Birth weight and school-age disabilities: A population-based study. *American Journal of Epidemiology, 154,* 895–901.

Aylward, G.P. (2002a). Cognitive and neuropsychological outcomes: More than IQ scores. *Mental Retardation and Developmental Disabilities Research Reviews, 8,* 234–240.

Aylward, G.P. (2002b). Methodological issues in outcome studies of at-risk infants. *Journal of Pediatric Psychology, 27,* 37–45.

Aylward, G.P. (2005). Neurodevelopmental outcomes of infants born prematurely. *Journal of Developmental and Behavioral Pediatrics, 26,* 427–440.

Aylward, G.P., Pfeiffer, S.I., Wright, A., & Verhulst, S.J. (1989). Outcome studies of low birth weight infants published in the last decade: A metaanalysis. *Journal of Pediatrics, 115,* 515–520.

Baker, J.P. (2000). The incubator and the medical discovery of the premature infant. *Journal of Perinatology, 20,* 321–328.

Barker, D.J., Eriksson, J.G., Forsen, T., & Osmond, C. (2002). Fetal origins of adult disease: Strength of effects and biological basis. *International Journal of Epidemiology, 31,* 1235–1239.

Barrington, K., & Finer, N. (2006). Inhaled nitric oxide for respiratory failure in preterm infants. *Cochrane Database of Systematic Reviews,* (1), CD000509.

Battaglia, F.C., & Lubchenco, L.O. (1967). A practical classification of newborn infants by weight and gestational age. *Journal of Pediatrics, 71,* 159–163.

Bhushan, V., Paneth, N., & Kiely, J.L. (1993). Impact of improved survival of very low birth weight infants on recent secular trends in the prevalence of cerebral palsy. *Pediatrics, 91,* 1094–1100.

Bhutta, A.T., Cleves, M.A., Casey, P.H., Cradock, M.M., & Anand, K.J. (2002). Cognitive and behavioral outcomes of school-aged children who were born preterm: A meta-analysis. *JAMA, 288,* 728–737.

Bjerager, M., Steensberg, J., & Greisen, G. (1995). Quality of life among young adults born with very low birthweights. *Acta Paediatrica, 84,* 1339–1343.

Botting, N., Powls, A., Cooke, R.W., & Marlow, N. (1997). Attention deficit hyperactivity disorders and other psychiatric outcomes in very low birthweight children at 12 years. *Journal of Child Psychology and Psychiatry, 38,* 931–941.

Botting, N., Powls, A., Cooke, R.W., & Marlow, N. (1998). Cognitive and educational outcome of very-low-birthweight children in early adolescence. *Developmental Medicine and Child Neurology, 40,* 652–660.

Bracewell, M., & Marlow, N. (2002). Patterns of motor disability in very preterm children. *Mental Retardation and Developmental Disabilities Research Reviews, 8,* 241–248.

Breslau, N. (1995). Psychiatric sequelae of low birth weight. *Epidemiologic Reviews, 17,* 96–106.

Breslau, N., Chilcoat, H., DelDotto, J., Andreski, P., & Brown, G. (1996). Low birth weight and neurocognitive status at six years of age. *Biological Psychiatry, 40,* 389–397.

Breslau, N., DelDotto, J.E., Brown, G.G., Kumar, S., Ezhuthachan, S., Hufnagle, K.G., et al. (1994). A gradient relationship between low birth weight and IQ at age 6 years. *Archives of Pediatrics and Adolescent Medicine, 148,* 377–383.

Breslau, N., Klein, N., & Allen, L. (1988). Very low birthweight: Behavioral sequelae at nine years of age. *Journal of the American Academy of Child and Adolescent Psychiatry, 27,* 605–612.

Brion, L.P., Bell, E.F., & Raghuveer, T.S. (2003). Vitamin E supplementation for prevention of morbidity and mortality in preterm infants. *Cochrane Database of Systematic Reviews,* (4), CD003665.

Brion, L.P., & Soll, R.F. (2001). Diuretics for respiratory distress syndrome in preterm infants. *Cochrane Database of Systematic Reviews,* (2), CD001454.

Brooks-Gunn, J., & Duncan, G.J. (1997). The effects of poverty on children. *Future of Children, 7,* 55–71.

Buck, G.M., Msall, M.E., Schisterman, E.F., Lyon, N.R., & Rogers, B.T. (2000). Extreme prematurity and school outcomes. *Paediatric and Perinatal Epidemiology, 14,* 324–331.

Budin, P. (1907). *The nursling.* London: Caxton.

Caravale, B., Tozzi, C., Albino, G., & Vicari, S. (2005). Cognitive development in low risk preterm infants at 3–4 years of life. *Archives of Disease in Childhood: Fetal and Neonatal Edition, 90,* F474–F479.

Cavalier, S., Escobar, G.J., Fernbach, S.A., Quesenberry, C.P., Jr., & Chellino, M. (1996). Postdischarge utilization of medical services by high-risk infants: Experience in a large managed care organization. *Pediatrics, 97,* 693–699.

Clerihew, L., & McGuire, W. (2004). Systemic antifungal drugs for invasive fungal infection in preterm infants. *Cochrane Database of Systematic Reviews,* (4), CD003953.

Cooke, R.W. (2004). Health, lifestyle, and quality of life for young adults born very preterm. *Archives of Disease in Childhood, 89,* 201–206.

Crowley, P. (2000). Prophylactic corticosteroids for preterm birth. *Cochrane Database of Systematic Reviews,* (1), CD000065.

Crowther, C.A., & Harding, J. (2003). Repeat doses of prenatal corticosteroids for women at risk of preterm birth for preventing neonatal respiratory disease. *Cochrane Database of Systematic Reviews,* (2), CD003935.

Crowther, C.A., & Henderson-Smart, D.J. (2001). Vitamin K prior to preterm birth for preventing neonatal periventricular haemorrhage. *Cochrane Database of Systematic Reviews,* (1), CD000229.

Crowther, C.A., & Henderson-Smart, D.J. (2003). Phenobarbital prior to preterm birth for preventing neonatal periventricular haemorrhage. *Cochrane Database of Systematic Reviews,* (3), CD000164.

Crowther, C.A., Hiller, J.E., & Doyle, L.W. (2002). Magnesium sulphate for preventing preterm birth in threatened preterm labour. *Cochrane Database of Systematic Reviews,* (4), CD001060.

Crowther, C.A., Hiller, J.E., Doyle, L.W., & Haslam, R.R. (2003). Effect of magnesium sulfate given for neuroprotection before preterm birth: A randomized controlled trial. *JAMA, 290,* 2669–2676.

Dammann, O., Kuban, K.C.K., & Leviton, A. (2002). Perinatal infection, fetal inflammatory response, white matter damage, and cognitive limitations in children. *Mental Retardation and Developmental Disabilities Research Reviews, 8,* 46–50.

Dammann, O., & Leviton, A. (1999). Brain damage in preterm newborns: Might enhancement of developmentally regulated endogenous protection open a door for prevention? *Pediatrics, 104,* 541–550.

Dammann, O., & Leviton, A. (2000). Brain damage in preterm newborns: Biological response modification as a strategy to reduce disabilities. *Journal of Pediatrics, 136,* 433–438.

Dammann, O., Leviton, A., Gappa, M., & Dammann, C.E. (2005). Lung and brain damage in preterm newborns, and their association with gestational age, prematurity subgroup, infection/inflammation and long term outcome. *BJOG, 112*(Suppl. 1), 4–9.

Dammann, O., Phillips, T.M., Allred, E.N., O'Shea, T.M., Paneth, N., Van Marter, L.J., et al. (2001). Mediators of fetal inflammation in extremely low gestational age newborns. *Cytokine, 13,* 234–239.

Dammann, O., Walther, H., Allers, B., Schroder, M., Drescher, J., Lutz, D., et al. (1996). Development of a regional cohort of very-low-birthweight children at six years: Cognitive abilities are associated

with neurological disability and social background. *Developmental Medicine and Child Neurology, 38,* 97–106.

de Vries, L.S., & Groenendaal, F. (2002). Neuroimaging in the preterm infant. *Mental Retardation and Developmental Disabilities Research Reviews, 8,* 273–280.

Dewey, D.G., Crawford, S.G., Creighton, D.E., & Sauve, R.S. (1999). Long-term neuropsychological outcomes in very low birth weight children free of sensorineural impairments. *Journal of Clinical and Experimental Neuropsychology, 21,* 851–865.

Doyle, L.W. (2001). Outcome at 5 years of age of children 23 to 27 weeks' gestation: Refining the prognosis. *Pediatrics, 108,* 134–141.

Doyle, L.W., & Anderson, P.J. (2005). Improved neurosensory outcome at 8 years of age of extremely low birthweight children born in Victoria over three distinct eras. *Archives of Disease in Childhood: Fetal and Neonatal Edition, 90,* F484–F488.

Doyle, L.W., Faber, B., Callanan, C., & Morley, R. (2003). Blood pressure in late adolescence and very low birth weight. *Pediatrics, 111,* 252–257.

Doyle, L.W., Ford, G., & Davis, N. (2003). Health and hospitalisations after discharge in extremely low birth weight infants. *Seminars in Neonatology, 8,* 137–145.

Drillien, C.M. (1961). The incidence of mental and physical handicaps in school-age children of very low birth weight. *Pediatrics, 27,* 452–464.

Drillien, C.M. (1967). The incidence of mental and physical handicaps in school age children of very low birth weight. II. *Pediatrics, 39,* 238–247.

Drillien, C.M., Thomson, A.J., & Burgoyne, K. (1980). Low-birthweight children at early school-age: A longitudinal study. *Developmental Medicine and Child Neurology, 22,* 26–47.

Dubowitz, L., Ricciw, D., & Mercuri, E. (2005). The Dubowitz neurological examination of the full-term newborn. *Mental Retardation and Developmental Disabilities Research Reviews, 11,* 52–60.

Dubowitz, L.M., Bydder, G.M., & Mushin, J. (1985). Developmental sequence of periventricular leukomalacia: Correlation of ultrasound, clinical, and nuclear magnetic resonance functions. *Archives of Disease in Childhood, 60,* 349–355.

Dubowitz, L.M., Dubowitz, V., Palmer, P.G., Miller, G., Fawer, C.L., & Levene, M.I. (1984). Correlation of neurologic assessment in the preterm newborn infant with outcome at 1 year. *Journal of Pediatrics, 105,* 452–456.

Education for All Handicapped Children Act of 1975, PL 94-142, 20 U.S.C. §§ 1400 *et seq.*

Einspieler, C., & Prechtl, H.F. (2005). Prechtl's Assessment of General Movements: A diagnostic tool for the functional assessment of the young nervous system. *Mental Retardation and Developmental Disabilities Research Reviews, 11,* 61–67.

El Metwally, D., Vohr, B., & Tucker, R. (2000). Survival and neonatal morbidity at the limits of viability in the mid 1990s: 22 to 25 weeks. *Journal of Pediatrics, 137,* 616–622.

Emsley, H.C., Wardle, S.P., Sims, D.G., Chiswick, M.L., & D'Souza, S.W. (1998). Increased survival and deteriorating developmental outcome in 23 to 25 week old gestation infants, 1990–4 compared with 1984–9. *Archives of Disease in Childhood: Fetal and Neonatal Edition, 78,* F99–F104.

Ericson, A., & Kallen, B. (1998). Very low birthweight boys at the age of 19. *Archives of Disease in Childhood: Fetal and Neonatal Edition, 78,* F171–F174.

Escobar, G.J., Joffe, S., Gardner, M.N., Armstrong, M.A., Folck, B.F., & Carpenter, D.M. (1999). Rehospitalization in the first two weeks after discharge from the neonatal intensive care unit. *Pediatrics, 104,* e2.

Escobar, G.J., Littenberg, B., & Petitti, D.B. (1991). Outcome among surviving very low birthweight infants: A meta-analysis. *Archives of Disease in Childhood, 66,* 204–211.

Escobar, G.J., McCormick, M.C., Zupancic, J.A., Coleman-Phox, K., Armstrong, M.A., Greene, J.D., et al. (2006). Unstudied infants: Outcomes of moderately premature infants in the neonatal intensive care unit. *Archives of Diseases in Childhood: Fetal and Neonatal Edition, 91,* F238–F244.

Finer, N.N., Higgins, R., Kattwinkel, J., & Martin, R.J. (2006). Summary proceedings from the Apnea-of-Prematurity Group. *Pediatrics, 117,* S47–S51.

Fiscella, K. (2005). Race, genes and preterm delivery. *Journal of the National Medical Association, 97,* 1516–1526.

Fowlie, P.W., & Davis, P.G. (2002). Prophylactic intravenous indomethacin for preventing mortality and morbidity in preterm infants (Cochrane Review). *Cochrane Database of Systematic Reviews, (3),* CD000174.

Francis-Williams, J., & Davies, P.A. (1974). Very low birthweight and later intelligence. *Developmental Medicine and Child Neurology, 16,* 709–728.

Gardner, M.O., Goldenberg, R.L., Cliver, S.P., Tucker, J.M., Nelson, K.G., & Copper, R.L. (1995). The origin and outcome of preterm twin pregnancies. *Obstetrics and Gynecology, 85,* 553–557.

Gesell, A.L., & Amatruda, C.S. (1945). *The embryology of behavior.* New York: Harper & Brothers.

Goldenberg, R.L., Culhane, J.F., & Johnson, D.C. (2005). Maternal infection and adverse fetal and neonatal outcomes. *Clinics in Perinatology, 32,* 523–559.

Gosselin, J., Gahagan, S., & Amiel-Tison, C. (2005). The Amiel-Tison Neurological Assessment at Term: Conceptual and methodological continuity in the course of follow-up. *Mental Retardation and Developmental Disabilities Research Reviews, 11,* 34–51.

Goyen, T.A., Lui, K., & Woods, R. (1998). Visual-motor, visual-perceptual, and fine motor outcomes in very-low-birthweight children at 5 years.

Developmental Medicine and Child Neurology, 40, 76–81.

Green, N.S., Damus, K., Simpson, J.L., Iams, J., Reece, E.A., Hobel, C.J., et al. (2005). Research agenda for preterm birth: Recommendations from the March of Dimes. *American Journal of Obstetrics and Gynecology, 193,* 626–635.

Gross, S.J., Slagle, T.A., D'Eugenio, D.B., & Mettelman, B.B. (1992). Impact of a matched term control group on interpretation of developmental performance in preterm infants. *Pediatrics, 90,* 681–687.

Grunau, R.E., Whitfield, M.F., & Davis, C. (2002). Pattern of learning disabilities in children with extremely low birth weight and broadly average intelligence. *Archives of Pediatrics and Adolescent Medicine, 156,* 615–620.

Grunau, R.E., Whitfield, M.F., & Fay, T.B. (2004). Psychosocial and academic characteristics of extremely low birth weight (< or = 800 g) adolescents who are free of major impairment compared with term-born control subjects. *Pediatrics, 114,* e725–e732.

Guyer, B., Freedman, M.A., Strobino, D.M., & Sondik, E.J. (2000). Annual summary of vital statistics: Trends in the health of Americans during the 20th century. *Pediatrics, 106,* 1307–1317.

Hack, M. (2006). Young adult outcomes of very-low-birth-weight children. *Seminars in Fetal and Neonatal Medicine, 11,* 127–137.

Hack, M., & Fanaroff, A.A. (1999). Outcomes of children of extremely low birthweight and gestational age in the 1990's. *Early Human Development, 53,* 193–218.

Hack, M., Fanaroff, A.A., & Merkatz, I.R. (1979). Current concepts: The low-birth-weight infant—evolution of a changing outlook. *New England Journal of Medicine, 301,* 1162–1165.

Hack, M., Flannery, D.J., Schluchter, M., Cartar, L., Borawski, E., & Klein, N. (2002). Outcomes in young adulthood for very-low-birth-weight infants. *New England Journal of Medicine, 346,* 149–157.

Hack, M., Schluchter, M., Cartar, L., & Rahman, M. (2005). Blood pressure among very low birth weight (<1.5 kg) young adults. *Pediatric Research, 58,* 677–684.

Hack, M., Taylor, H.G., Drotar, D., Schluchter, M., Cartar, L., Wilson-Costello, D., et al. (2005). Poor predictive validity of the Bayley Scales of Infant Development for cognitive function of extremely low birth weight children at school age. *Pediatrics, 116,* 333–341.

Hack, M., Taylor, H.G., Klein, N., Eiben, R., Schatschneider, C., & Mercuri-Minich, N. (1994). School-age outcomes in children with birth weights under 750 g [see comments]. *New England Journal of Medicine, 331,* 753–759.

Hack, M., Taylor, H.G., Klein, N., & Mercuri-Minich, N. (2000). Functional limitations and special health care needs of 10- to 14-year-old children weighing less than 750 grams at birth. *Pediatrics, 106,* 554–560.

Hack, M., Wilson-Costello, D., Friedman, H., Taylor, G.H., Schluchter, M., & Fanaroff, A.A. (2000). Neurodevelopment and predictors of outcomes of children with birth weights of less than 1000 g: 1992–1995. *Archives of Pediatrics and Adolescent Medicine, 154,* 725–731.

Hack, M., Youngstrom, E.A., Cartar, L., Schluchter, M., Taylor, G.H., Flannery, D.J., et al. (2005). Predictors of internalizing symptoms among very low birth weight young women. *Journal of Developmental and Behavioral Pediatrics, 26,* 93–104.

Hadders-Algra, M. (2002). Two distinct forms of minor neurological dysfunction: Perspectives emerging from a review of data of the Groningen Perinatal Project. *Developmental Medicine and Child Neurology, 44,* 561–571.

Hagberg, B., Hagberg, G., Beckung, E., & Uvebrant, P. (2001). Changing panorama of cerebral palsy in Sweden. VIII. Prevalence and origin in the birth year period 1991–94. *Acta Paediatrica, 90,* 271–277.

Hagberg, B., Hagberg, G., Olow, I., & van Wendt, L. (1996). The changing panorama of cerebral palsy in Sweden. VII. Prevalence and origin in the birth year period 1987–90. *Acta Paediatrica, 85,* 954–960.

Hagberg, H., Mallard, C., & Jacobsson, B. (2005). Role of cytokines in preterm labour and brain injury. *BJOG, 112*(Suppl. 1), 16–18.

Hagberg, H., Wennerholm, U.B., & Savman, K. (2002). Sequelae of chorioamnionitis. *Current Opinion in Infectious Diseases, 15,* 301–306.

Hakansson, S., Farooqi, A., Holmgren, P.A., Serenius, F., & Hogberg, U. (2004). Proactive management promotes outcome in extremely preterm infants: A population-based comparison of two perinatal management strategies. *Pediatrics, 114,* 58–64.

Hall, A., McLeod, A., Counsell, C., Thomson, L., & Mutch, L. (1995). School attainment, cognitive ability and motor function in a total Scottish very-low-birthweight population at eight years: A controlled study. *Developmental Medicine and Child Neurology, 37,* 1037–1050.

Halliday, H.L. (2001). Postnatal steroids: A dilemma for the neonatologist. *Acta Paediatrica, 90,* 116–118.

Halliday, H.L. & Ehrenkranz, R.A. (2001a). Delayed (>3 weeks) postnatal corticosteroids for chronic lung disease in preterm infants. *Cochrane Database of Systematic Reviews,* (1), CD001145.

Halliday, H.L., & Ehrenkranz, R.A. (2001b). Moderately early (7–14 days) postnatal corticosteroids for preventing chronic lung disease in preterm infants. *Cochrane Database of Systematic Reviews,* (1), CD001144.

Halliday, H.L., Ehrenkranz, R.A., & Doyle, L.W. (2004). Early postnatal (<96 hours) corticosteroids for preventing chronic lung disease in pre-

term infants (Cochrane Review). *Cochrane Database of Systematic Reviews,* (1), CD001146.

Halsey, C.L., Collin, M.F., & Anderson, C.L. (1996). Extremely low-birth-weight children and their peers: A comparison of school-age outcomes. *Archives of Pediatrics and Adolescent Medicine, 150,* 790–794.

Hansen, B.M., & Greisen, G. (2004). Is improved survival of very-low-birthweight infants in the 1980s and 1990s associated with increasing intellectual deficit in surviving children? *Developmental Medicine and Child Neurology, 46,* 812–815.

Hediger, M.L., Overpeck, M.D., Ruan, W.J., & Troendle, J.F. (2002). Birthweight and gestational age effects on motor and social development. *Paediatric and Perinatal Epidemiology, 16,* 33–46.

Henderson-Smart, D.J., Bhuta, T., Cools, F., & Offringa, M. (2003). Elective high frequency oscillatory ventilation versus conventional ventilation for acute pulmonary dysfunction in preterm infants. *Cochrane Database of Systematic Reviews,* (4), CD000104.

Henderson-Smart, D.J., & Davis, P.G. (2000). Prophylactic methylxanthines for extubation in preterm infants. *Cochrane Database of Systematic Reviews,* (1), CD000139.

Hess J.H. (1953). Experiences gained in a thirty year study of prematurely born infants. *Pediatrics, 11,* 425–434.

Hille, E.T., den Ouden, A.L., Bauer, L., van den Oudenrijn, C., Brand, R., & Verloove-Vanhorick, S.P. (1994). School performance at nine years of age in very premature and very low birth weight infants: Perinatal risk factors and predictors at five years of age. Collaborative Project on Preterm and Small for Gestational Age (POPS) Infants in the Netherlands. *Journal of Pediatrics, 125,* 426–434.

Hintz, S.R., Kendrick, D.E., Vohr, B.R., Poole, W.K., & Higgins, R.D. (2005). Changes in neurodevelopmental outcomes at 18 to 22 months' corrected age among infants of less than 25 weeks' gestational age born in 1993–1999. *Pediatrics, 115,* 1645–1651.

Ho, S., & Saigal, S. (2005). Current survival and early outcomes of infants of borderline viability. *NeoReviews, 6,* e123–e132.

Hofman, P.L., Regan, F., Jackson, W.E., Jefferies, C., Knight, D.B., Robinson, E.M., et al. (2004). Premature birth and later insulin resistance. *New England Journal of Medicine, 351,* 2179–2186.

Huddy, C.L., Johnson, A., & Hope, P.L. (2001). Educational and behavioural problems in babies of 32–35 weeks gestation. *Archives of Disease in Childhood: Fetal and Neonatal Edition, 85,* F23–F28.

Huppi, P.S., Murphy, B., Maier, S.E., Zientara, G.P., Inder, T.E., Barnes, P.D., et al. (2001). Microstructural brain development after perinatal cerebral white matter injury assessed by diffusion tensor magnetic resonance imaging. *Pediatrics, 107,* 455–460.

Huxley, R., Neil, A., & Collins, R. (2002). Unravelling the fetal origins hypothesis: Is there really an inverse association between birthweight and subsequent blood pressure? *Lancet, 360,* 659–665.

Inder, T.E., Anderson, N.J., Spencer, C., Wells, S., & Volpe, J.J. (2003). White matter injury in the premature infant: A comparison between serial cranial sonographic and MR findings at term. *American Journal of Neuroradiology, 24,* 805–809.

Inder, T.E., Warfield, S.K., Wang, H., Huppi, P.S., & Volpe, J.J. (2005). Abnormal cerebral structure is present at term in premature infants. *Pediatrics, 115,* 286–294.

Inder, T.E., Wells, S.J., Mogridge, N.B., Spencer, C., & Volpe, J.J. (2003). Defining the nature of the cerebral abnormalities in the premature infant: A qualitative magnetic resonance imaging study. *Journal of Pediatrics, 143,* 171–179.

Institute of Medicine, Committee on Understanding Premature Birth and Assuring Healthy Outcomes. (2006). *Preterm birth: Causes, consequences and prevention.* Washington, D.C.: National Academies Press.

An international classification of retinopathy of prematurity. The Committee for the Classification of Retinopathy of Prematurity (1984). *Archives of Ophthalmology, 102,* 1130–1134.

Irving, R.J., Belton, N.R., Elton, R.A., & Walker, B.R. (2000). Adult cardiovascular risk factors in premature babies. *Lancet, 355,* 2135–2136.

Jacob, S.V., Coates, A.L., Lands, L.C., MacNeish, C.F., Riley, S.P., Hornby, L., et al. (1998). Long-term pulmonary sequelae of severe bronchopulmonary dysplasia. *Journal of Pediatrics, 133,* 193–200.

Jones, R.A., Cummins, M., & Davies, P.A. (1979). Infants of very low birthweight: A 15-year analysis. *Lancet, 1,* 1332–1335.

Jongmans, M., Mercuri, E., de Vries, L., Dubowitz, L., & Henderson, S.E. (1997). Minor neurological signs and perceptual-motor difficulties in prematurely born children. *Archives of Disease in Childhood: Fetal and Neonatal Edition, 76,* F9–F14.

Keith, L.G., Cervantes, A., Mazela, J., Olesazuk, J.J., & Papiernick, E. (1998). Multiple births and preterm delivery. *Prenatal and Neonatal Medicine, 3,* 129.

Khadilkar, V., Tudehope, D., Burns, Y., O'Callaghan, M., & Mohay, H. (1993). The long-term neurodevelopmental outcome for very low birthweight (VLBW) infants with 'dystonic' signs at 4 months of age. *Journal of Paediatrics and Child Health, 29,* 415–417.

Kitchen, W.H., Ryan, M.M., Rickards, A., McDougall, A.B., Billson, F.A., Keir, E.H., et al. (1980). A longitudinal study of very low-birthweight infants. IV: An overview of performance at eight years of age. *Developmental Medicine and Child Neurology, 22,* 172–188.

Klebanov, P.K., Brooks-Gunn, J., & McCormick, M.C. (1994). School achievement and failure in very low birth weight children. *Journal of Developmental and Behavioral Pediatrics, 15,* 248–256.

Kogan, M.D., Alexander, G.R., Kotelchuck, M., MacDorman, M.F., Buekens, P., Martin, J.A., et al. (2000). Trends in twin birth outcomes and prenatal care utilization in the United States, 1981–1997. *JAMA, 284,* 335–341.

Kogan, M.D., Alexander, G.R., Kotelchuck, M., MacDorman, M.F., Buekens, P., & Papiernik, E. (2002). A comparison of risk factors for twin preterm birth in the United States between 1981–82 and 1996–97. *Maternal and Child Health Journal, 6,* 29–35.

Lawn, C.J., Weir, F.J., & McGuire, W. (2005). Base administration or fluid bolus for preventing morbidity and mortality in preterm infants with metabolic acidosis. *Cochrane Database of Systematic Reviews,* (2), CD003215.

Lefebvre, F., Bard, H., Veilleux, A., & Martel, C. (1988). Outcome at school age of children with birthweights of 1000 grams or less. *Developmental Medicine and Child Neurology, 30,* 170–180.

Lefebvre, F., Mazurier, E., & Tessier, R. (2005). Cognitive and educational outcomes in early adulthood for infants weighing 1000 grams or less at birth. *Acta Paediatrica, 94,* 733–740.

Liebling, A.F. (1939). A patron of the preemies. *The New Yorker, 15,* 20–24.

Lorenz, J.M., Paneth, N., Jetton, J.R., den Ouden, L., & Tyson, J.E. (2001). Comparison of management strategies for extreme prematurity in New Jersey and the Netherlands: Outcomes and resource expenditure. *Pediatrics, 108,* 1269–1274.

Lubchenco, L. O., Delivoria-Papadopoulos, M., & Searls, D. (1972). Long-term follow-up studies of prematurely born infants. II. Influence of birth weight and gestational age on sequelae. *Journal of Pediatrics, 80,* 509–512.

Lubchenco, L.O., Horner, F.A., Reed, L.H., Hix, I.E., Jr., Metcalf, D., Cohig, R., et al. (1963). Sequelae of premature birth: Evaluation of premature infants of low birth weights at ten years of age. *American Journal of Diseases of Children, 106,* 101–115.

Lubchenco, L.O., Searls, D.T., & Brazie, J.V. (1972). Neonatal mortality rate: Relationship to birth weight and gestational age. *Journal of Pediatrics, 81,* 814–822.

MacDorman, M.F., Martin, J.A., Mathews, T.J., Hoyert, D.L., & Ventura, S.J. (2005). Explaining the 2001–2002 infant mortality increase in the United States: Data from the linked birth/infant death data set. *International Journal of Health Services, 35,* 415–442.

Marlow, N., Roberts, L., & Cooke, R. (1993). Outcome at 8 years for children with birth weights of 1250 g or less. *Archives of Disease in Childhood, 68,* 286–290.

Marlow, N., Wolke, D., Bracewell, M.A., & Samara, M. (2005). Neurologic and developmental disability at six years of age after extremely preterm birth. *New England Journal of Medicine, 352,* 9–19.

Martens, P.J., Derksen, S., & Gupta, S. (2004). Predictors of hospital readmission of Manitoba newborns within six weeks postbirth discharge: A population-based study. *Pediatrics, 114,* 708–713.

Martin, J.A., Hamilton, B.E., Sutton, P.D., Ventura, S.J., Menacker, F., & Munson, M.L. (2005). Births: Final data for 2003. *National Vital Statistics Reports, 54,* 1–116.

Martin, J.A., Kochanek, K.D., Strobino, D.M., Guyer, B., & MacDorman, M.F. (2005). Annual summary of vital statistics—2003. *Pediatrics, 115,* 619–634.

McCormick, M.C., Brooks-Gunn, J., Workman-Daniels, K., Turner, J., & Peckham, G.J. (1992). The health and developmental status of very low-birth-weight children at school age. *JAMA, 267,* 2204–2208.

Ment, L.R., Vohr, B., Allan, W., Katz, K.H., Schneider, K.C., Westerveld, M., et al. (2003). Change in cognitive function over time in very low-birth-weight infants. *JAMA, 289,* 705–711.

Ment, L.R., Vohr, B., Allan, W., Westerveld, M., Sparrow, S.S., Schneider, K.C., et al. (2000). Outcome of children in the indomethacin intraventricular hemorrhage prevention trial. *Pediatrics, 105,* 485–491.

Ment, L.R., Vohr, B.R., Makuch, R.W., Westerveld, M., Katz, K.H., Schneider, K.C., et al. (2004). Prevention of intraventricular hemorrhage by indomethacin in male preterm infants. *Journal of Pediatrics, 145,* 832–834.

Mercuri, E., Ricci, D., Pane, M., & Baranello, G. (2005). The neurological examination of the newborn baby. *Early Human Development, 81,* 947–956.

Mikkola, K., Ritari, N., Tommiska, V., Salokorpi, T., Lehtonen, L., Tammela, O., et al. (2005). Neurodevelopmental outcome at 5 years of age of a national cohort of extremely low birth weight infants who were born in 1996–1997. *Pediatrics, 116,* 1391–1400.

Msall, M.E., Buck, G.M., Rogers, B.T., & Catanzaro, N.L. (1992). Kindergarten readiness after extreme prematurity. *American Journal of Diseases of Children, 146,* 1371–1375.

Msall, M.E., Phelps, D.L., DiGaudio, K.M., Dobson, V., Tung, B., McClead, R.E., et al. (2000). Severity of neonatal retinopathy of prematurity is predictive of neurodevelopmental functional outcome at age 5.5 years. Behalf of the Cryotherapy for Retinopathy of Prematurity Cooperative Group. *Pediatrics, 106,* 998–1005.

Msall, M.E., Rogers, B.T., Buck, G.M., Mallen, S., Catanzaro, N.L., & Duffy, L.C. (1993). Functional status of extremely preterm infants at kindergarten entry [see comments]. *Developmental Medicine and Child Neurology, 35,* 312–320.

Msall, M.E., & Tremont, M.R. (2000). Functional outcomes in self-care, mobility, communication, and learning in extremely low-birth weight infants. *Clinics in Perinatology, 27,* 381–401.

Murphy, B.P., Inder, T.E., Huppi, P.S., Warfield, S., Zientara, G.P., Kikinis, R., et al. (2001). Impaired cerebral cortical gray matter growth after treatment with dexamethasone for neonatal chronic lung disease. *Pediatrics, 107,* 217–221.

Nadeau, L., Tessier, R., Lefebvre, F., & Robaey, P. (2004). Victimization: A newly recognized outcome of prematurity. *Developmental Medicine and Child Neurology, 46,* 508–513.

National Institute of Child Health and Human Development. (1994). Report of the Consensus Development Conference on the Effect of Corticosteroids for Fetal Maturation on Perinatal Outcomes (NIH Publication No. 95-3784). Bethesda, MD: National Institute of Child Health and Human Development.

Nelson, N.M. (2000). A decimillennium in neonatology. *Journal of Pediatrics, 137,* 731–735.

O'Callaghan, M.J., Burns, Y.R., Gray, P.H., Harvey, J.M., Mohay, H., Rogers, Y.M., et al. (1996). School performance of ELBW children: A controlled study. *Developmental Medicine and Child Neurology, 38,* 917–926.

Ornstein, M., Ohlsson, A., Edmonds, J., & Asztalos, E. (1991). Neonatal follow-up of very low birthweight/extremely low birthweight infants to school age: A critical overview. *Acta Paediatrica Scandinavica, 80,* 741–748.

Osborn, D.A. (2001). Thyroid hormones for preventing neurodevelopmental impairment in preterm infants. *Cochrane Database of Systematic Reviews,* (4), CD001070.

O'Shea, T.M. (2002). Cerebral palsy in very preterm infants: New epidemiological insights. *Mental Retardation and Developmental Disabilities Research Reviews, 8,* 135–145.

Palta, M., Sadek-Badawi, M., Evans, M., Weinstein, M.R., & McGuinnes, G. (2000). Functional assessment of a multicenter very low-birth-weight cohort at age 5 years. Newborn Lung Project. *Archives of Pediatrics and Adolescent Medicine, 154,* 23–30.

Peterson, B.S., Vohr, B., Kane, M.J., Whalen, D.H., Schneider, K.C., Katz, K.H., et al. (2002). A functional magnetic resonance imaging study of language processing and its cognitive correlates in prematurely born children. *Pediatrics, 110,* 1153–1162.

Peterson, B.S., Vohr, B., Staib, L.H., Cannistraci, C.J., Dolberg, A., Schneider, K.C., et al. (2000). Regional brain volume abnormalities and long-term cognitive outcome in preterm infants. *JAMA, 284,* 1939–1947.

Pharoah, P.O., Stevenson, C.J., Cooke, R.W., & Stevenson, R.C. (1994a). Clinical and subclinical deficits at 8 years in a geographically defined cohort of low birthweight infants. *Archives of Disease in Childhood, 70,* 264–270.

Pharoah, P.O., Stevenson, C.J., Cooke, R.W., & Stevenson, R.C. (1994b). Prevalence of behaviour disorders in low birthweight infants [see comments]. *Archives of Disease in Childhood, 70,* 271–274.

Pinto-Martin, J., Whitaker, A., Feldman, J., Cnaan, A., Zhao, H., Bloch, J.R., et al. (2004). Special education services and school performance in a regional cohort of low-birthweight infants at age nine. *Paediatric and Perinatal Epidemiology, 18,* 120–129.

Pinto-Martin, J.A., Riolo, S., Cnaan, A., Holzman, C., Susser, M.W., & Paneth, N. (1995). Cranial ultrasound prediction of disabling and nondisabling cerebral palsy at age two in a low birth weight population. *Pediatrics, 95,* 249–254.

Postnatal corticosteroids to treat or prevent chronic lung disease in preterm infants. (2002). *Pediatrics, 109,* 330–338.

Powls, A., Botting, N., Cooke, R.W., & Marlow, N. (1995). Motor impairment in children 12 to 13 years old with a birthweight of less than 1250 g. *Archives of Disease in Childhood: Fetal and Neonatal Edition, 73,* F62–F66.

Repka, M.X. (2002). Ophthalmological problems of the preterm infant. *Mental Retardation and Developmental Disabilities Research Reviews, 8,* 249–257.

Rickards, A.L., Kitchen, W.H., Doyle, L.W., & Kelly, E.A. (1989). Correction of developmental and intelligence test scores for premature birth. *Australian Paediatrics Journal, 25,* 127–129.

Rogers, B., Msall, M., Owens, T., Guernsey, K., Brody, A., Buck, G., et al. (1994). Cystic periventricular leukomalacia and type of cerebral palsy in preterm infants. *Journal of Pediatrics, 125,* S1–S8.

Rydhstrom, H. (1990). Prognosis for twins with birth weight less than 1500 gm: The impact of cesarean section in relation to fetal presentation. *American Journal of Obstetrics and Gynecology, 163,* 528–533.

Saigal, S. (2000). Follow-up of very low birthweight babies to adolescence. *Seminars in Neonatology, 5,* 107–118.

Saigal, S., Hoult, L.A., Streiner, D.L., Stoskopf, B.L., & Rosenbaum, P.L. (2000). School difficulties at adolescence in a regional cohort of children who were extremely low birth weight. *Pediatrics, 105,* 325–331.

Saigal, S., Rosenbaum, P., Stoskopf, B., & Sinclair, J.C. (1984). Outcome in infants 501 to 1000 gm birth weight delivered to residents of the McMaster Health Region. *Journal of Pediatrics, 105,* 969–976.

Saigal, S., Rosenbaum, P., Szatmari, P., & Campbell, D. (1991). Learning disabilities and school problems in a regional cohort of extremely low birth weight (less than 1000 g) children: A comparison with term controls. *Journal of Developmental and Behavioral Pediatrics, 12,* 294–300.

Saigal, S., Stoskopf, B., Streiner, D., Boyle, M., Pinelli, J., Paneth, N., et al. (2006). Transition of extremely low-birth-weight infants from adolescence to young adulthood: Comparison with normal birth-weight controls. *JAMA, 295,* 667–675.

Saigal, S., Stoskopf, B.L., Streiner, D.L., & Burrows, E. (2001). Physical growth and current health status of infants who were of extremely low birth weight and controls at adolescence. *Pediatrics, 108,* 407–415.

Saigal, S., Szatmari, P., Rosenbaum, P., Campbell, D., & King, S. (1990). Intellectual and functional status at school entry of children who weighed 1000 grams or less at birth: A regional perspective of births in the 1980s. *Journal of Pediatrics, 116,* 409–416.

Saint-Anne Dargassies, S. (1977). *Neurological development of the full-term and premature neonate.* Amsterdam: Elsevier/North-Holland Biomedical Press.

Sanders, M.R., Donohue, P.K., Oberdorf, M.A., Rosenkrantz, T.S., & Allen, M.C. (1995). Perceptions of the limit of viability: Neonatologists' attitudes toward extremely preterm infants [see comments]. *Journal of Perinatology, 15,* 494–502.

Saugstad, O.D. (2006). Oxygen and retinopathy of prematurity. *Journal of Perinatology, 26*(Suppl. 1), S46–S50.

Sauve, R.S., Robertson, C., Etches, P., Byrne, P.J., & Dayer-Zamora, V. (1998). Before viability: A geographically based outcome study of infants weighing 500 grams or less at birth. *Pediatrics, 101,* 438–445.

Schmidt, B., Asztalos, E.V., Roberts, R.S., Robertson, C.M., Sauve, R.S., & Whitfield, M.F. (2003). Impact of bronchopulmonary dysplasia, brain injury, and severe retinopathy on the outcome of extremely low-birth-weight infants at 18 months: Results from the trial of indomethacin prophylaxis in preterms. *JAMA, 289,* 1124–1129.

Schmidt, B., Davis, P., Moddemann, D., Ohlsson, A., Roberts, R.S., Saigal, S., et al. (2001). Long-term effects of indomethacin prophylaxis in extremely-low-birth-weight infants. *New England Journal of Medicine, 344,* 1966–1972.

Screening examination of premature infants for retinopathy of prematurity. (2006). *Pediatrics, 117,* 572–576.

Shalev, B., Farr, A.K., & Repka, M.X. (2001). Randomized comparison of diode laser photocoagulation versus cryotherapy for threshold retinopathy of prematurity: Seven-year outcome. *American Journal of Ophthalmology, 132,* 76–80.

Silverman, W.A. (1979). Incubator-baby side shows (Dr. Martin A. Couney). *Pediatrics, 64,* 127–141.

Silverman, W.A. (1980). *Retrolental fibroplasia: A modern parable.* Monographs in Neonatology. New York: Grune & Stratton.

Slattery, M.M., & Morrison, J.J. (2002). Preterm delivery. *Lancet, 360,* 1489–1497.

Sola, A., Wen, T.C., Hamrick, S.E., & Ferriero, D.M. (2005). Potential for protection and repair following injury to the developing brain: A role for erythropoietin? *Pediatric Research, 57,* 110R–117R.

Soll, R.F. (2000). Prophylactic synthetic surfactant for preventing morbidity and mortality in preterm infants. *Cochrane Database of Systematic Reviews,* (2), CD001079.

Sommerfelt, K., Troland, K., Ellertsen, B., & Markestad, T. (1996). Behavioral problems in low-birthweight preschoolers. *Developmental Medicine and Child Neurology, 38,* 927–940.

Stanley, F.J., & Watson, L. (1992). Trends in perinatal mortality and cerebral palsy in Western Australia, 1967 to 1985. *BMJ, 304,* 1658–1663.

Stewart, A.L., Costello, A.M., Hamilton, P.A., Baudin, J., Townsend, J., Bradford, B.C., et al. (1989). Relationship between neurodevelopmental status of very preterm infants at one and four years. *Developmental Medicine and Child Neurology, 31,* 756–765.

Stromme, P., & Hagberg, G. (2000). Aetiology in severe and mild mental retardation: A population-based study of Norwegian children. *Developmental Medicine and Child Neurology, 42,* 76–86.

Symington, A., & Pinelli, J. (2006). Developmental care for promoting development and preventing morbidity in preterm infants. *Cochrane Database of Systematic Reviews,* (2), CD001814.

Szatmari, P., Saigal, S., Rosenbaum, P., Campbell, D., & King, S. (1990). Psychiatric disorders at five years among children with birthweights less than 1000g: A regional perspective. *Developmental Medicine and Child Neurology, 32,* 954–962.

Taylor, H.G., Klein, N., Minich, N.M., & Hack, M. (2000). Middle-school-age outcomes in children with very low birthweight. *Child Development, 71,* 1495–1511.

Tideman, E., Ley, D., Bjerre, I., & Forslund, M. (2001). Longitudinal follow-up of children born preterm: Somatic and mental health, self-esteem and quality of life at age 19. *Early Human Development, 61,* 97–110.

Van Marter, L.J. (2005). Strategies for preventing bronchopulmonary dysplasia. *Current Opinion in Pediatrics, 17,* 174–180.

Vohr, B.R., & Allen, M. (2005). Extreme prematurity—the continuing dilemma. *New England Journal of Medicine, 352,* 71–72.

Vohr, B.R., & Garcia Coll, C.T. (1985). Neurodevelopmental and school performance of very low-birth-weight infants: A seven-year longitudinal study. *Pediatrics, 76,* 345–350.

Vohr, B.R., Wright, L.L., Dusick, A.M., Mele, L., Verter, J., Steichen, J.J., et al. (2000). Neurodevelopmental and functional outcomes of extremely low birth weight infants in the National Institute of Child Health and Human Development Neonatal Research Network, 1993–1994. *Pediatrics, 105,* 1216–1226.

Vohr, B.R., Wright, L.L., Dusick, A.M., Perritt, R., Poole, W.K., Tyson, J.E., et al. (2004). Center differences and outcomes of extremely low birth weight infants. *Pediatrics, 113,* 781–789.

Vohr, B.R., Wright, L.L., Poole, W.K., & McDonald, S.A. (2005). Neurodevelopmental outcomes of extremely low birth weight infants <32 weeks' gestation between 1993 and 1998. *Pediatrics, 116,* 635–643.

Walsh, M.C., Morris, B.H., Wrage, L.A., Vohr, B.R., Poole, W.K., Tyson, J.E., et al. (2005). Extremely low birthweight neonates with protracted ventilation: Mortality and 18-month neurodevelopmental outcomes. *Journal of Pediatrics, 146,* 798–804.

Walsh, M.C., Szefler, S., Davis, J., Allen, M., Van Marter, L., Abman, S., et al. (2006). Summary proceedings from the Bronchopulmonary Dysplasia Group. *Pediatrics, 117,* S52–S56.

Walther, F.J., den Ouden, A.L., & Verloove-Vanhorick, S.P. (2000). Looking back in time: Outcome of a national cohort of very preterm infants born in the Netherlands in 1983. *Early Human Development, 59,* 175–191.

Wang, M.L., Dorer, D.J., Fleming, M.P., & Catlin, E.A. (2004). Clinical outcomes of near-term infants. *Pediatrics, 114,* 372–376.

Watterberg, K.L., Gerdes, J.S., Cole, C.H., Aucott, S.W., Thilo, E.H., Mammel, M.C., et al. (2004). Prophylaxis of early adrenal insufficiency to prevent bronchopulmonary dysplasia: A multicenter trial. *Pediatrics, 114,* 1649–1657.

Watterberg, K.L., Gerdes, J.S., & Cook, K.L. (2001). Impaired glucocorticoid synthesis in premature infants developing chronic lung disease. *Pediatric Research, 50,* 190–195.

Weisglas-Kuperus, N., Baerts, W., Fetter, W.P., Hempel, M.S., Mulder, P.G., Touwen, B.C., et al. (1994). Minor neurological dysfunction and quality of movement in relation to neonatal cerebral damage and subsequent development. *Developmental Medicine and Child Neurology, 36,* 727–735.

Weisglas-Kuperus, N., Baerts, W., Fetter, W.P., & Sauer, P.J. (1992). Neonatal cerebral ultrasound, neonatal neurology and perinatal conditions as predictors of neurodevelopmental outcome in very low birthweight infants. *Early Human Development, 31,* 131–148.

Whitelaw, A. (2001a). Intraventricular streptokinase after intraventricular hemorrhage in newborn infants. *Cochrane Database of Systematic Reviews,* (4), CD000498.

Whitelaw, A. (2001b). Postnatal phenobarbitone for the prevention of intraventricular hemorrhage in preterm infants. *Cochrane Database of Systematic Reviews,* (4), CD001691.

Whitelaw, A., Kennedy, C.R., & Brion, L.P. (2001). Diuretic therapy for newborn infants with posthemorrhagic ventricular dilatation. *Cochrane Database of Systematic Reviews,* (2), CD002270.

Whitfield, M.F., Grunau, R.V., & Holsti, L. (1997). Extremely premature (< or = 800 g) schoolchildren: Multiple areas of hidden disability. *Archives of Disease in Childhood: Fetal and Neonatal Edition, 77,* F85–F90.

Wilson-Costello, D., Friedman, H., Minich, N., Fanaroff, A.A., & Hack, M. (2005). Improved survival rates with increased neurodevelopmental disability for extremely low birth weight infants in the 1990s. *Pediatrics, 115,* 997–1003.

Wood, N.S., Marlow, N., Costeloe, K., Gibson, A.T., & Wilkinson, A.R. (2000). Neurologic and developmental disability after extremely preterm birth. EPICure Study Group. *New England Journal of Medicine, 343,* 378–384.

10

Congenital Infections

NANCY J. ROIZEN AND DANIEL C. JOHNSON

Congenital infections are an important cause of developmental disabilities, especially mental retardation, hearing loss, and vision loss. Congenital infections, which are frequently asymptomatic at birth, become more difficult to diagnose after the neonatal period. An alert clinician can increase the chances of making the diagnosis by considering epidemiological factors and clinical manifestations. In addition to the classic list of congenital infections, human immunodeficiency virus (HIV) and varicella should be added. A mnemonic that includes these two new additions is TV CHaiRS (*t*oxoplasmosis, *v*aricella, *cy*tomegalovirus, *h*erpes simplex, HIV [*a*cquired *i*mmunodeficiency syndrome], *r*ubella, and *s*yphilis). Recognizing the pattern of illness created by each of the infecting agents will help to ensure that evaluating someone for a "TV CHaiRS" infection does not become a spin of the dial but represents selective observation. Some comparisons are presented in Table 10.1. The epidemiology, clinical manifestations, diagnosis, treatment, and prognosis of all of these diseases except HIV are discussed in this chapter.

CONGENITAL CYTOMEGALOVIRUS INFECTION

Epidemiology

The incidence of congenital cytomegalovirus (CMV) infection ranges from 0.2% to 2.4% of all live births (Stagno, 2004), making it the most common congenital infection. In pregnant women, high-income groups compared with low-income groups are more seronegative (64.5% vs. 23.4%), have fewer primary infections (1.6% vs. 3.7%) and have fewer fetuses with congenital infections, but they have a higher percentage of primary infections (63% vs. 25%) (Stagno et al., 1986). Women who are young, unmarried, and of lower income are almost 4 times more likely to deliver a CMV-infected newborn than those who do not have all three of these factors (Fowler & Pass, 1991). In primary infections, the rate of intrauterine transmission increases from 36% in the first trimester to 77.6% in the third trimester (Bodeus, Hubinont, & Goubau, 1999). In contrast, congenital infection from seropositive mothers ranges from 0.2% to 1.5% (Stagno & Whitley, 1985).

Clinical Manifestations

Ten percent of newborns with congenital CMV infection present with symptoms. The systemic symptoms that are most frequent are petechiae (76%), jaundice (67%), hepatosplenomegaly (60%), and neurological findings, including microcephaly (53%), lethargy/hypotonia (27%), poor suck (19%), and seizures (7%). Thirty-four percent are premature, and 50% are small for gestational age (Boppana, Pass, Britt, Stagno, & Alford, 1992). Sequelae in children with symptomatic congenital CMV infection include the following: sensorineural hearing loss (58%), microcephaly (38%), seizures (23%), moderate to severe visual impairment (22%), paralysis (13%), and death (6%) (Coats et al., 2000; Pass, Fowler, & Boppana, 1991).

Ninety percent of newborns with congenital CMV infection are asymptomatic. In a study of 28 children who were asymptomatic at birth, at 1 year of age, 6% of the children had

Table 10.1. Congenital infections

	Cytomegalovirus	Herpes simplex	Rubella	Syphilis	Toxoplasma	Varicella
Percentage of babies infected	0.2–2.2	0.01–0.04	?	0.005	0.004–0.04	0.005
Percentage symptomatic	< 10	100	50	33–66	10	50
Transmission rate from primary infection (%)	24	50	?	50	40	24
Findings						
Intellectual disabilities (%)	4/70[a]	25–50	17–60	30	13/89[a]	31
Hearing loss (%)	5/61[a]	NA	68–93	3	10/20[a]	0
Vision loss (%)	2/14[a]	NA	2–18	NA	88/90[a]	62
Calcifications (%)	?/33[a]	Rare	Rare	0	10/?[a]	0
Other	—	—	Heart malformation	Bony and dental abnormalities	—	Limb hypoplasia
Treatment	Ganciclovir (experimental)	Acyclovir	—	Penicillin	Pyrimethamine and sulfadiazine	—

[a] Asymptomatic/symptomatic.

one or more complications at follow-up. Sequelae in this group included sensorineural hearing loss (5%), psychomotor retardation (4%), microcephaly (4%), and chorioretinitis or optic atrophy (2%) (Williamson et al., 1990). In another study of 307 children with asymptomatic congenital CMV infection, hearing loss was identified in 7.2% in infancy, with 50% of these hearing losses progressing. By a median age of 27 months, an additional 18.2% of the children had delayed-onset sensorineural hearing loss. The sensorineural hearing loss was fluctuating in 22.7% (Fowler et al., 1997). Ophthalmological problems are rare (Coats et al., 2000).

Diagnosis

Diagnosis of congenital CMV infection is usually accomplished by obtaining a suitable specimen from either urine or saliva for direct identification of the virus. A positive test from a specimen obtained within the first 2–3 weeks of life confirms intrauterine infection. Specimens obtained and tested after the infant is 3 weeks of age are suspect because perinatal infection can lead to positive cultures at 3 weeks of life and beyond (Stagno, 2001). Therefore, the diagnosis of congenital CMV infection should be pursued soon after birth. In the 85% of children who are asymptomatic at birth, the diagnostic evaluation usually does not occur until after the first month of life. Labeling these patients with a firm diagnosis of congenital CMV infection is nearly impossible unless a stored specimen obtained prior to 2–3 weeks of life is available. It is possible to exclude the diagnosis of congenital CMV infection with negative serology or culture or both.

Classic findings of congenital CMV infection at birth strongly support the diagnosis. Because of the large viral burden in congenitally infected infants, a CMV culture commonly turns positive within 1 week of plating (Stagno et al., 1975). Because cultures from postnatally infected patients take longer than 1 week to grow, presumptive diagnosis of congenital CMV infection can be made if a standard culture becomes positive within 1 week.

Standard culture techniques or the more rapid shell vial assay performed on urine and saliva specimens have a sensitivity that approaches 100% (Demmler, 1991; Rabella & Drew, 1990) as long as the laboratory is reliable and the specimens are handled properly. Polymerase chain reaction (PCR) testing, although less sensitive than culture, has proven to be sensitive on urine (93.2%), saliva (90.6%), and blood (81%–100%) samples with excellent specificity (> 97%) (Demmler, Buffone, Schimbor, & May, 1988; Warren, Balcarek, Smith, & Pass, 1992). PCR offers the advantage of using very small amounts of specimen for diagnosis, including as small an amount as that obtained on stored filter-paper newborn screening cards (Binda et al., 2004). Thus, retrospective diagnosis is possible for children thought to have congenital CMV who are identified after the first 3 weeks of life. Caution must be taken, however, to ensure that the stored filter-paper cards do not come into contact with another specimen because DNA may be transferred from one card to another (Johansson et al., 1997).

If specimens are sent for culture, serological testing for congenital CMV is not required or desirable. A negative CMV-specific immunoglobulin (Ig) G titer effectively rules out the diagnosis, whereas a positive IgG titer in the first year of life merely confirms the mother's infection. The presence of CMV-specific IgM may confirm infection, but knowledge of when the specimen was obtained and the methodology employed is crucial. IgM determination by immunofluorescent antibody technique may have poor sensitivity and false positives secondary to background fluorescence. Radioimmunoassay and enzyme-linked immunosorbent assay techniques are more sensitive, and specificity may approach 100% as long as the laboratory dilutes out rheumatoid factor and IgG prior to running the assay (Demmler, 1991). Presence of IgM after the first 3 weeks of life neither confirms nor denies the diagnosis because infection could have been acquired at the time of delivery.

When evaluating patients for the diagnosis of congenital CMV, laboratory studies should include a complete blood count, platelet count, liver enzyme and bilirubin determinations, computed tomography (CT) scan or magnetic resonance imaging (MRI) of the head, and a retinal examination performed by an ophthalmologist. In congenitally infected patients, retinal examinations should take place at least yearly until such time as the patient is able to describe visual field changes.

Treatment

Treatment of congenital CMV remains a conundrum. Drugs shown to improve the outcome of CMV infection in immunosuppressed hosts other than newborns include ganciclovir, valganciclovir, cidofovir, and foscarnet (Demmler, 2004). Only ganciclovir has received significant study for the treatment of congenital disease. In the largest of these studies, 100 infants with evidence of central nervous system (CNS) disease were randomized to either treatment with 6 weeks of intravenous ganciclovir at a dose of 6 mg/kg once daily or no therapy. Only 43 children had follow-up data at 1 year or more of life. Hearing loss either improved or did not worsen in 84% of children who received ganciclovir versus 41% for the nontreatment group when followed up at 6 months. At 12 months, the children in the ganciclovir group had not changed, while another 22% in the nontreatment group showed deterioration. The improved hearing parameters persisted beyond 12 months of life in those children available for testing. Ganciclovir treatment also reduced the duration of hepatitis, and ganciclovir recipients were temporarily better on the growth parameters of weight and head circumference. Neutropenia was seen in 63% of the children receiving ganciclovir versus 21% of the control group. Three ganciclovir recipients had catheter infections related to their indwelling intravenous catheter (Kimberlin et al., 2003). Behavioral and cognitive function was not evaluated. Therefore, the use of ganciclovir should be considered in newborns with evidence of CNS disease. A Phase I study of valganciclovir, an oral antiviral agent with good absorption, is in progress, and data is expected to publish soon. Investigators are moving toward a collaborative Phase II study comparing 6 weeks versus 6 months of oral valganciclovir for the treatment of congenital CMV.

Prevention

Prevention of congenital CMV infection remains the best option. Women who have seroconverted prior to conception rarely deliver a child with significant sequelae from congenital CMV infection. Pregnant seronegative women should practice good hand washing technique and consider avoiding mucous membrane contact with saliva and urine whenever possible. Studies have failed to show a statistically significant higher risk of seroconversion than in the general population among nursing staff in pediatric wards, intensive care units, or dialysis units. Workers in child care centers have perhaps the highest occupational risk (Pass & Stagno, 1988).

Development of live virus CMV vaccines are in progress, but theoretical concerns regarding oncogenesis and reactivation suggest that it will be many years before they are commercially available. Subunit vaccines are also in development. The most successful candidate vaccine to date contains purified protein B (Pass et al., 1999). It is safe and immunogenic in toddlers but has yet to undergo testing in neonates (Mitchell, Holmes, Burke, Duliege, & Adler, 2002).

Prognosis

The long-term prognosis of symptomatic congenital CMV infection reveals a bimodal distribution of intellectual outcomes. In follow-up at 6 years of age in a group of 32 children with symptomatic infection, the mean IQ score was 68; 41% had an IQ score of less than 70 and a mean IQ score of 29, and 59% had a mean IQ score of 92. Low IQ score was associated with microcephaly, neurological abnormalities, and chorioretinitis, which were apparent in the first year, and was not associated with the severity of neonatal reticuloendothelial disease or hearing loss (Conboy et al., 1987). The presence of CMV by DNA PCR in cerebrospinal fluid (CSF) samples obtained near birth correlated with abnormal neurological outcome (Troendle-Atkins et al., 1994). The 80% of children with asymptomatic CMV infection who do not develop hearing loss or other impairment have a prognosis comparable with that of uninfected children (Hanshaw, 1995). Children with congenital CMV infection with normal development at 12 months of age are unlikely to be at increased risk of subsequent intellectual impairment (Ivarsson, Lernmark, & Svanberg, 1997).

PERINATAL HERPES SIMPLEX INFECTION

Epidemiology

Neonatal herpes simplex virus (HSV) infection is a rare but potentially fatal disease. The incidence of neonatal HSV infection is estimated to range from 1 in 3,000 to 1 in 20,000 live births (American Academy of Pediatrics [AAP], 2003a). The seroprevalence of HSV type 2 (HSV-2) among women in the United States from 1988 to 1994 was 25.6%. Independent predictors of HSV-2 seropositivity were female sex, black race or Mexican American ethnic background, older age, less education, poverty, cocaine use, and a greater lifetime number of sexual partners (Fleming et al., 1997). In a study of more than 7,000 pregnant women, 2% of initially seronegative women acquired HSV-2 (Brown et al., 1997). Most cases of neonatal herpes occur as a result of maternal infection during delivery, and approximately 75% are HSV-2. In about 5% of cases, intrauterine infection occurs. About 10% of infants acquire their infection postpartum and not always from the mother; other sources include another contact shedding HSV (often type 1) from fever blisters or lesions on other sites (Kohl, 2004). The estimated risks of maternal-fetal transmission based on maternal infection are as follows (Mertz, 1993; Nahmias et al., 1971; Prober et al., 1987; Sweet & Gibbs, 1990):

1. Primary or nonprimary first episode with active lesions at delivery—50%

2. Asymptomatic first episode—33%

3. Recurrent HSV with active lesion—3%–4%

4. Asymptomatic recurrence—0.04%

Clinical Manifestations

Perinatal infection manifests in the first month of life, with 9% of cases symptomatic on the first day and 40% by the first week. Localized infection and disseminated infection occur at a mean of 5–6 days postpartum, and CNS infection occurs later, at a mean of 8–12 days postpartum (Kohl, 2004). Neonatal HSV infection presents clinically as 1) a disseminated infection in 51% of cases, 2) encephalitis in 32% of cases, and 3) localized infection in 17% of cases. Disseminated disease presents with fever or hypothermia, hepatosplenomegaly, vesicular skin lesions (80%), anorexia, vomiting, lethargy, respiratory distress, cyanosis, and circulatory collapse. Encephalitis-type disease usually presents with seizures, irritability, poor feeding, thermal instability, bulging fontanel, and pyramidal tract signs. Localized infections present with bullous lesions of the mouth and skin, keratoconjunctivitis, or chorioretinitis. Infections acquired in utero, mainly from first-trimester primary infections, can be manifested by skin vesicles, cutaneous scars and calcifications, absence of scalp skin, microcephaly, cerebral atrophy, hydranencephaly, cerebral and cerebellar necrosis, intracranial calcifications, hepatosplenomegaly, chorioretinitis, microphthalmia, keratoconjunctivitis, cataracts, retinal dysplasia, short digits, and bone abnormalities (Freij & Sever, 1988).

Diagnosis

Culture remains the "gold standard" for the diagnosis of mucocutaneous neonatal HSV infection. The neonate's body should be carefully examined for the presence of vesicular lesions, especially on the scalp if an intrauterine scalp electrode was used during labor. Ideally, culture specimens are obtained by scraping the base of a vesicle located on the skin or mucous membranes. In the absence of a vesicle, sites from which to gather surface specimens for culture include the conjunctival, genital, oral, nasopharyngeal, and rectal areas. Cultures usually turn positive within 1 week and generally within 1–3 days. Because the quality and site of the specimen influence the likelihood of obtaining a positive culture, a negative culture, considered by itself, cannot exclude the diagnosis of neonatal herpes infection. Positive surface cultures in the first 24 hours of life may represent transient presence of the virus and not true infection.

If culture is not available, then a direct fluorescent antibody stain or the less specific and less sensitive examination for intranuclear inclusions and multinucleated giant cells can be performed using cells from a scraping. Direct fluorescent antibody staining offers the advantages of sensitivity, specificity, and rapidity. Examination for intranuclear inclusions and multinucleated giant cells has a sensitivity of 60%–70% but is not specific for HSV. Staining methods include those of Papanicolaou, Giemsa, Wright, or Tzanck, but only the Papanicolaou or Wright stain is likely to demonstrate intranuclear inclusions (Arvin & Whitley, 2001).

Serology has some value for retrospective confirmation of the diagnosis of neonatal HSV infection but has almost no value when evaluating a neonate for the acute diagnosis of HSV infection. Present technology does not allow for reliable differentiation between maternal- and infant-derived HSV-specific IgG. In the first week following onset of symptoms, HSV-specific IgG will be negative in almost one half of infants with neonatal HSV infection (Whitley, Nahmias, Visintine, Fleming, & Alford, 1980). IgM-specific antibody may not become positive for several weeks after infection (Nahmias et al., 1969). Serology cannot be used to exclude the diagnosis of neonatal herpes in the acute setting.

The diagnosis of HSV encephalitis must be considered in any infant with seizures and fever in the neonatal period. Because as many as 40% of infants with herpes encephalitis do not have skin lesions, the diagnosis often rests on a high index of suspicion, associated maternal factors, and laboratory findings. Maternal diagnostic factors include a positive culture from the mother's genital tract, presence of maternal lesions, or a very recent history of lesions. Supporting laboratory diagnostic data consistent with HSV infection include an abnormal electroencephalogram (EEG), CT scan, or MRI of the head (see Chapter 24, this volume). CT scan and, less frequently, MRI of the head may be normal in the acute stages of HSV

encephalitis. A normal CSF examination is obtained in 3%–20% of cases. The EEG is usually the most sensitive noninvasive laboratory study (Whitley et al., 1982). A classic EEG pattern has been described involving the temporal lobe, but often other EEG patterns are seen involving the temporal or frontal lobes (Mizrahi & Tharp, 1982).

All infants suspected to have HSV, including those with only clinical evidence of mucocutaneous disease, must undergo a diagnostic lumbar puncture. In addition to sending spinal fluid for cell count, differential, and glucose and protein determinations, a PCR for HSV must be performed. PCR is sensitive (76%–100%) and specific for the presence of HSV in the spinal fluid, but a negative PCR does not exclude the diagnosis. It has been positive in patients with only mucocutaneous lesions and no other overt evidence of CNS disease (Kimberlin, Lakeman, et al., 1996; Troendle-Atkins, Demmler, & Buffone, 1993). The advent of PCR testing has nearly eliminated the need for brain biopsy in most clinical settings to make the diagnosis of HSV of the brain.

The initial evaluation of all patients in whom the diagnosis of neonatal HSV infection is considered should include a complete blood count, differential smear, platelet count, liver enzyme and bilirubin determinations, lumbar puncture (with CSF sent for cell count, differential smear, protein and glucose determinations, and HSV PCR), and viral culture. Herpes culture specimens should be obtained as noted previously. A CT scan or MRI or both of the head, an eye examination by an ophthalmologist, and an EEG should be performed. Other infections that may present with similar symptoms, including sepsis, must also be sought and excluded. Studies for HSV can rule in the diagnosis of neonatal HSV, but the absence of a positive test cannot, in itself, rule out HSV infection. Clinical and laboratory data must be combined to exclude the presence of HSV disease.

Treatment

Because of the rapidity of onset and disease progression, most patients with the possible diagnosis of neonatal herpes infection should receive antiviral therapy while the evaluation is in progress. Because of its overall effectiveness and safety profile, acyclovir is now the agent of choice for treatment of neonatal HSV infection. All neonatal patients with disseminated and encephalitic neonatal HSV infection should receive intravenous treatment with acyclovir, 60 mg/kg/day divided into three doses, for a minimum of 21 days. Those with disease confined to mucocutaneous surfaces and with a negative spinal fluid PCR can be treated for only 14 days (AAP, 2003a).

Patients unable to tolerate acyclovir may be treated with foscarnet (AAP, 2003a). Those with evidence of ocular disease should also receive topical ophthalmic antiviral drops such as idoxuridine, vidarabine, trifluridine, or acyclovir. Especially because high doses of acyclovir are used, good hydration must be maintained to limit the risk of acyclovir-induced nephrotoxicity.

Many patients who receive treatment experience mucocutaneous relapse within weeks to months after cessation of therapy. These patients should receive treatment for relapses up to the age of 6 months to reduce the risk of future sequelae (Kimberlin, Powell, et al., 1996).

Prevention

A meta-analysis in pregnant women with either recurrent or first-time episodes of genital herpes supported the use of prophylactic acyclovir starting at 36 weeks' gestation. Although the analysis was unable to prove acyclovir use could reduce the incidence of neonatal HSV, its use appears to reduce the presence of maternal HSV-related genital lesions, asymptomatic viral shedding, and the cesarean section rate (Sheffield, Hollier, Hill, Stuart, & Wendel, 2003). To date, the American College of Obstetricians and Gynecologists states that the use of acyclovir to suppress recurrent HSV infection in pregnancy is a reasonable option (Baker, 1999).

Prevention of neonatal HSV infection requires identification of the at-risk infant at or prior to delivery. If maternal lesions are present at the time of delivery and membranes are intact or have been ruptured for 4–6 hours or less, the risk of HSV transmission to the neonate is lessened by cesarean section. Prophylactic treatment with acyclovir of infants delivered through an infected canal is controversial. Some authors advocate prophylactic treatment in high-risk infants, defined as infants of mothers with primary HSV infection, infants with instrument-assisted deliveries, and those with prolonged or significant exposure to large quantities of virus (Overall, Whitley, Yeager, McCracken, & Nelson, 1984). If the infant is asymptomatic, other authors advocate a wait-and-see response based on whether surface cultures performed at birth, cultures performed after 24–48 hours, or serial weekly cultures until 4 weeks of life are positive, citing the poor immunological response seen in some patients treated with acyclovir and the recognition that patients have experienced CNS relapse after acyclovir treatment (Arvin & Whitley, 2001). If cultures turn positive, then a full evaluation is performed and treatment initiated. Infants with neonatal HSV infection should be placed in contact isolation.

Prognosis

In neonatal HSV infection, mortality is highest in the disseminated presentation (57%), less in the encephalitic presentation (15%), and not reported when localized to the skin, mouth, or eyes. Relative risk of death increases with coma (5.2), disseminated intravascular coagulation (3.8), prematurity (3.7), and disseminated disease with HSV pneumonitis (3.6). In survivors, morbidity is increased in children with HSV-2 (4.9), encephalitis (4.4), seizures, (3.0), and disseminated infections (2.1) (Whitley et al., 1991). With treatment, the mortality is 31% in disseminated disease and 6% in those with CNS disease (Kohl, 2004). The majority of children with the disseminated presentation, and 40% of children with the encephalitic presentation, have long-term neurological impairment. In cases in which infection is confined to the skin, mouth, or eyes and there are three or more recurrences of vesicles, 25% of children have neurological impairment (Whitley et al., 1991).

CONGENITAL LYMPHOCYTIC CHORIOMENINGITIS SYNDROME

Epidemiology

Lymphocytic choriomeningitis virus (LCMV) is an underdiagnosed fetal teratogen that causes a congenital syndrome that can include choreoretinitis, macrocephaly with and without hydrocephalus, microcephaly, intracranial calcifications, and associated intellectual disabilities (Barton & Mets, 2001). Congenital infection with LCMV was initially recognized in 1955 in England (Komrower, Williams, & Stones, 1955) and in 1992 in the United States (Barton et al., 1993). Human cases of LCMV are sporadic, and outbreaks have been reported after exposure to pet hamsters (Jenson, 2004). In a Chicago study to elucidate the spectrum of LCMV, ophthalmologists performed ophthalmological surveys of all residents of a home for people with severe intellectual disabilities and prospectively evaluated all patients with chorioretinitis or chorioretinal scars during a 3-year period at a large children's hospital (Mets, Barton, Khan, & Ksiazek, 2000). Sera for patients demonstrating chorioretinal scars were tested for *Toxoplasma gondii*, rubella virus, CMV, HSV, and LCMV antibodies. Four of 95 patients examined at the home had chorioretinal scars, and 2 were negative for all but LCMV titers. Three of 14 cases of chorioretinitis at the hospital were negative for all but LCMV titers. The researchers concluded that LCMV may be a more common cause of congenital chorioretinitis than previously believed.

Clinical Manifestations

Infection with LCMV during the first trimester of pregnancy appears to be associated with abortion. In the second and third trimesters, fetal infection results in intrauterine or early neonatal death and, in live-born infants, hydrocephalus, macrocephaly, microcephaly, and chorioretinitis (Enders, Varho-Gobel, Lohler, Terletskaia-Ladwig, & Eggers, 1999). A review of 26 infants with serologically confirmed congenital LCMV infection revealed that 22 were products of a full-term gestation. Twenty-one infants (88%) had chorioretinopathy, 10 (43%) had macrocephaly at birth, and

3 (13%) had microcephaly. Hydrocephalus or intracranial calcifications were documented in 5 infants, 9 (35%) infants died, and 10 (58%) of the 17 survivors had severe neurological sequelae, including spastic quadriparesis, seizures, visual loss, and intellectual disabilities (Wright et al., 1997). In a review of 28 affected eyes in 45 LCMV-infected infants, abnormal ophthalmic findings included chorioretinitis (generalized in 20 cases [71%] and macular scars in 10 [36%]), optic atrophy in 6 cases (21%), nystagmus in 3 (10%), esotropia in 1 (4%), microphthalmos in 1 (4%), and cataract in 1 (4%) (Barton & Mets, 2001).

Diagnosis

A high index of suspicion is the first necessary step to making the diagnosis of congenital LCMV. Often it is pursued in an infant when a diagnostic workup for congenital infection, especially toxoplasmosis, is negative and LCMV is then raised as a possible diagnosis. Maternal history of exposure to mice, hamsters, or gerbils is often elicited, because these animals are natural reservoirs of the organism. Serology or virus isolation or detection is used to make the diagnosis of LCMV infection. Detection of LCMV-specific IgG and IgM in either serum or CSF is diagnostic; testing is usually by indirect fluorescent antibody titer because it is commercially available and both sensitive and specific (Barton & Mets, 2001). PCR has been used to diagnose congenital LCMV, but it is not commercially available, and the ideal primers are not known at this time (Enders et al., 1999).

Treatment

There is currently no known treatment for LCMV infection. Therefore, emphasis is placed on developing an interdisciplinary team to treat the sequelae of infection in an attempt to reduce future morbidity.

Prevention

Limiting or excluding exposure to rodents that carry LCMV is the only known effective way to prevent congenital LCMV. There are no vaccines to prevent LCMV infection.

Prognosis

Because most cases of LCMV are identified as a result of chorioretinitis, macrocephaly, or microcephaly and negative TORCH (toxoplasmosis, other infections, rubella, CMV, and HSV) titers, the limited numbers of cases identified are a biased sample. A review of several case studies of LCMV revealed 15 (38%) of 40 infants with microcephaly at birth, 10 (34%) of 29 with macrocephaly, and 17 (89%) of 19 in whom imaging studies were done with hydrocephalus or intracranial, periventricular calcifications. Of 38 surviving infants, 32 (84%) had neurological sequelae, including cerebral palsy, intellectual disabilities, seizures, and decreased visual acuity (Barton & Mets, 2001). No prospective investigations are available that allow for complete description of the congenital LCMV syndrome.

CONGENITAL RUBELLA SYNDROME

Epidemiology

In the United States before the introduction of rubella vaccine in 1969, rubella was most prevalent in the 5- to 14-year-old age group, with a total of 58,000 cases reported in 1969 (Cooper & Alford, 2001). During the period from 1994 to 1996, 567 rubella cases were reported, with 422 (75.2%) in people ages 15–44 years and 171 (30.5%) in women of childbearing age (15–44 years), with 5 pregnant at the time of rash onset (Centers for Disease Control and Prevention [CDC], 1997). The ethnic distribution of rubella cases has shifted in recent years to about 75% or more occurring in Hispanics, who may have migrated from other countries to the United States (Reef et al., 2001). A review of the 49 infants with congenital rubella syndrome (CRS) born in California from 1990 to May 1999 identifies some demographic high-risk characteristics. Maternal demographics revealed that, compared with other California births, the mothers were younger (mean age of 23 years), more likely to identify themselves as Hispanic (73%) and foreign-born (60%), more likely to be pregnant for the first time (50%), and less likely to receive any prenatal care or receive no care until the third trimester (26%) (Reef et al., 2001).

Clinical Manifestations

Estimates of defects are affected by serological status and age at evaluation of the child. The most important determination of fetal outcome is gestational age at the time of infection. In a study of 258 seropositive infants, the risk of defects was 85% if infection occurred in the first 12 weeks, 35% in weeks 13–16, and none after 16 weeks (Miller, Cradock-Watson, & Pollock, 1982). Congenital rubella infection encompasses all outcomes associated with intrauterine rubella infection, including miscarriage, stillbirth, abortion, infection only, or combinations of birth defects termed *congenital rubella syndrome*. Clinical features group into three categories: 1) transient manifestations in newborns and infants; 2) permanent manifestations that may be present at birth or become apparent during the first year of life; and 3) developmental and late-onset manifestations, which may appear and progress through childhood, adolescence, and adulthood.

Forty percent of newborns with congenital rubella infection have clinical manifestations in the newborn period. Transient manifestations result from active infection and are self-limited but are diagnostically and prognostically important. In one group of newborns with symptomatic CRS, transient manifestations included purpura or "blueberry muffin" appearance (86%), hepatomegaly (72%), splenomegaly (69%), adenopathy (22%), bone lesions (22%), hepatitis (19%), and anemia (17%) (Cooper, Green, Krugman, Gioles, & Mirick, 1965). In children with neonatal thrombocytopenia, the mortality was 35%. Extreme prematurity, gross cardiac lesions or myocarditis, hepatitis, meningoencephalitis, and fulminant interstitial pneumonitis were factors that contributed to the high mortality rate (Cooper, 1985).

Permanent manifestations are structural defects that result from defective organogenesis and tissue destruction and scarring. They include the classic triad of hearing loss, cardiac and eye defects, and developmental disabilities. Analysis of 11 prospective studies that included 113 subjects with CRS conducted from 1969 to 1996 around the world revealed hearing impairment as the most frequent clinical manifestation of CRS (60%) and the defect more likely to present as a single defect than were the eye or heart defects (Reef et al., 2000). The hearing loss is usually uniform across all frequencies, equal in both ears, and severe, averaging 93 dB across the range from 250 to 4000 Hz (Wild, Sheppard, Smithells, Holzel, & Jones, 1989). Heart defects (45%), the second most common defects, were most frequently patent ductus arteriosis (20%) and peripheral pulmonic stenosis (12%) (Reef et al., 2000). Eye defects are the third most common defect. A study of 328 children with CRS revealed that 54 (16%) had cataracts, 78 (24%) had retinopathy, and 58 (18%) had strabismus (Wolff, 1973).

Late-onset manifestations include health problems, developmental disabilities, and progressive hearing loss. Late-onset health problems include insulin-dependent diabetes mellitus in 20% of adults; thyroid dysfunction (5%); late-onset ocular defects such as glaucoma, keratic precipitates, keratoconus, corneal hydrops, and spontaneous lens absorption; hypertension from renal artery and aortic stenosis; and subretinal neovascularization (Cooper & Alford, 2001). Children with CRS are at high risk for having multiple developmental disorders, including cerebral palsy, intellectual disabilities, and seizures. Developmental disabilities that may not be apparent in the first year include autism, which occurs with a frequency of approximately 6% (Cooper, 1985). In the second decade of life, a rare progressive rubella panencephalitis has been reported, manifested by ataxia, seizures, and progressive loss of mental function (Townsend et al., 1979).

Diagnosis

Direct culture of the virus from clinical specimens most often confirms the diagnosis of congenital rubella. Nasopharyngeal specimens provide the best yield, but cultures of CSF, conjunctiva, feces, and urine are also frequently positive. Pharyngeal fluid obtained in the first month of life has a better than 84% likelihood of being culture positive, but the yield on specimens tested in the first year of life declines steadily, reaching 11% by 1 year of age. Be-

cause congenital rubella is a chronic infection, positive cultures from an infant without a recent rubella-type rash are diagnostic for intrauterine infection. Postnatally acquired rubella viral cultures are rarely positive more than 2 weeks after the onset of rash (Cooper & Alford, 2001).

Serological diagnosis of congenital rubella generally depends on identifying the presence of rubella-specific IgM in the infant's blood. Several IgM assays are available commercially, but false positives can result if IgG and rheumatoid factor are not removed (Cubie & Edmond, 1985; Leinikki, Shekarchi, Dorsett, & Sever, 1978). The solid-phase immunosorbent technique is unaffected by rheumatoid factor (Mortimer, Tedder, Hambling, Shafi, & Burkhardt, 1981). Published experience has documented the presence of rubella-specific IgM in 48 (96%) of 50 congenitally infected infants ages birth to 6 months and in 11 (29%) of 38 congenitally infected infants ages 6.5 months to 2 years (Cradock-Watson & Ridehalgh, 1976). IgM levels wane over time, and IgM may be delayed in its development; therefore, a negative IgM test does not absolutely exclude the diagnosis of congenital rubella (Enders, 1985).

If the index of suspicion is high for the diagnosis of congenital rubella, serial measurement of rubella-specific IgG should be performed. To accurately confirm titer results, the specimens collected over time must be analyzed using the same assay performed at the same time. After 6–12 months of age, a persistently high IgG titer is presumptive evidence of congenital infection in an unimmunized child without a history of postnatal rubella (Enders, 1985).

After 1 year of age, diagnosis of congenital rubella by serological or culture methods is extremely difficult, and diagnosis is generally based on clinical criteria. Cultures rarely remain positive beyond 2 years of life. Only one patient has been reported to have had persistent rubella-specific IgM in the CSF (Vesikari, Meurman, & Maki, 1980). Rubella-specific antibody formation in children who receive rubella vaccine at 12–15 months of age further complicates retrospective diagnosis.

Laboratory evaluation for patients considered to have congenital rubella should include a complete blood count, differential smear of white blood cells, platelet count, liver enzyme and bilirubin determinations, long bone radiographs, chest radiograph, lumbar puncture (with CSF sent for glucose and protein determinations, cell count, and differential smear), retinal examination performed by an ophthalmologist, echocardiogram, and renal ultrasound. Retinal examination, thyroid function studies, and screening for diabetes mellitus must be repeated as the child ages because manifestations may not become evident until 2 years of age and beyond. Patients should also have age-appropriate hearing examinations and developmental testing repeated every few years.

Treatment

Treatment of congenital rubella is supportive. No antiviral therapy has proven to be successful in altering the natural history of congenital infection. Anecdotal reports using amantadine and interferon were not encouraging (Arvin, Schmidt, Cantell, & Merigan, 1982; Plotkin, Klaus, & Whitely, 1966). Emphasis is placed on developing an interdisciplinary team to treat the sequelae of infection in an attempt to reduce morbidity.

Prevention

Active immunization with a live virus vaccine currently provides immunity for greater than 90% of individuals vaccinated and lasts for at least 15 years (CDC, 1990). Although such immunization has been highly successful at dramatically reducing the incidence of congenital rubella, the incidence can vary from one year to the next (CDC, 1991). Vaccination is usually performed in childhood, but women of childbearing age may safely receive the vaccine. Women should be counseled not to become pregnant for 3 months after vaccination and should not be vaccinated while pregnant. If vaccination occurs during the period from 3 months prior to 3 months after conception, evidence to date suggests that risk to the fetus is low. A study of mothers vaccinated during this 6-month interval failed to identify any child with malformations consistent with congenital rubella on follow-up of 324 infants. Statistical evaluation of these data suggests that the risk to the fetus is on the order of 0%–1.6% (CDC, 1990).

Diagnosis of maternal rubella should be based on serologies and clinical findings. If the diagnosis of maternal rubella is made in the first or second trimester, termination of the pregnancy should be considered. If termination is not a viable option, then limited data suggest that high doses of immunoglobulin may prevent or modify infection in an exposed susceptible person. Protection of the fetus cannot be guaranteed because mothers treated in this fashion have delivered congenitally infected infants (AAP, 2003b).

Prognosis

Of those children with congenital rubella who survive to adolescence, one third will be in typical classes without resource help, one third will have mild to moderate cognitive deficits, and one third will have severe cognitive deficits (Desmond et al., 1985). One longitudinal study of growth found that intellectual disabilities correlated with a slowing of the growth rate. Children with a steady growth rate were less likely to have intellectual disabilities than were children whose growth rate slowed such that their final height was in less than the fifth percentile (Chiriboga-Klein et al., 1989). In the United Kingdom, 1,116 individuals born since 1965 are registered with the National CRS Programme. Of the 871 infants with confirmed or compatible rubella, one third of 220 who were initially diagnosed with congenital rubella infection are now categorized at last follow-up (mean age, 9 years) as having CRS. About 10% have died (75% of these as infants), with the cause of death most frequently complications associated with heart defects. Seven each have developed cancer, thyroid disorders, and diabetes mellitus (Tookey & Peckham, 1999).

CONGENITAL SYPHILIS
Epidemiology

Primary and secondary syphilis had a resurgence in the 1980s in the United States, peaked in 1989, and have continued to decline as a result of targeted public health efforts. The incidence of congenital syphilis has had a parallel course. In 2000, 529 congenital syphilis cases were reported, for a rate of 13.4 per 100,000 live-born infants. The rate was highest in the South (18.8) and lowest in the Midwest (9.1). In 2000, racial/ethnic minority populations had the highest congenital syphilis rates per 100,000, with 49.3 among blacks compared with 1.5 among non-Hispanic whites. Mothers who delivered at less than 19 years of age had the highest rate (16.0). Lack of prenatal care, late or limited prenatal care, and maternal use of illicit drugs are associated with congenital syphilis. In 2000, 82% of the cases were due to untreated, inadequately treated, or undocumented treatment of maternal syphilis before or during pregnancy (CDC, 2001). The untreated syphilitic pregnant mother can transmit the *Treponema pallidum* at any time during the pregnancy or at birth. In women with untreated early syphilis, 40% of pregnancies result in spontaneous abortion, stillbirth, or perinatal death. The rate of transmission is 60% to 100% during secondary syphilis and slowly decreases with time (AAP, 2003c).

Clinical Manifestations

The symptoms of congenital syphilis are divided into early manifestations, which are revealed before 2 years of age, and late manifestations, which are revealed after 2 years of age. In a study of 50 cases of early congenital syphilis, 39% were premature, 38% were of low birth weight, and 62% were symptomatic at birth. Clinical findings in the newborn period included the following: cutaneous lesions (41%), hepatosplenomegaly (38%), lymphadenopathy (9%), jaundice (9%), snuffles or rhinitis (7%), neurological signs (7%), pneumonia (7%), ascites (7%), and mucous patches (2%). Of the 50 patients, 9 died: 3 prenatally, 4 in the neonatal period, and 2 after a long, intensive hospitalization (Mascola, Pelosi, Blount, Alexander, & Cates, 1985).

Early manifestations can affect the liver, skin, and hematopoietic system. Liver involvement includes bile stasis, fibrosis, and extramedullary hematopoiesis. Hematopoietic findings include lymphadenopathy, Coombs-negative hemolytic anemia, and thrombocytopenia. Dermatological abnormalities may present with erythematous maculopapular or bullous lesions followed by desquamation of the hands and feet. Mucous membranes may exhibit mucous patches, rhinitis (snuffles), and condylomatous lesions. Roentgenographic abnormalities include often painful osteochondritis at the wrists, elbows, ankles, and knees and periostitis of the long bones. Nephritis and nephritic syndrome are also common (Azimi, 2004).

Late manifestations result primarily from chronic inflammation of bone, teeth, and the CNS. Persistent periostitis and associated thickening of the bone results in frontal bossing, thickening of the sternoclavicular portion of the clavicle, anterior bowing of the midportion of the tibia, and scaphoid scapula. Dental abnormalities include Hutchinson teeth, which are peg- or barrel-shaped upper central incisors; abnormal enamel with a resulting notch on the biting surface; and mulberry molars with a small biting surface and an excessive number of cusps. A saddle nose with a depression of the nasal root and possibly a perforated septum results from syphilitic rhinitis that destroys the adjacent bone and cartilage. Rhagades are linear scars that extend in a spoke-like pattern from previous mucocutaneous fissures of the mouth, anus, and genitalia (Azimi, 2004).

Some late manifestations may represent a hypersensitivity phenomenon. These may include interstitial keratitis with photophobia and lacrimation for weeks or months followed by corneal opacification and complete blindness. Other ocular manifestations may include choroiditis, optic atrophy, retinitis, and vascular occlusion. Eighth nerve deafness may appear at any age and presents initially as vertigo and high-tone hearing loss that progresses to permanent deafness. The Clutton joint is a synovitis involving the lower extremities, which presents as a painless joint swelling usually with spontaneous remission (Azimi, 2004).

Diagnosis

Infants should be evaluated for congenital syphilis if they were born to a nontreponemal (by Venereal Disease Research Laboratory [VDRL] or rapid plasma reagin [RPR] test) seropositive mother and the mother has untreated syphilis, received syphilis treatment with erythromycin, received standard treatment within 1 month of delivery, received standard treatment at any other time during pregnancy but failed to show a fourfold or greater drop in nontreponemal antibody titer, *or* failed to have documentation of the treatment (AAP, 2003c).

A definitive diagnosis of congenital infection can be made if the organism is identified on darkfield examination of a skin lesion or placenta. Because this type of testing is rarely performed, diagnosis usually rests on serological studies. Neonates, or their mothers, with positive nontreponemal serological titers must have specific treponemal serologies performed so as to confirm the origin of the nontreponemal antibody. *Treponema*-specific studies include the fluorescent treponemal antibody test, absorbed by nonpallidum treponemes (FTA-ABS), and the microhemagglutination–*T. pallidum* (MHA-TP) test. The latter is no longer available commercially and has been widely replaced by the *T. pallidum* particle agglutination (TP-PA) test. Unlike the nontreponemal tests, the treponemal antibody titers do not correlate with disease activity and, once becoming reactive, remain so for the life of the patient.

The presence of passively acquired maternal IgG in the neonate complicates the ability to definitively diagnose newborns with congenital syphilis by serology alone. Ideally, a sensitive and specific IgM assay or PCR test would allow differentiation between newborns who are merely exposed to, but not infected with, syphilis and those who are congenitally infected (Sanchez, 1998). Unfortunately, neither is currently commercially available.

Congenital syphilis is usually divided into two major diagnostic categories for epidemiological purposes: confirmed and presumptive (CDC, 1993). A confirmed diagnosis requires that *T. pallidum* be directly identified from specimens of lesions, placenta, umbilical cord, and/or autopsy material. Rarely is a confirmed diagnosis achieved in clinical practice. More commonly, patients are given a diagnosis of presumptive congenital syphilis. The presumptive

case definition requires fulfillment of either of the two following criteria:

1. Any case in which the infant's mother was untreated or inadequately treated for syphilis. Inadequate treatment includes any nonpenicillin therapy or penicillin treatment within 30 days prior to delivery.

2. Any case in which the infant or child has a reactive treponemal test for syphilis *and* any one of the following is present: a) any signs of congenital syphilis on physical examination, b) any long bone radiographic abnormality consistent with congenital syphilis, c) reactive CSF VDRL test, d) elevated CSF cell count or protein without an alternative etiology, e) VDRL or RPR serological titer in the infant that is fourfold or greater that of the mother when both specimens are drawn at birth and run in parallel, or f) reactive treponemal antibody test after 9–12 months of age.

Practically speaking, when considering treatment options, a third category, possible congenital syphilis, should be added to the list. This "diagnosis" is made when an infant has a positive RPR or VDRL titer in the absence of another clinical abnormality and has normal CSF and radiographic examinations, the mother received appropriate treatment, but the ability to assure newborn follow-up after discharge is uncertain.

The evaluation of patients for congenital syphilis can include many laboratory studies because the symptoms of congenital syphilis involve so many different organ systems. Patients with confirmed, presumptive, or possible congenital syphilis should have a quantitative nontreponemal serological test, complete blood count with differential smear, platelet count, and liver enzyme and bilirubin determinations. Long bone radiographs, lumbar puncture (with CSF sent for VDRL test, cell count, differential, and glucose and protein determinations), and an eye examination performed by an ophthalmologist are usually recommended but may only be required in symptomatic patients to define extent of disease because all patients with confirmed, presumptive, or possible congenital syphilis are treated similarly. Because of the epidemiological association between syphilis and HIV infection, all infants born to mothers with syphilis should have HIV antibody testing.

Serological studies on CSF should only be performed using the VDRL test. Studies such as the RPR or specific treponemal antibody studies are not recommended for CSF because of the possibility of false-positive results and the uncertainty of how to interpret these tests. Unfortunately, the CSF VDRL is relatively insensitive for neurosyphilis. It is currently impossible to use routine laboratory tests to exclude the diagnosis of neurosyphilis in the neonate (Ikeda & Jenson, 1990).

Treatment

The decision to treat infants born to mothers with positive serology for syphilis is based on the infant's diagnostic category. Because patients may not return for appropriate follow-up and the long-term consequences of untreated congenital syphilis are severe, a conservative approach to treatment has become the standard of care.

Patients with confirmed, presumptive, and possible congenital syphilis often receive identical treatment. Treatment recommendations are based on the CDC's (1993) guidelines. Treatment regimens use penicillin G, either in the form of crystalline penicillin G at a dose of 100,000–150,000 units/kg/day administered in divided doses every 8–12 hours for 10–14 days, or procaine penicillin G, 50,000 units/kg/day administered once daily intramuscularly for 10–14 days. All patients with confirmed or presumptive congenital syphilis receive either of these treatment courses rather than the single dose of benzathine penicillin G that was recommended in previous years. Because of the inability to exclude neurosyphilis definitively, all patients with confirmed or presumptive congenital syphilis receive a 10- to 14-day course of treatment with the understanding that some patients may be overtreated in the interest of ensuring that no patient with neurosyphilis receives insufficient treatment.

Because of uncertainty regarding their availability for follow-up, many of the infants in the "possible diagnosis" category also receive a 10- to 14-day course of treatment; however, infants with a "possible diagnosis" designation are at very low risk for actually being infected and may be treated with a single dose of benzathine penicillin G, 50,000 units/kg administered intramuscularly. Alternatively, if the mother is seronegative for HIV, has received adequate treatment during pregnancy for syphilis, and has serological confirmation of the success of that treatment and follow-up can be ensured, the infant could just be followed and not receive any treatment (AAP, 2003c).

Serological follow-up is important in all patients regardless of their treatment regimen. Infants successfully treated for congenital syphilis should have a VDRL titer that declines over time. Follow-up serology should be performed at 3-month intervals until the first birthday. Patients with proven neurosyphilis should have a follow-up lumbar puncture performed at 6 months of life to confirm that their indices have all returned to normal. If indices are still abnormal, retreatment is recommended.

Prevention

Identifying maternal syphilis during pregnancy easily prevents congenital syphilis. Serological screening is recommended when the mother presents for prenatal care and at 28 weeks' gestation if the mother is judged to be at high risk. Repeat serology should be performed on all mothers at the time of delivery.

Prognosis

Although treatment may cure the infection, the prognosis depends on the damage done before treatment. If treatment is prenatal or occurs in the first 3 months of life, before stigmata appear, most manifestations can be prevented. Studies show that treponemal organisms may remain in the eye, the CSF, and the lymphatic system. The question remains as to what happens if, later in life, the person becomes immunosuppressed (Ingall & Sanchez, 2001).

CONGENITAL TOXOPLASMOSIS
Epidemiology

In the United States, the incidence of congenital toxoplasmosis has been estimated to be 1 in

1,000 to 1 in 10,000 live births (AAP, 2003d). Rates of seropositivity of pregnant women with *Toxoplasma gondii* vary depending on factors such as age, dietary practices, and geography (Freij & Sever, 1991). Infection may be related to eating raw eggs or meat; unprotected exposure to cat feces through litter box changing, sandboxes, or gardening; or exposure in horse stables (McLeod & Remington, 2004). With primary maternal infection during pregnancy, the frequency of fetal infection in one study of 144 pregnant women was 21% at 6–20 weeks, 63% at 21–30 weeks, and 89% after 30 weeks (Foulon et al., 1999).

Clinical Manifestations

Infants with congenital toxoplasmosis infection are asymptomatic at birth in 70%–90% of cases (AAP, 2003d). Data and treatment have evolved over the last 40 years. In a 1960s study of 152 untreated children with congenital toxoplasmosis, 108 had neurological disease and 44 had generalized disease. Of the children with neurological disease, 94% had chorioretinitis, 51% had anemia, 50% had convulsions, 50% had intracranial calcifications, and 29% had jaundice. Of the children with generalized disease, 90% had hepatomegaly, 80% had jaundice, 68% had lymphadenopathy, 66% had chorioretinitis, and 77% had anemia. At 4 years of age, 9% of the children in the neurological disease group were typically developing, 89% had intellectual disabilities, 83% had convulsions, 76% had spasticity and palsies, 69% had severe visual impairment, and 44% had hydrocephalus or microcephalus. In the generalized group, 16% of the children were normal, and 81% had intellectual disabilities, 77% had convulsions, 58% had spasticity and palsies, 42% had severely impaired vision, and 6% had hydrocephalus or microcephalus (Eichenwald, 1960).

In a 1984 review of 210 infants with congenital toxoplasmosis infection identified by a serological screening program for pregnant women, outcomes were improved. This study probably underestimated the relative frequency of severe congenital infection because some women were treated in utero with spiramycin, many of the pregnancies with acute acquired infections diagnosed early during pregnancy were terminated, and only 13 infants had CT brain scans. The most frequent signs and symptoms found in the infants were the following: chorioretinitis (21.8%), prematurity (10.9%), icterus (10.0%), intrauterine growth retardation (6.2%), psychomotor retardation (5.2%), and convulsions (3.8%) (Couvreur, Desmonts, Tournier, & Szusterkac, 1984).

In a more recent 1995 study, 36 infants with congenital toxoplasmosis were identified and treated in the first few months of life with pyrimethamine and sulfadiazine for approximately 1 year. At 1 year of age on the Bayley Scales of Infant Development (Bayley, 1969), 79% had a mean Mental Developmental Index (MDI) of 102 and 21% had an MDI of less than 50. Neurological exams were normal for 45% and revealed abnormal tone in 33% and permanent neurological abnormalities in 22%. Seventy-eight percent had no seizure history, 11% had nonrecurring seizures, and 11% were on anticonvulsants after 2.5 months of age (Roizen et al., 1995). In a study of treatment of toxoplasmosis during pregnancy, 44% of 144 women gave birth to a congenitally infected infant. Antibiotic therapy did not reduce the transmission rate but did reduce the rate of sequelae among the infected infants evaluated at 1 year of age. Sequelae were found in 13%: 6% were severe, and 7% were mild sequelae. These sequelae included intrauterine death ($n = 3$), neurological abnormalities ($n = 2$), hydrocephalus and cerebral calcifications leading to death ($n = 1$), chorioretinal scars with severe visual impairment ($n = 1$), and hydrocephalus ($n = 1$) (Foulon et al., 1999).

Diagnosis

As with most congenital infections, history of exposure should be sought, but, in many patients with congenital *Toxoplasma* infection, a definitive history of exposure will not be found. Questions directed at exposure should include inquiries regarding cleaning of cat litter boxes; contact with sites where infected animals might defecate, including sandboxes, stables, and gardens; consumption of raw or undercooked meats; and consumption of raw eggs or unpasteurized milk. Many maternal infections go unrecognized. Concern regarding *Toxoplasma* is often raised only during pregnancy in the woman with afebrile lymphadenopathy and fatigue (Remington, McLeod, Thulliez, & Desmonts, 2001).

Diagnosis of congenital *Toxoplasma* infection is usually based on serological studies but is complicated by the fact that these studies have poor sensitivity and specificity. It is critical to use a reference laboratory because of the complexity of the testing and the high rate of false-positive and false-negative results from many of the available commercial kits. Serological test methods include the Sabin-Feldman dye test, complement fixation, indirect hemagglutination, immunofluorescent antibody, double-sandwich enzyme-linked immunosorbent assay, and immunosorbent agglutination assay (Desmonts, Naot, & Remington, 1981; Naot, Desmonts, & Remington, 1981; Naot & Remington, 1980). Although diagnosis is usually based on serological studies, histological examination or culture of the placenta, of newborn or cord blood, or of both at birth may be diagnostic (Remington et al., 2001). A thorough discussion of all of these tests is beyond the scope of this chapter, and the interested reader is directed to the cited references for further details of test methodology.

Because of the need to use a reference laboratory to diagnose congenital toxoplasmosis, for practical purposes preliminary screening at a commercial laboratory is usually performed prior to sending specimens to a reference laboratory. When there is a low index of suspicion, screening the infant or mother or both for the presence of *Toxoplasma*-specific IgG is usually performed. A negative IgG screen effectively rules out the diagnosis, and other etiologies for the patient's symptoms should be sought. In patients in whom the index of suspicion is high or the infant or mother or both have a positive *Toxoplasma*-specific IgG screen, blood specimens should be sent to a reference laboratory looking for *Toxoplasma*-specific IgG, IgM, IgA, and IgE. Presence of IgM, IgA, IgE, or any combination of the three is diagnostic when performed by a reference laboratory. Unfortunately, as many as 25% of congenitally infected infants have a negative IgM screen, and 10%

have negative results for IgA and IgE, even when testing is performed by a reference laboratory (Stepick-Biek, Thulliez, Araujo, & Remington, 1990; Wong et al., 1993). Therefore, negative screens for IgM, IgA, and IgE do not rule out the diagnosis of *Toxoplasma* infection, and follow-up serology is crucial to document decay of the infant's maternally acquired IgG. Treatment may delay the synthesis of infant-derived antibody so that measurement of infant-derived IgG may not be possible until several months after treatment is stopped (Remington et al., 2001).

PCR is an evolving diagnostic tool for congenital toxoplasmosis. Although the best use of PCR, as well as its sensitivity or specificity, are still uncertain, positive PCR results have been documented in CSF and urine specimens in symptomatic neonates (Filisetti, Gorcii, Pernot-Marino, Villard, & Candolfi, 2003; Fuentes et al., 1996).

Additional laboratory and clinical evaluations should include a complete blood count; platelet count; lumbar puncture for cell count, differential smear, and protein and glucose determinations; liver enzyme and bilirubin determinations; and either CT scan or MRI of the head (see Chapter 24, this volume). Eye examination is crucial for identifying chorioretinitis and can aid in confirming the diagnosis of congenital toxoplasmosis. In congenitally infected patients, retinal examinations should take place at least yearly until such time as the patient is able to describe visual field changes.

Treatment

The ideal drug regimen and duration of treatment for congenital toxoplasmosis remain to be determined. Treatment with combination therapy of pyrimethamine and sulfonamide preparations (either sulfadiazine or trisulfapyrimadines) for a duration of 1 year is currently recommended. Treatment with pyrimethamine should include folinic acid to prevent bone marrow suppression. Corticosteroid treatment should be added to the regimens of patients with active chorioretinitis, intense meningeal inflammation, or both until the inflammation has subsided. Treatment with 1 year of pyrimethamine and sulfadiazine reduces audiological complications and improves the developmental outcome of patients with congenital toxoplasmosis (McLeod, Wisner, & Boyer, 1992; Roizen et al., 1995).

Prevention

Prevention of congenital toxoplasmosis starts with awareness of the potential sources of exposure and avoidance of these sources. Pregnant women should be counseled to not clean litter boxes, to consume only well-cooked meats, and to avoid sandboxes and gardening when practical. Use of gloves when working in the garden or a sandbox or when cleaning litter boxes limits the risk of exposure (Frenkel, 1985).

Screening pregnant women for *Toxoplasma* antibody is controversial. Seroconversion prior to conception effectively eliminates the risk to the fetus with the exception of HIV-infected women or those otherwise significantly immunosuppressed. Although at low frequency, the latter groups have been documented to deliver congenitally infected newborns despite seroconversion prior to conception (European Collaborative Study, 1996; Mitchell et al., 1990). The availability of a reliable screening test and the ability to introduce treatment determine the cost-effectiveness of screening. If a women seroconverts during pregnancy or near the time of conception, her fetus is at risk for congenital toxoplasmosis. Management options include treatment with spiramycin during pregnancy, which reduces the likelihood of complications (Daffos et al., 1988), or termination of the pregnancy.

Prognosis

The long-term prognosis in congenital toxoplasmosis has been greatly improved by the introduction of antibiotic treatment from birth or in utero. In utero identification is not routine, and not all infants with congenital toxoplasmosis are identified early in infancy.

CONGENITAL VARICELLA SYNDROME

Epidemiology

In the United States, varicella during pregnancy is estimated to occur in 5–10 per 10,000 pregnancies, with some indications that there is an upward trend since the 1980s in the absolute number and the proportion of cases occurring in adults ages 15–44 years (Nathwani, Maclean, Conway, & Carrington, 1998). In 1947, the first case was reported of congenital defects following maternal infection with varicella (Laforet & Lynch, 1947). For the succeeding 20 years, the literature had no reports, and then 17 cases were reported between 1967 and 1984. Maternal varicella at any stage of pregnancy can result in intrauterine death or neonatal or infantile zoster. Congenital varicella syndrome has been reported almost exclusively when maternal varicella infection has occurred in the first 20–26 weeks of gestation (Gershon, 2001), with a risk of 2% and a mortality of 30% (Sauerbrei & Wutzler, 2001). Varicella in the third trimester places the mother at 10%–20% risk for pneumonia, which has a 10%–45% mortality. Varicella near term may result in neonatal varicella, which has 0%–3% mortality if it develops 0–4 days after birth and 20% mortality if it develops between 5 and 10–12 days after birth (Sauerbrei & Wutzler, 2001). A composite of 10 prospective studies conducted between 1960 and 1997 placed the prevalence of congenital varicella syndrome at 1.8% in 718 pregnancies (Gershon, 2001).

The largest published prospective study with comprehensive follow-up involved 347 women with varicella infection during pregnancy. This study included pregnant women enrolled at 10 perinatal centers and specialists examining the eyes, hearing, and physical and developmental features at three points in time up to 19–30 months after delivery. In this study, the prevalence of fetal varicella syndrome was 0.4%, with one case in the 347 women with primary varicella and none in the 15 women with herpes zoster (Harger et al., 2002). Two cases involved fetal death at 20 weeks and fetal hydrops at 17 weeks after maternal infection. Herpes zoster has been reported in infants whose mothers had varicella in pregnancy (Enders, Miller, Cradock-Watson, Boiley, & Ridehalgh, 1994). No studies have identified infants with fetal varicella syndrome whose mothers experienced varicella-zoster infection during their pregnancies.

Clinical Manifestations

The clinical manifestations of congenital varicella syndrome are believed to be due to the neurotrophic properties of the virus (Higa, Dan, & Manabe, 1987). In Alkalay, Pomerance, and Rimonin's (1987) study of 30 infants with congenital varicella, 85% of the infants were female, 38% were premature, and 39% were small for gestational age. In a review of 22 infants with congenital varicella syndrome, skin lesions were found in 100%, and initially some looked like skin loss but within a few months became cicatricial in a dermatome distribution. Other frequent manifestations of fetal varicella syndrome were neurological anomalies (77%), with 18% of those being intellectual disabilities; eye anomalies (68%), with 60% of those being chorioretinitis; and skeletal anomalies (68%), with 80% of those being hypoplasia of the upper/lower extremities (Alkalay et al., 1987). Ophthalmological manifestations include Horner's syndrome, choreoretinitis cataracts, microphthalmos, and atrophy or hypoplasia of the optic discs (Lambert, Taylor, Kriss, Holzel, & Heard, 1989). CNS manifestations include cortical atrophy, encephalitis, intellectual disabilities, and seizures. Limb findings include hypoplastic limbs with extremity bone or muscle loss or atrophy or hypoplastic or missing fingers.

Diagnosis

Diagnosis of fetal varicella syndrome is based on history, physical examination, and laboratory data. A history of maternal chickenpox between 8 and 20 weeks of gestation is associated with the fetal varicella syndrome. Rarely does maternal varicella infection after the 20th week of gestation cause symptomatic fetal infection (Gershon & LaRussa, 1992). The physical examination of the newborn should yield manifestations of the syndrome described previously.

As with all intrauterine infections, the presence of specific IgG antibody in congenitally exposed infants at birth merely confirms previous infection of the mother. Congenitally infected infants will usually have persistent varicella-specific IgG after 8 months of life. Passively acquired maternal antibody will have dissipated by that age (Gershon, Raker, Steinberg, Topf-Olstein, & Drusin, 1976). Unfortunately, studies have not clarified whether negative serology after 8 months of life rules out the diagnosis of congenital varicella. The literature contains reports of patients with presumed fetal varicella syndrome who have negative serology (Gershon, 2001). These reported patients either were misdiagnosed or failed to mount a measurable immunological response to their in utero varicella infection. Diagnosis in this latter group is based solely on clinical criteria. The diagnosis of fetal varicella can also be substantiated by the development of zoster in the first 1 or 2 years of life (Brunell, 1992).

Unless active varicella lesions are present at the time of delivery, cultures of the newborn for varicella to prove the diagnosis of fetal infection are futile. Because essentially all cases of developmentally disabling varicella infection of the fetus occur prior to the 20th week of gestation (Gershon, 2001), active lesions are not likely to be present. IgM serology has been used in one published report to support the diagnosis of fetal varicella syndrome. PCR has also proved the presence of varicella in a case report (Sauerbrei, Muller, Eichhorn, & Wutzler, 1996).

Prenatal varicella does occur and can lead to death as a result of a sepsis-like syndrome, pneumonia, hepatitis, and/or hemorrhagic disease, especially if onset of the neonate's rash is between 5 and 10 days after delivery. Diagnosis of perinatal varicella rests on maternal history of varicella within 21 days of delivery, characteristic lesions on examination, and identification of varicella by culture or direct immunofluorescence of epithelial cells from skin lesions. Although no data exist confirming the utility of acyclovir in this setting, infants with perinatal varicella are usually treated with intravenous acyclovir if there are active lesions (AAP, 1994e).

Patients with fetal varicella syndrome should have laboratory studies performed, including baseline serology, CT scan or MRI of the head, and an eye examination performed by an ophthalmologist checking for evidence of abnormalities.

Treatment

Because no evidence exists that infants with fetal varicella syndrome have an active viral infection, treatment with antiviral agents is not indicated. In infants with active lesions at the time of delivery or who go on to develop varicella within the first 10 days of life, antiviral therapy with intravenous acyclovir is the recommended treatment.

Prevention

Prevention of fetal varicella syndrome can be accomplished by prevention of maternal exposure to varicella during the first and early second trimester. Active immunization of all seronegative women of childbearing age with the varicella vaccine prior to conception would prevent the occurrence of fetal varicella syndrome. Its use during pregnancy is contraindicated. The efficacy of varicella-zoster immune globulin (VZIG) and acyclovir in the prevention or modification of the development of fetal varicella syndrome in a fetus whose seronegative mother is exposed to varicella is unknown; however, the Committee on Infectious Diseases of the AAP (2003e) recommends that pregnant women with a negative history for varicella receive VZIG within 48 hours and not more than 96 hours following exposure. If antibody is present, there is no need for VZIG administration. The Committee on Infectious Diseases (AAP, 2003e) further recommends VZIG administration if maternal rash occurs within 5 days prior to delivery or 48 hours following delivery. Pregnant women have received treatment with acyclovir without drug-induced complications (Brunell, 1992).

Prognosis

Early mortality is increased in fetal varicella syndrome, with one review reporting that 32% of affected infants died between 36 hours and 2 months of age as a result of recurrent aspiration pneumonia secondary to bulbar dysphagia, severe gastroesophageal reflux, or seizures (Meyers, 1974). Gershon and LaRussa (1992) reported a correlation between hypoplastic extremities and severe brain damage or death. In one study, the long-term developmental outcome for more mildly involved children improved over time (Enders, 1984). Congenital varicella syndrome represents a spectrum of involvement, with most cases in the severe range (Gershon, 2001).

CONCLUSION

Although a great deal of progress has been made in relation to congenital infections by almost completely preventing congenital rubella, in treating congenital toxoplasmosis in utero, and in preventing congenital syphilis with public health measures, we still have not developed effective measures with our most common congenital infection, cytomegalovirus. The clinician still needs to be suspicious of congenital infections as the cause of developmental disabilities, especially intellectual disabilities, hearing loss, and chorioretinitis, and to make the diagnosis and treat when possible.

REFERENCES

Alkalay, A.L., Pomerance, J.J., & Rimonin, D.L. (1987). Fetal varicella syndrome. *Journal of Pediatrics, 111,* 320–323.

American Academy of Pediatrics, Committee on Infectious Diseases. (2003a). Herpes simplex. In *Red book* (26th ed., pp. 344–353). Elk Grove Village, IL: Author.

American Academy of Pediatrics, Committee on Infectious Diseases. (2003b). Rubella. In *Red book* (26th ed., pp. 536–541). Elk Grove Village, IL: Author.

American Academy of Pediatrics, Committee on Infectious Diseases. (2003c). Syphilis. In *Red book* (26th ed., pp. 595–607). Elk Grove Village, IL: Author.

American Academy of Pediatrics, Committee on Infectious Diseases. (2003d). *Toxoplasma gondii* infections (Toxoplasmosis). In *Red book* (26th ed., pp. 631–636). Elk Grove Village, IL: Author.

American Academy of Pediatrics, Committee on Infectious Diseases. (2003e). Varicella-zoster infections. In *Red book* (26th ed., pp. 672–686). Elk Grove Village, IL: Author.

Arvin, A.M., Schmidt, N.J., Cantell, K., & Merigan, T.C. (1982). Alpha interferon administration to infants with congenital rubella. *Antimicrobial Agents and Chemotherapy, 21,* 259–261.

Arvin, A.M., & Whitley, R.J. (2001). Herpes simplex virus infections. In J.S. Remington & J.O. Klein (Eds.), *Infectious diseases of the fetus and newborn infant* (5th ed., pp. 425–446). Philadelphia: W.B. Saunders.

Azimi, P. (2004). Syphilis (*Treponema pallidum*). In R.R. Behrman, R.M. Kliegman, & H.B. Jenson (Eds.), *Nelson textbook of pediatrics* (17th ed., pp. 978–982). Philadelphia: W.B. Saunders.

Baker, D.A. (1999). Management of herpes in pregnancy. *ACOG Practice Bulletin 8.* Washington, DC: American College of Obstetrics and Gynecology.

Barton, L.L., Budd, S.C., Morfitt, W.S., Peters C.J., Ksiazek, T.G., Schindler, R.F., et al. (1993). Congenital lymphocytic choriomeningitis virus infection in twins. *Pediatric Infectious Disease Journal, 12,* 942–946.

Barton, L.L., & Mets, M.B. (2001). Congenital lymphocytic choriomeningitis virus infection: Decade of rediscovery. *Emerging Infections, 33,* 370–374.

Bayley, N. (1969). *Bayley Scales of Infant Development: Birth to two years.* New York: Harcourt Assessment.

Binda, S., Caroppo, S., Dido, P., Primache, V., Veronesi, L., Calvario, A., et al. (2004). Modification of CMV DNA detection from dried blood spots for diagnosing congenital CMV infection. *Journal of Clinical Virology, 30,* 276–279.

Bodeus, M., Hubinont, C., & Goubau, P. (1999). Increased risk of cytomegalovirus transmission in utero during late gestation. *Obstetrics and Gynecology, 93,* 658–660.

Boppana, S., Pass, R.F., Britt, W.S., Stagno, S., & Alford, C.A. (1992). Symptomatic congenital cytomegalovirus infection: Neonatal morbidity and mortality. *Pediatric Infectious Disease Journal, 11,* 93–99.

Brown, Z.A., Selke, S., Zeh, J., Kopelman, J., Maslow, A., Ashley, R.L., et al. (1997). The acquisition of herpes simplex virus during pregnancy. *New England Journal of Medicine, 337,* 509–515.

Brunell, P.A. (1992). Varicella in pregnancy, the fetus, and the newborn: Problems in management. *Journal of Infectious Diseases, 166*(Suppl. 1), S42–S47.

Centers for Disease Control. (1990). Rubella prevention: Recommendations of the Immunizations Practices Advisory Committee (ACIP). *MMWR: Morbidity and Mortality Weekly Report, 39,* 1–18.

Centers for Disease Control. (1991). Increase in rubella and congenital rubella syndrome—United States, 1988–1990. *MMWR: Morbidity and Mortality Weekly Report, 40,* 93–99.

Centers for Disease Control and Prevention. (1993). 1993 sexually transmitted diseases treatment guidelines. *MMWR: Morbidity and Mortality Weekly Report, 42,* 39–43.

Centers for Disease Control and Prevention. (1997). Rubella and congenital rubella syndrome—United States, 1994–1997. *MMWR: Morbidity and Mortality Weekly Report, 46,* 350–354.

Centers for Disease Control and Prevention. (2001). Congenital syphilis—United States, 2000. *MMWR: Morbidity and Mortality Weekly Report, 50,* 573–577.

Chiriboga-Klein, S., Oberfield, S.E., Casullo, A.M., Holahan, N., Fedun, B., Cooper, L.Z., et al. (1989). Growth in congenital rubella syndrome and correlation with clinical manifestations. *Journal of Pediatrics, 115,* 251–255.

Coats, D.K., Demmler, G.J., Paysse, E.A., Du, L.T., & Libby, C., for the Congenital CMV Longitudinal Study Group. (2000). Ophthalmologic findings in children with congenital cytomegalovirus infection. *Journal of the American Association for Pediatric Ophthalmology and Strabismus, 4,* 110–116.

Conboy, T.J., Pass, R.F., Stagno, S., Alford, C.A., Myers, G.J., Britt, W.J., et al. (1987). Early clinical manifestations and intellectual outcome in children with symptomatic congenital cytomegalovirus infection. *Journal of Pediatrics, 111,* 343–348.

Cooper, L.Z. (1985). The history and medical consequences of rubella. *Reviews in Infectious Diseases, 7*(Suppl. 1), S1–S10.

Cooper, L.Z., & Alford, C.A. Jr. (2001). Rubella. In J.S. Remington & J.O. Klein (Eds.), *Infectious diseases of the fetus and newborn infant* (5th ed., pp. 347–388). Philadelphia: W.B. Saunders.

Cooper, L.Z., Green, R.H., Krugman, S., Giles, J.P., & Mirick, G.S. (1965). Neonatal thrombocytopenic purpura and other manifestations of rubella contracted in utero. *American Journal of Diseases of Children, 110,* 416–427.

Couvreur, J., Desmonts, G., Tournier, G., & Szusterkac, M. (1984). A homogeneous series of 210 cases of congenital toxoplasmosis in 0–11 mo old infant detected prospectively. *Annals of Pediatrics (Paris), 31,* 815–819.

Cradock-Watson, I.E., & Ridehalgh, M.K.S. (1976). Specific immunoglobulins in infants with the congenital rubella syndrome. *Journal of Hygiene, 76,* 109–123.

Cubie, H., & Edmond, E. (1985). Comparison of five different methods of rubella IgM antibody testing. *Journal of Clinical Pathology, 38,* 203–207.

Daffos, F., Forestier, F., Capella-Pavlovsky, M., Thulliez, P., Aufrant, C., Valenti, D., et al. (1988). Prenatal management of 746 pregnancies at risk for congenital toxoplasmosis. *New England Journal of Medicine, 318,* 271–275.

Demmler, G.J. (1991). Summary of a workshop on surveillance for congenital cytomegalovirus disease. *Review of Infectious Disease, 13,* 315–329.

Demmler, G.J. (2004). Cytomegalovirus. In R.D. Feigin, J.D. Cherry, G.J. Demmler, & S.L. Kaplan (Eds.), *Textbook of pediatric infectious diseases* (5th ed., pp. 1912–1932). Philadelphia: W.B. Saunders.

Demmler, G.J., Buffone, G.J., Schimbor, C.M., & May, R.A. (1988). Detection of cytomegalovirus in urine from newborns by using polymerase chain reaction DNA amplification. *Journal of Infectious Diseases, 158,* 1177–1184.

Desmond, M.M., Wilson, G.S., Vorderman, A.L., Murphy, M.A., Thurber, S., Fisher, E.S., et al. (1985). The health and educational status of adolescents with congenital rubella syndrome. *Developmental Medicine and Child Neurology, 27,* 721–729.

Desmonts, G., Naot, Y., & Remington, J.S. (1981). Immunoglobulin M-immunosorbent agglutination assay for diagnosis of infectious diseases: Diagnosis of acute congenital and acquired toxoplasma infections. *Journal of Clinical Microbiology, 14*, 486–491.

Eichenwald, H.F. (1960). A study of congenital toxoplasmosis with particular emphasis on clinical manifestations, sequelae and therapy. In J.C. Siim (Ed.), *Human toxoplasmosis* (pp. 41–49). Copenhagen: Munksgaard.

Enders, G. (1984). Varicella-zoster virus infection in pregnancy. *Progress in Medical Virology, 29*, 166–196.

Enders, G. (1985). Serologic test combinations for safe detection of rubella. *Review of Infectious Diseases, 2*(Suppl. 1), S113–S122.

Enders, G., Miller, E., Cradock-Watson, J., Boiley, I., & Ridehalgh, M. (1994). Consequences of varicella and herpes zoster in pregnancy: Prospective study of 1739 cases. *Lancet, 343*, 1547–1550.

Enders, G., Varho-Gobel, M., Lohler, J., Terletskaia-Ladwig, E., & Eggers, M. (1999). Congenital lymphocytic choriomeningitis virus infection: An under-diagnosed disease. *Pediatric Infectious Disease Journal, 18*, 652–655.

European Collaborative Study and Research Network on Congenital Toxoplasmosis. (1996). Low incidence of congenital toxoplasmosis in children born to women infected with human immunodeficiency virus. *European Journal of Obstetrics, Gynecology and Reproductive Biology, 68*, 93–96.

Filisetti, D., Gorcii, M., Pernot-Marino, E., Villard, O., & Candolfi, E. (2003). Diagnosis of congenital toxoplasmosis: Comparison of targets for detection of *Toxoplasma gondii* by PCR. *Journal of Clinical Microbiology, 41*, 4826–4828.

Fleming, D.T., McQuillan, G.M., Johnson, R.E., Nahmias, A.J., Aral, S.O., Lee, F.K., et al. (1997). Herpes simplex virus type 2 in the United States, 1976 to 1994. *New England Journal of Medicine, 337*, 1105–1111.

Foulon, W., Villena, I., Stray-Pedersen, B., Decoster, A., Lappalainen, M., Pinon, J.M., et al. (1999). Treatment of toxoplasmosis during pregnancy: A multicenter study of impact on fetal transmission and children's sequelae at age 1 year. *American Journal of Obstetrics and Gynecology, 180*, 410–415.

Fowler, K.B., McCollister, F.P., Dahle, A.J., Boppana, S., Britt, W.J., & Pass, R.F. (1997). Progressive and fluctuating sensorineural hearing loss in children with asymptomatic congenital cytomegalovirus infection. *Journal of Pediatrics, 130*, 624–630.

Fowler, K.B., & Pass, R.F. (1991). Sexually transmitted diseases in mothers of neonates with congenital cytomegalovirus infection. *Journal of Infectious Diseases, 164*, 259–264.

Freij, B.J., & Sever, J.L. (1988). Herpesvirus infections in pregnancy: Risks to embryo, fetus, and neonate. *Clinics in Perinatology, 15*, 2008–2015.

Freij, B.J., & Sever, J.L. (1991). Toxoplasmosis. *Pediatrics in Review, 12*, 227–236.

Frenkel, J.K. (1985). Toxoplasmosis. *Pediatric Clinics of North America, 32*, 917–932.

Fuentes, I., Rodriguez, M., Domingo, C.J., del Castillo, F., Juncosa, T., & Alvar, J. (1996). Urine sample used for congenital toxoplasmosis diagnosis by PCR. *Journal of Clinical Microbiology, 34*, 2368–2371.

Gershon, A.A. (2001). Chickenpox, measles, and mumps. In J.S. Remington & J.O. Klein (Eds.), *Infectious diseases of the fetus and newborn infant* (5th ed., pp. 683–732). Philadelphia: W.B. Saunders.

Gershon, A.A., & LaRussa, P. (1992). Varicella-zoster virus infections. In S. Krugman, S.L. Katz, A.A. Gershon, & C.M. Wilfert (Eds.), *Infectious diseases of children* (pp. 587–614). St. Louis: Mosby–Year Book.

Gershon, A.A., Raker, R., Steinberg, S., Topf-Olstein, B., & Drusin, L.M. (1976). Antibody to varicella zoster virus in parturient women and their offspring during the first year of life. *Pediatrics, 58*, 692–696.

Hanshaw, J.B. (1995). Cytomegalovirus infections. *Pediatrics in Review, 16*, 43–48.

Harger, J.H., Ernest, J.M., Thurnau, G.R., Moawad, A., Thom, E., Landon, M.B., et al. (2002). Frequency of congenital varicella syndrome in a prospective cohort of 347 pregnant women. *Obstetrics and Gynecology, 100*, 260–265.

Higa, K., Dan, K., & Manabe, H. (1987). Varicella-zoster virus infections during pregnancy: Hypothesis concerning the mechanisms of congenital malformation. *Obstetrics and Gynecology, 69*, 214–222.

Ikeda, M.K., & Jenson, H.B. (1990). Evaluation and treatment of congenital syphilis. *Journal of Pediatrics, 117*, 843–852.

Ingall, D., & Sanchez, P.J. (2001). Syphilis. In J.S. Remington & J.O. Klein (Eds.), *Infectious diseases of the fetus and newborn infant* (5th ed., pp. 643–681). Philadelphia: W.B. Saunders.

Ivarsson, S.-A., Lernmark, B., & Svanberg, L. (1997). Ten-year clinical, developmental, and intellectual follow-up of children with congenital cytomegalovirus infection without neurologic symptoms at one year of age. *Pediatrics, 99*, 800–803.

Jenson, H.B. (2004). Lymphocytic choriomeningitis virus. In R.E. Behrman, R.M. Kliegman, & H.B. Jenson (Eds.), *Nelson textbook of pediatrics* (17th ed., pp. 1099–1100). Philadelphia: W.B. Saunders.

Johansson, P.J., Jonsson, M., Ahlfors, K., Ivarsson, S.A., Svanberg, L., & Guthenberg, C. (1997). Retrospective diagnostics of congenital cytomegalovirus infection performed by polymerase chain reaction in blood stored on filter paper. *Scandinavian Journal of Infectious Diseases, 29*, 465–468.

Kimberlin, D.W., Lakeman, F.D., Arvin, A.M., Prober, C.G., Corey, L., Powell, D.A., et al. (1996). Application of the polymerase chain reaction to the diagnosis and management of neonatal herpes simplex virus disease. National Institute of Allergy and Infectious Diseases Collaborative Antiviral Study Group. *Journal of Infectious Diseases, 174,* 1162–1167.

Kimberlin, D.W., Lin, C.Y., Sanchez, P.J., Demmler, G.J., Dankner, W., Shelton, M., et al., for the National Institute of Allergy and Infectious Diseases Collaborative Antiviral Study Group. (2003). Effect of ganciclovir therapy on hearing in symptomatic congenital cytomegalovirus disease involving the central nervous system: A randomized, controlled trial. *Journal of Pediatrics, 143,* 16–25.

Kimberlin, D., Powell, D., Gruber, W., Diaz, P., Arvin, A., Kumar, M., et al. (1996). Administration of oral acyclovir suppressive therapy after neonatal herpes simplex virus disease limited to the skin, eyes and mouth: Results of a Phase I/II trial. *Pediatric Infectious Disease Journal, 15,* 247–254.

Kohl, S. (2004). Herpes simplex virus. In R.G. Behrman, R.J. Kliegman, & H.B. Jenson (Eds.), *Nelson textbook of pediatrics* (17th ed., pp. 1051–1057). Philadelphia: W.B. Saunders.

Komrower, G.M., Williams, B.L., & Stones, P.B. (1955). Lymphocytic choriomeningitis in the newborn: Probable transplacental infection. *Lancet, 1,* 697–698.

Laforet, E.G., & Lynch, C.L. (1947). Multiple congenital defects following maternal varicella. *New England Journal of Medicine, 236,* 5334–5337.

Lambert, S.R., Taylor, D., Kriss, A., Holzel, H., & Heard, S. (1989). Ocular manifestations of the congenital varicella syndrome. *Archives of Ophthalmology, 107,* 52–56.

Leinikki, P.O., Shekarchi, I., Dorsett, P., & Sever, J.L. (1978). Determination of virus-specific IgM antibodies by using ELISA: Elimination of false-positive results with protein A-Sepharose absorption and subsequent IgM antibody assay. *Journal of Laboratory and Clinical Medicine, 92,* 849–857.

Mascola, L., Pelosi, R., Blount, J.H., Alexander, C.E., & Cates, W. Jr. (1985). Congenital syphilis revisited. *American Journal of Diseases of Children, 139,* 575–580.

McLeod, R., & Remington, J.S. (2004). Toxoplasmosis (*Toxoplasma gondii*). In R.E. Behrman, R.M. Kliegman, & H.B. Jenson (Eds.), *Nelson textbook of pediatrics* (17th ed., pp. 1144–1154). Philadelphia: W.B Saunders.

McLeod, R., Wisner, J., & Boyer, K. (1992). Toxoplasmosis. In S. Krugman, S.L. Katz, A.A. Gershon, & C.M. Wilfert (Eds.), *Infectious diseases of children* (pp. 388–397). St. Louis: Mosby–Year Book.

Mertz, G. (1993). Epidemiology of genital herpes infections. *Infectious Disease Clinics of North America, 4,* 825–837.

Mets, M.B., Barton, L.L., Khan, A.S., & Ksiazek, T.G. (2000). Lymphocytic choriomeningitis virus chorioretinitis mimicking ocular toxoplasmosis in two otherwise normal children. *American Journal of Ophthalmology, 130,* 209–215.

Meyers, J.D. (1974). Congenital varicella in term infants: Risk reconsidered. *Journal of Infectious Diseases, 129,* 215–217.

Miller, E., Cradock-Watson, J.E., & Pollock, T.M. (1982). Consequences of confirmed maternal rubella at successive stages of pregnancy. *Lancet, 2,* 781–784.

Mitchell, C.D., Erlich, S.S., Mastrucci, M.T., Hutto, S.C., Parks, W.P., & Scott, G.B. (1990). Congenital toxoplasmosis occurring in infants perinatally infected with human immunodeficiency virus 1. *Pediatric Infectious Diseases Journal, 9,* 512–518.

Mitchell, D.K., Holmes, S.J., Burke, R.L., Duliege, A.M., & Adler, S.P. (2002). Immunogenicity of a recombinant human cytomegalovirus gB vaccine in seronegative toddlers. *Pediatric Infectious Disease Journal, 21,* 133–138.

Mizrahi, E.M., & Tharp, B.R. (1982). A characteristic EEG pattern in neonatal herpes simplex encephalitis. *Neurology, 32,* 1215–1220.

Mortimer, P.P., Tedder, R.S., Hambling, M.H., Shafi, M.S., & Burkhardt, F. (1981). Antibody capture radioimmunoassay for anti-rubella IgM. *Journal of Hygiene, 86,* 139–153.

Nahmias, A.J., Dowdle, W.R., Josey, W.E., Naib, Z.M., Painter, L.M., & Luce, C. (1969). Newborn infection with herpesvirus hominis types 1 and 2. *Journal of Pediatrics, 75,* 1194–1203.

Nahmias, A.J., Josey, W.E., Naib, Z.M., Freeman, M.G., Fernandez, R.J., & Wheeler, J.H. (1971). Perinatal risk associated with maternal genital herpes simplex virus infections. *American Journal of Obstetrics and Gynecology, 110,* 825–837.

Naot, Y., Desmonts, G., & Remington, J.S. (1981). IgM enzyme-linked immunosorbent assay test for the diagnosis of congenital toxoplasma infection. *Journal of Pediatrics, 98,* 32–36.

Naot, Y., & Remington, J.S. (1980). An enzyme linked immunosorbent assay for detection of IgM antibodies to *Toxoplasma gondii:* Use for diagnosis of acute acquired toxoplasmosis. *Journal of Infectious Diseases, 142,* 757–766.

Nathwani, D., Maclean, A., Conway, S., & Carrington, D. (1998). Varicella infections in pregnancy and the newborn: A review prepared for the UK Advisory Group on Chickenpox on behalf of the British Society for the Study of Infection. *Journal of Infection, 36,* 59–71.

Overall, J.C., Whitley, R.J., Yeager, A.S., McCracken, G.H., & Nelson, J.D. (1984). Prophylactic or anticipatory antiviral therapy for newborns exposed to herpes simplex infection. *Pediatric Infectious Diseases, 3,* 193–195.

Pass, R.F., Duliege, A.M., Boppana, S., Sekulovich, R., Percell, S., Britt, W., et al. (1999). A subunit cytomegalovirus vaccine based on recombinant envelope glycoprotein B and a new adjuvant. *Journal of Infectious Diseases, 180,* 970–975.

Pass, R.F., Fowler, K.B., & Boppana, S. (1991). Progress in cytomegalovirus research. In M.P. Landini (Ed.), *Proceedings of the Third International Cytomegalovirus Workshop, Bologna, Italy* (pp. 3–10). London: Excerpta Medica.

Pass, R.F., & Stagno, S. (1988). Cytomegalovirus. In L.G. Donowitz (Ed.), *Hospital acquired infection in the pediatric patient* (pp. 174–187). Baltimore: Williams & Wilkins.

Plotkin, S.A., Klaus, R.M., & Whitely, J.P. (1966). Hypogammaglobulinemia in an infant with congenital rubella syndrome: Failure of l-adamantanamine to stop virus excretion. *Journal of Pediatrics, 69,* 1085–1091.

Prober, C.G., Sullender, W.M., Yasukawa, L.L., Au, D.S., Yeager, A.S., & Arvin, A.M. (1987). Low risk of herpes simplex virus infections in neonates exposed to the virus at the time of vaginal delivery to mothers with recurrent genital herpes simplex virus infections. *New England Journal of Medicine, 316,* 240–244.

Rabella, N., & Drew, W.L. (1990). Comparison of conventional and shell vial cultures for detecting cytomegalovirus infection. *Journal of Clinical Microbiology, 28,* 806–807.

Reef, S.E., Plotkin, S., Cordero, J.F., Katz, M., Cooper, L., Schwartz, B., et al. (2000). Preparing for elimination of congenital rubella syndrome (CRS): Summary of a workshop on CRS elimination in the United States. *Clinical Infectious Diseases, 31,* 85–95.

Reef, S.E., Plotkin, S., Cordero, J.F., Katz, M., Cooper, L., Schwartz, B., et al. (2001). Neonatal varicella. *Journal of Perinatology, 21,* 545–549.

Remington, J.S., McLeod, R., Thulliez, P., & Desmonts, G. (2001). Toxoplasmosis. In J.S. Remington & J.O. Klein (Eds.), *Infectious diseases of the fetus and newborn infant* (5th ed., pp. 205–346). Philadelphia: W.B. Saunders.

Roizen, N., Swisher, C.N., Stein, M.A., Hopkins, J., Boyer, K.M., Holfels, E., et al. (1995). Neurologic and developmental outcome in treated congenital toxoplasmosis. *Pediatrics, 95,* 11–20.

Sanchez, P.J. (1998). Laboratory tests for congenital syphilis. *Pediatric Infectious Disease Journal, 17,* 70–71.

Sauerbrei, A., Muller, D., Eichhorn, U., & Wutzler, P. (1996). Detection of varicella-zoster virus in congenital varicella syndrome: A case report. *Obstetrics and Gynecology, 88*(4 Pt. 2), 687–689.

Sauerbrei, A., & Wutzler, P. (2001). Neonatal varicella. *Journal of Perinatology, 21,* 545–549.

Sheffield, J.S., Hollier, L.M., Hill, J.B., Stuart, G.S., & Wendel, G.D. (2003). Acyclovir prophylaxis to prevent herpes simplex virus recurrence at delivery: A systematic review. *Obstetrics and Gynecology, 102,* 1396–1403.

Stagno, S. (2001). Cytomegalovirus. In J.S. Remington & J.O. Klein (Eds.), *Infectious diseases of the fetus and newborn infant* (5th ed., pp. 389–424). Philadelphia: W.B. Saunders.

Stagno, S. (2004). Cytomegalovirus. In R.E. Behrman, R.M. Kliegman, & H.B. Jenson (Eds.), *Nelson textbook of pediatrics* (17th ed., pp. 1066–1069). Philadelphia: W.B. Saunders.

Stagno, S., Pass, R.F., Cloud, G., Britt, W.J., Henderson, R.E., Walton, P.D., et al. (1986). Primary cytomegalovirus infection in pregnancy: Incidence, transmission to fetus, and clinical outcome. *Journal of the American Medical Association, 256,* 1904–1908.

Stagno, S., Reynolds, D.W., Tsiantos, A., Fuccillo, D.A., Long, W., & Alford, C.A. (1975). Comparative serial virologic and serologic studies of symptomatic and subclinical congenitally and natally acquired cytomegalovirus infections. *Journal of Infectious Diseases, 132,* 568–577.

Stagno, S., & Whitley, R.J. (1985). Herpesvirus infections of pregnancy. Part II: Herpes simplex virus and varicella-zoster virus infections. *New England Journal of Medicine, 313,* 1327–1330.

Stepick-Biek, R., Thulliez, R., Araujo, F.G., & Remington, J.S. (1990). IgA antibodies for diagnosis of acute congenital and acquired toxoplasmosis. *Journal of Infectious Diseases, 162,* 270–273.

Sweet, R.L., & Gibbs, R.S. (1990). Herpes simplex infection. In *Infectious diseases of the female genital tract* (2nd ed., pp. 144–150). Baltimore: Williams & Williams.

Tookey, P.A. & Peckham, C.S. (1999). Surveillance of congenital rubella in Great Britain 1971–1969. *British Medical Journal, 318,* 769–770.

Townsend, J.J., Baringer, J.B., Wolinsky, J.S., Malamud, N., Mednick, J.P., Panitch, H.S., et al. (1979). Progressive rubella panencephalitis late onset after congenital rubella. *New England Journal of Medicine, 292,* 990–993.

Troendle-Atkins, J., Demmler, G.J., & Buffone, G.J. (1993). Rapid diagnosis of herpes simplex virus encephalitis by using the polymerase chain reaction. *Journal of Pediatrics, 123,* 376–380.

Troendle-Atkins, J., Demmler, G.J., Williamson, W.D., McDonald, J.M., Istas, A.S., & Buffone, G.J. (1994). Polymerase chain reaction to detect cytomegalovirus DNA in the cerebrospinal fluid of neonates with congenital infection. *Journal of Infectious Diseases, 169,* 1334–1337.

Vesikari, T., Meurman, O.H., & Maki, R. (1980). Persistent rubella-specific IgM-antibody in the cerebrospinal fluid of a child with congenital rubella. *Archives of Disease in Childhood, 55,* 46–48.

Warren, W.P., Balcarek, K., Smith, R., & Pass R.F. (1992). Comparison of rapid methods of detection of cytomegalovirus in saliva with virus isolation in tissue culture. *Journal of Clinical Microbiology, 30,* 786–789.

Whitley, R.J., Arvin, A., Prober, C., Corey, L., Burchett, S., Plotkin, S., et al. (1991). Predictors of morbidity and mortality in neonates with herpes simplex virus infections. *New England Journal of Medicine, 324,* 450–454.

Whitley, R.J., Nahmias, A.J., Visintine, A.M., Fleming, C.L., & Alford, C.A. (1980). The natural history of herpes simplex virus infection of mother and newborn. *Pediatrics, 66,* 489–494.

Whitley, R.J., Seng-Jaw, S., Linneman, C., Liu, C., Pazin, O., &Alford, C.A., for the National Institute of Allergy and Infectious Diseases Collaborative Antiviral Study Group. (1982). Herpes simplex encephalitis. *Journal of the American Medical Association, 247,* 317–320.

Wild, N.J., Sheppard, S., Smithells, R.W., Holzel, H., & Jones, G. (1989). Onset and severity of hearing loss due to congenital rubella infection. *Archives of Disease in Childhood, 64,* 1280–1283.

Williamson, W.D., Percy, A.K., Yow, M.D., Gerson, B., Catlin, F.I., Koppelman, M.L., et al. (1990). Asymptomatic congenital cytomegalovirus infection: Audiologic, neuroradiologic and neurodevelopmental abnormalities during the first year. *American Journal of Diseases of Children, 144,* 1365–1368.

Wolff, S.M. (1973). The ocular manifestations of congenital rubella: A prospective study of 328 cases of congenital rubella. *Journal of Pediatric Ophthalmology and Strabismus, 10,* 101–141.

Wong, S.Y., Hajdu, M.P., Ramirez, R., Thulliez, P., McLeod, R., & Remington, J.S. (1993). Role of specific immunoglobulin E in diagnosis of acute toxoplasma infection and toxoplasmosis. *Journal of Clinical Microbiology, 31,* 2952–2959.

Wright, R., Johnson, D., Neumann, M., Ksiazek, T.G., Rollin, P., Keech, R.V., et al. (1997). Congenital lymphocytic choriomeningitis virus syndrome: A disease that mimics congenital toxoplasmosis or cytomegalovirus infection. *Pediatrics, 100,* E9.

11

Children Born to Drug-Dependent Mothers

HAROLYN M.E. BELCHER AND SONJA JOHNSON-BROOKS

Drug use during pregnancy remains one of the leading preventable causes of adverse infant and child outcomes. The spectrum of adverse outcomes includes health, cognitive, and behavioral sequelae. This chapter focuses on infant and child neurodevelopmental and neurobehavioral outcomes following fetal tobacco and illicit drug exposure. Fetal alcohol exposure is covered in Chapter 12 in this volume.

INCIDENCE AND PREVALENCE

The latest National Survey of Drug Use and Health, formerly called the National Household Survey, estimated that 19.7 million U.S. citizens (8.1% of the population) ages 12 years and older were current users of illicit drugs (Substance Abuse and Mental Health Services Administration, 2006). Another 126 million and 71.5 million U.S. citizens, ages 12 and older, were current users of alcohol and tobacco, respectively. The highest rate of illicit drug use, 20.2%, was reported among young adults ages 18–25 years. It was estimated that 22 million U.S. citizens met criteria for alcohol or drug dependence. Native Americans and individuals of multiracial heritage had the highest percentages of drug dependence—21.0% and 10.9%, respectively. White and African American individuals had a similar rate of dependence (9.3% and 8.5%, respectively). Asian Americans had the lowest rates of dependence (4.5%), and the rate for Hispanic Americans was 9.3%.

Among pregnant women ages 15–44 years, 3.9% (representing slightly more than 97,000 births per year) reported using illicit drugs in the month prior to interview, a rate significantly lower than the rate among women who were not pregnant (9.9%) (Substance Abuse and Mental Health Services Administration, 2006). In 2005, marijuana was the most widely used illicit drug among pregnant women (2.8% of pregnant women). One percent of all U.S. pregnant women used illicit drugs other than marijuana, including cocaine (or crack), heroin, hallucinogens, inhalants, or any nonmedical use of prescription-type psychotherapeutic drugs. Alcohol and tobacco use continue to remain significant preventable threats to favorable birth and offspring neurodevelopmental outcomes. Among pregnant women ages 15–44 years, 3.9% reported binge alcohol ingestion (five or more drinks at the same time or within a couple of hours of each other) on at least 1 day within the month prior to the survey. Seventeen percent of pregnant women smoked cigarettes within the month prior to the survey.

CHALLENGES TO DRAWING CONCLUSIONS FROM OUTCOME STUDIES OF CHILDREN WITH INTRAUTERINE DRUG EXPOSURE

Many factors should be considered when reviewing the literature on neurodevelopmental outcome of children with intrauterine drug exposure. Drug dependence is the result of a complex, often multigenerational, interplay between the individual, the drug, and the environment. At the individual level, having a parent with a history of drug dependence may impart genetic and environmental risk factors that contribute to poor neurobehavioral and neurodevelopmental outcomes in children (Block, Block, & Keyes, 1988; Conners et al., 2004; Luthar, Cushing, & Rounsaville, 1996; Wilens, 2004). There is a higher incidence of attention-deficit/hyperactivity disorder and conduct disorder in individuals with alcohol and illicit drug dependence compared to those without substance abuse disorders (Hovens, Cantwell, & Kiriakos, 1994; Milin, Halikas, Meller, & Morse, 1991). Women who become alcohol and drug dependent have higher rates of depression, suicidal behavior, anxiety, and withdrawn behaviors during childhood (Wilsnack, Wilsnack, Kristjanson, Vogeltanz-Holm, & Windle, 2004). In addition, individuals who abuse drugs are more likely to have experienced physical abuse and sexual abuse than their non–drug-dependent peers (Dube et al., 2003; Wilsnack, Vogeltanz, Klassen, & Harris, 1997).

Each drug has chemical properties that are associated with its addictive potential and has neurophysiological effects on the individual as well as the fetus. Frequently, infants are exposed to more than one potentially neurotoxic drug. The environment of the drug-dependent parent may expose the child to risk factors that are associated with poor neurodevelopmental outcome. Lack of parental supervision, family chaos, increased duration of child self-care, community drug trafficking, and peer influences may all play pivotal roles in infant, child, and adolescent outcomes (Block et al., 1988; Chilcoat & Anthony, 1996; Chilcoat, Dishion, & Anthony, 1995; Crum, Lillie-Blanton, & Anthony, 1996; Kandel, Simcha-Fagan, & Davies, 1986; National Institute on Drug Abuse, 1995; Richardson et al., 1989). Many of the aforementioned factors are challenging to compensate for, even using complex statistical models, and thus confound outcome results. Yet, given these caveats, the following information can be gleaned from the literature.

SPECTRUM OF HEALTH, BEHAVIOR, AND NEURODEVELOPMENTAL OUTCOMES FOR CHILDREN EXPOSED TO DRUGS

Tobacco

History Indigenous peoples of the Western Hemisphere introduced Christopher Columbus to tobacco in the 1490s (Ray & Ksir, 1996d). Tobacco has an interesting history in the early U.S. colonies; by the 1600s, tobacco was one of the major exports to England. Although there are more than 60 species of *Nicotiana,* two are most widely used: *Nicotiana tobacum,* the large-leafed plant grown in more than 100 countries, and *Nicotiana rustica,* the small-leafed plant indigenous to South America.

Chemical and Neuropharmacological Properties Nicotine, a colorless liquid alkaloid, is the active ingredient in tobacco. Ninety percent of nicotine is absorbed from inhalation, and the liver subsequently metabolizes 80%–90% of the nicotine. The physiological effects of smoking one cigarette are similar to injecting 1 mg of nicotine intravenously. Nicotine is one the most toxic drugs known. In humans, the lethal dose of nicotine is 60 mg (Ray & Ksir, 1996d).

Nicotine may adversely affect multiple neurotransmitter pathways. Nicotine stimulates and then occupies the cholinergic receptors, thereby inactivating the receptor sites. Thus, although nicotine exposure is known to affect multiple neurotransmitter systems, including those of serotonin (5-hydroxytryptamine, 5-HT), norepinephrine, and dopamine, it appears that the cholinergic neurotransmitter system is most affected (Law et al., 2003; Xu, Seidler, Ali, Slikker, & Slotkin, 2001). For example, Xu et al. (2001) found that nicotine administered to pregnant rats resulted in an increase in the binding of paroxetine in the midbrain, causing damage to serotonergic systems and creating a pattern of reactive sprouting at the 5-HT cell bodies. It is postulated that the damage to 5-HT neuronal and synaptic activity resulting from nicotine exposure may contribute to the onset of depression in tobacco-exposed children. Other animal models demonstrated that rats exposed to the nicotine equivalent of one pack of cigarettes per day via implantable osmotic mini-pumps had abnormal fetal brain development. Nicotine binds to the nicotinic acetylcholine receptors in the fetal brain, causing disruption of synaptic activity, cell loss, and neuronal damage. It has been determined that fetuses in the second and third trimesters are particularly susceptible to the negative effects of tobacco exposure because the number of nicotine receptor binding sites tends to significantly increase during these time periods (Cornelius, Ryan, Day, Goldschmidt, & Willford, 2001).

Other biological studies indicate that carbon monoxide and nicotine lower maternal uterine blood flow by up to 38% (Law et al., 2003). This, in turn, reduces the concentration of oxygen in maternal tissues and fetal cord blood, thereby leading to fetal hypoxia and malnutrition. This chronic hypoxia may disrupt neuronal pathways and impair cognitive development (Albrecht et al., 2004; DiFranza, Aligne, & Weitzman, 2004).

Nicotine causes the release of catecholamines. It also produces tolerance, physical dependence, and withdrawal symptoms, including irritability, anxiety, hunger, and craving, in cigarette smokers (Jarvik & Schneider, 1992).

Perinatal Health Impact The teratogenic effects of smoking tobacco and passive transmission through environmental tobacco smoke are extensively documented in the literature. Children exposed to nicotine in utero have an increased risk for low birth weight, defined as birth weight of less than 2,500 g (Jaakkola & Gissler, 2004). This increased risk, resulting from intrauterine growth retardation, demonstrates a dose–response relationship at the rate of 5% weight reduction per pack of cigarettes smoked per day (DiFranza et al., 2004). These infants weigh approximately 150–250 g less than non–tobacco-exposed infants and account for 20%–30% of all low-birth-weight babies (Law et al., 2003).

Inadequate fetal lung development and poor neonatal pulmonary functioning are associated with prenatal exposure to tobacco (DiFranza et al., 2004). Jakkola and Gissler (2004) tested the causal effect of maternal smoking during pregnancy on asthma development in childhood in a population-based cohort of Finnish singleton births ($N = 58,841$). These authors postulated that the direct effect of prenatal smoking on the risk for development of asthma in the first 7 years of life would be partially mediated by the presence of intrauterine growth retardation and preterm delivery. The results show that children whose mothers smoked more than 10 cigarettes per day during gestation had a 36% higher chance of developing asthma in the first 7 years of life. There appeared to be a small reduction in the direct effect when intrauterine growth retardation and preterm delivery were added to the model, suggesting that these mediating factors account for only a small portion of the effect.

Neurodevelopmental Outcome Law et al. (2003) examined the effects of smoking during pregnancy on neurobehavioral functioning in newborns. The NICU Network Neurobehavioral Scale (Lester & Tronick, 2005) was completed on 56 neonates 48 hours after birth (Boukydis & Lester, 1999). Examiners were blind to the prenatal smoking exposure status of the infants. Maternal smoking was measured using a timeline follow-back interview of smoking and alcohol use during pregnancy (Brown, Burgess, Sales, Evans, & Miller, 1998) and salivary cotinine bioassay. The results suggested neurotoxic effects of in utero tobacco exposure on neurobehavior. Specifically, the exposed infants showed evidence of increased excitability, hypertonia, and stress/abstinence symptoms in the central nervous system (CNS), gastrointestinal system, and visual field. These findings were demonstrated at a lower dose rate (6 cigarettes per day) than the 10 cigarettes per day that is traditionally cited in the literature on the dose–response relationship. The authors noted that establishing these neuroteratogenic effects at birth may provide compelling evidence for the role of prenatal tobacco exposure, over and above postnatal contextual factors, in the development of long-term deficits such as lower IQ and attention-deficit/hyperactivity disorder.

Cornelius et al. (2001) examined the longitudinal effects of prenatal smoking on neuropsychological functioning in a sample of 593 children. Participants were followed prospectively from the fourth month of gestation to 10 years. Neuropsychological tests were conducted at the 10-year follow-up to assess the impact of gestational smoking on learning, memory, problem solving, mental flexibility, attention, and hand–eye coordination. Results from longitudinal studies demonstrated an adverse effect of gestational smoking on learning, memory, problem solving, and hand–eye coordination. These results remained statistically significant even while accounting for other prenatal and current maternal substance abuse, demographic, psychological, and environmental variables. Fried, Watkinson, and Gray (2003) found that prenatal cigarette exposure continued to be negatively associated with overall intelligence, as measured by the short form of the Wechsler Intelligence Scale for Children (Wechsler, 1991), in a sample of 145 teenagers 13–16 years old.

Prenatal nicotine exposure is also associated with deficits in language development (DiFranza et al., 2004). Results from the Ottawa Prenatal Prospective Study (OPPS) showed that children prenatally exposed to cigarettes had decreased responsiveness on auditory-related items on the Bayley Scales of Infant Development (Bayley, 1969) at 12 and 24 months of age. Delays in language development continued to exist at age 4. Cognitive deficits, specifically on measures of verbal intelligence, reading, and language, continued to persist into early adolescence, providing further evidence for the dose-dependent response noted at earlier ages (Fried, Watkinson, & Siegel, 1997).

The literature clearly demonstrates that prenatal tobacco exposure is a risk factor for development of behavior problems, specifically aggressive and antisocial behaviors (Maughan, Taylor, Caspi, & Moffitt, 2004; Silberg et al., 2003). This relationship also seems to follow a dose–response effect between the amount of prenatal exposure and the emergence of behavior problems (DiFranza et al., 2004). Although researchers have attempted to account for confounding factors when analyzing the statistical relationship between prenatal exposure and childhood conduct problems, the strength of the association relies primarily on correlational data. The strength of the associa-

tion is reduced when other known confounding factors are analyzed. Maughan et al. (2004) identified three sources of confounding: 1) prenatal smoking exposure is more common among mothers with risk factors predisposing children to conduct problems; 2) women with antisocial traits are more likely to smoke; and 3) exposure to prenatal smoking, a behavior that is partly heritable, may be a genetic risk factor for conduct problems.

Silberg et al. (2003) tested the causal association between prenatal tobacco exposure and childhood conduct disorder in a sample of 538 Caucasian male twins. General linear models were used to examine the direct effect of prenatal smoking on childhood conduct disorder. Mother's conduct disorder symptoms in childhood were included as an operationalization of the latent variable "antisociality." The effects of prenatal smoking were significantly reduced (from $p = .03$ to $p = .18$) when mother's childhood conduct disorder symptoms and age were included in the model. Further latent variable modeling indicated a significant association between the latent transmission variable and childhood conduct disorder. Excluding the direct path between prenatal smoking and child conduct disorder did not worsen the model fit, suggesting a stronger association between maternal conduct symptoms and child behavior than tobacco exposure and child behavior.

Cocaine

History   Cocaine is a stimulant derived from the leaves of the *Erythroxylon coca* plant that thrives at 2,000–8,000 ft above sea level in the Andes mountains of Bolivia and Peru (Ray & Ksir, 1996c). Known cultivation of coca leaves dates back over 800 years, when the Incas of Peru used the coca leaves in religious ceremonies and later treated the leaves like money. Early Europeans imported coca leaves for many products, including coca lozengers, coca tea, and coca wine. In the United States, from the 1880s until 1903, coca leaf extract was used in Coca-Cola, to give Coke it's "lift." Sigmund Freud was a proponent of using cocaine to treat psychiatric illness and narcotic withdrawal, until a close friend developed cocaine psychosis while Dr. Freud treated his friend's morphine addiction. Today, cocaine continues to be used as a local anesthetic for otolaryngology and endoscopy procedures.

Chemical and Neuropharmacological Properties Cocaine blocks the presynatic reuptake of dopamine and serotonin. In addition, cocaine inhibits the nicotinic acetylcholine receptors located in the plasma membrane of nerve and muscle cells (Karpen, Aoshima, Abood, & Hess, 1982; Karpen & Hess, 1986). Cocaine has a binding site located on the dopamine transporter of the nerve terminal (Giros, Jaber, Jones, Wightman, & Caron, 1996).

Cocaine produces many cardiac effects, including tachycardia, arrythmia, elevations in blood pressure, myocardial infarction, and asystole. Cocaine's cardiac effects are attributed to stimulation of alpha receptors, its local anesthetic properties, and blockade of calcium–sodium channels (Crumb & Clarkson, 1990; Jones & Tackett, 1990). Cocaine can induce seizures, psychosis, and paranoia and can worsen depression (Gold, 1992; Merriam, Medalia, & Levine, 1988; Ray & Ksir, 1996c).

Using readily available ingredients, including baking soda, it was discovered that cocaine could be distilled into a concentrated smokable form of cocaine base that produced an intense and rapid "high." By the 1980s, this stable, highly addictive form of cocaine, known as "crack," made cocaine readily available, not only to the rich and famous, but to residents of inner city areas as well (Ray & Ksir, 1996c). Thus, the crack epidemic of the mid-1980s began.

Perinatal Health Impact Cocaine use during pregnancy is associated with an increase in adverse outcomes, including higher risk of sexually transmitted disease (36% vs. 1%, $p = .000$), premature rupture of membranes (23% vs. 0%, $p = .000$), abruption of the placenta (4% vs. 0%, $p = .007$), and fetal demise (5% vs. 0%, $p = .004$), when compared with women without a history of cocaine use (Hladky, Yankowitz, & Hansen, 2002). In a case–control study of 400 mother–infant dyads (200 with maternal cocaine use and 200 without drug use) (Ogunyemi & Hernandez-Loera, 2004), infants born to mothers with a history of cocaine use had a significantly higher risk of having respiratory distress syndrome (14% vs. 4%, $p = .001$), congenital syphilis (12% vs. 1%, $p = .000$), and prolonged hospital stay (10 vs. 3 days, $p = .000$).

Neurodevelopmental Outcome Early case reports led to many premature conclusions about neurodevelopmental outcome of children with intrauterine cocaine exposure. One meta-analysis of 118 studies of children with intrauterine cocaine exposure demonstrated that the majority of studies (92%) included children with polydrug exposure, including alcohol, tobacco, marijuana, and opiates (Lester, 1998). Over time, more sophisticated techniques were developed to identify and quantify cocaine and other drug use, and data collection and statistical analyses improved.

Impairment of brain growth in children with intrauterine drug exposure (IUDE) is documented in multiple studies (Azuma & Chasnoff, 1993; Bandstra, Morrow, Anthony, Accornero, & Fried, 2001; Butz et al., 1999; Chasnoff, 1992; Hurt, Brodsky, Braitman, & Giannetta, 1995). Disturbances of neuronal migration and differentiation have been reported in human infants exposed to cocaine during their gestation (Dominguez, Aguirre Vila-Coro, Slopis, & Bohan, 1991; Gomez-Anson & Ramsey, 1994; Heier et al., 1991; Kaufmann, 1990). The most common neurological anomaly found in children with cocaine/polydrug exposure is microcephaly (Frank et al., 1990).

In a study of children with cocaine/polydrug exposure, mean birth head circumference for infants with cocaine-only exposure was 1.71 standard deviations below the mean, and head circumference was 1.0 and 1.52 standard deviations below the mean for opiate-only and cocaine and opiate–exposed infants, respectively (Butz et al., 1999). Preliminary data from a small case–control magnetic resonance imaging (MRI) study suggest smaller white matter volumes in the frontal lobes of children with cocaine/polydrug exposure compared with children without drug exposure (z-score, 2.2; $p < .05$) (Belcher et al., 2004).

Midline prosencephalic developmental abnormalities, including agenesis of the corpus callosum, septo-optic dysplasia, and absence of the septum pellucidum, have been reported (Dominguez et al., 1991) in case studies of children with intrauterine cocaine exposure. Cranial ultrasound data, collected during the neonatal period, demonstrated that 35% of infants with intrauterine cocaine/polydrug exposure had one or more intracranial abnormalities (Dogra et al., 1994). Ultrasound findings were suggestive of degenerative changes or focal infarctions of the basal ganglia. In addition, schizencephaly and neuronal heterotopias are documented in children born to cocaine-dependent mothers (Gomez-Anson & Ramsey, 1994; Heier et al., 1991).

Differences in attention, distractibility, and visual memory have been reported in infants with cocaine/polydrug exposure (Bandstra et al., 2001; Jacobson, Jacobson, Sokol, Martier, & Chiodo, 1996; Pulsifer et al., 2002; Pulsifer, Radonovich, Belcher, & Butz, 2004; Struthers & Hansen, 1992). Studies of early school-age children with IUDE document significantly higher externalizing (e.g., inattention, aggression, disruptive behavior) and internalizing (e.g., withdrawn, anxious behaviors) behavior problems (Butz et al., 2000, 2001; Chasnoff et al., 1989). Delaney-Black et al. (2004) demonstrated gender- and duration-specific effects of prenatal cocaine, finding that behavior in school-age boys was more significantly and negatively affected by cocaine exposure than was behavior in girls. In a study of 145 children (111 with IUDE and 34 nonexposed children) by Butz et al. (2000), parents/caregivers of children with IUDE reported significantly more overall behavior problems, especially anxious/depressed behaviors. In addition, parenting stress was higher in caregivers of children with IUDE. Children with IUDE had significantly more deficits in attention compared with children without drug exposure (Butz, Pulsifer, Leppert, Rimrodt, & Belcher, 2003). A longitudinal case–cohort study of 476 children (253 cocaine-exposed and 223 non–cocaine-exposed infants) documented performance deficiencies on measures of visual attention in 7-year-old children with intrauterine cocaine exposure, after adjusting for

medical and sociodemographic variables and alcohol, marijuana, and tobacco exposure.

A recent meta-analysis of 36 studies that met stringent criteria, including using only prospective controlled studies whose evaluators were masked to drug of exposure and whose participants included children with cocaine exposure without substantial opiate, amphetamine, or phencyclidine exposure (Frank, Augustyn, Knight, Pell, & Zuckerman, 2001), concluded that, if exposure to other drugs was controlled, statistically or in the study design, prenatal cocaine exposure did not contribute to growth retardation. In addition, the majority of studies that controlled for other drug exposure did not find an association between intrauterine cocaine exposure and adverse cognitive and language outcomes. Half of the studies analyzed (three of six) demonstrated deficient motor skills in the first 7 months. Most notably, studies do support an association between cocaine exposure and less affective expression during infancy and early childhood, as well as less optimal scoring on behavior ratings scales and tests of sustained attention.

The Maternal Lifestyle Study (MLS) is a prospective, longitudinal, multisite study funded by the National Institute of Child Health and Human Development; the National Institute on Drug Abuse; the Administration on Children, Youth and Families; and the Center for Substance Abuse Treatment to determine the association between cocaine and opiate exposure and developmental and behavioral outcome, controlling for a host of medical and psychosocial covariates (Lester, 1998). In Phase I, conducted between 1993 and 1995, 19,079 mother–infant dyads were screened for enrollment from Brown University, University of Miami, Wayne State University, and the University of Tennessee at Memphis medical centers; 16,988 mother–infant dyads met criteria and 11,811 mothers consented to participate. Meconium samples were collected from the infants for enzyme-multiplied immunoassay for cocaine, opiates, tetrahydrocannabinol, amphetamines, and phencyclidine followed by gas chromatography/mass spectroscopy confirmation. In Phase II, 1,388 mother–infant dyads with and without drug exposure matched for race, gender, and gestational age were developed from the pool of 11,811. Results from the 1-month evaluation demonstrated subtle but consistent differences following adjustment for other drug exposure, including lower arousal, poorer quality of movement and self-regulation, increased hypertonia on the NICU Network Neurobehavioral Scale (Lester & Tronick, 2005), and longer interpeak I–III and interpeak III–V latencies on auditory brain response testing (Lester et al., 2002, 2003). At 3 years of age, cocaine exposure was not associated with Bayley Scales of Infant Development II (Bayley, 1993) Mental Development Index (MDI), Psychomotor Development Index (PDI), or Behavior Record Score scores (Messinger et al., 2004).

In sum, although a direct causal effect between cocaine and cognitive deficits was not apparent in this large prospective study, cocaine exposure was associated with factors such as low birth weight, disruptions in maternal care, low socioeconomic status, and low vocabulary scores that may place the child at risk for lower academic functioning (Messinger et al., 2004).

Marijuana

History   The most widely used illicit drug during pregnancy is marijuana (Office of Applied Studies, 2004). Marijuana is produced from the leaf of the *Cannabis* plant. George Washington grew *Cannabis* at Mt. Vernon, most probably to use for making rope or for "medicinal uses" (Ray & Ksir, 1996a).

Chemical and Neuropharmacological Properties   Marijuana's primary active ingredient is $\Delta 9$-tetrahydrocannabinol; however, marijuana is composed of more than 400 other chemical compounds (Ray & Ksir, 1996a). Sixty-one of these chemicals are unique to the *Cannabis* plant and are thus termed *cannabinoids*. Marijuana is considered a sedative-hypnotic.

Perinatal Health Impact   One large prospective study of more than 7,000 pregnant women found no associations between marijuana use and low birth weight, preterm delivery, or abruptio placentae obstetric outcome

from marijuana use during pregnancy (Shiono et al., 1995). Another study of more than 700 infants found no increased incidence of pregnancy, labor, or delivery complications associated with marijuana use during pregnancy (Richardson, Day, & McGauhey, 1993). In addition to the aforementioned study, two large prospective studies—the OPPS (Fried & O'Connell, 1987) and the Maternal Health Practices and Child Development Projects (MHPCD) (Richardson et al., 1993)—provide much of our knowledge on the effects of intrauterine marijuana exposure. Initiated in 1978, the OPPS is an ongoing longitudinal investigation of 190 children born to middle-class, primarily college-educated women with ($n = 140$) and without ($n = 50$) a history of marijuana use during pregnancy (Fried, Watkinson, Dillon, & Dulberg, 1987). From 1983 to 1985, the MHPCD recruited 763 primarily low-income women from Pittsburgh during their fourth month of gestation to monitor the developmental outcome of their children with and without exposure to marijuana and alcohol. These studies, along with others (Jacobson et al., 1994), found that marijuana use during pregnancy was not associated with fetal growth retardation.

Neurodevelopmental Outcome   Neonatal findings reported in infants with prenatal marijuana exposure include increased tremors and startles, abnormal sleep patterns characterized by decreased quiet sleep, and poorer habituation to light (Fried & Makin, 1987; Richardson et al., 1993). Interestingly, in a prospective study of 24 Jamaican infants with marijuana exposure compared to nonexposed neonates, there were no differences between the groups on day 3, when the infants were assessed with the Neonatal Assessment Scale (Brazelton, 1984) and at 1 month. Infants with heavy marijuana exposure demonstrated improved autonomic stability and quality of alertness, less irritability, and better self-regulation (Dreher, Nugent, & Hudgins, 1994). The Dreher et al. study is important to note because these neonates were generally exposed to higher potency marijuana and were less likely to be exposed to other drugs compared with neonates in U.S. and Canadian studies.

Outcome evaluation of 12- and 24-month-old children with intrauterine marijuana exposure enrolled in the OPPS study found no association between Bayley Scales of Infant Development (Bayley, 1969) scores and marijuana exposure after controlling for the home environment (Fried & Watkinson, 1988). Marijuana exposure was negatively correlated with the home environment. Findings of unadjusted hierarchical regression analyses of early elementary school–age children with second-trimester intrauterine marijuana exposure found that children exposed to marijuana had more errors of commission on the Continuous Performance Test (Lindgren & Lyons, 1984), suggesting increased impulsivity in marijuana-exposed children compared with children with no exposure (Leech, Richardson, Goldschmidt, & Day, 1999). At 10 years of age, children with heavy marijuana exposure during the first trimester had lower scores on the design memory and screening index of the Wide Range Assessment of Memory and Learning (Sheslow & Adams, 1990); in addition, the finding of increased commission errors persisted (Richardson, Ryan, Willford, Day, & Goldschmidt, 2002). The magnitude of the marijuana effects was small at this age, and, on structural equation modeling, there were no significant associations between marijuana exposure and neuropsychological domains. Recent functional MRI studies of young adults (18–21 years of age) with prenatal marijuana exposure demonstrated increased neural activity in the bilateral prefrontal cortex and right premotor cortex and decreased cerebellar activation during response inhibition (Smith, Fried, Hogan, & Cameron, 2004). More commission errors continued to be present in young adults exposed to marijuana.

In summary, intrauterine marijuana exposure appears to be associated with persistent deficits in prefrontal lobe functioning as evidenced by both the MHPCD and OPPS longitudinal studies. Specifically, children with intrauterine marijuana exposure were noted to have deficiencies in the stability of attention (e.g., the ability to maintain attention over time) (Fried & Watkinson, 2001). Clinically, increased impulsivity versus inattention is noted in children with fetal marijuana exposure (Leech et al., 1999).

Opiates

History   Opiates refer to a group of drugs derived from the juice of the *Papaver somniferum* (poppy) plant. The juice is only produced for about a week each year, after the petals drop and before the seeds mature. The use of opium can be traced back to 1500 B.C., when the Ebers papyrus documents the use of opium for excessive crying in children (Ray & Ksir, 1996b).

Chemical and Neuropharmacological Properties   Opium's primary medicinal uses include analgesia, cough suppression, and as an antidiarrheal. In the United States, there are more than 20 opioid drugs, including agents such as opium, morphine (the primary active ingredient of opium), codeine (the second most important alkaloid derivative), heroin (derived from morphine with two acetyl groups added to increase lipid solubility), methadone (a synthetic narcotic analgesic), and α-ʟ-methadyl acetate (levomethadyl acetate) (one of the longest acting synthetic opiates).

Opioids exert their effects through the multiple opioid receptors located in the brain, spinal cord, neural plexuses in the gastrointestinal tract and other parts of the autonomic nervous system, and white blood cells (Jaffe, 1992). Opioid receptors, including mu, kappa, delta, and lambda, serve different physiological functions. Mu and delta receptors are associated with mood, reinforcing effects, respiration, pain, blood pressure, and endocrine and gastrointestinal function. Opioids may act as either neurotransmitters, changing transsynaptic potential by acting at the presynaptic terminal, or neuromodulators, modulating the release of neurotransmitter at the postsynaptic site.

Perinatal Health Impact   The majority of studies suggest that infants with intrauterine opiate exposure weigh less and have smaller head circumferences than their non–drug-exposed peers (Fulroth, Phillips, & Durand, 1989; Kelly, Davis, & Henschke, 2000; Naeye,

Blanc, Leblanc, & Khatamee, 1973; Rosen & Johnson, 1982; Wilson, Desmond, & Wait, 1981). Infants with fetal opiate exposure have been reported to have a higher incidence of respiratory distress and infections, as well as longer hospitalizations resulting from withdrawal-related and non–withdrawal-related morbidity.

One of the major morbidities in infants with in utero opiate exposure is neonatal abstinence syndrome (NAS) or neonatal drug withdrawal syndrome. NAS is characterized by CNS and gastrointestinal symptoms, including irritability, tremors, disrupted sleep patterns, rigidity, seizures, poor suck, vomiting, diarrhea, dehydration, poor weight gain, temperature instability, and diaphoresis (Desmond & Wilson, 1975; Finnegan, Connaughton, Kron, & Emich, 1975; Kandall et al., 1977; "Neonatal drug withdrawal," 1998). NAS varies in frequency and onset depending on the dose and type of maternal opiate use (Fulroth et al., 1989; Kaltenbach & Finnegan, 1986; Kelly et al., 2000). Because of methadone's 15- to 57-hour half-life (Jaffe, 1992), neonatal withdrawal may not be seen until 72 hours after birth; however, onset may be protracted and can occur up to 4 weeks (Kandall & Gartner, 1974) after birth. In contrast, withdrawal from heroin is usually evident within 24–72 hours. Symptoms of NAS may be measured by a variety of instruments, including those developed by Finnegan et al. (1975) and Lipsitz (1975), to determine whether pharmacological management is necessary.

Probably the most common pharmacological agents used to control the adverse effects of NAS are tincture of opium (10 mg morphine equivalent/mL), paregoric (containing anhydrous morphine, 0.4 mg/mL), methadone, and phenobarbital. Tincture of opium is preferred for treatment of NAS because, not only does tincture of opium substitute for the opiate causing the withdrawal symptoms, but it also contains fewer additives and less alcohol than paregoric. Tincture of opium is usually diluted 25-fold (diluted tincture of opium [DTO]) so that DTO has the same concentration of morphine equivalent as paregoric. Initial DTO dosage is 0.1 mL/kg (2 drops/kg) every 4 hours with feedings. This dosage may be increased by

2 drops/kg every 4 hours until NAS symptoms are controlled. Dosage is gradually tapered by decreasing the dose amount, not by increasing dosing interval ("Neonatal drug withdrawal," 1998).

Paregoric is one of the earliest and most efficacious agents used to treat neonatal withdrawal ("Neonatal drug withdrawal," 1998; Tunis, Webster, Izes, & Finnegan, 1984). Fewer seizures and more physiological sucking was noted when infants were treated with paregoric compared with diazepam (Herzlinger, Kandall, & Vaughan, 1971; Kron, Litt, Eng, Phoeniz, & Finnegan, 1976). Paregoric use has declined, replaced by DTO, because of its many potentially toxic additives, including isoquinoline derivatives, camphor, 44% ethanol concentration, and benzoic acid.

Phenobarbital and diazepam have also been used to treat NAS. Phenobarbital reduces the irritability and tremulousness of NAS but does not control gastrointestinal symptoms. Poor feeding, weight gain, and feeding time were noted during phenobarbital therapy for NAS compared with paregoric (Kron et al., 1976). In addition, phenobarbital may cause CNS depression. In a study by Kaltenbach and Finnegan (1986), infants with NAS initially treated with phenobarbital were more likely to require a second drug to control NAS when compared with paregoric. A phenobarbital loading dose of 16 mg/kg over 24 hours, with a maintenance dosage of 2–8 mg/kg/day, controlled most narcotic symptoms (Finnegan, Mitros, & Hopkins, 1979). One to 2 mg of diazepam every 8 hours may result in rapid suppression of NAS signs; however, diazepam may result in CNS depression, poor sucking, and late-onset seizures (Kandall & Gartner, 1974). In addition, in one study, diazepam was never successful as a single agent to treat NAS.

Neurodevelopmental Outcome The MLS prospective, multisite study of auditory brain stem responses of 1,031 infants (477 cocaine/opiate-exposed infants and 554 non–drug-exposed infants) demonstrated longer latency to peak V at 50 dB with and without adjustment for covariates and longer peak III–V interpeak latency in unadjusted analysis (Lester et al., 2003). Covariates included socioeconomic status, gestational age, conceptional age, maternal age, study site, and other drug use. Earlier studies of opiate-exposed infants also demonstrated longer latencies to peak V and longer III–V interpeak latency (McPherson, Madden, & Payne, 1989; Trammer, Aust, Koser, & Obladen, 1992). These findings are thought to be associated with delayed maturation of the inferior colliculus in the midbrain (Krumholtz, Felix, Goldstein, & McKenzie, 1985; Murray, 1988).

Results of a study comparing paregoric, phenobarbital (loading), phenobarbital (titration), diazepam, and no treatment (for infants with mild NAS symptomatology) for infants with opiate exposure demonstrated no differences among the groups on 6-month Bayley Scales of Infant Development (Bayley, 1969) MDI score (Kaltenbach & Finnegan, 1986). In a longitudinal study of 39 infants (16 methadone-exposed and 23 non–drug-exposed) using partial-order scalogram analyses to study the differences among the scores on the subtests of the Infant Behavior Rating, only motor coordination distinguished between the methadone and non–drug-exposed infants at 4 months, after adjusting for family and medical risk factors. By 12 months, the attention subtest distinguished between the two groups of infants (Marcus, Hans, & Jeremy, 1984). One study that documents statistically significant differences in developmental outcome during infancy was done by Rosen and Johnson (1982), who studied 64 infants (41 methadone-exposed and 23 non–drug-exposed) at 6, 12, and 18 months. At 12 and 18 months, significant differences favoring the non–drug-exposed infants were found in mean MDI ($p < .05$) and PDI scores ($p < .05$) on the Bayley Scales of Infant Development.

The MLS study of children with cocaine and opiate exposure evaluated 1,227 infants (474 with cocaine exposure, 50 with opiate exposure, and 48 with cocaine and opiate exposure) through 3 years of age (Messinger et al., 2004). Opiate exposure was not associated with overall MDI at 2 or 3 years of age. Unadjusted mean PDI was 3.9 points lower than in infants not exposed to opiates ($p = .003$). Once analysis models were adjusted for covariates (study site, infant age, infant birth weight, ma-

ternal care, Home Observation for Measurement of the Environment Inventory [Caldwell & Bradley, 1984] score, and ethnicity), opiate exposure was no longer associated with PDI at 3 years of age. There were no cocaine-by-opiate interactions found in these analyses. In addition, there were no increases in clinically significant Behavior Rating Scale scores.

In summary, opiate exposure is associated with significant neonatal morbidity, including NAS, low infant growth parameters, and increased infections (Fulroth et al., 1989; Kelly et al., 2000; Wilson et al., 1981). Studies of infants with intrauterine opiate exposure now document potential maturation delays in midbrain development (Lester et al., 2003). The most recent longitudinal prospective data suggest no differences in MDI, PDI, and evaluator-rated behavior measures in children 2 and 3 years of age with opiate exposure compared to children without drug exposure (Messinger et al., 2004).

TREATMENT AND PREVENTION

Research to date on children with IUDE has focused primarily on examining their developmental trajectory. Studies demonstrate that risk factors associated with prenatal substance exposure may be a potential contributor to negative neurodevelopmental outcomes. Given this information, early intervention strategies are being developed to detect and prevent the onset of these problems and reduce their negative impact. Interventions geared toward treating the associated risk factors of IUDE may improve the quality of life for these children.

Home-based nursing interventions are one type of community-based educational intervention used for women who are drug dependent and their children. Home-based interventions seek to promote the health and well-being of children and families at risk for poor developmental outcomes by providing education, access to services, and enrichment experiences in the natural environment. Nurses are especially suited to provide intervention because of their expertise in the areas of women's and children's health, their capacity to handle complex clinical issues, and their ability to teach health awareness while improving access to medical care (Olds, 2002). Black et al. (1994) examined the impact of a home intervention designed to positively support parenting and child development through the first 18 months postpartum. Modest improvements were noted on measures of recovery, emotional responsiveness of the mother, and attitudes toward parenting for the women in the intervention. There were no developmental differences between the intervention and control children at the 18-month follow-up. The findings reveal only modest changes on measures of drug use and parenting behaviors resulting from the home intervention. In another randomized study of home-based nursing intervention in a cohort of 200 children with IUDE (Butz et al., 2001), mothers perceived that children who received home-based nursing intervention had significantly fewer behavior problems. Hofkosh et al. (1995) found a similar pattern of results, noting that the developmental capabilities of the children in their home-based clinical intervention were age appropriate at 1 year. These authors noted that the ability of the mother to provide a developmentally supportive environment most significantly affected child development.

Schuler, Nair, Black, and Kettinger (2000) conducted a home-based nursing intervention for 131 women with active substance abuse problems up to 24 months postdelivery. A pre–post randomized control design was used, with follow-up assessments at 6-month intervals through 24 months and yearly thereafter. The program was divided into two components. The parent component focused on teaching the parent to identify and to appropriately utilize family, community, and social systems for a range of services, including public assistance, domestic violence, and drug treatment. The child component focused on enhancing mother–child relationships by teaching parents how to play with their children in order to promote age-appropriate developmental skills. This home-based nursing intervention used a combination of the Infant Health and Development Program (''Enhancing the outcomes,'' 1990) and the HELP at Home curriculum from the Hawaii Early Learning Profile (Furuno, O'Reilly, Hosaka, Inatsuka, & Zeisloft-Falbey, 1991) that was modified to apply specifically to substance-abusing mothers and their children.

Results indicate that children in the early intervention group demonstrated significant improvements in motor and mental development compared with children in the control group up to 18 months. There were no differences between the groups on language development. Intervention mothers and mothers in the control group had similar rates of ongoing drug use (43% and 36%, respectively). There was no significant effect of the home-based intervention on mother–child relationships as operationalized by maternal competence and observed child responsiveness during mother–child interactions at the 18-month follow-up (Schuler, Nair, & Black, 2002). A sample of 108 cocaine-abusing mothers using the same home-based intervention (Schuler, Nair, & Kettinger, 2003) showed significant improvements in cognitive scores on the Bayley Scales of Infant Development (Bayley, 1969) following the home-based intervention; however, ongoing maternal drug use was associated with poor infant cognitive developmental outcomes through 18 months postpartum. These results suggest that ongoing maternal drug use is a critical environmental factor that appears to adversely affect the outcome of intervention trials in children exposed to IUDE.

Results of the home-based interventions have mixed outcomes. Overall, the findings suggest that these interventions result in some improvement of knowledge of parenting strategies, development of more positive attitudes toward parenting, and enhancement of the quality of mother–child relationships. Studied interventions demonstrate varied results on child development.

Other types of treatment approaches to improve mother–child relationships with drug-dependent mothers have focused on including multiple treatment methods within one model to provide a more comprehensive and holistic drug treatment approach. McComish et al. (2003) evaluated the efficacy of a family-focused residential drug treatment program for drug-dependent women and their children. Significant improvements in the mother's parenting knowledge and treatment retention were noted. This study demonstrated the importance of inclusion of children in early intervention with drug-dependent mothers. Though the children in the intervention did not initially show signs of developmental delay, longitudinal data demonstrated signs of motor and language delay for some of the children in the intervention group. Thus, early detection and consequently early treatment of developmental delays occurred in the children as a result of their participation in this comprehensive residential program.

In a qualitative analysis of mothers' attitudes toward holistic treatment approaches, Sword, Niccols, and Fan (2004) found that mothers with drug dependence noted several perceived benefits to this model of substance abuse treatment. New Choices, an interdisciplinary substance abuse treatment program, offered mothers with drug dependence the following services: addictions treatment, nutrition counseling, parenting education, children's programs, prenatal and postpartum services, and access to a family physician. Participants indicated that the program provided unique opportunities to positively affect several areas of their lives, including increasing positive health outcomes, providing better access to community-based services, enhancing parenting skills, and improving child behavior and development. They specifically attributed changes in their children's motor, social, and language skills to participation in the enhanced children's program. Likewise, Luthar and Suchman (2000) found significant quantitative results supporting the inclusion of a supportive psychotherapy group designed to enhance abstinence, parenting skills, and mother–child relationships as an adjunct to a traditional methadone maintenance program offering drug treatment and access to medical care. Children whose mothers participated in the comprehensive drug-treatment program had a lower risk for child maltreatment and spent more interactive time with their mothers immediately following the intervention.

Although most studies have focused on adult mothers, substance abuse among young mothers (younger than 20 years) is also an important public health concern. Studies show that young drug-abusing mothers are at increased risk for parenting problems as a result of a variety of factors, including lack of parenting experience, less education, and lack of fiscal resources. Furthermore, these mothers may have their own problems understanding and developing basic psychoemotional developmental skills such as learning to trust, problem solving, and impulse control (Baldwin, Rawlings, Marshall, Conger, & Abbott, 1999). Field et al. (1998) examined the effect of a multimodal intervention for adolescent mothers and their children with IUDE. The participants in this study attended a 4-month treatment program located within their vocational school. Mothers received drug and social rehabilitation, parenting and vocational courses, and relaxation therapy. Infants were placed in a nursery while their mothers attended high school or GED preparation classes. The mothers volunteered as teacher-aid trainees in the nursery and learned parenting skills while tending to their babies. At the 6-month follow-up, the mothers and infants in the treatment group looked similar to a non–drug-exposed control group on measures of mother–child interactions and child developmental outcomes.

The Mom Empowerment, Too (ME2) program combined community-based nursing and drug treatment using a participatory action research model for a young adult population. Participatory action research allows researchers to collect outcome data while modifying aspects of the intervention in response to the feedback of the participants (Rains & Ray, 1995). Public health nurses used a variety of treatment modalities to provide case management services; access to drug treatment, medical care, and social services; educational and parenting classes; group therapy; and life skills training. The children (ages birth to 5) took part in developmental and health-promoting exercises while their parents attended their sessions. The investigators documented improvements in taking responsibility and learning to trust. Both areas of improvement are related to effective parenting.

The studies presented in this chapter delineate the potential neurobiological effects of IUDE on child health, neurodevelopment, and behavior. The lack of research on programs specifically focused on prevention of poor behavior and developmental outcomes in children with IUDE underscores the need for empirically validated interventions. Such interventions should ideally begin during pregnancy and continue throughout childhood, both to prevent the onset of negative outcomes and to address the risk of behavioral and developmental deficits. A few promising prevention and treatment approaches continue to undergo rigorous and systematic study: inclusion of drug treatment for mothers to prevent relapse (Schuler et al., 2002), clinic- and home-based parent training in combination with live coaching (Barnard & McKeganey, 2004), and providing a holistic approach to treatment where multiple services and providers are within the same location (McComish et al., 2003; McMurtrie, Rosenberg, Kerker, Kan, & Graham, 1999; Sword et al., 2004).

CONCLUSION

Intrauterine tobacco and illicit drug exposure are associated with adverse infant health outcomes. Studies suggest that infants exposed to these substances are at risk for attention and behavioral deficits during childhood. Data suggest that nicotine exposure places the child at risk for poorer cognitive outcome. Less conclusive data exist on the causal associations between illicit drug exposure and cognitive outcomes. At-risk environmental exposures, such as poverty, community violence, neglect, and maltreatment, as well as genetics may contribute to adverse outcomes of children with IUDE. More research is necessary to develop comprehensive prevention and intervention programs for this vulnerable population.

REFERENCES

Albrecht, S.A., Maloni, J.A., Thomas, K.K., Jones, R., Halleran, J., & Osborne, J. (2004). Smoking cessation counseling for pregnant women who smoke: Scientific basis for practice for AWHONN's SUCCESS project. *Journal of Obstetric, Gynecologic, and Neonatal Nursing, 33,* 298–305.

Azuma, S.D., & Chasnoff, I.J. (1993). Outcome of children prenatally exposed to cocaine and other drugs—a path-analysis of 3-year data. *Pediatrics, 92,* 396–402.

Baldwin, J.H., Rawlings, A., Marshall, E.S., Conger, C.O., & Abbott, K.A. (1999). Mom Empowerment,

Too! (ME2): A program for young mothers involved in substance abuse. *Public Health Nursing, 16,* 376–383.

Bandstra, E.S., Morrow, C.E., Anthony, J.C., Accornero, V.H., & Fried, P.A. (2001). Longitudinal investigation of task persistence and sustained attention in children with prenatal cocaine exposure. *Neurotoxicology and Teratology, 23,* 545–559.

Barnard, M., & McKeganey, N. (2004). The impact of parental problem drug use on children: What is the problem and what can be done to help? *Addiction, 99,* 552–559.

Bayley, N. (1969). *Bayley Scales of Infant Development: Birth to two years.* New York: Harcourt Assessment.

Bayley, N. (1993). *Bayley Scales of Infant Development—Second Edition manual.* New York: Harcourt Assessment.

Belcher, H.M.E., Kraut, M.A., Slifer, K.J., Cataldo, M.D., Stern, S.S., Sparks, B.F., et al. (2004). Children with in-utero drug exposure: Preliminary MRI findings. *Pediatric Research, 55,* 82A.

Black, M.M., Nair, P., Kight, C., Wachtel, R., Roby, P., & Schuler, M. (1994). Parenting and early development among children of drug-abusing women: Effects of home intervention. *Pediatrics, 94,* 440–448.

Block, J., Block, J.H., & Keyes, S. (1988). Longitudinally foretelling drug usage in adolescence: Early childhood personality and environmental precursors. *Child Development, 59,* 336–355.

Boukydis, C.F., & Lester, B.M. (1999). The NICU Network Neurobehavioral Scale: Clinical use with drug exposed infants and their mothers. *Clinics in Perinatology, 26,* 213–230.

Brazelton, T.B. (1984). *Neonatal Behavioral Assessment Scale: Clinics in developmental medicine.* (2nd ed.) Philadelphia: Lippincott-Raven.

Brown, R.A., Burgess, E.S., Sales, S.D., Evans, D.M., & Miller, I.W. (1998). Reliability and validity of a smoking timeline follow-back interview. *Psychology of Addictive Behaviors, 12,* 101–112.

Butz, A.M., Kaufmann, W.E., Royal, R., Kolodner, K., Pulsifer, M., Lears, M.K., et al. (1999). Opiate and cocaine exposed newborns: Growth outcomes. *Journal of Child and Adolescent Substance Abuse, 8,* 1–16.

Butz, A.M., Pulsifer, M.B., Leppert, M., Rimrodt, S., & Belcher, H. (2003). Comparison of intelligence, school readiness skills, and attention in in-utero drug-exposed and nonexposed preschool children. *Clinical Pediatrics (Philadelphia), 42,* 727–739.

Butz, A.M., Pulsifer, M., Marano, N., Belcher, H., Lears, M.K., & Royall, R. (2001). Effectiveness of a home intervention for perceived child behavioral problems and parenting stress in children with in utero drug exposure. *Archives of Pediatrics and Adolescent Medicine, 155,* 1029–1037.

Butz, A.M., Pulsifer, M., Marano, N., Lang, M.E., Belcher, H.M.E., Lears, M.K., et al. (2000). Effectiveness of home intervention for children with behavior problems and parenting stress in children with in-utero drug exposure (IUDE). *Pediatric Research, 47,* 178A.

Caldwell, B., & Bradley, R. (1984). *Home Observation for Measurement of the Environment.* Little Rock: University of Arkansas at Little Rock.

Chasnoff, I.J. (1992). Cocaine, pregnancy, and the growing child. *Current Problems in Pediatrics, 22,* 302–321.

Chasnoff, I.J., Anson, A., Hatcher, R., Stenson, H., Iaukea, K., & Randolph, L.A. (1989). Prenatal exposure to cocaine and other drugs. In J.A. Harvey & B.E. Kosofsky (Eds.), *Cocaine: Effects on the developing brain* (pp. 314–328). New York: New York Academy of Sciences.

Chilcoat, H.D., & Anthony, J.C. (1996). Impact of parent monitoring on initiation of drug use through late childhood. *Journal of the American Academy of Child and Adolescent Psychiatry, 35,* 91–100.

Chilcoat, H.D., Dishion, T.J., & Anthony, J.C. (1995). Parent monitoring and the incidence of drug sampling in urban elementary school children. *American Journal of Epidemiology, 141,* 25–31.

Conners, N.A., Bradley, R.H., Mansell, L.W., Liu, J.Y., Roberts, T.J., Burgdorf, K., et al. (2004). Children of mothers with serious substance abuse problems: An accumulation of risks. *American Journal of Drug and Alcohol Abuse, 30,* 85–100.

Cornelius, M.D., Ryan, C.M., Day, N.L., Goldschmidt, L., & Willford, J.A. (2001). Prenatal tobacco effects on neuropsychological outcomes among preadolescents. *Journal of Developmental and Behavioral Pediatrics, 22,* 217–225.

Crum, R.M., Lillie-Blanton, M., & Anthony, J.C. (1996). Neighborhood environment and opportunity to use cocaine and other drugs in late childhood and early adolescence. *Drug and Alcohol Dependence, 43,* 155–161.

Crumb, W.J., Jr., & Clarkson, C.W. (1990). Characterization of cocaine-induced block of cardiac sodium channels. *Biophysical Journal, 57,* 589–599.

Delaney-Black, V., Covington, C., Nordstrom, B., Ager, J., Janisse, J., Hannigan, J.H., et al. (2004). Prenatal cocaine: Quantity of exposure and gender moderation. *Journal of Developmental and Behavioral Pediatrics, 25,* 254–263.

Desmond, M.M., & Wilson, G.S. (1975). Neonatal abstinence syndrome: Recognition and diagnosis. *Addictive Diseases, 2,* 113–121.

DiFranza, J.R., Aligne, C.A., & Weitzman, M. (2004). Prenatal and postnatal environmental tobacco smoke exposure and children's health. *Pediatrics, 113,* 1007–1015.

Dogra, V.S., Shyken, J.M., Menon, P.A., Poblete, J., Lewis, D., & Smeltzer, J.S. (1994). Neurosonographic abnormalities associated with maternal history of cocaine use in neonates of appropriate size for their gestational age. *AJNR: American Journal of Neuroradiology, 15,* 697–702.

Dominguez, R., Aguirre Vila-Coro, A., Slopis, J.M., & Bohan, T.P. (1991). Brain and ocular abnormalities in infants with in utero exposure to cocaine and other street drugs. *American Journal of Diseases of Children, 145,* 688–695.

Dreher, M.C., Nugent, K., & Hudgins, R. (1994). Prenatal marijuana exposure and neonatal outcomes in Jamaica: An ethnographic study. *Pediatrics, 93,* 254–260.

Dube, S.R., Felitti, V.J., Dong, M., Chapman, D.P., Giles, W.H., & Anda, R.F. (2003). Childhood abuse, neglect, and household dysfunction and the risk of illicit drug use: the adverse childhood experiences study. *Pediatrics, 111,* 564–572.

Enhancing the outcomes of low-birth-weight, premature infants: A multisite, randomized trial. The Infant Health and Development Program (1990). *Journal of the American Medical Association, 263,* 3035–3042.

Field, T.M., Scafidi, F., Pickens, J., Prodromidis, M., Pelaez-Nogueras, M., Torquati, J., et al. (1998). Polydrug-using adolescent mothers and their infants receiving early intervention. *Adolescence, 33,* 117–143.

Finnegan, L.P., Connaughton, R.E., Kron, R., & Emich, J. (1975). Neonatal abstinence syndrome: Assessment and Management. *Addictive Diseases: An International Journal, 2,* 141–158.

Finnegan, L.P., Mitros, T.F., & Hopkins, L.E. (1979). Management of neonatal narcotic abstinence utilizing a phenobarbital loading dose method. *NIDA Research Monograph, 27,* 247–253.

Frank, D.A., Augustyn, M., Knight, W.G., Pell, T., & Zuckerman, B. (2001). Growth, development, and behavior in early childhood following prenatal cocaine exposure: A systematic review. *Journal of the American Medical Association, 285,* 1613–1625.

Frank, D.A., Bauchner, H., Parker, S., Huber, A.M., Kyei-Aboagye, K., Cabral, H., et al. (1990). Neonatal body proportionality and body composition after in utero exposure to cocaine and marijuana. *Journal of Pediatrics, 117,* 622–626.

Fried, P.A., & Makin, J.E. (1987). Neonatal behavioural correlates of prenatal exposure to marihuana, cigarettes and alcohol in a low risk population. *Neurotoxicology and Teratology, 9,* 1–7.

Fried, P.A., & O'Connell, C.M. (1987). A comparison of the effects of prenatal exposure to tobacco, alcohol, cannabis and caffeine on birth size and subsequent growth. *Neurotoxicology and Teratology, 9,* 79–85.

Fried, P.A., & Watkinson, B. (1988). 12- and 24-month neurobehavioural follow-up of children prenatally exposed to marihuana, cigarettes and alcohol. *Neurotoxicology and Teratology, 10,* 305–313.

Fried, P.A., & Watkinson, B. (2001). Differential effects on facets of attention in adolescents prenatally exposed to cigarettes and marihuana. *Neurotoxicology and Teratology, 23,* 421–430.

Fried, P.A., Watkinson, B., Dillon, R.F., & Dulberg, C.S. (1987). Neonatal neurological status in a low-risk population after prenatal exposure to cigarettes, marijuana, and alcohol. *Journal of Developmental and Behavioral Pediatrics, 8,* 318–326.

Fried, P.A., Watkinson, B., & Gray, R. (2003). Differential effects on cognitive functioning in 13- to 16-year-olds prenatally exposed to cigarettes and marihuana. *Neurotoxicology and Teratology, 25,* 427–436.

Fried, P.A., Watkinson, B., & Siegel, L.S. (1997). Reading and language in 9- to 12-year olds prenatally exposed to cigarettes and marijuana. *Neurotoxicology and Teratology, 19,* 171–183.

Fulroth, R., Phillips, B., & Durand, D.J. (1989). Perinatal outcome of infants exposed to cocaine and/or heroin in utero. *American Journal of Diseases of Children, 143,* 905–910.

Furuno, S., O'Reilly, K.A., Hosaka, C.M., Inatsuka, T.T., & Zeisloft-Falbey, B. (1991). *HELP at home: Hawaii Early Learning Profile.* Palo Alto, CA: VORT Corp.

Giros, B., Jaber, M., Jones, S.R., Wightman, R.M., & Caron, M.G. (1996). Hyperlocomotion and indifference to cocaine and amphetamine in mice lacking the dopamine transporter. *Nature, 379,* 606–612.

Gold, M.S. (1992). Cocaine and "crack": Clinical aspects. In J.H. Lowinson, P.D. Ruiz, R.B. Millman, & J.G. Langrod (Eds.), *Substance abuse: A comprehensive textbook* (2nd ed., pp. 205–221). Baltimore: Williams & Wilkins.

Gomez-Anson, B., & Ramsey, R.G. (1994). Pachygyria in a neonate with prenatal cocaine exposure: MR features. *Journal of Computer Assisted Tomography, 18,* 637–639.

Heier, L.A., Carpanzano, C.R., Mast, J., Brill, P.W., Winchester, P., & Deck, M.D. (1991). Maternal cocaine abuse: The spectrum of radiologic abnormalities in the neonatal CNS. *AJNR: American Journal of Neuroradiology, 12,* 951–956.

Herzlinger, R.A., Kandall, S.R., & Vaughan, H.G. (1971). Neonatal seizures associated with narcotic withdrawal. *Journal of Pediatrics, 91,* 638–641.

Hladky, K., Yankowitz, J., & Hansen, W.F. (2002). Placental abruption. *Obstetrical and Gynecological Survey, 57,* 299–305.

Hofkosh, D., Pringle, J.L., Wald, H.P., Switala, J., Hinderliter, S.A., & Hamel, S.C. (1995). Early interactions between drug-involved mothers and infants: Within-group differences. *Archives of Pediatrics and Adolescent Medicine, 149,* 665–672.

Hovens, J.G., Cantwell, D.P., & Kiriakos, R. (1994). Psychiatric comorbidity in hospitalized adolescent substance abusers. *Journal of the American Academy of Child and Adolescent Psychiatry, 33,* 476–483.

Hurt, H., Brodsky, N.L., Braitman, L.E., & Giannetta, J. (1995). Natal status of infants of cocaine users and control subjects: A prospective comparison. *Journal of Perinatology, 15,* 297–304.

Jaakkola, J.J., & Gissler, M. (2004). Maternal smoking in pregnancy, fetal development, and childhood asthma. *American Journal of Public Health, 94,* 136–140.

Jacobson, J.L., Jacobson, S.W., Sokol, R.J., Martier, S.S., Ager, J.W., & Shankaran, S. (1994). Effects of alcohol use, smoking, and illicit drug use on fetal growth in black infants. *Journal of Pediatrics, 124,* 757–764.

Jacobson, S.W., Jacobson, J.L., Sokol, R.J., Martier, S.S., & Chiodo, L.M. (1996). New evidence for neurobehavioral effects of in utero cocaine exposure. *Journal of Pediatrics, 129,* 581–590.

Jaffe, J.H. (1992). Opiates: Clinical aspects. In J.H. Lowinson, P. Ruiz, R.B. Millman, & J.G. Langrod (Eds.), *Substance abuse: A comprehensive textbook* (2nd ed., pp. 186–194). Baltimore: Williams & Wilkins.

Jarvik, M.E., & Schneider, N.G. (1992). Nicotine. In J.H. Lowinson, P. Ruiz, R.B. Millman, & J.G. Langrod (Eds.), *Substance abuse: A comprehensive textbook* (2nd ed., pp. 334–356). Baltimore: Williams & Wilkins.

Jones, L.F., & Tackett, R.L. (1990). Central mechanisms of action involved in cocaine-induced tachycardia. *Life Sciences, 46,* 723–728.

Kaltenbach, K., & Finnegan, L.P. (1986). Neonatal abstinence syndrome, pharmacotherapy and developmental outcome. *Neurobehavioral Toxicology and Teratology, 8,* 353–355.

Kandall, S.R., Albin, S., Gartner, L.M., Lee, K.S., Eidelman, A., & Lowinson, J. (1977). The narcotic-dependent mother: Fetal and neonatal consequences. *Early Human Development, 1,* 159–169.

Kandall, S.R., & Gartner, L.M. (1974). Late presentation of drug withdrawal symptoms in newborns. *American Journal of Diseases of Children, 127,* 58–61.

Kandel, D.B., Simcha-Fagan, O., & Davies, M. (1986). Risk factors for delinquency and illicit drug use from adolescence to young adulthood. *Journal of Drug Issues, 16,* 67–90.

Karpen, J.W., Aoshima, H., Abood, L.G., & Hess, G.P. (1982). Cocaine and phencyclidine inhibition of the acetylcholine receptor: Analysis of the mechanisms of action based on measurements of ion flux in the millisecond-to-minute time region. *Proceedings of the National Academy of Sciences of the United States of America, 79,* 2509–2513.

Karpen, J.W., & Hess, G.P. (1986). Cocaine, phencyclidine, and procaine inhibition of the acetylcholine receptor: Characterization of the binding site by stopped-flow measurements of receptor-controlled ion flux in membrane vesicles. *Biochemistry, 25,* 1777–1785.

Kaufmann, W.E. (1990). Developmental cortical abnormalities after prenatal exposure to cocaine. *Society of Neuroscience Abstracts, 16,* 305.

Kelly, J.J., Davis, P.G., & Henschke, P.N. (2000). The drug epidemic: Effects on newborn infants and health resource consumption at a tertiary perinatal centre. *Journal of Paediatrics and Child Health, 36*, 262–264.

Kron, R.E., Litt, M., Eng, D., Phoeniz, M.D., & Finnegan, L.P. (1976). Neonatal narcotic abstinence: Effects of pharmacotherapeutic agents and maternal drug usage on nutritive sucking behavior. *Journal of Pediatrics, 88*, 637–641.

Krumholtz, A., Felix, J., Goldstein, P., & McKenzie, E. (1985). Maturation of the brain-stem evoked potential in preterm infants. *Electroencephalography and Clinical Neurophysiology, 62*, 124–134.

Law, K.L., Stroud, L.R., Lagasse, L.L., Niaura, R., Liu, J., & Lester, B.M. (2003). Smoking during pregnancy and newborn neurobehavior. *Pediatrics, 111*, 1318–1323.

Leech, S.L., Richardson, G.A., Goldschmidt, L., & Day, N.L. (1999). Prenatal substance exposure: Effects on attention and impulsivity of 6-year-olds. *Neurotoxicology and Teratology, 21*, 109–118.

Lester, B. (1998). The Maternal Lifestyles Study. *Annals of the New York Academy of Sciences, 846*, 296–305.

Lester, B.M., Lagasse, L., Seifer, R., Tronick, E.Z., Bauer, C.R., Shankaran, S., et al. (2003). The Maternal Lifestyle Study (MLS): Effects of prenatal cocaine and/or opiate exposure on auditory brain response at one month. *Journal of Pediatrics, 142*, 279–285.

Lester, B.M., & Tronick, E.Z. (2005). *NICU Network Neurobehavioral Scale (NNNS)*. Baltimore: Paul H. Brookes Publishing Co.

Lester, B.M., Tronick, E.Z., Lagasse, L., Seifer, R., Bauer, C.R., Shankaran, S., et al. (2002). The Maternal Lifestyle Study: Effects of substance exposure during pregnancy on neurodevelopmental outcome in 1-month-old infants. *Pediatrics, 110*, 1182–1192.

Lindgren, S., & Lyons, D. (1984). *Pediatric Assessment of Cognitive Efficiency (PACE)*. Iowa City: University of Iowa, Department of Pediatrics.

Lipsitz, P.J. (1975). A proposed narcotic withdrawal score for use with newborn infants: A pragmatic evaluation of efficacy. *Clinical Pediatrics, 14*, 592–594.

Luthar, S.S., Cushing, G., & Rounsaville, B.J. (1996). Gender differences among opioid abusers: Pathways to disorder and profiles of psychopathology. *Drug and Alcohol Dependence, 43*, 179–189.

Luthar, S.S., & Suchman, N.E. (2000). Relational Psychotherapy Mothers' Group: A developmentally informed intervention for at-risk mothers. *Development and Psychopathology, 12*, 235–253.

Marcus, J., Hans, S.L., & Jeremy, R.J. (1984). A longitudinal study of offspring born to methadone-maintained women. III. Effects of multiple risk factors on development at 4, 8, and 12 months. *American Journal of Drug and Alcohol Abuse, 10*, 195–207.

Maughan, B., Taylor, A., Caspi, A., & Moffitt, T.E. (2004). Prenatal smoking and early childhood conduct problems: Testing genetic and environ-mental explanations of the association. *Archives of General Psychiatry, 61*, 836–843.

McComish, J.F., Greenberg, R., Ager, J., Essenmacher, L., Orgain, L.S., & Bacik, W.J., Jr. (2003). Family-focused substance abuse treatment: A program evaluation. *Journal of Psychoactive Drugs, 35*, 321–331.

McMurtrie, C., Rosenberg, K.D., Kerker, B.D., Kan, J., & Graham, E.H. (1999). A unique drug treatment program for pregnant and postpartum substance-using women in New York City: Results of a pilot project, 1990–1995. *American Journal of Drug and Alcohol Abuse, 25*, 701–713.

McPherson, D.L., Madden, J.D., & Payne, T.F. (1989). Auditory brainstem-evoked potentials in term infants born to mothers addicted to opiates. *Journal of Perinatology, 9*, 262–267.

Merriam, A.E., Medalia, A., & Levine, B. (1988). Partial complex status epilepticus associated with cocaine abuse. *Biological Psychiatry, 23*, 515–518.

Messinger, D.S., Bauer, C.R., Das, A., Seifer, R., Lester, B.M., Lagasse, L.L., et al. (2004). The Maternal Lifestyle Study: Cognitive, motor, and behavioral outcomes of cocaine-exposed and opiate-exposed infants through three years of age. *Pediatrics, 113*, 1677–1685.

Milin, R., Halikas, J.A., Meller, J.E., & Morse, C. (1991). Psychopathology among substance abusing juvenile offenders. *Journal of the American Academy of Child and Adolescent Psychiatry, 30*, 569–574.

Murray, A.D. (1988). Newborn auditory brainstem evoked responses (ABRs): Prenatal and contemporary correlates. *Child Development, 59*, 571–588.

Naeye, R.L., Blanc, W., Leblanc, W., & Khatamee, M.A. (1973). Fetal complications of maternal heroin addiction: Abnormal growth, infections, and episodes of stress. *Journal of Pediatrics, 83*, 1055–1061.

National Institute on Drug Abuse. (1995). *Drug use among racial/ethnic minorities*. Bethesda, MD: National Institutes of Health.

Neonatal drug withdrawal. (1998). *Pediatrics, 101*, 1079–1088.

Office of Applied Studies. (2002). *Illicit drug use in the past month among females aged 15 to 44, by pregnancy status and demographic characteristics: Percentages*. Rockville, MD: Substance Abuse and Mental Health Services Administration.

Office of Applied Studies. (2004). *The National Survey on Drug Use and Health report: Pregnancy and substance abuse*. Rockville, MD: Substance Abuse and Mental Health Services Administration.

Ogunyemi, D., & Hernandez-Loera, G.E. (2004). The impact of antenatal cocaine use on maternal characteristics and neonatal outcomes. *Journal of Maternal-Fetal and Neonatal Medicine, 15*, 253–259.

Olds, D.L. (2002). Prenatal and infancy home visiting by nurses: From randomized trials to community replication. *Prevention Science, 3*, 153–172.

Pulsifer, M.B., Radonovich, K., Belcher, H.M.E., & Butz, A.M. (2004). Intelligence and school readiness skills in preschool children with prenatal drug exposure. *Child Neuropsychology, 10,* 89–101.

Pulsifer, M.B., Radonovich, K., Hoffman, J., O'Reilly, M., Belcher, H.M.E., & Butz, A.M. (2002). *Effects of prenatal drug exposure on cognitive functioning in young children.* Abstract presented at the International Neuropsychological Society.

Rains, J.W., & Ray, D.W. (1995). Participatory action research for community health promotion. *Public Health Nursing, 12,* 256–261.

Ray, O., & Ksir, C. (1996a). Marijuana and hashish. In O. Ray & C. Ksir (Eds.), *Drugs, society, and human behavior* (7th ed., pp. 403–427). New York: McGraw-Hill.

Ray, O., & Ksir, C. (1996b). Opiates. In O. Ray & C. Ksir (Eds.), *Drugs, society, and human behavior* (7th ed., pp. 336–367). New York: McGraw-Hill.

Ray, O., & Ksir, C. (1996c). Stimulants. In O. Ray & C. Ksir (Eds.), *Drugs, society, and human behavior* (7th ed., pp. 134–163). New York: McGraw-Hill.

Ray, O., & Ksir, C. (1996d). Tobacco. In O. Ray & C. Ksir (Eds.), *Drugs, society, and human behavior* (7th ed., pp. 266–290). New York: McGraw-Hill.

Richardson, G.A., Day, N.L., & McGauhey, P.J. (1993). The impact of prenatal marijuana and cocaine use on the infant and child. *Clinical Obstetrics and Gynecology, 36,* 302–318.

Richardson, G.A., Ryan, C., Willford, J., Day, N.L., & Goldschmidt, L. (2002). Prenatal alcohol and marijuana exposure: Effects on neuropsychological outcomes at 10 years. *Neurotoxicology and Teratology, 24,* 309–320.

Richardson, J.L., Dwyer, K., McGuigan, K., Hansen, W.B., Dent, C., Johnson, C.A., et al. (1989). Substance use among eighth-grade students who take care of themselves after school. *Pediatrics, 84,* 556–566.

Rosen, T.S., & Johnson, H.L. (1982). Children of methadone-maintained mothers: Follow-up to 18 months of age. *Journal of Pediatrics, 101,* 192–196.

Schuler, M.E., Nair, P., & Black, M.M. (2002). Ongoing maternal drug use, parenting attitudes, and a home intervention: Effects on mother-child interaction at 18 months. *Journal of Developmental and Behavioral Pediatrics, 23,* 87–94.

Schuler, M.E., Nair, P., Black, M.M., & Kettinger, L. (2000). Mother–infant interaction: Effects of a home intervention and ongoing maternal drug use. *Journal of Clinical Child Psychology, 29,* 424–431.

Schuler, M.E., Nair, P., & Kettinger, L. (2003). Drug-exposed infants and developmental outcome: Effects of a home intervention and ongoing maternal drug use. *Archives of Pediatrics and Adolescent Medicine, 157,* 133–138.

Sheslow, W., & Adams, W. (1990). *Manual for the Wide Range Assessment of Memory and Learning.* Wilmington, DE: Jastak Associates.

Shiono, P.H., Klebanoff, M.A., Nugent, R.P., Cotch, M.F., Wilkins, D.G., Rollins, D.E., et al. (1995). The impact of cocaine and marijuana use on low birth weight and preterm birth: A multicenter study. *American Journal of Obstetrics and Gynecology, 172,* 19–27.

Silberg, J.L., Parr, T., Neale, M.C., Rutter, M., Angold, A., & Eaves, L.J. (2003). Maternal smoking during pregnancy and risk to boys' conduct disturbance: An examination of the causal hypothesis. *Biological Psychiatry, 53,* 130–135.

Smith, A.M., Fried, P.A., Hogan, M.J., & Cameron, I. (2004). Effects of prenatal marijuana on response inhibition: An fMRI study of young adults. *Neurotoxicology and Teratology, 26,* 533–542.

Struthers, J.M. & Hansen, R.L. (1992). Visual recognition memory in drug-exposed infants. *Journal of Developmental and Behavioral Pediatrics, 13,* 108–111.

Substance Abuse and Mental Health Services Administration. (2006). *Results from the 2005 National Survey on Drug Use and Health: National findings* (DHHS Publication No. 06-4194). Rockville, MD: Office of Applied Statistics.

Sword, W., Niccols, A., & Fan, A. (2004). "New Choices" for women with addictions: Perceptions of program participants. *BMC Public Health, 4,* 10. Retrieved November 22, 2006, from http://www.biomedcentral.com/1471-2458/4/10

Trammer, R.M., Aust, G., Koser, K., & Obladen, M. (1992). Narcotic and nicotine effects on the neonatal auditory system. *Acta Paediatrica, 81,* 962–965.

Tunis, S.L., Webster, D.M., Izes, J.K., & Finnegan, L.P. (1984). Maternal drug use and the effectiveness of pharmacotherapy for neonatal abstinence. *Pediatric Research, 18,* 396.

Wechsler, D. (1991). *Wechsler Intelligence Scale for Children* (3rd ed.). New York: Harcourt Assessment.

Wilens, T.E. (2004). Attention-deficit/hyperactivity disorder and the substance use disorders: The nature of the relationship, subtypes at risk, and treatment issues. *Psychiatric Clinics of North America, 27,* 283–301.

Wilsnack, S.C., Vogeltanz, N.D., Klassen, A.D., & Harris, T.R. (1997). Childhood sexual abuse and women's substance abuse: National survey findings. *Journal of Studies on Alcohol, 58,* 264–271.

Wilsnack, S.C., Wilsnack, R.W., Kristjanson, A.F., Vogeltanz-Holm, N.D., & Windle, M. (2004). Alcohol use and suicidal behavior in women: Longitudinal patterns in a U.S. national sample. *Alcoholism: Clinical and Experimental Research, 28,* 38S–47S.

Wilson, G.S., Desmond, M.M., & Wait, R.B. (1981). Follow-up of methadone-treated and untreated narcotic-dependent women and their infants: Health, developmental, and social implications. *Journal of Pediatrics, 98,* 716–722.

Xu, Z., Seidler, F.J., Ali, S.F., Slikker, W., Jr., & Slotkin, T.A. (2001). Fetal and adolescent nicotine administration: Effects on CNS serotonergic systems. *Brain Research, 914,* 166–178.

12

Fetal Alcohol Syndrome and Related Disorders

JOAN E. PELLEGRINO AND LOUIS PELLEGRINO

The connection between maternal alcohol consumption and deleterious fetal effects was first brought to light in the English-language medical literature by Jones, Smith, Ulleland, and Streissguth in 1973. Children with *fetal alcohol syndrome* (FAS) were recognized to have a characteristic pattern of dysmorphic features, physical anomalies, and abnormalities of growth and development that could be related to a history of maternal alcohol consumption during pregnancy. Subsequent research has successfully and conclusively established the causal link between prenatal alcohol exposure and the constellation of features associated with FAS (Allebeck & Olsen, 1998). FAS has now been recognized as a major cause of cognitive and psychosocial disability in the general population, and, by extension, as a major public health issue (Riley et al., 2003). This chapter reviews what is known about FAS and the effects of prenatal alcohol exposure more generally and highlights efforts to establish the pathogenesis of the disorder with a view toward developing strategies for prevention and remediation.

DEFINITIONS AND DIAGNOSIS

As noted previously, FAS is characterized by a constellation of clinical findings, including characteristic facial features, growth abnormalities, and central nervous system (CNS) manifestations associated with a history of prenatal alcohol exposure (Table 12.1). After the initial description of FAS, there was a gradual recognition that the effects of prenatal alcohol exposure were broader, and sometimes subtler, than could be captured by the more narrowly defined, classic FAS. The term *fetal alcohol effect* emerged and was quickly adopted as a way to characterize this broader group of people who seemed to have clinically significant problems related to prenatal alcohol exposure but who did not have the dysmorphia associated with FAS.

With time it became clear, however, that the term lacked clarity and consistency in application and could not be used reliably for epidemiological purposes. In 1996, the Institute for Medicine published its findings summarizing recommendations for a change in terminology (Stratton, Howe, & Battaglia, 1996). In this scheme, "classic" FAS was again recognized as a distinct diagnostic entity associated with characteristic facial dysmorphisms, growth anomalies, and CNS dysfunction. The broader effects of prenatal alcohol exposure were captured by the terms *alcohol-related birth defects* (ARBDs) and *alcohol-related neurodevelopmental disorder* (ARND).

ARBDs include a wide variety of congenital malformations that have been associated both clinically and scientifically with fetal alcohol exposure (Table 12.2). This category explicitly recognizes that individuals exist who do not meet criteria for FAS but who have a clear history of prenatal alcohol exposure and specific congenital anomalies that are not otherwise explained. Similarly, the category ARND recognizes that individuals exist with a variety of CNS anomalies, motor control difficulties, and neuropsychological impairments that are

Table 12.1. Features of fetal alcohol syndrome

Facial dysmorphisms

Eyes: short palpebral fissures; epicanthal folds; ptosis

Premaxillary zone: maxillary hypoplasia, small nose, thin vermillion border, smooth philtrum

Minor ear anomalies

Growth retardation

Low birth weight for gestational age

Decelerating weight gain unrelated to nutrition

Weight disproportionately low relative to height

Central nervous system manifestations

Decreased cranial size at birth

Structural brain abnormalities:

- Microcephaly
- Partial or complete agenesis of the corpus callosum
- Cerebellar hypoplasia
- Other cerebral abnormalities

Abnormalities on neurological examination:

- "Hard signs" (e.g., sensorineural hearing loss)
- "Soft signs" (e.g., poor tandem gait, poor hand–eye coordination)

Adapted from Stratton, K., Howe, C., and Battaglia, F. (Eds.). (1996). *Fetal alcohol syndrome: Diagnosis, epidemiology, prevention and treatment.* Washington, DC: National Academies Press.

Table 12.2. Birth defects associated with prenatal alcohol exposure

Cardiac

Atrial septal defects

Ventricular septal defects

Aberrant great vessels

Tetralogy of Fallot

Skeletal

Hypoplastic nails

Shortened fifth digits; clinodactyly

Radioulnar synostosis

Flexion contractures

Camptodactyly

Klippel-Feil sequence*

Hemivertebrae

Scoliosis

Renal

Aplastic, dysplastic, or hypoplastic kidneys

Ureteral duplications

Hydronephrosis

Ocular

Strabismus

Retinal vascular anomalies

Micropthalmia with associated refractive errors

Auditory

Conductive or sensorineural hearing loss

Other

Many anomalies described; alcohol-related etiology uncertain

Adapted from Stratton, K., Howe, C., and Battaglia, F. (Eds.). (1996). *Fetal alcohol syndrome: Diagnosis, epidemiology, prevention and treatment.* Washington, DC: National Academies Press.
*Klippel-Feil sequence: short neck, low hairline, limited head movement related to cervical vertebral anomaly.

best explained by prenatal alcohol exposure, despite the absence of the other features of FAS. More recently, the term *fetal alcohol spectrum disorder* has emerged to characterize the variety of outcomes that have come to be associated with prenatal fetal alcohol exposure (Sokol, Delaney-Black, & Nordstrom, 2003).

Despite these efforts to better characterize the range of effects of prenatal alcohol exposure, significant diagnostic uncertainties have remained. Most important, consistent and reliably reproducible criteria for classic FAS itself have been lacking. In 2002, the U.S. Congress mandated the Centers for Disease Control and Prevention (CDC), acting through the National Center on Birth Defects and Developmental Disabilities and in coordination with the National Task Force on Fetal Alcohol Syndrome and Fetal Alcohol Effect, to develop guidelines for the diagnosis of FAS and other disorders related to prenatal alcohol exposure. The result of these efforts was published in 2004 (Bertrand et al., 2004); the consensus diagnostic criteria for FAS from this report are summarized in Table 12.3. The proposed diagnostic criteria are limited to the full fetal alcohol syn-

drome, with the intent that the guidelines will be expanded and refined to include other alcohol-related disorders in the future.

Facial Dysmorphisms

As previously noted, a variety of dysmorphic features (see Table 12.1) and congenital anomalies (see Table 12.2) have been reported in individuals with FAS. Facial dysmorphisms include short palpebral fissures, epicanthal folds, ptosis, maxillary hypoplasia, small nose, thin vermillion border, smooth philtrum, and minor ear anomalies. For the purposes of the new guidelines, only three of these dysmorphic features are considered and all three must be present in order to fulfill the diagnostic criteria for FAS. A *smooth philtrum* and *thin vermillion*

Table 12.3. Consensus diagnostic criteria for fetal alcohol syndrome (FAS)

Facial dysmorphisms (based on racial norms; all three characteristics must be present)

Smooth philtrum (University of Washington Lip-Philtrum Guide rank 4 or 5)

Thin vermillion (University of Washington Lip-Philtrum Guide rank 4 or 5)

Small palpebral fissures (at or below the 10th percentile)

Growth problems

Confirmed prenatal or postnatal height or weight that measure at or below the 10th percentile

Central nervous system abnormalities

Structural

- Head circumference at or below the 10th percentile
- Clinical significant brain abnormalities

Neurological

- Neurological problems such as seizures, "soft" neurological signs

Functional

Either

- Global cognitive/intellectual impairment (below the 3rd percentile or 2 standard deviations below the mean of accepted standardized measures of intellectual ability)

Or

- Functional deficits below the 16th percentile (1 standard deviation below the mean of accepted standardized measures) in at least 3 of the following domains:

  Cognitive or developmental deficits or discrepancies

  Executive functioning

  Motor functioning

  Attention or hyperactivity

  Social skills

  Other functional domains (e.g., sensory issues, pragmatic language dysfunction, short-term memory deficits)

Maternal alcohol exposure

Defined as confirmed or unknown; *confirmation of exposure is not required for the diagnosis of FAS*

From Betrand, J., Floyd, R., Weber, M., O'Connor, M., Filey, E., Johnson, K., et al. (2004). *Fetal alcohol syndrome: Guidelines for referral and diagnosis.* Atlanta: Centers for Disease Control and Prevention.

border must be noted, and each must measure 4 or 5 on the Lip-Philtrum Guide developed at the University of Washington (Astley & Clarren, 1999, 2000) (Figure 12.1). *Small palpebral fissures* (measuring at or below the 10th percentile according to age and racial norms) must also be observed.

Growth Problems

Impairments in height, weight, or both are needed in order to fulfill the criteria. Because most children with FAS are symmetrical for height and weight (Jacobson & Jacobson, 2002), deficiencies in either height *or* weight, but not height *for* weight, were included in the criteria. The severity of growth restriction was defined as at or below the 10th percentile, documented at any one point in time either prenatally or postnatally (adjusted for age, sex, gestational age, and race or ethnicity).

Central Nervous System Abnormalities

To meet the FAS diagnostic criteria for CNS abnormality, there must be documentation of either a structural, neurological, or functional deficit, or a combination of these. A *structural* deficit is defined as small or diminished overall head circumference at or below the 10th percentile, adjusted for age and gender. For children with overall growth deficiency, the head circumference should be disproportionately small compared with the overall size (less than or equal to the 3rd percentile). A clinically significant brain abnormality observed through imaging would also fulfill the criteria (see section on CNS manifestations later in the chapter). A *neurological* deficit is defined as docu-

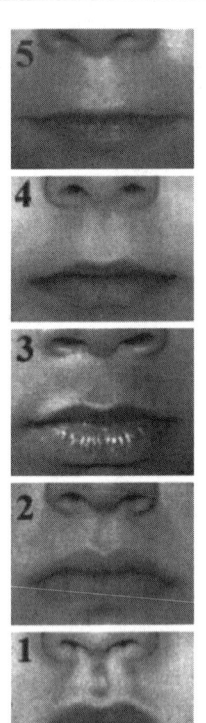

Figure 12.1. The University of Washington Lip-Philtrum Scale provides a 5-point Lickert scale to assess vermillion border and philtrum appearance. Grade 1 demonstrates a full, typically arched upper lip and well-demarcated philtrum. Grades 4 and 5 demonstrate the flattening and thinning of the vermillion border and smoothing of the philtrum, with loss of demarcations, that are characteristic of FAS. (From Astley, S.J., & Clarren, S.K., Diagnosing the full spectrum of fetal alcohol-exposed individuals: introducing the 4-digit diagnostic code. Alcohol & Alcoholism, 2000, 35(4), 400–410, by permission of Oxford University Press.)

mented evidence of neurologic damage. This could include seizures not caused by postnatal insult or fever, or soft neurological signs on physical examination. Criteria for a *functional* deficit can be met in one of two ways: a global cognitive deficit may be identified (or a significant developmental delay in children too young for an intelligence quotient [IQ] assessment), *or* deficits in three or more specific functional domains may be demonstrated. Specific functional domains include executive function, motor skills, attention and impulse control, and social skills (sensory dysfunction, pragmatic language deficits, memory deficits, and difficulty responding appropriately to commonly used parenting practices are also mentioned as other areas of potential difficulty). In the assessment of either global cognitive function or specific functional domains,

norm-referenced, standardized measures should be used whenever possible and should be administered by appropriately trained professionals using reliable and validated instruments. For global cognitive deficits, scores that fall 2 standard deviations below the mean (below the 3rd percentile) are considered significant. For specific functional domains, scores falling 1 standard deviation below the mean (below the 16th percentile) in three areas are considered significant.

Maternal Alcohol Exposure

Documentation of prenatal alcohol exposure should be sought and should include the consumption patterns of the mother during the pregnancy based on observation, self-report, report by a reliable informant, or medical records. This information, however, is often difficult to obtain and may not be reliable. Exposure is often unknown because of adoption or conflicting evidence. Therefore, confirmed prenatal alcohol exposure is not required to fulfill the diagnostic criteria for FAS. Confirmed absence of alcohol exposure would rule out a diagnosis of FAS.

EPIDEMIOLOGY

Establishing the exact frequency of FAS and related disorders has been challenging for several reasons. As mentioned previously, lack of clarity related to inconsistent application of diagnostics terms has contributed to these difficulties. There have also been discrepancies among various studies with regard to case ascertainment methods. Studies by the CDC (1995, 1997, 2002) report prevalence rates ranging from 0.2 to 1.5 cases per 1,000 live births across various populations. A recent review of the literature suggests a prevalence estimate of 0.5 to 2.0 cases per 1,000 (May & Gossage, 2001). Attempts to estimate the prevalence of the wider spectrum of fetal alcohol effects provide even greater difficulties. Based on the best available information, another recent review provided an estimate of the prevalence of all alcohol-related effects (FAS plus ARBD plus ARND) as 9.1 per 1,000 (Sampson et al., 1997).

Specific population subgroups have also been identified as being at particularly high risk for FAS. Higher rates of FAS have been reported among low socioeconomic and minority groups. Black children are 5 times more likely and Native Americans are 16 times more likely than whites to exhibit classic FAS (Chavez, Cordero, & Becerra, 1988; Egeland et al., 1998; May, Hymbaugh, Aase, & Samet, 1983). Poverty has also been associated with increased risk of maternal alcohol use and subsequent FAS (Abel, 1995). In the future, larger, population-based studies may eventually result in a revision of many of these estimates, but even allowing for imperfections in our current prevalence estimates, it remains clear that the rates of fetal alcohol–related sequelae are unacceptably high and represent a major public health concern.

ALCOHOL AS A TERATOGEN

Alcohol is a known human teratogen. Like most teratogens, it can produce a wide spectrum of fetal effects depending on the amount, frequency, timing, and duration of exposure. In 1999, more than 50% of women of childbearing age reported alcohol consumption in the past month (Ebrahim, Anderson, & Floyd, 1999), and 15% of these could be classified as moderate or heavy drinkers (Hanson, Streissguth, & Smith, 1978; Wilsnack, Wilsnack, & Hiller-Sturmhofel, 1994). National survey data indicate that 13% of women continue to use alcohol during pregnancy (CDC, 1999). Based on these data, and the fact that 50% of pregnancies are unintended, an estimated 2% of women could be at risk for an alcohol-exposed pregnancy annually (Project CHOICES Research Group, 2002).

Exposure early in gestation is more likely to cause the broadest effects, including the dysmorphisms and congenital anomalies associated with FAS. Exposure in the third trimester has been associated with growth retardation. The lack of dysmorphic features, however, is not predictive of the neurobehavioral deficits that occur in children exposed to alcohol prenatally. Both the first and third trimesters are times of vulnerability to the fetus. Although the true threshold of exposure has not been adequately defined, the peak blood alcohol concentration seems to be more significant than the total alcohol dose in producing microcephaly (Pierce & West, 1986); yet, low-level exposure of one drink per week has been associated with aggression and externalizing behaviors in exposed children at age 6–7 years (Sood et al., 2001). Both the American Academy of Pediatrics (2000) and the American College of Obstetricians and Gynecologists recommend abstinence during pregnancy.

Basic research is beginning to shed light on possible molecular mechanisms explaining the clinical effects of prenatal alcohol exposure. Alcohol has been found to affect multiple aspects of brain development and function. Alcohol causes synaptic degradation and neuronal apoptosis in many different regions of the developing brain, possibly related to its N-methyl-D-aspartate (NMDA) antagonist and γ-aminobutyric acid (GABA)-mimetic properties (Olney, Ishimaru, Bittigau, & Ikonomidou, 2000). Alcohol also interferes with other aspects of nerve cell development and functioning. It has been shown that it disrupts L1-mediated cell adhesion; individuals with deleterious mutations of the L1 gene show brain pathological features similar to those of individuals with prenatal alcohol exposure (Bearer, 2001). Alcohol can also influence the synthesis, release, receptor binding, and signaling of a variety of neurotransmitters. Effects on the serotonergic system have been of particular interest. Prenatal alcohol exposure decreases the production of serotonin in the brain stem, with concomitant reductions in serotonergic innervation of the cortex. This may have direct implications with regard to some of the neurobehavioral characteristics associated with FAS (Druse, Kuo, & Tajuddin, 1991; Tajuddin & Druse, 1999). Alcohol is also known to adversely affect the fetal white matter (Ozer, Sarioglu, & Gure, 2000), and specifically retards the development of the radial glia, which is suspected to contribute to abnormalities of the corpus callosum (Guizzetti, Catlin, & Costa, 1997; Valles et al., 1996). Alcohol increases oxidative stress in fetal nervous tissue; use of antioxidants as part of a broader FAS prevention program has been suggested (Cohen-Kerem & Koren, 2003) (see later).

GENETIC SUSCEPTIBILITY

The effects of prenatal alcohol exposure on the fetus vary considerably and are only partly explained by the degree and frequency of maternal alcohol consumption. Studies have shown that alcohol absorption varies considerably for the same woman at different times, depending on whether alcohol is consumed on a full or empty stomach (Riley et al., 2003). Alcohol is metabolized to acetaldehyde by alcohol dehydrogenase (ADH) and the cytochrome P-450 isoenzyme 2E1, and then oxidized by aldehyde dehydrogenase (ALDH) to acetate. The deleterious effects of alcohol on the fetus are related to the action of alcohol itself, as well as its metabolites. Functional variants have been identified in the genes for both ADH and ALDH. Specific variants have been identified in the Asian population that have been found to be protective against alcoholism (Thomasson et al., 1991). Another variant of ADH, found specifically in the African American population, appears to be protective against the effects of prenatal alcohol exposure on the fetus (McCarver, Thomasson, Martier, Sokol, & Li, 1997).

CENTRAL NERVOUS SYSTEM MANIFESTATIONS

Prenatal alcohol exposure is known to have a wide variety of effects on the developing brain. Early autopsy studies often focused on the most severe cases and revealed severe anomalies in nearly every region of the brain (Roebuck, Mattson, & Riley, 1998). In recent years, brain imaging studies have clarified our understanding of the effects of alcohol on the developing brain considerably. These studies have confirmed earlier pathological and clinical findings with regard to the more nonspecific manifestations of prenatal alcohol exposure. Micrencephaly (small brain size) associated with clinically significant microcephaly (small head size) has been consistently observed (Swayze et al., 1997). Ventriculomegaly, loss of normal cortical asymmetry, and proportional loss of white matter volume relative to gray matter volume have been reported (Archibald et al., 2001; Henkenius, Riley, Jernigan, & Toga, 2002; Swayze et al., 1997).

Neuroimaging has also provided evidence that specific brain regions are particularly vulnerable to the effects of prenatal alcohol exposure. For example, the basal ganglia, the cerebellum, and the hippocampus have been implicated in several studies (Archibald et al., 2001; Mattson et al., 1996; Roebuck et al., 1998). A convergence of data from several studies has provided convincing evidence for a particular vulnerability of the corpus callosum and other midline brain structures (Bookstein, Sampson, Connor, & Streissguth, 2002; Bookstein, Sampson, Streissguth, & Connor, 2001; Bookstein, Streissguth, Sampson, Connor, & Barr, 2002; Roebuck, Mattson, & Riley, 2002; Swayze et al., 1997). Reduction in the size of the corpus callosum has been correlated with the presence of facial dysmorphic features and with specific evidence for deficits in interhemispheric transfer of information. Functional imaging studies have further extended our understanding of the sometimes subtle consequences of fetal alcohol exposure. Studies of less severely affected individuals (individuals with relatively mild cognitive impairments) have demonstrated regions of reduced brain metabolic activity (e.g., the basal ganglia, thalamus, and various regions of the cortices), even in the absence of observable structural brain abnormalities (Bhatara et al., 2002; Clark, Li, Conry, Conry, & Loock, 2000; Riikonen, Salonen, Partanen, & Verho, 1999), lending credence to the notion that a wide spectrum of neurological effects may result from prenatal alcohol exposure.

NEURODEVELOPMENTAL OUTCOMES

FAS and related disorders have long been associated with significant adverse neurodevelopmental outcomes. As with FAS, estimates of the prevalence of specific neurodevelopmental disorders connected with ARND and ARBD have varied widely across studies (one such estimate is presented in Table 12.4) (Burd, Cotsonas-Hassler, Martsolf, & Kerbeshian, 2003). There is general agreement, however, that prenatal alcohol exposure results in both generalized intellectual impairment and specific neuropsychological deficits and that these deleterious effects have lifelong consequences for the individual and manifold consequences for society (Bertrand et al., 2004).

Table 12.4. Estimated prevalence of neuro-developmental disorders in fetal alcohol syndrome

Mental retardation: 15–20%

Learning disorders: 25%

Speech and language disorders: 30%

Attention-deficit/hyperactivity disorder: 40%

Sensory impairment: 30%

Cerebral palsy: 4%

Epilepsy: 8–10%

Reprinted from *Neurotoxicology and Teratology, 25*, Burd, L., Cotsonas-Hassler, T.M., Martsolf, J.T., & Kerbeshian, J., Recognition and management of fetal alcohol syndrome, 681–688, Copyright 2003, with permission from Elsevier.

Intellectual and Learning Disabilities

Prenatal exposure to alcohol is known to have the potential for generalized deleterious effects on cognition and learning. As in the general population, learning disabilities are more common than generalized cognitive impairment in individuals with FAS, but both are seen with increased frequency in people with FAS. This observation is directly correlated with increased requirements for special education services (Aronson & Hagberg, 1998; Autti-Ramo, 2000; Greenbaum, Nulman, Rovet, & Koren, 2002) and long-term psychosocial dysfunction (Roebuck, Mattson, & Riley, 1999; Streissguth & O'Malley, 2000).

Specific Neurocognitive Impairments A host of studies suggest that specific neurocognitive functions may be adversely affected by prenatal alcohol exposure above and beyond what can be accounted for by general decrements in intellectual ability. Children and adults with FAS are known to have difficulties with planning, goal-directed activity, and response inhibition, all qualities associated with executive function (Connor, Sampson, Bookstein, Barr, & Streissguth, 2000; Mattson, Goodman, Caine, Delis, & Riley, 1999). Attention-deficit/hyperactivity disorder (ADHD) is frequently diagnosed in these individuals (Coles, 2001; O'Malley & Nanson, 2002), but the clinical manifestations of the disorder are distinct. Children with FAS tend to present at a younger age with the symptoms of ADHD and are more likely to have a host of associated comorbid learning, behavioral, and emotional problems. They are also less predictable in their

response to pharmacological interventions (Oesterheld et al., 1998). Various studies have highlighted specific problems with language and verbal function (Greenbaum et al., 2002; Kerns, Don, Mateer, & Streissguth, 1997; Mattson & Riley, 1998; Mattson & Roebuck, 2002), visual-perceptual and visuospatial function (Aronson & Hagberg, 1998; Kaemingk, Mulvaney, & Halverson, 2003; Meyer, 1998; Uecker & Nadel, 1998), and short-term memory (Aronson & Hagberg, 1998; Korkman, Kettunen, & Autti-Ramo, 2003; Mattson, Riley, Gramling, Delis, & Jones, 1998). It should, therefore, not be surprising, given the variety and frequency of specific neurocognitive impairments and generalized intellectual and learning disabilities, that children with FAS are much more likely to experience academic difficulties, grade retention, and the need for special education services (Autti-Ramo, 2000).

Psychosocial Dysfunction Prenatal alcohol exposure has specific detrimental effects on social cognition and social behavior (Autti-Ramo, 2000; Greenbaum et al., 2002). These effects can be seen at every stage of development from infancy through adulthood. Infants demonstrate increased irritability and dysfunctional attachments to caregivers (Coles & Platzman, 1993; Kelly, Day, & Streissguth, 2000), as well as problems with state regulation (e.g., dysfunctional sleep–wake cycles). Young children show early difficulties with impulsive and sometimes aggressive behavior and continue to have difficulties with state regulation. They also exhibit general social immaturity and poor social cognition, inappropriate choices of friends, and inappropriate sexual behavior. Preteens and adolescents tend to be isolated from their peers and are more likely to engage in antisocial and risky behavior, including an increased tendency to abuse alcohol and drugs (Olson, Feldman, Streissguth, Sampson, & Bookstein, 1998; Olson et al., 1997). Adults have significant problems establishing satisfactory long-term relationships and are more likely to have problems finding and holding onto jobs (Streissguth et al., 1991). A disproportionate number of individuals in jail show features of FAS (Fast, Conry, & Loock, 1999).

Psychiatric Disorders Individuals with FAS are at increased risk for the development of significant emotional difficulties and frank mental illness. As previously mentioned, children exposed to alcohol in utero are much more likely to be diagnosed with ADHD and concomitant disruptive behavioral disorders, such as oppositional defiant disorder and conduct disorder (Coles, 2001; Oesterheld et al., 1998; O'Malley & Nanson, 2002). Adolescents and adults are known to have an increased risk for a variety of psychiatric disorders, including alcohol or drug dependence, depression, psychotic disorders, and personality disorders (Burd, Klug, Martsolf, & Kerbeshian, 2003; Famy, Streissguth, & Unis, 1998).

STRATEGIES FOR INTERVENTION AND REMEDIATION

Several key observations must be recognized when attempts are made to intervene on behalf of individuals with FAS. As noted previously, the effects of prenatal alcohol exposure are lifelong; they are also extremely variable. It is not possible or advisable to define monolithic strategies for intervention and remediation that would apply to all individuals with FAS. Having said this, it is possible and necessary to define a framework for intervention that recognizes the special characteristics and issues attendant on the FAS diagnosis. The following discussion represents an attempt to define such a framework.

Diagnosis: The Beginning of Remediation

Accurate and early diagnosis of FAS itself, as well as the diagnosis of associated disability, is the critical first step in the process of establishing a plan for intervention and remediation. Even in instances when the diagnosis of FAS itself is delayed, it is often possible to recognize individuals at risk for adverse outcomes, either on the basis of known prenatal alcohol exposure or on the basis of recognized developmental delays or functional deficits. The early diagnosis of FAS itself becomes critical in situations in which a child does not meet the functional criteria for early intervention or special education services. Children with milder neurocognitive manifestations of prenatal alcohol exposure may "fall through the cracks" of existing educational and therapeutic systems and frequently flounder for several years before significant academic and social difficulties are fully recognized.

Establishing a Basis for Intervention: Recognizing Individual Variation

Although individuals with FAS have a number of psychological and behavioral characteristics in common, these commonalities are not sufficiently consistent or specific across individuals to allow for the definition of universal strategies for remediation. It is necessary to define very specific neurodevelopmental profiles for each individual before it will be possible to establish rational strategies for intervention. Given the variety and complexity of the variables involved, it will not be possible for any one professional to fully define such a profile. Multidisciplinary programs exist in some locales that provide the means to define an actionable profile of skills based on the input of several relevant professional disciplines at a single point in time. In most locales, however, the same objective may be achieved over a period of time across a variety of diagnostic and therapeutic settings. For example, a primary care pediatrician may be the first person to recognize the characteristics of FAS, a medical specialist (e.g., medical geneticist, neurologist, or developmental pediatrician) may confirm the diagnosis, and a variety of therapists and educational specialists may provide the necessary data to establish a functional profile for the development of an intervention plan.

Under either scenario, having a single person who provides service coordination becomes critical. This function is often served by a proactive and involved parent but may also be served by interested and involved professionals. Primary care physicians, teachers, and social workers are often strategically positioned to serve this function.

Interventions Across Multiple Settings

Bronfenbrenner (1979) defined the concept of the developmental setting and identified this as the nexus and engine of developmental change and the proper venue for the creation of effective interventions for change. Developmental settings typically include the home, the school, and the workplace but may vary from place to place and from culture to culture. A complex dynamic exists within and across these various settings that strongly influences the effects of any particular intervention.

Early intervention efforts for children with FAS are usually focused on the provision of services and supports in the home environment. Having a stable and nurturing home is known to be protective with respect to long-term functional outcomes for individuals with FAS (Coles & Platzman, 1993). Unfortunately, many children with FAS find themselves on shifting sands when it comes to getting settled in a stable home situation. This relates in part to the challenging temperamental and behavioral characteristics of these children. Helping caregivers understand the neurodevelopmental consequences of FAS can provide the basis for teaching and supporting effective parenting strategies. At the societal level, it must be recognized that children with FAS are much more likely to find themselves in foster care. One study estimates that children in foster care are 10 to 15 times more likely than the general population to exhibit features of FAS (Astley, Stachowiak, Clarren, & Clausen, 2002). Community-level efforts to support at-risk families are a necessary complement to the provision of traditional early intervention services.

After the home, the school provides the most important developmental setting for children with FAS. Many of these children will experience significant academic and social difficulties in school. Every effort should be made to strike a balance between creating opportunities for typical social experiences and providing needed specialized educational and therapeutic supports. Even in circumstances in which a nearly ideal intervention regimen is defined, many children with FAS will still experience significant embarrassment and discouragement requiring some form of counseling support. For children with cognitive and learning difficulties, the value of "extracurricular activities" is often underestimated. These types of activities may provide a child with the experience of success and accomplishment that usually eludes them in the academic domain. Parents play a particularly important role in helping academically challenged children find those special strengths and competencies that will form the basis for work-related and recreational activities during the adult years.

Finding the means and methods for intervention on behalf of adults with FAS is challenging. Many people find that the availability of services and supports drops off precipitously with the 18th birthday. Efforts to create bridges between the developmental settings that characterize childhood and those that characterize adulthood have increased in recent years, but much more is still needed.

Pharmacological Interventions

In addition to educational, psychological, and therapeutic interventions, some individuals with FAS will benefit from medications directed at behavioral symptoms. Little specific information currently exists in the medical literature about the effects of psychotropic medications on individuals with FAS, however. Studies suggest that some children and adults with FAS may benefit from the use of stimulant medications but also suggest that the effects of these drugs may be less predictable compared with the effects observed in the general population (Oesterheld et al., 1998; O'Malley & Nanson, 2002). Other psychotropic medications may be considered judiciously (e.g., selective serotonin reuptake inhibitors, alpha agonists, antianxiolytics, and neuroleptics), but information about safety and efficacy in children is limited, and many of these medications must still be prescribed "off label." In general, medications are directed toward ameliorating specific target symptoms (e.g., inattention, anxiety, behavioral rigidity, explosive-aggressive behavior). Many medications should be started at a low dose, and slowly increased while monitoring carefully for the emergence of side effects. In general, it is best to avoid the use of multiple psychotropic agents in the same individual. Before a medication is started, anticipated outcomes should be defined, and a plan for confirming efficacy should be clearly stated. At this time, the use of these medications in individuals with FAS remains very much an art awaiting the arrival of confirmatory science.

STRATEGIES FOR PREVENTION

In 1981, the U.S. Surgeon General established clear guidelines that women who are pregnant or who are at risk for becoming pregnant should abstain entirely from alcohol consumption ("Surgeon General's advisory," 1981). These guidelines arise from the recognition that FAS would cease to exist if it were possible to prevent alcohol consumption in anticipation of each conception and pregnancy. Given the level of alcohol consumption among women of childbearing age (Ebrahim et al., 1999), prevention efforts have necessarily focused on identifying women at risk and creating practical and effective behavior-based interventions to reduce the likelihood of fetal alcohol exposure.

Populations at Risk

A number of studies have identified subpopulations at special risk for alcohol consumption during pregnancy (Abel & Hannigan, 1995; Flynn, Marcus, Barry, & Blow, 2002; Gladstone, Nulman, & Koren, 1996; Kvigne et al., 2003; O'Connor & Whaley, 2003). Women of lower socioeconomic status, smokers, and women who are unmarried or who have multiple sexual partners are at increased risk. Ethnic groups at increased risk include African Americans, American Indians, and Native Alaskans. Women with a history of drug use, mental illness, or physical or sexual abuse or who have been hospitalized for drug treatment or mental illness are also at increased risk. A number of local and national prevention efforts have specifically targeted these at-risk groups (Bertrand et al., 2004).

Screening Instruments

A number of screening instruments have been developed to help identify individuals at specific risk for alcohol consumption during pregnancy. In general, these screening tests incorporate quantity-frequency measures (designed

to assess general or average patterns of alcohol consumption) or maximum quantity measures (designed to assess the frequency of binge drinking), or a combination of both. The Alcohol Timeline Followback (TLFB) (Sobell & Sobell, 2000) is a particularly reliable measure, but its use has been confined mainly to research settings, in part because of the length of time required for administration.

Several measures have been developed that are tailored to particular clinical situations; many of these tests have names that are acronyms based on question content designed to aid in recall (Table 12.5). On the 4-question CAGE questionnaire (Ewing, 1984), items are scored as 1 point for a "yes" answer and 0 points for a "no" answer; a total of 2 or more points is considered clinically significant. The CAGE has been found to be most useful for screening nonpregnant women and for detecting patterns of alcohol use and dependency (Fiellin, Ried, & O'Connor, 2000). The AUDIT is a 10-item questionnaire that is also used to screen nonpregnant women and is superior to the CAGE in identifying current, clinically significant drinking patterns (Saunders, Oasland, Babor, De LaFuente, & Grant, 1993). The T-ACE and the TWEAK are questionnaires specifically developed for use in screening pregnant women (Russell, 1994; Sokol, Martier, & Ager, 1989). The specificity of the TWEAK is high across all ethnic groups, but the sensitivity varies greatly across ethnic groups (O'Connor & Whaley, 2003). The CRAFFT questionnaire (Knight, Shrier, & Bravender, 1999) was developed to screen for drug and alcohol use in adolescents; its questions are specifically targeted to this population.

Techniques for Intervention

Several effective techniques have been developed for the purpose of reducing or eliminating alcohol consumption during pregnancy. *Brief intervention* is a technique that uses time-limited self-help strategies to reduce alcohol use or, in cases of alcohol dependence, help identify the need for referral for more intensive services (Babor & Higgins-Biddle, 2000; Fleming, 2003). The technique has been shown to be more effective than no treatment, and in

Table 12.5. Screening instruments for individuals at risk for alcohol consumption during pregnancy

CAGE Questionnaire
C—Have you ever felt that you should CUT down on your drinking?
A—Have people ever ANNOYED you by criticizing your drinking?
G—Have you ever felt GUILTY about your drinking?
E—Have you ever had a drink in the morning as an EYE OPENER?

T-ACE Questionnaire
T—TOLERANCE to alcohol
A—ANNOYANCE at criticism about drinking
C—Self-identified need to CUT down on alcohol consumption
E—History of having a morning drink or EYE OPENER

TWEAK Questionnaire
T—TOLERANCE
W—WORRY expressed by family or friends
E—Morning EYE OPENER
A—AMNESIA or "blackouts" related to drinking
K—Need to "CUT" down on drinking

CRAFFT Questionnaire
C—A history of riding in a CAR with a driver under the influence of drugs or alcohol
R—Use of drugs or alcohol to help the individual RELAX or "fit in"
A—History of drinking or using drugs ALONE
F—FORGETS things that happen while using drugs or alcohol
F—FAMILY or FRIENDS express concern about alcohol or drug use
T—A history of the individual getting into TROUBLE related to drug or alcohol use

some cases is just as effective as more comprehensive programs. Cognitive-behavioral techniques are employed, and nonspecialists are frequently trained to administer the program. Clinically, the technique has most often been used as an intervention for populations not considered at high risk for alcohol dependence. *Motivational interviewing* is another technique that uses empathetic counseling methods to encourage behavioral change by enhancing an individual's awareness of choices regarding alcohol use (Miller & Rollnick, 1991). A limitation of the technique relates to the requirement for specialized clinicians and training to allow proper administration of the elements of the motivational interview.

The CDC has funded and, at the time of this writing, is piloting a variant of brief intervention that employs motivational interview techniques and is called Project CHOICES (Ingersoll, Floyd, Sobell, & Velasquez, 2003). Initial results of the project are promising and suggest significant reductions in alcohol use during pregnancy.

Limiting the Deleterious Effects of Prenatal Alcohol Exposure

Although eliminating prenatal alcohol exposure entirely remains the ideal and primary target of prevention efforts, a body of research exists that attempts to discover strategies for limiting the teratogenic effects of alcohol exposure when it does occur. Oxidative stress has been identified as one of the mechanisms by which alcohol creates damage in various body tissues. Animal studies suggest that antioxidants may be protective in this regard, but this has not been confirmed in humans (Cohen-Kerem & Koren, 2003). Similarly, neuroprotective peptides derived from astrocytes have been found to reduce the rate of fetal demise after high-dose alcohol exposure in mice (Brenneman et al., 2004). These early research findings may eventually lead to the development of a second tier of preventative strategies aimed at limiting the deleterious effects of alcohol on the fetus in cases in which primary efforts to eliminate prenatal alcohol exposure altogether are incompletely effective.

CONCLUSION

Much still needs to be done in our efforts to understand, remediate, and prevent FAS and related disorders. Recent advances in developing consistent and reliable diagnostic criteria for FAS must be followed by improvements in our ability to diagnosis the broader range of fetal alcohol–related disorders. We are also in the early stages of understanding the pathogenesis of FAS, particularly with reference to the development of treatment strategies aimed at reducing or eliminating the toxic effects of alcohol on the fetus. Finally, there is a need to improve community-based efforts to identify at-risk mothers and to provide effective interventions to reduce maternal alcohol consumption. With all of the important advances in the science of FAS described in this chapter, the simple fact remains that the prevention of fetal alcohol exposure in the first place is the only absolutely effective strategy available to us for dealing with FAS.

RESOURCES FOR FAMILIES

Web Sites

- *National Organization on Fetal Alcohol Syndrome*—http://www.nofas.org

- *CDC website on FAS; contains FAS Guidelines for Referral and Diagnosis* (Bertrand et al., 2004)—http://www.cdc.gov/ncbddd/fas

- *FAS site for families*—http://www.fetalalcoholsyndrome.org

- *FAS site for families*—http://kidshealth.org/parent/medical/brain/fas.html

- *National Institute of Health FAS site*—http://www.nlm.nih.gov/medlineplus/fetalalcoholsyndrome.html

Further Reading

- Kulp, L., & Kulp, J. (2000). *The best I can be: Living with fetal alcohol syndrome—effects*. Brooklyn Park, MN: Better Endings New Beginnings.

- Steissguth, A. (1997). *Fetal alcohol syndrome: A guide for families and communities*. Baltimore: Paul H. Brookes Publishing Co.

REFERENCES

Abel, E.L. (1995). An update on the incidence of FAS: FAS is not an equal opportunity birth defect. *Neurotoxicology and Teratology, 17,* 437–443.

Abel, E.L., & Hannigan, J.H. (1995). Maternal risk factors in Fetal Alcohol Syndrome: Provocative and permissive influences. *Neurotoxicology and Teratology, 17,* 445–462.

Allebeck, P., & Olsen, J. (1998). Alcohol and fetal damage. *Alcoholism: Clinical and Experimental Research, 22*(7 Suppl.), 329S–332S.

American Academy of Pediatrics, Committee on Substance Abuse and Committee on Children with Disabilities. (2000). Fetal alcohol syndrome and alcohol-related neurodevelopmental disorders. *Pediatrics, 106*(2 Pt 1), 358–361.

Archibald, S.L., Fennema-Notestine, C., Gamst, A., Riley, E.P., Mattson, S.N., & Jernigan, T.L. (2001). Brain dysmorphology in individuals with severe prenatal alcohol exposure. *Developmental Medicine and Child Neurology, 43,* 148–154.

Aronson, M., & Hagberg, B. (1998). Neuropsychological disorders in children exposed to alcohol during pregnancy: A follow-up study of 24 children to alcoholic mothers in Goteborg, Sweden. *Alcoholism: Clinical and Experimental Research, 22,* 321–324.

Astley, S.J., & Clarren, S.K. (1999). *Diagnostic guide for fetal alcohol syndrome and related conditions* (2nd ed.). Seattle: University Publication Services.

Astley, S.J., & Clarren, S.K. (2000). Diagnosing the full spectrum of fetal alcohol-exposed individuals: Introducing the 4-digit diagnostic code. *Alcohol and Alcoholism, 35,* 400–410.

Astley, S.J., Stachowiak, J., Clarren, S.K., & Clausen, C. (2002). Application of the fetal alcohol syndrome facial photographic screening tool in a foster care population. *Journal of Pediatrics, 141,* 712–717.

Autti-Ramo, I. (2000). Twelve-year follow-up of children exposed to alcohol in utero. *Developmental Medicine and Child Neurology, 42,* 406–411.

Babor, T., & Higgins-Biddle, J. (2000). Alcohol screening and brief intervention: Dissemination strategies for medical practice and public health. *Addiction, 95,* 677–686.

Bearer, C.F. (2001). L1 cell adhesion molecule signal cascades: Targets for ethanol developmental neurotoxicity. *Neurotoxicology, 22,* 625–633.

Bertrand, J., Floyd, R., Weber, M., O'Connor, M., Riley, E., Johnson, K., et al. (2004). *Fetal alcohol syndrome: Guidelines for referral and diagnosis*. Atlanta: Centers for Disease Control and Prevention.

Bhatara, V.S., Lovrein, F., Kirkeby, J., Swayze, V., II, Unruh, E., & Johnson, V. (2002). Brain function in fetal alcohol syndrome assessed by single photon emission computed tomography. *South Dakota Journal of Medicine, 55*(2), 59–62.

Bookstein, F.L., Sampson, P.D., Connor, P.D., & Streissguth, A.P. (2002). Midline corpus callosum is a neuroanatomical focus of fetal alcohol damage. *Anatomical Record, 269,* 162–174.

Bookstein, F.L., Sampson, P.D., Streissguth, A.P., & Connor, P.D. (2001). Geometric morphometrics of corpus callosum and subcortical structures in the fetal-alcohol-affected brain. *Teratology, 64,* 4–32.

Bookstein, F.L., Streissguth, A.P., Sampson, P.D., Connor, P.D., & Barr, H.M. (2002). Corpus callosum shape and neuropsychological deficits in adult males with heavy fetal alcohol exposure. *Neuroimage, 15,* 233–251.

Brenneman, D.E., Spong, C.Y., Hauser, J.M., Abebe, D., Pinhasov, A., Golian, T., et al. (2004). Protective peptides that are orally active and mechanistically nonchiral. *Journal of Pharmacology and Experimental Therapeutics, 309,* 1190–1197.

Bronfenbrenner, U. (1979). *The ecology of human development: Experiments by nature and design.* Cambridge, MA: Harvard University Press.

Burd, L., Cotsonas-Hassler, T.M., Martsolf, J.T., & Kerbeshian, J. (2003). Recognition and management of fetal alcohol syndrome. *Neurotoxicology and Teratology, 25,* 681–688.

Burd, L., Klug, M.G., Martsolf, J.T., & Kerbeshian, J. (2003). Fetal alcohol syndrome: Neuropsychiatric phenomics. *Neurotoxicology and Teratology, 25,* 697–705.

Centers for Disease Control and Prevention. (1995). Update: Trends in fetal alcohol syndrome—United States, 1979–1993. *MMWR: Morbidity and Mortality Weekly Report, 44,* 249–251.

Centers for Disease Control and Prevention. (1997). Surveillance for fetal alcohol syndrome using multiple sources—Atlanta, Georgia, 1981–1989. *MMWR: Morbidity and Mortality Weekly Report, 46,* 1118–1120.

Centers for Disease Control and Prevention. (1999). Alcohol use among women of childbearing age—United States. *MMWR: Morbidity and Mortality Weekly Report, 51,* 273–276.

Centers for Disease Control and Prevention. (2002). Fetal alcohol syndrome—Alaska, Arizona, Colorado, and New York, 1979–1993. *MMWR: Morbidity and Mortality Weekly Report, 51,* 433–435.

Chavez, G., Cordero, J., & Becerra, J. (1988). Leading major congenital malformations among minority groups in the United States of America, 1981–1986. *MMWR: Morbidity and Mortality Weekly Report, 37*(SS-3), 17–24.

Clark, C.M., Li, D., Conry, J., Conry, R., & Loock, C. (2000). Structural and functional brain integrity of fetal alcohol syndrome in nonretarded cases. *Pediatrics, 105,* 1096–1099.

Cohen-Kerem, R., & Koren, G. (2003). Antioxidants and fetal protection against ethanol teratogenicity: I. Review of the experimental data and implications to humans. *Neurotoxicology and Teratology, 25,* 1–9.

Coles, C.D. (2001). Fetal alcohol exposure and attention: Moving beyond ADHD. *Alcohol Research & Health, 25,* 199–203.

Coles, C.D., & Platzman, K.A. (1993). Behavioral development in children prenatally exposed to drugs and alcohol. *International Journal of the Addictions, 28,* 1393–1433.

Connor, P.D., Sampson, P.D., Bookstein, F.L., Barr, H.M., & Streissguth, A.P. (2000). Direct and indirect effects of prenatal alcohol damage on executive function. *Developmental Neuropsychology, 18,* 331–354.

Druse, M., Kuo, A., & Tajuddin, N. (1991). Effects of in utero ethanol exposure on the developing serotonergic system. *Alcoholism, 15,* 678–684.

Ebrahim, S., Anderson, A., & Floyd, R. (1999). Alcohol consumption by reproductive-aged women in the USA: An update on assessment, burden and prevention in the 1990's. *Prenatal and Neonatal Medicine, 4,* 419–430.

Egeland, G.M., Katherin, P., Gessner, B.D., Ingle, D., Berner, J.E., & Middaugh, J.P. (1998). Fetal alcohol syndrome in Alaska, 1977 through 1992: An administrative prevalence derived from multiple data sources. *American Journal of Public Health, 88,* 781–786.

Ewing, J. (1984). The CAGE questionnaire. *JAMA, 252,* 1905–1907.

Famy, C., Streissguth, A.P., & Unis, A.S. (1998). Mental illness in adults with fetal alcohol syndrome or fetal alcohol effects. *American Journal of Psychiatry, 155,* 552–554.

Fast, D.K., Conry, J., & Loock, C.A. (1999). Identifying fetal alcohol syndrome among youth in the criminal justice system. *Journal of Developmental and Behavioral Pediatrics, 20,* 370–372.

Fiellin, D., Ried, M., & O'Connor, P. (2000). Screening for alcohol problems in primary care: A systematic review. *Archives of Internal Medicine, 160,* 1977–1989.

Fleming, M. (2003). Brief interventions and the treatment of alcohol use disorders: Current evidence. *Recent Developments in Alcoholism, 16,* 375–390.

Flynn, H., Marcus, S., Barry, K., & Blow, F. (2002). Rates and correlates of alcohol use among pregnant women in obstetrics clinics. *Alcoholism: Clinical and Experimental Research, 27,* 81–87.

Gladstone, J., Nulman, I., & Koren, G. (1996). Reproductive risk of binge drinking during pregnancy. *Reproductive Toxicology, 10,* 3–13.

Greenbaum, R., Nulman, I., Rovet, J., & Koren, G. (2002). The Toronto experience in diagnosing alcohol-related neurodevelopmental disorder: A unique profile of deficits and assets. *Canadian Journal of Clinical Pharmacology, 9,* 215–225.

Guizzetti, M., Catlin, M., & Costa, L.G. (1997). The effects of ethanol on glial cell proliferation: Relevance to the fetal alcohol syndrome. *Frontiers in Bioscience, 2,* e93–e98.

Hanson, J.W., Streissguth, A.P., & Smith, D. (1978). The effect of moderate alcohol consumption during pregnancy on fetal growth and morphogenesis. *Journal of Pediatrics, 92,* 457–460.

Henkenius, A.L., Riley, E.P., Jernigan, T.L., & Toga, A.W. (2002). Mapping cortical gray matter asymmetry patterns in adolescents with heavy prenatal alcohol exposure. *Neuroimage, 17,* 1807–1819.

Ingersoll, K., Floyd, L., Sobell, M., & Velasquez, M.M., for the Project Choices Intervention Research Group. (2003). Reducing the risk of alcohol-exposed pregnancies: A study of a motivational intervention in community settings. *Pediatrics, 111*(5 Pt. 2), 1131–1135.

Jacobson, J.L., & Jacobson, S.W. (2002). Effects of prenatal alcohol exposure on child development. *Alcohol Research and Health, 26,* 282–286.

Jones, K.L., Smith, D.W., Ulleland, P., & Streissguth, A.P. (1973). Pattern of malformation in offspring of chronic alcoholic mothers. *Lancet, 1,* 1267–1271.

Kaemingk, K.L., Mulvaney, S., & Halverson, P.T. (2003). Learning following prenatal alcohol exposure: Performance on verbal and visual multitrial tasks. *Archives of Clinical Neuropsychology, 18,* 33–47.

Kelly, S.J., Day, N., & Streissguth, A.P. (2000). Effects of prenatal alcohol exposure on social behavior in humans and other species. *Neurotoxicology and Teratology, 22,* 143–149.

Kerns, K.A., Don, A., Mateer, C.A., & Streissguth, A.P. (1997). Cognitive deficits in nonretarded adults with fetal alcohol syndrome. *Journal of Learning Disabilities, 30,* 685–693.

Knight, J., Shrier, L., & Bravender, T. (1999). A new brief screen for adolescent substance abuse. *Archives of Pediatrics and Adolescent Medicine, 153,* 591–596.

Korkman, M., Kettunen, S., & Autti-Ramo, I. (2003). Neurocognitive impairment in early adolescence following prenatal alcohol exposure of varying duration. *Child Neuropsychology, 9,* 117–128.

Kvigne, V.L., Leonardson, G.R., Borzelleca, J., Brock, E., Neff-Smith, M., & Welty, T.K. (2003). Characteristics of mothers who have children with fetal alcohol syndrome or some characteristics of fetal alcohol syndrome. *Journal of the American Board of Family Practice, 16,* 296–303.

Mattson, S.N., Goodman, A.M., Caine, C., Delis, D.C., & Riley, E.P. (1999). Executive functioning in children with heavy prenatal alcohol exposure. *Alcoholism: Clinical and Experimental Research, 23,* 1808–1815.

Mattson, S.N., & Riley, E.P. (1998). A review of the neurobehavioral deficits in children with fetal alcohol syndrome or prenatal exposure to alcohol. *Alcoholism: Clinical and Experimental Research, 22,* 279–294.

Mattson, S.N., Riley, E.P., Gramling, L., Delis, D.C., & Jones, K.L. (1998). Neuropsychological comparison of alcohol-exposed children with or without physical features of fetal alcohol syndrome. *Neuropsychology, 12,* 146–153.

Mattson, S.N., Riley, E.P., Sowell, E.R., Jernigan, T.L., Sobel, D.F., & Jones, K.L. (1996). A decrease in the size of the basal ganglia in children with fetal alcohol syndrome. *Alcoholism: Clinical and Experimental Research, 20,* 1088–1093.

Mattson, S.N., & Roebuck, T.M. (2002). Acquisition and retention of verbal and nonverbal information in children with heavy prenatal alcohol exposure. *Alcoholism: Clinical and Experimental Research, 26,* 875–882.

May, P.A., & Gossage, J.P. (2001). Estimating the prevalence of fetal alcohol syndrome: A summary. *Alcohol Research and Health, 25,* 159–167.

May, P.A., Hymbaugh, K., Aase, J.M., & Samet, J. (1983). Epidemiology of fetal alcohol syndrome among American Indians of the Southwest. *Social Biology, 30,* 374–387.

McCarver, D.G., Thomasson, H., Martier, S., Sokol, R.J., & Li, T.K. (1997). Alcohol dehydrogenase-2*3 allele protects against alcohol-related birth defects among African Americans. *Journal of Pharmacology and Experimental Therapeutics, 283,* 1095–1101.

Meyer, M.J. (1998). Perceptual differences in fetal alcohol effect boys performing a modeling task. *Perceptual and Motor Skills, 87*(3 Pt. 1), 784–786.

Miller, W., & Rollnick, S. (1991). *Motivational interviewing: Preparing people to change addictive behavior.* New York: The Guilford Press.

O'Connor, M., & Whaley, S.E. (2003). Alcohol use in pregnant low-income women. *Journal of Studies on Alcoholism, 64,* 773–783.

Oesterheld, J.R., Kofoed, L., Tervo, R., Fogas, B., Wilson, A., & Fiechtner, H. (1998). Effectiveness of methylphenidate in Native American children with fetal alcohol syndrome and attention deficit/ hyperactivity disorder: A controlled pilot study. *Journal of Child and Adolescent Psychopharmacology, 8,* 39–48.

Olney, J.W., Ishimaru, M.J., Bittigau, P., & Ikonomidou, C. (2000). Ethanol-induced apoptotic neurodegeneration in the developing brain. *Apoptosis, 5,* 515–521.

Olson, H.C., Feldman, J.J., Streissguth, A.P., Sampson, P.D., & Bookstein, F.L. (1998). Neuropsychological deficits in adolescents with fetal alcohol syndrome: Clinical findings. *Alcoholism: Clinical and Experimental Research, 22,* 1998–2012.

Olson, H.C., Streissguth, A.P., Sampson, P.D., Barr, H.M., Bookstein, F.L., & Thiede, K. (1997). Association of prenatal alcohol exposure with behavioral and learning problems in early adolescence. *Journal of the American Academy of Child and Adolescent Psychiatry, 36,* 1187–1194.

O'Malley, K.D., & Nanson, J. (2002). Clinical implications of a link between fetal alcohol spectrum disorder and attention-deficit hyperactivity disorder. *Canadian Journal of Psychiatry, 47,* 349–354.

Ozer, E., Sarioglu, S., & Gure, A. (2000). Effects of prenatal ethanol exposure on neuronal migration, neuronogenesis and brain myelination in the mice brain. *Clinical Neuropathology, 19,* 21–25.

Pierce, D.R., & West, J.R. (1986). Blood alcohol concentration: A critical factor for producing fetal alcohol effects. *Alcohol, 3,* 269–272.

Project CHOICES Research Group. (2002). Alcohol-exposed pregnancy: Characteristics associated with risk. *American Journal of Preventive Medicine, 23,* 166–173.

Riikonen, R., Salonen, I., Partanen, K., & Verho, S. (1999). Brain perfusion SPECT and MRI in fetal alcohol syndrome. *Developmental Medicine and Child Neurology, 41,* 652–659.

Riley, E.P., Guerri, C., Calhoun, F., Charness, M.E., Foroud, T.M., Li, T.-K., et al. (2003). Prenatal alcohol exposure: Advancing knowledge through international collaboration. *Alcoholism: Clinical and Experimental Research, 27,* 118–135.

Roebuck, T.M., Mattson, S.N., & Riley, E.P. (1998). A review of the neuroanatomical findings in children with fetal alcohol syndrome or prenatal exposure to alcohol. *Alcoholism: Clinical and Experimental Research, 22,* 339–344.

Roebuck, T.M., Mattson, S.N., & Riley, E.P. (1999). Behavioral and psychosocial profiles of alcohol-exposed children. *Alcoholism: Clinical and Experimental Research, 23,* 1070–1076.

Roebuck, T.M., Mattson, S.N., & Riley, E.P. (2002). Interhemispheric transfer in children with heavy prenatal alcohol exposure. *Alcoholism: Clinical and Experimental Research, 26,* 1863–1871.

Russell, M. (1994). New assessment tools for drinking in pregnancy: T-ACE, TWEAK, and others. *Alcohol Health and Research World, 18,* 55–61.

Sampson, P.D., Streissguth, A.P., Bookstein, F.L., Little, R.E., Clarren, S.K., Dehaene, P., et al. (1997). Incidence of fetal alcohol syndrome and prevalence of alcohol-related neurodevelopmental disorder. *Teratology, 56,* 317–326.

Saunders, J., Oasland, O., Babor, T., De LaFuente, J., & Grant, M. (1993). Development of the Alcohol Use Disorders Identification Test (AUDIT): WHO Collaborative Project on Early Detection of persons with harmful alcohol consumption–II. *Addiction, 88,* 791–804.

Sobell, L., & Sobell, M. (2000). Alcohol timeline followback (TLFB). In *Handbook of psychiatric measures* (pp. 477–479). Washington, DC: American Psychiatric Association.

Sokol, R.J., Delaney-Black, V., & Nordstrom, B. (2003). Fetal alcohol spectrum disorder. *JAMA, 290,* 2996–2999.

Sokol, R.J., Martier, S., & Ager, J.W. (1989). The T-ACE questions: Practical prenatal detection of risk-drinking. *American Journal of Obstetrics and Gynecology, 160,* 863–868.

Sood, B., Delaney-Black, V., Covington, C., Nordstrom-Klee, B., Ager, J., Templin, T., et al. (2001). Prenatal alcohol exposure and childhood behavior at age 6 to 7 years: I. Dose-response effect. *Pediatrics, 108,* E34.

Stratton, K., Howe, C., & Battaglia, F. (Eds.). (1996). *Fetal alcohol syndrome: Diagnosis, epidemiology, prevention and treatment.* Washington, DC: National Academies Press.

Streissguth, A.P., Aase, J.M., Clarren, S.K., Randels, S.P., LaDue, R.A., & Smith, D.F. (1991). Fetal alcohol syndrome in adolescents and adults. *JAMA, 265,* 1961–1967.

Streissguth, A.P., & O'Malley, K. (2000). Neuropsychiatric implications and long-term consequences of fetal alcohol spectrum disorders. *Seminars in Clinical Neuropsychiatry, 5,* 177–190.

Surgeon General's advisory on alcohol and pregnancy. (1981). *FDA Drug Bulletin, 11*(2), 9–10.

Swayze, V.W., II, Johnson, V.P., Hanson, J.W., Piven, J., Sato, Y., Giedd, J.N., et al. (1997). Magnetic resonance imaging of brain anomalies in fetal alcohol syndrome. *Pediatrics, 99,* 232–240.

Tajuddin, N.F., & Druse, M.J. (1999). In utero ethanol exposure decreased the density of serotonin neurons: Maternal ipsapirone treatment exerted a protective effect. *Brain Research: Developmental Brain Research, 117,* 91–97.

Thomasson, H., Edenberg, H., Crabb, D., Mai, X., Jerome, R., Li, T., et al. (1991). Alcohol and aldehyde dehydrogenase genotypes and alcoholism in Chinese men. *American Journal of Human Genetics, 48,* 677–681.

Uecker, A., & Nadel, L. (1998). Spatial but not object memory impairments in children with fetal alcohol syndrome. *American Journal of Mental Retardation, 103,* 12–18.

Valles, S., Sancho-Tello, M., Minana, R., Climent, E., Renau-Piqueras, J., & Guerri, C. (1996). Glial fibrillary acidic protein expression in rat brain and in radial glia culture is delayed by prenatal ethanol exposure. *Journal of Neurochemistry, 67,* 2425–2433.

Wilsnack, S., Wilsnack, R., & Hiller-Sturmhofel, S. (1994). How women drink: Epidemiology of women's drinking and problem drinking. *Alcohol Health and Research World, 18,* 173–181.

13

Plumbism

Elevated Lead Levels

CECILIA T. DAVOLI

Plumbism (elevated lead level) puts a child at risk for a wide range of developmental disabilities. The developing brain is potentially susceptible to damage from lead exposure, and this damage may not be reversible. Although we have developed the ability to effectively identify and treat children with elevated lead levels, the primary goal of management for plumbism is prevention.

BACKGROUND/ HISTORICAL PERSPECTIVE

Lead is a metal that has no noticeable appearance, smell, or taste in the small quantities that can cause plumbism. There is no human nutritional or biochemical requirement for lead and no physiological mechanism for its breakdown. It has been utilized for myriad medicinal and technological purposes over the centuries (Needleman, 1992). Plumbism is, therefore, found in both industrialized and developing countries and can affect individuals in all ethnic, racial, and socioeconomic groups.

The first clinical description of plumbism was by the Greek physician Nikander in the second century B.C. (Major, 1932). In the late 1700s, Benjamin Franklin commented on the "dry gripes" (colic) and "dangles" (wristdrop) that were observed in tinkers, typesetters, and painters who were exposed to lead (Needleman, 1992). During the 1800s, workers in other lead-related occupations developed chronic symptoms (National Research Council, 1993), and plumbism was recognized as a clini-

cal entity with the potential for long-lasting sequelae.

Childhood plumbism was first described in 1892 by a resident at the Children's Hospital in Brisbane, Australia (Turner, 1892). He reported on four children who presented with recurrent emesis, headache, and ocular neuritis and concluded that they had localized basal meningitis. He and his chief cared for numerous children with similar symptoms over the next several years. In addition to ocular symptoms, many of these children suffered from muscle wasting, wristdrop, and footdrop. In 1897, both physicians published articles that ascribed these children's symptoms to lead. Although galvanized water storage tanks were first postulated to be responsible for causing the plumbism, the powdery old paint on house railings and porches was ultimately identified as the lead source (Gibson, 1904).

In the United States, the first documentation of pediatric plumbism was a 1914 case report of a child with recurrent meningitis, seizures, and coma (Thomas & Blackfan, 1914). The etiology of the illness remained obscure until the boy was noted to have the narrow blue-black "lead line" on the margin of his gums that can sometimes be seen in cases of chronic, severe lead exposure. Environmental assessment revealed that the railings of his bedstead were covered with chipped paint.

Prior to the 1940s, it was believed that children who recovered from acute plumbism were "cured" and had no permanent sequelae. This premise was challenged in a 1943 account of 20 children who had been treated for symptomatic plumbism in infancy and early child-hood (Byers & Lord, 1943). Serial psychomet-ric assessment revealed deficits in visual-motor function, language skills, and behavior, and 19 of the children encountered significant school difficulties. This was the first time that follow-up data were used to demonstrate the potential long-term sequelae of childhood lead expo-sure.

SOURCES OF LEAD EXPOSURE

Lead is ubiquitous, and lead exposure can occur almost anywhere in the world. In the vast majority of cases, children with plumbism have multiple lead sources in their environ-ment. Table 13.1 lists many of the potential sources of lead exposure for children.

In urban U.S. locations, paint is frequently the principal source of lead exposure. Paint containing lead can be found in most U.S. homes built before 1950, and in some built as late as the 1970s. In 1978, the U.S. Consumer Product Safety Commission banned lead in paint for residential use. Lead continues to be added to paint for cars, boats, bridges, and other industrial structures.

Peeling and crumbling lead-based paint may disintegrate into dust particles and fall onto the floor and other surfaces in a home.

Table 13.1.   Potential lead sources for children

Residential paint in pre-1978 homes
Industrial paint
Lead-contaminated dust/soil
Painted toys/furniture
Renovations/abatement
Vinyl mini-blinds
Industrial point sources
Leaded gasoline
Leaded solder/plumbing
Seams in food cans
Leaded crystal
Glazed pottery
Adult occupational/hobby exposure
Folk remedies/medicinals
Ingestion of a foreign body containing lead
Hair dye
Cosmetics
Calcium supplements
Placental transfer
Breast milk

Disintegration of paint frequently occurs when there is repetitive friction, such as when sash-type windows are raised and lowered. Young children can be exposed to lead-contaminated dust through hand-to-mouth activities such as thumb sucking and mouthing of objects that have been on the floor. Older toys and furni-ture, such as cribs and playpens, may have been painted with leaded paint and may be mouthed. Children may also be exposed to lead through ingestion or inhalation while living in a home containing leaded paint if that home is being renovated or abated (undergoing re-moval of lead paint). Such exposure can also occur if nearby buildings in the neighborhood are being renovated.

Lead that has been deposited in dust and soil is another potential source of lead expo-sure. Some of this lead represents fallout from leaded gasoline and industrial point sources (e.g., lead smelters, incinerators). The dust and soil around older, deteriorating housing may contain large amounts of lead particles, which can potentially be tracked into the house. Lead in dust and soil poses a greater risk to children during the spring and summer months, when they spend more time playing outside and the soil is drier and more mobile (Haley & Talbot, 2004).

Leaded gasoline continues to be used in some parts of the world, thereby contributing to a certain proportion of the lead in air, dust, soil, and water in those areas. Lead was phased out of gasoline in the United States in a step-wise fashion, beginning in 1978. The decline in the use of leaded gasoline was paralleled by a decline in the mean blood lead concentration in the U.S. population.

Another potential lead source is water that is conducted through pipes with lead-soldered joints and fittings or collected in lead-lined rainwater tanks (Centers for Disease Control and Prevention [CDC], 2004a). Lead pipes can still be found in some parts of the United States in homes built before the 1920s. Acidic (soft) water can potentially leach higher amounts of lead from such pipes.

Lead can contaminate the food supply via several means. Food cans containing lead-soldered seams were previously very common in this country and contributed to 25%–40%

of human lead ingestion in the 1970s. Today, it is unusual to find cans with lead-soldered seams in the United States, unless they have been imported from another country. Lead crystal containers and lead-glazed vessels may expose entire families to lead if used to store acidic beverages such as wine or citrus juice. Many imported pieces of pottery contain leaded glaze or may not have been properly fired (CDC, 2004b). Produce grown in soil with a high lead content can be contaminated with lead.

Adults employed in smelters, battery plants, radiator repair shops, bridge painting, and numerous other lead-related occupations have potential exposure to lead. Hobbies such as stained glass work, pottery, home renovations, and furniture refinishing may pose a risk of lead exposure. Childhood plumbism from these sources can be avoided if the adults wear protective clothing, change clothes before returning home, and wash contaminated clothing separately from that of other family members.

Since antiquity, lead and lead compounds have been prescribed for a wide variety of ailments, and many cultures continue to use folk remedies that contain lead. Examples of lead-containing medicinals include Mexican Azarcon or Greta, which are used to treat abdominal distress, and Asian Pay-loo-ah, which is used to treat fever. Immigrants frequently bring their traditional folk remedies with them from their homeland and may not be aware that these might contain lead.

Ingestion of a leaded foreign body such as lead shot, curtain/fishing weights, or jewelry can result in an extreme elevation in blood lead level (VanArsdale, Leiker, Kohn, Merritt, & Horowitz, 2004). Additional unusual sources of lead exposure include ingestion of hair dye containing lead and burning of paper that is printed with ink containing leaded pigments. Some cosmetics contain lead, such as the eye makeup Surma or Kohl, which is used by Indian and Middle Eastern peoples. Lead has also been found in bone meal and dolomite, which are often used as calcium supplements (Scelfo & Flegal, 2000).

Lead freely crosses the placenta and can be transmitted via breast milk; therefore, pregnant and lactating women should not be exposed to potential lead sources (Ettinger et al., 2004). Fetal plumbism was first widely reported among 19th century women who were employed in industries involving lead exposure. It was noted that these women experienced sterility, miscarriage, stillbirth, and premature delivery at a higher rate than expected (National Research Council, 1993). Maternal lead exposure can also result from any of the sources listed previously. If fetal or neonatal plumbism is suspected, a careful environmental history for maternal lead exposure should be undertaken.

DIAGNOSIS OF PLUMBISM

The blood lead level, measured in micrograms per deciliter (mcg/dL), is the definitive screening and diagnostic test for childhood plumbism. The CDC (1991) has defined 10 mcg/dL and above as an elevated blood lead level in a child (Table 13.2). Screening for plumbism is important because most children with elevated blood lead levels are asymptomatic. A venous lead level is preferred because capillary specimens may be inaccurate due to skin contamination and inconsistent technique. Not all screening sites can perform venipuncture, so a capillary sample is frequently obtained as an initial screening test. Follow-up venipuncture is indicated to confirm any elevated capillary blood lead level. The timing/frequency of subsequent blood tests is dependent on the individual child's age, initial blood lead level, and risk of ongoing lead exposure.

Before 1960, the diagnosis of plumbism was established by clinical signs such as lead lines on the gums or acute neurological find-

Table 13.2. Centers for Disease Control and Prevention classification of childhood plumbism

Class	Blood lead level (mcg/dL)
I	Less than or equal to 9
IIA	10–14
IIB	15–19
III	20–44
IV	45–69
V	≥ 70

Adapted from Centers for Disease Control. (1991). *Preventing lead poisoning in young children.* Atlanta, GA: Author.

ings. Long bone radiographs with dark lines at the epiphyses were often used to confirm the diagnosis. As knowledge accumulated about the potential long-term sequelae of subclinical plumbism, formal blood screening programs were established. Screening was previously done using the blood free erythrocyte proto-porphyrin (FEP) level, which can be elevated due to plumbism. The FEP level is no longer used because it is not a sufficiently sensitive indicator of plumbism at lower blood lead levels, and it can also be elevated because of other effects on the developing erythrocyte.

Table 13.3 lists the factors that the CDC (1997) has determined will place a child at greater risk for lead exposure. Blood lead screening is indicated for children who are determined to have at least one risk factor or those whose history reveals potential exposure to the sources described in the preceding section. Current screening programs focus primarily on children between ages 9 months and 6 years, who are at highest risk of lead exposure. Blood lead screening is also indicated for any child, adolescent, or young adult whose medical, environmental, developmental, and/or psychosocial history places him or her at high risk for lead exposure/ingestion. Several studies have shown good sensitivity and negative predictive value of screening questionnaires to guide a child's history and blood lead

Table 13.3. High risk factors for childhood lead exposure

Sibling, housemate, or playmate of child with plumbism

Residence in or regular visitation to pre-1950 home

Residence in or regular visitation to pre-1978 home with recent or ongoing renovations

Residence in region that contains 27% of housing that is pre-1950

Residence in region that contains 12% of children with a blood lead level greater than or equal to 10 mcg/dL

Receipt of services from a public assistance program (e.g., Medicaid)

Member of racial/ethnic minority group

Parent/adult household member with occupational lead exposure

Any other characteristic of a group with increased risk of lead exposure

Adapted from Centers for Disease Control and Prevention (1997). *Screening young children for lead poisoning: Guidance for state and local public health officials.* Atlanta, GA: Author.

testing (Schaffer, Szilagyi, & Weitzman, 1994; Tejeda, Wyatt, Rostek, & Solomon, 1994).

In reality, the blood lead level is a poor estimate of the total body burden of lead because this screening method is only able to quantify lead that is located in the bloodstream. Blood lead probably represents a combination of 1) lead absorbed within the preceding 72 hours, 2) lead absorbed within the preceding 3–4 months, and 3) lead that was absorbed many years earlier and is being remobilized from other body tissues, including bone. Serial blood lead levels can be obtained to monitor the slow decrease in blood lead level that occurs as a child grows older. The rate of this lead level decrease is theoretically more affected by the chronicity of a child's lead exposure than by the peak level but is probably most related to a child's individual nutritional state and metabolism. There is no way to predict or quantify the rate of fall in blood lead level in an individual child as he or she naturally diureses lead from the body.

If a child with an elevated blood lead level does have symptoms, they are initially nonspecific and may include irritability and behavior changes (e.g., hyperactivity, crankiness). These symptoms may be normal behavioral variants for any specific child and are too vague to be diagnostic of lead exposure. If the blood lead level increases further, a child may develop chronic or intermittent abdominal pain, often accompanied by intermittent vomiting, constipation, and anorexia. Some children will demonstrate lassitude, slowed acquisition or loss of developmental skills, or decreased activity level. Headaches, ataxia, or other overt neurological disturbances may manifest themselves.

As the blood lead level passes 70 mcg/dL, a child is at increasing risk for developing acute encephalopathy. This usually presents as intractable vomiting and lethargy, quickly progressing to stupor and coma. Seizures are quite common in children with lead encephalopathy. If there is a delay in diagnosis, or if appropriate emergency medical care and chelation therapy are not given promptly in an intensive care setting, encephalopathy can progress to death.

In some children, plumbism may be identified as a secondary diagnosis. Children who demonstrate pica (ingestion of non-nutritive substances) and other hand-to-mouth activities (e.g., thumb sucking, mouthing of toys) are at particularly high risk for lead exposure. Children with cognitive delay may engage in excessive pica or other hand-to-mouth activities that are not age appropriate. In this case, a blood lead level determination should be done, even if the child is over the age level delineated by the CDC guidelines. Girls adopted from China comprise another group with increased risk of plumbism because of their significant airborne industrial lead exposure (Miller & Hendrie, 2000).

It is not possible to prove what potential effect(s) a specific lead level may have on an individual child, nor is it possible to prove a direct causal relationship between a specific lead level and a developmental disability. Nonetheless, the body of accumulated evidence supports the tenet that lead has the potential to cause damage to the developing brain (Pocock, Smith, & Baghurst, 1994).

CLINICAL EFFECTS OF LEAD

Central Nervous System Effects

Lead has no physiological use in the human body, and it is postulated that potential harmful effects can occur at blood lead levels below the CDC action level of 10 mcg/dL (Canfield et al., 2003). In children, the developing central nervous system is the site of potential damage, especially during the first few years of life. The potential sequelae may be long lasting and may not become clinically evident until the child demonstrates school difficulties or behavior problems. Nonetheless, it is not possible to definitively identify lead as the cause of or contributor to an individual child's specific symptoms.

Following ingestion, lead enters the bloodstream via gastrointestinal absorption and is carried via a calcium transport mechanism. Lead is initially transported within the erythrocytes, then diffuses into the plasma, then moves into the remainder of the body. Although lead's potential to cause damage to the central nervous system is not completely understood, various biochemical mechanisms are theorized to contribute to aberrant neuro-

development. Multiple studies have suggested that lead's activation of protein kinase C plays some role in disruption of cellular function (Kim, Chakraborti, Goldstein, Johnston, & Bressler, 2002). At high levels, lead can disrupt the normal capillary function of the endothelial cells in the blood–brain barrier, resulting in vasogenic edema (Hossain et al., 2004). It is also theorized that lead interferes with vitamin D metabolism, which may alter the body's absorption and transport of calcium, resulting in disruption of intracellular calcium-dependent processes.

In the developing brain, synaptic connections increase rapidly within the first 2 years of life. Toddlers have twice the number of synaptic brain connections and activity as adults, with the composition of the adult synaptic network being derived by selective "pruning" of synapses during early childhood. It is postulated that childhood lead exposure somehow alters the activity and efficiency of the brain's developing synaptic network, resulting in a qualitative difference in the normal synaptic pruning process (Goldstein, 1992). In addition, lead's adverse effects on the brain's N-methyl-D-aspartate receptors may contribute to its potential to cause deficits in learning, attention, behavior, and intelligence (Toscano & Guilarte, 2005).

Many clinical studies have documented the potential long-term sequelae of early lead exposure. In a landmark paper published in 1979, it was shown that 6- and 7-year-old children with higher concentrations of lead in their teeth scored lower on the Wechsler Intelligence Scale for Children–Revised (Wechsler, 1974) than did those with lower lead levels (Needleman et al., 1979). Long-term follow-up of these children demonstrated persistent problems with neurobehavioral and academic function (Needleman, Schell, Bellinger, Leviton, & Allred, 1990). A study on lead exposure and intelligence quotient (IQ) in British schoolchildren yielded similar results (Yule, Lansdown, Millar, & Urbanowicz, 1981).

These apparent neurodevelopmental differences have been documented earlier in life. Elevated umbilical cord blood lead levels have been shown to correlate with decreased scores on cognitive tests during the first 2 years of life

(Bellinger, Leviton, Waternaux, Needleman, & Rabinowitz, 1987). This was primarily found in children with ongoing postnatal exposure, as evidenced by elevated blood lead levels at 24 months of age. Subsequent follow-up of the children to age 10 years showed academic performance deficits in those with elevated lead levels (Bellinger, Stiles, & Needleman, 1992). Similar work was done in a cohort of children who lived near a lead-smelting factory in Port Pirie, Australia (Baghurst et al., 1992). Both Bellinger's work and the Port Pirie study showed that these early cognitive deficits have the potential to persist into childhood.

Plumbism has potential adverse effects on other areas of neurobehavioral development. Language skills such as verbal processing, sentence repetition, and verbal comprehension have all been noted to be impaired in children with elevated lead levels (Mayfield, 1983). Lead has been shown to have an impact on auditory processing abilities (Dietrich, Succop, Berger, & Keith, 1992), which could affect both receptive and expressive language development. In a case report series of six children with autism, the most severe form of communication disorder, it has been suggested that lead exposure may accelerate or exacerbate symptoms (Accardo, Whitman, Caul, & Rolfe, 1988).

Clinical studies of children with plumbism have also assessed other cognitive functions, including academic achievement, visual-motor skills, behavior, and attention. In all of these areas, children with higher lead levels had worse performance than those with lower lead levels. Needleman et al. (1979) showed that teachers who were blinded to their students' lead status consistently identified maladaptive behavior patterns in those children with elevated lead levels. The frequency of problem behaviors appeared to increase with increasing lead level, in a dose–response relationship. Examples of identified behavior deficits included distractibility, hyperactivity, impulsivity, inability to follow directions, and impaired attention span. All of these behavior characteristics are potentially long lasting and may contribute to the subsequent school difficulties and academic underachievement that have been observed in some children with lead exposure.

Other Clinical Effects

Lead has potential adverse effects on other biochemical processes in the body. Each cell in the body synthesizes its own heme enzymes, and lead partially inhibits heme synthesis in all cell types that have been studied. Blood lead levels of 15–18 mcg/dL are the threshold for elevation of the red blood cell FEP. Anemia due to lead exposure can occur at blood lead levels over 60 mcg/dL. A shortened red blood cell life span has also been demonstrated in adults with similar blood lead levels.

Several studies have shown that children with lead exposure have diminished growth, both ponderal and linear (Schwartz, Angle, & Pitcher, 1986; Shukla, Dietrich, Bornschein, Berger, & Hammond, 1991). This growth deficit can be seen in neonates whose mothers had excessive exposure to lead as indicated by elevated umbilical cord lead levels. Many of these women will bear preterm or small-for-gestational-age infants. Growth retardation appears to continue postnatally if the children continue to be exposed to high levels of lead during infancy and early childhood. It is recommended that evaluation for lead exposure be included in the workup for children with failure to thrive.

Acute and chronic lead exposure have the potential to adversely affect renal function in several ways. Both animal and human studies have demonstrated a correlation between elevated blood lead levels and hypertension (Needleman, 1992). Children with blood lead levels greater than 150 mcg/dL can develop an acquired Fanconi syndrome, with impaired proximal tubule reabsorption and resultant glycosuria, phosphaturia, and aminoaciduria. If acute, Fanconi syndrome is usually fully reversible by chelation therapy.

Lead has also been shown to alter the ratios of peripheral blood lymphocytes in children (Li, Zhengyan, Rong, & Hanyun, 2005). It is postulated that lead may have functionally significant adverse effects on the immune system at various life stages (Dietert, Lee, Hussain, & Piepenbrink, 2004). It is possible that lead may have potential influence on childhood asthma and autoimmune diseases.

PREVENTION OF LEAD EXPOSURE

Prevention of childhood lead exposure usually involves multiple agencies and individuals whose efforts should be coordinated. The most successful prevention strategies involve the family, the medical community, the local public health system, social services agencies, and state/federal legislative measures. Families who are educated about potential lead sources can also learn how to minimize their children's lead exposure in a number of ways.

Initial preventive efforts are usually focused on appropriate housecleaning techniques to remove lead-contaminated dust. Sweeping and vacuuming are discouraged, because both of these activities stir up a great deal of dust. Wet-cleaning techniques, such as using a mop or damp cloth, are preferable. It is often recommended that a high-phosphate detergent be used instead of a regular cleanser or soap because phosphate can form a chemical bond with lead. Most household cleansers do not contain a high percentage of phosphate, but it can be found in trisodium phosphate (TSP; available in hardware stores) and some powdered automatic dishwasher detergents. Similar wet-cleaning techniques can be used for all surfaces in the home.

Another effective technique is use of a high-efficiency particulate air (HEPA) vacuum cleaner, which is capable of trapping dust particles as small as 0.3 microns in diameter. Lead particles are found in highest proportion in smaller dust particles, which are usually not captured by common household vacuum cleaners. The HEPA vacuum is an integral part of the cleanup effort that must be undertaken in a home after renovation or abatement is complete.

Abatement is the process by which lead (especially lead paint) is permanently removed or encapsulated. It should be carried out only by qualified individuals who have been specifically trained in safe techniques. Household belongings should be stored off-site or encased in plastic before abatement begins. Workers must be protected by specialized clothing, headware, and respirators with HEPA filters. Painted surfaces should not be sanded or burned because both techniques will create dangerous amounts of lead dust and fumes. If complete abatement cannot be done, measures such as encapsulation of walls will assist with prevention of lead exposure. Window and door frames can be completely replaced with vinyl/metal ones that do not contain lead paint. Meticulous cleanup must be done after any work is completed to ensure that there will be no exposure to lead-contaminated debris. The entire family (including pets) must vacate a home that is undergoing renovation or abatement and should not return to the home until all of the work and cleanup have been completed.

Young children should be carefully monitored to keep them away from peeling paint and crumbling plaster. Their cribs or beds should not be placed against a wall that has peeling paint on it. If they are playing or hiding in an area with peeling paint, the area should be cleaned and their access to that wall should be blocked until appropriate repairs can be made. Their toys and pacifiers should be washed frequently. Hand washing should be carried out before meals, snacks, and naps and after playing outside. Children should be encouraged to play in grassy areas instead of areas containing dust that may be contaminated with lead. They should not be given antique toys or use old cribs that may be painted with lead paint. Other leaded objects should be removed from their immediate environment.

Because of the danger of exposure to lead solder in some imported food cans, these cans should not be used for heating or storage of food. Acidic foods leach more lead from a metal can, so it is best to buy fruits, juices, tomatoes, and sodas that have been packaged in glass, plastic, or cardboard containers. Pottery and ceramic containers should not be used to store or cook food because these may contain leaded glazes. When using water for drinking or cooking in a house with old plumbing, it is best to run the water for several minutes to flush the pipes. Cold tap water should be used for making baby formula or juice because hot tap water will pick up more lead from the pipes or solder. Boiling the water will not remove the lead from it.

Good nutrition is an essential component of primary prevention of lead exposure. Parents should be encouraged to give their children well-balanced meals and use good hygiene during food preparation. Healthy snacks are important because gastrointestinal absorption of lead is increased if the stomach is empty. Fried foods and foods with a high fat content will increase the absorption of lead. The skin and fat should be removed from meat, and foods should be cooked via low-fat techniques such as baking or boiling. Children with low calcium or iron stores will have enhanced lead absorption. Iron deficiency must be medically corrected, and the child's diet should be rich in foods that contain iron and calcium. Foods high in vitamin C assist with iron absorption, whereas tea given with a meal decreases the body's absorption of iron.

TREATMENT (CHELATION)

Chelation is the process by which a metal is chemically bound in a form that is easily excreted by the human body. When a child's blood lead level is 45 mcg/dL or higher, chelation is used to lower the level quickly. This is essential in cases of neurologically symptomatic plumbism and the presence of a blood lead level over 70 mcg/dL, which are considered medical emergencies. Chelating agents enhance the natural diuresis of lead from the body through renal excretion. Natural diuresis ordinarily requires months to years, whereas chelating agents can accomplish the same degree of diuresis in days to weeks. Chelation therapy is only able to remove lead directly from the most accessible and mobile body compartment, the bloodstream. As lead is removed from the bloodstream, lead from other body compartments (e.g., soft tissues) can be mobilized and shifted into the bloodstream for removal. More than 70% of the body's lead burden is stored in bone, where it is not available for chelation.

Acute lead encephalopathy is a medical emergency, and treatment must occur in an intensive care setting (Gordon, Roberts, Amin, Williams, & Paloucek, 1998). Initial chelation therapy is provided by intramuscular British antilewisite (BAL; dimercaprol) and intravenous calcium disodium versenate (CaNa$_2$EDTA). Dimercaprol has the potential to cause hemolysis in children with glucose-6-phosphate dehydrogenase deficiency, and so

must be used with extreme caution in that setting. Parenteral fluid therapy is given at a rate that ensures continued urine flow without causing overhydration, except in cases in which cerebral edema requires fluid restriction. Diazepam and other anticonvulsants may be required for management of acute seizures.

In January 1991, the Food and Drug Administration approved an oral chelating agent for the treatment of childhood plumbism: *meso*-2,3-dimercaptosuccinic acid (also referred to as DMSA, succimer, or Chemet). This agent is chemically related to dimercaprol, but is more lead specific and water soluble and has fewer side effects than other chelating agents. The succimer treatment regimen lasts 19 days, with careful periodic laboratory monitoring of renal, hepatic, and hematological function. Children who do not respond to succimer or who have sulfur sensitivity may be treated with a 5-day course of intramuscular CaNa$_2$EDTA.

It is imperative that chelation be carried out in a lead-safe environment because all of these agents have the potential to enhance gastrointestinal absorption of ingested lead. In most cases, chelation occurs in a hospital setting to ensure that the child remains in a lead-safe environment. Rarely, chelation may be given in an outpatient setting such as a lead-safe home. The family of any child undergoing outpatient treatment must be able to achieve medication compliance, adhere to environmental guidelines, and return frequently for monitoring blood work.

Medical treatment of plumbism is not a substitute for primary preventive measures. The goal of medical management in childhood plumbism is lowering of the blood lead level as quickly as possible. Despite the fact that we have the ability to lower a child's lead level pharmacologically, chelation does not appear to have any ameliorating effect on a child's ultimate neuropsychological outcome (Rogan et al., 2001).

REMEDIATION

According to the 1997 CDC guidelines, children with elevated blood lead levels should be referred to a specialty center that is experienced in treating children with plumbism. An important part of the evaluation is a thorough developmental assessment, which would ideally include 1) formal neuropsychological evaluation of both verbal and nonverbal intelligence; 2) evaluation of expressive and receptive language skills; 3) screening of hearing, with formal audiology assessment if deficits are suspected; and 4) measures of behavior, attention, and memory. As children enter the late preschool and early school-age years, assessment of readiness skills and academic abilities becomes important, especially in children who are experiencing difficulties.

Because plumbism is a diagnosis that places a child at risk for developmental disabilities, a child may qualify for early intervention services whether or not any deficits have been identified. Therefore, young children with lead exposure should routinely be referred for early intervention services, such as a Head Start program. Older children may benefit from special education services if they are determined to have specific learning disabilities.

CONCLUSION

The causes and potential adverse consequences of childhood lead exposure have been definitively known for more than a century. There is a quick, accurate technique for measuring blood lead levels in children and clear guidelines for screening and monitoring are available. Effective preventive measures can be taught to families, and safe abatement procedures have been developed. In children with lead levels at or above 45 mcg/dL, effective chelating agents are available for treatment. Children with a history of plumbism are at potential risk for subsequent manifestation of developmental disabilities and may benefit from intervention/remediation.

REFERENCES

Accardo, P., Whitman, B., Caul, J., & Rolfe, U. (1988). Autism and plumbism. *Clinical Pediatrics, 27,* 41–44.

Baghurst, P.A., McMichael, A.J., Wigg, N.R., Vimpani, G.V., Robertson, E.F., Roberts, R.J., et al. (1992). Environmental exposure to lead and children's intelligence at the age of seven years. *New England Journal of Medicine, 327,* 1279–1284.

Bellinger, D., Leviton, A., Waternaux, C., Needleman, H., & Rabinowitz, M. (1987). Longitudinal analyses of prenatal and postnatal lead exposure and early cognitive development. *New England Journal of Medicine, 316,* 1037–1043.

Bellinger, D.C., Stiles, K.M., & Needleman, H.L. (1992). Low-level lead exposure, intelligence and academic achievement: A long-term follow-up study. *Pediatrics, 90,* 855–861.

Byers, R.K., & Lord, E.E. (1943). Late effects of lead poisoning on mental development. *American Journal of Diseases of Children, 66,* 471–494.

Canfield, R.L., Henderson, C.R., Cory-Slechta, D.A., Cox, C., Jusko, T.A., & Lanphear, B.P. (2003). Intellectual impairment in children with blood lead concentrations below 10 mcg per deciliter. *New England Journal of Medicine, 348,* 1517–1526.

Centers for Disease Control. (1991). *Preventing lead poisoning in young children.* Atlanta, GA: Author.

Centers for Disease Control and Prevention. (1997). *Screening young children for lead poisoning: Guidance for state and local public health officials.* Atlanta, GA: Author.

Centers for Disease Control and Prevention. (2004a). Blood lead levels in residents of homes with elevated lead in tap water—District of Columbia, 2004. *MMWR: Morbidity and Mortality Weekly Report, 53,* 268–270.

Centers for Disease Control and Prevention. (2004b). Childhood lead poisoning from commercially manufactured French ceramic dinnerware—New York City, 2003. *MMWR: Morbidity and Mortality Weekly Report, 53,* 584–586.

Dietert, R.R., Lee, J.E., Hussain, I., & Piepenbrink, M. (2004). Developmental immunotoxicology of lead. *Toxicology and Applied Pharmacology, 198,* 86–94.

Dietrich, K.N., Succop, P.A., Berger, O.G., & Keith, R.W. (1992). Lead exposure and the central auditory processing abilities and cognitive development of urban children: The Cincinnati Lead Study Cohort at age 5 years. *Neurotoxicology and Teratology, 14,* 51–56.

Ettinger, A.S., Tellez-Rojo, M.M., Amarasiriwardena, C., Bellinger, D., Peterson, K., Schwartz, J., et al. (2004). Effect of breast milk lead on infant blood lead levels at 1 month of age. *Environmental Health Perspectives, 112,* 1381–1385.

Gibson, J.L. (1904). A plea for painted railings and painted walls of rooms as the source of lead poisoning amongst Queensland children. *Australasian Medical Gazette, 23,* 149–153.

Goldstein, G.W. (1992). Neurologic concepts of lead poisoning in children. *Pediatric Annals, 21,* 384–388.

Gordon, R.A., Roberts, G., Amin, Z., Williams, R.H., & Paloucek, F.P. (1998). Aggressive approach in the treatment of acute lead encephalopathy with an extraordinarily high concentration of lead. *Archives of Pediatrics and Adolescent Medicine, 152,* 1100–1104.

Haley, V.B., & Talbot, T.O. (2004). Seasonality and trend in blood lead levels of New York State children. *BMC Pediatrics, 4,* 8.

Hossain, M.A., Russell, J.C., Miknyoczki, S., Ruggeri, B., Lal, B., & Laterra, J. (2004). Vascular endothelial growth factor mediates vasogenic edema in acute lead encephalopathy. *Annals of Neurology, 55,* 660–667.

Kim, K.A., Chakraborti, T., Goldstein, G., Johnston, M., & Bressler, J. (2002). Exposure to lead elevates induction of ZIF268 and ARC mRNA in rats after electroconvulsive shock: The involvement of protein kinase C. *Journal of Neuroscience Research, 69,* 268–277.

Li, S., Zhengyan, Z., Rong, L., & Hanyun, C. (2005). Decrease of CD4 + T-lymphocytes in children exposed to environmental lead. *Biological Trace Element Research, 105*(1–3), 19–25.

Major, R.H. (1932). *Classic descriptions of disease.* Baltimore: Charles C Thomas.

Mayfield, S.A. (1983). Language and speech behaviors of children with undue lead absorption: A review of the literature. *Journal of Speech and Hearing Research, 26,* 362–368.

Miller, L.C., & Hendrie, N.W. (2000). Health of children adopted from China. *Pediatrics, 105,* 76–82.

National Research Council. (1993). *Measuring lead exposure in infants, children, and other sensitive populations.* Washington, DC: National Academy Press.

Needleman, H.L. (1992). *Human lead exposure.* Boca Raton, FL: CRC Press.

Needleman, H.L., Gunnoe, C., Leviton, A., Reed, R., Peresie, H., Maher, C., et al. (1979). Deficits in psychologic and classroom performance of children with elevated dentine lead levels. *New England Journal of Medicine, 300,* 689–695.

Needleman, H.L., Schell, A., Bellinger, D., Leviton, A., & Allred, E.N. (1990). The long-term effects of exposure to low doses of lead in childhood. *New England Journal of Medicine, 322,* 83–88.

Pocock, S.J., Smith, M., & Baghurst, P. (1994). Environmental lead and children's intelligence: A systematic review of the epidemiological evidence. *British Medical Journal, 309,* 1189–1197.

Rogan, W.J., Dietrich, K.N., Ware, J.H., Dockery, D.W., Salganik, M., Radcliffe, J., et al. (2001). The effect of chelation therapy with succimer on neuropsychological development in children exposed to lead. *New England Journal of Medicine, 344,* 1421–1426.

Scelfo, G.M., & Flegal, A.R. (2000). Lead in calcium supplements. *Environmental Health Perspectives, 108,* 309–313.

Schaffer, S.J., Szilagyi, P.G., & Weitzman, M. (1994). Lead poisoning risk determination in an urban population through the use of a standardized questionnaire. *Pediatrics, 93,* 159–163.

Schwartz, J., Angle, C., & Pitcher, H. (1986). Relationship between childhood blood lead levels and stature. *Pediatrics, 77,* 281–288.

Shukla, R., Dietrich, K.N., Bornschein, R.L., Berger, O., & Hammond, P.B. (1991). Lead exposure and growth in the early preschool child: A follow-up report from the Cincinnati Lead Study. *Pediatrics, 88,* 886–892.

Tejeda, D.M., Wyatt, D.D., Rostek, B.R., & Solomon, W.B. (1994). Do questions about lead exposure predict elevated lead levels? *Pediatrics, 93,* 192–194.

Thomas, H.M., & Blackfan, K.D. (1914). Recurrent meningitis, due to lead, in a child of five years. *American Journal of Diseases of Children, 8,* 377–380.

Toscano, C.D., & Guilarte, T.R. (2005). Lead neurotoxicity: From exposure to molecular effects. *Brain Research: Brain Research Reviews, 49,* 529–554.

Turner, A.J. (1892). A form of cerebral disease characterised by definite symptoms, probably a localised basic meningitis. In *Transcript of the Intercolonial Medical Congress of Australasia* (pp. 98–100). Sydney: Intercolonial Medical Congress of Australasia.

VanArsdale, J.L., Leiker, R.D., Kohn, M., Merritt, T.A., & Horowitz, B.Z. (2004). Lead poisoning from a toy necklace. *Pediatrics, 114,* 1096–1099.

Wechsler, D. (1974). *Wechsler Intelligence Scale for Children–Revised.* New York: Harcourt Assessment.

Yule, W., Lansdown, R., Millar, I.B., & Urbanowicz, M.A. (1981). The relationship between blood lead concentrations, intelligence and attainment in a school population: A pilot study. *Developmental Medicine and Child Neurology, 23,* 567–576.

IV

Assessment

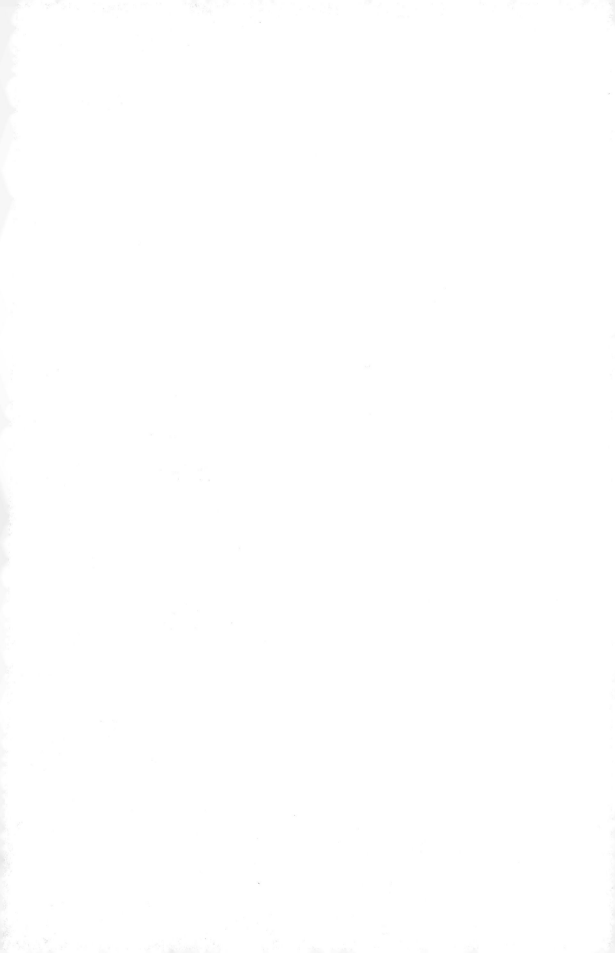

14

The Developmental History

TONI M. WHITAKER AND FREDERICK B. PALMER

A complete developmental assessment requires a comprehensive pediatric and developmental history and a detailed physical and neurodevelopmental examination. The goals of the complete hands-on developmental assessment, and therefore the developmental history, are

1. To define and delineate the nature, chronology, breadth, and topography of the developmental symptoms, including associated disabilities, that is, to detail the developmental profile of disability

2. To identify where possible a general or specific etiology of developmental disorder (this should always include consideration of a neurodegenerative etiology)

3. To address issues of prognosis

4. To identify additional factors (medical, social, community) that may influence prognosis favorably or unfavorably

5. To suggest potential interventions

The developmental history should also serve as a vehicle to identify points of special focus for the pediatric and neurodevelopmental examinations, imaging or laboratory investigations, and interdisciplinary examinations. Given the time constraints of the clinical setting and the varying cooperation of the pediatric patient, the developmental history may provide the majority of useful data obtained from a "complete" assessment.

This chapter summarizes a general approach for use by faculty, fellows, and pediatric residents for obtaining the developmental history. The approach is adaptable to inpatient and outpatient settings and can be used with children of all ages. It is used as part of extensive interdisciplinary assessments and focused developmental pediatric consultations. It should be approached with careful thought rather than as a session for rote data collection. Although protocols are helpful as reminders, especially for the beginner, they discourage thoughtful adaptation of an interview based on the emerging story provided by the caregiver.

Attention to the child's and family's cultural background has become increasingly important. The developmentalist must understand the special and sometimes unique stresses of migration, acculturation, and refugee status as well as culturally specific responses a family may have to their child with a disability. Availability and skilled use of translators is essential (Lynch & Hanson, 1992; Misra-Hebert, 2003).

Usually the history is taken immediately following initial introductions to the patient and family. It is important to realize that the first few minutes of contact with the family may strongly influence the pediatrician–family relationship. The parents will usually have major realistic or unrealistic concerns and anxieties about their child and his or her future. Immediately prior to meeting the physician, they may have dealt with necessary but un-

This work is supported in part by grant 90-DD-0578 from the U.S. Department of Health and Human Services, Administration for Children and Families, and by grant MC-00038 from the Health Resources and Services Administration's Maternal and Child Health Bureau.

pleasant administrative and financial aspects of the evaluation. The initial contact with the pediatrician must convey a direct and strong interest in the child and in the parents' concerns independent of time constraints, cultural differences, and nature or severity of the child's problems. It must enlist the parents in the evaluation process. By summarizing the evaluation process, and reviewing what is hoped to be accomplished during the visit, the pediatrician can often allay some anxiety as well as focus the parents on their role as historians.

CHIEF COMPLAINT

The interview should begin with elicitation of the chief complaint. This should be a general, open-ended series of questions designed to provide an overview of the breadth of developmental, medical, and related concerns and complaints. It must include the primary concerns of the parents independent of concerns of the referring source. The pediatrician should also develop a general impression of the nature of the parents' reaction to the evaluation. Are they similarly concerned? How have they adapted to the suspicion of developmental abnormality in their child? Do they deny its existence? Are they guilty or angry? Do they convey hopeless resignation? Are they eager to address the issues?

Although answers to these questions may become more apparent (or change) later in the interview, initial information about them will often be provided during earliest questioning. It is often helpful to ask the parents what they believe is wrong with their child and what others have told them. Their responses may provide insight into their notions of the child's problems and may suggest ways in which diagnoses and recommendations should be presented to the parents at the conclusion of the assessment process. Parents often recognize their child's delayed development but may not appreciate the scope of the problem. For example, it is common for parents to report only speech and language delay in a child in whom evaluation reveals global cognitive delay (intellectual disabilities).

Age of referral for initial developmental evaluation is closely related to the nature of the complaint and the initial developmental diagnosis (Lock, Shapiro, Ross, & Capute, 1986). Not surprisingly, referrals for motor delay are most common during the first 6–18 months of life. In the early preschool years, language delay is the common referring complaint. Later in the preschool years, behavior problems supervene as the major cause for referral. Academic difficulties become the focus in the early school years. Accordingly, children with cerebral palsy are most often diagnosed in the first 2 years of life, followed by those with intellectual disabilities, autism spectrum disorders, or communication disorders, and then by those with attention-deficit/hyperactivity disorder or learning disability. By exploring all possible complaints rather than focusing the evaluation on the single referral complaint, however, the physician may be able to detect "presymptomatic" abnormalities in other development streams. This can lead to earlier complete diagnosis of disability than might otherwise occur. For example, the infant with cerebral palsy, however mild, may also have other developmental symptoms. Thus, a comprehensive history is indicated in almost all referral situations.

Upon completion of the chief complaint portion of the interview, it is usually helpful to begin with the pregnancy and birth history and to proceed chronologically, delineating development to the current time. The traditional concept of "present illness" is not useful when the onset of illness is unclear. At best it may be confusing, and at worst it may lead the physician to see the onset of developmental problems as the time the parents first became concerned about developmental symptoms, thereby obscuring earlier related presymptomatic abnormalities. By beginning with gestational history and proceeding chronologically, the parents may be helped to see the child's problems in the context of overall development rather than as a limited grouping of current symptoms.

PRENATAL AND PERINATAL/NEONATAL HISTORY

The gestational, birth, and neonatal history should include a cataloguing of important events and indicators beginning prior to conception and continuing through the neonatal

Table 14.1.   Prenatal and perinatal history

Gestational history
Maternal age
Paternal age
Parity
Length of gestation
Maternal weight gain
Fetal activity (onset, quality, cessations)
Previous or subsequent maternal obstetric problems
Prenatal monitoring or diagnostic procedures
Complicating factors:
• Bleeding/spotting
• Rash/infection/exposures/fever
• Toxemia
• Blood group incompatibility
• Diabetes
• Trauma
• Medications (during or prior)
• Illicit drug use (during or prior)
• Alcohol use
• Tobacco use
• Radiation exposure
• "At risk" sexual behaviors or partners
• Multiple gestation
• Other
 	
Labor and delivery history
Hospital
Duration of labor
Monitoring
Analgesia/sedation
Presentation
Apgar scores
Problems:
• Preterm labor (and type/duration of treatment)
• Premature rupture of membranes
• Maternal fever, infection
	• Toxemia
	• Abnormal bleeding
	• Failure of labor to progress
	• Labor induced
	• Cesarean section
	• Forceps/instrumentation
	• Resuscitation
	• Abnormalities noted at birth
	• Abnormal placenta
	• Other
	
	Neonatal history
	Growth parameters (including percentile for
	   gestational age)
	• Weight
	• Length
	• Head circumference
	Duration of hospitalization
	Problems:
	• Respiratory distress syndrome
	• Apnea
	• Cyanosis
	• Oxygen therapy, asphyxia
	• Symptoms of hypoxic-ischemic encephalopathy
	  (seizures, irritability, hypotonia, coma, stupor)
	• Infections
	• Jaundice
	• Congenital abnormalities
	• Feeding problems
	• Screening abnormalities (neonatal screening
	  measures vary among states)
	• Brain imaging (hemorrhage, hydrocephalus,
	  structural anomaly)
	• Eye/retinal exam(s)
	• Hearing screening
	• Other

period. Specific items that should be included are summarized in Table 14.1. It is important to remember that "abnormal" gestation, birth, and neonatal occurrences place an infant at risk for adverse developmental outcome; however, with some exceptions, they rarely allow the diagnosis to be made on the basis of risk factors alone. For the individual child, most profiles of risk will be insufficient to make definitive diagnostic or prognostic statements. When followed longitudinally, such an infant would be identified for careful developmental monitoring, with further evaluations planned if abnormality were suspected.

When a child with a developmental disability is seen for evaluation, risk factors assume a somewhat different role. Rather than being markers of developmental diagnosis or prognosis, they may suggest an etiology for the present developmental disability. For example, the presence of multiple pregestational or gestational abnormalities suggests a prenatal onset of abnormality. This should be noted even when perinatal difficulties are also present. The prenatal abnormalities may have been compounded by the perinatal problems or even have led to them directly.

Prenatal History

Prenatal history queries (see Table 14.1) should address possible indicators in several categories. *Infectious* etiologies should be sought by questioning about symptoms, immunity, and exposures related to common congenital infections, including toxoplasmosis, cytomegalovirus, rubella, varicella, syphilis, and herpes. Congenital parvovirus infection may result in hydrops and spontaneous abortion (Al-Khan, Caligiuri, & Apuzzio, 2003). Evidence for human immunodeficiency virus (HIV) infection, exposure, or risk behaviors should be sought. A high index of suspicion is necessary. HIV infection may be associated with any of a wide range of neurodevelopmental manifestations, from minimal abnormality to severe progressive encephalopathy (see also Chapter 10 in this volume).

Evidence for *toxic exposures* should be explored, including use of medications, illicit drugs, and tobacco and consumption of alcohol. The extent of adverse effect, if any, on the fetus may be difficult to determine even when such substances are known to have been present during the pregnancy. Inquiries about exposure to environmental toxins, including lead, may be pursued, though an individual's recognition of such exposure may be limited.

Any *maternal illness* (particularly if febrile), *symptoms of toxemia*, or suggestion of *placental or fetal compromise* may be important. Maternal genitourinary tract infections and chorioamnionitis are associated with increased risk of developmental disorders, including cerebral palsy (Dammann, Kuban, & Leviton, 2002; Nelson, 2003; Wu, 2002). Maternal factors such as preeclampsia may affect placental function and result in compromise of varying degrees to the fetus (Cheng, Chou, Tsou, Fang, & Tsao, 2004). Abnormalities of fetal movement are nonspecific but useful indicators of fetal abnormality. Fetal movement is usually perceived by the mother by 12–16 weeks' gestation. Late onset of fetal activity (later than 20 weeks) may alert the clinician to fetal abnormalities. Quantitative abnormalities of fetal movements may also be reported. Hypotonic infants often have a history of late onset or paucity of fetal movement and related abnormal presentations at delivery (breech). It is common for the mother of a hyperactive preschooler to report "intrauterine hyperactivity." Recognizing this may assist the physician

in convincing the family of the "organic" basis for their child's hyperactivity.

Perinatal History

Perinatal history queries (see Table 14.1) should be directed at identifying potential perinatal brain insult as well as identifying markers of prenatal abnormality. The most important markers are the intrauterine growth parameters of weight, length, and head circumference. Growth parameters that are small for gestational age suggest deprivation of placental supply to the fetus (i.e., blood flow, gas exchange, nutrients) or abnormality of the fetus itself (i.e., anomaly, congenital infection, effects of toxins). The former fetus is likely to have catch-up growth following delivery, whereas the latter is likely to show persistent postnatal growth failure. Special attention should be given to head circumference measurements. Birth microcephaly denotes a prenatal contribution to abnormality despite perinatal history. Although studies have not consistently identified intrauterine growth retardation alone as a marker for subsequent developmental delays, there is an increased risk of long-term cognitive deficits in infants who are born small for gestational age (Larroque, Bertrais, Czernichow, & Leger, 2001; O'Keeffe, O'Callaghan, Williams, Najman, & Bor, 2003).

Perinatal hypoxia-ischemia is difficult to measure historically. Apgar scores are routinely obtained at 1 and 5 minutes after delivery and may be good discriminators for early mortality, but they are not clearly predictive of specific neurological abnormalities or of long-term neurodevelopmental disabilities (Caravale, Allemand, & Libenson, 2003; Casey, McIntire, & Leveno, 2001). Low late Apgar scores are uncommon but more meaningful (Nelson & Ellenberg, 1981); however, evidence of perinatal asphyxia (from Apgar or other measure) accompanied by clinical signs and symptoms of hypoxic-ischemic encephalopathy is very predictive. Evidence has consistently shown that asphyxiated term infants with symptoms such as hypotonia, depressed consciousness, abnormal primitive reflexes, and seizures have an increasingly poor prognosis with increasing severity of symptoms

(Robertson & Finer, 1985; Sarnat & Sarnat, 1976). In contrast, infants with less significant symptoms such as jitteriness or hypertonus may have suffered only mild asphyxia. Although it has been shown that mildly asphyxiated infants have a better overall prognosis, they are at increased risk for early developmental delays, later sequelae such as school-age learning and behavior problems, or both (Dixon et al., 2002; Robertson, Finer, & Grace, 1989). Information about perinatal brain imaging in term and preterm children is especially helpful (Kuban & Leviton, 1994). Abnormal neuroimaging and electroencephalograms may be helpful in predicting neurological complications (de Vries & Groenendaal, 2002; Ment et al., 2002).

Premature birth itself, with or without the multitude of medical complications that may be associated, is a risk factor for developmental delays and long-term disabilities (Allen, 2002; Msall & Tremont, 2002). It has been historically difficult to fully delineate the role of early-gestation birth versus the roles of socioeconomic and medical factors in delay and disability (see Chapter 9 in this volume).

Neonatal History

Information about treatments for neonatal complications may be helpful in assessing developmental risk status for a child. Therapeutic interventions during the neonatal period have evolved over the years and continue to advance as information emerges on efficacy and potential safety issues (including those related to developmental disabilities). Recent studies have suggested that long-term neurodevelopmental complications are associated with early postnatal steroid treatment for prevention of chronic lung disease in premature infants (LeFlore, Salhab, Broyles, & Engle, 2002; Yeh et al., 2004). Standards for routine monitoring and treatment of neonatal jaundice have changed in response to a historical decline in cases of kernicterus (as a result of successful management of its common etiologies); however, with recent trends toward shorter neonatal hospital stays and potential increased rates of hyperbilirubinemia, there is renewed discussion about potential long-term neurode-

Table 14.2. Problems in early infancy

Excessive quietness
Hyperactivity/irritability
Colic (after 2 months)
Altered sleep–wake cycle
Feeding problems
Floppiness
Stiffness (difficulty diapering)
Other

velopmental complications of more moderate elevations of bilirubin, particularly in preterm and near-term infants (American Academy of Pediatrics, 2004; Newman, Xiong, Gonzales, & Escobar, 2000; Shapiro, 2003).

Questioning about the infant's adaptation to extrauterine existence during the first few months logically follows from perinatal questioning and easily leads into the detailed questioning about developmental milestones that will form the core of the developmental history. Problems in early infancy are usually reported as problems with physiological adaptation or unusual state of arousal (Table 14.2). Persistent slow or difficult feeding may suggest brain abnormality. Severe or persistent "colic," gastroesophageal reflux, and difficulty with swallowing, aspiration, or congestion during feeding may have a central nervous system basis. Seldom should it take more than 15 or 20 minutes to feed an infant. The infant who regularly takes longer or needs to be awakened for feeds may be showing early symptoms of a developmental disorder. The excessively irritable infant or the infant with temperamental characteristics outside the normal range of variation is also of concern. Most of these markers in early infancy are nonspecific. They may be transient or persistent, and seen by the parent as trivial or problematic, but they offer the clinician early insight into the integrity of the infant's nervous system.

DEVELOPMENTAL MILESTONES

Developmental milestones are the cornerstone of the developmental history. They allow the clinician to identify delay or confirm normality. When delay is present, they provide a quantitative measure to supplement formal testing of current functioning. They allow detection of subtle qualitative deviancies in developmental progress that are useful in identifying the milder developmental disabilities. When progress in "separate" development streams is compared, uneven or dissociated patterns suggest particular developmental diagnoses. Milestone questioning should include a careful description of current functioning but must also include a retrospective survey of previous developmental progress. Careful attention to patterns of development allows the detection of developmental plateau or loss of skills that may suggest progressive disease, subclinical seizures, or other unrecognized accompanying disability.

It has been recognized for decades that careful questioning of parents will result in better recall of development details (McGraw & Molloy, 1941). Thus, the clinician must be prepared to define developmental landmarks in understandable terms, clarifying where needed or giving examples. When pressed, parents can often give an interval during which a milestone occurred or will date it from a familiar holiday or family event. Rote elicitation of milestones from a checklist is often unrewarding. Even with careful questioning, there will be some parents who cannot give a meaningful developmental history. The experienced physician will recognize this early and move on to other areas.

It is usually most helpful to organize milestone questioning into the separate streams of motor (gross and fine), language (receptive and expressive), adaptive (self-help skills), and neurobehavioral development. Usually parents will find it easiest to describe the child's current level of functioning initially and then proceed to retrospective recall of milestones. In almost all situations, initial questioning should include a request for the parents to estimate the child's current level of functioning (e.g., "How old a child does Arnold act like?"). This may result in a global estimate or a series of stream-specific estimates if the parents recognize differences between types of abilities. This estimate is often very accurate, even when parents are entirely naive. It also offers insight into the parents' current level of concern and understanding of the child's disability. This may provide information on how the results of the

completed evaluation should be communicated to the parents.

Motor Assessment

Gross motor milestones (Table 14.3) are the easiest to recall for most parents and are a nonthreatening point to begin questioning. Using age of attainment of individual milestones, rate of progress is best reflected as a motor quotient, defined as motor age divided by chronological age (Capute & Shapiro, 1985). As a general clinical rule of thumb, a gross motor quotient below 50 in infants with nonprogressive conditions ultimately will be associated with functional motor disability; a gross motor quotient of 50 or above is unlikely to be associated with long-term disability. Exceptions include children with hemiplegia, who may have only mild delays in gross motor milestones but may have substantial qualitative disability in gross and fine motor function.

Table 14.3. Age of achievement of major motor milestones

Milestone	Mean age (months)
Gross motor	
Lifts head only	1
Lifts head prone to wrists	4
Rolls over (prone to supine)	4
Rolls over (supine to prone)	5
Sits supported	5
Sits alone	6
Comes to sit	8
Crawls	8
Pulls to stand	9
Cruises	9
Walks alone	12
Runs	15
Fine motor	
Opens fists	3
Brings objects to midline	4
Transfers	5
Reaches unilaterally and grasps	6
Makes pincer movement (mature)	10–11
Releases voluntarily	12
Displays handedness	24

Adapted from Capute, A.J., Palmer, F.B., Shapiro, B.K., Wachtel, R.C., Ross, A. and Accardo, P.J. (1984). Primitive reflex profile: A quantitation of primitive reflexes in infancy. *Developmental Medicine and Child Neurology, 26,* 375–383, published by Blackwell Publishing.

Motor development should never be used as a quantitatively specific marker for cognitive development. Excellent motor development may be seen in children with severe intellectual disabilities; by contrast, many children and adults with frank cerebral palsy are of normal or above-normal intelligence and extremely productive. Nevertheless, despite the absence of useful quantitative prediction, there is a qualitative relationship between motor and cognitive development. Motor abnormalities serve as useful markers of nonmotor developmental abnormality. As has been demonstrated repeatedly, intellectual disabilities and other nonmotor developmental disabilities may initially present with motor abnormality before the more functionally significant disability is apparent. This is true even when the motor abnormalities are minor and nondisabling (Drillien & Drummond, 1983; Nelson & Ellenberg, 1982; Samsom, de Groot, Bezemer, Lafeber, & Fetter, 2002).

Language Assessment

Language assessment is among the most difficult and complex aspects of the developmental pediatric evaluation; yet, it is the key to the detection, diagnosis, classification, habilitation, and monitoring of a wide variety of developmental disorders, including intellectual disabilities, hearing loss, preschool language disorders, specific learning disabilities, and autism spectrum disorders. The normal orderly progression of language development from the prelinguistic markers of infancy, through early language acquisition and refinement in the preschooler, to mastery of written language in the school child should be seen as a function of the complex interplay between experience and neurological maturation. Severe environmental insults such as hearing impairment or profound deprivation are necessary to cause disabling alterations of this progression, whereas seemingly mild or otherwise inapparent neurological abnormalities are associated with a wide range of language disability. Recognition and characterization of delay or deviations in the orderly progression of language development is the goal of language assessment.

Developmental pediatric assessment of language development in infancy and the pre-school years is based on observation and parental report of the child's age of attainment and quality of performance on individual receptive and expressive language milestones. Many milestone batteries have been published, but all derive primarily from the work of Gesell (Gesell & Amatruda, 1941; Gesell et al., 1940) and Sheridan (Sheridan, 1964, 1968).

The Clinical Linguistic and Auditory Milestone Scale (CLAMS) is composed of language milestones in receptive and expressive categories (Accardo & Capute, 2005; Capute & Accardo, 1978; Capute et al., 1986) (see Chapter 19 in this volume). Although for some milestones this scale is somewhat arbitrary, its use is an essential step in recognizing disordered language. Mean ages of attainment of milestones for the CLAMS are shown in Table 14.4. These data represent information collected through standard questioning of parents about their child's age of first attainment of a given skill. Sample questions are presented in Table 14.5. These questions may require elaboration or examples to assist parents' recall and are intended as guidelines. It is essential for questioning to be as specific and focused as possible. When carefully elicited, milestone language performance is closely related to cognitive abilities as measured concurrently by formal psychometric measures in children referred for delay (Kube, Wilson, Petersen, & Palmer, 2000).

Prelinguistic Development The "prelinguistic" phase of development is marked by easily recognizable milestones prior to the emergence of true words at about 12 months of age. These prelinguistic milestones can best be viewed as the earliest representation of the subsequent and more familiar receptive and expressive language stream.

Expressive milestones begin with decline of guttural noises and the onset of cooing at about 6 weeks of age. They progress through the raspberry, repetitive babbling, and duplicated consonant pairs, some of which may, with time, be used meaningfully (e.g., discriminate use of "dada" or "mama" at 10 months). By 12 months, the onset of jargon usually coincides with the first expressive use of true words and marks the culmination of the prelinguistic period.

Table 14.4. Age of achievement of major receptive and expressive language milestones

	Standard deviation (in months)	Mean age (in months)
Receptive		
Alerts to sound	1.1 weeks	1.3 weeks
Smiles socially	5.0 weeks	2.2 weeks
Orients (voice)	2.8	1.2
Gestures	8.6	1.5
Follows one-step command with gesture	11.1	1.7
Follows one-step command without gesture	13.6	2.1
Identifies five body parts	16.7	2.8
Identifies eight body parts	19.0	3.2
Expressive		
Coos	6.5 weeks	2.7 weeks
Ah-goos	4.0	1.6
Razzes	4.4	1.6
Babbles	6.3	1.4
Says "mama/dada" indiscriminately	7.7	1.7
Says "dada" discriminately	10.5	2.5
Says "mama" discriminately	11.1	2.7
Says first word	11.3	2.3
Utters immature jargon	12.2	2.1
Utters second word	12.4	2.2
Utters third word	13.2	2.2
Uses 4–6 words	14.7	2.5
Uses mature jargon	16.5	2.9
Uses 7–20 words	16.9	2.9
Uses 2-word combinations	19.2	3.0
Uses 2-word sentences	20.6	3.0
Uses 50 words	20.9	3.2
Preschool receptive		
Follows two-step command	24	
Knows gender	30	
Knows full name	36	
Knows age	36	
Uses prepositional commands (under, behind, in front of)	36	
Identifies three colors	36	
Knows what to do when "hungry," "tired," "cold"	36	
Follows three-step commands	54	
Knows home address	60	

Sources: Capute and Accardo (1978), Capute et al. (1986), Gesell and Amatruda (1941), Gesell et al. (1940), and Sheridan (1964, 1968).

Note: Receptive milestones elicited during examination may be more accurate than those reported by the parents.

Prelinguistic receptive language skills of auditory alerting and orienting should be seen as neurosensory in nature. To develop, they require intact peripheral auditory functioning as well as age-appropriate central nervous system maturation. Their value is greatest in recognizing abnormalities of the latter. At birth, the infant should have an elicitable response to sound. This may be an obvious motor response or be more subtle, such as a change in respiratory rate. This initial "alerting" response is followed by the more mature auditory "orienting" responses in which the infant turns to the source of sound. These milestones may be difficult to elicit from some parents; however, their presence or absence is usually easily dem-

Table 14.5. Sample questions from the Clinical Linguistic and Auditory Milestone Scale (CLAMS)

Milestone	Sample question
Alert	When did your infant recognize presence of sound by blinking, startling, or moving any part of the body?
Social smile (communicative smile)	When did your infant smile at you when you talked to him or her or stroked his or her face? When could you get him or her to smile?
Coo	When did your infant produce long vowel sounds in a musical fashion?
Orient to voice	When you enter a room and the baby doesn't see you at first, does he or she turn immediately to the correct side when you speak to him or her, or does he or she search for you sometimes, looking first in the right direction and sometimes not?
Ah-goo	When did the baby first say "ah-goo?"
Razz	When did your baby first give you the "raspberry?"
Babble	When did your infant first babble (demonstrate repetitive strings of consonants)?
Gesture language	When did your infant wave bye-bye or play Pat-a-Cake?
Mama/dada (indiscriminately)	When did your child first say "dada" and "mama" but without reference to the mother or the father?
Mama/dada (discriminately)	When did your child first refer to the father as "dada"? When did your child first refer to the mother as "mama"?
First word	When did your child say his or her first word other than "dada," "mama," or family names? Name it.
Second word	When did your child have two words? Name them.
Third word	When did your child have three words? Name them.
One-step command without gesture	When did your child first follow simple commands such as "give me _____" or "bring me _____," not accompanied by a gesture?
Four to six words	When did your child have a four- to six-word vocabulary? Name them.
Immature jargon	When did your child begin to jargon—to run unintelligible words together in an attempt to make a "sentence"? (Demonstrate.)
Seven to 20 words	When did your child have a 7- to 20-word vocabulary?
Mature jargon	When did your child's jargon begin to include intelligible words? (Demonstrate.)
Body parts	How many body parts can your child point to when named? Which ones? When could he or she point to five? Eight?
Two-word phrases	When did your child start to put two words together in a phrase (not a sentence, frequently both nouns)?
Fifty words	When did your child have a 50-word vocabulary?
Two-word sentences	When did your child put a noun and a verb together in a sentence?

From Capute, A.J., Palmer, F.B., Shapiro, B.K., Watchel, R.C., Schmidt, S., and Ross, A. (1986). Clinical Linguistic and Auditory Milestone Scale: Prediction of cognition in infancy. *Developmental Medicine and Child Neurology, 28,* 762–771, published by Blackwell Publishing.

onstrated on examination. Although these neurosensory skills are useful in assessing receptive language, they should not be used to exclude hearing loss.

Linguistic Development Expressive linguistic milestones include measures of increasing vocabulary size from a few single words at 12–15 months to 50 words by 24 months and rapid increases thereafter. Care should be taken that all reported words are used with meaning and are not just rote repetition of words without comprehension (echolalia). It is helpful to ask parents of a child younger than 2 years of age to list the infant's words to determine the size and quality of the vocabulary. Words will be primarily nouns initially but should progress rapidly to include verbs and modifiers before 2 years. A vocabulary that is age appropriate in size but consists of little variety in content (e.g., all zoo animals or cartoon characters) may indicate an underlying deficit in language comprehension. By 24 months, the first use of personal pronouns is apparent, but the infant will often use them inconsistently or interchangeably. By 30 to 36 months, all personal pronouns should be used frequently and consistently.

Phrase length is the second major parameter of early expressive milestone development. Until about 18 months, single-word utterances are used exclusively. Single recognizable words may be scattered in long jargon utterances (mature jargon), but true two-word phrases do not yet occur. Soon after the onset of two-word phrases ("night-night mommy," "daddy car"), longer utterances and true sentences appear ("daddy go car," "want milk now").

Phonological errors may interfere with accurate assessments of expressive capabilities if the child cannot be easily understood. For children who use or understand more than one language, overall language abilities are best represented by the combined skills from each language. Complex aspects of functional communication such as semantics, prosody, and pragmatic use of language may need to be specifically explored, though these are somewhat more difficult for the pediatrician to objectively measure.

It is tempting to rely solely on expressive milestones in language. They are readily recalled and easily understood; however, a satisfactory profile of language development or disorder is incomplete without an understanding of receptive language development. The presence of receptive delay in the child with expressive delay is a poor prognostic indicator, compared to the prognosis for a child with expressive delay only. Early receptive language skills include pointing to body parts, following simple commands, pointing to pictures, and demonstrating comprehension by response to questions. Sample preschool receptive language markers are noted at the bottom of Table 14.4. The ages of attainment shown are traditional.

When is language delayed? Although cutoffs are inevitably arbitrary, it is useful to be *concerned* about any infant or child who shows consistent milestone attainment that is 1 full standard deviation below the mean. This reflects a developmental rate or language quotient of 70–85. Such infants should be followed closely for language, cognitive, behavioral, or learning disorders. Any additional concerns about hearing acuity should be pursued with pure tone or brain stem audiometry. When milestones are attained at a rate slower than 2 standard deviations below the mean, representing a language quotient less than 70, a full evaluation is indicated, including an etiological search, psychometric evaluation of intelligence, audiometry, and usually speech and language evaluation. With greater delays, the presence of moderate or greater intellectual disabilities or a severe communication disorder is very likely. Such disorders will generally not be missed by the developmentalist. They are usually detected by the primary physician in the context of developmental screening; however, complete assessment to characterize the profile of abnormalities and their implications for habilitation may be extremely difficult and can represent a challenge to even the most sophisticated clinician.

Milder delays are more common and are represented in the majority of children referred for language problems. Approximately 6%–8% of preschoolers will be identified as having delayed or disordered acquisition of language. Of this group, 36%–48% will have an IQ score in the *low*-normal range or below at age 7, more than 40% will have reading delay, and 25%–30% will have teacher-reported behavior problems (Silva, 1987).

Once language delay is recognized and quantified (language quotient), it is necessary to compare the *rate* of language acquisition with the rate of acquisition of skills in other developmental domains to make a developmental diagnosis. In uncomplicated intellectual disabilities, cognitive development as measured by language *and* nonlanguage (visual problem-solving) development are *both* delayed; however, comparison with motor development will indicate clear cognitive-motor *dissociation,* with motor skills developing at a more normal rate. This dissociation may be obvious in the older child with intellectual disabilities but is the key to the initial diagnosis of uncomplicated intellectual disabilities in the infant with a chief complaint of "possible developmental delay." If motor delay is also present, the language and problem-solving delay may still indicate intellectual disabilities, but it is necessary to be certain that the motor abnormality has not so compromised expressive language and fine motor capacities as to give a falsely low estimation of intelligence. Generally, careful attention to receptive language skills will reveal the most accurate picture of language ability in a child with additional impairment.

When there is dissociation between language and visual-motor measures of cognition with visual skills falling in the normal range, the child has a communication disorder, not intellectual disabilities. This may be due to hearing loss, central nervous system dysfunction (developmental language disorder, autism spectrum disorder), or both. The language abnormality may be subtle, as in the preschooler with mild expressive language delay, or severe and associated with other developmental abnormalities, as in autism. When superimposed on general cognitive delay (intellectual disabilities *with* communication disorder), it may go unrecognized and thereby interfere with adequate habilitation.

Consideration must be given to an autism spectrum disorder in a child with delays or deviation in language acquisition (often with associated delays in general cognition) who has limited reciprocal social interaction, restricted or stereotypic behavior patterns, or both. A child with an autism spectrum disorder and higher cognitive functioning, such as in Asperger syndrome, may have an adequate number of words in his or her vocabulary and be able to use words in phrases and sentences but have difficulty with functional communication nevertheless (see Chapters 29–32 in Volume II).

Neurobehavioral Assessment

Behavioral disturbances in children with developmental disabilities are extremely common and diverse. They range from mild noncompliance to severe self-injurious behaviors. The general interview approach should be twofold:

1. The clinician should probe for atypical or deviant behaviors usually thought of as neurological symptoms, such as self-stimulatory behaviors, hyperactivity, attention aberrations, tics, and repetitive or stereotypic behaviors. In infancy, nonspecific problems such as irritability or poor responsiveness may presage later neurobehavioral abnormality. Frequency, severity, setting, impact on daily functioning, and modifying influences should be noted where possible. These variables will be important in deciding whether to intervene and in choosing the most appropriate interventions (see Chapter 8 in this volume).

2. Problematic behaviors that are more clearly due to environmental influences also should be noted. These may include perceived noncompliance with inappropriately complex commands or simple school refusal in a child with learning disability. Some of these behaviors may be responsive to reviewing appropriate expectations with the parents or other simple environmental manipulations.

It may be helpful to use certain standard inventories of behavior abnormalities to further investigate complaints. Multiple behavior rating scales have been developed for use by parents, teachers, or examiners. Inventories may be broad in scope to elucidate a wide variety of behavioral issues, or may be narrower in scope to address specific concerns such as an autism spectrum disorder or attention-deficit/hyperactivity disorder. Many behaviors will be due to both neurological and environmental factors and may require a coordinated neuropharmacological and environmental treatment approach.

Adaptive Functioning Assessment

Performance of individual self-help skills requires skill-specific minimal competence in cognitive, motor, and neurobehavioral areas (Table 14.6). Success in performing a given self-help skill generally implies cognitive performance at that level or higher. Therefore, a child who self-initiates toileting has at least some cognitive skills at the 18-month level; however, a child not yet toilet trained may have the cognitive requisites but not yet have the motor, behavioral, or experiential requisites. Thus, failure to accomplish a given self-help skill does not indicate cognitive skills below that level. If adaptive functioning does not appear to be at the child's level of cognitive functioning and no other obvious impediments exist, a functional therapy program directed at that milestone may be warranted.

Informal questioning about fine-motor play activities may offer general information

Table 14.6. Age of attainment of major adaptive (self-help) skill milestones

Milestone	Mean age of attainment (months)
Feeding*	
Feeds self with fingers	7
Uses spoon	15
Uses cup	15
Spears with fork	30
Spreads with knife	60–72
Dressing	
Helps with dressing	12
Undresses partially (shoes, socks)	24
Undresses completely	36
Buttons	48
Dresses self completely	48
Ties shoes	60
Toilet training	
Voids or defecates when placed	By 12
Initiates toileting	18

*Clinician should also ask, "Does the child experience gagging? Vomiting? Tongue thrust? Drooling? What is the child's current diet? Any difficulties advancing?"

about visual problem-solving abilities but is not a substitute for actual "hands-on" assessment of these skills (see Chapter 22 in this volume). Objective measures of functional independence have been developed and can supplement the history of adaptive development (Msall, DiGaudio, & Duffy, 1993).

PAST MEDICAL HISTORY

The past medical history should include all previous illnesses (particularly those that have been recurrent or severe), injuries, evaluations, procedures, and issues in well-child care as would be included in any complete pediatric history. Parents who have difficulty recalling the details of specific medical complaints or complicated conditions will often at least be able to provide names or specialties of physicians seen in the past. Current and recent medication use may also provide a gauge for severity of a particular problem. Parents should be asked if they have concerns about sensory deficits and if their child's vision or hearing, or both, have been screened. Targeted screening for groups at risk of environmental exposure to lead is recommended but may not have occurred during routine well-child care (Canfield

et al., 2003; Meyer et al., 2003). Completion of a review of systems may uncover minor or significant concerns that may or may not directly relate to behavior or developmental problems but will provide insight into the parents' overall view of the child's health.

Special attention should be directed to any previous developmental screening or assessment performed by the primary care physician, school, community agency, or other provider.

FAMILY HISTORY

The primary goal of the family history is to identify any possible genetic etiology (see Chapter 4 in Volume I; Chapters 17–24 in Volume II). Autosomal dominant conditions often have variable expression, so a high index of suspicion for partially expressed syndromes is necessary. Advanced maternal or paternal age at the time of conception may be a clue to the presence of chromosomal or single-gene disorders, respectively (Glaser & Jabs, 2004; Kuhnert & Nieschlag, 2004). Nonspecific indicators of familial disease are also important. These include history of fetal loss; difficulties conceiving; unexplained infant or childhood deaths; and nonspecific emotional, behavior, or academic problems. The parents' educational level should be determined. The family history also offers an opportunity to learn of the family's experience with disability, which may greatly influence their abilities to adapt to their own family member's developmental needs.

SOCIAL HISTORY

Elicitation of the social history should focus on the resources the family has available to cope with the problems presented by a youngster with a developmental disability. These resources (or constraints) may be financial, legal, community, extended family, and/or religious. Family and marital discord, if present, needs to be identified and sensitively explored.

CONCLUSION

On completion of the developmental history, the physician should have an initial picture from the parent's perspective of the nature, topography, and severity of the referring developmental complaint and any associated disabilities or medical problems. General categories of etiology and the possibility of a progressive condition should have been explored. Specific foci for the physical, neurological, and developmental examinations should have been identified. The pediatrician–caregiver relationship will have been initiated and in many cases firmly established. The level of the parents' understanding and adjustment to their child's developmental symptoms should be apparent. Available resources and current impediments to implementing eventual recommendations and follow-up will be identified.

REFERENCES

Accardo, P.J., & Capute, A.J. (2005). *The Capute Scales: Cognitive Adaptive Test/Clinical Linguistic and Auditory Milestone Scale (CAT/CLAMS)*. Baltimore: Paul H. Brookes Publishing Co.

Al-Khan, A., Caligiuri, A., & Apuzzio, J. (2003). Parvovirus B-19 infection during pregnancy. *Infectious Diseases in Obstetrics and Gynecology, 11*, 175–179.

Allen, M.C. (2002). Preterm outcomes research: A critical component of neonatal intensive care. *Mental Retardation and Developmental Disabilities Research Reviews, 8*, 221–233.

American Academy of Pediatrics. (2004). Management of hyperbilirubinemia in the newborn infant 35 or more weeks of gestation. *Pediatrics, 114*, 297–316.

Canfield, R.L., Henderson, C.R., Jr., Cory-Slechta, D.A., Cox, C., Jusko, T.A., & Lanphear, B.P. (2003). Intellectual impairment in children with blood lead concentrations below 10 microg per deciliter. *New England Journal of Medicine, 348*, 1517–1526.

Capute, A.J., & Accardo, P.J. (1978). Linguistic and auditory milestones during the first two years of life: A language inventory for the practitioner. *Clinical Pediatrics (Philadelphia), 17*, 847–853.

Capute, A.J., Palmer, F.B., Shapiro, B.K., Wachtel, R.C., Ross, A., & Accardo, P.J. (1984). Primitive reflex profile: A quantitation of primitive reflexes in infancy. *Developmental Medicine and Child Neurology, 26*, 375–383.

Capute, A.J., Palmer, F.B., Shapiro, B.K., Wachtel, R.C., Schmidt, S., & Ross, A. (1986). Clinical Linguistic and Auditory Milestone Scale: Prediction of cognition in infancy. *Developmental Medicine and Child Neurology, 28*, 762–771.

Capute, A.J., & Shapiro, B.K. (1985). The motor quotient: A method for the early detection of motor delay. *American Journal of Diseases of Children, 139*, 940–942.

Caravale, B., Allemand, F., & Libenson, M.H. (2003). Factors predictive of seizures and neurologic outcome in perinatal depression. *Pediatric Neurology, 29*, 18–25.

Casey, B.M., McIntire, D.D., & Leveno, K.J. (2001). The continuing value of the Apgar score for the assessment of newborn infants. *New England Journal of Medicine, 344*, 467–471.

Cheng, S.W., Chou, H.C., Tsou, K.I., Fang, L.J., & Tsao, P.N. (2004). Delivery before 32 weeks of gestation for maternal pre-eclampsia: Neonatal outcome and 2-year developmental outcome. *Early Human Development, 76*, 39–46.

Dammann, O., Kuban, K.C., & Leviton, A. (2002). Perinatal infection, fetal inflammatory response, white matter damage, and cognitive limitations in children born preterm. *Mental Retardation and Developmental Disabilities Research Reviews, 8*, 46–50.

de Vries, L.S., & Groenendaal, F. (2002). Neuroimaging in the preterm infant. *Mental Retardation and Developmental Disabilities Research Reviews, 8*, 273–280.

Dixon, G., Badawi, N., Kurinczuk, J.J., Keogh, J.M., Silburn, S.R., Zubrick, S.R., et al. (2002). Early developmental outcomes after newborn encephalopathy. *Pediatrics, 109*, 26–33.

Drillien, C., & Drummond, M. (1983). *Developmental screening and the child with special needs: A population study of 5,000 children* (Clinics in Developmental Medicine, No. 86). Philadelphia: J. B. Lippincott.

Gesell, A., & Amatruda, C.S. (1941). *Developmental diagnosis*. New York: Hoeber.

Gesell, A., Halverson, H.B., Thompson, H., Ilg, F.L., Castner, B.M., Ames, L.B., et al. (1940). *The first five years of life: A guide to the study of the preschool child*. New York: Harper.

Glaser, R.L., & Jabs, E.W. (2004, January 21). Dear old dad. *Science of Aging Knowledge Environment, 2004*(3), re1. Retrieved from November 27, 2006, http://sageke.sciencemag.org/cgi/content/full/2004/3/re1

Kuban, K.C., & Leviton, A. (1994). Cerebral palsy. *New England Journal of Medicine, 330*, 188–195.

Kube, D.A., Wilson, W.M., Petersen, M.C., & Palmer, F.B. (2000). CAT/CLAMS: Its use in detecting early childhood cognitive impairment. *Pediatric Neurology, 23*, 208–215.

Kuhnert, B., & Nieschlag, E. (2004). Reproductive functions of the ageing male. *Human Reproduction Update, 10*, 327–339.

Larroque, B., Bertrais, S., Czernichow, P., & Leger, J. (2001). School difficulties in 20-year-olds who were born small for gestational age at term in a regional cohort study. *Pediatrics, 108*, 111–115.

LeFlore, J.L., Salhab, W.A., Broyles, R.S., & Engle, W.D. (2002). Association of antenatal and postnatal dexamethasone exposure with outcomes in extremely low birth weight neonates. *Pediatrics, 110*(2, Pt. 1), 275–279.

Lock, T.M., Shapiro, B.K., Ross, A., & Capute, A.J. (1986). Age of presentation in developmental disability. *Journal of Developmental and Behavioral Pediatrics, 7,* 340–345.

Lynch, E.W., & Hanson, M.J. (1992). *Developing cross-cultural competence: A guide for working with young children and their families.* Baltimore: Paul H. Brookes Publishing Co.

McGraw, M.B., & Molloy, L.B. (1941). The pediatric anamnesis: Inaccuracies in eliciting developmental data. *Child Development, 12,* 55.

Ment, L.R., Bada, H.S., Barnes, P., Grant, P.E., Hirtz, D., Papile, L.A., et al. (2002). Practice parameter. Neuroimaging of the neonate: Report of the Quality Standards Subcommittee of the American Academy of Neurology and the Practice Committee of the Child Neurology Society. *Neurology, 58,* 1726–1738.

Meyer, P.A., Pivetz, T., Dignam, T.A., Homa, D.M., Schoonover, J., & Brody, D. (2003). Surveillance for elevated blood lead levels among children—United States, 1997–2001. *Morbidity and Mortality Weekly Report: CDC Surveillance Summaries, 52*(10), 1–21.

Misra-Hebert, A.D. (2003). Physician cultural competence: Cross-cultural communication improves care. *Cleveland Clinic Journal of Medicine, 70,* 289, 293, 296–288.

Msall, M.E., DiGaudio, K.M., & Duffy, L.C. (1993). Developmental aspects of functional assessment in children: Use of the WeeFIM in children with developmental disabilities. *Rehabilitation Clinics of North America, 4,* 517–527.

Msall, M.E., & Tremont, M.R. (2002). Measuring functional outcomes after prematurity: Developmental impact of very low birth weight and extremely low birth weight status on childhood disability. *Mental Retardation and Developmental Disabilities Research Reviews, 8,* 258–272.

Nelson, K.B. (2003). Can we prevent cerebral palsy? *New England Journal of Medicine, 349,* 1765–1769.

Nelson, K.B., & Ellenberg, J.H. (1981). Apgar scores as predictors of chronic neurologic disability. *Pediatrics, 68,* 36–44.

Nelson, K.B., & Ellenberg, J.H. (1982). Children who "outgrew' cerebral palsy. *Pediatrics, 69,* 529–536.

Newman, T.B., Xiong, B., Gonzales, V.M., & Escobar, G.J. (2000). Prediction and prevention of extreme neonatal hyperbilirubinemia in a mature health maintenance organization. *Archives of Pediatrics and Adolescent Medicine, 154,* 1140–1147.

O'Keeffe, M.J., O'Callaghan, M., Williams, G.M., Najman, J.M., & Bor, W. (2003). Learning, cognitive, and attentional problems in adolescents born small for gestational age. *Pediatrics, 112,* 301–307.

Robertson, C., & Finer, N. (1985). Term infants with hypoxic-ischemic encephalopathy: Outcome at 3.5 years. *Developmental Medicine and Child Neurology, 27,* 473–484.

Robertson, C.M., Finer, N.N., & Grace, M.G. (1989). School performance of survivors of neonatal encephalopathy associated with birth asphyxia at term. *Journal of Pediatrics, 114,* 753–760.

Samsom, J.F., de Groot, L., Bezemer, P.D., Lafeber, H.N., & Fetter, W.P. (2002). Muscle power development during the first year of life predicts neuromotor behaviour at 7 years in preterm born high-risk infants. *Early Human Development, 68,* 103–118.

Sarnat, H.B., & Sarnat, M.S. (1976). Neonatal encephalopathy following fetal distress: A clinical and electroencephalographic study. *Archives of Neurology, 33,* 696–705.

Shapiro, S.M. (2003). Bilirubin toxicity in the developing nervous system. *Pediatric Neurology, 29,* 410–421.

Sheridan, M.D. (1964). Development of auditory attention and language symbols in young children. In G. Refrew & K. Murphy (Eds.), *The child who does not talk* (Clinics in Developmental Medicine, No. 13, pp. 1–10). London: Spastics International Medical Publications.

Sheridan, M.D. (1968). *Developmental progress in infants and young children.* London: Her Majesty's Stationery Office.

Silva, P.A. (1987). Epidemiology, longitudinal course and some associated factors: An update. In W. Yule & M. Rutter (Eds.), *Language development and disorders* (Clinics in Developmental Medicine, No. 101/102, pp. 1–15). Philadelphia: J.B. Lippincott.

Wu, Y.W. (2002). Systematic review of chorioamnionitis and cerebral palsy. *Mental Retardation and Developmental Disabilities Research Reviews, 8,* 25–29.

Yeh, T.F., Lin, Y.J., Lin, H.C., Huang, C.C., Hsieh, W.S., Lin, C.H., et al. (2004). Outcomes at school age after postnatal dexamethasone therapy for lung disease of prematurity. *New England Journal of Medicine, 350,* 1304–1313.

15

The Dysmorphology Examination

THOMAS R. MONTGOMERY

The spectrum of neurodevelopmental disabilities encompasses a number of possible etiologies, many of which are of prenatal origin. Physical differences—dysmorphic features—serve as clues to abnormal prenatal development. These clues may be associated with abnormalities in neurodevelopment with resultant disability. Although an interrelationship between physical and neurodevelopmental disorders is not always as well defined as it is in Down syndrome, the relationship between congenital anomalies and intellectual disabilities has been well established (Croen, Grether, & Selvin, 2001; Jelliffe-Pawlowski, Shaw, Nelson, & Harris, 2003; Summit, 1969). The incidence of congenital anomalies in cerebral palsy is much greater than in the general population (Coorssen, Msall, & Duffy, 1991; Croen, Grether, Curry, & Nelson, 2001; Torfs, van den Berg, Oechsli, & Cummins, 1990), and children with learning disabilities have an increased incidence of congenital anomalies (Accardo, Tomazic, Morrow, Haake, & Whitman, 1991), as do children with autism (Bertrand et al., 2001; Hultman, Sparen, & Cnattingius, 2002).

Whenever a child is diagnosed as having a significant neurodevelopmental disorder, the parents wish to know why this happened to their child and if it will recur. Through a careful dysmorphology examination, disorders with a chromosomal, genetic, and/or environmental etiology often can be identified, allowing accurate recurrence risk counseling. In addition, determination as to the developmental pathogenesis of the defect can be made, which also can be important relative to recurrence risk counseling as well as to discussions with the family about prognosis.

An ever-increasing number of genetic markers continue to be identified in children with neurodevelopmental disorders. It is not practical to order a wholesale assay of all possible fluorescent in situ hybridization studies of gene deletions or duplications. Rather, the clinician can narrow the search by combining clinical findings on the dysmorphology examination with a reasonable differential diagnosis list of possible syndromes that may have a genetic marker. Likewise, high-resolution karyotyping can provide evidence of some genetic deletions and duplications, but the cytogenetist will be greatly assisted when alerted to clinical signs that suggest specific chromosomal sites to search.

CLASSIFICATION OF ERRORS OF PHYSICAL DEVELOPMENT

Errors in physical development leading to congenital anomalies can be divided into four types based on developmental pathogenesis: malformation, disruption, deformation, and dysplasia (Figure 15.1). Each has different mechanisms of action and different implications relative to recurrence risk.

Malformation

A malformation is an intrinsic defect in development whereon an arrest occurred at a normal stage of development. For example, the lip normally closes at 35 days of gestation. If an arrest occurs in its normal closure, a cleft lip results. Cleft palate, ventricular septal defect, and meningomyelocele are further examples of malformations. Malformations occur singly or as one feature of a multiple malformation

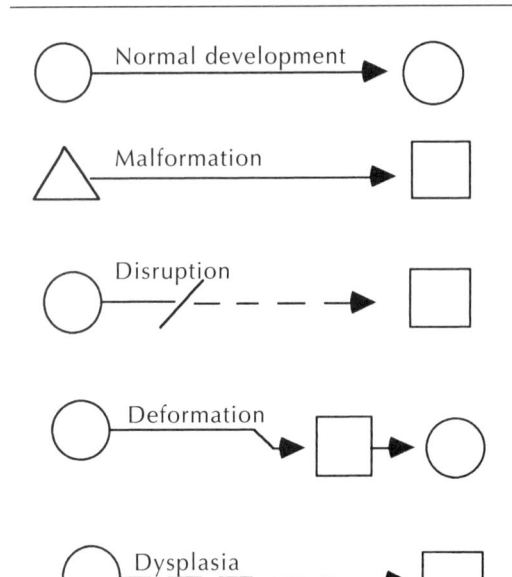

Figure 15.1. Errors of morphological development. (Reprinted from *Journal of Pediatrics, 100,* Sprangler, J., et al., Errors of morphogenesis: Concepts and terms, 160–165, Copyright © 1982, with permission from Elsevier.)

syndrome. The recurrence risk for most situations in which a single isolated malformation occurs in an otherwise normal child is 3%–5%. In cases in which a malformation is one feature of a multiple malformation syndrome, the recurrence risk becomes specific to the syndrome itself and not the single malformation.

Disruption

A disruption is a defect caused by destruction of, or interference with, a structure that previously had developed normally. Disruptions are caused by factors such as teratogens, vascular accidents, amniotic bands, infection, and ischemia. By definition, disruptions began with normal organogenesis and thus are not heritable conditions. Disruptions can mimic malformations, making it crucial to determine the difference. Malformations have a strong genetic and heritable nature, and thus the risk for recurrence is great. Disruptions lack this genetic implication, and the genetic risk for recurrence is minimal. It is important to determine the etiology of the disruption. Amniotic bands do not tend to be recurrent; for example, a disruption to a developing hand by an amniotic band resulting in loss of the hand has a very low recur-

rence risk. Conversely, when a vascular accident to the limb bud resulting in a loss of the hand occurs because of vasoconstriction caused by maternal cocaine use, there may be a high recurrence risk for other vascular accidents in future pregnancies if the mother continues to use cocaine during future pregnancies.

Deformation

A deformation is an abnormality of shape or function that occurs as a result of external forces applied to body parts that previously have developed normally. No genetic or primary abnormality of the underlying tissue or organ system has occurred. Once the external forces are removed, there is a possibility for correction of the deformed part. Intrauterine constraint is the most common factor leading to deformational defects. Once the child has been removed from the constraining forces imposed by the uterus, the defects usually rapidly recover. Some, such as an equinovarus foot caused by malposition of the fetus, are deformations that may require casting and, in some cases, surgery. Plagiocephaly from excessive supine positioning during early infancy is a common example of a postnatal deformity. This is frequently seen in hypotonic children who are late to roll over. It needs to be differentiated from the malformation of craniosynostosis, which also causes plagiocephaly. The treatment for plagiocephaly varies greatly depending on the cause—positioning deformation or craniosynostosis malformation.

Dysplasia

Dysplasia is the abnormal organization of cells into tissues. A dysplasia may have a genetic origin, such as the dysplasia of connective tissue in Marfan syndrome. Isolated hemangiomas are an example of nongenetic dysplasias. Some dysplasias have their clinical onset postnatally, such as the dysplasia caused by storage disorders. Like malformations, dysplasias may be part of a broader syndrome and thus will have recurrence risks related to the specific syndrome, as in the case of the telangiectasias in ataxia-telangiectasia.

SEQUENCES, SYNDROMES, AND ASSOCIATIONS

The four mechanisms that lead to structural defects can, and often do, interact with one another. A malformation may cause disruptive or deforming defects, or both, through a cascade of events termed a *sequence* (Figure 15.2). If the initiating event is a malformation, then it is a malformation sequence. Likewise, there are disruption sequences, deformation sequences, and dysplasia sequences, all named for the initiating event. If a malformation is involved but the initiating event cannot be determined, the ultimate structural defects are labeled malformations. This maintains the possible heritable nature of the disorder.

Meningomyelocele is a malformation sequence that involves, as the initiating event, a malformation in closure of the neural tube. There is subsequent lower extremity paresis with muscle wasting and equinovarus foot deformation. The Arnold-Chiari brain malformation leads to obstructive hydrocephalus. The Pierre Robin sequence has as its initiating event hypoplasia of the mandible. This event results in a relative deficiency of space for the tongue, which drops back (glossoptosis), blocking palatal closure. Thus, the palatal defect in the Pierre Robin sequence is not a primary malformation. Rather, it is a deformation as part of a malformation sequence.

A *syndrome* represents a pattern of structural defects that have a single underlying origin (see Figure 15.2). The origin can be of a chromosomal, genetic, or teratogenic nature. The most well-recognized syndrome is Down syndrome. The underlying origin of the multiple malformations that make up this frequently diagnosed neurodevelopmental disability is the chromosomal abnormality of trisomy 21.

The term *association* describes a pattern of malformations that occur at a rate that is inconsistent with chance alone. This represents a nonrandom association of structural defects, the origin of which is not known (see Figure 15.2). Associations are descriptions of patterns of defects that may, with time and better understanding, become syndromes. VATER association is an example of defects that occur together with sufficient frequency that chance alone does not explain them. The acronym stands for the major findings of *v*ertebral anomaly, *a*nal anomaly, *t*racheo*e*sophageal fistula, and *r*enal or *r*adial anomaly. The grouping of VATER association and hydrocephalus has been identified as a syndrome. This pattern has been found to occur as an autosomal recessive disorder (Iafolla, McConkie-Rosell, & Chen, 1991). The CHARGE association—*c*oloboma of the eye, *h*eart anomaly, *a*tresia choanae, *r*etardation of mental and somatic development, *g*enital hypoplasia, and *e*ar anomaly/deafness—has a variant, CHARGE-like syndrome, that is X-linked recessive (Abruzzo & Erickson, 1989). The primary difference is the appearance of a cleft palate in the X-linked syndrome that is not present in the classic association. Genetic research will continue to change the designation of association to that of syndrome as etiologies are found for all or a subgroup of the defects that comprise an association.

Careful dysmorphology examination of children with neurodevelopmental disabilities will help to determine whether structural defects that may be present fit into one of the previously described categories. If so, the neurodevelopmental disability itself may be de-

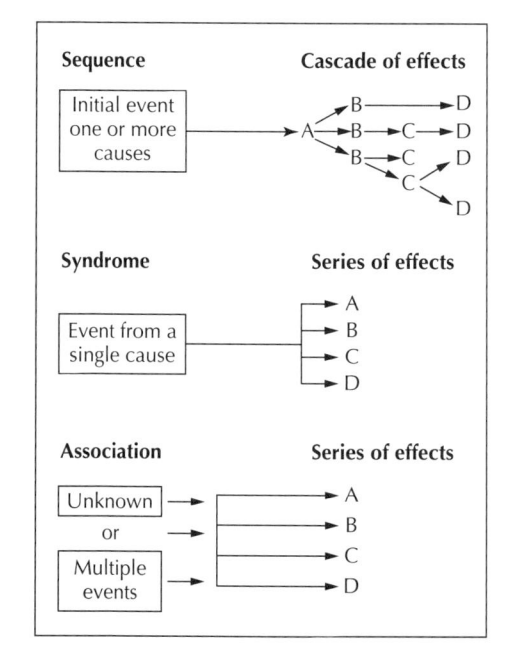

Figure 15.2. Sequence, syndrome, and association. (Reprinted from *Journal of Pediatrics, 100,* Sprangler, J., et al., Errors of morphogenesis: Concepts and terms, 160–165, Copyright © 1982, with permission from Elsevier.)

scribed as an integral part of the sequence, association, or syndrome. The failure to diagnose a specific syndrome, association, or sequence, however, does not eliminate the possibility of a prenatal etiology for any existing neurodevelopmental disorder.

MAJOR MALFORMATIONS

Major malformations are life threatening or have serious medical or cosmetic complications. A single major malformation occurs at a rate of approximately 3% of the population. Thus, 3% of the population with neurodevelopmental disabilities would be expected to have an unrelated major anomaly; however, epidemiological studies have identified 19%–40% of children with cerebral palsy as having at least one major malformation (Croen, Grether, Curry, et al., 2001; Torfs et al., 1990).

Cleft lip and palate, congenital heart defects, meningomyelocele, and primary brain abnormalities, including absent corpus callosum and Arnold-Chiari malformation, are examples of major malformations. Many major malformations are obvious, or their effect is obvious. Although one cannot see a malformed heart, the effect may be obvious based on the presence of cyanosis or signs of heart failure. Conversely, many malformations of the heart do not present with dramatic signs, although a murmur may be present. Malformations of the brain may be more obvious from the effect on neurodevelopment than the effect on head size or shape, although midline brain defects do contribute to abnormal midline facial development that will be obvious on examination.

MINOR MALFORMATIONS

Recognizable patterns of malformations primarily consist of multiple minor malformations in development, so the search for structural defects is in reality a search for trifles. Minor anomalies can be defined as structural defects that have no serious medical or cosmetic consequences. Any specific minor anomaly occurs in about 4% of the general population; however, in a study reported by Marden, Smith, and McDonald (1964), it was determined that 14% of newborn babies have a single minor anomaly, 0.8% have two, and 0.5%

have three. Thus, 0.5% of children with neurodevelopmental disabilities will be expected to have three or more minor anomalies if the neurodevelopmental disability is unrelated to the occurrence of the anomalies.

Studies of neurodevelopmental disabilities indicate that the number of anomalies in affected children far exceeds that expected by chance alone. In children with cerebral palsy, 32%–73% have multiple minor anomalies (Miller, 1989; Torfs et al., 1990). Studies of children with intellectual disabilities have reported that 30%–50% have dysmorphic or chromosomal disorders (Kirby, 2002), and Bertrand et al. (2001) reported that 30% of autistic children have dysmorphic features. Children with learning disabilities have been found to have statistically significantly higher rates of minor malformations than controls or patients with abnormal behavior but no learning disability (Accardo et al., 1991).

Many minor anomalies found on visual inspection involve the skin and hair. These structures are of ectodermal origin. Because the central nervous system also is of ectodermal origin, such minor malformations found in children with neurodevelopmental disabilities are significant and imply an early embryological interrelationship. Most of the skin lesions in the neurocutaneous syndromes listed in Table 15.1 are minor malformations. When found, they re-

Table 15.1.   Skin lesions in neurocutaneous syndromes

Neurofibromatosis
Café au lait spots
Lisch nodules (of iris)
Neurofibromas
Axillary freckling
Perianal freckling

Tuberous sclerosis
Hypopigmented macules (ash-leaf spots)
Adenoma sebaceum (facial angiofibromas)
Shagreen patch
Café au lait spots
Periungual fibromas

Sturge-Weber syndrome
Facial port-wine stain
Extension of lesion to body

Ataxia-telangiectasia
Scleral telangiectasias
Telangiectasias of pinnae, face, and nose

quire careful investigation to determine if one of the neurocutaneous syndromes is present.

The examination of the head, extremities, and skin will identify three fourths of minor anomalies. Table 15.2 lists frequently found minor malformations. These should be sought during the physical examination in all children suspected of having a neurodevelopmental disorder.

Down Syndrome as a Model for Dysmorphic Development

The child with Down syndrome is recognized easily by physicians and the public as having features that are distinct from those of other children and other family members. This pertains to children of all races and ethnic backgrounds. Although the visual effect of Down

Table 15.2. Minor malformations in neurodevelopmental disorders

Cranium	**Face and mouth**	Hypoplasia of digits
Large fontanels (especially posterior)	Micrognathia	Hypoplastic nails
Frontal bossing	Narrow maxilla	Narrow hyperconvex nails
Flat brow	Broad maxillary alveolar ridges	Thick dermal pads
Flat occiput	Shallow malar eminences	Proximal placement of thumb
Prominent occiput	Shallow orbital ridges	Camptodactyly
Third saggital fontanel	Ridged central palate	Asymmetry of length of digits
Metopic suture open to bregma	Cleft uvula	Single flexion crease of fifth digit
Scalp defect	Long philtrum	Extra flexion creases
Parietal foramina	Short philtrum	
	Simple philtrum	**Foot**
Eyes	Angular lip pits	Syndactyly of toes
Inner epicanthal folds	Narrow vermilion border	Overlapping toes
Slanting of palpebral fissures	Tooth hypoplasia	Recessed toe
Brushfield spots	Short lingual frenulum	Hypoplastic nails
Heterochromia iridis		Dorsiflexion of halux
Ptosis	**Skin**	Asymmetric length
Freckled iris	Skin tags	Crease between halux and
Hypotelorism	Skin sinuses	second digit
Hypertelorism	Webbed neck	
Coloboma	Lax skin	**Body**
	Abnormally placed dimples	Single umbilical artery
Nose	Café au lait spots	Short neck
Flat nasal bridge	Depigmented spots	Anal tag
Prominent nasal bridge	Unusual lesions/nevi/	Sacral dimple
Anteverted nostrils	"birthmarks"	Shield chest
Long nasal septum	Supernumerary nipples	
Bulbous nasal tip		**Genitals**
Hypoplastic alae nasae	**Hair**	Glandular hypospadias
	Alopecia > 0.3 cm of scalp	Shawl scrotum
Auricle	Hirsutism	Vaginal tag
Preauricular tags	Excess scalp hair whorls	Hypoplasia of labia majora
Preauricular pits	Absent scalp hair whorls	
Incomplete helix	Excess widow's peak hair pattern	**Dermatoglyphics**
Absent lobes	Synophrys	Distal axial palmar triradius
Low-set ears	Low hairline on neck	Open field in hallucal area
Notched lobes	White forelock	Lack of ridges
Bifid lobe		High frequency of low arch
Lop ear	**Hand**	patterns of fingertips
Cup-shaped ear	Simian crease	High frequency of whorl patterns
Helix attached to scalp	Bridged simian crease	
Excess tissue to helix	Brachydactyly	
Slanted away from eye	Clinodactyly	

Sources: Aase (1992); Jones (1988); Leppig, Werler, Cann, Cook, and Holmes (1987); and Smith and Bostian (1964).

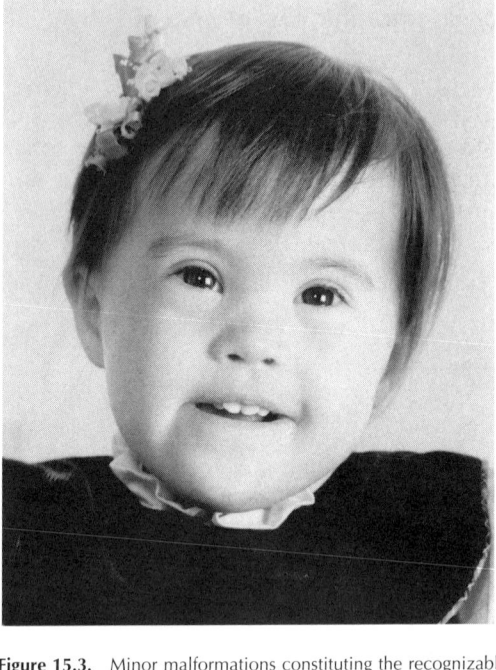
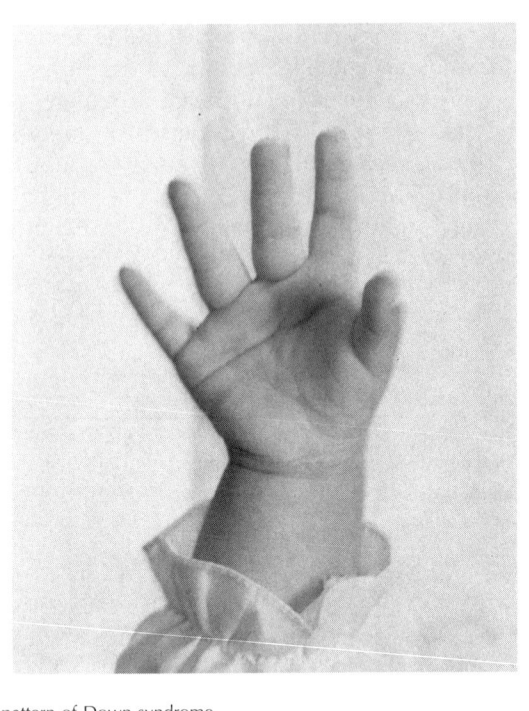

Figure 15.3.   Minor malformations constituting the recognizable pattern of Down syndrome.

syndrome is readily apparent (Figure 15.3), this disorder is in fact a composite of minor malformations that form a classic pattern (Table 15.3). Taken individually, each malformation is insignificant. No single minor malformation is pathognomonic for Down syndrome. Each occurs in normal individuals at varying percentages, but none occurs in greater than 4% of the normal population (Pueschel & Pueschel, 1992).

The major malformations found in Down syndrome are also characteristic but not pathognomonic. Congenital heart defects occur in approximately 50% of children with Down syndrome. The persistent atrioventricular canal is quite characteristic for Down syndrome, but it is not the only congenital heart defect found. Gastrointestinal defects throughout the intestinal tract occur with significantly increased frequency when compared with the general population, with duodenal atresia being the most common and characteristic of Down syndrome. Other major malformations reported with increased frequency in Down syndrome, but that are not pathognomonic, include tracheoesophageal fistula, incomplete fusion of vertebrae, cryptorchidism, and athyrosis.

THE DYSMORPHOLOGY HISTORY

An important element in the neurodevelopmental assessment is the portion of the history devoted to possible prenatal or genetic etiology. This is part of the dysmorphology history. Careful inquiry into the family history, with the construction of a pedigree, will help to determine if other family members have been affected similarly. Autosomal recessive disorders may be more common in a pedigree that reflects consanguinity. Autosomal dominant disorders may be readily apparent if one of the parents is affected similarly; however, the parent may not have been diagnosed previously. Wide variability of expression is the rule for autosomal dominant disorders. A parent may be only mildly affected while the child who has the same disorder is severely affected. It is not uncommon to diagnose a parent with neurofibromatosis at the time of diagnosis of the child. This may also happen with Noonan syndrome and other autosomal dominant syndromes. The physician finds not one but two patients—the parent and the child—with the new diagnosis.

X-linked recessive disorders will be reflected in the maternal pedigree. Fragile X syn-

Table 15.3. Minor malformations of Down syndrome

Head and face

Brachycephaly
Midface hypoplasia
Intraorbital distance reduced
Depressed nasal bridge
Upslanting palpebral fissures
Epicanthal folds
Brushfield spots
Small pinnae
Overfolding of the helix
Prominent antihelix
Absent or attached earlobes
Prominent lips
Protruding tongue
Papillary hypertrophy
Excessive fissuring of tongue
Short neck
Broad base of neck

Extremities

Shortened distal extremities
Broad and stubby hands and feet
Clinodactyly
Brachydactyly
Hypoplastic middle phalanx
Simian creases
Syndactyly
Wide space between first and second toes
Plantar crease between first and second toes

Sources: Jones (1988); Pueschel and Pueschel (1992).

drome, which cytogenetically has excessive strings of triplet nucleic acids and methylation of the acids, represents a disorder in which the pattern of inheritance does not conform to mendelian genetic concepts. The pedigree may appear to be that of a classic X-linked recessive disorder, but about 20% of males who have the mutation on their X chromosome show no physical or mental features of the disorder, whereas approximately one third of carrier females have some evidence of intellectual disabilities. Likewise, the degree of excessive repeats and the presence of methylation is correlated to the degree of symptoms found. The longer the string of triplet repeats, the more severe the neurodevelopmental impairment will be.

A history of abnormal past pregnancies may indicate possible intrauterine abnormalities. A high incidence of fetal loss may represent undiagnosed genetic abnormalities, and advanced maternal age is associated with an increased incidence of chromosomal anomalies.

Determining exposure to teratogens can be vexing. Mothers generally are willing to discuss their multiple minor exposures to over-the-counter medications or to household agents such as cleansers; however, they may be very reluctant to discuss exposure to the most serious of teratogens—alcohol. A careful history of fetal exposure to alcohol may be the most important discussion concerning teratogens. Prenatal exposure to alcohol is the most common preventable cause of neurodevelopmental disability and should be sought in every history. Other unusual exposures, including exposure to illicit drugs, may shed light on the potential etiology of a neurodevelopmental disorder. Cocaine is a potent vasoconstrictor that may result in disruptions caused by vasoocclusion but not in primary malformations. Complications of gestation, especially bleeding and abnormalities of fetal movement, indicate abnormalities that may have neurodevelopmental and dysmorphic consequences.

Postnatal growth and development have direct implications as to possible dysmorphic conditions. A review of growth charts can be helpful in identifying and timing disorders associated with microcephaly and macrocephaly. A prenatal history of growth disturbances may indicate problems occurring prior to any perinatal events; however, defects in brain development of prenatal onset often are associated with poor transition from intrauterine to extrauterine life, leading to abnormalities of labor and delivery. These perinatal problems should not overshadow the fact that there were prenatal abnormalities. Catastrophic perinatal events leading to neurodevelopmental disabilities will first result in an acute encephalopathy and prolong the newborn nursery hospitalization.

PHYSICAL EXAMINATION

The dysmorphology examination begins with anthropometric measurements. Supine length for children younger than 3 years and standing height for those older than 3 years must be taken accurately and plotted on age- and sex-specific growth charts. Length or height less than the 5th percentile for age and sex is considered short stature and requires explanation. Constitutional short stature, chronic illness, endocrine disorders, and short stature syndromes are all possible explanations. Likewise, tall stature—length or height greater than the 95th percentile for age and sex—requires evaluation and explanation. Overgrowth or tall stature syndromes such as fragile X or Weaver syndrome should be considered when growth is excessive.

Weight percentiles need to be compared with length/height percentiles, with discrepancies for unusually heavy or unusually light children explained. Failure to thrive, chronic illness, and malformation syndromes may contribute to a child being underweight. Obesity is usually exogenous; however, obesity syndromes such as Prader-Willi or Beckwith syndrome often present as short stature and obesity in children.

Abnormal head size—microcephaly and macrocephaly—should be determined by graphing head circumference on the Nelhaus curve (Nelhaus, 1968). This chart is age and sex specific from birth to 18 years. Microcephaly is defined as a head circumference greater than 2 standard deviations below the mean. Macrocephaly is a head circumference greater than 2 standard deviations above the mean. As the degree of microcephaly or macrocephaly increases, the possibility for neurodevelopmental disability increases. Abnormal head shape, or plagiocephaly, is seen in many syndromes involving craniosynostosis, such as Crouzon and Apert syndromes. Dolichocephaly, or long and narrow skull shape, is typically observed in premature infants but is also caused by sagittal suture craniosynostosis.

Overall posture and body appearance of the child may be an important observation with regard to dysmorphic conditions. Does the child appear to be properly proportioned? Are the head and body proportions normal? Does the top half of the body seem to fit with the lower half? Are the extremities appropriate for the trunk or do they appear too long or too short? If there appears to be an abnormality of proportion, then further anthropomorphic measurements are needed. Upper segment and lower segment trunk measurements taken from the pubic symphysis will determine lower

extremity proportions. Arm span as compared with height will determine whether the upper extremities are appropriately proportionate to the body. Hand and foot sizes can be measured and charted on age-specific curves. As abnormalities of proportion appear, further investigation will be necessary. Normal values for body measurements are available in the handbook by Hall, Froster-Iskenius, and Allanson (1989).

Abnormalities in facial proportions cause unusual appearance. Hypertelorism and hypotelorism can be determined accurately by comparing measurements of the inner canthal distance, the outer canthal distance, and the inner pupillary distance (Figure 15.4). Palpebral fissure length also can be measured. Small palpebral fissures are found in several dysmorphic syndromes, including fetal alcohol syndrome. An abnormal-appearing philtrum can be measured and the measurement plotted on normal curves. Likewise, the position of ears that appear to be low set can be determined accurately by extending a line between the inner canthi out to the sides of the head. Low-set ears are defined as falling below this line. The appearance of low-set ears may be the consequence of macrocephaly or of a misshapen skull. This causes a greater-than-usual cranial mass to extend above normally set ears. Abnormality of ear rotation can also occur, with posteriorly rotated ears being abnormal when the axis of the auricle is more than 15 degrees from perpendicular. Abnormalities of morphogenesis gen-

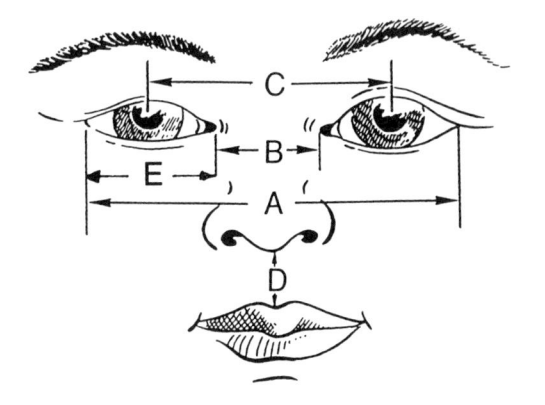

Figure 15.4. Facial measurements. (Reprinted from *Smith's recognizable patterns of human malformation* [4th ed.], K.L. Jones, p. 669, Copyright 1988, with permission from Elsevier.) (*Key:* A, outer canthal distance; B, inner canthal distance; C, inner pupillary distance; D, philtrum length; E, palpebral fissure length.)

erally result in low-set and posteriorly rotated ears because this is the position of the auricle in fetal development.

Other abnormalities of body proportion include an abnormally short or long neck. A short neck may prompt radiographic investigation for cervical vertebral anomalies as seen in the Klippel-Feil anomaly. Webbing of the neck is a common feature of Noonan, Turner, Down, and other syndromes that have neurodevelopmental consequences.

The careful search for minor malformations is the essence of the dysmorphology examination. One minor malformation is insignificant, but a pattern of multiple minor malformations may indeed be the defining characteristic of a specific disorder or syndrome. Even if no readily identifiable syndrome exists, a pattern of minor malformations indicates that prenatal development was not appropriate. This suggests that any existing neurodevelopmental disability also may be due to inappropriate prenatal development.

RADIOGRAPHY, NEUROIMAGING, AND GENETICS STUDIES

The presence of three or more minor malformations increases the risk that an occult major malformation may also be present. An appropriate evaluation includes a radiographic examination for bony anomalies, especially when abnormalities of size or proportion are present (see Chapter 24, this volume). This includes lateral skull, spine, rib, long bone, and hand radiographs. Radiographs of the hands should include an evaluation of bone age. Severely delayed bone age is found in the dysmorphic sequence caused by hypothyroidism. Asymmetry of bone maturation is characteristic of Sotos syndrome. Neuroimaging is necessary for the investigation of microcephaly, macrocephaly, and plagiocephaly. Special bone window studies on computed tomography may be the best study when craniosynostosis is suspected.

High-resolution karyotyping and cytogenetic markers (fluorescent in situ hybridization assays) have expanded our knowledge of the variation of presentations of many dysmorphic syndromes. Prior to discovery of a specific genetic marker, only those patients with classic signs were diagnosed with a specific syndrome. Specific genetic markers have been found in patients with less than classic clinical findings in almost all syndromes, including Williams syndrome, Angelman syndrome, Prader-Willi syndrome, and tuberous sclerosis. Clinical suspicion based on the dysmorphology examination, however, continues to be essential in determining which patients are to have specific testing performed. As the number of genetic markers increases, it is necessary to use continuously updated references, such as the web sites Online Medelian Inheritance in Man and GeneTest to determine the availability of a genetic marker for a suspected syndrome.

Tissue culture for enzyme analysis for metabolic or storage diseases may be indicated in patients in whom the possibility of such a disorder is high based on findings on the physical examination. These are not indicated as routine studies searching for occult malformations (see Chapter 5, this volume). Whenever a specific syndrome or dysmorphic disorder is diagnosed, an expanded battery of laboratory tests and subspecialty consultations may become necessary.

CONCLUSION

The examination for dysmorphic features remains an important aspect of the complete neurodevelopmental assessment of children. The presence of malformations, deformations, dysplasias, or disruptions will help to determine the etiology of the disability. This may be a defined syndrome or an association diagnosed by the pattern of abnormalities found. Even if the pattern of abnormalities is not classic for a defined syndrome, there may be enough evidence to warrant obtaining specific genetic assays. The increasing array of genetic testing available, however, has not precluded the need for a careful dysmorphology examination. Equally important, the pattern of abnormalities found on examination may not result in a specific diagnosis but may indicate the timing and potential genetic influence of accompanying disabilities.

REFERENCES

Aase, J.M. (1992). Dysmorphic diagnosis for the pediatric practitioner. *Pediatric Clinics of North America, 39,* 135–156.

Abruzzo, M.A., & Erickson, R.P. (1989). Re-evaluation of new X-linked syndrome for evidence of CHARGE syndrome or association. *American Journal of Medical Genetics, 34,* 397–400.

Accardo, P.J., Tomazic, T., Morrow, J., Haake, C., & Whitman, B.Y. (1991). Minor malformations, hyperactivity, and learning disabilities. *American Journal of Diseases of Children, 145,* 1184–1187.

Bertrand, J., Mars, A., Boyle, C., Bove, F., Yeargin-Allsopp, M., & Decoufle, P. (2001). Prevalence of autism in a United States population: The Brick Township, New Jersey, investigation. *Pediatrics, 108,* 1155–1161.

Coorssen, E.A., Msall, M.A., & Duffy, L.C. (1991). Multiple minor malformations as a marker for prenatal etiology of cerebral palsy. *Developmental Medicine and Child Neurology, 33,* 730–736.

Croen, L.A., Grether, J.K., Curry, C.J., & Nelson, K.B. (2001). Congenital anomalies among children with cerebral palsy: More evidence for prenatal antecedents. *Journal of Pediatrics, 138,* 804–810.

Croen, L.A., Grether, J.K., & Selvin, S. (2001). The epidemiology of mental retardation of unknown cause. *Pediatrics, 107,* e86.

Hall, J.G., Froster-Iskenius, U.G., & Allanson, J.E. (1989). *Handbook of normal physical measurements.* Oxford, England: Oxford Medical Publications.

Hultman, C.M., Sparen, P., & Cnattingius, S. (2002). Perinatal risk factors for infantile autism. *Epidemiology, 13,* 417–423.

Iafolla, A.K., McConkie-Rosell, A., & Chen, Y.T. (1991). VATER and hydrocephalus: A distinct syndrome? *American Journal of Medical Genetics, 38,* 46–51.

Jelliffe-Pawlowski, L.L., Shaw, G.M., Nelson, V., & Harris, J.A. (2003). *Archives of Pediatrics and Adolescent Medicine, 157,* 545–550.

Jones, K.L. (Ed.). (1988). *Smith's recognizable patterns of human malformation* (4th ed.). Philadelphia: W.B. Saunders.

Kirby, R.S. (2002). Co-occurrence of developmental disabilities with birth defects. *Mental Retardation and Developmental Disabilities Research Reviews, 8,* 182–187.

Leppig, K.A., Werler, M.M., Cann, C.L., Cook, C.A., & Holmes, L.B. (1987). Predictive value of minor anomalies: I. Association with major malformations. *Journal of Pediatrics, 110,* 520–537.

Marden, P.M., Smith, D.W., & McDonald, M.J. (1964). Congenital anomalies in the newborn infant, including minor variations. *Journal of Pediatrics, 64,* 357–360.

Miller, G. (1989). Minor congenital anomalies and ataxic cerebral palsy. *Archives of Disease in Childhood, 64,* 557–562.

Nelhaus, G. (1968). Head circumference from birth to 18 years: Practical composite international and interracial graphs. *Pediatrics, 41,* 106–114.

Pueschel, S.M., & Pueschel, J.K. (1992). *Biomedical concerns in persons with Down syndrome.* Baltimore: Paul H. Brookes Publishing Co.

Smith, D.W., & Bostian, K.E. (1964). Congenital anomalies associated with idiopathic mental retardation. *Journal of Pediatrics, 65,* 189–196.

Sprangler, J., Benirschke, K., Hall, J.G., Lenz, W., Lowry, R.B., Opitz, J.M., et al. (1982). Errors of morphogenesis: Concepts and terms. *Journal of Pediatrics, 100,* 160–165.

Summit, R.L. (1969). Cytogenetics in mentally defective children with anomalies: A controlled study. *Journal of Pediatrics, 74,* 58–66.

Torfs, C.P., van den Berg, B.J., Oechsli, F.W., & Cummins, S. (1990). Prenatal and perinatal factors in the etiology of cerebral palsy. *Journal of Pediatrics, 116,* 615–619.

16

The Amiel-Tison and Gosselin Neurological Assessment from Birth to 6 Years of Age

CLAUDINE AMIEL-TISON AND JULIE GOSSELIN

In every domain explored by the neurological assessment of infants and young children, responses evolve developmentally with brain maturation, which is very rapid in the first year of life and continues at a slower pace in the following years. Chasing after neurological signs through maturative changes is discouraging for clinicians, who instead often choose to rely on the functional consequences of cerebral impairment, more specifically on motor milestones within the first 2 years of life. This methodological error is often misleading when dealing with moderate and mild cases because apparent normalization of gross motor function by the end of the second year is the most common trajectory. Despite this apparent normalization, repeated systematic neurological examinations in high-risk populations have shown that neurological and cranial signs progressively emerge within the first 2 years of life and persist as a permanent clue to perinatal cerebral insult. From this perspective, neurological assessment cannot be replaced by the developmental assessment, which must be considered complementary.

Our objective has been to devise a neurological instrument based on a fixed set of observations and maneuvers (Amiel-Tison & Gosselin, 2001). The results are scored individually according to the child's age. The determination of the neurological status is based on the notion of symptomatic clusters and deviant profiles instead of a global score, which provides less qualitative information. Our recent data (Gosselin, Amiel-Tison, Infante-Rivard, Fouron, & Fouron, 2002; Gosselin, Fouron, & Amiel-Tison, 2006) support the construct validity of this categorization, which reflects the continuum from mild, to moderate, to severe neurological involvement at the corrected age of 2 years in children at risk for hypoxic-ischemic damage. These results also demonstrate the predictive validity of the evaluation for anticipation of later difficulties in higher cerebral function at school age among these children.

This evaluation is formatted for use in both clinical and research settings. It is simple and easy to perform routinely and can be completed in 10–15 minutes. The use of a single conceptual framework from 40 weeks' gestation (Amiel-Tison, 2002) to 6 years of age avoids the pitfalls associated with methodological changes in the course of neurodevelopmental surveillance throughout childhood. It allows early targeting of the children who are at the highest risk of experiencing learning difficulties. Finally, by distinguishing neurological signs from their functional impact, it also helps the parents to better understand the developmental trajectory of their child.

HISTORICAL BACKGROUND AND CONCEPTUAL FRAMEWORK

In her very first week as a resident in the neonatal unit of Port-Royal-Baudelocque, one of us (C.A.T.) admitted a full-term neonate with status epilepticus secondary to acute fetal asphyxia during labor. Facing such a disaster, it became evident that a structured follow-up was needed for children such as this one beginning at discharge and continuing for several years without interruption. This child was included in a first cohort of 41 full-term newborn infants with hypoxic-ischemic damage born between 1962 and 1965 (Amiel-Tison, 1969). Because of the absence of any standardized neurological assessment for infants and young children at that time, the outcome was initially categorized by degrees of disability. Since then, our goal has been to devise a neurological assessment integrating both André Thomas's conception of muscle tone (Thomas & de Ajuriaguerra, 1949) and the method for analytical evaluation of passive muscle tone in limbs developed by his followers (Saint-Anne Dargassies, 1977; Stamback & de Ajuriaguerra, 1958). Successive steps in the elaboration of the assessment presented here can be summarized as follows:

1. Identification of the different components of axial tone in normal and abnormal development (Amiel-Tison, 1975; Amiel-Tison, Korobkin, & Esque-Vaucouloux, 1977)

2. Didactic description of each selected item and interpretation of results according to maturational stages within the first year of life, with a chart to gather monthly data (Amiel-Tison, 1976; Amiel-Tison & Grenier, 1986)

3. Interpretation of normal and abnormal results (Amiel-Tison, 1985) in light of the anatomic and physiological correlates presented by Sarnat (1984), allowing pediatricians to become fully aware of the clinical significance of their observations

4. Integration of cranial data as an indispensable component of the systematic neurological assessment (Amiel-Tison, Gosselin, &

Infante-Rivard, 2002; Amiel-Tison & Stewart, 1994)

5. Conceptual distinction between neurological impairment associated with brain damage and disabilities evolving with maturation (Amiel-Tison & Stewart, 1989)

6. Description of the specific procedures for administration and scoring (Amiel-Tison & Gosselin, 2001; Amiel-Tison & Stewart, 1989) applicable to the neurological assessment both at 40 weeks of gestation (Amiel-Tison, 2002; Gosselin, Gahagan, & Amiel-Tison, 2005) and up to 6 years, thereby preventing any methodological breakdown in the follow-up of high-risk populations

7. Identification of a five-level classification based on absence/presence of clusters of signs reflecting the complete spectrum from normal to disabling cerebral palsy (CP) (Gosselin et al., 2002)

8. Demonstration of the validity of the neurological assessment for predicting long-term outcome, especially with regard to higher cerebral function at school age in children at risk of hypoxic-ischemic damage (Couture, 2005; Gosselin et al., 2002)

9. Training of pediatricians for widespread use of the standardized assessment in primary care (Rozé et al., 2004)

ANATOMICAL AND PHYSIOLOGICAL FOUNDATIONS

Pediatricians became fully aware of the clinical significance of their observations (Amiel-Tison, 1985) after Sarnat (1984) reviewed anatomic and physiological correlates of early neurological development. It was then possible to clinically follow the individual development of both lower and upper motor control systems. The lower system, consisting of the brainstem and cerebellum, matures early (beginning at 24 weeks' gestational age) in an ascending wave. Its essential role is to maintain posture against gravity and maintain flexor tone in the limbs. The upper system, consisting of the cerebral hemispheres and basal ganglia, matures

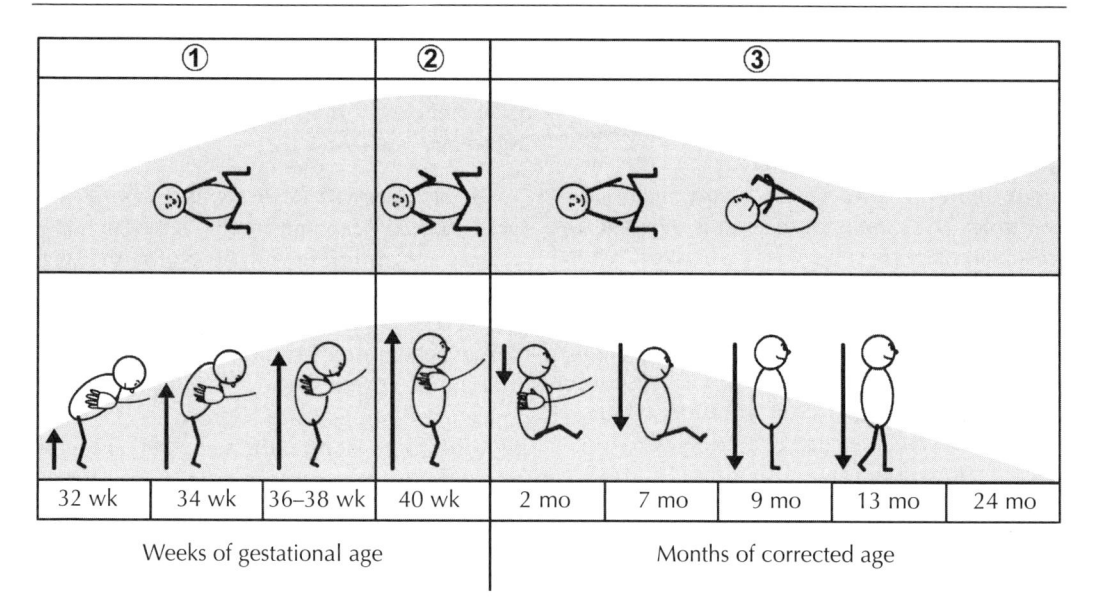

Figure 16.1. Evolution of passive muscle tone in limbs and gross motor milestones from birth through the first 2 years of age. 1) During the prenatal period, as exhibited in infants born prematurely (32, 34, and 36–38 weeks' gestation). 2) At term (40 weeks' gestation). 3) During the first 2 years of life (corrected ages in months for preterm infants). (From Gosselin, J., & Amiel-Tison, C. [2007]. *Évaluation neurologique de la naissance à 6 ans.* Montréal, Canada: Éditions du CHU Ste-Justine; reprinted by permission.)

later (beginning at 32 weeks' gestational age) and rapidly in the first 2 years in a descending wave. Its essential role is to control the lower motor system, to achieve relaxation of the limbs and control of antigravity forces, finally allowing erect posture, walking, and fine motor skills (Figure 16.1). This distinction became even more relevant after pathological and radiological data had shown that brain damage in the neonate is mainly located in the cerebral hemispheres in the full-term neonate with hypoxic-ischemic encephalopathy or in the premature newborn with periventricular leukomalacia. Consequently, the best predictors of injury should be found in responses that depend on the upper motor control system and not responses that depend mainly on brainstem activity. These signs are not specific to any cause: They may accompany hypoxic-ischemic damage or infectious or toxic insults, as well as genetic disorders (Garcia-Cazoria et al., 2004).

DESCRIPTION OF THE METHOD

Domains Explored

The Amiel-Tison and Gosselin Neurological Assessment from Birth to 6 Years is largely traditional in nature, including head growth measurement, assessment of passive muscle tone,

observation of motor activity, and elicitation of deep tendon reflexes, primitive reflexes, and postural reactions. Gross and fine motor performances are observed separately because they represent functional milestones. Qualitative abnormalities concerning these performances as well as secondary deformations are also noted. Terminology as well as a few technical points are discussed here to clarify the underlying conceptual framework.

Passive Muscle Tone Passive tone, also called extensibility, refers to muscle resistance at rest and is assessed in the limbs, segment by segment, with a number of maneuvers evaluating the range of a *slow movement executed by the examiner while the subject remains passive.* Results are usually expressed as an angle, estimated but not measured. The normal range varies greatly in the first 2 years of life because of the spectacular changes in tone occurring with maturation. In the body axis, the appreciation of muscle tone implies the comparison of slow ventral and dorsal incurvations. Normally flexion is greater than or equal to extension: More extension than flexion is abnormal at any age. The maneuvers are easy to perform on an infant or young child lying on the examination table. The results provide valuable information on upper motor control (see later).

Resistance to Rapid Stretching   When the brain is intact, rapid stretching of one segment of a limb does not cause an increase in resistance: The range of motion is identical to the one obtained by the slow maneuver. When upper motor control is altered, the response to the rapid maneuver is modified; two abnormal responses enable the examiner to differentiate between two degrees of severity. One response (*phasic*) is brisk and of short duration, whereas the other (*tonic*) is more marked and protracted. These abnormal responses, often associated with excessive deep tendon reflexes and clonus, allow confirmation of spasticity and suggest damage in the upper motor control. These signs of spasticity are not present at birth but emerge in the first months depending on progressive maturation, the more subtle occurring the latest.

Motor Activity   The French school has extensively documented the assessment of motor activity in the neonate under the term *active tone*. This notion has been used in particular to describe the active movement of the head against gravity during the raise-to-sit maneuver and its reverse in the term neonate. The terminology of "active tone" is then used to clearly indicate that the child him- or herself is actively performing, this active performance being completely different from the passive drop of the head due to gravity. By 2 months of corrected age, maturation is such that the response to the raise-to-sit maneuver and its reverse cannot be separated anymore. Head control, defined as the ability to maintain the head steady within the axis of the trunk for at least 15 seconds, is then demonstrated when the child is held upright, sitting on the examination table. This first gross motor milestone will be followed later by independent sitting and walking.

Therefore, after the neonatal period, the term *active tone* becomes not only useless but misleading because the examiner becomes progressively an observer as the child begins to self-initiate motor performance. This explains why "active tone" is present in our neonatal assessment but absent in the assessment applied through childhood. Gross motor mile-

stones are then scored as present or absent (with or without delay in timing), and their quality of execution is further analyzed according to age.

Head Growth Patterns and Cranial Sutures Status   Damage in the cerebral hemispheres may interfere with head growth. Magnetic resonance imaging (MRI) studies have shown that, up to 6 years, head circumference is an excellent predictor of brain volume (Bartholomeusz, Courchesne, & Karns, 2002). In typical conditions, head growth follows a smooth progression on the same percentile on the standard curve as the height and weight parameters, with appropriate *head–body proportionality*. Various deviant situations can be identified during the first 2 years of follow-up. Mainly because of the unique and temporary capacity of the skull to adapt to brain volume, catch-up growth or decline can be observed; however, facing the lack of a universal definition of catch-up growth or decline, each team has its own standards for classifying these parameters, preventing any valid comparison between various cohort studies. From the available literature, the following definitions appear to be reasonable: 1) *decline* refers to a decrease of 1 standard deviation (SD) or more, not followed by a catch-up; and 2) *catch-up* refers to an increase of 1 SD or more, whether preceded by a postnatal decline or not. Two patterns of catch-up may be identified: complete catch-up with return to the initial percentile and incomplete catch-up with an increase (1 SD) that does not reach the initial value by 2 years of corrected age (Amiel-Tison et al., 2002). According to the head growth pattern during the first 2 years of life, several categories, including normocephaly, microcephaly, and macrocephaly, may be defined.

Normocephaly is crudely defined as head circumference at $\pm$ 2 SD from the mean. Based on the previous considerations, it becomes easy to understand that such a wide range of normal head growth does not necessarily reflect normal brain growth. *Microcephaly* may be absolute or relative. There are two types of absolute microcephaly: 1) primary, defined as 2 SD below the mean since birth; and 2) secondary, defined as 2 SD below the mean, postnatally acquired. From a semantic point of view, it is interesting to note that the term *microcephaly* (literally "small head") is used to designate both a small head and a small brain (*micrencephaly*, which literally means small brain, is rarely used). *Relative microcephaly, postnatally acquired* results from a continuous decline of more than 50 centiles between birth and 2 years of corrected age in children whose head circumference at birth was above the 52nd centile. This pattern may also be referred as "suboptimal head growth." *Macrocephaly* is currently defined as head circumference 2 SD above the mean. Mostly of genetic origin, this sign may be present from birth or appear progressively during the first year of life. From a semantic point of view, the term *macrocephaly* (enlarged head) is not synonymous with *megalencephaly* (enlarged brain) because the brain may or may not fill the skull, as shown on MRI.

Considering that head growth is mainly passive in early childhood as a result of the rapid volumetric increase of cerebral hemispheres, the cranial suture status constitutes a valuable complement to head growth pattern. The mobility of cranial bones at the suture level allows overlapping or distention, related to underlying insufficient or excessive hemispheric growth (after exclusion of hydrocephaly). The anatomic description of cranial sutures is summarized elsewhere (Amiel-Tison et al., 2002). The squamous suture, with its distinctive bevel shape, can be considered as a junction between cranial vault and cranial base. Because of its shape and location, its sensitivity is specific: This suture is the last to distend in cases of volumetric increase and the first to overlap in cases of cerebral atrophy, even when head circumference remains within normal limits. Because cranial suture status often represents more subtle brain growth impairments, its evaluation should be an integrated component of the neurological assessment.

Data Collection and Scoring System

The examination chart for the Amiel-Tison and Gosselin Neurological Assessment from Birth to 6 Years (Gosselin & Amiel, 2007) includes four sections along with a profile summary sheet with a classification at 2 years of age and subsequent annual profiles up to 6 years of age.

The first section is general in content and is completed at each examination. The next three sections are to be used during neurological examinations according to age and take into account the changes in muscle tone, primary reflexes, and postural reactions resulting from maturation. The scoring system is as follows:

- A score of 0 indicates a typical result for that age, within the normal range.

- A score of 1 indicates a moderately abnormal result for that age.

- A score of 2 indicates a definite abnormal result for that age.

For certain items, scoring is considered inappropriate, and examiners circle an "X" to indicate examination results (e.g., the presence of primitive reflexes during the fourth, fifth, and sixth month of age). For these items, no conclusions should be made regarding the normal or abnormal nature of results. A gray shaded area in a column on the test form indicates that the item does not have to be tested for that particular age (e.g., comparison of slow and rapid dorsiflexion angles of the foot during the first 3 months of life).

Two main studies have tested the interrater reliability of the items. McCarraher-Wetzel and Wetzel (1984), who used the original version known as the Neurological Evaluation of the Newborn and the Infant (Amiel-Tison, 1976), mainly studied the agreement between examiners with regard to passive muscle tone expressed in angles. They reported an overall agreement of 90% for the entire assessment. This rate was maintained after 1 year. More specifically, they obtained an agreement of 90% for the scarf sign, 80% for foot dorsiflexion, and 73% for popliteal angle. A more recent study involving three independent examiners (Deschênes, Gosselin, Couture, & Lachance, 2004), testing 35 infants, was done with the Amiel-Tison Neurological Assessment at Term (Amiel-Tison, 2002). This neonatal assessment is based on the same methodology and shares most of its content with the neurological assessment from birth to 6 years. Among the 29 items, 16 showed excellent reliability, with kappa coefficients higher than 0.75; kappa coefficients ranging between 0.40 and 0.75 were obtained for 11 items, and kappa coefficients lower than 0.40 were found for 2 items. The overall reliability was 0.76, confirming the very good interrater reliability of the assessment.

Summary Impressions Following Each Assessment

At the end of each assessment, the examiner is asked to provide his or her overall opinion concerning the responses obtained. This step-by-step synthesis is not based on a total computed score. Within the first 6 months, signs and symptoms are rather nonspecific; as the child grows older, the clinical picture becomes more specific, and clusters of signs usually emerge. Within the same period, etiological clues become more definite and the type of brain damage better identified with complementary investigations.

Categorization at 2 Years of Corrected Age

Two years of corrected age appears to be the right time for a "short-term" synthesis of results because the period of rapid brain maturation is over. In severe cases, the neuromotor and cranial findings are conspicuous enough to confirm a diagnosis of CP based on the characteristic abnormalities of movement and postural tone. In moderate cases, however, the age of acquisition of independent walking must be included to allow the distinction between disabling and nondisabling CP, depending on the absence or presence of independent walking by 2 years. It is difficult for the neurologist to ignore independent walking because this ability is so particular to human beings. Categorization by independent walking is consistent with clinical experience and corroborates the work of Pinto-Martin et al. (1995). The exception is children with hemiplegic CP, who usually walk before 2 years. At 2 years of corrected age, topographic and symptomatic varieties of CP can already be labelled precisely. In the following years, the functional impact on gross motor function will progressively become more precise.

Based on the application of this clinical method over many years with children at risk of minor or moderate hypoxic-ischemic brain damage, a categorization has emerged to classify the most significant minor neurological signs. A five-level scale of neurological status categorized according to association and severity of neurological and cranial signs, including specific clusters of signs and their severity, has been developed (Table 16.1). Three neurocranial signs have emerged as part of a symptomatic cluster (Amiel-Tison & Stewart, 1994). Two of these three signs test passive tone and should be particularly helpful in revealing impairment of the corticospinal system: abnormal stretch reflex in the triceps surae obtained by rapid dorsiflexion of the foot, and imbalance of passive axial tone with predominance of extensor tone (Figure 16.2). The third sign is a ridge over the squamous sutures reflecting a deceleration in hemispheric growth following

Table 16.1. Categorization according to association and severity of neurological and cranial signs

Categories	Neurological signs
Disabling cerebral palsy	Uni- or bilateral tonic stretch reflex ± other abnormalities
	Absence of independent walking at 2 years of corrected age
Nondisabling cerebral palsy	Uni- or bilateral tonic stretch reflex ± other abnormalities
	Independent walk before 2 years of corrected age
Neurocranial triad	Uni- or bilateral phasic stretch reflex
	Imbalance of passive axial tone
	Squamous ridges
Intermediate	One or two signs of the neurocranial triad or nonspecific signs such as hypotonia
Normal	No neurological signs or isolated squamous ridges

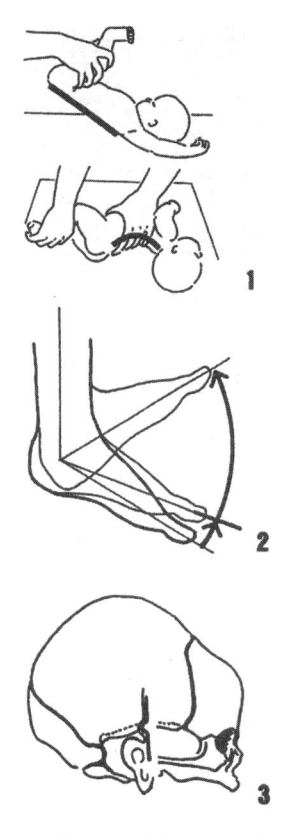

Figure 16.2.   Triad of neurocranial signs: 1) imbalance in passive muscle tone of the trunk with excessive extension; 2) phasic stretch during rapid dorsiflexion of the foot; and 3) squamous ridge (may disappear after the age of 4 years). These three signs (or at least the first two) are only significant when clustered together. (From Gosselin, J., & Amiel-lison, C. [2007]. *Évaluation neurologique de la naissance à 6 ans.* Montréal, Canada: Éditions du CHU Ste-Justine; reprinted by permission.)

the perinatal insult. All signs usually appear within the first 2 years of life. The first two signs are persistent, whereas the squamous ridge may be permanent or regressive with re-molding after 4 years of age (Amiel-Tison et al., 1996); cranial signs cannot be taken into consideration when found in isolation.

The triad of neurocranial signs includes mild signs but cannot be labeled as "soft signs" because they are believed to be part of a well-defined neurological syndrome of damage to the upper motor control structures. In fact, the clustering of any kind of mild signs should eliminate the use of *soft signs,* a meaningless term that masks methodological imprecision.

Assessment from 2 to 6 Years

In the course of neurodevelopmental follow-up, the neurological assessment may be re-peated yearly using the same method. The stability with regard to the neurological status defined on the previously described five-level scale was analyzed in a recent prospective study on a cohort of children at risk of hypoxic-ischemic insult (Gosselin & Amiel-Tison, 2004). The same examiner tested 78 children between 2 and 6 years of age without access to previous results of the neurological assessment. The neurological status was stable in 49 children (62.8%) and unstable in 29 (37.2%). Most of the children with recorded changes (24 of 29) belonged to the intermediate group at 2 years of corrected age: One third (8 of 24) of the intermediate group developed normal neurological status by the later examinations, whereas two thirds (16 of 24) showed consolidation of the initial signs into the neurocranial triad. These preliminary data suggest either late emergence or late detection of minor neurological signs. Nevertheless, they show stability of the neurological status in a majority of children.

Training

Training pediatricians and other professionals to perform the assessment is much easier today because of our better understanding of the underlying neurophysiology. The availability of pictures, drawings, and videotapes facilitates the transmission of manual skills (Amiel-Tison & Gosselin, 2001; Amiel-Tison & Grenier, 1986; Amiel-Tison & Lafaurie-Levêque, 2001). A master–apprentice situation is the most efficient method of training. Our recent experience in the transmission of this method as part of a regional program to evaluate perinatal care seems to support the feasibility of extending the use of the instrument to primary care setting (Rozé et al., 2004).

CORRELATIONS WITH LONG-TERM OUTCOME

Over the last decade, a prospective study was initiated to validate the neurological status defined on the five-level scale among a population of children at risk for hypoxic-ischemic insult as a result of uteroplacental insufficiency.

Developmental performance at preschool age (Gosselin et al., 2002) and intellectual performance at school age (Couture, 2005; Gosselin & Amiel-Tison, 2004) were analyzed according to neurological status. We noted that no child with disabling CP was found in this cohort of 72 children. Signs compatible with nondisabling CP were found in 8 children (11%), and the neurocranial triad was detected in 15 children (21%). The signs were intermediate in 20 children (28%). Finally, normal neurological status was found in 29 children (40%). The observed progressive increase in the number of children in each group, from CP to normal, supports the concept of a lesional continuum across the categories.

At preschool age (mean age = 3.7 ± 1.2 years), Griffiths Mental Development Scales (Griffiths, 1996) scores in all six domains showed an inverse association with the severity of neurocranial signs. The differences were statistically significant ($p < .05$) with a negative gradient related to the severity of the neurological status in three of the six domains assessed: coordination, language, and reasoning. There was also an interesting and statistically significant association between laterality of the abnormal stretch reflex and the language and reasoning scores. For the language scores, the performance of the children with a right stretch reflex was significantly lower than the scores of those with a left stretch reflex or a normal neurological examination. The performance of the children with bilateral stretch reflexes was the lowest, clearly different from the other three groups, with a mean of 87 ($p < .05$).

At school age (mean 6.6 years), 50 of the 72 children were tested for intelligence quotient (IQ) with the Wechsler Intelligence Scale for Children, Third Edition (WISC-III; Wechsler, 1991). The results from the neurological assessment completed at 2 years of age were used to categorize the children. Significant differences were found between groups for Verbal IQ score ($p < .001$), Full Scale IQ score ($p = .012$), and Verbal Comprehension Index ($p = .001$), clearly demonstrating the relationship between early specific neurocranial signs and higher functions, especially verbal skills.

Another study of 81 preschool children (46 boys, 35 girls; mean age 4.6 years) with language impairment was recently completed. A battery of standardized tests, including the neurological assessment, was administered. Only 32 of 81 children (39.5%) were considered to be without any neurological findings. Among the 49 children with abnormal neurological status, 26 (32.1%) showed isolated signs (mostly hypotonia and asymmetry), 8 (9.9%) showed the neurocranial triad, and 15 (18.5%) had signs compatible with nondisabling CP (Beausoleil, 2004). These preliminary results support the use of the neurological assessment to provide etiological clues in a cohort of children presenting with language impairment.

COMMON PITFALLS IN APPLICATION

An overview of the recent literature reveals that neurological assessment of any kind is rarely used in high-risk newborn follow-up studies. Why is this so? The impression that this examination is excessively sophisticated and therefore excessively burdensome may be a possible explanation; however, an underlying lack of understanding of the pathophysiology could be the real reason for avoiding the integration of the neurological assessment into systematic follow-up programs. This renunciation of the neurological examination is reflected in a shift toward the use of functional outcome measures instead. This trend may lead to an accessory role for the pediatrician, who becomes a coordinator rather than contributing directly to the evaluation of the child. Being conscious of the challenge involved in the use of a standardized neurological assessment, it seems important to review the most common pitfalls that occur in practice. They can be summarized into three categories.

1. *Temptation to simplify the method by using a short version or a few items from different assessments.* This practice can be compared with a psychologist selecting several items from a few different standardized developmental tests to assess developmental performance and compute a developmental quotient. Although this would be unacceptable for developmental testing, it is

often done for neurological testing. In the worst-case scenario, no method is delineated and instead a vague description of the neurological examination, such as "a physical assessment was performed by an experienced neurologist or neonatologist," is given. In most cases, these approaches have not been submitted to the type of validation process that underlies standardized assessments. Validation is indispensable to guarantee the quality of the data and the subsequent inferences.

2. *Temptation to dichotomize the results into normal and abnormal or to compute a total score on a continuous scale to facilitate presentation of follow-up outcome.* When the neurological status is dichotomous, abnormal status usually refers to severe sequelae (CP, intellectual disabilities, epilepsy, neurosensory impairments) and the children with more moderate or mild neurological impairment are classified as normal. Such a dichotomy constitutes a real deprivation by ignoring the whole spectrum of neurological impairments. Conversely, the use of a total score may be hazardous as well. Appealing because of its application to statistical analyses, such a score could also lead to the loss of relevant information concerning specific findings or clusters of signs. As recommended by Rapin (1996), these scores should always be complemented by personal clinical impressions; however, qualitative impressions remain difficult to use for statistical inferences.

3. *Temptation to make premature diagnoses before 2 years of corrected age.* In a clinical context, the pressure comes mainly from the need to allocate limited intervention resources for more severe cases. In a research context, the pressure for premature diagnoses is often linked to grant duration and the need to publish; however, such a practice leads to two opposing misconceptions about long-term outcome. The first misconception is that children can "outgrow" CP between 1 and 7 years of age (Nelson & Ellenberg, 1982), giving the fallacious impression of improvement. The second misconception is that children can be con-

sidered within normal limits at 12 months and considered to have cognitive impairments at 30 months (Miller et al., 2002), giving the fallacious impression of deterioration. The apparent instability in the outcome of these children can be avoided by waiting until 2 years of corrected age to categorize the outcome on a neurological basis. Based on categorization at 2 years, it becomes possible to identify the risk group for later cognitive disabilities. From this perspective, the age of 2 years constitutes the minimal age before which any type of short-term conclusion is hazardous.

CONCLUSION

In the field of developmental neurology, no assessment is perfect; each method results from a compromise between excessive simplification and excessive sophistication, in order to fulfill the needs of both clinicians and researchers (Hadders-Algra, 2005). As usual, the extremes are easy to define: absence of neurological and cranial findings or else a severe pathological condition, with general agreement on their definitions. Between the normal and the severely abnormal situations, mild and moderate findings should be identified because most of these children will later experience various types of dysfunction that could have been anticipated.

For the time being, application in this field is clearly insufficient for several reasons, already well stated by Alfred Strauss more than 50 years ago (Strauss & Lehtinen, 1947; as cited in Accardo, 1997). Strauss mentioned three types of difficulties in detecting minor brain damage in young children: 1) lack of knowledge of developmental neurology, 2) incomplete developmental history of the child, and 3) lack of short neurological screening tools. The first two points are remediable if pediatricians receive comprehensive training in normal development and perinatal neurology. We have tried to remediate point 3 by providing pediatricians with a short, easy-to-handle neurological assessment. Accurately identifying minor brain damage as early as possible could undoubtedly be beneficial to the children and their families. Developing standards of care that reflect this knowledge could result in largely improved "best practices."

REFERENCES

Accardo, P. (1997). The "expanded" Strauss syndrome. In P.J. Accardo, B.K. Shapiro, & A.J. Caputo (Eds.), *Behavior belongs in the brain* (pp. 3–16). Timonium, MD: York Press.

Amiel-Tison, C. (1969). Cerebral damage in full-term newborn: Aetiological factors, neonatal status and long term follow-up. *Biologia Neonatorum, 14,* 234–250.

Amiel-Tison, C. (1975). Neurologic evaluation of the small neonate: The importance of head straightening. In L. Gluck (Ed.), *Modern perinatal medicine* (pp. 347–357). Chicago: Year Book Medical Publishers.

Amiel-Tison, C. (1976). A method for neurologic evaluation within the first year of life. *Current Problems in Pediatrics, 7,* 1–50.

Amiel-Tison, C. (1985). Pediatric contribution to the present knowledge on the neurobehavioral status of infant at birth. In J. Mehler & R. Fox (Eds.), *Neonate cognition, beyond the blooming buzzing confusion* (pp. 365–380). Mahwah, NJ: Lawrence Erlbaum Associates.

Amiel-Tison, C. (2002). Update of the Amiel-Tison Neurologic Assessment for the Term Neonate or at 40 weeks corrected age. *Pediatric Neurology, 27,* 196–212.

Amiel-Tison, C., & Gosselin, J. (2001). *Neurological development from birth to 6 years.* Baltimore: The Johns Hopkins University Press.

Amiel-Tison, C., Gosselin, J., & Infante-Rivard, C. (2002). Head growth and cranial assessment as part of the neurological examination in infancy. *Developmental Medicine and Child Neurology, 44,* 643–648.

Amiel-Tison, C., & Grenier, A. (1986). *Neurologic assessment within the first year of life.* New York: Oxford University Press.

Amiel-Tison, C., Korobkin, R., & Esque-Vaucouloux, M. (1977). Neck extensor hypertonia: A clinical sign of insult to the central nervous system of the newborn. *Early Human Development, 1,* 181–190.

Amiel-Tison, C., & Lafaurie-Levêque, M. (2001). *Examen neurologique du nouveau-né à terme.* Paris: AP-HP Secteur Audiovisuel.

Amiel-Tison, C., Njiokiktjien, C., Vaivre-Douret, L., Verschoor, C.A., Chavanne, E., & Garel, M. (1996). Relation of early neuromotor and cranial signs with neuropsychological outcome at 4 years. *Brain and Development, 18,* 280–286.

Amiel-Tison, C., & Stewart, A. (1989). Follow-up studies during the first five years of life: A pervasive assessment of neurological function. *Archives of Disease in Childhood, 64,* 496–502.

Amiel-Tison, C., & Stewart, A. (1994). Apparently normal survivors: Neuromotor and cognitive function as they grow older. In C. Amiel-Tison & A. Stewart (Eds.), *The newborn infant: One brain for life* (pp. 227–237). Paris: Editions INSERM.

Bartholomeusz, H.H., Courchesne, E., & Karns, C.M. (2002). Relationship between head circumference and brain volume in healthy normal toddlers, children and adults. *Neuropediatrics, 33,* 239–241.

Beausoleil, P.A. (2004). *Profil de développement neuropsychique chez des enfants d'âge préscolaire présentant des difficultés langagières: Mémoire de maîtrise.* Montreal: Université de Montréal.

Couture, M. (2005). *Signes neurologiques mineurs et persistants et rendement cognitif à l'âge scolaire chez des enfants à risque de difficultés d'apprentissage.* Doctoral thesis, Université de Montréal, Montreal, Quebec, Canada.

Deschênes, G., Gosselin, J., Couture, M., & Lachance, C. (2004). Interobserver reliability of the Amiel-Tison Neurological Assessment at Term. *Pediatric Neurology, 30,* 190–194.

Garcia-Cazoria, A., Sans, A., Baquero, M., Garcia-Bargo, M.D., Arellano, M., Poo, P., et al. (2004). White matter alterations associated with chromosomal disorders. *Developmental Medicine and Child Neurology, 46,* 148–153.

Gosselin, J., & Amiel-Tison, C. (2004). Évaluation de la fonction neuromotrice de la naissance à 6 ans: Catégorisation à 2 ans d'âge corrigé; corrélation avec le QI à 6 ans. In *Progrès en néonatalogie* (pp. 15–28). Paris: Société Française de Néonatalogie.

Gosselin, J., & Amiel-Tison, C. (2007). *Évaluation neurologique de la naissance á 6 ans.* Montréal, Canada: Éditions du CHU Ste-Justine.

Gosselin, J., Amiel-Tison, C., Infante-Rivard, C., Fouron, C., & Fouron, J.C. (2002). Minor neurological signs and developmental performance in high risk children at preschool age. *Developmental Medicine and Child Neurology, 44,* 323–328.

Gosselin J., Fouron, J.C., & Amiel-Tison, C. (2006). Uteroplacental insufficiency and neurodevelopmental outcome. *Neoreviews, 7*(4), e202–e207.

Gosselin, J., Gahagan, S., & Amiel-Tison, C. (2005). The Amiel-Tison Neurological Assessment at Term: Conceptual and methodological continuity in the course of follow-ups. *Mental Retardation and Developmental Disabilities Research Reviews, 11,* 34–51.

Griffiths, R. (1996). *Griffiths Mental Development Scales: 1996 revision (revised by M. Huntley).* Henley-on-Thames, England: The Test Agency

Hadders-Algra, M. (2005). The neuromotor examination of the preschool child and its prognostic significance. *Mental Retardation and Developmental Disabilities Research Reviews, 11,* 180–188.

McCarraher-Wetzel, A.P., & Wetzel, R.C. (1984). A review of the Amiel-Tison neurologic evaluation of the newborn and infant. *American Journal of Occupational Therapy, 38,* 585–593.

Miller, S.P., Newton, N., Ferriero, D.M., Partridge, J.C., Glidden, D.V., Barnwell, A., et al. (2002). Predictors of 30-month outcome after perinatal depression: Role of proton MRS and socioeconomic factors. *Pediatric Research, 52*, 71–77.

Nelson, K.B., & Ellenberg, J.H. (1982). Children who "outgrew" cerebral palsy. *Pediatrics, 69*, 529–536.

Pinto-Martin, J.A., Riolo, S., Cnaan, A., Holzman, C., Susser, M.W., & Paneth, N. (1995). Cranial ultrasound prediction of disabling and nondisabling cerebral palsy at age two in a low birth weight population. *Pediatrics, 95*, 249–254.

Rapin, I. (1996). Neurological examination. In I. Rapin (Ed.), *Preschool children with inadequate communication* (Clinics in Developmental Medicine, No. 139, pp. 98–122). London: MacKeith Press.

Rozé, J.C., N'Guyen, S., Bureau-Rouger, V., Beucher, A., Gosselin, J., & Amiel-Tison, C. (2004). Follow-up network for newborns with a handicap risk: Experience of the Pays-de-la-Loire network. *Journal de Gynécologie Obstétrique et Biologie de Reproduction, 33*(1 Suppl), S54–S60.

Saint-Anne Dargassies, S. (1977). *Neurological development in the full-term and premature neonate.* Amsterdam: Excerpta Medica.

Sarnat, H.B. (1984). Anatomic and physiologic correlates of neurological development in prematurity. In H.B. Sarnat (Ed.), *Topics in neonatal neurology* (pp. 1–25). Orlando, FL: Grune & Stratton.

Stambak, M., & de Ajuriaguerra, J. (1958). Évolution de l'extensibilité musculaire depuis la naissance jusqu'à l'âge de 2 ans. *Presse Médicale, 66*, 24–36.

Thomas, A., & de Ajuriaguerra, J. (1949). *Étude sémiologique du tonus musculaire.* Paris: Éditions Médicales Flammarion.

Wechsler, D. (1991). *Wechsler Intelligence Scale for Children, Third Edition (WISC-III).* San Antonio, TX: Psychological Corp.

17

The Neonatal
Neurodevelopmental Examination

MARILEE C. ALLEN

For many years, there was little interest in neonatal neurodevelopmental examinations because of the prevailing opinion that newborns, with their immature, dormant central nervous systems (CNSs), had no voluntary movements or meaningful responses. Although excellent pathological studies described the structural development of the human CNS, there was little interest in describing its functional development. Assessment of a child's functional abilities entailed tracking developmental milestones through infancy into childhood (Illingworth, 1972).

The first real interest in neonatal development was sparked by a fascination with the more primitive aspects of CNS function (i.e., reflexes), but subsequent work resulted from recognizing the impact of muscle tone on movement and posture and the neonate's active participation in parent–infant interactions. Neonates are exquisitely sensitive to tactile, olfactory, and kinesthetic cues; their responses elicit important parental caregiving behaviors, including cuddling, warming, and breast feeding. Their hearing is excellent, and they see faces best when held in the crook of a parent's arm. Their facial expressions provide important feedback to parents. Most important, their eager responses to positive human interactions promote bonding with parents and caregivers.

The newborn infant is therefore *not* passive, but an active, vigorous, responsive person with a rapidly maturing CNS that is vulnerable to a variety of environmental and perinatal insults. Birth is a traumatic process that abruptly severs the placental supply of nutrients and ox-

ygen and requires that complex physiological systems be fully functional for maintaining extrauterine life. Infants born preterm rely on immature organ systems that are not yet fully functional. Growth and development of all the organ systems, especially the CNS, requires uninterrupted supplies of nutrients and oxygen. The fact that fetal development, birth, and neonatal development generally proceed as normally as they do is nothing short of miraculous. It is not surprising that neurodevelopmental disabilities arise from malformations of and injury to the developing CNS.

Neuromaturation is the functional development of the CNS, a dynamic process resulting from continuous interactions between the genome and the environment (first the intrauterine environment, then the extrauterine environment). The neonatal neurodevelopmental examination is a window onto the neuromaturation of an individual neonate at one point in time. Understanding the dynamic nature of neuromaturation and how examination findings typically change over time is essential for identifying deviations from the norm. Discerning their *significance* is more difficult. Many factors influence examination findings, including environmental conditions and stimuli; the infant's state of alertness; his or her metabolic, fluid, and electrolyte status; malformation or abnormal development of part or all of the CNS; and injuries to the CNS during fetal, perinatal, and neonatal life. A single examination of a stable awake infant at term yields a great deal of information. Multiple serial examinations enhance assessment of neuromaturation and interpretation of examination findings.

At present, neither neonatal neurodevelopmental assessments nor neuroimaging studies of brain structure can predict with certainty the impact of an injured or malformed CNS on a child's functional abilities, or how the CNS will remodel over time. They can be used, separately or together, not for diagnosis but to identify high-risk infants most likely to benefit from comprehensive neurodevelopmental followup and early intervention services, especially when these resources are limited. Normal neonatal functional assessments and neuroimaging studies are very reassuring. Current technology cannot predict how an individual child will function in the future on a variety of complex tasks.

This chapter provides a historical perspective of clinical neurodevelopmental assessments, an appreciation of factors that influence the neonate's examination and responses, descriptions of components of a comprehensive neonatal neurodevelopmental examination, discussions of abnormal examination findings and their significance, and suggestions for using neonatal functional assessments.

HISTORY OF NEONATAL ASSESSMENT

Early in the 20th century, an interest in examining newborns was sparked by the recognition that many of the reflexes described in experiments on adult decorticate animals are easily elicited in normal newborns. Full-term neonates have many pathological reflexes (e.g., Babinski's reflex) and primitive reflexes that influence posture and movement (e.g., Moro reflex). Peiper (1963) catalogued many of the reflexes and autonomic, sensory, and physiological reactions observed in infants and children. Many of the primitive reflexes elicited in healthy full-term infants persist in neonates with CNS injury and can be an early indicator of cerebral palsy (Paine, 1960, 1964; Paine et al., 1964; Stern, 1971). Capute and colleagues quantified strength and completeness of a number of primitive reflexes (Grades 0–4, and described their suppression with higher cortical control during the first year in typically developing full-term infants (Capute, 1979; Capute et al., 1982, 1984). This grading system was subsequently used to describe the emergence

of selected primitive reflexes prior to term in preterm infants in a neonatal intensive care unit (NICU) (Allen & Capute, 1986b, 1990).

Several authors have detailed typical findings on neonatal neurological examination (Illingworth, 1972; Paine, 1960; Prechtl, 1977; Saint-Anne Dargassies, 1977). Full-term neonates have brisk deep tendon reflexes and an increased reflexogenic zone, as well as many pathological and primitive reflexes. Unsustained clonus can frequently be elicited, especially at the ankles. When teaching, Capute frequently stated, "all newborns are born with cerebral palsy; it is just that most outgrow it" to emphasize that full-term newborns demonstrate many examination findings indicative of brain injury in older children and adults. Hyperreflexia and the pathological and primitive reflexes are suppressed with evolution of higher cortical function during the first year, as voluntary movement emerges.

Muscle tone (i.e., the tightness or looseness of muscles, as controlled by the brain) has always been difficult to precisely describe. Adult neurologist André-Thomas capped a distinguished career by focusing on newborns; he distinguished passive from active muscle tone and devised methods for describing tone (André-Thomas, Chesni, & Saint-Anne Dargassies, 1960). Passive tone reflects the extensibility of the muscles, and active tone is observed with active movement (e.g., when pulling an infant from supine to a supported sitting position). Saint-Anne Dargassies and Amiel-Tison furthered this work by describing typical and atypical development of passive and active tone in full-term neonates, asphyxiated infants, and preterm infants as they approach term (Amiel-Tison, 1968, 1974, 2003; Amiel-Tison & Grenier, 1986; Amiel-Tison, Maillard, Lebrun, Breart, & Papiernik, 1999; Paine, 1960; Saint-Anne Dargassies, 1977).

Strong upper and lower extremity flexor tone is characteristic of full-term neonates. This degree of flexor hypertonia is abnormal at any other time of life. As they approach term, initially hypotonic extremely preterm infants develop flexor tone in a caudocephalad manner, first in their lower extremities, then in their upper extremities (Allen & Capute, 1990; Amiel-Tison, 2002; Saint-Anne Dargassies,

1977). Development of tone and reflexes proceeds in an orderly manner according to postmenstrual age (PMA; the infant's gestational age at birth plus chronological age at the time of the examination). For the most part, examination findings are similar in preterm infants examined at a given PMA, whether they were just born or were born much earlier.

Amiel-Tison contributed to this work by adding descriptions of active tone through the axis of the body (i.e., neck and trunk) (Amiel-Tison, 1974, 2002, 2003; Amiel-Tison & Grenier, 1986; Amiel-Tison, Korobkin, & Esque-Vaucouloux, 1977; Amiel-Tison et al., 1999). She described methods of assessing active neck extensor and flexor tone, and identified neck extensor hypertonia as a clinical sign of CNS injury or increased intracranial pressure. She described neurological examinations through infancy and early childhood, and developed a simplified examination (the Neurological Examination, and a later version known as the Neurologic Assessment at Term) for routine use by health care providers to follow development from term to 6 years (Amiel-Tison & Gosselin, 2001; Gosselin, Gahagan, & Amiel-Tison, 2005). It takes only 5–10 minutes to perform and focuses on patterns of development, not on scores.

Amiel-Tison also demonstrated how the evolution of neurodevelopmental examination findings reflects anatomical and physiological development of CNS in the fetus and neonate (Amiel-Tison, 2002; Sarnat, 1984, 1989). The lower subcortical pathway maintains posture against gravity and limb flexion. It originates in the brain stem (reticular formation, vestibular nuclei, and tectum), and connects to the thalamus and cerebellum. Its development from 24 to 32 weeks' gestation or PMA is reflected in the emergence of reflexes and muscle tone. Higher corticospinal pathways originate in the motor and premotor cortex of the cerebral hemispheres, connect to the basal ganglia, cross at the medulla, and descend laterally in the spinal cord. Myelination of the corticospinal tract begins at 32 weeks' gestation or PMA, proceeding from the pons upward to the cortex and downward through the spinal cord. Its maturation is reflected in the neonate's gradual improvement in head control and axial tone. The corticospinal system suppresses the subcortical system; enables erect posture, walking, and fine motor control; and does not completely develop until adolescence.

The Dubowitz Neurological Examination of the Full-Term Newborn was developed over 20 years as a practical, easy-to-learn examination for health care providers to incorporate into their routine clinical assessments of preterm and full-term infants, even during the first few days after birth (Dubowitz & Dubowitz, 1981; Dubowitz, Dubowitz, & Mercuri, 1999; Dubowitz, Mercuri, & Dubowitz, 1998; Dubowitz, Ricciw, & Mercuri, 2005). The revised examination takes 10–15 minutes to perform and includes 34 items subdivided into six categories (tone, tone patterns, reflexes, movements, abnormal signs, and behavior). It was standardized in 224 low-risk full-term neonates. Interrater reliability is above 96%. Although patterns of performance are the clinical focus of the examination, researchers have derived an optimality score that was standardized on full-term infants.

Brazelton designed a Newborn Behavioral Assessment Scale (NBAS) for describing a newborn's behavioral repertoire as he or she adapts to the extrauterine environment, thereby demonstrating his or her competencies and responsiveness to parents (Brazelton, 1973; Brazelton & Nugent, 1995). The NBAS requires attention to the infant's organized behavioral states of alertness during the examination. It is also used to compare infants from different cultures or racial/ethnic groups, and it was revised to enhance its usefulness for high-risk infants. It requires specific training, certification, and recertification every 3 years.

The Assessment of Preterm Infants' Behavior (APIB) is "based in ethological-evolutionary thought and focuses on the assessment of mutually interacting behavioral subsystems in simultaneous interaction with the environment" (Als, Butler, Kosta, & McAnulty, 2005, p. 94). The examiner presents a specified sequence of sensory challenges to preterm or full-term infants (from birth to 1 month after term) and carefully observes infant responses and competence. Infant competence is defined as "the degree of differentiation of subsystem function and degree of modulation of subsystem balance at any stage in infant development" (Als et al., 2005, p. 94). A skilled examiner may take an hour to perform the examination and another 30–45 minutes to score it. It requires extensive training. Interrater reliability and concurrent and construct validity have been established. There are specifications for timing of the examination, the room, and how the examiner should be dressed. The APIB is primarily used to guide developmental support strategies as part of the Neonatal Individualized Developmental Care and Assessment Program (NIDCAP) (Als, 1998; Als, Duffy, & McAnulty, 1996; Als & Gilkerson, 1997).

The Einstein Neonatal Neurobehavioral Assessment Scale (ENNAS) was developed at Albert Einstein University to evaluate the neurobehavioral organization of full-term infants (Kurtzberg et al., 1979; Majnemer & Snider, 2005). It assesses tone, primitive reflexes, orientation to sensory stimuli, and behavioral state organization. Examiners require some expertise in neonatal assessment. The ENNAS takes 20–30 minutes to administer and correlates highly with formal neurological examinations (kappa = 0.94, 97% agreement). Good interrater reliability ($r = .97$) has been established.

Korner developed the Neurobehavioral Assessment of the Preterm Infant (NAPI) to measure the progression of neurobehavioral performance in preterm infants from 32 weeks' to 40 weeks' PMA (Hyman, Snider, Majnemer, & Mazer, 2005; Korner, Constantinou, Dimiceli, Brown, & Thom, 1991; Korner et al., 1987; Majnemer & Snider, 2005; Snider et al., 2005). It evaluates developmental change in seven neurobehavioral domains: motor development/vigor, scarf sign, popliteal angle, alertness/orientation, irritability, percent asleep, and cry quality. Test–retest reliability and interrater reliability have been established. It has been validated against an index of medical complications and measures of neonatal physiology.

The Test of Infant Motor Performance (TIMP) was developed to evaluate motor control and organization of posture and movement for functional activities in preterm and full-term infants (Campbell & Hedeker, 2001;

Campbell, Kolobe, Osten, Lenke, & Girolami, 1995; Campbell, Wright, & Linacre, 2002). It can be used in preterm infants at 32 weeks' PMA and extends to 4 months after term. Functional activities include the way the infant interacts, communicates needs, and explores and adapts to the environment. The examiner carefully observes 27 spontaneous behaviors and elicits infant responses on 25 items. Test–retest, intrarater, and interrater reliability have been established.

The National Institute of Child Health and Human Development NICU Network Neurobehavioral Scale (NNNS) was developed to measure neurological integrity, behavioral function, and processes of behavioral organization influenced by risk factors (Boukydis, Bigsby, & Lester, 2004; Lester & Tronick, 2004; Lester, Tronick, & Brazelton, 2004; Salisbury, Fallone, & Lester, 2005). The NNNS has three parts: 1) neurological assessment of tone and primitive reflexes; 2) behavioral assessment of state, sensory, and interactive responses; and 3) items that measure stress and document withdrawal from narcotics. It takes 30 minutes to administer and 15 minutes to score. Examiners must complete a training program. Its primary use to date has been in a large multicenter study to measure effects of intrauterine drugs on child outcomes (Lester, Tronick, LaGasse, et al., 2004).

Prechtl's Assessment of General Movements is a new approach that assesses spontaneous infant movements (Einspieler & Prechtl, 2005; Einspieler, Prechtl, Bos, Ferrari, & Cioni, 2004; Einspieler, Prechtl, Ferrari, Cioni, & Bos, 1997; Prechtl, 1997). It involves videotaping spontaneous movements of awake, quiet infants, followed by careful analysis of the type and quality of the infant's movements. Trained examiners evaluate videotapes based on global visual Gestalt perception. Interrater agreement ranges from 89% to 93%, and kappa is 0.88. Specific recommendations regarding analysis of videotapes address examiner fatigue. Results on the Assessment of General Movements correlate highly with neurological examination results.

The type and quality of infant movements reflect the development of higher cortical control over central pattern generator networks in the brain stem and spinal cord (Einspieler & Prechtl, 2005). Injury to the corticospinal tract results in movements that are less complex, variable, and fluid and more monotonous, rigid, abrupt, and chaotic. Persistence of cramped-synchronized movements and absence of fidgety movements by 9–20 weeks from term are associated with CNS injury. Cramped-synchronized movements are rigid contractions of limb and trunk muscles. Fidgety movements, characterized by small-amplitude, moderate-speed movements of the neck, trunk, and limbs in all directions and with variable acceleration, typically emerge at 6–9 weeks after term.

Many examiners use abnormal, high-pitched infant cries and difficulty with sucking as clinical indicators of CNS injury despite a lack of reliable, valid, easy-to-use, precise clinical measures (Lagasse, Neal, & Lester, 2005; Rogers & Arvedson, 2005). Computer analysis of a recording of an infant's cry can generate a digital spectrogram or calculations of cry characteristics. Although eliciting the cry by applying a standardized pain stimulus requires little training, analyzing cry characteristics and interpreting the data require expertise and are quite time consuming. Current cry measures are limited by poor specificity. Despite a paucity of reliable, standardized clinical measures of sucking, much progress has been made in technological analyses of a neonate's ability to suck and swallow. These include manometric analyses, videofluoroscopy, ultrasonography, flexible endoscopy, and respiratory measures during feedings.

Maturity and age are not synonymous: Just as children can be more or less mature for their ages, there is also normal individual variation in maturity at each week of gestation. In addition to genetic variability, neuromaturation is influenced by first the intrauterine, then the extrauterine environment. A number of examinations' items have been used to assess gestational age and maturity, so my colleagues and I combined many tone, reflex, and behavior items into a Maturity Score as a method of following neuromaturation in individual preterm infants prior to term (Allen, 2005; Allen & Capute, 1986a, 1986b, 1990; Allen & Donohue, 2005; Amiel-Tison, 1968,

2002, 2003; Amiel-Tison et al., 1999). In a sample of low-risk, extremely preterm infants in an NICU, Maturity Scores demonstrate individual variability but nonetheless increase linearly with gestational/postmenstrual age. These and other measures of neuromaturation can be used to follow early development. Research studies of these and other measures of neuromaturation have the potential to provide insight into causes of CNS injury, mechanisms for recovery, and effects of neuroprotective factors (Institute of Medicine, 2006).

Since the 1970s, many methods have been developed for assessing CNS function in preterm and full-term neonates. Some methods require little training, whereas others require attending workshops or training sessions that are even more extensive. Some can be performed in 5 minutes or less, and some require an hour or more. Some have no or few specifications for how, where, and when the examination should be performed, whereas others have multiple specific requirements. Clinicians and researchers need to decide what questions they are asking when examining the neonate, in order to select the appropriate method and the most important aspects of the examination.

FACTORS INFLUENCING THE NEONATAL NEURODEVELOPMENTAL EXAMINATION

Infant responses during an examination are influenced not only by degree of neuromaturation and CNS integrity, but also by the infant's medical status and internal regulatory systems and the environment. Interpretation of the significance of examination findings requires attention to all contributing factors.

Infant's Medical Status

An infant's medical condition can have a profound influence on tone, reflexes, and sensory responses. Infants acutely ill with respiratory distress, hypotension, necrotizing enterocolitis, and/or sepsis are generally markedly hypotonic, weak, and less responsive. During recovery from acute illness, the infant may continue to demonstrate hypotonia and weakness. Exercise intolerance—manifest by exhaustion and increased work of breathing with handling and feeding—is a frequent finding in infants recovering from acute illness (especially respiratory illness). The exercise intolerance, weakness, and hypotonia of infants with chronic lung disease/bronchopulmonary dysplasia (CLD/BPD) often improve as their lung disease improves. Nevertheless, many children with CLD/BPD have residual hypotonia, with motor delay consistent with either cerebral palsy or minor neuromotor dysfunction.

The infant's level of alertness, tone, and reflexes can be profoundly influenced by metabolic, fluid, and electrolyte disturbances. These include hypoglycemia, hypocalcemia, hypercalcemia, hyponatremia, hypernatremia, hyperkalemia, hypermagnesemia, and hyperammonemia. Hyperbilirubinemia may contribute to lethargy. Even if they have no specific vitamin or mineral deficiencies, infants with poor nutrition may be weak and hypotonic. Occasionally, undernourished infants demonstrate hypertonia with increased extensor tone, which improves as their nutritional status improves. Episodes of neck extensor hypertonia and arching of the trunk are not unusual in infants with acute or severe gastrointestinal reflux.

Anything that causes CNS irritability, including drug withdrawal, increased intracranial pressure (i.e. from cerebral edema or hydrocephalus), or meningeal irritation, can cause extensor hypertonia, hyperreflexia, jitteriness, and seizures. Some infants with chronic severe hydrocephalus are profoundly weak and hypotonic, poorly responsive, and unable to nipple feed. These findings can dramatically improve when intracranial pressure is reduced.

Medications can also influence neurological findings. Phenobarbital (Luminal), sedatives, and narcotics generally make an infant more sleepy and lethargic, with lower tone and responsiveness. Hypomagnesemia, often from antenatal magnesium sulfate (Epsom Salt) used to treat tocolysis or preeclampsia, makes an infant lethargic, hypotonic, and hyporeflexic. Caffeine or theophylline (e.g., Theo-Dur) toxicity is manifested by jitteriness, irritability, hyperreflexia, and even seizures. The β-adrenergic stimulators (e.g., albuterol [e.g.,

Proventil]), used to treat reactive airways in infants with CLD/BPD, can cause jitteriness, tremors, and hyperreflexia.

Infants withdrawing from in utero exposure or NICU treatment with narcotics can have abnormalities on examination. The well-described syndrome of withdrawal from heroin and methadone is characterized by marked jitteriness, irritability, hypertonia, poor feeding, poor weight gain, and diarrhea. These symptoms can persist for 4–6 months, and may last longer with intrauterine exposure to methadone. Withdrawal from cocaine may cause irritability, jitteriness, and marked hypertonia.

Infant's Internal Regulatory Systems

An essential component of any neonatal examination is assessment of an infant's behavior, arousal, and ability to regulate states and transition from state to state during the course of the examination. Infants' states of alertness include deep sleep, light sleep, drowsiness, quiet alertness, fussiness, and vigorous crying. The infant's degree of arousal and ability to regulate states of alertness are not only important aspects of CNS function but must be taken into account when evaluating the significance of examination findings. This is difficult to teach. The ability to interpret examination findings in light of the infant's state of alertness requires experience with multiple examinations of typical neonates, as well as infants with abnormal neurodevelopmental examinations.

The infant's state of alertness should be noted at the beginning, during the course, and at the end of a comprehensive neurodevelopmental examination. Full-term neonates and preterm infants at term demonstrate well-organized patterns of quiet and active sleep, wakefulness, and crying that cycle over time. Individual infants vary in amount of time spent crying or awake. Immediately after birth, the typical full-term neonate tends to be in a quiet alert state, which promotes bonding, but subsequently he or she spends much of the time sleeping.

Like us all, infants who are sleeping are generally more hypotonic than at other times. Deep tendon, pathological, and primitive reflexes are generally easier to elicit during sleep or drowsy states, primarily because the underlying muscle tone is lower and there is less interference with movement. Stretching on awakening should not be interpreted as extremity extensor tone (unless the extension persists throughout the examination).

Infants who are crying tend to be more hypertonic than they are at other times. Normal crying infants generally maintain tight flexor extremity tone with fisting. The crying infant may be more hyperreflexic than at other times, and crying may bring out jitteriness. There are some neonates who demonstrate neck extensor hypertonia, extremity extensor tone, or both with intense crying. This is less worrisome if it is only manifested with crying, with a return to flexion and a head-neutral position when consoled. Persistent neck extensor hypertonia or extremity extensor tone or both is an abnormal finding and is worrisome evidence of CNS dysfunction.

Infants who are markedly irritable or lethargic are also worrisome. Infants who go from sleeping to crying, but do not demonstrate a quiet alert state, are irritable. Every attempt should be made to console the infant, and how much intervention is required to console the infant should be noted. Infants who are sleeping or drowsy throughout the examination, with poor responses to arousal attempts, are lethargic. Both irritability and lethargy may signal CNS abnormality or may be due to medications, underlying medical conditions, or environmental circumstances.

Because evaluation of an infant's responsiveness to touch, sound, and visual stimuli is such an important aspect of the neonatal neurodevelopmental examination, it is important to recognize factors underlying responses. These include the infant's ability to perceive the stimulus, make some movement in response to it, self-regulate following it, and habituate to it. Perception can be appreciated by observation of movement in response to an auditory or visual stimulus. This should be recorded but should not replace essential evaluations independent of the neurodevelopmental examination (e.g., auditory brain stem responses, ophthalmological evaluation). Evidence of self-regulation following a stimulus varies from a change in state (e.g., from drowsy

to quiet alert, from quiet alert to crying) or movement without changing states to symptoms suggestive of stress (e.g., eye blinking, gaze aversion, yawn) or physiological instability (e.g., mottled skin, oxygen desaturation, bradycardia).

Habituation, which can be observed as early as 25–26 weeks' gestation, is a response reduction with repeated presentations of unvarying stimuli (Allen & Capute, 1986b). The ability of an infant to habituate to repeated stimuli and a preference for novel stimuli should be evaluated and will have implications for how an examination is performed. For example, if the examiner does not recognize all aspects of the Moro reflex when it is first elicited, it should not be repeated immediately, but should be elicited again during a subsequent portion of the examination.

Environmental Issues

Consideration should be given to the environment in which an infant is examined. The examiner should be relaxed and have room to place the infant in prone, supine, supported sitting, ventral suspension (holding the infant horizontally across one's hand), and vertical suspension (holding the infant upright). Many examination items can be administered while holding the infant on a parent's lap or one's own lap. The temperature of the room should be comfortable enough to remove the infant's clothes without concern for hypothermia, but not so warm as to engender discomfort or sleep. Brightly lit rooms discourage an infant from opening his or her eyes and should be avoided. There should be enough diffuse light to allow the examiner to recognize not only infant responses but also physiological changes (e.g., cyanosis, mottling of the skin).

The timing of the infant's examination with respect to feeding and sleep cycles can influence the examination. Hungry infants tend to be irritable and may be jittery. Infants tend to go to sleep at the end of feedings. At the end of a long period of being awake, a drowsy infant may be perceived as lethargic or an overstimulated, crying infant may seem to be irritable. Progressive attempts to arouse a sleeping infant should be made, starting with very gentle ones (e.g., light touch, talking).

NEONATAL NEURODEVELOPMENTAL EXAMINATION

The neonatal neurodevelopmental examination focuses on the development of muscle tone, reflexes, sensory responses, and behavior. Examinations typically begin with careful observation of the infant before any handling or sensory stimulation is introduced. Then, infant responses to a variety of examination maneuvers provide additional information about CNS function. All infants should be handled gently, avoiding sudden movements and carefully evaluating the infant's physiological stability, position, and ability to tolerate handling. Signs of physiological instability or significant distress are indications for delaying or deferring the examination. Although this chapter details many aspects of the neonatal examination, nothing can replace the experience gained by examining many infants.

General Physical Examination

Both review of the medical history and a general physical examination should be performed to evaluate the infant's medical condition, nutritional status, and presence of abnormalities or anomalies. In addition to ascertaining the presence of any acute or chronic illnesses, pertinent details of the infant's medical history include demographic, antenatal, perinatal, and neonatal risk factors (see Chapter 14, this volume). General physical examinations detect evidence of chronic lung or heart disease, physiological instability, poor growth, congenital anomalies, musculoskeletal defects, and increased intracranial pressure. Signs of respiratory distress include color changes (to grey, dusky, or blue), apnea, increased work of breathing (substernal, suprasternal, or intercostal retractions with labored breathing), and weakness. Dysmorphic features and congenital anomalies suggest genetic syndromes or chromosomal disorders. A narrow, high-arched palate suggests abnormal tongue movement during pregnancy, since tongue and oropha-

ryngeal movements help shape a fetus's palate. An infant may have tremulous tongue movements with crying, but fasciculations on the periphery of the tongue of a quiet infant raise concerns about neuromuscular disease (e.g., Werdnig-Hoffmann disease) or CNS injury.

The examiner should pay special attention to the skeletal system, noting any malformations, deformations, or contractures. Deformations occur in utero with oligohydramnios and multiple gestations and toward the end of pregnancy. The most common deformations are torticollis, plagiocephaly, and foot deformities. After birth, inattention to how very sick infants in a NICU are positioned may lead to acquired contractures. Prolonged positioning of a sick and/or hypotonic infant in prone or supine with hips widely abducted can lead to iliotibial band contractures (with resistance to hip adduction). Many infants demonstrate a preference to turn their head to one side, and if positioning them reinforces this head preference, they can develop plagiocephaly with ipsilateral asymmetrical flattening of the occiput or torticollis.

Standard growth parameters (i.e., weight, height, head circumference) are compared with published norms for an overall assessment of nutritional status. Skull size and shape reflect brain growth; therefore, it is important to measure the head, examine the skull, and palpate the cranial sutures. Head circumference should be measured several times and the maximum value recorded. If a caput succedaneum or cephalohematoma is present, the infant's head should be measured again after several days. Overlapping sutures initially after birth is an adaptation to labor and delivery, but if it persists beyond the first week, it suggests poor brain growth. If a bulging fontanel and widely split sutures are detected, a neuroimaging study is indicated to differentiate between increased intracranial pressure and rapid brain growth. Of all the cranial sutures (i.e., lambdoidal, coronal, sagittal, metopic, and squamous sutures), the squamous suture is especially sensitive and informative of increased intracranial pressure (Amiel-Tison, 2002; Gosselin et al., 2005). It is palpated just above the ears, at the junction of the parietal and temporal bones and the base of the cranium.

Assessment of Posture and Movement

Observing an infant's posture and movements provides a substantial amount of information about CNS function (Amiel-Tison, 2002; Prechtl, 1997; Saint-Anne Dargassies, 1977). The infant's movements and posture in prone, supine, and sidelying positions reflect an infant's underlying muscle tone, state of alertness (see previous discussion), and degree of higher cortical control of movement. An example of an abnormal neurological sign is a cortical thumb, which occurs when the fisted hand encloses the thumb because of inability to abduct the thumb.

The flexor hypertonia of full-term neonates is reflected in their tendency to return their limbs to flexion after movement. Although muscle tone is relaxed in sleep, the full-term infant generally maintains a flexed posture. When agitated, full-term infants often return to full flexion (less than a 90-degree popliteal angle) of their upper and lower extremities. Typical full-term infants have tight hip adduction, as well as flexion, with elevation of their buttocks in prone. In the supine position, a typical full-term infant's legs are generally flexed at the hip and knee, with the hips adducted so that the knees do not touch the bed.

A preterm or sick infant's posture reflects hypotonia. Although these infants often demonstrate some limb flexion (or semiflexion) at rest, return of their limbs to full flexion after movement is less likely and less brisk than in full-term infants. Even when hypotonic infants manifest some hip flexion, they are often frog-legged: hip adductor tone is insufficient to overcome gravity, and the knees touch the bed. Severely hypotonic or weak infants passively lie in whatever position they are placed, including limb extension.

Persistent extension of a neonate's extremities is abnormal, except in infants with prolonged breech posture in utero. Intermittent extension may be seen when an infant is stretching but is generally brief. Persistent posture with extremities extended should prompt a careful examination of tone, to distinguish between neonates with abnormal extensor hypertonia and hypotonic infants inadvertently positioned with limbs extended. Therefore, the infant who demonstrates extremity extension should be carefully examined several times to assess whether extremity extension is temporary or state related, or a persistent abnormality.

Full-term infants, when placed in the supine position, should have no space between the bed and the back of their neck (Amiel-Tison, 1974; Amiel-Tison et al., 1977). Preterm infants are frequently dolichocephalic (with long, narrow heads) and may have space between the bed and the back of their necks, but they should not have any space between the bed and their shoulders and upper back. Increased space between the bed and the neck or shoulders is an indicator of neck extensor hypertonia. Lying with the neck extended and head turned to the side is termed *retrocollis*, and extension or arching of the whole body is termed *opisthotonus*. Increased neck and trunk extensor tone makes lying flat in supine difficult or impossible, necessitating a lateral decubitus position. Neck and trunk extensor hypertonia is an abnormal neurological finding that is associated with an increased risk for cerebral palsy (Nelson & Ellenberg, 1979).

Spontaneous movements express neural activity and are important forces in fetal and neonatal development. Prechtl and colleagues have provided systematic descriptions of the complexity, variability, and coordination of spontaneous general movements of typically developing, awake preterm and full-term infants in no distress (Einspieler & Prechtl, 2005; Einspieler et al., 2004; Prechtl, 1997). General movements are complex, variable movements of the extremities, trunk, and neck that begin gradually and wax and wane in intensity, force, and speed. The movement patterns of preterm infants are similar to fetal patterns, but their movements are faster with larger amplitude (Cioni & Prechtl, 1990). With neuromaturation, infant movements become more fluent, complex, and elegant, with more rotations along the axis of the limbs and small changes in direction. The typical full-term neonate in a quiet alert state makes frequent smooth, symmetrical, variable movements with small to moderate amplitude and slow to moderate speed, as well as isolated complex finger movements. These movements stop briefly in response to external stimuli (e.g., alert to a novel sound). At 6–9 weeks from term, fidgety movements emerge as small-amplitude movements of the neck, trunk, and limbs with moderate speed and variable acceleration and in all directions.

Abnormal movements include persistent tremors; slow stereotyped movements; and repetitive limb flexion and extension, chewing, or in-and-out mouth movements. Many preterm infants, infants withdrawing from narcotics, and infants with brain injury are jittery (frequent small-amplitude movements of the extremities). Of all the major movement patterns, absence of fidgety movements at 9–20 weeks from term are most predictive of later cerebral palsy (Einspieler & Prechtl, 2005; Einspieler et al., 2002, 2004; Prechtl et al., 1997).

Persistently asymmetrical posture or movement should be noted. Asymmetrical facies suggest facial nerve palsy or a dysmorphic syndrome. A neonate with asymmetrical arm movement should be examined for evidence of a brachial plexus injury. Neonates may demonstrate a lateral head preference, preferring to turn their head to one side more than the other (to the right is more common), which may influence subsequent motor development (Konishi, Kuriyama, Mikawa, & Suzuki, 1987; Konishi, Mikawa, & Suzuki, 1986; Konishi et al., 1997). The asymmetrical tonic neck reflex (ATNR) is a primitive reflex that promotes an asymmetrical posture and is frequently strong in early infancy. With the ATNR, the limbs on the side of the infant's face extend and the limbs on the opposite side flex (i.e., fencing posture). Positioning preterm or sick NICU infants so that the caregiver always comes from one side probably contributes to the asymmetries frequently seen in preterm infants.

Muscle Tone

Individuals have underlying *muscle tone*, which is the tightness or looseness of muscles as controlled by the brain. Assessment of underlying muscle tone is a critical component of every physical examination because it provides a window onto CNS function. State of alertness, movement, emotion, illness, metabolic distur-

bances (hypocalcemia, hypomagnesemia), and medications (e.g., phenobarbital, narcotics) influence tone. Muscle tone is an important component of the ability to stay upright, move, and perform delicate tasks with one's hands. Individuals with spasticity demonstrate an imbalance of tone that interferes with motor function. Experience is required to recognize how muscle tone differs among individuals and how muscle tone within an individual changes over time and in different circumstances (e.g., sleep, changes in emotion). Hypotonia often accompanies medical illness (e.g., sepsis, respiratory distress syndrome), and it is often difficult to distinguish between hypotonia and weakness.

On examination, one evaluates an infant's muscle tone by observing his or her posture and movement (see previous discussion), feeling the resistance offered with passive movement, changing his or her position and observing subsequent movement (active tone), and evaluating how tone changes with changes in state. The examination maneuvers that André-Thomas devised to describe tone facilitate measuring and communicating an infant's muscle tone, and how his or her tone changes with different states and with serial examinations over time (André-Thomas et al., 1960).

Extremity Muscle Tone The strong flexor tone of the typical newborn, termed *flexor hypertonia* in recognition that it is abnormal at any other point in life, is an important adaptation for fetal growth in the crowded uterus. Flexor extremity tone is strongest immediately after birth, and the mechanical effects of intrauterine crowding dissipate over the ensuing week. Flexor hypertonia can hamper drawing blood from the antecubital fossa because it is so difficult to fully extend a full-term infant's arms. Some full-term neonates have mild flexion contractures at the elbows or knees that wane in the months following birth. Even at term, preterm infants do not manifest this degree of flexor hypertonia.

There are several methods for assessing extremity tone (Amiel-Tison, 2002; Andre-Thomas et al., 1960; Saint-Anne Dargassies, 1977). Subjective assessment entails alternately flexing and extending a limb and feeling resistance to flexion (normally a lot) and resistance to extension (normally very little). When held upright in vertical suspension, extremity flexor tone maintains flexed legs, overcoming gravity. The popliteal angle, the heel-to-ear maneuver, and recoil measure passive lower extremity flexor tone, and recoil is used to determine upper extremity flexor tone. The foot dorsiflexion angle and the square window at the wrist do not measure tone but have been used in gestational age measures because they reflect hormones the mother secretes to promote laxity of her pelvic ligaments as her pregnancy approaches term.

Correct interpretation of examination results depends on the examiner's care in performing the examination and observing infant responses. The popliteal angle is the angle behind the knee, made by the thigh and calf, and this maneuver does not assess range of movement. To assess the popliteal angle, the infant's legs should be flexed at the hips and the knees, and then gently extended at the knee (keeping it flexed at the hip) until one meets resistance or the infant starts to cry. Typical full-term neonates have a popliteal angle of less than 90 degrees. The heel-to-ear maneuver is similar in that the infant's legs are flexed at the hips and gently extended at the knees toward the head. By term, a typical infant's feet cannot be brought anywhere near the head. This maneuver is not meant to assess trunk tone, so the infant's buttocks should be flat on the bed. Recoil is assessed by first flexing the infant's arm or leg for 5 seconds, then extending the limb for 5 seconds, then releasing it and observing the extent and rapidity of return to flexion. The typical full-term infant demonstrates brisk return to marked flexion (less than 90-degree antecubital and popliteal angles), and this brisk recoil is generally not inhibited by prolonged extension holding the limb in extension for 30 seconds.

Extremely preterm infants born before 28 weeks' gestation are strikingly hypotonic, offering no resistance to alternately flexing and extending their limbs (Allen & Capute, 1990; Amiel-Tison, 1968, 2002, 2003; Saint-Anne Dargassies, 1977). Although they may demonstrate recoil immediately after birth, this is due to mechanical effects of their intrauterine posture and dissipates over several days. They

have nearly full extension with passive measures of tone and with recoil. In extremely preterm infants, extremity flexor tone evolves with neuromaturation in a caudocephalad direction: first in the lower extremities, then in the upper extremities. Both the caudocephalad direction and the time line mirror the evolution of flexor tone in the fetus in utero. Although the strength of their flexor tone also peaks at term (i.e., 38–40 weeks' PMA), preterm infants at term generally have less flexor hypertonia than full-term neonates. Positioning NICU infants with extremity flexion is a reasonable attempt to mimic the intrauterine mechanical effects on development of flexor hypertonia (Aucott, Donohue, Atkins, & Allen, 2002). In both preterm infants at term and full-term neonates, flexor hypertonia gradually diminishes during the next few months.

Deviations from the norm include delayed development of flexor hypertonia, generalized or focal hypotonia, extremity extensor tone, and asymmetries. Multiple, serial examinations over time help to determine the significance of deviations in muscle tone. Persistent abnormalities are more worrisome than transient ones. In preterm infants in an NICU, serial examinations not only help determine how persistent tonal abnormalities are, but also allow determination of the infant's rate of development of flexor tone (Allen, 2005). Delay in acquisition of flexor hypertonia is less worrisome than persistent hypotonia. Generalized hypotonia may be seen with any number of medical conditions, including respiratory distress, sepsis, necrotizing enterocolitis, and poor nutrition. There may be some delay in improvement of the hypotonia when the infant's medical condition improves, but persistent hypotonia beyond convalescence is worrisome.

Persistent extensor tone in any extremity is abnormal in neonates. Intermittent extensor tone with stretching or crying, especially in the lower extremities, is not an uncommon finding during an examination. Extremity extensor tone that predominates during the examination is very worrisome, especially if accompanied by neck extensor hypertonia, increased shoulder retraction, or both. Persistence of these findings signals the need for comprehensive neurodevelopmental follow-up and early intervention, with careful attention to positioning and range of movement.

During the examination, the examiner should look for any evidence of asymmetrical muscle tone. When evaluating tone symmetry, the infant's head should be kept in midline. Even if neonates do not demonstrate consistent changes in posture, the ATNR can profoundly influence underlying muscle tone (Allen & Caput, 1986b, 1990; Caputo et al., 1982). Inattention to head position can account for transient right–left asymmetries of tone in many neonates. Persistently positioning an infant with lateral rotation of the head to one side contributes to persistent asymmetries that can influence later motor function (Konishi et al., 1987; Konishi et al., 1986; Konishi et al., 1997). Consistent and persistent asymmetries of posture, movement, tone, and reflexes may signal an underlying intracranial lesion (e.g., unilateral middle cerebral artery infarction or intraparenchymal hemorrhage) that can be diagnosed with neuroimaging studies. The risk of cerebral palsy, especially hemiplegia, is high in these infants. Less dramatic asymmetries diminish with neuromaturation or persist as signs of subtle CNS dysfunction.

Axial Muscle Tone *Axial tone* is the muscle tone through the axis of the body. It has a profound influence on stabilizing the upright body while sitting, standing, or walking. Like flexor tone, axial tone emerges in a caudocephalad direction, first in the trunk, then in the neck. Head control continues to develop in the months following term.

Draping the prone infant over the examiner's hand (i.e., ventral suspension) and noting the range of trunk flexibility in the supine and sidelying positions are maneuvers that assess trunk tone. With ventral suspension, trunk tone is manifested by the degree of draping over the examiner's hand (while prone). An infant whose trunk forms a straight horizontal line in ventral suspension has good trunk tone. This maneuver should be performed on an awake infant because trunk tone also decreases with sleep. An infant with marked truncal hypotonia forms an upsidedown *U*. The extremely preterm infant develops progressively increasing trunk tone, form-

ing more of a sideways "C" over the examiner's hand, and by term, a horizontal line. A tendency toward an upward "U" shape is indicative of increased trunk extensor tone.

The relative balance between trunk extensor and flexor tone is assessed by observing degree of incurvation with dorsal extension and ventral flexion of the trunk in sidelying and supine. After placing one palm against the back of an infant in the sidelying position, the examiner holds the infant's pelvis and thighs, gently extends the infant's trunk until meeting resistance, and observes the degree of dorsal curvature of the spine. Degree of ventral flexion is assessed by holding a supine infant's legs and pelvis and determining the maximal curvature of the spine when gently pushing the legs toward the chest and head. Degree of ventral flexion normally exceeds degree of dorsal extension. The typical full-term neonate has a moderate degree of trunk flexion and very little trunk extension. Infants with truncal hypotonia demonstrate both pronounced dorsal extension and ventral flexion. Infants with trunk extensor hypertonia (as seen in opisthotonus) have a greater degree of dorsal extension than ventral flexion.

The examiner can easily recognize marked neck hypotonia while handling the infant, especially when changing the infant's position. Danger of hyperextending the infant's neck prohibits any maneuvers to demonstrate marked neck hypotonia. Hyperextension of the neck must be avoided in all infants at risk for atlanto-occipital or any head–neck instability, including infants with trisomy 21 (Down syndrome). The examiner should therefore take the time to evaluate the infant's underlying neck tone with gentle handling before performing specific maneuvers to assess it.

When placed in an upright, supported sitting position, typical full-term neonates can at least briefly hold their heads upright. They may have difficulty bringing the head to an upright position and sustaining it there. When the examiner holds the infant's shoulders and pulls him or her from supine to a supported sitting position, the typical full-term infant has a mild initial head lag, but then active contractions of the neck flexors bring the head forward before gravity would. Pulling an infant to a sitting position using the hands engages the arms and shoulders and interferes with assessment of neck muscles. In a seated upright position, gentle movements of the typical full-term neonate's trunk demonstrate relatively equal balance between neck flexors and extensors, with active symmetrical movements to attempt to keep the head upright.

Hypotonia, or a relative imbalance of neck extensors and flexors, constitutes an abnormal finding for full-term infants. Preterm or hypotonic infants demonstrate a more pronounced head lag when being pulled to a sitting position and have difficulty bringing the head forward against gravity and keeping the head in the midline axis (i.e., the head rolls to the side as it moves forward). When gently tilted in a supported sitting position, the head moves passively in all directions, with gravity. An excessive movement of the head backward and insufficient efforts to keep the head upright or pull it forward demonstrate neck extensor hypertonia, an imbalance of neck tone with neck extensors predominating over neck flexors. When pulled to a sitting position, the infant with neck extensor hypertonia demonstrates a marked head lag followed by persistent neck extension even when the infant is tilted forward and gravity should bring the head forward. An infant with mild neck extensor hypertonia only has delayed forward movement of the head when pulled to a sitting position from supine.

Neck, trunk, and lower extremity extensor hypertonia constitutes opisthotonus, which is a sign of CNS injury. An abnormally strong tonic labyrinthine reflex, a primitive reflex in which the lower extremities extend and the shoulders retract with neck extension, contributes to opisthotonic posture. Severe neck extensor hypertonia on neonatal and infant examinations has been associated with an increased risk of cerebral palsy (Nelson & Ellenberg, 1979). Conversely, typical infants may demonstrate mild and transient neck extensor hypertonia when crying vigorously. Positioning an intubated infant in neck extension by placing a roll beneath the neck has been associated with neck extensor posturing, and many of these infants also have increased shoulder retraction and lower extremity extension. In-

fants with severe gastroesophageal reflux have been noted to have increased neck extension and arching of the trunk. Determination of the significance of neck extensor hypertonia therefore requires an assessment of all contributing factors. This is especially difficult in sick infants with CLD/BPD, who required prolonged mechanical ventilation, and have severe gastroesophageal reflux and signs of CNS injury on neuroimaging studies.

Hip and Shoulder Tone Hip flexor and adductor tone and shoulder tone gradually emerge in the fetus and preterm infant, beginning at 32–36 weeks' PMA. The extremely preterm infant is initially hypotonic, and with neuromaturation develops hip flexor tone, then hip adductor tone, followed by shoulder tone. The late preterm or near-term infant, at 34–26 weeks' PMA, has frog-legged posture, with hips flexed but still quite abducted. By term, infants have hip adductor tone strong enough to counteract gravity and maintain hip adduction in the supine and prone positions. When the examiner alternately abducts and adducts the legs, there is resistance to full abduction and an easy return to hip adduction.

Infants who have frog-legged posture for prolonged periods can develop iliotibial band contractures. Iliotibial band contractures limit hip adduction, which can interfere with rolling over. If the contractures persist, infants sit with their legs widely adducted, and this interferes with their ability to roll on their side and get into and out of a sitting position. Prevention of this deformity begins in the NICU, with careful attention to positioning sick and preterm infants with their legs flexed and adducted, and later swaddling them with their legs flexed and knees together (Downs, Edwards, McCormick, Roth, & Stewart, 1991).

The anterior scarf sign, posterior scarf sign, and slip-through at the shoulders measure degree of shoulder tone. For the anterior scarf sign, the examiner brings the infant's arm across the chest and notes the position of the elbow with respect to the sternum. A typical full-term neonate's elbow comes nowhere near his or her sternum, while an extremely preterm infant's elbow crosses the sternum and may go past his or her axilla. The posterior scarf sign signifies severe hypotonia, when an infant's elbows can be positioned to touch behind the back. Shoulder tone can also be assessed by lifting an infant to an upright position by placing the examiner's hands under the infant's upper arms at the shoulders. An infant with low shoulder tone "slips through" the examiner's hands unless the examiner encircles and holds the infant's chest. The typical full-term neonate has enough shoulder tone to be lifted with the examiner's hands just under the arms at the axilla. With neuromaturation, the "typical" extremely preterm infant first loses the posterior scarf sign, followed by the anterior scarf sign closer to term. As many as 30% of preterm infants still had slip-through at the shoulders when examined at 37–41 weeks' PMA (Allen & Capute, 1990).

Overall Assessment of Muscle Tone

The typical full-term neonate has symmetrical flexor hypertonia, trunk tone sufficient to keep the trunk horizontal on ventral suspension, active neck flexion when pulled to a sitting position from supine, strong hip adductor tone, and no scarf signs or slip-through at the shoulders. The initially hypotonic extremely preterm infant progressively develops extremity flexor, trunk, neck, hip, and shoulder tone in a caudocephalad direction. Typical full-term neonates have a higher degree of flexor hypertonia than preterm infants do at term.

Abnormalities of muscle tone include hypotonia, extensor hypertonia, and asymmetries of tone. Some infants have generalized hypotonia with extremity, neck, trunk, hip, and shoulder hypotonia. Generalized hypotonia can be caused by medical illness, metabolic disturbances, medications, CNS injury, and neuromuscular disorders. The infant with hypotonia of one arm should be evaluated for brachial plexus injury. Following perinatal asphyxia, tone abnormalities are common, especially axial and upper extremity hypotonia and neck, trunk, and extremity extensor hypertonia. Even in the absence of a history of perinatal asphyxia, extensor hypertonia of the neck, trunk, and/or extremities is a worrisome abnormality that indicates a need for comprehensive neurodevelopmental follow-up and early intervention. Persistent markedly asymmetri-

cal tone may signal unilateral CNS injury that can lead to cerebral palsy, especially spastic hemiplegia. Careful attention to how NICU infants are positioned promotes symmetry and avoids misinterpretation of mild asymmetries on examination.

Reflexes

Typical full-term neonates have strong, complete deep tendon, pathological, and primitive reflexes. Most reflexes are absent or weak at less than 26–28 weeks' gestation. With neuromaturation, they become stronger and more complete, demonstrating the same caudocephalad pattern as they emerge as does muscle tone.

Deep Tendon Reflexes

Full-term neonates are generally quite hyperreflexic, with easily elicited brisk deep tendon reflexes. Preterm infants born before 28 weeks' gestation are generally hypotonic and subsequently develop deep tendon reflexes in a caudocephalad direction. Generally by 32–33 weeks' gestation or PMA, deep tendon reflexes are easily elicited. Preterm infants at term are just as hyperreflexic as their term counterparts. At term, full-term and preterm infants are so hyperreflexic that they have an increased reflexogenic zone (i.e., reflexes are easily elicited with taps anywhere on their limbs). Unsustained clonus is common at term, especially at the ankles.

The common practice of trying to elicit the deep tendon reflexes with the examiner's fingertips provides an inconsistent stimulus that may miss the extent of the infant's hyperreflexia. (The fact that reflexes can be elicited in this manner speaks to the degree of hyperreflexia normally present at term.) The examiner should use a small reflex hammer to elicit reflexes at the pectoralis (elicited by striking over the pectoralis muscle), biceps, brachioradialis, knees, and ankles. The triceps reflex is inconsistent in neonates. Ankle jerks can also be appreciated by holding the infant's foot with the thumb and behind the infant's calf with the fingers, and tapping the examiner's thumb. Ankle jerks elicited in this manner are felt rather than seen, and this method does not require locating the Achilles tendon in small infants.

Pathological Reflexes The pathological reflexes (i.e., Babinski's reflex, Chaddock's reflex, mass reflex, crossed adduction) are normally present in the full-term neonate, develop in a caudocephalad direction, and should be symmetrical. These examination findings are normally present in early infancy but are abnormal at any other time of life (hence, the term *pathological reflexes*).

The Babinski, Chaddock, Gordon, and Oppenheim reflexes are all maneuvers that elicit the same response: extension and upward movement of the big toe and an outward fanning of the other toes. If the Babinski reflex test is performed in the classical manner, stroking along the lateral aspect of the sole from heel to toes, then curving to stroke along the base of the toes, neonates flex their toes as part of the very strong lower extremity grasp reflex. Babinski's reflex is best elicited in neonates by lateral stroking only, avoiding the base of the toes. Chaddock's reflex is similar to Babinski's, but the examiner strokes along the side of the infant's foot, arcing around the lateral maleolus and then upward to the toes. Some prefer Chaddock's reflex in neonates because it avoids eliciting the lower extremity grasp reflex. Gordon's reflex is elicited by squeezing the infant's gastrocnemius muscle. Oppenheim's reflex is elicited by running the examiner's knuckles along the infant's shin, downward from the knee to the foot. (The Gordon and Oppenheim reflex tests are seldom used.)

Both the mass reflex and crossed adduction are overflow phenomena from the increased reflexogenic zone seen in neonates. The mass reflex is elicited by putting the examiner's fingertips over the infant's symphysis pubis and tapping the fingertips gently with a reflex hammer. A positive mass reflex is seen when both of the infant's legs immediately adduct. Crossed adduction can be elicited by tapping the infant's patella with a reflex hammer and observing an immediate but brief adduction of the opposite leg. It can also be elicited by tapping over the adductors of one leg and observing adduction of the contralateral leg.

Primitive Reflexes The primitive reflexes are complex, stereotyped, automatic movement patterns that emerge during fetal and preterm life, are present in full-term infants, peak in the months following birth, and become more difficult to elicit during the first year as voluntary motor control dramatically improves (Allen & Capute, 1986a, 1990; Capute et al., 1982; Capute et al., 1984). Primitive reflexes are useful components of the neonatal neurodevelopmental examination because they are easily elicited in full-term neonates, progressively develop during fetal and preterm neuromaturation, and often persist in infants with cerebral palsy (Allen & Capute, 1986b, 1989; Capute, 1979; Milani-Comparetti & Gidoni, 1967; Paine, 1964; Paine et al., 1964; Stern, 1971). Most primitive reflexes emerge by 30 to 32 weeks' gestation or PMA and are strong and complete by 34–36 weeks' gestation or PMA.

The earliest primitive reflexes are the grasps and rooting, in that elements of these primitive reflexes have been elicited in fetuses as early as 11–12 weeks' gestation, they are usually present (but weak) in the most immature preterm survivors, and they become stronger and more complete with neuromaturation (Allen, 2005; Allen & Capute, 1986b, 1990; Amiel-Tison, 2002; Gesell & Amatruda, 1945; Saint-Anne Dargassies, 1977). Gentle pressure on the soles of the infant's feet, at the base of the toes, elicits toe flexion, or the lower extremity grasp reflex. Applying pressure to the infant's palms and gently pulling up elicits the upper extremity grasp reflex. The full-term neonate demonstrates tight finger flexion, and upward traction results in strong elbow flexion as well (this component is also termed the *traction response*). Some full-term neonates have such strong reflexes that the examiner may lift the infant off the bed with the upper extremity grasp reflex and traction response. Rooting is also termed the *four cardinal points reflex* and can be elicited by gentle pressure on the infant's upper lip or lower lip or on either side of the mouth. The complete response is characterized by turning the head, sticking out the tongue, and starting to suck on the examiner's finger, a pacifier, or a nipple.

The Moro reflex is the classic neonatal primitive reflex because it is easily elicited and recognized. It can be elicited by any sudden, startling stimulus (e.g., a loud sound) or movement (e.g., bumping the isolette). The preferred method is to lift the infant's head and shoulders slightly off the bed and gently allow them to fall back against the examiner's hand. The full Moro reflex response is initial arm abduction and arm and finger extension, followed by arm adduction and flexion. The latter component is accompanied by either finger flexion or a *C* or *O* configuration of the thumb and first finger. A full-term neonate with flexor hypertonia may demonstrate a more muted response than the preterm infant, with less initial full-arm extension, whereas the preterm infant often does not demonstrate full adduction and flexion with the second component of the Moro reflex.

The ATNR is elicited with either active or passive turning of the infant's head to one side. The limbs on the face side tend to extend, and the limbs on the occiput side tend to flex. The changes in posture may be very brief and with only a small amplitude. If changes in posture are not observed, the examiner should feel for tone changes as the head is turned from one side to the other. The flexor hypertonia of the full-term neonate may inhibit the ATNR, which may be manifest only in changes in muscle tone.

Other primitive reflexes that can be elicited by moving the infant's head and observing limb movements are the tonic labyrinthine and the symmetrical tonic neck reflexes. Generally, they evolve prior to term but, like the ATNR, are often inhibited by normal flexor hypertonia. With the tonic labyrinthine reflex, the infant is placed in supine and the head is gently flexed, then extended (but not hyperextended). With neck extension, infants extend their legs and retract their shoulders; with neck flexion, they flex their legs and protract their shoulders. This is an exaggerated primitive reflex in infants with abnormal neck extensor hypertonia, leading to the retracted shoulders, arching of the trunk, and extended legs seen with opisthotonus. The symmetrical tonic neck reflex is not as prominent but can be observed in some neonates, especially in preterm infants. With neck extension, the infant tends to

extend the arms and flex the legs; with neck flexion, the arms flex and the legs extend (therefore competing with effects of the tonic labyrinthine reflex).

With the infant in ventral suspension, Galant's, or the trunk incurvature, reflex is elicited by gently stroking the infant's back just lateral to the spine. The infant's lower back curves to the side that was stimulated. The infant may also demonstrate hip elevation at the same time as trunk incurvature. Components of this reflex can be elicited very early in gestation (e.g., 25 weeks' gestation), and the reflex becomes stronger by 30 weeks' gestation (Allen & Capute, 1986b).

Several reflexes that require the examiner to hold the infant in vertical suspension do not emerge until 33–36 weeks' gestation or PMA (Allen & Capute, 1986b, 1990). Lower extremity placing is elicited by holding the infant in vertical suspension and bringing the lower shin and the dorsal aspect of the foot in contact with the edge of a bed or table. In response to this pressure, the infant first flexes the lower extremity and then extends it (as if "placing" the foot on the table). Stepping is elicited by holding the infant upright and placing some weight on the plantar aspect of the feet, then leaning the infant forward, alternately tilting him or her from side to side. This may elicit reciprocal flexion then extension, in an alternating fashion, simulating walking or stepping; however, not more than half of full-term neonates and preterm infants at term demonstrate stepping (Paine et al., 1964).

The primary value of the primitive reflexes is in recognizing asymmetries. The Moro reflex, grasps, ATNR, Galant's reflex, placing, and stepping are all useful for detecting asymmetries. The infant with a brachial plexus injury may have the initial arm extension and abduction with the Moro reflex, but not the subsequent flexion and adduction in the affected arm. Absent or very weak primitive reflexes, especially the grasp reflexes, are worrisome findings suggestive of CNS injury. The hypertonic, irritable infant with CNS injury may demonstrate extremely strong or even obligatory primitive reflexes. The upper and lower extremity grasps and Galant's reflex are normally very strong and complete by term (and symmetrical), but other primitive reflexes are obligatory if a strong complete response is elicited every time, with no interference from spontaneous movements. For example, an infant has an obligatory ATNR if, whenever the head is turned to one side, he or she maintains the fencing posture until the head is turned back to midline.

Postural Responses

The early postural responses are attained with neuromaturation during the first year, serve to keep the infant's head and body upright, and form the basis of functional motor abilities. Active leg, trunk, and neck tone are necessary for Amiel-Tison's body righting reaction (Amiel-Tison, 2002). The examiner holds the infant in an upright position, supporting the trunk with one hand and allowing the feet to touch a horizontal surface. The mature response of a typical full-term neonate is to contract the extensor muscles that allow the infant to "stand" upright briefly, even raising his or her head and supporting his or her own weight for a few seconds. Excessive extension with righting, with neck extension, arching of the trunk, or both, is abnormal, as is no response. In preterm infants, this righting reaction begins with lower extremity extension, followed by progressively more involvement of the trunk with increasing PMA.

Lateral head righting is present but still immature in the full-term newborn. When held in supported sitting and gently tilted to the side, full-term neonates typically rotate their heads away from the tilted side. Lateral head rotation can also be elicited in preterm infants at term. Asymmetrical responses should be noted. Within several months from term, typical infants have mature lateral head righting, as demonstrated by prompt lateral neck flexion when tilted to the side, to keep their heads upright. With neuromaturation during the first year, subsequent postural reactions develop, including lateral flexion of the trunk and the use of countermovements (e.g., extending an arm or leg on the side opposite to the tilt) to maintain an upright position.

Cranial Nerve Assessment

Although it is more difficult than in older children, it is possible to assess cranial nerve function in the neonate. Unless there are specific concerns about an infant's cranial nerves, the examiner does not need to evaluate the corneal reflexes or the gag reflex. The corneal reflex tests cranial nerve V. When the examiner gently touches a wisp of cotton to the infant's sclera, the infant immediately blinks. The gag reflex is elicited by touching the posterior pharynx or tongue. Cranial nerve I is seldom routinely tested, but full-term neonates demonstrate remarkable abilities to discriminate odors including recognizing their own mother's breast milk by smell, within several days after birth. All infants should have their hearing screened after birth, but the examiner may choose to evaluate cranial nerve VIII function by observing the infant's alerting response to sound. The infant alerts if there is any movement immediately after a sound stimulus (e.g., rattle, bell). If the infant was moving or sucking at the time of the stimulus, he or she may cease all movements in response to a sudden sound.

Assessment of cranial nerve II requires an infant to be in a quiet alert state. Visual ability can be assessed by evaluating an infant's ability to fixate on and track a face or paper with a bull's-eye target (i.e., black-and-white concentric circles on glossy paper). A normal full-term neonate has a fixed focal length of 20–30 cm (8–12 inches), and anything closer or farther away is more difficult for him or her to see. When the infant fixates his or her gaze on the stimulus, the examiner slowly moves it from side to side and observes the infant's eye and head movements. For the Amiel-Tison examination, once the infant fixates on a circular black-and-white bull's-eye, the examiner moves it twice to the right and then twice to the left, four times in a row. The normal full-term infant should follow this movement with both eyes and turn the head. Preterm infants have poorer visual acuity and shorter attention spans than full-term infants, but these progressively improve as the infant approaches term. Some infants require multiple attempts to get them to fixate and follow and need repeated efforts to bring their attention back to the stimulus. Absence of response is abnormal. Researchers have used the ability of full-term neonates to discriminate visual patterns and a marked preference for novel patterns to evaluate visual acuity in preterm and full-term infants. Similarly, typical full-term neonates and preterm infants at term demonstrate optokinetic nystagmus when alternating black-and-white stripes are moved across their visual field (e.g., using an optokinetic nystagmus drum that spins on a central pole) (Allen & Capute, 1986a).

Eye movements are controlled by cranial nerves III (oculomotor), IV (trochlear), and VI (abducens). Observation of eye movements when assessing the infant's ability to fixate and follow is sufficient, as long as full extraocular movements are observed. If the infant does not follow a visual stimulus, the doll's-eye maneuver may be used to elicit eye movements. Some intermittent dysconjugate gaze or nystagmus may be observed in newborns, but these findings are worrisome if persistent.

Careful observations of an infant's sucking, swallowing, spontaneous movements, and responses can assess whether cranial nerves V, VII, IX, X, and XII are intact. Cranial nerve V is the trigeminal nerve and controls facial sensation and jaw movement. Cranial nerve VII, the facial nerve, also controls facial movement. They can be assessed by observing the infant's rooting and sucking responses. The infant roots when the upper or lower lip or corner of the mouth is touched, and he or she turns the head, opens the mouth, and starts to suck. Peripheral facial nerve palsies are not uncommon in newborns and are often transient. An infant may demonstrate subtle asymmetries of facial expression, especially of the eyes or mouth, only when crying. With nonnutritive sucking, the infant should have not only an up-and-down movement of the jaw but also a stripping action of the tongue (i.e., anterior-posterior tongue movements) and the creation of a vacuum. Neonates often do not yet have a good lip seal and may dribble milk while feeding. Coordinated sucking, swallowing, and breathing does not generally occur until approximately 34 weeks' PMA. Abnormal findings include absence of suck, uncoordinated sucking or swallowing, immature suck/swallow pat-terns for PMA, hyperactive gag reflex, and strong tongue thrust. A gag reflex is hyperactive when a strong gag reflex is elicited even with touching the anterior aspect of the tongue. Tongue thrust is characterized by abnormally strong tongue extension and protrusion when a nipple is inserted into the infant's mouth. Inability to protect the airway is a very serious symptom that requires immediate investigation and intervention.

Cranial nerve XI controls the sternocleidomastoid muscle, which rotates and nods the head. This can be assessed by observation of the infant's spontaneous movements. In addition, an intact cranial nerve XI is necessary for lateral head rotation in response to being tilted to one side, the earliest form of the lateral head righting postural response.

Summary

Neuromaturation typically proceeds in a orderly manner, whether it occurs in utero or in an NICU. It is characterized by evolution from hypotonia to tight flexor extremity tone and gradual improvement of axial tone; progression of deep tendon reflexes to hyperreflexia; evolution of the pathological and primitive reflexes to being strong, complete, and symmetrical; improved visual attention and responsiveness to the environment; and better organization of internal regulatory systems. Knowledge of typical development, and of variations from it, is a necessary tool for neonatal neurodevelopmental assessment, but experience is necessary for determining the significance of atypical findings. Further research on the neuromaturation and neurodevelopment of high-risk preterm and full-term neonates has the potential to further our understanding of the relationships between structure and function of the developing CNS and to provide insight into mechanisms of and recovery from CNS injury.

USE OF NEONATAL NEURODEVELOPMENTAL ASSESSMENTS

As discussed previously, the various methods devised to assess neonatal CNS function reflect a variety of approaches and goals. Objectives vary from demonstrating a neonate's competencies to parents, to obtaining information needed for individualizing developmental interventions, to detecting abnormalities and predicting later neurodevelopmental disability. Neonatal assessments have been studied in many different populations: full-term newborns, infants with neonatal encephalopathy, extremely preterm infants, infants with chronic lung disease, neonates with intrauterine growth restriction, and infants with signs of malformation of or injury to the CNS. A single assessment is sufficient for many methods, and this is generally performed at term, when the infant is stable. Other assessments appraise the dynamic nature of neuromaturation by relying on serial evaluations.

Comparisons Among Neonatal Assessments

How much overlap is there between the various published neonatal assessment methods? Only a few studies have addressed this issue. A study of 32 neonates with congenital heart disease found similarities between two neurobehavioral assessments, the ENNAS and the NAPI, with correlations in similar clusters ranging from .35 to .65 (Limperopoulos et al., 1997).

Several studies have evaluated the relationship between Prechtl's Assessment of General Movements and various neurological examinations. A study of 45 preterm infants with risk factors for brain injury established 96% agreement between the Amiel-Tison Neurologic Assessment at Term and General Movements at term, with a kappa of 0.87 (Paro-Panjan, Sustersic, & Neubauer, 2005). When performed at 3 months from term, agreement was 82% with a kappa of 0.54, and all the children with normal examinations demonstrated normal fidgety movements. In a sample of 58 high-risk preterm and full-term infants, overall agreement between the Dubowitz Neurological Assessment examination and General Movements was 80% and ranged from 73% in infants assessed before 37 weeks' PMA up to 93% at 57–65 weeks' PMA (i.e., 2 months after term) (Cioni, Prechtl, et al., 1997).

Prechtl's Assessment of General Movements and his Neurological Examination did not correlate well during the first 2 weeks after birth in asphyxiated full-term infants, but correlations improved during the next few months (Prechtl, Ferrari, & Cioni, 1993).

It is reassuring that very different methods of assessing neonatal CNS function correlate as well as they do. Each method has its limitations, and one wonders how they could be used in conjunction with each other and with neuroimaging to enhance prediction of neurodevelopmental outcomes. Further study of their differences may also provide insight into factors that influence neuromaturation and how the CNS recovers from injury.

Evidence of CNS Injury or Malformation

Severe perinatal asphyxia is associated with high mortality and morbidity rates, but it is difficult to define and to distinguish from other causes of neonatal encephalopathy (e.g., metabolic) (Dixon et al., 2002; Ishikawa, Ogawa, Kanayama, & Wada, 1987). Sarnat and Sarnat (1976) graded severity of neonatal encephalopathy as mild, moderate, and severe based on its various signs (e.g., altered consciousness, reflexes and tone, autonomic dysfunction, seizures). The more abnormal the neurological examination and the higher the grade of encephalopathy, the higher the risk of death and neurodevelopmental disability (Brown, Purvis, Forfar, & Cockburn, 1974; Dixon et al., 2002; Finer, Robertson, Richards, Pinnell, & Peters, 1981; Robertson, Finer, & Grace, 1989; Thompson et al., 1997).

Infants with signs of brain injury frequently have abnormal neonatal neurological examinations. Neck extensor hypertonia is seen with increasing frequency as severity of encephalopathy increases from mild (6%), to moderate (37%), to severe (70%) (Amiel-Tison et al., 1977). In a study of 52 full-term neonates with multiple risk factors for brain injury, abnormal examinations were highly correlated with abnormalities on cranial ultrasound, electroencephalography (EEG), and cerebral function monitoring (Paro-Panjan, Sustersic, et al., 2005). Infants with structural brain abnormalities or dysmorphic features (suggesting possible prenatal insult) were most likely to have a static profile with no changes in the examination over time, and examination findings suggestive of prenatal onset (e.g., high-arched palate, cortical thumbs, suture ridges).

Other studies have demonstrated strong correlations between signs of brain injury and abnormalities on the Dubowitz Neurological Examination. A study of 58 full-term neonates with encephalopathy found that infants with normal magnetic resonance imaging (MRI) scans had only mild tone abnormalities after the first week, whereas infants with severe lesions (e.g., basal ganglia lesions) had persistent, diffuse abnormalities on MRI examination (Mercuri et al., 1999). Infants with signs of white matter injury but no basal ganglia lesions demonstrated improvement in behavior, tone, and feeding. Another study at term of 66 preterm infants with birth weights below 1,500 g found that both white and gray matter abnormalities on MRI were strongly associated with Dubowitz scores (especially with tone and tone pattern subscores) (Woodward, Mogridge, Wells, & Inder, 2004). In a study that found abnormalities on cranial ultrasound in as many as 20% of 177 *apparently well neonates* born between 36 and 42 weeks' gestation, it was noted that many had deviant patterns on the Dubowitz examination (Mercuri, Dubowitz, Brown, & Cowan, 1998).

In addition to tonal abnormalities, infants with brain injury demonstrate abnormal posture, spontaneous movements, and behavior. A study of nine infants with brain malformations on neuroimaging studies demonstrated that they had poorer behavioral state organization and abnormal General Movements (Ferrari et al., 1997). Many (6 of 9) had excessive wakefulness and lacked one or two movement patterns found in typically developing infants. A study of 26 full-term neonates with mild to severe encephalopathy noted hypokinesis in many immediately after birth, followed by a period of abnormal-quality General Movements (Prechtl et al., 1993). In a study of 21 preterm infants with periventricular echodensities on cranial ultrasound scans, echodensities that persisted beyond 14 days were associated with abnormal General Movements (Bos,

Martijn, Okken, & Prechtl, 1998). In 40 infants born before 35 weeks' gestation, abnormalities on cranial ultrasound correlated only with General Movements at 52 weeks' PMA, not at 34 weeks' or 40 weeks' PMA (Garcia, Gherpelli, & Leone, 2004).

Prediction of Neurodevelopmental Outcome

The ability to more accurately predict neurodevelopmental outcome in high-risk neonates provides better information for parent counseling and allocating limited comprehensive developmental follow-up and early intervention resources. By providing more immediate feedback regarding functional CNS effects, such prediction could improve safety of randomized clinical trials of obstetrical, NICU, and developmental interventions. It is highly unlikely that any test will predict the future with 100% certainty. Not only can a child with initially typical development suffer subsequent brain injury, but also the child with CNS injury has the potential for recovering some or all function or for learning to cope with or circumvent remaining deficits.

Using the neurological examination described by Paine (1960) in the U.S. National Collaborative Perinatal Project, as many as 11% of approximately 40,000 infants born from 1959 to 1966 had abnormal neurological examinations (Nelson & Ellenberg, 1979). At 7 years, 1% of those children had cerebral palsy, compared with 0.3% of children with normal neonatal neurological examinations. Extremity or axial hypotonia or hypertonia, jerky or myoclonic movements, abnormal upper or lower extremity grasps, and nystagmus all had relative risks above 20 for cerebral palsy. The clinician's overall impression of abnormal brain function, including neonatal seizures, was noted in only 0.5% of neonates but carried a relative risk of 99.

Early studies of full-term neonates with signs of severe perinatal asphyxia/encephalopathy noted high mortality and morbidity rates, and many had severe multiple disabilities (e.g., disabling cerebral palsy, severe cognitive impairment, sensory impairments, seizures, microcephaly) (Brown et al., 1974; De Souza &

Richards, 1978; Finer et al., 1981; Robertson et al., 1989). The more neurological signs that were present, the higher the risk of neurodevelopmental disability. A high mortality rate was associated with severe persistent hypotonia, whereas initial hypotonia followed by extensor hypertonia was highly associated with severe neurodevelopmental disability.

In the Groningen Perinatal Project that used Prechtl's (1977) Neurological Examination, 80 of 1,655 full-term infants (5%) born from 1975 to 1977 were identified as abnormal (Bierman-van Eendenburg, Jurgens-van der Zee, Olinga, Huisjes, & Touwen, 1981; Hadders-Algra, 1987; Hadders-Algra, Touwen, & Huijes, 1986). When evaluated at 6 years, more children with abnormal neonatal examinations had died (5% vs. 2%), had severe disabilities (8% vs. 0), and had minor neurological dysfunction (29% vs. 5%) than children with normal neonatal examinations. Behavior problems were also more common in the children with abnormal neonatal examinations.

The overwhelming majority of neurodevelopmental outcomes studies (Table 17.1) establish the reassuring nature of normal neonatal assessments (Allen & Capute, 1989; Amess et al., 1999; Amiel-Tison & Stewart, 1991; Bierman-van Eendenburg et al., 1981; Brown et al., 1974; Downs et al., 1991; Dubowitz et al., 1984; Gross, Kosmetatos, Grimes, & Williams, 1978; Hadders-Algra, 1987; Hadders-Algra et al., 1986; Lacey, Rudge, Rieger, & Osborn, 2004; Paro-Panjan, Neubauer, Kodric, & Batanic, 2005; Paro-Panjan, Sustersic, & et al., 2005; Stewart, 1988; Stewart, Thorburn, Lipscomb, & Amiel-Tison, 1983; Stewart et al., 1988; Thompson et al., 1997; Weisglas-Kuperus, Baerts, Fetter, & Sauer, 1992; Weisglas-Kuperus, Baerts, & Sauer, 1993; Weisglas-Kuperus et al., 1994). For the most part, full-term and preterm infants with normal neonatal assessments have normal neurodevelopmental outcomes, which is reflected in the generally high negative predictive values (82%–100%) reported.

Abnormalities on neonatal neurodevelopmental assessments are strong predictors of neurodevelopmental outcome in full-term infants, neonates with encephalopathy, and preterm infants at term. The more severe and the higher the number of abnormalities on examination, the higher the risk of neurodevelopmental disability (Allen & Capute, 1989; Bierman-van Eendenberg et al., 1981; Brown et al., 1974; Dubowitz et al., 1984; Hadders-Algra, 1987; Marlow, Wolke, Bracewell, & Samara, 2005; Robertson et al., 1989; Thompson et al., 1997). Examinations of preterm infants before 34 weeks' PMA are less predictive than examinations at term (Kolobe, Bulanda, & Susman, 2004; Lacey et al., 2004).

In a study of 210 high-risk preterm infants examined at term with the comprehensive neurodevelopmental examination described previously, infants with abnormal examinations had a higher incidence of cerebral palsy (36% vs. 6%; $p < .00001$), minor neuromotor dysfunction (27% vs. 13%; $p < .05$), and cognitive impairment (36% vs. 15%; $p < .0005$) than infants with normal neonatal examinations (Allen & Capute, 1989). The strong relationship between an abnormal neonatal neurodevelopmental examination and motor impairment persisted even when subgroups of infants with chronic lung disease, intracranial hemorrhage, and gestational age below 28 weeks were analyzed separately.

Several studies have demonstrated the value of the Amiel-Tison Neurologic Assessment at Term in predicting neurodevelopmental outcome in preterm infants and in full-term infants with encephalopathy or multiple risk factors for brain injury (Amess et al., 1999; Paro-Panjan, Neubauer, et al., 2005; Paro-Panjan, Sustersic, et al., 2005; Stewart et al., 1988). Agreement between the Amiel-Tison examination and neurological outcome at 12–15 months is excellent in full-term infants and preterm infants at 3 months from term but is much less in preterm infants at term (kappas of 0.83, 0.77, and 0.39, respectively). Serial Amiel-Tison examinations improve agreement and specificity by allowing the examiner to detect patterns or clinical profiles for individual infants. In a similar manner, the low sensitivity of the Test of Infant Motor Performance (TIMP) performed at term for predicting motor performance at 4–5 years improves when performed at 3 months (33%–72%) (Kolobe et al., 2004).

Prechtl's Assessment of General Movements is also most predictive (see Table 17.1) when performed weeks to months after birth

Table 17.1. Prediction of neurodevelopmental outcome with neonatal assessments

Study	Sample	Number	Exam	Age/PMA	Age at follow-up	Outcome	Sensitivity	Specificity	Positive predictive value	Negative predictive value
Paro-Panjan, Neubauer, Kodric, and Bratanic (2005)	Preterm	45	Amiel-Tison	Term	12–15 months	Neurologic	92%	45%	—	—
	Preterm	45	Amiel-Tison	3 months	12–15 months	Neurologic	100%	75%	—	—
	Preterm	45	General Movements	Term	12–15 months	Neurologic	96%	40%	—	—
	Preterm	45	General Movements	3 months	12–15 months	Neurologic	100%	35%	—	—
Lacey, Rudge, Rieger, and Osborn (2004)	GA < 31 weeks	138	Abnormal	PMA > 33 weeks	3 years	Cerebral palsy	52%	98%	88%	88%
	GA < 31 weeks	138	Unusual/Abnormal	PMA > 33 weeks	3 years	Cerebral palsy	86%	83%	57%	96%
	GA < 31 weeks	65	Unusual/Abnormal	PMA < 33 weeks	3 years	Cerebral palsy	57%	90%	40%	95%
Garcia, Gherpelli, and Leone (2004)	GA < 35 weeks	33	General Movements	PMA < 37 weeks	12–19 months	Denver	100%	44%	36%	100%
	GA < 35 weeks	39	General Movements	PMA 37–42 weeks	12–19 months	Denver	78%	50%	47%	80%
	GA < 35 weeks	26	General Movements	PMA 49–56 weeks	12–19 months	Denver	75%	67%	60%	80%
Kolobe, Bulanda, and Susman (2004)	High risk	61	TIMP	30 days after term	4–5 years	Peabody motor	33%	94%	60%	83%
	High risk	61	TIMP	60 days after term	4–5 years	Peabody motor	50%	86%	55%	84%
	High risk	61	TIMP	90 days after term	4–5 years	Peabody motor	72%	91%	75%	91%
Ferrari et al. (2002)	GA < 37 weeks	83	Dubowitz	PMA 28–37 weeks	2–3 years	Cerebral palsy	58%	45%	54%	48%
	GA < 37 weeks	79	Prechtl	PMA 38–42 weeks	2–3 years	Cerebral palsy	68%	63%	66%	65%
	GA < 37 weeks	70	Touwen	PMA 43–46 weeks	2–3 years	Cerebral palsy	89%	52%	67%	84%
	GA < 37 weeks	84	Touwen	PMA 47–60 weeks	2–3 years	Cerebral palsy	95%	70%	77%	93%

Study	Group	N	Assessment	Age at assessment	Age at outcome	Outcome				
Maas et al. (2000)	GA < 37 weeks	83	General Movements	PMA 28–37 weeks	2–3 years	Cerebral palsy	100%	38%	63%	100%
	GA < 37 weeks	79	General Movements	PMA 38–42	2–3 years	Cerebral palsy	100%	41%	63%	100%
	GA < 37 weeks	70	General Movements	PMA 43–46 weeks	2–3 years	Cerebral palsy	100%	55%	55%	100%
	GA < 37 weeks	84	General Movements	PMA 47–60 weeks	2–3 years	Cerebral palsy	82%	86%	86%	100%
	GA < 30 weeks	100	Prechtl	Term	2 years	Touwen exam	44%	90%	31%	94%
	GA < 30 weeks	100	Prechtl	Term	2 years	Bayley MDI	25%	89%	23%	90%
	GA < 30 weeks	100	Prechtl	Term	2 years	Bayley PDI	29%	90%	33%	88%
	GA < 30 weeks	80	General Movements	Term	2 years	Touwen exam	71%	53%	13%	95%
	GA < 30 weeks	80	General Movements	Term	2 years	Bayley MDI	60%	53%	15%	90%
	GA < 30 weeks	80	General Movements	Term	2 years	Bayley PDI	55%	52%	16%	88%
Amess et al. (1999)	FTNB	19	Amiel-Tison	0–2 days	11–15 months	Griffiths	100%	53%	31%	100%
	FTNB	14	Amiel-Tison	3–25 days	11–15 months	Griffiths	91%	71%	71%	91%
Cioni et al. (1997)	GA < 37 weeks	65	Dubowitz	PMA < 38 weeks	2 years	Griffiths	75%	48%	58%	67%
	GA < 37 weeks	60	Prechtl	PMA 38–42 weeks	2 years	Griffiths	79%	71%	72%	78%
	GA < 37 weeks	61	Amiel-Tison	PMA 43–47 weeks	2 years	Griffiths	93%	90%	90%	90%
	GA < 37 weeks	66	Amiel-Tison	PMA 48–56 weeks	2 years	Griffiths	94%	67%	74%	92%
	GA < 37 weeks	61	Amiel-Tison	PMA 57–65 weeks	2 years	Griffiths	93%	90%	91%	93%
	GA < 37 weeks	65	General Movements	PMA < 38 weeks	2 years	Griffiths	58%	58%	67%	67%
	GA < 37 weeks	65	General Movements	PMA 38–42 weeks	2 years	Griffiths	91%	58%	67%	86%
	GA < 37 weeks	60	General Movements	PMA 38–42 weeks	2 years	Griffiths	100%	72%	64%	100%
	GA < 37 weeks	61	General Movements	PMA 43–47 weeks	2 years	Griffiths	100%	79%	74%	100%

(continued)

Table 17.1. (continued)

Study	Sample	Number	Exam	Age/PMA	Age at follow-up	Outcome	Sensitivity	Specificity	Positive predictive value	Negative predictive value
Prechtl, Ferrari, and Cioni (1993)	GA < 37 weeks	66	General Movements	PMA 48–56 weeks	2 years	Griffiths	100%	85%	87%	100%
	GA < 37 weeks	61	General Movements	PMA 57–65 weeks	2 years	Griffiths	97%	97%	97%	97%
	FTNB	26	Prechtl	0–2 weeks	17–24 months	Griffiths	100%	23%	56%	100%
	FTNB	26	Prechtl	15–22 weeks	17–24 months	Griffiths	100%	85%	87%	100%
	FTNB	26	General Movements	0–2 weeks	17–24 months	Griffiths	100%	46%	65%	100%
	FTNB	26	General Movements	15–22 weeks	17–24 months	Griffiths	85%	85%	85%	85%
Allen and Capute (1989)	GA < 37 weeks	210	Allen Neurodev exam	PMA 34–44 weeks	1–5 years	Cerebral palsy	80%	69%	38%	94%
	GA < 37 weeks	210	Allen Neurodev exam	PMA 34–44 weeks	1–5 years	Motor dysfunction	69%	77%	65%	81%
	GA < 37 weeks	210	Allen Neurodev exam	PMA 34–44 weeks	1–5 years	Developmental disability	63%	78%	69%	73%
Stewart (1988)	GA < 33 weeks	65	Amiel-Tison	PMA 38–42 weeks	1 year	Major disability	61%	67%	—	—
	GA < 33 weeks	65	Amiel-Tison	PMA 38–42 weeks	1 year	Any disability	67%	80%	—	—
	GA < 33 weeks	56	Exam plus ultrasound	PMA 38–42 weeks	1 year	Major disability	62%	100%	—	—
	GA < 33 weeks	56	Exam plus ultrasound	PMA 38–42 weeks	1 year	Any disability	60%	95%	—	—

Key: Amiel-Tison, Amiel-Tison Neurological Assessment; Bayley, Bayley Scales of Infant Development; Denver, Denver Developmental Screening Test; Dubowitz, Dubowitz Neurological Examination of the Full-Term Newborn; FTNB, full-term newborn; GA, gestational age; General Movements, Prechtl's Assessment of General Movements; Griffiths, Griffiths Mental Development Scales; Peabody motor, Peabody Developmental Motor Scales; MDI, mental development index; Peabody motor, Peabody Developmental Motor Scales; PDI, psychomotor development index; PMA, postmenstrual age; Prechtl, Prechtl's Neurological Examination of the Full-Term Newborn Infant; TIMP, Test of Infant Motor Performance; Touwen, Touwen's Examination of the Child with Minor Neurological Dysfunction.

or term (Einspieler & Prechtl, 2005; Einspieler et al., 2004; Ferrari et al., 2002; Prechtl et al., 1993). At 6–9 weeks after birth or term, fidgety movements generally replace the writhing movements seen earlier. The quality of fidgety movements, not their quantity, is most predictive of neurodevelopmental outcome. If fidgety movements are not observed from 9 to 20 weeks after term or the infant demonstrates consistent cramped synchronized movements, or both, the risk of neurological impairment, especially cerebral palsy, is high (Einspieler et al., 2002; Prechtl et al., 1997). A multicenter longitudinal study of general movements in high-risk preterm and full-term infants has provided a wealth of data regarding prediction. Specificity is lowest prior to and at term but increases to 82% for absence of fidgety movements at 47–60 weeks' PMA (i.e., 2–5 months after term) and to 100% for cramped synchronized movements by 43–46 weeks, PMA (i.e., 3–6 weeks after term). Asymmetrical movements at 2–3 months from term or birth may signal spastic hemiplegia (Guzzetta et al., 2003). The trajectory of General Movements can refine prediction of types of cerebral palsy (Cioni, Prechtl, et al., 1997). A study of 52 children followed for 4–9 years found that definitely abnormal general movements were associated with cerebral palsy, whereas mildly abnormal general movements were associated with minor neurological dysfunction, attention-deficit/hyperactivity disorder, and aggressive behavior (Hadders-Algra & Groothuis, 1999). The authors of two studies were not impressed with the ability of General Movements to predict 2- to 4-year neurodevelopmental outcome (Maas et al., 2000; Wildschut et al., 2005).

Several studies have evaluated the relationship between the Einstein Neonatal Neurobehavioral Assessment Scale (ENNAS) and later neurodevelopment. One study of 51 high-risk neonates and 23 healthy controls found that normal ENNAS results accurately predicted normal cognitive and neurological outcome at 1 and 3 years (Majnemer, Rosenblatt, & Riley, 1994). Positive predictive values were low, but they were higher when more subtle developmental impairments were detected at 3 years than they had been at 1 year.

Even at school age, however, there were many false positives (Majnemer & Rosenblatt, 2000). Another study found an association between the ENNAS visual and auditory items and cognitive scores at both 1 and 6 years, and between active motility items and cognitive scores at 1 year (Wallace, Rose, McCarton, Kurtzberg, & Vaughan, 1995).

There is little agreement as to which neonatal assessment method best predicts neuromotor or cognitive outcome. One study found that Prechtl's Assessment of General Movements was consistently a slightly better predictor of 2-year neurological outcome than the Dubowitz Neurological Examination for preterm infants and Prechtl's examination for full-term infants (Cioni, Ferrari, et al., 1997). A study of the Amiel-Tison Neurologic Assessment and Prechtl's Assessment of General Movements at term found that both had excellent sensitivity for predicting motor and cognitive abilities at 12–15 months, but relatively low specificity (45% vs. 40%) (Paro-Panjan, Sustersic, et al., 2005). When evaluated at 3 months from term, specificity, and agreement improved for the Amiel-Tison examination, but not for General Movements (specificity 75% vs. 35%, kappa 0.77 vs. 0.37). Another study of preterm infants evaluated at 3 months after term found just the opposite (Seme-Ciglenecki, 2003), with General Movements a better predictor of cerebral palsy at 2 years than the earlier version of the Amiel-Tison Neurological Examination (Amiel-Tison & Grenier, 1986). Another comparison study in 100 infants born before 30 weeks' gestation found that the Prechtl Neurological Examination and cranial ultrasonography, but not General Movements, predicted 2-year neuromotor and cognitive outcome (Maas et al., 2000).

Studies have uniformly demonstrated strong relationships between neonatal measures of CNS structure (on neuroimaging studies) and function (clinical assessments), and each measure is an independent predictor of later neurodevelopmental outcomes. Several studies have demonstrated how clinical neonatal assessments improve prediction when used in conjunction with neuroimaging studies. We found that our comprehensive neonatal neurodevelopmental examination predicted cerebral palsy in preterm infants with intracranial hemorrhage (Allen & Capute, 1989). In another study of high-risk preterm children, cranial ultrasound scans best predicted cerebral palsy and cognitive abilities at 3.6 years, but the neonatal neurodevelopmental examination further enhanced prediction, especially in children with ventriculomegaly (Weisglas-Kuperus et al., 1992).

The Amiel-Tison Neurological Examination correlates highly with cranial ultrasound scans (0.97), EEGs (0.89), and cerebral function monitoring (0.88); predicts 12- to 15-month motor and cognitive outcome; and also can provide clues regarding etiology and timing of CNS injuries (Amiel-Tison, 2002; Paro-Panjan, Sustersic, et al., 2005). Stewart et al. (1988) found that the combination of cranial ultrasound scans and the Amiel-Tison Neurological Examination predicted normal neurodevelopmental progress at 1 year better than either did alone. No infant with normal examination and ultrasound developed major disability, and only 2% developed minor problems (e.g., strabismus, mild neurological signs). A study of cerebral magnetic resonance spectroscopy of preterm infants at term found that the Amiel-Tison Neurological Examination had a higher sensitivity (91% vs. 79%) but lower specificity (71% vs. 93%) for predicting neurological and cognitive outcome at 12 months from term (Amess et al., 1999). There were more false positives with the examination. Prediction improved dramatically when the cerebral magnetic resonance spectroscopy was used in combination with the examination (sensitivity 89%–100%, specificity 100%, positive predictive value 100%, and negative predictive value 90%–100%).

In conclusion, the preponderance of evidence confirms strong relationships between various clinical methods of assessing CNS integrity in neonates and later neurodevelopmental outcome. Prediction can be enhanced with serial assessments during the first few weeks and months and when used in conjunction with neuroimaging studies. There may be even greater value in using neonatal examinations to screen populations of infants in resource-poor settings (McGready et al., 2000). A normal neonatal assessment is very reassuring, and infants with abnormalities should receive comprehensive neurodevelopmental follow-up and early intervention during infancy and childhood.

Guiding Developmental Interventions

Neonatal assessments of CNS function can be used to counsel parents and to guide developmental support and early interventions, both in the NICU and after discharge home to the community. Although some have used Brazelton's Neonatal Behavioral Assessment Scale (NBAS) cluster scores to predict neurodevelopmental disability, its primary value is in demonstrating the capacity a neonate has for responding to interactions with his or her parents (Lowman, Stone, & Cole, 2006; Parker, Zahr, Cole, & Brecht, 1992). Als' Newborn Individualized Developmental Care and Assessment Program (NIDCAP) depends on the Assessment of Preterm Infants' Behavior (APIB) to individualize care plans for infants in an NICU, based on the infant's current functioning and ability to handle sensory input and handling (Als, 1998; Als & Gilkerson, 1997). The goal of this assessment and program is to estimate an infant's strengths, vulnerabilities, and thresholds for signs of disorganization, and for caregivers and families to provide care that enhances the infant's stability and competence. Although there is some evidence of small differences in neurobehavior and CNS structure with NIDCAP, more research is needed to ascertain long-term neurodevelopmental outcomes and to determine efficacy (Als et al., 2004; Symington & Pinelli, 2006).

Many examination methods provide important information for guiding developmental support. Hypotonic preterm infants positioned with hip support for flexion and adduction in an NICU are less likely to be frog-legged or develop hip adduction contractures (Downs et al., 1991). Recognizing prominent asymmetries or neck extensor hypertonia with shoulder retraction on examination indicates a need to pay careful attention to how the infant is positioned (de Groot, Hopkins & Touwen, 1995; Georgieff & Bernbaum, 1986; Konishi et al., 1987).

Comprehensive assessments of convalescing infants assist in planning for discharge from the NICU. This is an excellent time to review with parents their infant's hospital course, health status, and neonatal assessment findings (including hearing screenings). Results from neonatal assessments and neuroimaging studies assist in planning for specialty follow-up and community resources to support their infant's development.

Research

There is a need for much more clinical research to answer questions raised when working with preterm and full-term infants in an NICU. How does the intrauterine environment influence development of CNS structure and function? How does this process change with preterm birth and subsequent development in an NICU? Although the preterm infant at term has many similarities to full-term neonates on examination, some recognized neuromotor and neurobehavioral differences emphasize differences between intrauterine and NICU environments (Amiel-Tison, 2003; Kurtzberg et al., 1979; Majnemer, Brownstein, Kadanoff, & Shevell, 1992). More studies are needed to address how prenatal, perinatal, and neonatal illnesses influence the development of CNS structure and function. Furthermore, how can NICUs be modified to better support CNS development?

How does early CNS function reflect early CNS anatomical and physiological development? Studies that compare findings on different clinical neonatal functional assessments, increasingly sophisticated neuroimaging technology, and neurophysiological measures (e.g., EEG, auditory brain stem responses) can provide insight into how the CNS is injured and how it recovers from injury. What experience is necessary for normal neuromaturation? A small study of General Movements in 14 blind neonates raises questions about how proprioceptive and vestibular systems are calibrated. Although initially normal, these infants had poorer head control and more exaggerated fidgety movements by 2 months from term, followed by a long period of ataxia (Prechtl, Cioni, Einspieler, Bos, & Ferrari, 2001).

The long time period required to determine neurodevelopmental outcome has contributed to delayed recognition of inadvertent side effects of treatments or medications studied in randomized controlled trials (Allen, 2002). Prolonged courses of high-dose dexamethasone (e.g., Decadron, Hexadrol) were used for 15 years to treat chronic lung disease in preterm NICU infants before an increase in cerebral palsy and cognitive impairments was noted in children treated with this regimen. A study of the general movements in 15 preterm infants with chronic lung disease found a transient reduction of quantity of spontaneous movements after dexamethasone was started, as well as reduced speed and amplitude of general movements (Bos, Martijn, van Asperen, et al., 1998). Such a finding in an early trial would emphasize the importance of careful neurodevelopmental follow-up before use of the medication became widespread.

CONCLUSION

As measures of early brain function, neonatal neurodevelopmental examinations and assessments can tell us a great deal about CNS integrity. Some neonatal neurological examinations (i.e., the Amiel-Tison Neurologic Assessment at Term and the Dubowitz Neurological Examination of the Full-Term Newborn) have been simplified over 20 years as quick, efficient examinations of neonates and are easy to learn and score. Other examinations are more detailed, and some require special equipment. Some examinations require a great deal of training and expertise. Although much research still needs to be done on how medical illness and other prenatal, perinatal, and neonatal factors influence each assessment, and how findings should be interpreted, assessment of a neonate's CNS function is both possible and practical.

Except for the extreme cases of brain injury or malformation, neither clinical assessments nor neuroimaging studies can be used to diagnose neurodevelopmental disability in the neonatal period. They can be used to identify neonates at high risk for neurodevelopmental disability who require comprehensive neurodevelopmental follow-up and individualized developmental support through infancy. The more abnormal the examination is, the higher the risk of disability. Evidence suggests that use of clinical neonatal assessments in conjunction with neuroimaging studies refines prediction of neurodevelopmental disabilities. Nonetheless, the ability of some newborns with abnormal clinical assessments and neuroimaging studies to recover function is a tribute to the resilience and plasticity of the neonatal CNS.

Neonatal assessments are useful in focusing neurodevelopmental support and intervention efforts, especially in this era of limited resources. It is neither feasible nor necessary to provide all infants with all developmental interventions. Clinical neonatal assessments provide the information necessary for individualizing developmental support and intervention strategies. Research is needed to determine which infants most benefit from specific developmental interventions. Moreover, much of the care and many of the medications used in the NICU not been systematically studied regarding efficacy. By providing more immediate feedback in randomized clinical trials, neonatal assessments of CNS function can improve their safety and even provide insight into how these intervention might be improved. There is no doubt that much research is needed to determine methods of improving the outcomes of high-risk neonates (Institute of Medicine, 2006).

Meaningful use of neonatal assessments requires an understanding of the concept of risk, a knowledge of typical development of full-term and preterm infants, recognition of any deviations from typical development, understanding their significance, and an appreciation of the enormous complexity of development processes and remodeling of the fetal and infant CNS.

REFERENCES

Allen, M.C. (2002). Preterm outcomes research: A critical component of neonatal intensive care. *Mental Retardation and Developmental Disabilities Research Review, 8*, 221–233.

Allen, M.C. (2005). Assessment of gestational age and neuromaturation. *Mental Retardation and Developmental Disabilities Research Review, 11*, 21–33.

Allen, M.C., & Capute, A.J. (1986a). Assessment of early auditory and visual abilities of extremely premature infants. *Developmental Medicine and Child Neurology, 28*, 458–466.

Allen, M.C., & Capute, A.J. (1986b). The evolution of primitive reflexes in extremely premature infants. *Pediatric Research, 20*, 1284–1289.

Allen, M.C., & Capute, A.J. (1989). Neonatal neurodevelopmental examination as a predictor of neuromotor outcome in premature infants. *Pediatrics, 83*, 498–506.

Allen, M.C., & Capute, A.J. (1990). Tone and reflex development before term. *Pediatrics, 85*, 393–399.

Allen, M.C., & Donohue, P.K. (2005). Maturation and neuromaturation of multiples. In I. Blickstein & L.G. Keith (Eds.), *Multiple pregnancy: Epidemiology, gestation and perinatal outcomes* (2nd ed., pp. 758–767). New York: Taylor and Francis.

Als, H. (1998). Developmental care in the newborn intensive care unit. *Current Opinion in Pediatrics, 10*, 138–142.

Als, H., Butler, S., Kosta, S., & McAnulty, G. (2005). The Assessment of Preterm Infants' Behavior (APIB): Furthering the understanding and measurement of neurodevelopmental competence in preterm and full-term infants. *Mental Retardation and Developmental Disabilities Research Review, 11*, 94–102.

Als, H., Duffy, F.H., & McAnulty, G.B. (1996). Effectiveness of individualized neurodevelopmental care in the newborn intensive care unit (NICU). *Acta Paediatrica: Supplement, 416*, 21–30.

Als, H., Duffy, F.H., McAnulty, G.B., Rivkin, M.J., Vajapeyam, S., Mulkern, R.V., et al. (2004). Early experience alters brain function and structure. *Pediatrics, 113*, 846–857.

Als, H., & Gilkerson, L. (1997). The role of relationship-based developmentally supportive newborn intensive care in strengthening outcome of preterm infants. *Seminars in Perinatology, 21*, 178–189.

Amess, P.N., Penrice, J., Wylezinska, M., Lorek, A., Townsend, J., Wyatt, J.S., et al. (1999). Early brain proton magnetic resonance spectroscopy and neonatal neurology related to neurodevelopmental outcome at 1 year in term infants after presumed hypoxic-ischaemic brain injury. *Developmental Medicine and Child Neurology, 41*, 436–445.

Amiel-Tison, C. (1968). Neurological evaluation of the maturity of newborn infants. *Archives of Disease in Childhood, 43*, 89–93.

Amiel-Tison, C. (1974). Neurological evaluation of the small neonate: The importance of head straightening reactions. In L. Gluck (Ed.), *Modern perinatal medicine* (pp. 347–357). Chicago: Year Book.

Amiel-Tison, C. (2002). Clinical assessment of the infant nervous system. In M.I. Levene, F.A. Chervenak, M.J. Whittle, M.J. Bennett, & J. Punt (Eds.), *Fetal and neonatal neurology and neurosurgery*

(3rd ed., pp. 99–120). London: Churchill Livingstone.

Amiel-Tison, C. (2003). Neurologic maturation of the neonate. *NeoReviews, 4,* e199–e206.

Amiel-Tison, C., & Gosselin, J. (2001). *Neurologic development from birth to six years.* Baltimore: The Johns Hopkins University Press.

Amiel-Tison, C., & Grenier, A. (1986). *Neurologic assessment during the first year of life.* New York: Oxford University Press.

Amiel-Tison, C., Korobkin, R., & Esque-Vaucouloux, M.T. (1977). Neck extensor hypertonia: A clinical sign of insult to the central nervous system of the newborn. *Early Human Development, 1,* 181–190.

Amiel-Tison, C., Maillard, F., Lebrun, F., Breart, G., & Papiernik, E. (1999). Neurological and physical maturation in normal growth singletons from 37 to 41 weeks' gestation. *Early Human Development, 54,* 145–156.

Amiel-Tison, C., & Stewart, A. (1991). Neurologic versus behavioral neonatal assessment after birth asphyxia. *American Journal of Obstetrics and Gynecology, 165,* 1157–1158.

André-Thomas, Chesni, Y., & Saint-Anne Dargassies, S. (1960). *The neurological examination of the infant* (Little Club Clinics in Developmental Medicine, No. 1). London: National Spastics Society.

ARICD. (1996). *Ruth Griffiths Mental Development Scales for Babies: Birth to 2 years* (manual rev.). Henley, England: Test Agency.

Aucott, S., Donohue, P.K., Atkins, E., & Allen, M.C. (2002). Neurodevelopmental care in the NICU. *Mental Retardation and Developmental Disabilities Research Review, 8,* 298–308.

Bierman-van Eendenburg, M.E., Jurgens-van der Zee, A.D., Olinga, A.A., Huisjes, H.H., & Touwen, B.C. (1981). Predictive value of neonatal neurological examination: A follow-up study at 18 months. *Developmental Medicine and Child Neurology, 23,* 296–305.

Bos, A.F., Martijn, A., Okken, A., & Prechtl, H.F. (1998). Quality of general movements in preterm infants with transient periventricular echodensities. *Acta Paediatrica, 87,* 328–335.

Bos, A.F., Martijn, A., van Asperen, R.M., Hadders-Algra, M., Okken, A., & Prechtl, H.F. (1998). Qualitative assessment of general movements in high-risk preterm infants with chronic lung disease requiring dexamethasone therapy. *Journal of Pediatrics, 132,* 300–306.

Boukydis, C.F., Bigsby, R., & Lester, B.M. (2004). Clinical use of the Neonatal Intensive Care Unit Network Neurobehavioral Scale. *Pediatrics, 113,* 679–689.

Brazelton, T.B. (1973). *Neonatal Behavioral Assessment Scale.* Philadelphia: J.B. Lippincott.

Brazelton, T.B., & Nugent, J.K. (1995). *Neonatal Behavioral Assessment Scale* (3rd ed.) London: MacKeith Press.

Brown, J.K., Purvis, R.J., Forfar, J.O., & Cockburn, F. (1974). Neurological aspects of perinatal asphyxia.

Developmental Medicine and Child Neurology, 16, 567–580.

Campbell, S.K., & Hedeker, D. (2001). Validity of the Test of Infant Motor Performance for discriminating among infants with varying risk for poor motor outcome. *Journal of Pediatrics, 139,* 546–551.

Campbell, S.K., Kolobe, T.H., Osten, E.T., Lenke, M., & Girolami, G.L. (1995). Construct validity of the test of infant motor performance. *Physical Therapy, 75,* 585–596.

Campbell, S.K., Wright, B.D., & Linacre, J.M. (2002). Development of a functional movement scale for infants. *Journal of Applied Measurement, 3,* 190–204.

Capute, A.J. (1979). Identifying cerebral palsy in infancy through study of primitive-reflex profiles. *Pediatric Annals, 8,* 589–595.

Capute, A.J., Palmer, F.B., Shapiro, B.K., Wachtel, R.C., Ross, A., & Accardo, P.J. (1984). Primitive reflex profile: A quantitation of primitive reflexes in infancy. *Developmental Medicine and Child Neurology, 26,* 375–383.

Capute, A.J., Shapiro, B.K., Accardo, P.J., Wachtel, R.C., Ross, A., & Palmer, F.B. (1982). Motor functions: associated primitive reflex profiles. *Developmental Medicine and Child Neurology, 24,* 662–669.

Cioni, G., Ferrari, F., Einspieler, C., Paolicelli, P.B., Barbani, M.T., & Prechtl, H.F. (1997). Comparison between observation of spontaneous movements and neurologic examination in preterm infants. *Journal of Pediatrics, 130,* 704–711.

Cioni, G., & Prechtl, H.F. (1990). Preterm and early postterm motor behaviour in low-risk premature infants. *Early Human Development, 23,* 159–191.

Cioni, G., Prechtl, H.F., Ferrari, F., Paolicelli, P.B., Einspieler, C., & Roversi, M.F. (1997). Which better predicts later outcome in full-term infants: Quality of general movements or neurological examination? *Early Human Development, 50,* 71–85.

de Groot, L., Hopkins, B., & Touwen, B. (1995). Muscle power, sitting unsupported and trunk rotation in pre-term infants. *Early Human Development, 43,* 37–46.

De Souza, S.W., & Richards, B. (1978). Neurological sequelae in newborn babies after perinatal asphyxia. *Archives of Disease in Childhood, 53,* 564–569.

Dixon, G., Badawi, N., Kurinczuk, J.J., Keogh, J.M., Silburn, S.R., Zubrick, S.L. et al. (2002). Early developmental outcomes after newborn encephalopathy. *Pediatrics, 109,* 26–33.

Downs, J.A., Edwards, A.D., McCormick, D.C., Roth, S.C., & Stewart, A.L. (1991). Effect of intervention on development of hip posture in very preterm babies. *Archives of Disease in Childhood, 66,* 797–801.

Dubowitz, L., & Dubowitz, V. (1981). *The neurological assessment of the preterm and full-term newborn infant* (Clinics in Developmental Medicine, Vol. 79). Philadelphia: J.B. Lippincott.

Dubowitz, L., Mercuri, E., & Dubowitz, V. (1998). An optimality score for the neurologic examination of the term newborn. *Journal of Pediatrics, 133,* 406–416.

Dubowitz, L., Ricciw, D., & Mercuri, E. (2005). The Dubowitz neurological examination of the full-term newborn. *Mental Retardation and Developmental Disabilities Research Review, 11,* 52–60.

Dubowitz, L.M., Dubowitz, V., Palmer, P.G., Miller, G., Fawer, C.L., & Levene, M.I. (1984). Correlation of neurologic assessment in the preterm newborn infant with outcome at 1 year. *Journal of Pediatrics, 105,* 452–456.

Dubowitz, L.M.S., Dubowitz, V., & Mercuri, E. (1999). *The neurological assessment of the preterm and full-term newborn infant* (Clinics in Developmental Medicine, Vol. 148). London: MacKeith Press.

Einspieler, C., Cioni, G., Paolicelli, P.B., Bos, A.F., Dressler, A., Ferrari, F., et al. (2002). The early markers for later dyskinetic cerebral palsy are different from those for spastic cerebral palsy. *Neuropediatrics, 33,* 73–78.

Einspieler, C., & Prechtl, H.F. (2005). Prechtl's Assessment of General Movements: A diagnostic tool for the functional assessment of the young nervous system. *Mental Retardation and Developmental Disabilities Research Review, 11,* 61–67.

Einspieler, C., Prechtl, H.F., Ferrari, F., Cioni, G., & Bos, A.F. (1997). The qualitative assessment of general movements in preterm, term and young infants—review of the methodology. *Early Human Development, 50,* 47–60.

Einspieler, C., Prechtl, H.F.R., Bos, A.F., Ferrari, F., & Cioni, G. (2004). *Prechtl's method on the qualitative assessment of general movements in preterm, term and young infants* (Clinics in Developmental Medicine, Vol. 167). London: MacKeith Press.

Ferrari, F., Cioni, G., Einspieler, C., Roversi, M.F., Paolicelli, P.B., Ranzi, A., et al. (2002). Cramped synchronized general movements in preterm infants as an early marker of cerebral palsy. *Archives of Pediatrics and Adolescent Medicine, 156,* 460–467.

Ferrari, F., Prechtl, H.F., Cioni, G., Einspieler, C., Gallo, C., Paolicelli, P.B., et al. (1997). Posture, spontaneous movements, and behavioural state organisation in infants affected by brain malformations. *Early Human Development, 50,* 87–113.

Finer, N.N., Robertson, C.M., Richards, R.T., Pinnell, L.E., & Peters, K.L. (1981). Hypoxic-ischemic encephalopathy in term neonates: Perinatal factors and outcome. *Journal of Pediatrics, 98,* 112–117.

Garcia, J.M., Gherpelli, J.L.D., & Leone, C.R. (2004). The role of spontaneous general movement assessment in the neurological outcome of cerebral lesions in preterm infants. *Journal of Pediatrics (Rio de Janeiro), 80,* 296–304.

Georgieff, M.K., & Bernbaum, J.D. (1986). Abnormal shoulder girdle muscle tone in premature infants during their first 18 months of life. *Pediatrics, 77,* 664–669.

Gesell, A.L., & Amatruda, C.S. (1945). *The embryology of behavior.* New York: Harper & Brothers.

Gosselin, J., Gahagan, S., & Amiel-Tison, C. (2005). The Amiel-Tison Neurological Assessment at Term: Conceptual and methodological continuity in the course of follow-up. *Mental Retardation and Developmental Disabilities Research Review, 11,* 34–51.

Gross, S.J., Kosmetatos, N., Grimes, C.T., & Williams, M.L. (1978). Newborn head size and neurological status: Predictors of growth and development of low birth weight infants. *American Journal of Diseases of Children, 132,* 753–756.

Guzzetta, A., Mercuri, E., Rapisardi, G., Ferrari, F., Roversi, M.F., Cowan, F., et al. (2003). General movements detect early signs of hemiplegia in term infants with neonatal cerebral infarction. *Neuropediatrics, 34,* 61–66.

Hadders-Algra, M. (1987). *Correlates of brain dysfunction in children—a followup study.* Groningen: Drukkerij van Denderen B.V.

Hadders-Algra, M., & Groothuis, A.M.C. (1999). Quality of general movements in infancy is related to neurological dysfunction, ADHD, and aggressive behavior. *Developmental Medicine and Child Neurology, 41,* 381–391.

Hadders-Algra, M., Touwen, B.C., & Huisjes, H.J. (1986). Neurologically deviant newborns: neurological and behavioural development at the age of six years. *Developmental Medicine and Child Neurology, 28,* 569–578.

Hyman, C., Snider, L.M., Majnemer, A., & Mazer, B. (2005). Concurrent validity of the Neurobehavioural Assessment for Pre-term Infants (NAPI) at term age. *Pediatric Rehabilitation, 8,* 225–234.

Illingworth, R.S. (1972). *The development of the infant and young child—normal and abnormal.* Baltimore: Williams & Wilkins.

Institute of Medicine. (2006). *Preterm birth: Causes, consequences and prevention.* Washington, DC: National Academies Press.

Ishikawa, T., Ogawa, Y., Kanayama, M., & Wada, Y. (1987). Long-term prognosis of asphyxiated full-term neonates with CNS complications. *Brain and Development, 9,* 48–53.

Kolobe, T.H., Bulanda, M., & Susman, L. (2004). Predicting motor outcome at preschool age for infants tested at 7, 30, 60, and 90 days after term age using the Test of Infant Motor Performance. *Physical Therapy, 84,* 1144–1156.

Konishi, Y., Kuriyama, M., Mikawa, H., & Suzuki, J. (1987). Effect of body position on later postural and functional lateralities of preterm infants. *Developmental Medicine and Child Neurology, 29,* 751–757.

Konishi, Y., Mikawa, H., & Suzuki, J. (1986). Asymmetrical head-turning of preterm infants: some effects on later postural and functional lateralities. *Developmental Medicine and Child Neurology, 28,* 450–457.

Konishi, Y., Takaya, R., Kimura, K., Takeuchi, K., Saito, M., & Konishi, K. (1997). Laterality of finger movements in preterm infants. *Developmental Medicine and Child Neurology, 39,* 248–252.

Korner, A.F., Constantinou, J., Dimiceli, S., Brown, B.W., Jr., & Thom, V.A. (1991). Establishing the reliability and developmental validity of a neurobehavioral assessment for preterm infants: A methodological process. *Child Development, 62,* 1200–1208.

Korner, A.F., Kraemer, H.C., Reade, E.P., Forrest, T., Dimiceli, S., & Thom, V.A. (1987). A methodological approach to developing an assessment procedure for testing the neurobehavioral maturity of preterm infants. *Child Development, 58,* 1478–1487.

Kurtzberg, D., Vaughan, H.G., Jr., Daum, C., Grellong, B.A., Albin, S., & Rotkin, L. (1979). Neurobehavioral performance of low-birthweight infants at 40 weeks conceptional age: Comparison with normal fullterm infants. *Developmental Medicine and Child Neurology, 21,* 590–607.

Lacey, J.L., Rudge, S., Rieger, I., & Osborn, D.A. (2004). Assessment of neurological status in preterm infants in neonatal intensive care and prediction of cerebral palsy. *Australian Journal of Physiotherapy, 50,* 137–144.

Lagasse, L.L., Neal, A.R., & Lester, B.M. (2005). Assessment of infant cry: Acoustic cry analysis and parental perception. *Mental Retardation and Developmental Disabilities Research Review, 11,* 83–93.

Lester, B.M., & Tronick, E.Z. (2004). History and description of the Neonatal Intensive Care Unit Network Neurobehavioral Scale. *Pediatrics, 113,* 634–640.

Lester, B.M., Tronick, E.Z., & Brazelton, T.B. (2004). The Neonatal Intensive Care Unit Network Neurobehavioral Scale procedures. *Pediatrics, 113,* 641–667.

Lester, B.M., Tronick, E.Z., LaGasse, L., Seifer, R., Bauer, C.R., Shankaran, S., et al. (2004). Summary statistics of Neonatal Intensive Care Unit Network Neurobehavioral Scale scores from the Maternal Lifestyle Study: A quasinormative sample. *Pediatrics, 113,* 668–675.

Limperopoulos, C., Majnemer, A., Rosenblatt, B., Shevell, M.I., Rohlicek, C., & Tchervenkov, C. (1997). Agreement between the neonatal neurological examination and a standardized assessment of neurobehavioural performance in a group of high-risk newborns. *Pediatric Rehabilitation, 1,* 9–14.

Lowman, L.B., Stone, L.L. & Cole, J.G. (2006). Using developmental assessments in the NICU to empower families. *Neonatal Network, 25,* 177–186.

Maas, Y.G.H., Mirmiran, M., Hart, A.A.M., Koppe, J.G., Ariagno, R.L. & Spekreijse, H. (2000). Predictive value of neonatal neurologic tests for developmental outcome of preterm infants. *Journal of Pediatrics, 137,* 100–106.

Majnemer, A., Brownstein, A., Kadanoff, R., & Shevell, M.I. (1992). A comparison of neurobehavioral performance of healthy term and low-risk preterm infants at term. *Developmental Medicine and Child Neurology, 34,* 417–424.

Majnemer, A., & Rosenblatt, B. (2000). Prediction of outcome at school age in neonatal intensive care unit graduates using neonatal neurologic tools. *Journal of Child Neurology, 15,* 645–651.

Majnemer, A., Rosenblatt, B., & Riley, P. (1994). Predicting outcome in high-risk newborns with a neonatal neurobehavioral assessment. *American Journal of Occupational Therapy, 48,* 723–732.

Majnemer, A., & Snider, L. (2005). A comparison of developmental assessments of the newborn and young infant. *Mental Retardation and Developmental Disabilities Research Review, 11,* 68–73.

Marlow, N., Wolke, D., Bracewell, M.A., & Samara, M. (2005). Neurologic and developmental disability at six years of age after extremely preterm birth. *New England Journal of Medicine, 352,* 9–19.

McGready, R., Simpson, J. Panyavudhikrai, S., Loo, S., Mercuri, E., Haataja, L., et al. (2000). Neonatal neurological testing in resource-poor settings. *Annals of Tropical Paediatrics, 20,* 193–204.

Mercuri, E., Dubowitz, L., Brown, S.P., & Cowan, F. (1998). Incidence of cranial ultrasound abnormalities in apparently well neonates on a postnatal ward: Correlation with antenatal and perinatal factors and neurologic status. *Archives of Disease in Childhood: Fetal and Neonatal Edition, 79,* F185–F189.

Mercuri, E., Guzzetta, A., Haataja, L., Cowan, F., Rutherford, M., Counsell, S., et al. (1999). Neonatal neurological examination in infants with hypoxic-ischemic encephalopathy: Correlation with MRI findings. *Neuropediatrics, 30,* 83–89.

Milani-Comparetti, A., & Gidoni, E.A. (1967). Pattern analysis of motor development and its disorders. *Developmental Medicine and Child Neurology, 9,* 625–630.

Nelson, K.B., & Ellenberg, J.H. (1979). Neonatal signs as predictors of cerebral palsy. *Pediatrics, 64,* 225–232.

Paine, R.S. (1960). Neurologic examination of infants and children. *Pediatric Clinics of North America, 7,* 471–510.

Paine, R.S. (1964). The evolution of infantile postural reflexes in the presence of chronic brain syndromes. *Developmental Medicine and Child Neurology, 6,* 345–361.

Paine, R.S., Brazelton, T.B., Donovan, D.E., Drorbaugh, J.E., Hubbell, J.P., Jr., & Sears, E.M. (1964). Evolution of postural reflexes in normal infants and in the presence of chronic brain syndromes. *Neurology, 14,* 1036–1048.

Parker, S.J., Zahr, L.K., Cole, J.G., & Brecht, M.L. (1992). Outcome after developmental intervention in the neonatal intensive care unit for mothers of preterm infants with low socioeconomic status. *Journal of Pediatrics, 120,* 780–785.

Paro-Panjan, D., Neubauer, D., Kodric, B.A., & Bratanic, B. (2005). Amiel-Tison Neurological Assessment at term age: Clinical application, correlation with other methods, and outcome at 12 to 15 months. *Developmental Medicine and Child Neurology, 47,* 19–26.

Paro-Panjan, D., Sustersic, B., & Neubauer, D. (2005). Comparison of two methods of neurologic assessment in neonates. *Pediatric Neurology, 33,* 317–324.

Peiper, A. (1963). *Cerebral function in infancy and childhood.* New York: Consultants Bureau Enterprises.

Prechtl, H.F. (1997). State of the art of a new functional assessment of the young nervous system: An early predictor of cerebral palsy. *Early Human Development, 50,* 1–11.

Prechtl, H.F., Cioni, G., Einspieler, C., Bos, A.F., & Ferrari, F. (2001). Role of vision on early motor development: Lessons from the blind. *Developmental Medicine and Child Neurology, 43,* 198–201.

Prechtl, H.F., Einspieler, C., Cioni, G., Bos, A.F., Ferrari, F., & Sontheimer, D. (1997). An early marker for neurological deficits after perinatal brain lesions. *Lancet, 349,* 1361–1363.

Prechtl, H.F., Ferrari, F., & Cioni, G. (1993). Predictive value of general movements in asphyxiated fullterm infants. *Early Human Development, 35,* 91–120.

Prechtl, H.F.R. (1977). *The neurological examination of the full-term newborn infant* (2nd ed.) (Clinics in Developmental Medicine, Vol. 63). London: Spastics International Medical Publications/William Heinemann.

Robertson, C.M.T, Finer, N.N., & Grace, M.G.A. (1989). School performance of survivors of neonatal encephalopathy associated with birth asphyxia at term. *Journal of Pediatrics, 115,* 753.

Rogers, B., & Arvedson, J. (2005). Assessment of infant oral sensorimotor and swallowing function. *Mental Retardation and Developmental Disabilities Research Review, 11,* 74–82.

Saint-Anne Dargassies, S. (1977). *Neurological development of the full-term and premature neonate.* Amsterdam: Elsevier/North-Holland.

Salisbury, A.L., Fallone, M.D., & Lester, B. (2005). Neurobehavioral assessment from fetus to infant: the NICU Network Neurobehavioral Scale and the Fetal Neurobehavior Coding Scale. *Mental Retardation and Developmental Disabilities Research Review, 11,* 14–20.

Sarnat, H.B. (1984). Anatomic and physiologic correlates of neurologic development in prematurity. In H.B. Sarnat (Ed.), *Topics in neonatal neurology* (pp. 1–24). New York: Grune & Stratton.

Sarnat, H.B. (1989). Do the corticospinal and corticobulbar tracts mediate functions in the human newborn? *Canadian Journal of Neurological Sciences, 16,* 157–160.

Sarnat, H.B., & Sarnat, M.S. (1976). Neonatal encephalopathy following fetal distress: A clinical and electroencephalographic study. *Archives of Neurology, 33,* 696–705.

Seme-Ciglenecki, P. (2003). Predictive value of assessment of general movements for neurological development of high-risk preterm infants: A com-

parative study. *Croatian Medical Journal, 44,* 721–727.

Snider, L., Tremblay, S., Limperopoulos, C., Majnemer, A., Filion, F., & Johnston, C. (2005). Construct validity of the Neurobehavioral Assessment of Preterm Infants. *Physical and Occupational Therapy in Pediatrics, 25,* 81–95.

Stern, R.M. (1971). The reflex development of the infant. *American Journal of Occupational Therapy, 25,* 155–158.

Stewart, A.L. (1988). Prediction of long-term outcome in high-risk infants: The use of objective measures of brain structure and function in the neonatal intensive care unit. *Bailliere's Clinical Obstetrics and Gynaecology, 2,* 221–236.

Stewart, A., Hope, P.L., Hamilton, P., Costello, A.M., Baudin, J., Bradford, B., et al. (1988). Prediction in very preterm infants of satisfactory neurodevelopmental progress at 12 months. *Developmental Medicine and Child Neurology, 30,* 53–63.

Stewart, A.L., Thorburn, R.J., Lipscomb, A.P., & Amiel-Tison, C. (1983). Neonatal neurologic examinations of very preterm infants: Comparison of results with ultrasound diagnosis of periventricular hemorrhage. *American Journal of Perinatology, 1,* 6–11.

Symington, A., & Pinelli, J. (2006). Developmental care for promoting development and preventing morbidity in preterm infants. *Cochrane Database of Systematic Reviews, 2,* CD001814.

Thompson, C.M., Puterman, A.S., Linley, L.L., Hann, F.M., van der Elst, C.W., Molrwno, C.D., et al. (1997). The value of a scoring system for hypoxic-ischemic encephalopathy in predicting neurodevelopmental outcome. *Acta Paediatrica, 86,* 757–761.

Wallace, I.F., Rose, S.A., McCarton, C.M., Kurtzberg, D., & Vaughan, H.G., Jr. (1995). Relations between infant neurobehavioral performance and cognitive outcome in very low birth weight preterm infants. *Journal of Developmental and Behavioral Pediatrics, 16,* 309–317.

Weisglas-Kuperus, N., Baerts, W., Fetter, W.P., Hempel, M.S., Mulder, P.G., Touwen, B.C., et al. (1994). Minor neurological dysfunction and quality of movement in relation to neonatal cerebral damage and subsequent development. *Developmental Medicine and Child Neurology, 36,* 727–735.

Weisglas-Kuperus, N., Baerts, W., Fetter, W.P., & Sauer, P.J. (1992). Neonatal cerebral ultrasound, neonatal neurology and perinatal conditions as predictors of neurodevelopmental outcome in very low birthweight infants. *Early Human Development, 31,* 131–148.

Weisglas-Kuperus, N., Baerts, W., & Sauer, P.J. (1993). Early assessment and neurodevelopmental outcome in very low-birth-weight infants: Implications for pediatric practice. *Acta Paediatrica, 82,* 449–453.

Wildschut, J., Feron, F.J.M., Hendriksen, J.G.M., van Hall, M., Gavilanes-Jiminez, D.W.D., Hadders-Algra, M., et al. (2005). Acid-base status at birth, spontaneous motor behaviour at term and 3 months and neurodevelopmental outcome at age 4 years in full-term infants. *Early Human Development, 81*, 535–544.

Woodward, L.J, Mogridge, N., Wells, S.W., & Inder, T.E. (2004). Can neurobehavioral examination predict the presence of cerebral injury in the very low birth weight infant? *Journal of Developmental and Behavioral Pediatrics, 25*, 326–334.

18

Neurodevelopmental Assessment of Infants and Young Children

BRUCE K. SHAPIRO AND HILARY GWYNN

RATIONALE AND GOALS

Developmental disorders are the manifestations of static, chronic neurological encephalopathy commencing in childhood. Frequently, they are associated with functional impairments that may lead to handicap. The major goal of the early detection of developmental disorders is to provide early intervention. The goal of early intervention is to maximize independence and minimize secondary disability. Although early intervention is usually viewed from the perspective of the individual with the developmental disorder, such intervention is not limited to the child, but affects the family and the community as well.

Cure is not the usual outcome of early identification. Early identification may result in primary prevention of neurodevelopmental disability, as with early identification and treatment of metabolic disorders such as phenylketonuria, branched-chain ketoaciduria, hypothyroidism, and galactosemia. Most commonly, however, the goal of early identification is to facilitate the child's reaching his or her potential by diminishing the effect of the impairment and preventing secondary disability by seeking alternative pathways that exploit the developmental plasticity of the young nervous system and by the use of assistive technologies and environmental modifications.

Identification at an early age is prerequisite to the institution of early intervention services, but the question "How early is early?" remains metaphysically elusive. The emergence of measurable skills or physiological states is age dependent. Early for one disorder may be late for another. For example, 6 weeks may be early for the identification of cerebral palsy but too late to prevent the adverse cognitive outcomes of hypothyroidism. We cannot yet diagnose cerebral palsy reliably at 6 weeks.

From the family's perspective, the process of early identification is an intervention that provides answers to questions that may be the source of anxiety and familial discord. Familial interventions frequently focus on optimizing the environment for the child with developmental disorders by providing anticipatory guidance and by helping the family to set realistic goals and to adapt to a member with functional limitations. Program monitoring and advocacy are additional roles that require early identification and diagnosis for successful performance.

Society has endorsed the early identification and provision of services as a means of enhancing the likelihood of a person with a developmental disorder achieving independent function and of diminishing secondary disability. As a result, the early identification and provision of services to children with, or at risk of, disabling conditions has been mandated by rules, regulations, and statutes, such as the Individuals with Disabilities Education Improvement Act of 2004 (PL 108-446). In addition, early identification allows the target population to be defined and thereby improves resource allocation and planning.

Current Practices

The American Academy of Pediatrics (AAP; Council on Children with Disabilities et al., 2006) has presented an algorithm for identifying children with developmental disorders. The authors recommended that developmental surveillance be a part of each well-child visit. If concerns are raised, then developmental screening/brief assessments should be performed. In the absence of concerns, screening/brief assessments should be undertaken at the 9-, 18-, and 30-month visits. If the screening/brief assessments are positive or concerning, then referral for further developmental and medical evaluations as well as early developmental intervention services is recommended. Existing data suggest that this may not be the most effective method of detecting developmental dysfunction.

Assumptions

Two basic assumptions form the foundation of early identification efforts:

1. Early detection leads to better outcome.

2. Once identified, children are able to receive effective therapeutic services.

Unfortunately, both basic assumptions may be unrealistic. The first posits that earlier service provision is associated with improved outcomes. Although anecdotal and clinical impressions abound, few controlled studies have been performed that compare treatments or assess the long-term effects on the child and family of early detection (Ramey & Ramey, 1998).

The second assumption is based on the belief that effective therapeutic services exist and that the children who require such services are able to receive them. The first part of this assumption is unproved. Because of the lack of defined outcomes, the clinical heterogeneity of the population, a reluctance to employ control groups, and the inability to separate therapeutic effect from maturational influences, we do not have developmental interventions that are of proven efficacy (see Chapter 26, this volume). PL 108-446, however, mandates a system of interagency collaboration between

health, education, and social services and seeks to ensure appropriate early intervention services to children with, or at risk of, developmental disorders.

Despite the availability of services, many potentially eligible children are not receiving early intervention. Barriers to receiving early intervention services are the result of complex interactions between state and locally administered delivery systems, insurance companies, providers, physicians, and families with children with developmental delays. Parent and child factors also may impede early intervention. Parents and providers note that high motivation and persistence are needed by families in order to receive services (Shannon, 2004).

Unless these assumptions can be satisfied, the existing gulf between science and practice will be maintained. Although current attempts at early identification are presumed to be of value, their tenuous theoretical foundation must not be forgotten. Well-meaning attempts to identify children with developmental disorders could preclude further advances in the treatment of these disorders if a single approach to detection, early treatment, and management is mandated.

APPROACHES TO IDENTIFICATION

Historical Risk

Historical risk is commonly used to determine eligibility for developmental follow-up projects or early identification efforts. The basis for the approach is that a child who experiences a risk factor is at substantially higher risk for developmental disorders. The data obtained from record review or other secondary sources are used to create a risk registry.

Unfortunately, the historical risk approach to early identification is incomplete because 1) most children with developmental disorders do not have identified risk factors that are followed routinely, and 2) most children with risk factors do not have developmental disorders. For example, in the National Perinatal Collaborative Project, a pediatrician's impression that a newborn had definite brain abnormality on discharge from the nursery carried a relative risk of 99 for cerebral palsy (Nelson & Ellenberg, 1979). This meant that surviving children identified as at risk had 99 times the normal chance of being diagnosed as having cerebral palsy by age 7. Because the prevalence of cerebral palsy was low, however, only 1 of 8 children with the factor developed cerebral palsy. Furthermore, of the children with cerebral palsy, only 22.7% had this risk factor. Thus, using a factor with a relative risk of 99 would lead us to miss a substantial number of children with cerebral palsy and to follow a large number of children who would not develop cerebral palsy. In addition to being limited by the classification abilities of the individual risk factors, the historical risk approach is further limited by overlapping factors that covary (e.g., teenage pregnancy, smoking, and low birth weight).

Care must be taken to choose appropriate risk factors. Children enrolled in risk registries must be followed to determine whether they develop the condition they are at risk of having. Incomplete follow-up may mean that some children with the disorder of interest will not be provided early intervention and that the cost to detect an affected child will escalate. In addition, if the risk factor is common but not specific enough, excessive resources will be expended in detection. For example, prematurity is associated with developmental disabilities, but trying to track all premature infants would require following approximately 10% of the population.

If there is a research interest in a particular group of children, then historical risk is an appropriate technique; however, historical risk would not appear to be used appropriately to enhance early identification of developmental disorders. Furthermore, historical risk yields little useful information about an individual child and therefore cannot replace assessment as a prelude to treatment.

Presymptomatic Presentations

Developmental disorders are multidimensional and frequently associated with other dysfunctions. Structural anomalies and dysmorphisms, metabolic abnormalities, and evidence of neurological dysfunction may permit the presymptomatic diagnosis of a developmental disorder before the child evidences failure to meet age-appropriate developmental expectations.

Prenatal diagnostic techniques may detect genetic syndromes and malformations that are associated with developmental disability. Among the tools used are chorionic villus sampling amniocentesis, ultrasound, fetal MRI, and fetoscopy. Cells obtained from amniocentesis or chorionic villus biopsy may be used for chromosomal analysis or grown in culture to determine metabolic/enzymatic capabilities. The composition of amniotic fluid may be measured directly, as in the case of α-fetoprotein and spina bifida.

Structural anomalies and dysmorphisms may predominate in the clinical picture early in life and lead to the early diagnosis of intellectual disability or other developmental disorder (see Chapter 15, this volume). The baby with Down syndrome is usually diagnosed on the basis of dysmorphisms rather than symptoms of developmental dysfunction. Such findings may also predominate in nonchromosomal conditions, as in fetal alcohol syndrome.

Metabolic abnormalities may present as acute physiological decompensation or as the insidious accumulation of metabolic intermediaries (see Chapter 5, this volume). Children with acute metabolic disturbances usually present with their primary dysfunction before developmental dysfunction is evident. Some children with metabolic abnormalities may not have a cyclical course but may have only a single episode of decompensation and have their resulting developmental disorder predominate, such as in glutaric aciduria. Children with progressive processes usually present with developmental dysfunction before the primary diagnosis is established.

Neurological dysfunction in childhood usually results from diffuse processes such as asphyxia, infection, metabolic disturbances, or primary brain anomalies. As a result, developmental disorders may present as major neurological syndromes such as seizures or coma or subtle neurological abnormalities such as abnormal muscle tone, jitteriness, or feeding dysfunction (see Chapter 17, this volume). Although the neurological signs may prove nondisabling, they serve as markers of other dysfunctions that are functionally important.

When present, associated dysfunctions assist the early identification of developmental disorders; however, the associated dysfunctions are relatively uncommon and, therefore, do not contribute substantially to early identification. More often, it is the presence of one developmental disorder (e.g., motor dysfunction) that leads to the diagnosis of the other developmental disorders.

Screening

One method suggested for the early identification of developmental disorders has been screening (see Chapter 20, this volume). This method is applied to asymptomatic children and seeks to identify children who are "at risk" for developmental disorders and will thus require a fuller or developmental assessment. Screening is based on the suppositions that the disorder is frequent, that the disorder can be readily detected at an early age, and that the early detection benefits the patient. It is only one step in the diagnostic and treatment process and not an end. The outcome of screening is the label "at risk." Symptomatic or at-risk children require diagnostic assessment.

Developmental screening utilizes the age of the child or the age of milestone achievement. By fixing either age, a criterion (critical value) can be defined that would place a child at risk. For example, all 15-month-old children should be walking; speaking in phrases should occur before 30 months.

Most children with developmental disorders come from the "normal" population, and most developmental disorders are not obvious to the casual observer; thus, screening for developmental disorders fails. Most children with impairments who present for developmental assessment are not detected by developmental screening performed by health care providers. The failure of the screening process results from two factors: lack of use of screening instruments by primary care providers and lack of appreciation of maternal assessments.

The initial detection of developmental disorders typically occurs when the child's parent decides that the child has failed to meet age-

Table 18.1. Developmental expectations by age

Age	Focus
Newborn	Physiological stability
	Dysmorphisms/structural anomalies
	Neurological syndromes
3–6 months	Environmental contact
	Vision
	Hearing
	Periodicity
	Prolonged colic
6–18 months	Gross motor abilities
24–36 months	Language abilities
24 months and up	Behavior
Preschool and up	School performance
	Cutting/writing/drawing
	Reading/spelling
	Arithmetic

appropriate expectations (Table 18.1). Usually there has been substantial "back fence" consultation before the mother decides to bring her concern to the physician's attention. Studies have shown high correlation between maternal estimates of the child's abilities and the results of formal psychometric testing. Thus, the proper action when a mother raises concerns about her infant is an assessment and not a screening test.

Primary physicians do not provide developmental surveillance routinely. Many pediatricians respond to parental concerns with comments as, "He's too young to tell," "He'll outgrow it," "If it is significant, it will become apparent later (as the child ages)," and "What can you do about it anyway?" Such attitudes were justified in the past, in part because of the failure of the early screening instruments and the lack of program availability for children and families identified as at risk. Such attitudes toward early identification must be revised to reflect current evidence and practices.

Because no screening instrument is entirely satisfactory for the detection of developmental disorders, the impact of placing a child in an "at-risk" category should not be underestimated (Wolfensberger, 1965). Nor should one take solace if a child screens as "normal." Application of the most researched developmental screening instrument, the Denver Developmental Screening Test (Frankenburg &

Dodds, 1969), to a hypothetical population of 10,000 with a 3% rate of intellectual disabilities (300 cases) demonstrated that approximately 2 children will be missed (213 cases) for each child correctly identified as having intellectual disabilities, and 1,164 of 9,700 normal children will be misclassified (Accardo & Caputo, 1979).

Although the reliability and validity of screening instruments to detect children with developmental disorders have been reported, whether screening improves detection of developmental disorders is unclear. Wide-ranging screening applied at a single point in time is destined to be unsuccessful: It will be applied too early for some disorders and too late for others. In the absence of screening, approximately half of motor disorders present before 1 year of age, communication disorders present at 32 months, and intellectual disabilities present at 27 months (Lock, Shapiro, Ross, & Caputo, 1986). Whether targeting symptoms of developmental failure is more effective than wide-ranging screening remains speculative.

Assessment

Development is an end product of neural function. The degree to which environment can influence early developmental achievement is not known. Developmental assessment, thus, can be viewed as an extension of the neurological examination. If the child is making appropriate developmental progress, then the nervous system is either working properly or making the necessary compensations. Early development is not a random process. By focusing on the end product, a developmental achievement or milestone, it is possible to chart patterns of developmental progress. Charting the patterns reveals fairly fixed developmental sequences. Children roll before sitting, stand before they walk, and say one word before they speak in phrases. The amount of time between achievements can be measured and compared with the amount of time a "typical" child requires to make the same transition.

The sequence of development is mapped by a series of developmental "milestones." The relationship between the age at which a milestone is achieved and the age at which the typical child achieves a milestone is usually expressed as a percentage, a developmental quotient, or a rate. For example, a 12-month-old who is functioning at a 6-month level is not simply 6 months behind but is functioning at a developmental rate of 50%.

In children without developmental disorders, development is a unified process. In children with developmental disorders, however, asynchronous development is common. As a result, development is conventionally divided into gross motor, fine motor/problem-solving, language, and social/adaptive streams. Independent rates of development are assigned for each of these streams. By observing patterns of strength and weakness, it is possible to reach an early diagnosis (Table 18.2).

The assessment of development is possible in the fetus and neonate (see Chapters 16 and 17, this volume, and Chapter 3, Volume II). Development is progressing before the time of birth. Developmental sequences exist for premature infants and serve as a means of defining gestational age. The availability of ultrasonic imaging has permitted observation of developmental movement patterns in utero that may prove to be important markers of prenatal integrity; however, early assessments are based on fewer parameters and may have less prognostic ability.

Developmental assessment is most frequently used as a prelude to diagnosis and

Table 18.2. Developmental dissociation and early diagnosis

	Motor	Problem solving	Language	Social/Adaptive
Cerebral palsy	−	±	±	±
Intellectual disabilities	±	−	−	−
Language disorder/Hearing disorder	±	±	−	±
Autism spectrum disorder	±	±	−	−

Note: By comparing areas of strength with areas of weakness, it is possible to arrive at early diagnosis. The areas of strength are relative because it is possible to have overlapping syndromes. This approach supports the primacy of language assessment as a method of early detection.

treatment. The purpose of assessment is to delineate the child's abilities and compare them with those of a typical child. In doing so, the examiner is able to develop a profile that can serve as the basis for a treatment program.

Developmental assessment is often criticized as not being applicable to young infants and children. Although the ability of testing to predict degrees of normality is poor for individual children, the ability of early assessment to define abnormal groups is much better (Knobloch & Pasamanick, 1963; VanderVeer & Schweid, 1974). Some investigators believe that the improved predictive value arises because there is less developmental variability exhibited by such groups relative to children without developmental disorders, whereas others have suggested that the degree of departure from typical is the main reason for improved prediction. Regardless of the mechanism, the greater a child's degree of developmental delay, the higher the predictive validity of an early diagnosis.

Developmental Milestones

Developmental milestones or achievements are the key parameters of developmental assessment. For proper assessment, milestones must have specific definitions, be clinically measurable, and have predictive validity. When confronted with a child suspected of having a developmental dysfunction, there is a tendency to list all of the child's accomplishments as reflective of his or her developmental status. This usually provides a good deal of information that is marginal for diagnosis, may be of no prognostic import, and is potentially confusing.

Developmental assessment does not concern itself with the mechanism of the milestone achievement but rather with whether and when the milestone was achieved. Statements such as "His brother does all of the talking for him" should be noted but should not detract from the fact that the child was not speaking his first word until age 2. Interpretation and conclusions can be accomplished better after the data are collected.

Milestones are the culmination of many interactive processes. Consequently, there is a need for precision in the application of developmental milestones. Each milestone may form its own spectrum. For example, in babbling, the child initially will say "ba" then "baba," followed by strings of the same vowel and consonant ("bababa"), and then different strings of vowels and consonants ("rarara") followed by differing vowel–consonant combinations ("rabada"). Although it is possible to delineate the spectrum further for each milestone, this is unnecessary for first-level assessment if precise definitions are used.

Imprecise milestone definitions may lead to missing a diagnosis by crediting a child with achievement of a milestone at too early an age. For example, the ability to play peek-a-boo is said to occur at 9 months; however, unless the milestone is clearly defined as the child *initiating* the peek-a-boo game, the child may be given credit incorrectly when any of the following are observed: social smile (occurs at 6 weeks), visual recognition of the mother (2 months), laughing out loud (4.5 months), pulling at an object (5 months), or anticipation of common events (approximately 7 months).

Developmental sequences are interrelated, and disordered development in one sequence may bring attention to other areas. For example, children with intellectual disabilities may present with nondisabling mild motor delays, but the relationship between developmental sequences is not close enough for one area to be substituted for another. Normal gross motor development is not a guarantee of normal cognition.

Graphic representation, criterion reference, and best performance are three ways that milestones may be used clinically. Graphic representation of developmental sequences permits charting of the child's development in a fashion similar to growth (Figure 18.1). Outliers are readily identified, as are children who are altering their rate of milestone achievement. Population-specific modifications, however, may be required to optimize referral. Using the age of milestone achievement or the child's age as the criterion of performance is the basis of screening (see previous discussion). Criterion-referenced approaches hold either the age of achievement or the function (milestone) constant to identify children who do not

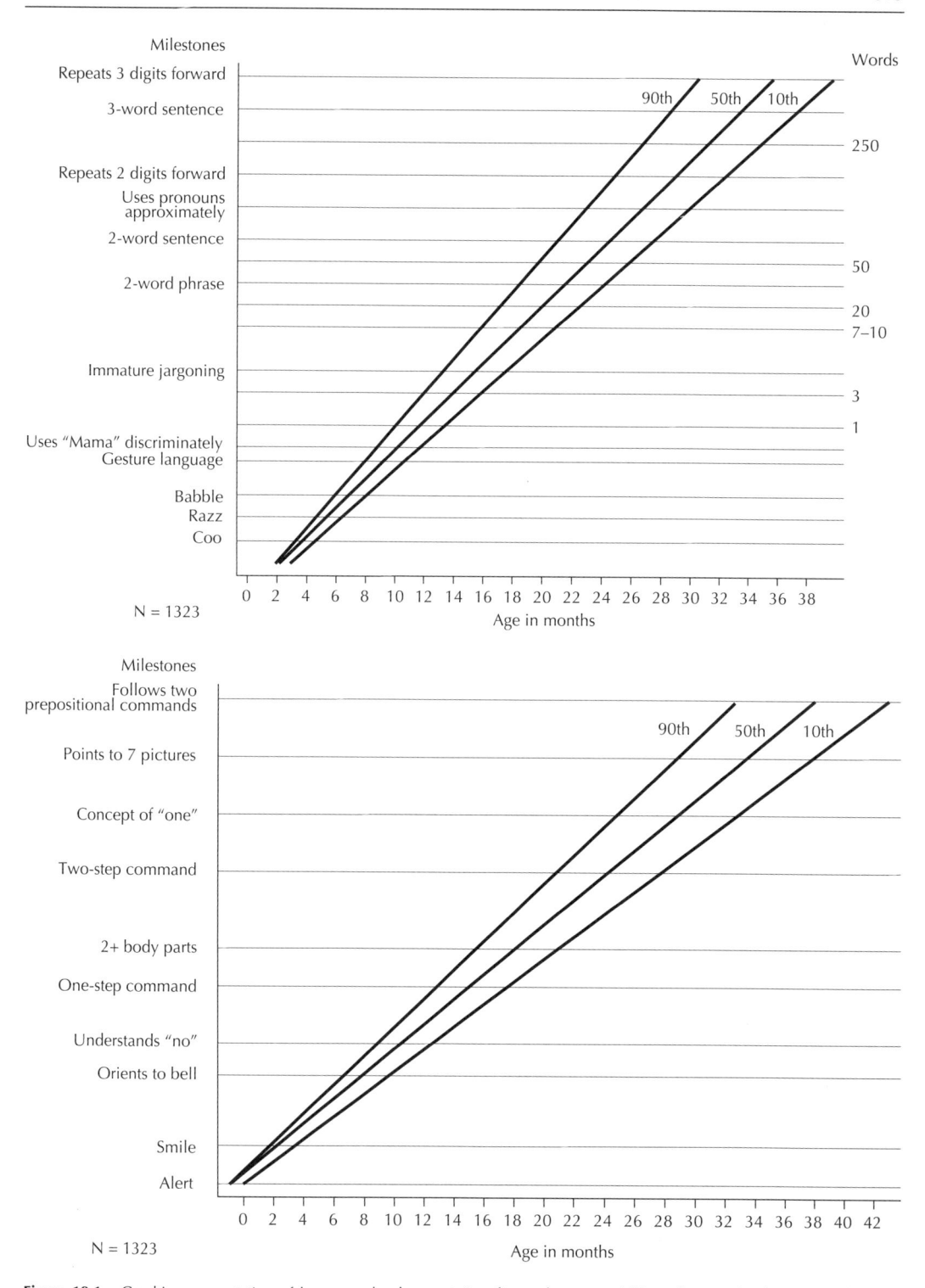

Figure 18.1. Graphic representation of language development. Top figure shows acquisition of expressive language milestones. Bottom figure shows acquisition of receptive language milestones. Data are derived from 1,323 typically developing children. (From Visintainer, P.F., & Bennett A. [2005]. Standardization of the Capute Scales. In P.J. Accardo & A.J. Capute [Eds.], *The Capute Scales: Cognitive Adaptive Test/Clinical Auditory & Linguistic Milestone Scale [CAT/CLAMS]* [p. 66]. Baltimore: Paul H. Brookes Publishing Co.; reprinted by permission.)

meet the critierion (e.g., all children who are not walking by 18 months). It is the basis for developmental screening. Best performance attempts to determine the child's highest level of accomplishment and to assign a rate of development to it. It is the basis for infant intelligence tests, but is limited because it does not permit one to determine how the child came to that point. Thus, subacute and chronic deterioration would not be detected by the best performance technique.

Although the best pediatric practice is the prospective collection of developmental data, usually retrospective methods are employed. This method has been challenged because of the interference of poor parental recall; however, in children with moderate to severe delays (rates of development of 50% or less), modest inaccuracy of parental recall does not alter milestone classification substantially. In addition, best performance techniques may be used to supplement retrospectively collected data.

Parental recall of developmental achievements can be improved by linking the child's progress to important family events (e.g., "Was she sitting by her first Christmas?"). The reliability of parent recall can be validated by use of the finding that children with developmental disorders tend to vary across milestones within a stream by no more than 10%. Developing rates for each milestone in a sequence can identify poorly recalled milestones readily. Finally, the use of developmental sequences to construct patterns of development diminishes the import of single milestones.

Motor Sequences Motor development is the major developmental focus of the latter part of the first year of life. Motor milestones are clearly observed and well remembered by parents. Table 18.3 lists the motor milestones and mean age of performance of 381 children without developmental disorders. Milestones were noted concurrently at each well-child visit during the first 2 years of life.

A motor quotient can be used to diagnose motor delay in children from 8 to 18 months of age. The motor quotient is calculated by dividing the child's motor age by his or her chronological age. The motor age is the age of the child's best motor performance before two milestones were missed. A motor quotient of

Table 18.3. Motor development milestones

Milestone	Mean age of achievement (months)
Roll prone to supine	4
Roll supine to prone	5
Sit (supported)	5
Sit (alone)	6
Creep (locomotion in prone)	7
Come to sit	8
Crawl (quadruped locomotion)	8
Pull to stand	8
Cruise	9
Walk (one hand held)	11
Walk (alone)	12

From Capute, A.J., & Shapiro, B.K. (1985). The Motor Quotient: A method for the early detection of motor delay. *American Journal of Diseases of Children, 139,* 941. Copyright © 1985 American Medical Association. All Rights reserved.

less than 50 will identify children who will walk later than 24 months with a sensitivity of 0.87 and a specificity of 0.89 (Capute & Shapiro, 1985). In a general pediatric population, a motor quotient of 70 corresponds to the 95th percentile and a quotient of 50 corresponds to the 99th percentile.

Motor delay is a common presentation for children with developmental disorders (Figure 18.2). The presence of motor delay in a young child merits a complete evaluation that should go beyond the motor examination and extend into language and cognitive areas. Motor delay is the *sine qua non* for the diagnosis of cerebral palsy. In cases in which the motor dysfunction is not disabling, motor delay is more commonly a marker for aberrant cognitive development. Although children with motor impairment may have normal intelligence, motor delay is a common presentation of intellectual disabilities and is frequently a precursor of later learning disabilities.

Language Sequences Language development is one of the most remarkable aspects of child development. Of all of the developmental sequences, language is most closely correlated with later cognitive development. Language delay is the most common presentation of developmental disorders between 2 and 4 years of age and is seen in both intellectual disabilities and the communicative/autistic/ processing disorder spectrum. Disordered lan-

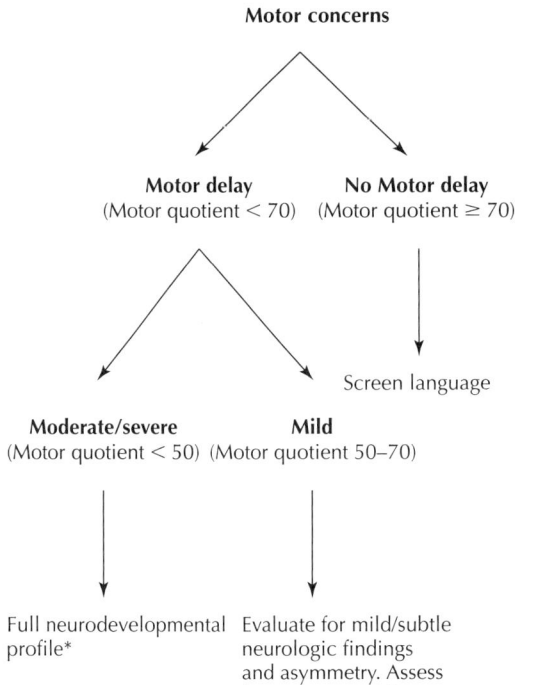

Figure 18.2. A clinical approach to motor delay. (*A full neurodevelopmental profile includes a complete neuromotor assessment that classifies the physiological and topographic distribution of the motor deficit and evaluates the presence of contractures and other orthopedic deformities [particularly of the hips and spine], cognitive processes, speech and language, special senses, and behavior.)

guage frequently is found in children with behavioral disturbances.

Although there are many schemata for language assessment, most commonly early language development is divided into that which is understood (receptive language) and that which is said (expressive language), and how it is said (speech). In addition, language development before the onset of words is called prelinguistic.

By the age of 7, most children are speaking in a mature fashion; however, it is in earliest life that infants make their most rapid progress. In the space of 2 years, infants progress from being marginally communicative to being able to make their needs known through gestural and verbal means. Despite this rapid progress, until recently infant language development had been overlooked as a means of detecting abnormal development. Prelinguistic language was largely ignored and interpreted incorrectly

as random, heavily environmentally influenced, and of little prognostic import until studies demonstrated a relationship between prelinguistic language development and later developmental outcomes. As the importance of prelinguistic development becomes more widely known and the clinical assessment of its milestones are more widely performed, it may become possible to detect mild intellectual disabilities in the first year of life.

Language disorders occur in 4%–6% of preschool children. Mild expressive language or speech delays tend to resolve; however, children with mixed dysfunctions have a more guarded prognosis. Many of these children are later recognized to have intellectual disabilities. Those who do not have intellectual disabilities are at risk for continuing difficulty with academic learning and later social adjustment (Klackenburg, 1980).

Although monitoring of early language development is important, it is difficult to assess language directly in the well-baby setting. Infants and toddlers may choose not to demonstrate their language capacity in the clinic, and time constraints may preclude the necessary cajoling. Parental report of the child's current activities, however, is an effective substitute for direct observation. The Clinical Linguistic and Auditory Milestone Scale (CLAMS) (Capute et al., 1986; Accardo & Capute, 2005) is one of several instruments that utilize parent reporting to monitor early language development (others include the Receptive-Expressive Emergent Language Test–3 [Bzoch, League, & Brown, 2003] and the Early Language Milestone Scale–2 [Coplan, 1993]). The CLAMS was standardized on 381 normal children. Milestone achievement data were collected at each well-child visit during the first 2 years. Milestones, age of achievement, and standard deviations are shown in Table 18.4. Figure 18.1 shows growth charts for expressive and receptive language milestones (Visintainer & Bennett, 2005).

The assessment of language is more difficult than the assessment of motor abilities. Motor development is dramatic, and the milestones are clearly delineated. Most parents require little explanation of a motor milestone. By contrast, most parents do not focus on early language development, and the milestones are

Table 18.4. Language development milestones

Milestone	Mean age of achievement	Standard deviation
Alert	1.1 weeks	1.3 weeks
Social smile	5.0	2.2
Coo	6.5	2.7
Orient (voice)	2.8 months	1.2 months
"Ah-goo"	4.0	1.6
Razz	4.4	1.6
Babble	6.3	1.4
"Mama"/"Dada" indiscriminately	7.7	1.7
Gesture	8.6	1.5
"Dada" discriminately	10.5	2.5
"Mama" discriminately	11.1	2.7
Command with gesture	11.1	1.7
First word	11.3	2.3
Immature jargon	12.2	2.1
Second word	12.4	2.2
Third word	13.2	2.2
Command without gesture	13.6	2.1
4–6 words	14.7	2.5
Mature jargon	16.5	2.9
5 body parts	16.7	2.8
7–20 words	16.9	2.9
8 body parts	19.0	3.2
2-word combinations	19.2	3.0
2-word sentences	20.6	3.0
50 words	20.9	3.2

Source: Capute et al. (1986).

less clearly differentiated. Consequently, there is a need for greater precision in the definitions of language accomplishments.

Even when the precise definitions are applied, it is not uncommon to see expressive language abilities being overestimated because of echolalia, programmed speech, or the use of "single-word" phrases (such as "Stop that!" or "Me want"). To diminish the likelihood of misinterpretation, it is necessary to ensure that the child uses language with communicative intent (demonstrating underlying comprehension), that the child is an active participant in the communication and simple repetition is not credited, and that novel combinations of words are used.

Language delay exists when the child's rate of language development approximates 75%. This is a somewhat higher cutoff than for motor delay because of the increased prevalence of language disorders over cerebral palsy. In the general population, a rate of 70% approximates the 95th percentile and a rate of

55% approximates the 99th percentile. A clinical approach to language delay is outlined in Table 18.5.

Fine Motor/Problem-Solving Sequences

Fine motor/problem-solving abilities are used as the basis of infant intelligence tests because of the difficulty in eliciting language in infants and toddlers and the previous lack of appreciation of prelinguistic development. These abilities are not used for routine developmental surveillance because delays in fine motor or problem-solving functions are not early presentations for developmental disorders. (The exception is seen when there is asymmetrical hand function.) In addition, fine motor/problem-solving abilities are not amenable to parental report because of the fine distinctions that must be made and the rigor required to define specific tasks. The assessment of fine motor/problem-solving abilities is needed to separate communicative disorders from intellectual disabilities.

Table 18.5. A clinical approach to language delay

1. Does language delay exist?
2. Is the child showing consistent progress but a slow rate of development?
3. Is this primarily an expressive delay or a mixed receptive/expressive delay?
4. Are other developmental sequences involved?
5. Is this a generalized process? Are other sequences involved to an equal degree? (Consider intellectual disabilities if problem-solving abilities are delayed similarly.)
6. Does the parent have any questions about the child's ability to hear?
7. Are there risk factors for developmental disorders?
8. What disorders (e.g., hearing loss, intellectual disabilities, language lags, articulation disorders, learning disorders, dyslexia, autism) exist in the family?
9. Does the child have any dysmorphisms (particularly growth disturbances and findings about the head and neck) or stigmata of metabolic dysfunction (e.g., goiter)?
10. Differential diagnosis and recommendations for further evaluation:
    a. If the child is losing language ability, careful documentation of baseline abilities is indicated as a prelude to evaluation for neurodegenerative processes.
    b. Most mild expressive delays are familial and resolve without treatment.
    c. Children with mixed receptive/expressive disorders or severe expressive delays (developmental quotients < 60) should receive a full psycholinguistic evaluation, including audiology, psychological testing, and speech and language evaluations.
    d. Infants with generalized processes or major risk factors should have a comprehensive neurodevelopmental evaluation that focuses on motor as well as psycholinguistic abilities.
    e. Audiological evaluation is indicated whenever a parent raises a question about the child's ability to hear.
    f. Dysmorphisms of the head and neck should raise the possibility of hearing loss.
    g. Dysmorphisms or stigmata of metabolic dysfunction should be further evaluated as indicated by the findings. Such findings may be associated with intellectual disabilities or other developmental disorders.

Fine motor/problem-solving abilities are the end result of the coupling of visual, motor, and cognitive functions. In the earliest part of the first year, visual interaction is the main focus. Between the second and last quarter of the first year, hand function is refined. It is in the last part of the first year and into the second year that problem-solving ability clearly emerges. As the child develops, fine motor/problem-solving ability evolves into visual perception and spatial organizing abilities. With increased language function, verbal equivalents of problem solving emerge and are able to be measured.

Table 18.6 lists sequences of fine motor/problem-solving abilities that occur during the first 2 years of life.

Delay, Dissociation, and Deviance in Diagnosis

Delay If the parameters measured in developmental assessment are the times of achievement of the developmental milestone sequences, then three adverse outcomes are possible. The first adverse outcome occurs when there is significant delay in the developmental sequences. Delay may occur across sequences or affect only a single stream of development. Delay brings children to attention.

Traditionally, delay has been defined as a developmental rate of less than 70%. More recently, delay has been defined as a rate of less than 75%. Although appropriate for language and problem-solving abilities because the rates of retardation and language disorders approximate 5%, this definition is not logical for motor functions when the rate of cerebral palsy is less than 1%. For motor abilities, it is probably more appropriate to consider a rate of 50%–60% to be delayed; however, because of the association between nondisabling motor dysfunction and communication disorders and intellectual disabilities, it is warranted to perform a language assessment on children whose rate of motor development is less than 70%.

J.R. is a 40-month-old boy who presented with a chief complaint of language delay. His language

Table 18.6. Major fine motor/problem-solving developmental milestones

Milestone	Mean age of achievement (months)
Visual	
Fixation (alerting)	Birth
Follows across midline (horizontal or vertical)	2
Follows in a circle	3
Visual threat	3
Notices pellet	5
Fine motor	
Hands open	3
Hands to midline	4
Transfers objects	5
Unilateral reach	6
Inferior pincer	9
Mature pincer	11
Voluntary release	12
Problem solving	
Inspects objects	7–8
Object constancy	
Looks over edge	9
Uncovers toy	10
Recovers cube under cup	11
Writing	
Marks paper	12
Scribbles in imitation	16
Scribbles spontaneously	18
Pellet/bottle tasks	
Places pellet in bottle	12
Dumps pellet in imitation	14
Spontaneously dumps pellet	16

development was notable for cooing at 5 months, babbling at 1 year, saying his first word at 18 months, and not putting words into sentences until 2 months ago. He uses "I" and "you" appropriately but occasionally misuses "me." J.R. does not use tense or plurals. He knew all of his primary body parts by 2½ and has recently stopped echoing. His mother thinks J.R. hears adequately. His early history did not reveal significant medical events. His other developmental milestones were also achieved later. He did not walk until 18 months and does not engage in interactive play, but feeds himself and can undress. Assessment of his language abilities found him to be functioning at approximately 2 years in expressive language and 2½ years in receptive language. His fine motor/problem-solving skills were at the 26-month level. J.R.'s delay was thought to be

global, and his mild intellectual disability was confirmed on psychological testing.

Developmental delay is a symptom and not a diagnosis. Some have advocated starting therapy but deferring a diagnosis to increase certainty and spare parents unnecessary grief. Developmental delays, however, result from a variety of causes. Treating delay without a diagnosis frequently results in incomplete habilitation, unrealistic goals, and frustrated children, parents, and therapists. In addition, treating delay without a diagnosis may impede proper therapy.

Dissociation Another adverse outcome of assessment is dissociation, which occurs when one stream of development is significantly out of phase with the other streams. By convention, dissociation exists when there is a 15% discrepancy in abilities. As mentioned previously, dissociation occurs commonly in children with developmental disorders and is a means of achieving early diagnoses (see Table 18.2). Cerebral palsy is associated with a language–motor dissociation with the motor abilities being significantly behind. Intellectual disability has depression of language and problem-solving abilities with better motor abilities. Communicative (and hearing) disorders show delay in language areas and sparing of problem-solving and motor areas. Because there may be multiple disorders in a single child, the areas of strength are relative and development evidenced in these areas may not be normal.

L.B. is a 13-month-old girl referred for failure to sit. Her gross motor milestones were delayed. She did not roll until 7 months and did so by "flipping." Sitting propped was accomplished at 10 months, but she has been unable to sit erect without arm support and cannot assume a sitting posture independently. Her past medical history revealed that she was born at 34 weeks' gestation and had suffered a grade 2 intraventricular hemorrhage and mild jaundice but was otherwise a perfectly healthy premature infant. By contrast to her motor delays, her language was precocious. She used 10 words, knew three primary body parts, and used directed pointing. Her parents reported that L.B. had a pincer grasp since 1 year of age but was not yet handed. The physical examination was notable for hypotonia to passive movement at the hips but spastic catches at the ankles. Some resistance to straight leg raising was noted.

Deep tendon reflexes were symmetrically increased in the legs, with an increased reflexogenic zone and unsustained clonus at the ankles. Toe signs were upgoing. L.B. had a strong positive supporting reflex but was not significantly restricted by other primitive reflexes. Propping responses were established anteriorly and laterally. This child showed a motor–language dissociation with motor abilities being further behind, and in addition had an upper extremity–lower extremity dissociation with more involvement in the legs. Thus, L.B. was diagnosed to have a spastic diplegia.

Deviance The third adverse outcome that may result from assessment is the nonsequential, or deviant, achievement of developmental milestones. This may be exemplified by children who skip milestones or do not follow the expected sequence (e.g., the child who never crawls, or the child who uses 75 words but does not yet use sentences). Children who show deviant development may also be delayed (e.g., early infantile autism), but more commonly they later manifest disorders of central processing/communication.

Etiological Evaluation

Unfortunately, there is no "standard workup" for children with developmental disorders. Practice parameters have been put forth by the American Academy of Neurology (AAN) (Shevell et al., 2003), the AAP (Moeschler, Shevell, & Committee on Genetics, 2006), and the American College of Medical Genetics (Curry et al., 1997) for the evaluation of the child with developmental delay or intellectual disability (Table 18.7). The AAN has published practice parameters for children with cerebral palsy.

Table 18.7. Suggested etiological evaluation of the child with delayed development

Test	Comment	Yield
In-depth history	Includes pre-, peri-, and postnatal events (including seizures); developmental attainments; and three-generation pedigree in family history	
Physical examination	Particular attention to minor/subtle abnormalities	
	Neurological examination for skull abnormalities, focality, and abnormalities of tone; primitive reflexes; and postural responses (in infants)	
	Behavioral phenotype	
Vision/hearing evaluation		
Karyotype		3.7%
Fragile X screen	Preselection on clinical grounds may increase yield to 7.6%	2.6%
Neuroimaging	MRI preferred	40%–55%
	Positives increased by abnormalities of skull contour or size, or focal neurological examination	
	Identification of specific etiologies is rare; most conditions that are found do not alter treatment plan	
	Need to weigh risk of sedation against possible yield	
Thyroid function (T_3, T_4, TSH levels)	Near 0% in settings with universal newborn screening program	~4%
Serum lead level	If there are identifiable risk factors for excessive environmental lead exposure	?
Metabolic testing	Urine organic acids, plasma amino acids, ammonia, lactate, and a capillary blood gas; focused testing based on clinical findings warranted	~1%
Subtelomeric deletion	Obtain in the presence of dysmorphisms with a normal karyotype and fragile X DNA study; higher in severe intellectual disability	6.6%
MECP2 for Rett syndrome	Females with severe intellectual disability	?
EEG	May be deferred in absence of history of seizures	~1%

Sources: Curry et al. (1997) and Shevell et al. (2003).
Key: EEG, electroencephalogram; MRI, magnetic resonance imaging; T_3, triiodothyronine; T_4, thyroxine; TSH, thyroid-stimulating hormone.

Such parameters do not provide a clinical cookbook. Instead, they note that inquiry related to genetic conditions or moderating factors, such as chronic disease states or metabolic/progressive neurological processes, is dictated by history and physical findings. Historical questions related to the pre-, peri-, and postnatal periods are found in standard pediatric texts. Special care must be taken when eliciting the developmental history to ensure that the child has not plateaued or deteriorated. The family history should focus on genetic and neurological diseases as well as developmental disorders (including learning disabilities). The physical examination should focus on structural abnormalities, dysmorphic findings, neurological abnormalities, and signs of metabolic storage disease (e.g., organomegaly). Further etiological evaluations may be wide ranging and include neuroimaging, chromosome analysis, sophisticated metabolic studies, and electrophysiological techniques. Such investigations have low yield but may be of great importance if a hereditary condition can be found.

Reevaluation is important if the initial assessment does not reveal an etiological diagnosis. This is because facial dysmorphisms may not be appreciated as a syndrome until the child ages, new disorders are being described (e.g., congenital disorders of glycosylation), and previously described disorders are found to have a broader expression in populations other than those initially described (e.g., fragile X syndrome in females and *MECP2* abnormalities in males).

DIAGNOSIS AND BEYOND

Assessment is a part of the diagnostic and therapeutic process. One result of assessment should be to arrive at a diagnosis. Developmental diagnoses are based on the most evident aspects of the child's dysfunction. They have been criticized because they are not related to etiology, are not grounded in neural mechanisms, are not sufficient to define a treatment program, and are of limited value in prognostication. Despite this, diagnosis remains the cornerstone of treatment for the fol-

lowing reasons (Shapiro, Wachtel, Palmer, & Camputo, 1987):

1. A full developmental diagnosis is necessary to establish a developmental profile with reasonable goals.

2. The provision of therapeutic services is dependent on the establishment of a diagnosis.

3. Lack of a diagnosis precludes genetic counseling.

4. Although limited, general prognostic statements can be derived from the diagnosis.

Diagnosis is not sufficient to define a treatment program. If a child is found to have a developmental disorder, a comprehensive evaluation should be performed to establish a developmental profile. A developmental profile may include assessments that measure a variety of different domains in addition to function. Anatomical measures such as joint angles and alignment may be evaluated in children who undergo orthopedic surgery. Dynamic measures such as those found in movement analysis may be used in assessment. Physical measures such as work, time, speed, or force may be used. Assessment may extend beyond the performance of an action and include measuring the desires of the patient or family to assist prioritization of treatment objectives. A developmental profile will determine the presence of additional impairments, identify the current needs, define the long-term goals, and attempt to discover the etiology of the dysfunctions.

The causes of neural dysfunction in childhood are diffuse, and because of the multiplicity of diagnoses and the wide variance within diagnostic categories, the resulting treatment program is likely to be unique to each individual child. Periodic reassessments are required to ensure that the treatment program is still valid. Reassessments should be performed whenever a child is not meeting expectations. Planned reassessments are usually performed quarterly in infancy, semiannually in early elementary school, and at times of transition (e.g., before entrance to middle school and high school, in the latter part of high school).

Reassessments yield valuable information about responses to treatment. Measuring developmental function at the start of therapy and at a later time can tell you whether the child is making progress relative to his or her developmental rate.

S.A. is 33 months old. She started speech and language therapy at 24 months. At the start of therapy, she had about 10 words and was jargoning (age equivalent, 18 months). She now has 50 words and uses some 2-word sentences (age equivalent, 24 months). Her parents are very happy that she is communicating so well.

At the start of therapy, S.A.'s rate of language development was 75% (18/24). At 33 months, her rate of language development was 73% (24/33). Even though S.A. is communicating more, her rate of development was not altered by her speech and language therapy.

Repeated assessments provide important information for long-term planning. If several evaluations reveal consistent rates of development, then it may be possible to use the information to prognosticate. For example, if a child is functioning at a 6-month level at 12 months, a 12-month level at 24 months, and an 18-month level at 36 months, one could expect that the child would maintain his or her rate of development and be functioning at an 8-year level at age 16 years.

In a broader context, assessment may result in identification of community characteristics that need to be modified to ensure full participation. For example, knowing the number of local children with severe behavior disturbance would influence planning and allocation of educational resources. Knowing the number of people with developmental disorders in the community who are unemployed because they lack transportation to get to work might result in changes in the public transportation system.

CONCLUSION

Early identification is a prerequisite to early intervention. Most children with developmental disorders present because of parental concerns relating to failure to achieve age appropriate expectations. Mild motor delay (motor quotient > 50) is not uncommon and usually is not associated with cerebral palsy. Motor delay is a marker for aberrant neurodevelopment

and may be associated with cognitive/linguistic dysfunction. Delayed language acquisition is the most common presenting sign of neurodevelopmental dysfunction in early childhood. Primary care providers should focus on language development and note achievement of language milestones as part of well-child, preventive health-care visits. The use of developmental rates to define the developmental phenomena of delay, dissociation, or deviance will enable the primary care provider to progress beyond recognition of language delay to the diagnosis of autism, intellectual disabilities, receptive-expressive language disorders, or hearing loss.

REFERENCES

Accardo, P.J., & Capute, A.J. (1979). *The pediatrician and the developmentally delayed child.* Baltimore: University Park Press.

Accardo, P.J., & Capute, A.J. (Eds.). (2005). *The Capute Scales: Cognitive Adaptive Test/Clinical Auditory & Linguistic Milestone Scale [CAT/CLAMS].* Baltimore: Paul H. Brookes Publishing Co.

Bzoch, K.R., League, R., & Brown, V.L. (2003). *Receptive-Expressive Emergent Language Test: A method for assessing the language skills of infants* (3rd ed.). Austin, TX: PRO-ED.

Capute, A.J., Palmer, F.B., Shapiro, B.K., Wachtel, R.C., Schmidt, S., & Ross, A. (1986). Clinical Linguistic and Auditory Milestone Scale: Prediction of cognition in infancy. *Developmental Medicine and Child Neurology, 28,* 762–771.

Capute, A.J., & Shapiro, B.K. (1985). The Motor Quotient: A method for the early detection of motor delay. *American Journal of Diseases of Children, 139,* 940–942.

Coplan, J. (1993). *Early Language Milestone Scale* (2nd ed.). Austin, TX: PRO-ED.

Council on Children with Disabilities, Section on Developmental Behavioral Pediatrics, Bright Futures Steering Committee, Medical Home Initiatives for Children with Special Needs Project Advisory Committee. (2006). Identifying infants and young children with developmental disorders in the medical home: An algorithm for developmental surveillance and screening. *Pediatrics, 118,* 405–420.

Curry, C.J., Stevenson, R.E., Aughton, D., Byrne, J., Carey, J.C., Cassidy, S., et al. (1997). Evaluation of mental retardation: Recommendations of a Consensus Conference: American College of Medical Genetics. *American Journal of Medical Genetics, 72,* 468–477.

Frankenburg, W.K., & Dodds, J.B. (1969). *The Denver Developmental Screening Test.* Denver: University of Colorado Medical Center.

Individuals with Disabilities Education Improvement Act of 2004, PL 108-446, 20 U.S.C. §§ 1400 *et seq.*

Klackenburg, G. (1980). What happens to children with retarded speech development at 3? *Acta Paediatrica Scandinavica, 69,* 681–685.

Knobloch, H., & Pasamanick, B. (1963). Predicting intellectual potential in infancy. *American Journal of Diseases of Childhood, 106,* 43–51.

Lock, T.M., Shapiro, B.K., Ross, A., & Capute, A.J. (1986). Age of presentation in developmental disability. *Journal of Developmental and Behavioral Pediatrics, 7,* 340–345.

Moeschler, J.B., Shevell, M., & Committee on Genetics. (2006). Clinical genetic evaluation of the child with mental retardation or developmental delays. *Pediatrics, 117,* 2304–2316.

Nelson, K.B., & Ellenberg, J.H. (1979). Neonatal signs as predictors of cerebral palsy. *Pediatrics, 64,* 225–232.

Ramey, C.T., & Ramey, S.L. (1998). Prevention of intellectual disabilities: Early interventions to improve cognitive development. *Preventive Medicine, 27,* 224–232.

Shannon, P. (2004). Barriers to family-centered services for infants and toddlers with developmental delays. *Social Work, 49,* 301–308.

Shapiro, B.K., Wachtel, R.C., Palmer, F.B., & Capute, A.J. (1987). Evaluation, diagnosis, treatment, and habilitation. In H.M. Wallace, R.F. Biehl, A.C. Oglesby, & L.T. Taft (Eds.), *Handicapped children and youth* (pp. 126–133). New York: Human Sciences Press.

Shevell, M., Ashwal, S., Donley, D., Flint, J., Gingold, M., Hirtz, D., et al. (2003). Practice parameter: Evaluation of the child with global developmental delay. Report of the Quality Standards Subcommittee of the American Academy of Neurology and the Practice Committee of the Child Neurology Society. *Neurology, 60,* 367–380.

VanderVeer, B., & Schweid, E. (1974). Infant assessment: Stability of mental functioning in young retarded children. *American Journal of Mental Deficiency, 79,* 1–4.

Visintainer, P.F., & Bennett, A. (2005). Standardization of the Capute Scales. In P.J. Accardo & A.J. Capute (Eds.), *The Capute Scales: Cognitive Adaptive Test/Clinical Auditory & Linguistic Milestone Scale (CAT/CLAMS).* Baltimore: Paul H. Brookes Publishing Co.

Wolfensberger, W. (1965). Diagnosis diagnosed. *Journal of Mental Subnormality, 11,* 62–70.

19

The Capute Scales

MARY L. O'CONNOR LEPPERT

The Capute Scales is one of the many contributions Arnold J. Capute made to the field of neurodevelopmental disabilities. Capute's intention was to "provide the pediatrician with a scale of expected linguistic and auditory milestones which can rapidly be applied within the constraints of a busy practice" (Capute & Accardo, 1978, p. 847). The language milestone scale, entitled the Clinical Linguistic and Auditory Milestone Scale (CLAMS), was quite useful in identifying language delay but could not differentiate language delay caused by disorders of communication from that caused by global cognitive disorders. Therefore, a second scale to measure nonverbal cognitive ability was added. This scale, The Clinical Adaptive Test (CAT), expanded Capute's test such that both cognitive streams of development (language and visual-motor abilities) could be assessed. The CAT/ CLAMS, now known as the Capute Scales (Accardo & Capute, 2005), rapidly differentiates communication disorders from intellectual disabilities as the cause of language delay in children younger than 36 months of age.

Accurate early differentiation and diagnosis of the cause of language delay is of great value to the child and his or her parents because accurate diagnosis provides direction for medical etiological workup, alerts the clinician to the presence of associated disorders, provides a factual foundation on which to base parent counseling, and gives direction for early intervention services and follow-up.

HISTORY

All modern developmental assessment measures are based in some degree on the pioneering work of Arnold Gesell. Gesell is credited for establishing the first norms of developmental milestones in five streams of child development: gross motor, visual motor, language, social, and adaptive. Gesell was assiduous in his recording of the timing and sequence of normal development. He observed that, in typically developing children, development is an orderly, timed, and sequential process that occurs with such regularity that it is quite predictable (Gesell & Amatruda, 1947). From his observations, Gesell published the first test of child development. The original test included a large number of test items, employed many instruments, and took quite some time to administer.

Cattell (1940) revised Gesell's original test in order to increase its efficiency. Cattell eliminated test items that were cumbersome, items that employed instruments that were used for very limited test ages, and those items that were subjective in interpretation. Gesell's works were later modified and employed in assessments by such notable authors as Illingsworth (1975), Sheridan (1968), Bayley (1969, 1993), and others.

Capute acknowledged that his tests were constructed as an amalgamation of developmental milestones drawn from a number of sources (Capute & Accardo, 1978). Capute and colleagues aimed to design a test that would

This chapter is adapted by permission from Accardo, P.J., & Capute, A.J. (Eds.). (2005). *The Capute Scales: Cognitive Adaptive Test and Clinical Linguistic and Auditory Milestone Scale (CAT/CLAMS)*. Baltimore: Paul H. Brookes Publishing Co.

minimize the number of test items and employ only items that covered a wide range of testing ages and were not subject to too much interpretation. The employment of test items that can be used across a range of ages minimizes the shifts between items, maintains the engagement of the child, and allows the examiner the opportunity to observe when a child reaches the limit of his or her ability on a test item.

Following the addition of the visual-motor portion of the test, the CAT/CLAMS was used in research with children with varying histories or conditions that put them at increased risk for developmental delay. The language scale was tested first in a group of children with motor impairment (Capute, Shapiro, Wachtel, Gunther, & Palmer, 1986), and then in children with suspected delay (Hoon, Pulsifer, Gopalan, Palmer, & Capute, 1993; Kube, Wilson, Petersen, & Palmer, 2000; Rossman et al., 1994; Wachtel, Shapiro, Palmer, Allen, & Capute, 1994), children with HIV infection (Wachtel, Teppert, Houck, McGrath, & Thompson, 1994), children with hypoplastic left heart syndrome (Rogers et al., 1995), and high-risk infants (Doig, Macias, Saulor, Craver, & Ingram, 1999). Finally, the Capute Scales were studied in a group of children with no known risk or suspicion of delay, in order to assess how well the Scales identified children with delay when compared with the Bayley Scales of Infant Development II (BSID-II) (Bayley, 1993; Leppert, Shank, Shapiro, & Capute, 1998). The Capute Scales correlated well with the BSID-II in this population, which suggested its usefulness in general pediatrics for well-child care. The Capute Scales were then standardized in a large normative population. The standardization (Visintainer, Leppert, Bennett, & Accardo, 2004) was a multicenter effort in which data were collected from 1,402 children tested at prescribed ages in the general pediatric setting. Some 1,055 protocols filled appropriate inclusion criteria to be used for data interpretation. Of the 1,402 children included, 53.5% were male and 63.7% were Caucasian.

Inclusion criteria for the standardization encompassed children who presented for well-child care and were born between 36 and 42 weeks' gestation, spoke English as the primary language in the home, and were within a defined age window at the time of the exam. Children were excluded from the standardization if they were of low birth weight, had a known or suspected developmental delay, had seizures, were from non–English speaking homes, or were not in the care of their birth parents. The standardization of the Capute Scales indicated that there was tremendous agreement between the language and visual-motor scores achieved by the normative sample of children at specific test ages and the milestones established on the Capute Scales at the same test ages.

PRINCIPLES OF THE CAPUTE SCALES

Language delay is a frequent concern of parents of children between the ages of 18 and 36 months of age. Symptoms include limited vocabulary, lack of phrase or sentence use at age-appropriate levels, failure to understand the spoken word, and failure to speak understandably. The differential diagnoses of these concerns include hearing impairment, communication disorders (expressive language disorders, receptive and expressive language disorders, autism, selective mutism, speech production disorders), and intellectual disabilities. The initial investigation for any child with delayed language should be an age-appropriate hearing assessment.

In the presence of adequate hearing, assessment turns to the two cognitive streams of development: language and visual-motor abilities. The Capute Scales measures each stream individually and employs the developmental quotient (DQ) to ascertain a rate of development in each stream. Once rates of development are established in individual streams, the rates are compared to determine if delay is pervasive, and therefore indicative of intellectual disabilities, or limited to the language stream, thereby indicating a disorder of communication.

Gesell clearly delineated the normal sequence and timing of milestone acquisition in each of the five streams of development that form the basis of all developmental assessment (Gesell & Amatruda, 1947). The regularity and predictability of normal development provide a paradigm by which abnormal development may be appreciated. Abnormal or atypical development may take any one or a combination of three patterns: delay, deviancy, or dissociation.

Developmental *delay* is defined as a slower rate of milestone acquisition than is normally expected, but one in which the normal order and sequence of milestone acquisition are maintained. Delay may be seen in a single stream of development or across several streams and is determined by the presence of a DQ that is less than 70–75. The pattern that a child's developmental rate takes over time may be of both diagnostic and prognostic value. Longitudinal assessments of development that portray a consistent, albeit delayed, developmental pattern are prognostic of future delay. A pattern of normal developmental rate followed by a plateau or regression in developmental rate raises etiological concerns of degenerative disorders. In addition, developmental rate may be used to monitor recovery or the response to therapy in a child who has previously demonstrated delay.

Deviancy is the nonsequential acquisition of milestones within a specific developmental stream. As an example, a parent may report that a child "rolls over" at 2 months (normal age expected for this milestone is 4–5 months), but examination indicates that the child's highest motor skill is propping up on his or her elbows in the prone position (normally a 3-month-age skill). This motor vignette is considered deviant in that propping up to the elbows, then to the wrists, in prone should precede rolling. In the language stream, deviancy is seen in the uncoupling of the rates of receptive and expressive milestones acquisition, or in the uncoupling of expressive milestones alone. The child reported to have a 100-word vocabulary (> 24-month age equivalent) but who cannot speak in phrases (< 21-month age equivalent) exemplifies expressive language deviancy. Unlike delay and dissociation, deviancy does not imply a diagnosis, but it does indicate to the clinician that there is likely to be an underlying pathology causing the deviancy within that stream that begs further assess-

ment, or, as in the case of language, a cautious review of the language history.

Dissociation is an uneven rate of milestone acquisition (disparate DQs) when comparing two or more streams of development. An example of dissociation is seen in a 24-month-old child with gross motor skills at a 12-month age equivalent (DQ = 50), but with language and visual-motor skills that approximate his or her chronological age (DQs near 100). In such an example, the child demonstrates significant motor delay that is dissociated from other streams of development, suggesting the possible presence of cerebral palsy or motor impairment, but normal cognitive skills. Dissociation, as it applies to the Capute Scales, is seen when there is a discrepancy between the two cognitive streams of development. Most frequently the dissociative pattern will be that of delayed language development in the presence of normal visual-motor abilities, indicating a communication disorder. When both language and visual-motor streams are delayed to a DQ less than 70, with little discrepancy or dissociation between the streams, intellectual disability is the implied diagnosis.

TEST ADMINISTRATION

The language battery of the Capute Scales relies almost exclusively on parental history in the first 18 months of life, then on a combination of parental history and clinical observation. The visual-motor battery requires direct observation of a child performing specific test items during the assessment. Capute often remarked that "Children love to show off." To ensure that a child has the opportunity to show off, and thus optimize cooperation with testing, all testing should begin at an age set several months lower than the child's estimated mental age. To that end, the Capute Scales scoring sheet begins with the question: "Like how old a child does your child act?" Maternal estimate of a child's developmental age is generally accurate (Pulsifer, Hoon, Palmer, Gopalan, & Capute, 1994) and provides the examiner with information that allows testing to begin at an age level that assures that a child will meet success from the start. By starting visual-motor testing below the estimated age of development, the examiner is assured that a basal age will be established during the evaluation. If a child is performing well on younger test items, and subsequently refuses to attempt test items or reverts to a younger use of the item (e.g., stacking blocks vertically when the examiner is demonstrating a horizontal four-cube train), it will be apparent to the examiner that a child's refusal is from his or her inability to perform, rather than his or her unwillingness to comply.

Testing is generally done in a setting with few distractions, with the parents seated next to the child but asked not to prompt the child during the testing. In the younger or reluctant child, it often behooves the examiner to have the child seated on a parent's lap for testing. The child is seated at a table of suitable height for testing, and the examiner sits across from the child with the testing items within reach, but preferably not on the testing surface. Infants younger than 5–6 months may be tested in the supine position. Language history is generally obtained using a standard set of questions for both receptive and expressive skills. Visual-motor skills are tested beginning below the child's estimated age ability, then advancing through all tests with the same item until the child reaches the limit of his or her ability with the item. For example, the examiner introduces the red ring to a child and observes that the child can follow the ring in a circle, then allows the child to reach for and pull down the ring. The ring is left with the child as the examiner observes the child's ability to transfer and possibly inspect the ring. If the child is successful in transfer and inspection, the examiner will test if the child will pull the ring by the string. The use of one test item continually from the basal level to the ceiling of the child's ability provides continuity during testing, lessens frustration over the removal of an interesting toy, and reduces the overall test time.

Language Scale Administration

The language battery relies almost exclusively on parental history of the language abilities in children younger than 18 months of age, but testing in the older child requires some participation and demonstration, particularly of receptive language abilities. The test items that require the child to perform during the assessment are marked with an asterisk (*) on the testing form (Table 19.1). Acquiring informa-

Table 19.1. Language test items and age in months

Age	Test item(s)
1	1. Alerts to sound (R*)
	2. Soothes when picked up (R)
2	1. Social smile (R*)
3	1. Cooing (E)
4	1. Orients to voice (R*)
	2. Laughs aloud (E)
5	1. Orients towards bell laterally (R*)
	2. Ah-goo (E)
	3. Razzing (E)
6	1. Babbling (E)
7	1. Orients towards bell (upwardly/indirectly) (R*)
8	1. "Dada" inappropriately (E)
	2. "Mama" inappropriately (E)
9	1. Orients toward bell (upward indirectly) (R*)
	2. Gesture language (E)
10	1. Understands "no" (R)
	2. Uses "dada" discriminately (E)
	3. Uses "mama" discriminately (E)
11	1. One word (other than "mama" and "dada") (E)
12	1. One-step command with gesture (R)
	2. Two-word vocabulary (E)
14	1. Three-word vocabulary (E)
	2. Immature jargoning (E)
16	1. Four- to six-word vocabulary (E)
	2. One-step command without gesture (R)
18	1. Mature jargoning (E)
	2. Seven- to 10-word vocabulary (E)
	3. Points to one picture (R*)
	4. Identifies two or more body parts (R)
21	1. 20-word vocabulary (E)
	2. Two-word phrases (E)
	3. Points to two pictures (R*)
24	1. 50-word vocabulary (E)
	2. Two-step command (R)
	3. Two-word sentences (E)
30	1. Uses pronouns appropriately (E)
	2. Concept of "one" (R*)
	3. Points to seven pictures (R*)
	4. Repeats two digits forward (E*)
36	1. 250-word vocabulary (E)
	2. Three-word sentence (E)
	3. Repeats three digits forward (E*)
	4. Follows two-prepositional commands (R*)

Key: *Should be performed by child; E, expressive language; R, receptive language.

tion about language milestones from the parents is expeditious and also eliminates the need for children to demonstrate verbal skills at an age when they are reluctant to speak to strangers. The cost of the reliance on parental history, however, is that the examiner must be assiduous in obtaining a detailed history and diligent in assuring the accuracy of milestones to avoid overestimating a child's verbal abilities. The examiner will be more successful in assessment if he or she defines the milestone in question. In particular, vocabulary, mature and immature jargon, phrases (noun and modifier), and sentences (noun and verb) often require definition by example for a parent to report accurately.

Vocabulary size is defined as the number of words or word approximations that are used consistently, specifically, and spontaneously, but vocabulary does not include proper nouns such as the names of family members. Word approximations are words that have some component of a single word but may have dropped a consonant or syllable (e.g., "bobble" for *bottle,* "at" for *cat*). A word approximation that is understandable to the parent and used specifically and consistently by the child may be considered part of the vocabulary. Spontaneous word use is important to stress in the history because children will echo words that they have just heard (echolalia) but may not be able to use the same word spontaneously when the appropriate time arises. Echolalia is a normal developmental phenomenon that consists of the repetition of a word or of a whole or a part of a sentence. Echolalia generally begins at about 18 months of age, peaks at 24 months of age, and should be considered abnormal after about 30 months of age.

Immature jargon is described as the use of spontaneous gibberish that reflects the tone, prosody, and inflection of mature language use but is completely nonsensical. Immature jargon is present at a developmental age when vocabulary consists of about 3 words (14 months). Mature jargon is a similar string of gibberish with tone and inflection, but the child will use a formed, understandable word in the midst of the nonsense. Mature jargoning is coincident with a vocabulary of approximately 7–10 words (18 months).

Two-word phrases are consistent with a vocabulary of about 20 words and are generally seen at a developmental level of about 21 months. It is prudent to define a 2-word phrase as a noun and a modifier such as "big truck" and "Daddy car." Often parents will credit children for the use of 2-word phrases that are actually single-word concepts, such as "thank you" or "hot dog." Two-word sentences generally occur at 24 months of age, require the use of both a noun and a verb, and are associated with a vocabulary of about 50 words.

Defining expressive language milestones helps reduce the overinflation of a child's expressive abilities. Further precision can be achieved if the examiner recognizes that the expressive skills can be paired to ensure accuracy. Using "Mama" and "Dada" specifically generally occurs with the acquisition of the first word. Immature jargoning is consistent with a 3-word vocabulary, mature jargoning is consistent with a 10-word vocabulary, 2-word phrases with 20 words, and 2-word sentences with 50 words; 3-word sentences and pronoun use are consistent with a 250-word vocabulary. An examiner aware of these paired milestones will make further inquiries to clarify the expressive language in a child whose paired milestones are discrepant. For instance, a child who is credited with a 20-word vocabulary but is not using any mature jargoning is deviant. Before accepting these conflicting milestones, one might ask the parent to list the words that make up the vocabulary and inquire again if the words are used spontaneously.

Receptive milestones in the first 18 months of life are also largely taken from parental reports. The ages at which a baby smiles, turns to Mom's voice, and understands "no" are some of the milestones noted in the first year by parental history. Responding to the bell (alerting at 1 month, and responses at 5, 7, and 9 months) requires observation of the child in the exam setting. Active participation in receptive language skills assessment begins at 18 months, when children begin to point to pictures on the picture test cards and point to facial body parts to demonstrate understanding. At 36 months, the child must demonstrate understanding of two separate prepositional commands in response to an examiner's directions

("Put this cube under the cup, and put this cube in front of the cup.").

As with the expressive language skills, clarity in the history taking of receptive language skills ensures accuracy of the developmental assessment. While inquiring about a child's ability to follow a two-step command, one must ensure the commands are not related. For example, "Get your shoes, and put them on" is a two-step command that can be accomplished by following only one command, "Put your shoes on." In contrast, "Put on your shoes, and shut the door" is a two-step command that requires two separate responses. All responses to the language battery are recorded on the scoring sheet as "yes" for items that the

child passes, and "no" for the items that the child fails. One begins the test about two age sets below the child's estimated level of abilities and proceeds until the child reaches a ceiling age, defined as the highest age set at which a child has any correct responses.

Visual-Motor Scale Administration

The visual-motor ability scale employs 11 test components that cover 57 milestones over 19 test ages (Table 19.2). Unlike the language battery, during the visual-motor assessment the child must successfully perform all of the test items, some spontaneously and some after demonstration by the examiner. Again, it is

Table 19.2. Visual-motor test items and age in months

Age	Test item	Age	Test item
1	1. Visually fixates momentarily on red ring 2. Chin off table in prone	12	1. Releases one cube in cup 2. Crayon mark
2	1. Visually follows ring horizontally and vertically 2. Chest off table in prone	14	1. Solves glass frustration 2. Out and in with peg 3. Solves pellet-bottle with demonstration
3	1. Visually follows ring in circle 2. Supports on forearms in prone 3. Visual threat response	16	1. Solves pellet-bottle spontaneously 2. Round block in formboard 3. Scribbles in imitation
4	1. Unfisted 2. Manipulates fingers 3. Supports on wrists in prone	18	1. Ten cubes in cup 2. Solves round hole in formboard reversed 3. Spontaneous scribbling with crayon 4. Pegboard completed spontaneously
5	1. Pulls down ring 2. Transfers 3. Regards pellet	21	1. Obtains object with stick 2. Solves square in formboard 3. Tower of three cubes
6	1. Obtains cube 2. Lifts cup 3. Radial rake	24	1. Attempts to fold paper 2. Horizontal four-cube train 3. Imitates stroke with crayon 4. Completes formboard
7	1. Attempts pellet 2. Pulls out peg 3. Inspects ring	30	1. Horizontal-vertical stroke with crayon 2. Formboard reversed 3. Folds paper with definite crease 4. Train with chimney
8	1. Pulls ring by string 2. Secures pellet 3. Inspects bell	36	1. Three-cube bridge 2. Draws circle 3. Names one color 4. Draw-a-Person with head plus one other body part
9	1. Scissors grasp (immature pincer) 2. Rings bell 3. Over the edge for toy		
10	1. Combines cube and cup 2. Uncovers bell 3. Fingers pegboard		
11	1. Mature overhand pincer movement 2. Solves cube under cup		

recommended that the testing begin with test items two age sets below the child's estimated level of function to ensure that a basal level is obtained and to help the examiner differentiate the child who can no longer perform advancing test items from the child who refuses to perform the test items. Testing continues sequentially through advancing test sets until a ceiling age is reached.

It is recommended that the test item in use on the visual-motor scale be used sequentially through advancing test ages until the child can no longer perform skills with the item. Cube use begins at 6 months. Initially, the child will attempt to obtain the cube with an immature raking movement. By 10 months, the child will secure the cube, then combine the cube and cup by banging them together, but the 10-month-old child will not release the cube into the cup, even with demonstration. By 11 months of age, the child will seek to find the cube hidden under the cup while the child is watching. (At a mental age younger than 11 months, the child will appear to lose attention to the hidden cube.) At 12 months, a child will voluntarily release one cube into the cup, and by 18 months, he or she will fill the cup with 10 cubes. The 21-month-old will stack a tower of three cubes after demonstration by the examiner. At 24 months, the child will replicate a four-cube horizontal train made by the examiner, and similarly will replicate a four-cube train with a chimney at 30 months. At 36 months, the child will imitate a three-cube bridge demonstrated by the examiner. Use of a single test item at consecutive test ages allows for continuous testing from 6 to 36 months of age without disruption or attention shifting.

The bell is also a test item that is used continually from age 8 to14 months. At 8 months, the child presented with a bell will accept the bell and inspect the bell and clapper with clear interest. By 9 months, the child will ring the bell, and by 10 months, a child who witnesses the bell being covered by a towel or handkerchief will uncover the bell in an effort to continue to play with it. At 14 months of age, the child will solve the glass frustration test. In this test item, a piece of Plexiglas is placed between the child and the bell. The child of 14 months' mental age will demonstrate the understanding that the glass is in the way, and will reach around or over the glass, or attempt to move the glass in order to obtain the bell. The child with cognitive skills younger than 14 months will try nearly to frustration (i.e., the glass frustration test), by swatting at the Plexiglas, to obtain the bell without understanding that the glass is in the way.

Like the cube, cup, and bell, the crayon and paper are used over a wide range of test ages. A child of 12 months of age who is presented with a crayon and paper will mark the paper, particularly after demonstration by the examiner. At 16 months, a child will scribble in imitation of the examiner, but at 18 months, the child given paper and a crayon will scribble spontaneously. At 24 months, the child will imitate a stroke with a crayon, and will attempt to fold a piece of paper in half following demonstration by the examiner. At 30 months, the child imitates horizontal and vertical strokes and will fold the paper with a definite crease after demonstration by the examiner. By 36 months, the child will draw a circle in imitation of one drawn before him or her and will draw a man on request by the examiner.

During all of the visual-motor testing, useful clinical information regarding subtle motor difficulties can be obtained by careful observation of the quality of hand and finger movement. Putting pegs in a pegboard and stacking or lining up cubes are activities in which handedness, tremor, and adventitious movements of the child's hand become quite obvious.

SCORING

It is recommended that testing on the Capute Scales always begin at an age level younger than the maternal estimation of the child's mental age. This ensures that the child will meet success in the early test items, will be more cooperative in testing, and will establish a basal score. The basal score is defined as the highest test age group at which the child successfully completes all of the test items within the age set. Once a basal age is obtained, the examiner will continue to administer test items until a child reaches a test age set in which he or she has no correct responses. The last age set at which a child has any success is considered the ceiling age of the test battery. To calculate the age equivalent, one starts with the basal age and adds the decimal value of each correctly scored item above the basal score to the basal score itself. The age equivalent is then divided by the child's chronological age and multiplied by 100 to determine the DQ. The DQ represents the rate of development in each stream measured. An illustration of the scoring and calculation of the age equivalent and DQ is given in Figure 19.1.

The interpretation of the results of the Capute Scales requires application of the previously discussed principles of delay, deviancy, and dissociation after the DQs for each of the test batteries are calculated and compared. In a typically developing child, the expectation is that

Table 19.3. Diagnostic interpretation of developmental quotients (DQs)

Language DQ	Visual-motor DQ	Diagnosis
Normal	Normal	Normal
Delayed	Delayed	Intellectual disability
Delayed	Normal	Communication disorder

both the language and visual-motor skill DQs are greater than 85 (no delay). In a child with intellectual disability, both of the cognitive streams will be delayed and have DQs of less than 70–75 (Table 19.3). Dissociation is commonly seen in communication disorders in which the language stream is delayed but the

	Yes	No
Eleven months		
1. Mature overhand pincer (0.5)	√	
2. Solves cube under cup (0.5)	√	
Twelve months		
1. Releases one cube in cup (0.5)	√	
2. Crayon mark (0.5)	√	
Fourteen months		
1. Solves glass frustration (0.6)	√	
2. Out and in with peg (0.6)	√	
3. Solves pellet-bottle with demonstration (0.6)		√
Sixteen months		
1. Solves pellet-bottle spontaneously (0.6)		√
2. Round block in formboard (0.6)	√	
3. Scribbles in imitation (0.6)		√
Eighteen months		
1. Ten cubes in cup (0.5)		√
2. Solves round hole in formboard reversed (0.5)		√
3. Spontaneous scribbling with crayon (0.5)		√
4. Pegboard completed spontaneously (0.5)		√

Age equivalent = Basal age (12 months) + 0.6 + 0.6 + 0.6 = 13.8 months
DQ = Age equivalent (13.8 months)/chronological age (20 months) × 100
DQ = 13.8/20 × 100 = 69

Figure 19.1.   Scoring sample.

Table 19.4. Interpretation of language testing

Expressive language	Receptive language	Diagnosis
Delayed	Delayed	Receptive and expressive language disorder
Delayed	Normal	Expressive language disorder

visual-motor stream is within normal limits. In the presence of dissociation between streams, the language stream should be closely scrutinized to determine if there is deviancy within the language stream. Deviancy is observed most often when receptive and expressive language abilities are developing at different rates. With rare exception, deviant language is marked by delayed expressive language skills relative to receptive language abilities (Table 19.4).

CAPUTE PEARLS OF WISDOM

The orderly and sequential manner in which milestones are acquired in each of the streams of development was well delineated by Arnold Gesell. Capute appreciated stages or phases within the individual streams of cognitive development (Capute, 1996). Expressive language milestones may be grouped into three phases during the first 2 years of life. The guttural phase, or the very beginning of language, is observed in the first 2 months of life. This phase is characterized by physiological noises (burping, sneezing, crying, yawning) that are in no way an attempt at social interaction.

The prelinguistic phase, or the pre–word utterance phase, begins with cooing at 2–3 months and lasts until about 11 months of age. The prelinguistic phase is characterized by social attempts to initiate or reciprocate language in a fashion that falls short of true word use. The prelinguistic phase begins with cooing, then advances to ah-gooing, razzing, and babbling. Babbling evolves from the 6-month vocalization of repetitive vowel–consonant combinations ("da-da-da-da") to the nonspecific or indiscriminate "dada" sound at about 8 months, which children use to label any person or object of their attention. Shortly thereafter, a child will use "dada" for familiar males, and ultimately "Dada" is used discriminately and specifically for the father figure at 10 months of life.

The prelinguistic phase gives way to the linguistic phase of development at about 11 months of life. The linguistic phase starts with the use of formed identifiable words, generally nouns. The use of the first word generally follows the specific use of "Dada" and "Mama." Single word acquisition is quite slow initially, with one word at about 1 year, and 50 words by 2 years, but expands very quickly to 250 words by 3 years. Children are capable of conveying affect and emotion even before a substantial expressive vocabulary is established. Immature and mature jargoning, seen at 14 and 18 months, respectively, are delivered with tone and expression that imply meaning and sentiment.

As with the language scales, Capute divided the visual-motor milestones of infancy into four stages. In the first month of life (Stage I), the infant uses the eyes only to momentarily fix on an object or person. In the second month (Stage II), the infant uses the eyes as well as head movement to fix and follow an object across the midline in the vertical and horizontal planes. In the third month (Stage III), the infant employs the eyes and head together in such a way that he or she can follow an object in a complete circle and will demonstrate a visual threat response. In Stage IV, at a chronological age of 4 months, the infant will use the eyes, head, and hands to fix, follow, and obtain objects presented in his or her field of vision.

From pulling down and transferring the ring at 5 months to the development of the mature pincer grasp at 11 months, the infant's ability to combine eye, head, and hand movement matures as the refinement of grasp occurs. Grasping and transferring the ring at 5 months requires both visual attention to the ring and reaching the hand to the ring by extension of the whole arm. Initially an infant will grasp an object placed on a surface before him or her or use a raking movement of the whole hand, which is supported by the ulnar border of the hand. By 6 months, an infant can secure an object using the radial rake. The radial rake uses a movement initiated by the index and middle fingers, but ulnar support is no longer required. By 9 months, a child will use an immature pincer grasp or the scissors grasp, which is the use of the thumb and two opposing fingers. By 11 months, the grasp is fully matured to a precise pincer movement recruiting only the thumb and index finger to secure even the smallest of objects.

CONCLUSION

The Capute Scales are a developmental assessment tool used to evaluate the cognitive (language and visual-motor) streams of development. Capute intended that this test be used to differentiate disorders of communication from intellectual disabilities in a child who presents with language delay by employing the developmental principles of delay and dissociation. Capute designed his test such that it could easily be used by pediatric practitioners of different training backgrounds, in a quick and efficient manner, so that it is conducive for use in the primary care setting. The relative paucity of testing items, the continual manner in which they are used, and the ability to rely on parental history of language milestone acquisition add to the expediency of the test.

The ability to quantify delay on the Capute Scales was an additional intention in the design of the test. The employment of the DQ allows the examiner to quantify delay at each assessment and track the rate of development on subsequent assessments. Consistent patterns of delay add certainty to prognosis of future development.

Nearly 30 years of clinical experience with the Capute Scales attest to the success of Capute's goal for this assessment tool. In many different pediatric populations, the tool has proven to be an efficient, accurate, and quantitative measure of cognitive development that is useful in differentiating the child who presents with language delay that is a consequence of a communication disorder from the child whose language delay is secondary to intellectual disabilities.

REFERENCES

Accardo, P.J., & Capute, A.J. (Eds.). (2005). *The Capute Scales: Cognitive Adaptive Test and Clinical Linguistic and Auditory Milestone Scale (CAT/CLAMS).* Baltimore: Paul H. Brookes Publishing Co.

Bayley, N. (1969). *Bayley Scales of Infant Development.* San Antonio, TX: Harcourt Assessment.

Bayley, N. (1993). *Bayley Scales of Infant Development* (2nd ed.). San Antonio, TX: Harcourt Assessment.

Capute, A.J. (1996). CAT/CLAMS pearls of wisdom. In *The Capute Scales: CAT/CLAMS instruction manual.* Baltimore: Author.

Capute, A.J., & Accardo, P.J. (1978). Linguistic and auditory milestones during the first two years of life. *Clinical Pediatrics, 17,* 847–853.

Capute, A.J., Shapiro, B.K., Wachtel, R.C., Gunther, V.A., & Palmer, F.B. (1986). The Clinical Linguistic and Auditory Milestone Scale (CLAMS) identification of cognitive defects in motor delayed children. *American Journal of Diseases of Children, 140,* 694–698.

Cattell, P. (1940). *The measurement of intelligence of infants and young children.* New York: The Psychological Corp.

Doig, K.B., Macias, M.M., Saulor, C.F., Craver, J.R., & Ingram, P.E. (1999). The Child Development Inventory: A developmental outcome measure for follow-up of the high-risk infant. *Journal of Pediatrics, 135,* 358–362.

Gesell, A., & Amatruda, C.S. (1947). *Developmental diagnosis: Normal and abnormal development.* New York: Paul B. Hoeber.

Hoon, A.H., Pulsifer, M.B., Gopalan, R., Palmer, F.B., & Capute, A.J. (1993). The CAT/CLAMS in early cognitive assessment. *Journal of Pediatrics, 123,* S1–S8.

Illingsworth, R.S. (1975). *The development of the infant and young child, normal and abnormal* (6th ed.). Baltimore: Williams & Wilkins.

Kube, D.A., Wilson, W.M., Petersen, M.C., & Palmer, F.B. (2000). CAT/CLAMS: Its use in detecting early childhood cognitive impairments. *Pediatric Neurology, 23,* 208–215.

Leppert, M.L., Shank, T.P., Shapiro, B.K., & Capute, A.J. (1998). The Capute Scales: CAT/CLAMS—a pediatric assessment tool for the early detection of mental retardation and communication disorders. *Mental Retardation and Developmental Disabilities Research Reviews, 4,* 14–19.

Pulsifer, M.B., Hoon, A.H., Palmer, F.B., Gopalan, R., & Capute, A.J. (1994). Maternal estimates of developmental age in preschool children. *Journal of Pediatrics, 125,* S18–S24.

Rogers, B.T., Msall, M.E., Buck, G.M., Lyon, N.R., Norris, M.K., Roland, J.M., et al. (1995). Neurodevelopmental outcomes of children with hypoplastic left heart syndrome. *Journal of Pediatrics, 126,* 496–498.

Rossman, M.J., Hyman, S., Rorabaugh, M.L., Berlin, L.E., Allen, M.C., & Modlin, J.F. (1994). The CAT/CLAMS assessment of early intervention services. *Clinical Pediatrics, 33,* 404–409.

Sheridan, M.D. (1968). *Developmental progress in infants and young children.* London: Her Majesty's Stationery Office.

Visintainer, P., Leppert, M., Bennett, A., & Accardo, P.J. (2004). The standardization of the Capute Scales: Methods and results. *Journal of Child Neurology, 19,* 967–972.

Wachtel, R.C., Shapiro, B.K., Palmer, F.B., Allen, M.C., & Capute, A.J. (1994). CAT/CLAMS: A tool for the pediatric evaluation of infants and young children with developmental delay. *Clinical Pediatrics, 33,* 410–415.

Wachtel, R.C., Tepper, B.J., Houck, D., McGrath, C.J., & Thompson, C. (1994). Neurodevelopment in pediatric HIV infection. *Clinical Pediatrics, 33,* 416–420.

20

Developmental Screening

The Pathway to Early Identification

MARY L. O'CONNOR LEPPERT AND ERIN M. ROSIER

The practice of medicine has changed from the classic role of diagnosis and management of illness to an expanded role of health supervision and disease prevention. The increased role of the pediatrician in screening is seen in the numerous policy statements on screening for newborn metabolic disorders, hearing, environmental lead exposure, blood pressure, vision, and other risk factors. The age at which screening measures are recommended is the balance of the optimal time for disease identification and, in many cases, a critical time period for effective intervention. Newborn screening includes evaluation of disorders such as hypothyroidism and phenylketonuria because early identification and immediate intervention for these disorders substantially change the outcome for the individual child and, indirectly, for society. Newborn hearing screens are now universally recommended because there is good evidence that children with hearing impairment who are identified and treated before 6 months of age have better outcomes on language measures than children identified and treated after 6 months (Yoshinaga-Itano, Sedey, Coulter, & Mehl, 1998).

Developmental screening provides a greater challenge for pediatricians because development is by definition a continuum. It is a process of milestone acquisition, which occurs at an expected rate and in an expected sequence. *Delay* is the term applied to a normal developmental sequence that is occurring at a slower-than-expected rate. The objective of developmental screening tools is to identify delay. Screens are cross-sectional analyses applied to whole populations to identify those individuals not meeting standard expectations for development or behavior at the time of screening. The interpretation of screening test results must then be put into context for each child in regard to that individual child's history and risk factors. Medical predisposition to developmental disorders (e.g., genetic disorders, metabolic disorders, a history of meningitis or prematurity, a family history of delays) or environmental risks such as lead exposure, malnutrition, poverty, and lower parental education level add perspective to the results of isolated screening measures.

Screening, then, must be a complement to a larger mission: *surveillance*. In contrast to screening, surveillance provides longitudinal analysis of behavior and development and does so with the knowledge of historical, environmental, and functional risk factors relevant to an individual child. The American Academy of Pediatrics (AAP) Policy Statement on Surveillance and Screening defined surveillance as a

Flexible, longitudinal, continuous and cumulative process whereby knowledgeable health care professionals identify children who may have developmental problems. There are five components of developmental surveillance: eliciting and attending to the parent's concerns about their child's development, documenting and maintaining a developmental history, making accurate observations of the child, identifying the risk and protective factors and maintaining an accurate record and documenting the process and findings. (2006, p. 408)

Screening, as a complement of the surveillance process, allows a broader perspective to the interpretation of developmental screening measures. A 10-month-old infant who fails a developmental screen because of the absence of canonical babbling is categorically delayed; however, a pediatrician with knowledge of the child's historical risk may appropriately choose to monitor further language acquisition in a child who was born 3 months prematurely or may refer to an audiologist a full-term child with a history of neonatal meningitis or a family history of hearing impairment.

Similarly, surveillance imparts a degree of flexibility to a process that is, by nature, a spectrum of time-dependent processes. Quantifiable delays in gross motor development are alarming in the first year of life but become of qualitative importance after functional walking is achieved. Conversely, qualitatively poor fine motor movement may be observed in toddlers but does not become of functional importance until later, when a child is expected to be able to button, snap, zip, and hold a pencil properly. Similarly, it is unreasonable to screen for learning disabilities until sufficient academic exposure permits appreciation of discrepancy from standard expectation. A pediatrician who has been doing periodic screening and surveillance and who has prior knowledge of risks for an individual child will anticipate age-specific or domain-specific delays, however. For example, one might anticipate fine motor difficulties in a child who was born extremely prematurely or reading disabilities in a child with a history of language delay or a family history of learning disabilities. It is clear that risk does not imply diagnosis but that risk adds an important dimension to the interpretation of signs and symptoms during the diagnostic process.

The concept of domain-specific screening at specific ages may provide more reasonable, more specific, and clearer recommendations to the pediatrician than the previous nebulous recommendation that pediatricians provide periodic screening of all infants and toddlers at preventive health care visits. Significant visual and hearing impairments can and should be identified in the first 6 months of life. Motor disorders are identified in the first year of life. Disorders of communication and cognition generally become evident between the first and third years of life. Difficulties with fine motor development often become evident in preschoolers, as they are expected to learn to button and zip. Disorders of social interactions and behavior are evident at all ages but must be put into context with the child's language, cognition, environment, and the like. The model of age- and domain-specific screening, under the broader task of surveillance, will likely provide the optimal approach to developmental and behavioral health supervision.

RATIONALE FOR SCREENING

The rationale for screening for developmental and behavioral disorders is clearly the early identification of disorders by the identification of developmental delay or failure. The purpose of early identification is fourfold. First, early identification of delay or deviant development within a single developmental stream alerts those doing surveillance to the increased risk of delay in other streams of development. The child diagnosed with a language disorder, for example, is at greater risk for disorders of behavior and social development. Second, early identification may provide strategies to prevent or reduce secondary disorders, such as reducing the cognitive disabilities in children with congenital hypothyroidism with early treatment with levothyroxine or reducing the degree of language disorder in children by early treatment of hearing impairment. Third, early identification of delay or disorder directs diagnostic testing and medical investigation of the etiology of the disorder, which in turn direct family counseling regarding prognosis and possible recurrence risks. Finally, early identification and subsequent definition of developmental delay direct the type and intensity of early intervention services. These benefits of early identification, as a result of screening and surveillance, have formed the bases of screening recommendations by different professional groups and directed federal legislation for early intervention services.

The AAP Committee on Children with Disabilities (2006) has recently updated its policy statement to include an algorithm for developmental surveillance and screening. Surveillance is recommended at every well-child preventative health care visit, and prompt screening employed for any child with whom concern is raised during the surveillance process. In children with whom there is no historical risk and with whom no concerns are raised during surveillance, standardized screening tests are recommended at 9-, 18-, and 30- month well-child visits. The designated ages of routine screening that are recommended focus the screening process on the specific domains most pertinent to the child's chronological age: the 9-month visit focuses on vision, hearing and motor development, as delays or disorders in these areas are generally identifiable at this age. The 18-month screen focuses on language and communication, and, therefore, autism screening is also recommended as part of this evaluation. By the 30-month visit, cognitive and language delays are readily detectable. The AAP's new policy statement continues to recommend that children with whom concerns are raised after screening have diagnostic developmental assessment, a medical evaluation to investigate the etiology of the developmental condition, and a referral to early intervention services.

Coincident with the evolving recommendations for screening and early identification, the federal government has mandated the availability of intervention services at earlier and earlier ages. The Education for All Handicapped Children Act of 1975 (PL 94-142) ensured free and appropriate educational services for school-age children with disabilities. The Individuals with Disabilities Education Act (IDEA) of 1990 (PL 101-476) followed PL 94-142 to provide intervention services for preschoolers. Subsequent amendments to IDEA in 1997 (Part C; PL 105-17) established federally mandated, state-operated early intervention programs from birth onward for infants and toddlers who exhibit disability, delay, or significant risk for delay. Early intervention programs (Part C programs) provide comprehensive, multidisciplinary evaluations; determine the eligibility of a child for services; and define the individual types and goals of services to eligible children from birth to 36 months of age. Primary care providers are encouraged to become familiar with the availability of early intervention services and how to access and col-laborate with these services and their providers. The AAP stated that "An environment should be created in which the physician, family and other service providers work together in a caring, collegial and compassionate atmosphere that ensures that early intervention services are of high quality, accessible, continuous, comprehensive and culturally competent" (2001b, p. 1157).

SCOPE OF THE PROBLEM

Estimates of the incidence of developmental problems diagnosed before 18 years of age range from 11.8% to 18% of children in the United States (Alyward, 1997; Boyle, Decoufle, & Yeargin-Allsopp, 1994; Newacheck et al., 1998); however, the age of a child at diagnosis varies with the type and severity of disability. Children with disorders of lower prevalence but higher severity, such as Down syndrome, cerebral palsy, and neurological disorders, appear to be more likely to be diagnosed early and by a physician than are children with disorders of higher prevalence but lesser severity, such as speech disorders, hyperactivity, and other developmental disorders (Palfrey, Singer, Walker, & Butler, 1987). These disorders of lower severity were also more likely to be diagnosed by nonphysicians than physicians and were more likely to be diagnosed closer to age 5. In the same study, Palfrey et al. found that only 29% of developmental disabilities were diagnosed before 5 years of age.

Data from the *Twenty-Fourth Annual Report to Congress on the Implementation of the Individuals with Disabilities Education Act* indicate that 2% of children between birth and 2 years of age were served under Part C during the 2000–2001 academic year (U.S. Department of Education, 2002). In the same year, 5% of preschoolers (age 3–5) were served under Part B, and 11.5% of children enrolled in preschool through grade 12 received services under the IDEA. Disability categories varied with the age of children served as well; under Part B, approximately 55% of children were diagnosed with speech and language impairments, 25% with developmental delay, 4.3% with intellectual disabilities, and 2.6% with autism. In the same 2000–2001 school year, approximately 50% of children in prekindergarten through twelfth grade were diagnosed with learning disability, 19% with speech and language impairment, 10.6% with intellectual disabilities, and 8% with emotional disturbance. This data set implies that early and effective surveillance for risks, and screening for delays in children from birth to 5 years, may identify at earlier ages a larger proportion of children who will later qualify for services and provide them the benefit of earlier interventions. Intervention for children with delay or risk of delay prior to school entry saves society an estimated $30,000 to $100,000 (Glascoe, 1999).

PRINCIPLES OF DEVELOPMENTAL SCREENING AND SURVEILLANCE

Periodic screening measures are administered to screen large populations of children with little risk for developmental disorders to identify developmental failure in one or more domains of development or behavior. In children who are considered "at risk" for developmental disorders, the screening and surveillance process is often modified. Children with known genetic risks such as Down syndrome require expanded medical and developmental surveillance to include medical issues such as thyroid disease, cardiac or gastrointestinal disorders, and spinal cord compression from atlantoaxial subluxation and also require focused developmental surveillance because of the anticipated difficulties with cognition and language. Biological risks such as congenital hypothyroidism, in utero alcohol or substance exposure, and environmental lead exposure should raise the suspicion level of the primary care provider to specific patterns of delays or disabilities. Historical risk of prematurity, low birth weight, intraventricular hemorrhage, periventricular leukomalacia, perinatal seizure, or postnatal events such as meningitis will direct developmental surveillance and screening measures to specific domains of development.

Environmental and social factors have additional well-documented influences on development. Factors affecting parent–child interaction and poverty have an effect on devel-

opment; children from lower-income homes or homes with diminished child stimulation are more likely to show a decline in cognitive performance in the first few years of life (Aylward, 1996). A subset of children will demonstrate both environmental and biological risks, thus further increasing their risks of developmental and behavioral disorders.

Surveillance of development and behavior in a medical home by a primary care provider who has knowledge of the medical, genetic, familial, and psychosocial background of an individual child gives a greater dimension to the interpretation of developmental screening tests. Screening of a child with a history of 28-week prematurity but no intracranial hemorrhage who is pulling to stand but is not yet walking or cruising will be interpreted differently from that of a term child who is crawling but has not made any effort to pull to stand or cruise at 12 months. Similarly, a child with a known history of a unilateral intrauterine stroke may pass standard motor and cognitive developmental screening measures at 12 months of age, but the knowledgeable clinician will be observant of asymmetry of motor use of the hands in late infancy because of the increased risk of hemiplegia.

Given the fluid nature of development, screening must be done periodically. Many developmental problems are age specific. The new policy statement of the AAP (2006) on screening and surveillance reflects the screening ages most appropriate for age specific developmental problems. Screening of gross motor development is paramount in the first year of life, but becomes less of a focus as a child ambulates well. Language and cognitive disorders come to the fore in the second and third years of life when anticipated vocabulary acquisition or clarity of speech fails to be demonstrated at age-appropriate levels. School-age difficulties such as learning disabilities and graphomotor problems are not recognized until there is occasion to employ the skills required for academics. Some delays or disabilities that are identified early present a second risk for delay or disability later in life. Language delay, particularly receptive and expressive delay, increases the risk of language-based learning disabilities later on and can guide the scope and intensity of future surveillance. It is important to be mindful of the increased risk of secondary disorders in children diagnosed early with more severe disorders. Children may be identified with cerebral palsy by the end of the first year of life, but cognitive, language, attentional, and behavioral disturbances are not identified until much later.

METHODS OF SCREENING

Screening measures take one of two formats: parent questionnaires and clinician-administered tests (Table 20.1). Questionnaires are completed by parents, teachers, or care providers to elicit concerns regarding an individual child that are based on their knowledge of the child's abilities and behaviors. Parent screening tools have a number of advantages that make them ideally suited to the first step in screening. Parent screening measures require very little time from the primary physician, as little as 5 minutes for scoring and counseling parents for normal screens. Questionnaires may be given to parents to complete in the waiting room, mailed to parents for completion prior to a preventive health visit, or given to the parents at a visit to return at a follow-up appointment. Parents who have difficulty with reading or language may require the aid of office staff to complete the questionnaire. Parent screening tools are often quite inexpensive and can cover a wide range of developmental streams. Evidence suggests that some standard parent screening tools meet the same level of sensitivity and specificity (70%–80%) at correctly identifying children with delay as do physician-administered screening tools (Glascoe, 1997). Glascoe (1998), using the Parents' Evaluation of Developmental Status (PEDS), found that parent reliability was not influenced by parent education, family income, or many other socioeconomic variables, and so the PEDS could safely be used in screening in populations of varied demographic characteristics. Finally, Glascoe suggested that the nature of parent concerns was predictive of developmental outcome. Concerns regarding language, global or cognitive skills, fine motor skills, and school skills were good predictors of developmental problems. Glascoe (1999) suggested that the nature of parent concerns could most appropriately direct further diagnostic assessment and intervention.

Numerous physician- or professional-administered screening measures are available, and they vary tremendously in the scope of the screen (general development vs. specific stream of development), in the time required to administer them, and in their psychometric properties (see Table 20.1). Ideally, general screening measures, given either by parent questionnaire or physician administration, that indicate concern in a particular area of development should be followed by an assessment measure of narrow scope that is valid, reliable, sensitive, and specific. To date, no specific screening tools are recommended for use in primary care, and no specific directives exist as to the advantage of parent questionnaires over direct screening measures or vice versa.

PROPERTIES OF SCREENING TESTS

Screening tests should meet basic psychometric standards for specificity, sensitivity, positive predictive value, validity, and reliability. Acceptable levels of specificity and sensitivity on measures of development and behavioral tools are 70%–80% (Glascoe, 2000). Sensitivity represents a procedure's ability to detect a disease if one is present (true positives) (Dawson & Trapp, 2004). Sensitivity, as it applies to developmental screens, is represented arithmetically as the number of positive identifications of delays divided by the number of children with delay, identified or unidentified.

Specificity is a measure of a procedure's ability to give a negative test result if no disease is present (true negatives) (Dawson & Trapp, 2004). Arithmetically, specificity is the number of children identified by the test as normal divided by the actual number of normal children, correctly or incorrectly identified by the test.

The predictive value of a positive test represents the proportion of times that a patient with a positive diagnostic test result actually has the disease being investigated. The predictive value of a negative test represents the proportion of times that a patient with a negative diagnostic test result does not have the disease being investigated (Dawson & Trapp, 2004).

Table 20.1.   Samples of developmental and behavioral screening measures

Ages and Stages Questionnaire (ASQ; Bricker & Squires, 1999)

http://www.brookespublishing.com

Age: 4–60 months

Time: 15 minutes

Format: Parent questionnaire

Description: Communication, gross motor, fine motor, problem solving, personal-social

Battelle Developmental Inventory, Second Edition (BDI-2; Newborg, 2004)

http://www.riverpub.com

Age: Birth to 8 years

Time: 10–30 minutes for screening test

Format: Clinician administered

Description: Personal-social, adaptive, motor, communication, cognition

Bayley Infant Neurodevelopmental Screener (BINS; Aylward, 1995)

http://www.harcourtassessment.com

Age: 3–24 months

Time: 5–10 minutes

Format: Clinician administered

Description: Auditory and visual receptive functions, verbal and expressive motor functions, cognitive processes

BRIGANCE Screens

http://www.curriculumassociates.com

Age:

- Infant and Toddler Screen (Brigance & Glascoe, 2002): Birth to 23 months
- Early Preschool Screen II (Brigance & Glascoe, 2005a): 2–2$\frac{1}{2}$ years
- Preschool Screen II (Brigance & Glascoe, 2005c): 3–4 years
- K & 1 Screen II (Brigance & Glascoe, 2005b): Kindergarten and first grade

Time: 10–15 minutes

Format: Clinician administered

Description: Age-specific domains that may include gross motor, fine motor, self-help, language, social, emotional, preacademics, general knowledge, graphomotor

Child Development Inventory (CDI; Ireton, 1992)

http://www.agsnet.com

Age: 15 months to 6 years

Time: 30–50 minutes

Format: Parent questionnaire

Description: Social, self-help, gross motor, fine motor, expressive language, language comprehension, letters, numbers, general development

Eyberg Child Behavior Inventory (ECBI; Eyberg, 1999)

http://www.parinc.com

Age: 2–16 years

Time: 5 minutes

Format: Clinician administered

Description: Conduct problems

Parents' Evaluation of Developmental Status (PEDS; Glascoe, 1998)

http://www.pedstest.com

Age: Birth to 8 years

Time: 2 minutes if conducted as interview

Format: Parent questionnaire or parent interview

Description: Wide range of developmental, behavioral, and family issues

Pediatric Symptom Checklist (PSC; Jellinek, Patel, Froehle, & Anglin, 2004)
http://www.massgeneral.org/allpsych/PediatricSymptomChecklist/psc_home.htm
Age: 4–16 years
Time: 5 minutes
Format: Parent questionnaire
Description: Psychosocial functioning, emotional and behavioral problems

Temperament and Atypical Behavior Scale (TABS; Bagnato, Neisworth, Salvia, & Hunt, 1999)
http://www.brookespublishing.com
Age: 11–71 months
Time: 15 minutes
Format: Parent-completed checklist
Description: Atypical behavior: detached, hypersensitive/active, underreactive, dysregulated

---

Other properties that a test should possess are validity and reliability. Validity indicates whether a test measures what it is intended to measure, and reliability indicates whether the results of a test measure are reproducible (Dawson & Trapp, 2004). Reliability may measure the consistency of test results done by different examiners on the same subject (intertest), or by the same examiner at different times (intratest), or it may refer to the consistency of the same measurement on different occasions (test–retest). Acceptable levels of reliability are 80% or higher. Reliability is generally expressed by use of the kappa statistic, defined as the agreement beyond chance divided by the amount of possible agreement beyond chance. The higher the kappa, the less likely that agreement of test results occurred by chance; the lower the kappa, the more likely that agreement of test results may have occurred by chance.

Properties of test measures that are more difficult to define but must be considered by the examiner include issues surrounding cultural bias, language barriers, and the validity of test measures in children with preexisting handicaps such as blindness, hearing impairment, and significant motor impairment.

To be useful in clinical practice, screening measures are ideally expeditious, use few instruments, test defined streams of development, and are valid, reliable measures with good sensitivity and specificity. Screening measures *are not* synonymous with assessment tools. Screening tools alert to the possibility of developmental delay, whereas assessment tools are expected to confirm the presence of delay, determine the degree of delay, and make inferences for diagnoses.

SCREENING IN PRACTICE

The precursor to the 2006 AAP recommendations for screening was a 2001 recommendation for performing periodic developmental screening of all infants and young children during preventative health care visits (AAP, 2001a). Despite this recommendation, the application of developmental screening in the practice setting of primary care providers for infants and children is inconsistent. A recent survey of pediatricians found that 71% of those polled identified potential developmental problems using clinical assessment (no standardized measures) (Sands et al., 2005). A separate study surveyed the practices of pediatricians and family practitioners with regard to developmental screening for delay at the 2-year routine examination. This study indicated that 53% of polled practitioners did not use any standardized instrument, and of the 47% who did use standardized instruments, the vast majority (38% of the 47%) used either the Denver Developmental Screening Test (Frankenburg & Dodds, 1969) or the Denver II (Frankenburg et al., 1992; Sices, Feudtner, McLaughlin, Drotar, & Williams, 2003). In contrast to the reported practices of the primary care providers, only 57% of parents of children 10–35 months of age reported that their child received a developmental assessment (Halfon et al., 2004).

CHALLENGES OF SCREENING IN PRIMARY CARE

A number of practical and perceived obstacles exist to routine screening with validated instruments in the primary care office. A periodic survey of AAP fellows who reported practice of developmental screening indicated that the vast majority of pediatricians use clinical judgment and nonstandardized means to identify delay (Sands et al., 2005). Parents seen in developmental clinics occasionally reported that their primary care physicians responded to developmental concerns with a "give it more time" attitude. This "wait and see" approach in response to parent concerns about development is perceived by some families and nonmedical professionals as an unnecessary obstruction to early access to intervention services (Shannon, 2004).

Eighty-three percent of pediatricians polled in the AAP Periodic Survey of Fellows thought that time was a significant barrier to routine screening, 49% reported insufficient staff to accommodate screening, and 46% reported that poor reimbursement was a barrier (Sands et al., 2005). The time required to administer, score, and counsel parents on developmental screening tools is a major consideration because the length of time added to a routine health maintenance visit can vary from just a few minutes with parent questionnaires to 30 minutes on some of the more formal screening tools.

Costs of assessment and reimbursement are also considerations in current practice settings. Dobrez et al. (2001) estimated the cost of various screening measures by estimating the average hourly wage of physicians and the proportion of an hour required to administer and to counsel on screening measures. The cost was least (approximately $11) for parent-completed questionnaires, which require only 5 minutes of physician consultation time for a normal screen, and greatest (highest estimate, $82) for screening and consultation for abnormal results on screening measures that require physician administration. In a separate study, Glascoe, Foster, and Wolraich (1997) estimated the cost of developmental screening based on the average hourly physician wage as

well as the cost of referral for formal developmental assessment for the positive screens. Glascoe et al. used four methods of screening to define those children who would be referred for assessment: 1) those whose parents expressed concerns, 2) those who had positive clinician-administered screens, 3) those with two-stage positive screening (parents expressed concerns and there was a positive clinician-administered screen), and 4) those with two-stage negative screening (no parent concerns were expressed, but there was a positive physician-administered screen). In this model, the two-stage negative screen proved to have the highest true-positive rate (95%), but the two-stage positive screen proved the least costly.

The AAP provides coding for developmental testing in primary care using Current Procedural Terminology (CPT) codes for limited developmental screens (code 96110), which Medicare reimburses at a rate of $13.64. Code 96110 is used for validated screening instruments at any routine preventive medical visits. Informal inquiry regarding developmental and behavioral concerns does not qualify for reimbursement under this code, but validated parent questionnaires and brief physician-administered screening tools are included. Extended developmental testing (code 96111) may be used when standardized tests for specific or general developmental concerns are deemed necessary. The use of code 96111 assumes that a validated test, requiring 1 hour or more to administer, is employed by a physician or other professional and is accompanied by a completed report. The Medicare reimbursement rate for code 96111 is approximately $145 (AAP, 2005).

CONCLUSION

Screening is a single aspect of a continuous process of developmental surveillance and the first step in the process of early identification. Screening tests are generally applied to whole populations of children to identify those children who are not meeting typical expectations for development or behavior. Once a child is identified by a screening measure as having atypical behavior or development, formal assessment with the goal of diagnosis and service determination should be undertaken. Screening, then, is the prelude to assessment, diagnosis, and therapeutic intervention.

REFERENCES

American Academy of Pediatrics. (2005). *Developmental screening/testing coding fact sheet for primary care pediatricians.* Elk Grove Village, IL: Author.

American Academy of Pediatrics, Committee on Children with Disabilities. (2001a). Developmental surveillance and screening of infants and young children. *Pediatrics, 108,* 192–196.

American Academy of Pediatrics, Committee on Children with Disabilities. (2001b). Role of the pediatrician in family-centered early intervention services. *Pediatrics, 107,* 1155–1157.

American Academy of Pediatrics, Policy Statement. (2006). Identifying infants and young children with developmental disorders in the medical home: An algorithm for developmental screening and surveillance. *Pediatrics, 118,* 405–420.

Aylward, G.P. (1995). *Bayley Infant Neurodevelopmental Screener (BINS).* San Antonio, TX: Harcourt Assessment.

Aylward, G.P. (1996). Environmental risk, intervention and developmental outcome. *Ambulatory Child Health, 2,* 161–170.

Aylward, G.P. (1997). Conceptual issues in developmental screening and assessment. *Developmental and Behavioral Pediatrics, 18,* 340–349.

Bagnato, S.J., Neisworth, J.T., Salvia, J., & Hunt, F.M. (1999). *Temperament and Atypical Behavior Scale (TABS): Early childhood indicators of developmental dysfunction.* Baltimore: Paul H. Brookes Publishing Co.

Boyle, C.A., Decoufle, P., & Yeargin-Allsopp, M. (1994). Prevalence and health impact of developmental disabilities in US children. *Pediatrics, 93,* 399–403.

Bricker, D., & Squires, J. (1999). *Ages and Stages Questionnaires (ASQ): A parent-completed, child-monitoring system* (2nd ed.). Baltimore: Paul H. Brookes Publishing Co.

Brigance, A., & Glascoe, F.P. (2002). *BRIGANCE Infant and Toddler Screen.* North Billerica, MA: Curriculum Associates.

Brigance, A., & Glascoe, F.P. (2005a). *BRIGANCE Early Preschool Screen II.* North Billerica, MA: Curriculum Associates.

Brigance, A., & Glascoe, F.P. (2005b). *BRIGANCE K & 1 Screen II.* North Billerica, MA: Curriculum Associates.

Brigance, A., & Glascoe, F.P. (2005c). *BRIGANCE Preschool Screen II.* North Billerica, MA: Curriculum Associates.

Dawson, B., & Trapp, R.G. (2004). *Basic and clinical biostatistics* (4th ed.). New York: Lange Medical Books/McGraw-Hill.

Dobrez, D., Sasso, A.L., Holl, J., Shalowitz, M., Leon, S., & Budetti, P. (2001). Estimating the cost of developmental and behavioral screening of preschool children in general pediatric practice. *Pediatrics, 108,* 913–922.

Education for All Handicapped Children Act of 1975, PL 94-142, 20 U.S.C. §§ 1400 *et seq.*

Eyberg, S. (1999). *Eyberg Child Behavior Inventory (ECBI).* Lutz, FL: Psychological Assessment Resources.

Frankenburg, W.K., & Dodds, J.B. (1969). *The Denver Developmental Screening Test.* Denver: University of Colorado Medical Center.

Frankenburg, W.K., Dodds, J.B., Archer, P., Bresnick, B., Maschka, P., Edelman, N., & Shapiro, H. (1992). *Denver II* (2nd ed.). Denver: Denver Developmental Materials.

Glascoe, F.P. (1997). Parents' concerns about children's development: Prescreening technique or screening test? *Pediatrics, 99,* 522–528.

Glascoe, F.P. (1998). *Collaborating with parents: Using Parents' Evaluation of Developmental Status (PEDS) to detect and address developmental and behavioral problems.* Nashville: Ellsworth & Vandemeer Press.

Glascoe, F.P. (1999). Using parents' concerns to detect and address developmental and behavioral problems. *Journal of the Society of Pediatric Nurses, 4,* 24–35.

Glascoe, F.P. (2000). Early detection of developmental and behavioral problems. *Pediatrics in Review, 21,* 272–279.

Glascoe, F.P., Foster, E.M., & Wolraich, M.L. (1997). An economic analysis of developmental detection methods. *Pediatrics, 99,* 830–837.

Halfon, N., Regalado, M., Sareen, H., Inkelas, M., Reuland, C.H.P., Glascoe, F.P., et al. (2004). Assessing development in the pediatric office. *Pediatrics, 113,* 1926–1933.

Individuals with Disabilities Education Act Amendments of 1997, PL 105-17, U.S.C. §§ 1400 *et seq.*

Individuals with Disabilities Education Act (IDEA) of 1990, PL 101-476, 20 U.S.C. §§ 1400 *et seq.*

Ireton, H.R. (1992). *Child Developmental Inventory (CDI).* Bloomington, MN: Pearson Assessments.

Jellinek, M., Patel, B.P., Froehle, M.C., & Anglin, T.M. (2004). *Bright Futures in practice: Mental health* (Vol. 2, Tool kit). Washington, DC: National Center for Education in Maternal and Child Health.

Newacheck, P.W., Strickland, B., Shonkoff, J.P., Perrin, J.M., McPherson, M., McManus, M., et al. (1998). An epidemiologic profile of children with special health care needs. *Pediatrics, 102,* 117–123.

Newborg, J. (2004). *Batelle Developmental Inventory* (2nd ed.). Rolling Meadows, IL: Riverside Publishing.

Palfrey, J.S., Singer, J.D., Walker, D.K., & Butler, J.A. (1987). Early identification of children's special needs: A study in five metropolitan communities. *Journal of Pediatrics, 111,* 651–659.

Sands, N., Silverstein, M., Glascoe, F.P., Gupta, V.B.,

Tonniges, T.P., & O'Connor, K.G. (2005). Pediatricians reported practices regarding developmental screening: Do guidelines work? Do they help? *Pediatrics, 116,* 174–179.

Shannon, P. (2004). Barriers to family-centered services for infants and toddlers with developmental delays. *Social Work, 49,* 301–308.

Sices, L., Feudtner, C., McLaughlin, J., Drotar, D., & Williams, M. (2003). How do primary care physicians identify young children with developmental delays? A national survey. *Developmental and Behavioral Pediatrics, 24,* 409–417.

U.S. Department of Education. (2002). *Twenty-fourth annual report to Congress on the implementation of the Individuals with Disabilities Education Act.* Washington, DC: Author.

Yoshinaga-Itano, C., Sedey, A.L., Coulter, D.K., & Mehl, A.L. (1998). Language of early and later-identified children with hearing loss. *Pediatrics, 102,* 1161–1171.

21

Neurodevelopmental Assessment of School-Age Children

THOMAS R. MONTGOMERY

School failure—due to behavior or learning disorder—is the most frequent presenting concern for the neurodevelopmentalist. A diagnostic evaluation can accurately assess the child with a neurodevelopmental disability and can identify those children whose school failure is due to emotional, psychiatric, or non-neurodevelopmental causes. The evaluation includes a careful search for etiology. Unlike the school system, which provides an academic evaluation, or specific therapists, who provide evaluations for their disciplines, the neurodevelopmentalist can conduct a comprehensive evaluation that will encompass all concerns and come to a diagnosis and etiology. For example, an occupational therapist is able to evaluate the motor coordination of a clumsy child and can determine quite accurately the need for treatment for motor planning problems. Determining that this motor planning problem may be part of a broader neurodevelopmental disorder, however, is beyond the scope of occupational therapy, but it is within the realm of a neurodevelopmentalist. Similarly, a partial medical evaluation that addresses only hyperactivity or only inattention may result in the behavioral diagnosis of attention-deficit/hyperactivity disorder (ADHD) when a learning disability exists. A treatment recommendation for stimulant medication may follow. Acting-out behavior caused by the unrecognized learning disability may lead to the erroneous conclusion that additional stimulant medication is needed. Meanwhile, the child's underlying learning disability remains undiagnosed.

The close relationships and interactions between the different streams or segments of development form the basis of the need for a comprehensive evaluation beyond the single presenting symptom of school, learning, or behavior problem. The five streams or segments of development that characterize the early years of life—language, problem solving, motor, adaptive, and social—evolve into manifestations of cognitive, academic, and performance development in the school-age child. Visual skills in infancy evolve through fine motor skills into problem-solving and early academic skills. Early motor development is related to overall neurodevelopment, and early language development is related to future intellectual development. Thus, a history of delay in achievement of milestones in early life is a strong indicator of the neurodevelopmental basis of a presenting problem with academic achievement. Also, difficulties in one stream of development often are accompanied by difficulties in the other areas. Cognitive problems, emerging from delays in language, frequently are accompanied by motor coordination difficulties (Berninger & Rutberg, 1992; Blondis, Snow, & Accardo, 1990). Both are associated with disorders in behavioral development. Likewise, abnormal early motor development is associated with abnormal cognitive and academic achievement (Nelson & Ellenburg, 1982).

The intimate interrelationships of development streams and the evolution of developmental disorders over time necessitate a comprehensive assessment. Thus, the child who is hyperactive or inattentive requires an evaluation that goes beyond a behavioral assessment, and the child with academic problems requires more than an educational evaluation. The following evaluation guidelines for the neurodevelopmentalist are based on these complex interrelationships in neurodevelopment.

MEDICAL HISTORY

The history can document the onset and progression of developmental problems. Also, it can narrow the etiological possibilities as well as exclude presumed and inappropriate etiological factors. A recent stress or other life event may have prompted the consultation, but the history will document an earlier onset of difficulties. For example, a recent divorce may be implicated as the etiology for a child's school failure, but the history may uncover developmental problems occurring several years before the divorce. Parents often voice their initial concerns coinciding with the child's entrance into formal education; however, behavior or developmental problems may have been present for years prior to kindergarten.

Chronic medical conditions may not be appreciated by the parent as important to the neurodevelopmentalist; thus, such conditions will require specific inquiry. Asthma, especially, can cause both persistent fatigue and frequent absenteeism and have a significant effect on academic achievement. Alternatively, some parents may give undue weight and significance to medical issues that in fact have little true influence on the child's school difficulties. An accurate history and assessment will help determine the importance of associated medical conditions and their treatments. Likewise, medications, including the bronchodilators for asthma and many of the allergy medications, can affect alertness or cause hyperactivity, or both. Specific questions should be posed to the parents regarding the effect of any medicines on the child's performance and behavior.

Although prenatal and perinatal events can provide important etiological information, maternal reports of perinatal complications must be interpreted cautiously. Mothers vividly recall the birth process. Any variation from the expected, even if medically inconsequen-

tial, often is given undue significance. Indeed, perinatal events may become greatly magnified in an attempt to establish a cause for the child's disorder. Although school and behavior problems are more common in low birth weight premature infants than in full-term infants, most children with learning disabilities do not have a perinatal etiology (Msall & Tremont, 2002). The single most important perinatal fact to document is the time of discharge from the nursery. If the baby went home the next day with the mother, the possibility of a significant perinatal event causing chronic neurodevelopmental disability is extremely unlikely.

The family history should specifically explore the early educational history of the parents and siblings. Regardless of ultimate level of academic achievement, a parent may have had significant early educational difficulties. It is important to explore any positive reports of neurodevelopmental disorders in the family history to determine the extent of a familial or genetic problem. Known genetic disorders, including neurofibromatosis and Noonan syndrome, may be present but undiagnosed in a parent and now present with learning disorders in the child. Genetic disorders such as fragile X syndrome and tuberous sclerosis have been reported in children with learning disabilities, rather than the classic presentation of intellectual disabilities.

The social history, current family constellation, and associated emotional diagnoses also may shed light on the etiology of the child's disorder as well as on planned interventions. The significance of these problems must be interpreted within the context of the entire evaluation. Viewed in isolation, social stresses can assume inappropriate dimensions. Some children can be impressively resistant to social stresses, whereas others can be affected to a great degree by what would otherwise be considered a relatively minor stress. There is always some stress that can be identified as the most important event in a child's life, but, in reality, it may not have a significant impact on the current school problem.

DEVELOPMENTAL HISTORY

The developmental history as delineated in Chapter 14 of this volume is a defining element

Table 21.1. Age of achievement of major developmental milestones

Milestone	Mean age of attainment (months)	Milestone	Mean age of attainment (months)
Gross motor		**Expressive language**	
Rolls over	5	Laughs	4
Sits	6	Babbles	6
Comes to sit	8	Says "Dada" inappropriately	8
Crawls	9	Says "Mama" inappropriately	10
Pulls to stand	10	Says "Dada" appropriately	10
Cruises	11	Says "Mama" appropriately	10
Walks	12		
Goes up stairs	21	Utters first word	11
Goes down stairs	27	Uses jargon	15
Pedals tricycle	36	Utters 2-word sentence	24
Skips	60	Uses pronouns	36
Pedals bicycle	72	Says name, age, gender	36
Fine motor/adaptive		**Receptive language**	
Reaches		Alert	1
Transfers	4	Recognizes Mom	3
Performs pincer grasp	5	Turns to voice	4
Eats with fingers	9	Understands "no"	9
Uses cup unaided	9	Gesture games	9
Uses spoon	12	Follows 1-step command	12
Uses fork	12	with gesture	15
Undresses	24	without gesture	17
Dresses	24	Follows 2-step command	24
Unbuttons	36		
Buttons	36		
Ties shoes	48		
Spreads with knife	60		
	72		

Sources: Capute et al. (1986), Doel (1965), and Illingworth (1985).

to a neurodevelopmental assessment. By meticulously chronicling milestones such as those listed in Table 21.1, an accurate assessment of the rate and flow of early development is possible. Accurate developmental history taking requires skill and experience. It is often necessary to provide parents with markers for orienting developmental milestones. Such markers may include birthdays, holidays, family moves, births of siblings, and other events of special significance to the family. By ascertaining what the child was doing at these special times, a log of milestones can be reconstructed.

Delay, dissociation, and deviancy are the abnormal elements sought in a developmental history. These elements will determine the extent and nature of the child's current problems as well. The child with learning disabilities characteristically has a history of language delay and motor deviance. The language delay also may reflect dissociation of slower language development from normal adaptive skills. The variations of delay, dissociation, and deviancy in the histories of children with learning disabilities reflect the variability of the disorders themselves. The presence of any of these abnormalities of development documents the early origin of the current neurodevelopmental disorder. The interrelationships between streams of development also can be identified.

An abnormal developmental history can help the family understand the extent and nature of their child's disorder. Because children with dyslexia characteristically have a language delay, discussing that with the family can help put the dyslexia into context of the child's overall neurodevelopment. Likewise, early fine motor problems, including difficulties with buttoning and tying shoes, frequently are identified in children with dysgraphia. Reminding the parent of this when discussing the diagnosis will reinforce the fine-motor control nature of the problem and de-emphasize other suspected issues, including inattention. A history of difficulties in performance, such as coloring or responding to questions in a timely manner, is found in children with difficulty in efficient output of information both verbally and in written work.

Precise descriptions of behavior problems are important because overgeneralizations such as "bad behavior" will not help establish a diagnosis. A checklist of behavior problems can be reviewed with the parents (Table 21.2). It is important for the parents and physician to agree on the definitions of behavioral terms. Examples of abnormal behavior can help clarify the significance of any reported problems. A history confirming behavior problems outside the home is important. The child's teacher is an important source of information, as are babysitters, coaches, and extended family members.

The use of formal behavior rating scales may lessen individual variation in the reporting of behavior problems. The Conners Scales, originally devised in 1969 (Conners, 1969), remain quite popular. A revised manual was published in 1989 (Conners, 1989). The Vanderbilt ADHD Diagnostic Parent Rating Scale (Wolraich et al., 2003) has become quite popular and has been used in large-scale studies; however, even the most objective of rating scales cannot replace the interview. The behavior descriptors on checklists are not unique to any specific behavioral diagnosis. Normally developing children will display many of these behaviors. It is the frequency and intensity of the behaviors that make them clinically abnormal, not the actual behavioral acts themselves. Therefore, questions to parents should focus on the degree of disruption the behavior is causing and not on the descriptive term—hyperactivity or lack of attention—itself. Many children are referred for a neurodevelopmental assessment because of the disruptive nature of their behavior and its effect on academic achievement. The referring complaint may be ADHD, but careful delineation of the disruptive behaviors may reveal that they are not specifically those of ADHD. Thus, different behavioral diagnoses need to be entertained.

Table 21.2. Checklist of behavior problems

Inattention
Distractibility
Impulsivity
Hyperactivity
Emotional lability
    Temper tantrums
    Excess crying or upset
Perseveration
    Head banging
    Rocking
Aggressiveness
Destructiveness
Violence
Noncompliance
Sibling problems
Peer problems
Stealing
Lying
Truancy
Cruelty to animals
Fire setting
Fearlessness
Lack of remorse
Self-injury
Pica
Encopresis
Enuresis
Mealtime problems
Bedtime problems

PHYSICAL EXAMINATION

Physical clues to the etiology and diagnosis may be found in the growth parameters. Evidence of chronic illness may manifest with poor growth. Many short stature syndromes are associated with learning disorders (Table 21.3), and some also have associated microcephaly. A finding of macrocephaly, suggesting hydrocephalus or Sotos syndrome (cerebral gigantism), may be present. Nelhaus (1968) head circumference curves are sex-specific graphs from birth through adolescence and are the preferred curves for plotting head circumference of school-age children.

Dysmorphic features of the head, body, and extremities (Table 21.4) (see also Chapter

Table 21.3. Short stature syndromes possibly associated with learning disabilities and without intellectual disabilities

Down mosaic syndrome[a]
Partial trisomy 8 syndrome
Turner syndrome
Turner mosaic syndrome
Tetra X syndrome
Aarskog syndrome
Dubowitz syndrome[a]
Noonan syndrome[a]
Opitz syndrome
Robinow syndrome
Russell-Silver syndrome
Williams syndrome[a]
Fetal alcohol syndrome[a]

Sources: Bergsma (1979) and Jones (1988).
[a]Microcephaly is a prominent finding.

15, this volume) may help determine the presence of a recognizable syndrome. Dysmorphic features, even without a specific syndrome diagnosis, imply a prenatal onset to a neurodevelopmental problem. There is an increase in minor congenital anomalies in children with learning disabilities (Accardo, Tomazic, Morrow, Haake, & Whitman, 1991). Body asymmetries may suggest a congenital growth abnormality or a secondary chronic neuromotor disorder, such as a subtle hemiplegia. Skin lesions of neurocutaneous syndromes may have gone unrecognized previously. The depigmented ash-leaf spots of tuberous sclerosis can be particularly difficult to detect in children with a fair complexion. Wood's lamp inspection of the body will exaggerate these pigment changes and should be employed if the suspicion of a neurocutaneous syndrome exists. Adenoma sebaceum and shagreen patches also may be present. The café au lait spots of neurofibromatosis usually are accompanied by other skin lesions, such as axillary freckling and Lisch nodules of the iris. Telangiectasias, unusual nevi, and other skin markings also should be noted because they may represent a nonspecific neurocutaneous disorder.

In rare instances, organ enlargement, such as hepatomegaly, will contribute to an etiological diagnosis. Hepatomegaly resulting from storage disorders usually is an associated finding with presenting symptoms of striking phys-

ical and neurodevelopmental impairments. Sanfilippo syndrome, however, can present with delayed development, hepatomegaly, and only subtle coarsening of the facial features.

An expanded neuromotor examination will identify subtle variations of tone, posture, and reflexes as well as abnormalities of fine motor coordination. The subtle nature of these asymmetries should not keep them from being recognized as important markers of mild central nervous system dysfunction. Inspection of stance and gait often will reveal the effect of tone abnormalities. The running gait stresses the motor system and thus exaggerates any abnormality. Other stressed gait tests include tandem walking, toe walking, heel walking, and stressed walking on the medial and lateral edges of the feet as described by Fog and Fog (1963). Tremor and involuntary movements during arm extension testing—chorea, athetosis, or drift—are abnormal and are not to be relegated to maturational delay.

As the abnormalities of tone and reflexes become more prominent, frank neuromotor disabilities, including mild cerebral palsy, may be diagnostic possibilities. There are no obvious dividing lines between normal motor function, clumsiness, and cerebral palsy. A spectrum of motor dysfunction exists, and the child with learning disabilities often falls on this spectrum in the zone of dysfunction without frank neuromotor disability. The child with attention deficit, a learning disability, or both may have a definite motor abnormality that could range from subtle abnormalities of fine finger movements, through mild hypotonia and apraxia, to obvious motor disability confirming the diffuse neurodevelopmental nature of the disorder (Mostofsky, Newschaffer, & Denckla, 2003; Viholainen, Ahonen, Cantell, Lyytinen, & Lyytinen, 2002).

The school-age child can be tested reliably for the motor functions listed in Table 21.5. Synkinesia, as assessed by a rapid finger-tapping task, and dysdiadochokinesia (impaired rapid alternating movements) are extinguished by 8 years in boys and by 7 years in girls. Graphesthesia is dependent on the child's being able to recognize written numbers. The examiner "draws" a number in the child's

Table 21.4. Dysmorphic features of the head, body, and extremities

Head and skull	Webbed
Microcephaly	Low hairline
Macrocephaly	Limited range of motion
Frontal bossing	**Chest and back**
Flat occiput	Pectus excavatum
Asymmetrical shape	Pectus carinatum
Plagiocephaly	Short sternum
Brachycephaly	Broad/shield chest
Face	Scoliosis
Asymmetrical, flat, broad, thin	**Genitalia**
Micrognathia	Cryptorchidism
Prognathia	Macroorchidism
Midface hypoplasia	Shawl scrotum
Eyes	Hypoplastic labia
Hypertelorism	**Limbs**
Hypotelorism	Asymmetrical/hemihypertrophy/hemiatrophy
Small palpebral fissures	Excessive or limited range of motion
Upward or downward palpebral slant	Increased carrying angle
Epicanthal folds	Disproportionate to trunk
Synophrys	**Hands and feet**
Iris speckling	Syndactyly
Ptosis	Polydactyly
Nose and mouth	Clinodactyly
Low nasal bridge	Brachydactyly
Broad nasal bridge	Arachnodactyly
Anteverted nostrils	Tapered digits
Lip pits	Broad digits
Cleft lip/palate	Proximal thumb/hallux
High-arched palate	Nail dysplasia/hypoplasia
Long or short philtrum	Simian crease
Smooth philtrum	Unusual dermatoglyphics
Carplike mouth	**Skin and hair**
Downturned lip	Tags, pits, dimples
Thin vermilion border	Café au lait spots
Abnormal dentition	Depigmented spots
Ears	Telangiectasias
Preauricular tags or pits	Sacral spots/hair
Low-set/posterior rotation	Cutis aplasia
Abnormal auricles	Hirsutism
Neck	Sparse hair
Short	Abnormal or absent hair whorls

Sources: Jones (1988); Keele (1985); and Leppig, Werler, Cann, Cook, and Holmes (1987).

palm and allows the child to identify the number by feel. Awkward upper extremity posturing on stressed gait testing is abnormal if it persists beyond 7 years.

The documentation of normal vision and hearing acuity also serves to dispel attempts at blaming a learning problem on a peripheral sensory disorder. If abnormalities of vision or hearing are detected, they must be addressed and corrected.

NEURODEVELOPMENTAL TESTING DATA

Neurodevelopmental assessment instruments are available to obtain objective data about the

Table 21.5. Motor function evaluation

Function	Description
Synkinesia	The presence of abnormal mirror movements or overflow of fine finger movements from one hand to the other
Diadochokinesia	The ability to perform rapid alternating movements, such as rapid pronation and supination of the hand
Tremor	Fine involuntary movements often seen on intention
Arm extension posturing	Involuntary movements observed in the outstretched hands and arms on performing the Romberg maneuver
Graphesthesia	The ability to recognize a number by feel when the number is traced on the palm of the hand
Finger localization	The ability to detect, with eyes closed, which fingers of a hand are touched
Lateral dominance	The establishment of dominant hand, foot, and eye
Right–left orientation	The ability to discriminate right from left on oneself and on the examiner
Random movements	The presence of extraneous motor movements when performing tasks, including arms extended, palms up; tongue protruded; or eyes closed
Stressed gait posturing	The presence of abnormalities, particularly of the upper extremities, when performing stressed gait maneuvers of tandem walking/running, heel and toe walking, and Fog test gaits
Toe tapping	The ability to perform rapid movements with the feet

child's overall cognitive functions, differences or dissociation between verbal abilities and visual problem-solving skills, and academic achievement in core areas. This includes assessment of perceptual skills in visual-motor ability and auditory processing. The instruments described in this section are readily available and can be administered by neurodevelopmentalists or trained assistants. They are not to be confused with formal neuropsychometric instruments that require interpretation by a licensed psychologist.

The Kaufman Brief Intelligence Test (K-BIT) Vocabulary subtest (Kaufman & Kaufman 1990) and the Peabody Picture Vocabulary Test, Third Edition (Dunn & Dunn, 1997) are two measures of verbal skills that provide standard scores as well as age levels of performance. Informal verbal assessments using age-graded vocabulary lists have been circulated and may be helpful, but most have not been standardized, thus limiting their results to an age-level score and not a standard score.

Motor-free visual problem-solving tests include the Matrices subtest of the K-BIT and the Test of Nonverbal Intelligence–3 (Brown, Sherbenou, & Johnsen, 1997). Both will generate a standard score and an age level of performance.

Four tests of visual-motor problem-solving skills for office use include the Draw-a-Man Test (Goodenough, 1926), the Gesell figures, the Bender Gestalt figures (Koppitz, 1963), and the Rey-Osterrieth complex figure (Accardo & Capute, 1979). For the Draw-a-Man Test (Table 21.6), the child is given a blank sheet of paper and is asked to draw the best possible picture of a man; there is no time limit. This test differs from the other three in that there is no model figure to copy; the child must generate the figure independently. The Gesell figures (Table 21.7) are particularly useful for the younger child or the child with more delays. Rather stringent criteria must be applied when interpreting the accuracy of the reproductions of the more advanced figures. The Bender Gestalt figures (Figure 21.1) are an excellent test of visual-motor skills for the child above 5 years of age. A detailed scoring system (Koppitz, 1963) allows for more objective grading and less individual interpretation than with the Gesell figures. The Rey-Osterrieth complex figure (Osterrieth, 1945) is another drawing test for the older child and adolescent. The child with a spatial orientation disorder has particular difficulty with this integration of figures into a complex design. The processes of drawing and of reconstructing figures may demonstrate abnormalities in pencil grasp, motor control, speed, efficiency, and attention to task. There may be deviancy in the construction itself. These problems may not be appreci-

Table 21.6.   Scoring the Goodenough Draw-a-Man Test

1. Head shown	26. Opposition of thumb shown
2. Legs shown	27. Hands shown distinct from fingers or arms
3. Arms shown	28. Arm joint shown; elbow, shoulder, or both shown
4. Trunk shown	
5. Length of trunk greater than breadth	29. Leg joint shown; knee, hip, or both shown
6. Shoulders indicated	30. Head in proportion
7. Both arms and legs attached to trunk	31. Arms in proportion
8. Legs attached to trunk; arms attached to trunk at correct point	32. Legs in proportion
	33. Feet in proportion
9. Neck shown	34. Both arms and legs in two dimensions
10. Neck outline continuous with head, trunk, or both	35. Heels shown
11. Eyes shown	36. Firm lines without overlapping at junctions
12. Nose shown	37. Firm lines with correct joining
13. Mouth present	38. Head outline more than a circle
14. Nose and mouth in two dimensions; lips shown	39. Trunk outline more than a circle
15. Nostrils indicated	40. Outline of arms and legs without narrowing at junction with body
16. Hair shown	
17. Hair nontransparent, over more than circumference	41. Features symmetrical and in correct position
	42. Ears shown
18. Clothing shown	43. Ears in correct position and proportion
19. Two articles of clothing nontransparent	44. Eyebrows or eyelashes shown
20. No transparencies, both sleeves and trousers shown	45. Pupil of eye shown
	46. Eye length greater than height
21. Four or more articles of clothing definitely indicated	47. Eye glance directed to front in profile
	48. Both chin and forehead shown
22. Costume complete, without incongruities	49. Projection of chin shown
23. Fingers shown	50. Profile with not more than one error
24. Correct number of fingers shown	51. Correct profile
25. Fingers in two dimensions, length greater than breadth, angle less than 180 degrees	

Adapted from Accardo P.J. and Capute A.J. (1979). *The pediatrician and the developmentally delayed child.* Baltimore: University Park Press.

Score 1 point for each correct item. Every 4 points equals 1 year above the basal year of 3.

Table 21.7.   Age norms for correct and objective copy of geometric forms

Form	Age (years)
Circle	3 (Gesell[a], Revised Stanford-Binet[b])
Triangle	5 (Gesell, Revised Stanford-Binet)
British flag	over 5 (Gesell)
Horizontal diamond	6 (Gesell)
Square	5 (Kuhlmann[c], Revised Stanford-Binet)
Vertical diamond	7 (Revised Stanford-Binet)

Reprinted by permission of the publisher from PSYCHOLOGICAL APPRIASAL OF CHILDREN WITH CEREBRAL DEFECTS by Edith Meyer Taylor, p. 332, Cambridge, Mass.: Harvard University Press, Copyright © 1959 by the Commonwealth Fund.

[a]Gesell, *op. cit.,* p. 169.

[b]Terman and Merrill, *op. cit.,* pp. 82, 92, 201, 219, 98, 230.

[c]Frederick Kuhlmann, *A Handbook of Mental Tests* (Baltimore: Warwick and York, 1922), p. 102.

ated if the child is not observed. For instance, the circle in the Gesell figures classically is drawn by beginning at the top and proceeding counterclockwise. A right-handed child with learning disabilities may well begin at the bottom and continue clockwise. The circle is indeed reproduced, and the item is passed, but it was done in a deviant fashion suggesting a possible visual-motor problem.

Assessment of graphomotor skills with these same tests can help to determine the presence of a writing performance disorder. Abnormalities in the speed, accuracy, and efficiency of construction of these tasks may relate directly to difficulties in written work affecting all areas of academic achievement. Disorders of performance may not be appreciated on many standardized assessment tools because there are no time limits when administering the test.

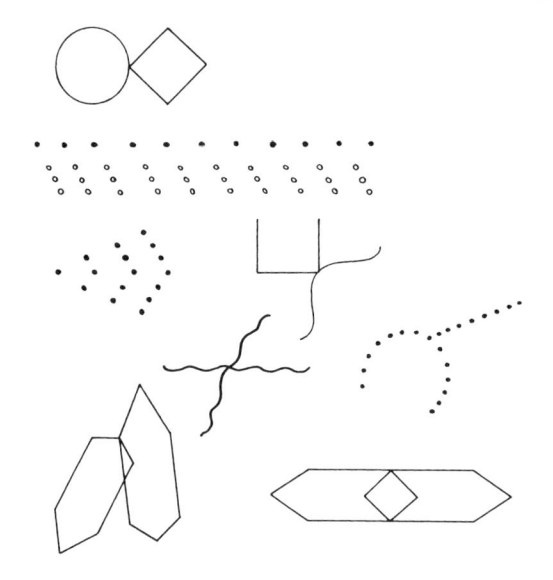

Figure 21.1. The Bender Gestalt figures. (From Bender, L. [1938]. *A visual motor Gestalt test and its clinical use.* New York: American Orthopsychiatric Association. Copyright © 1938; reprinted by permission of L. Bender's estate.)

Difficulties in construction need to be related to the assessment of speed and accuracy of handwriting as described later.

Processing of auditory memory can be assessed for digits forward, digits reversed, and sentences (Table 21.8). Some children with learning disabilities will have the cognitive power to reverse digits at an age-appropriate level but will not have the auditory memory to recite a longer string of digits forward. Thus, they paradoxically will achieve a lower age level for digits forward than for digits reversed. Likewise, such children clearly recall the meaning of a sentence but are unable to repeat the exact wording. Again, rote auditory memory skills are below the general cognitive level.

The Wide Range Achievement Test–Revised (WRAT-R) (Jastek & Jastek, 1984) provides standard scores and grade equivalents and covers spelling, math, and reading. The WRAT-R reading section, however, includes only word recognition, or decoding, and not comprehension. If the child can accurately decode words on the WRAT-R and there is a concern for reading comprehension, graded reading paragraphs can be used with questions pertaining to the paragraph read, thus tapping comprehension. In assessing decoding ability on the WRAT-R, special attention should be paid to the types of reading errors the child commits. One child may tend to have a pure phonetic approach, with the result not being an actual word. Another child with reading difficulty may pursue a purely visual approach and not have any phonetic capabilities whatsoever. Analysis of the process of reading, not just the ultimate level achieved, may identify the child's disorder best. Also, some children with significant reading disorder can decipher the content of a paragraph but cannot accurately decode single words when those words are not part of a sentence. An objective assessment of the phonetic aspects of decoding is the Woodcock-Johnson III Word Attack Test (McGrew & Woodcock, 2001). This test of reading nonsense words will exaggerate any phonetic problem that may be present.

An alternative to the WRAT-R in mathematics is to provide test items reflecting a progression of math facts—addition, subtraction, regrouping, multiplication, division, fractions, and exponents. The results can be listed by level of achievement and not by grade level. This generic approach to math skills eliminates confusion and significant discrepancy between national grade-level norms as assessed on the WRAT-R and math activities in the local school.

The Children's Handwriting Evaluation Scales (CHES and CHES-M) (Phelps & Stempel, 1987) for manuscript will provide a standard score for handwriting speed and accuracy. During testing, the child can be observed for pencil grasp, writing speed, spelling skills, spacing, motor planning, and overall organization of the task. Deficits in the output of written information are becoming manifest at earlier ages because of the significant increase in written work starting as early as kindergarten. This disorder of performance is often undiagnosed or is misdiagnosed as a lack of attention when in fact the child has graphomotor impairments and dysgraphia.

The data from these tests can be organized in tabular form for better inspection of delays and dissociations (discrepancies) (Figure 21.2). When available, standard scores can be compared, as can age levels and grade levels. Comparison of the data can be further achieved by creating developmental quotients (DQs) for

Table 21.8. Assessment of auditory memory from repetition of digits and sentences

Digits forward			
2½ years	47	63	58
3 years	641	352	837
4½ years	4729	3852	7261
7 years	31859	48372	96183
10 years	473296	429736	728394
Adult	7259483	4715396	4183582
Digits reversed			
7 years	295	816	473
8 years	8526	4837	3629
12 years	81379	68582	62518
Adult	471952	583694	752618
Sentences			
4 years	We are going to buy some candy for Mother.		
	Jack likes to feed the little puppies in the barn.		
5 years	Jane wants to build a big castle in her playhouse.		
	Tom has lots of fun playing ball with his sister.		
8 years	Fred asked his father to take him to see the clowns in the circus.		
	Billy made a beautiful boat out of wood with his sharp knife.		
11 years	At the summer camp, the children get up early in the morning and go swimming.		
	Yesterday, we went for a ride in our car along the road that crosses the bridge.		
13 years	The airplane made a careful landing in the space that had been prepared for it.		
	Tom Brown's dog ran quickly down the road with a huge bone in his mouth.		

tests that do not yield a standard score but do have a developmental age level. The DQ is calculated by dividing the age level achieved on the test by the child's chronological age and multiplying by 100. The DQ then can be expressed in units compatible with a standard score, or IQ score equivalent. Sometimes, the grade level attained on an academic test may be more informative than a standard score. For instance, a $9\frac{5}{12}$-year-old in the fourth grade with a reading standard score of 85 on the WRAT-R has a grade-level reading level of mid-second grade. The standard score may be thought to be adequate, but the child is actually two grade levels below expected in reading, a significant delay. Deviant development on testing will not be apparent from the table of data but can be determined from observing the child's performance.

EXAMINATION OF BEHAVIOR

The office examination of behavior is fraught with hazard. Some children are anxiety stricken and others are excessively well behaved, and only the most uninhibited will display their full repertoire of abnormal behavior for the physician. When abnormal behaviors are displayed, they should be discussed with the parents to determine if such behaviors are in fact the behaviors that are present at home or school.

LABORATORY TESTS

There is no routine battery of laboratory tests that is helpful in the diagnostic evaluation of learning disabilities. Multiple genetic markers may eventually become available for familial learning disabilities. Studies of large populations of children with fragile X syndrome have revealed several children who have fragile X and have learning disabilities without intellectual disabilities (Hagerman & Silverman, 2002). Additional genetic markers for neurodevelopmental disorders are being reported with increasing frequency. There have been no specific markers reported for learning disabilities or ADHD, but case reports of children with learning disabilities with an abnormal genetic marker that usually results in severe neurodevelopmental impairment, such as autism, are

Domain	Age level	Standard Score/DQ	Grade level
Verbal			
Visual problem solving			
Visual motor			
Auditory			
Reading: *Decoding*			
Comprehension			
Phonics			
Math			
Spelling			
Writing			
Notes related to performance:			

Figure 21.2. Sample format for organizing neurodevelopmental testing data. (*Key*: DQ, developmental quotient.)

appearing in the literature. These reports raise the level of concern about genetic testing for learning disabilities. Currently, the decision should be made in the context of a suspicious pedigree or a family member with a known genetic disorder.

Specific tests, including neuroimaging and electroencephalography, should be limited to individuals with additional signs and symptoms that would warrant such investigations. To date, electroencephalographic mapping and other neurophysiological studies have not been shown to be effective in making a diagnosis of learning disability.

DIAGNOSTIC FORMULATION

The display of data from the testing (see Figure 21.2) can be analyzed to arrive at a diagnosis from the differential diagnosis of specific learning disability, slow learning, intellectual disabilities, academic underachievement, performance disorder, or normal neurodevelopment (with or without behavior or emotional problems, or both, affecting school perfor-

mance). Usually, there are sufficient data and enough evidence from the neurodevelopmental assessment to be precise with the diagnosis. Documented discrepancies between normal cognitive functions and impaired academic achievement—the classic definition of a specific learning disability—are apparent by comparing standard scores and DQs and make for a straightforward diagnosis. As concepts of learning expand, the term *learning disability* is being applied to all academic underachievement. Treatment and outcome for a child with this broader spectrum of learning disability—the slow learner—are similar to those of classic discrepancy-model specific learning disability.

Disorders of performance, especially in written work, are often missed by the traditional school evaluation and should be sought out and diagnosed by the neurodevelopmental assessment. These children will have delayed scores in handwriting speed and accuracy that may be associated with delayed scores in visual-motor and visuospatial tests.

The diagnosis of attention deficit disorders and other behavior or emotional problems leading to school failure should be evident from the history and observations during the testing. Poor test scores should be carefully interpreted in these children and a determination made as to whether the child was unable to perform a test or was inattentive in performing the test. This difference is not always obvious because most children will become inattentive when they are forced to perform at a level above their capability. The 9-year-old who becomes inattentive when reading at the third-grade level but is quite attentive when reading at the first-grade level more likely has a reading disorder and not an attention disorder.

Characteristically, the child with a typical neurodevelopmentally based learning disability will have decreased motor coordination, cognitive variability (dissociation of skills), academic underachievement, and disorders of attention. The severity of each component can vary greatly, thus contributing to the wide spectrum of clinical presentations. One child may have significant motor incoordination and a serious learning disability with few problems with attention. Another may be quite inattentive and hyperactive, with relatively mild motor and cognitive problems.

Recommendations of strategies for remediation through special education are obvious necessities; however, strategies for circumvention of deficiencies by highlighting strengths must be pursued as well. It is not sufficient to recommend a special reading program for a child with a reading disability/dyslexia. The child needs to be able to function in a classroom in spite of impaired reading. Thus, verbal instruction, oral testing, verbal responses to testing, books on tape, and voice-activated computer systems may be necessary accommodations or circumvention techniques for the child to be successful. Children with disorders of performance, particularly difficulty with written work/dysgraphia, are most successful with accommodations such as multiple choice tests, dictation of homework answers to someone else for transcription, use of tape-recording devices, and keyboarding with a word-processing device or laptop computer in the classroom.

Medication, behavior modification, family and individual counseling, occupational therapy, speech and language therapy, and special education all must be considered within the context of the diagnosis. Any single recommendation must be made within the framework of all the other recommendations. The effect of one recommendation on another, and the effect of the total intervention plan, must be judged in relation to the impact on the lifestyle and functioning of the child, the family, and the school.

Occasionally the neurodevelopmental evaluation cannot be precise in its diagnosis, and further information may need to be collected. This may be more common with older children whose disabilities have evolved into a complex pattern of symptoms. Formal psychometric testing, psychiatric evaluation, or specific evaluations by an occupational therapist or speech-language pathologist may be necessary; however, the neurodevelopmental evaluation, unlike a school-based assessment, does not require that all children receive an evaluation from a fixed battery of professionals. Federal funding of special education services may demand that children receive a multidisciplinary evaluation to comply with bureaucratic guidelines and to prevent a loss of civil rights, but such an evaluation is not required by a neurodevelopmentalist in order to make a diagnosis. The neurodevelopmental evaluation, although comprehensive, can be complete when it is properly directed to the individual patient and to the signs and symptoms discovered during the evaluation.

CONCLUSION

Accurate neurodevelopmental assessment of the school-age child can be comprehensive without being multidisciplinary. The spectrum of developmental disabilities within this age group applies not only to the spectrum of severity of disability but also to the spectrum of interrelationships of disorders among the streams of development. This concept is fundamental to a neurodevelopmental evaluation and emphasizes the fact that abbreviated or limited evaluations will not reflect the child accurately or correctly diagnose the neurodevelopmental disorder.

REFERENCES

Accardo, P.J., & Capute, A.J. (1979). *The pediatrician and the developmentally delayed child.* Baltimore: University Park Press.

Accardo, P.J., Tomazic, T., Morrow, J., Haake, C., & Whitman, B.Y. (1991). Minor malformations, hyperactivity, and learning disabilities. *American Journal of Diseases of Childhood, 145,* 1184–1187.

Bender, L. (1938). *A visual motor Gestalt test and its clinical use.* New York: American Orthopsychiatric Association.

Bergsma, D. (1979). *Birth defects compendium* (2nd ed.). New York: Alan R Liss.

Berninger, V.W., & Rutberg, J. (1992). Relationship of finger function to beginning writing: Application to diagnosis of writing disabilities. *Developmental Medicine and Child Neurology, 34,* 198–215.

Blondis, T.A., Snow, J.H., & Accardo, P.J. (1990). Integration of soft signs in academically normal and academically at-risk children. *Pediatrics, 85,* 421–425.

Brown, L., Sherbenou, R.J., & Johnsen, S.K. (1997). *Test of Nonverbal Intelligence* (3rd ed.). Austin, TX: PRO-ED.

Capute, A.J, Palmer, F.B., Shapiro, B.K., Wachtel, R.C., Schmidt, S., & Ross, A. (1986). Clinical Linguistic and Auditory Milestone Scale: Prediction of cognition in infancy. *Developmental Medicine and Child Neurology, 28,* 762–771.

Conners, C.K. (1969). A teacher rating scale to use in drug studies with children. *American Journal of Psychiatry, 126,* 884–888.

Conners, C.K. (1989). *Manual for Conners' Rating Scales.* North Tonawanda, NY: Multihealth Systems.

Doel, E.A. (1965). *Vineland Social Maturity Scale.* Circle Pines, MN: American Guidance Service.

Dunn, L.M., & Dunn, L. K. (1997). *Peabody Picture Vocabulary Test* (3rd ed.). Circle Pines, MN: American Guidance Service.

Fog, E., & Fog, M. (1963). Cerebral inhibition examined by associated movements. In R. MacKeith & M. Bax (Eds.), *Minimal cerebral dysfunction* (pp. 52–57). London: Spastics Society Medical Publications in association with William Heinemann Medical Books.

Goodenough, F.L. (1926). *Measurement of intelligence by drawings.* New York: Harcourt, Brace and World.

Hagerman, R.J., & Silverman, A. (2002). *Fragile X syndrome: Diagnosis, treatment and research.* Baltimore: Johns Hopkins University Press.

Illingworth, R.S. (1985). *The development of the infant and young child, abnormal and normal.* Edinburgh: Churchill Livingston.

Jastek, J., & Jastek, S. (1984). *The Wide Range Achievement Test–Revised.* Wilmington, DE: Jastek Associates.

Jones, K.L. (1988). *Smith's recognizable patterns of human malformation.* Philadelphia: W.B. Saunders.

Kaufman, A.S., & Kaufman, N.L. (1990). *Kaufman Brief Intelligence Test.* Circle Pines, MN: American Guidance Service.

Keele, D.K. (1985). A diagnostic approach to the dysmorphic child. *Contemporary Pediatrics, 2,* 63–84.

Koppitz, E.M. (1963). *The Bender-Gestalt Test for Young Children.* New York: Grune & Stratton.

Leppig, K.A., Werler, M.M., Cann, C.I., Cook, C.A., & Holmes, L.B. (1987). Predictive value of minor anomalies: In association with major malformations. *Journal of Pediatrics, 110,* 531–537.

Mcgrew, K.S., & Woodcock, R.W. (2001). *Woodcock-Johnson III.* Itasca, IL: Riverside Publishing.

Mostofsky, S.H., Newschaffer, C.J., & Denckla, M.B. (2003). Overflow movements predict impaired response inhibition in children with ADHD. *Perceptual Motor Skills, 97,* 1315–1331.

Msall, M.E., & Tremont, M.R. (2002). Measuring functional outcomes after prematurity: Developmental impact of very low birth weight and extremely low birth weight status on childhood disability. *Mental Retardation and Developmental Disabilities Research Reviews, 8,* 258–272.

Nelhaus, G. (1968). Head circumference from birth to 18 years: Practical composite international and interracial graphs. *Pediatrics, 41,* 106–114.

Nelson, K.B., & Ellenberg, J.H. (1982). Children who ''outgrew'' cerebral palsy. *Pediatrics, 69,* 529–536.

Osterrieth, P.-A. (1945). Le test de copie d'une figure complexe: Contribution à l'étude de la perception. *Archives de Psychologie, 30,* 205–356.

Phelps, J., & Stempel, L. (1987). *The Children's Handwriting Evaluation Scales.* Dallas TX: Scottish Rite Hospital for Crippled Children.

Taylor, E.M. (1959). *Psychological appraisal of children with cerebral defects.* Cambridge, MA: Harvard University Press.

Terman, KM., & Merrill, M.A. (1973). *Stanford-Binet Intelligence Scale.* Boston: Houghton Mifflin.

Viholainen, H., Ahonen, T., Cantell, M., Lyytinen, P., & Lyytinen, H. (2002). Development of early motor skills and language in children at risk for familial dyslexia. *Developmental Medicine and Child Neurology, 44,* 761–769.

Wolraich, M.L., Lambert, W., Doffing, M.A., Bickman, L., Simmons, T., & Worley, K. (2003). Psychometric properties of the Vanderbilt ADHD Diagnostic Parent Rating Scale in a referred population. *Journal of Pediatric Psychology, 8,* 559–567.

22

Functional Assessment in Neurodevelopmental Disorders

MICHAEL E. MSALL AND EMILY R. MSALL

A variety of assessment tools are available to pediatric professionals for the developmental surveillance of motor, cognitive, communicative, and neurobehavioral impairments; however, few instruments can capture the impact of the spectrum of motor, cognitive, and communicative dysfunctions on degrees of disability in early and middle childhood and among children with substantial neurodevelopmental impairments. The purpose of this chapter is to provide a framework for the use of functional assessment in children with established neurodevelopmental disabilities and to describe functional measures applicable to pediatric populations.

Functional assessment is the process of determining as accurately as possible an individual's ability to perform the tasks of daily living and to fulfill the social roles expected of peers of the same age and culture. To understand the health context and to provide a broader perspective on functional assessment, several models of child disability are discussed. These include the neurodevelopmental spectrum model (Capute & Accardo, 1996a), the Institute of Medicine developmental kaleidoscope model (National Research Council and Institute of Medicine, 2004), and the International Classification of Functioning, Disability and Health (ICF) model (World Health Organization, 2001). Functional measures that encompass adaptive skills and health-related quality of life are highlighted with respect to their psychometric properties and utility for children with neurodevelopmental disorders.

SCOPE OF THE PROBLEM

The scope of children at risk for neurodevelopmental disability or with established neurodevelopmental disability is large. Among American children ages birth to 20 years, there are approximately 200,000 children with cerebral palsy, 400,000 with significant cognitive disability (intellectual and adaptive scores more than 3 standard deviations below the mean), 160,000 with autism spectrum disorders, 160,000 with sensorineural hearing loss worse than 50 db, and 40,000 with vision worse than 20/200 despite corrective lenses (Msall et al., 2003). More than 20 per 1,000 preschool children—approximately 400,000 in absolute number—have major neurodevelopmental disorders affecting mobility, cognitive-adaptive, or communicative skills (Msall, Tremont, & Ottenbacher, 2001). Major advances in genetics have allowed for the early identification of children with chromosomal disorders, inborn errors of metabolism, and

This research was supported by National Institute of Child Health and Human Development/National Center of Medical Rehabilitation Research Grant No. 1U01 HD37614 (NICHD Family and Child Well-Being Network: Child Disability.)

This chapter is dedicated to Herb Abelson for his lifelong commitment to enhancing health and developmental outcomes of children. Paula Jaudes, Steve Goldstein, and Nancy Schwartz provided ongoing support and a shared vision of biopsychosocial commitments to children at risk medically or socially. Shelly Field and Jen Park were invaluable with editing and technical assistance.

congenital malformations. These disorders involve 30 per 1,000 children and include 600,000 preschoolers and 1.2 million school-age children (Kirby, Brewster, Canino, & Pavin, 1995). Among children ages 6–21 years, 300,000 have recurrent seizures that have a substantial impact on cognitive, learning, and behavioral status.

The risks for neurodevelopmental disability are multidimensional and encompass socioeconomic and environmental conditions as well as biomedical factors. Children at risk for neurodevelopmental disorders include children living with psychosocial disadvantage because of poverty or confirmed child abuse, or those living with parents with mental illness or substance misuse or who did not finish high school. As many as 1 in 3 children have exposure to these socioeconomic and environmental risks (PRB/KIDS COUNT Special Report, 2002). Biomedical risks include low birth weight status and prematurity, failure to thrive, and lead exposure. In the past decade, more than 500,000 children have survived being born with very low birth weight (VLBW) status (1,001–1,500 g) or extremely low birth weight (ELBW) status (< 1,000 g). Furthermore, data from population surveys indicate that between 1 in 6 and 1 in 8 children have an ongoing developmental, behavior, or health condition that requires medical management, educational accommodations, and behavioral supports (Hogan, Rogers, & Msall, 2000; Newacheck et al., 1998). Given the scope of these risks and the importance of optimizing outcomes of children with disability, this review highlights advances in functional assessment using adaptive measures and multi-attribute pediatric health-related quality-of-life instruments.

MODELS OF CHILD FUNCTIONING, DISABILITY, PARTICIPATION, AND SUPPORTS

Three frameworks have been used to describe the complex web of children's health, development, and well-being. The first framework, the *neurodevelopmental spectrum model,* focuses on medical diagnosis of central nervous system dysfunction (Capute & Accardo, 1996). This clinical/medical tradition aims for accurate di-

agnosis, critical analysis of laboratory indicators, and use of optimal management strategies informed by intense medical cohort studies. In addition, this model quantifies delays in development or intensity of clusters of behavioral states and establishes criteria for 1) developmental motor, cognitive, social-emotional, or adaptive disorders; 2) communicative impairments; 3) coordination and perceptual impairments; 4) autism spectrum disorders; 5) specific learning disabilities; 6) attention-deficit/hyperactivity disorder; and 7) neurobehavioral disorders. The strength of the neurodevelopmental spectrum model is its reliance on comprehensive assessment of developmental and behavioral processes often involving several sessions of standardized interviewing and structured observation. The robust observational traditions of Gesell, Bayley, Illingworth, Griffiths, Neligan, and Capute allow for descriptions of a child's movements and hand skills, elicitation of problem-solving skills, and observation of neurobehavioral and communicative skills (Bayley, 1933; Capute & Biehl, 1973; Gesell et al., 1940; Griffiths, 1954; Illingworth, 1984; Neligan & Prudham, 1969). More recently, the MacArthur-Bates Communicative Development Inventories (CDI; Fenson et al., 2007), the Communication and Symbolic Behavior Scales Developmental Profile (Wetherby & Prizant, 2002), and the Capute Scales (Accardo & Capute, 2005) have demonstrated the value of gestures, nonverbal communication, and play as precursors of communicative and social skills in preschool children. In school-age children, direct observations of coordination, perceptual ability, memory, reading, and neurobehavioral maturity are required in conjunction with psychoeducational and neuropsychological assessments of higher cortical functioning and academic achievement (Aylward, 2002; Montgomery, 1988; Sattler, 2001, 2002; Shapiro, 2001).

Despite these strengths in providing a comprehensive and thorough description of medical diagnosis and disability, the neurodevelopmental spectrum model does not provide a complete framework for understanding the complex relationships that contribute to health and well-being. By focusing on a child's impairments, the neurodevelopmental spectrum model may not adequately account for a child's skill in performing daily living activities in his or her natural environments at home and in the community. For example, stating that a child has diplegic cerebral palsy at age 5 and does not perform the running task on the Gross Motor Function Measure (GMFM; Russell, Rosenbaum, Avery, & Lane, 2002) does not acknowledge the fact that the child may be able to execute many other important tasks such as walking, dressing, communicating, learning similar to peers, and maintaining continency at kindergarten entry. Similarly, describing a child with an autism spectrum disorder and a Clinical Evaluation of Language Fundamentals–4 (Semel et al., 2003) total language standard score of less than 70 at age 7 years does not acknowledge that the child can talk in sentences about concrete information, follow specific directions, learn in groups, perform basic calculations, and swim the backstroke on the YMCA swim team. Equally, to describe a child with fetal alcohol syndrome at the age of 8 as having a Wechsler Intelligence Scale for Children–IV (WISC-IV; Wechsler, 2003) Full Scale intelligence quotient (IQ) score of 75 does not indicate the child's ability to decode early paragraphs, construct a village of Legos, take a shower without assistance, and ride a two-wheel bike without training wheels on a community bike path.

Another shortcoming of the neurodevelopmental spectrum model is that a large number of children do not receive a combination of medical and developmental assessments over time that are informed by current best practices. Too often, explicit measures of spontaneous movements, postural skills, and adaptive and functional skills are not included. Thus, a child with cerebral palsy is only described with respect to difficulty with motor skills that peers perform easily and not with respect to self-mobility; postural control; manipulative hand skills; communicative understanding; and developmental style of curiosity, persistence, and problem-solving adaptability. This leads to misperceptions that neurodevelopmental diagnosis represents a categorical classification system that does not allow for progress and has uniform developmental trajectories over the life span.

The second framework, the *biopsychosocial model,* combines biological, psychological, and social perspectives on a child's health and well-being (Stein & Silver, 1999). This model takes into account the child's physical, behavioral, and developmental status as well as use of medical services (glasses, hearing aids, inhalation medications for asthma, anticonvulsants, nutrition supports); rehabilitative and compensatory services (physical therapy, occupational therapy, speech-language therapy, alternative mobility supports, augmentative communication, robotic assistants); educational supports (early intervention and special education services); and behavioral supports (counseling, psychopharmacology, applied behavioral analysis programs). This model also allows for descriptions of both developmental strengths and challenges with daily activities. This model can be applied to a heterogeneous population of children with complex medical, developmental, or behavioral impairments. The weakness of this model is that it measures each use of medications or services as a separate impairment. Thus, individuals with myopia, intermittent asthma, and attention-deficit/hyperactivity disorder can be described as having multiple impairments because of repeated use of medications and health services, despite the fact that their symptoms are readily controlled. The additional weakness of this model is its failure to recognize that many children with learning and behavioral disorders have an underlying neurodevelopmental impairment that is best managed by building on strengths, working toward achievable successes, and not overemphasizing deficit remediation.

In 2004, the National Research Council and the Institute of Medicine proposed a developmental kaleidoscope model of children's health that includes biology and behavior, physical and social environment, and policy and services. This model of children's health and well-being involves three domains: health impairments and illness, functioning in daily life, and health potential. The latter captures the development of assets and positive aspects of health such as competence, capacity, and developmental potential. The developmental ka-

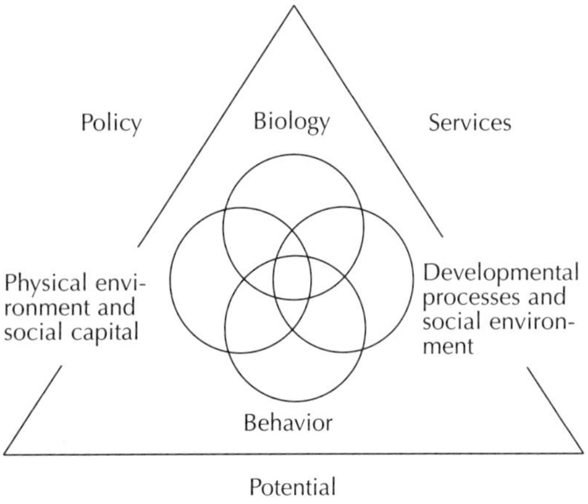

A 16-year-old girl with hemiplegia who is failing tenth grade 1 year after a stroke due to sickle cell disease

- *Biology*—vulnerability of teens with acquired brain injury to succeed in school.

- *Physical environment and social capital*—no neuropsychologist at school; mother did not finish high school; limited family supports and financial resources.

- *Behavior*—prior to her stroke, difficulty keeping up academically and completing school assignments because of frequent school absences.

- *Child health*—pediatrician frustrated in finding developmental psychologist who will work with her and school so that educational modifications and success can take place.

- *Policy*—gaps in mentoring vulnerable teens with degrees of learning difficulty and executive dysfunction to set goals for functional academics, vocational training, and community living.

- *Services*—after-school mentoring and tutoring program has scarce resources for adolescents in poverty; teen requires regular transfusions and desferoximine to prevent iron overload.

- *Potential*—without appropriate biopsychosocial management, teen will leave school and have limited employment opportunities and community successes.

Figure 22.1. Findings of the developmental kaleidoscope model of children's health, well-being, and potential in a 16-year-old girl with hemiplegia who is failing tenth grade 1 year after a stroke resulting from sickle cell disease.

leidoscope model is illustrated in Figure 22.1 for a 16-year-old girl with sickle cell anemia who has hemiplegia and difficulties in school after a stroke the previous year. Although the developmental kaleidoscope model takes into account the dynamic factors that contribute to overall health, the model assumes that the

major challenges to health are not neurodevelopmental but behavioral and that functional outcomes arise from a mismatch of individual child factors and community resources.

The third framework, the ICF model, describes a child's health and well-being in terms of four components: 1) body structures, 2) body functions, 3) activities, and 4) participation (World Health Organization, 2001). Body structures are anatomic parts of the body, such as organs and limbs, as well as structures of the nervous, sensory, and musculoskeletal systems. Body functions are the physiological functions of body systems, including psychological functions such as attending, remembering, and thinking. Activities are daily tasks, including communicating, walking, carrying, feeding, dressing, toileting, bathing, reading, preparing meals, shopping, and washing clothes. Participation reflects involvement in community life and includes relationships, education, work, and recreational, religious, civic, and social activities.

The ICF model also accounts for contextual factors in a child's life, including environmental and personal factors. Environmental factors, such as policy, social, and physical facilitators and barriers, include positive and negative attitudes of others, legal protections, and discriminatory practices. Personal factors include age, gender, interests, and sense of self-efficacy. Figure 22.2 illustrates how to apply the ICF model to a child with diplegic cerebral palsy. The strength of the ICF model is that it describes both functioning and enablement. Thus, it offers strong descriptions of both health and disability. Its current weakness is that it has not been widely used with children and does not have explicit indicators for all of the domains of the model. The model, however, does offer the promise of a much broader perspective with respect to children's activities and participation (Simeonsson, Lollar, Hollowell, & Adams, 2000). To illustrate the potential of this model, a variety of scenarios are described in Table 22.1.

FUNCTIONAL AND ADAPTIVE MEASURES

In using developmental assessment batteries for motor, communicative, adaptive, and be-

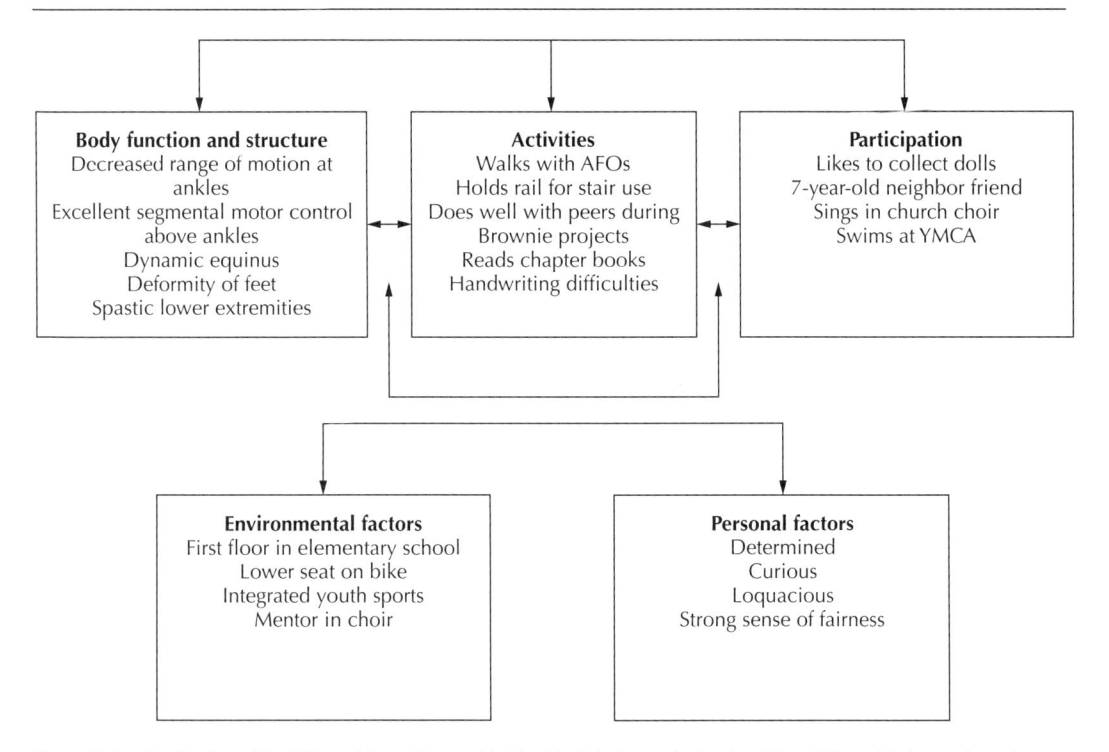

Figure 22.2. Application of the ICF model to a 7-year-old girl with diplegic cerebral palsy. (*Key:* AFOs, ankle-foot orthoses.)

havioral skills, the evaluator must understand the purpose of the measure (Kirschner & Guyatt, 1985). Discriminative instruments are designed to compare an individual child's performance with that of typically developing peers. Examples of discriminative instruments include the Bayley Scales of Infant Development, Third Edition (Bayley, 2005), the Peabody Developmental Motor Scales, Second Edition (Folio & Fewell, 2000), the Peabody Picture Vocabulary Test, Third Edition (Dunn & Dunn, 1997), the Preschool Language Scale, Fourth Edition (Zimmerman, Steiner, & Pond, 2002), the WISC-IV, and the Stanford-Binet Intelligence Scales, Fifth Edition (Roid, 2003). Although a WISC-IV Full Scale IQ score of 65 in a 10-year-old boy tells us that the child's performance was significantly delayed (i.e., more than 2 standard deviations below the mean compared with 10-year-old peers), the score does not indicate the child's basic skills in mobility, communication, self-care, functional academics, friendships, and community participation.

An evaluative instrument specifies criterion-related tasks (e.g., GMFM, Pediatric Eval-uation of Disability Inventory [PEDI; Haley, Coster, Ludlow, Haltiwanger, & Andrellos, 1992], Functional Independence Measure for Children [WeeFIM; Msall, DiGaudio, Rogers, LaForest, Lyon, et al., 1994]) and describes current levels of performance in key dimensions that are sensitive to change over time (Guyatt, Walter, & Norman, 1987). For example, the GMFM specifies an individual's performance in motor tasks of lying and rolling, sitting, crawling and kneeling, and standing, and upright mobility skills of walking, running, and jumping. In analyzing a diverse population of children with cerebral palsy, Rosenbaum's team (2002) found that there were certain functional categories that could describe appropriate goals and developmental trajectories and could be used to evaluate the impact of physical therapy, spasticity management, and surgical management.

A predictive measure is designed to assess key skills related to a future state. For example, Capute and Shapiro (1985) used the Gross Motor Quotient to predict who would be diagnosed with cerebral palsy in the preschool years based on the rate of early motor mile-

Table 22.1. International Classification of Functioning, Disability and Health (ICF) model scenarios in children with neurodevelopmental disorders

Dimension	Definition	2-year-old girl	4-year-old boy	7-year-old girl	10-year-old boy
Pathophysiology	Molecular/cellular mechanisms	800 g, 27 weeks' gestation, periventricular leukomalacia	Fragile X with CNS dysfunction and autism spectrum disorder	22q deletion with truncus arteriosus and cleft palate repair	Prenatal polydrug exposure with CNS dysgenesis
Body structures and body functions	Organ structure/function	Asthma; spastic diplegia; speech delays	Hypotonia; communication, neurobehavioral, and adaptive delays	Nasal speech; malocclusion; 90-db sensory hearing loss bilaterally	Microcephaly; hyperactivity; impulsivity
Activity (functional) strengths	Ability to perform essential activities: feed, dress, toilet, walk, talk	Indoor walking with AFOs; drinks with straw; likes to pretend play with dolls	Climbs slide and goes down easily; speaks 30 words; mesmerized by Elmo; imitates actions of others	Rides bike; open set speech recognition after cochlear implant; speaks in short sentences	Reads at second-grade level; excellent basketball skills
Activity (functional) limitations	Difficulty in performing essential activities	Unable to walk 50 ft or climb steps; unclear speech unless repeats	Decreased nonverbal skills; difficulty waiting; transitioning impulsive	Speech difficult to understand; inattentive in large groups; not reading	Difficulty with language skills, spelling, and attention
Participation	Involvement in community roles typical of peers	Plays in parallel with peers	Quality preschool services and behavioral management	Roller blades; ice-skates; in mime group	Guard on YMCA basketball team; excels in artwork
Participation restrictions	Difficulty in assuming roles typical of peers	Misses child care due to asthma; uses supplemental nutrition products	YMCA will not let him use playground because he bites	School does not have nonverbal curriculum for academics	Repeated first & third grades; initial IEP past year; mother died 2 years ago
Contextual factors: environmental facilitators	Attitudinal, legal, policy, and architectural facilitators	Has asthma care plan; participates in Hanen Group	Mother is unable to attend genetic support groups because she works outside the home	Community speech therapist works closely with teacher and school therapist	Adoptive foster parent insists he will learn; knows positive behavior management; attends church
Contextual factors: environmental barriers	Attitudinal, legal, policy, and architectural barriers	On waiting list for speech therapy; early intervention service coordinator just left program	Denied life insurance policy	First grade had signing as only education option	School will close for failure to meet standards

Key: AFOs, ankle-foot orthoses; CNS, central nervous system; IEP, individualized education program.

stone attainment. Rapin and colleagues demonstrated that children with autism spectrum disorders who had a preschool nonverbal IQ score greater than 80 were similar in middle childhood adaptive performance to children with developmental language disorders than to children with intellectual disability (IQ score < 70). Among children with autism spectrum disorder and a preschool nonverbal IQ score less than 80, performance in middle childhood was similar to children with intellectual disability (Rapin, 1996). It is in this criterion approach to assessment that adaptive and functional measures broaden our understanding of how the child with neurodevelopmental impairment performs in daily activities. Several representative instruments are summarized in Table 22.2 and in the following sections.

Pediatric Evaluation of Disability Inventory

The PEDI assesses functional activities in self-care, mobility, and social function, caregiver assistance, and modification of environment for children ages 6 months to 7.5 years (Feldman, Haley, & Coryell, 1990). Social function includes communication, problem solving, play, peer and adult interaction, memory, household chores, self-protection, and community safety. The PEDI has been used in children with traumatic brain injury, cerebral palsy, and spina bifida, and with children in preschool programs because of physical or developmental impairments (Haley, Fragala-Pinkham, Ni, Skrinar, & Kaye, 2004; Kothari, Haley, Gill-Body, & Dumas, 2003). The PEDI Caregiver Assistance and Modification Scale includes eight self-care items, seven mobility items, and five social function items. These categories take 15–20 minutes to administer, are available in a variety of languages, and have a computerized assisted interview format (Haley, Ni, Ludlow, & Fragala-Pinkham, 2006).

Functional Independence Measure for Children

The WeeFIM is an evaluative measure of basic functional skills that consists of 18 items encompassing three subscales: self-care, mobility,

and social cognition. There are eight items for self-care activities of daily living, five items for mobility, and five items for social cognitive functioning. The latter domain includes understanding verbal and nonverbal communication, use of language and gestures, social interaction, play, and memory of routines. The WeeFIM instrument has been normed on a population of more than 500 children in good health and without disability, ages 1–7 years, living in western New York, and has a robust correlation with chronological age for typically developing children between 18 and 48 months (Msall, DiGaudio, Duffy, et al., 1994). Initial validation studies included more than 700 children with neurodevelopmental disabilities including extreme prematurity, cerebral palsy, and genetic disorders. In preschool children with evolving motor, communicative, and developmental impairments, the WeeFIM proves to have excellent test–retest reliability as well as concurrent validity with psychological and educational measures of adaptive functioning, including the Battelle Developmental Screening Inventory (Newborg, Stock, Wnek, Guidubaldi, & Svinicki, 1988), the Vineland Adaptive Behavior Scales (VABS; Sparrow, Balla, & Cicchetti, 1984), and the Amount of Assistance Questionnaire (Msall et al., 2001; Ottenbacher et al., 1997, 1999, 2000a). The WeeFIM also has excellent equivalence reliability for face-to-face or telephone interviews (Ottenbacher et al., 1996). Most importantly, the WeeFIM demonstrated responsiveness to change over time in the preschool years in a diverse cohort of children with motor, communicative, health, and developmental challenges (Ottenbacher et al., 2000b).

The WeeFIM has been used in the longitudinal study of developmental, health, and functional outcomes in children with severe congenital heart disease (Limperopoulos et al., 2001), in children with spinal muscle atrophy (Chung, Wong, & Ip, 2004), in children with retinopathy of prematurity (Msall, Phelps, et al., 2000), in girls with severe disabilities as a result of Rett syndrome (Colvin et al., 2003), in a population sample of school-age children with Down syndrome (Leonard, Msall, Bower, Tremont, & Leonard, 2002), and in survivors of shaken baby–inflicted head trauma (Lowen,

Table 22.2. Adaptive-functional scales for childhood disabilities

	Pediatric Evaluation of Disability Inventory (PEDI; Haley, Coster, Ludlow, Haltiwanger, & Andrellos, 1992)	Functional Independence Measure for Children (WeeFIM; Msall, DiGaudio, Rogers, LaForest, Lyon, et al., 1994)	Warner Initial Developmental Evaluation of Adaptive and Functional Skills (WIDEA-FS; Gray et al., 2006)	Vineland Adaptive Behavior Scales, Second Edition (VABS-2), Survey Form (Sparrow, Balla, & Cicchetti, 2005)	Scales of Independent Behavior–Revised Early Developmental Form (SIB-R; Bruininks, Woodcock, Weatherman, & Hill, 1996)
Age range	6 months to 7 years	1.5–7 years	Birth to 36 months	Birth to 19 years	Birth to 5 years
Domains	Motor Self-care Social function Caregiver assistance (CA) Environmental modifications (EM)	Self-care Mobility Social cognition	Self-care Mobility Social cognition: verbal, gesture, play	Communication Daily living Socialization Motor	Adaptive skills Problem behaviors
Concurrent validity	Battelle WeeFIM Injury severity	Battelle VABS PEDI AAQ	Capute Scales Chronological age	VABS Kaufman ABC-II	Chronological age Early screening profiles
Disability samples	Children with brain injury, cerebral palsy, spinal injury, or juvenile arthritis	Children with cerebral palsy, prematurity, or congenital heart, sensory, genetic, developmental, learning, or attentional disorders	Children in early intervention, or with special health care needs	Children with autism spectrum disorders, intellectual disabilities, or developmental disabilities	Children with intellectual disabilities or developmental disabilities
Time to administer	45 minutes; 15 minutes for CA/EM scales	20 minutes	15 minutes	20–60 minutes	5 minutes
Future research	Computerized assisted version	Multicenter norms	U.S. centers for child disability	Use in early intervention	Prediction at 6–10 years

Key: AAQ, Amount of Assistance Questionnaire (Msall, DiGaudio, Rogers, LaForest, Lyon, et al., 1994); Batelle, Batelle Developmental Inventory (Newborg, Stock, Wnek, Guidubaldi, & Svinicki, 1988); Capute Scale, The Capute Scales (Accardo & Capute, 2005); Kaufman ABC-II, Kaufman Assessment Battery for Children, Second Edition (Kaufman & Kaufman, 2004); VABS, Vineland Adaptive Behavior Scales (Sparrow, Balla, & Cicchetti, 1984).

Msall, Jenny, et al., 2000). The WeeFIM has been translated into Japanese, Chinese, and Thai with both norms generated for children in good health and without disability as well as application to children with disability using appropriate developmental assessments (Jongjit, Komsopapong, & Chira-Adisai, 2002; Tsuji et al., 1999; Wong, Wong, Chan, & Wong, 2002).

There is a direct overlap between the Wee-FIM and the PEDI Caregiver Assistance Scale ratings. Concurrent validity across domains exceeds $\rho = .9+$ (Msall et al., 2001; Ziviani et al., 2001). Thus, one can use either the WeeFIM or PEDI Caregiver Assistance Scale if one wishes to measure functional strengths and limitations in toddlers and preschoolers. The strength of both the WeeFIM and the PEDI is that they reflect a rich tradition of measuring basic activities of daily living. An additional benefit of the PEDI is that it has been widely used among pediatric rehabilitation professionals in hospital and community settings and can be linked to a school function measure. The weakness of the WeeFIM instrument is that it was not designed by the distributors for outpatient pediatric surveillance, and, therefore, is hard to apply in preschool community settings. In addition, its norms are from only one American geographic region and thus may not reflect the diversity of the national population. Finally, there have been questions raised about whether its ceiling items in motor areas can fully capture the complexity of gait performance after orthopedic, spasticity management, or neurosurgical interventions.

Warner Initial Developmental Evaluation of Adaptive and Functional Skills

Because both the PEDI Caregiver Assistance and the WeeFIM items include several components of an activity, the test rating does not reflect partial success in particular skills. For this reason, Msall and colleagues have developed the Warner Initial Developmental Evaluation of Adaptive and Functional Skills (WIDEA-FS; Gray et al., 2006). The WIDEA-FS includes 50 items involving four domains: self-care (eating, dressing, and diaper awareness), mobility (roll, sit, scoot, crawl, cruise,

walk unassisted or with aids), communication, and social cognition. Initial standardization involved more than 300 children ages 2–30 months seen in pediatric primary care during well-child visits. Robust construct validity occurred between the pilot 43 items of the WIDEA-FS and the Capute Scales, and between child age and progression of adaptive skills (Msall et al., 2001). Interdisciplinary feedback from nursing, speech, occupational therapy, psychology, and pediatrics professionals has resulted in the addition of seven items to clarify the complexity of early communication and play skills. Multicenter normative and early intervention field testing has recently been completed on the 50-item WIDEA-FS (Gray et al., 2006)

Vineland Adaptive Behavior Scales

The VABS and VABS-2 (Sparrow, Balla, & Cicchetti, 2005) are interview surveys for assessing adaptive behavior. In children younger than 6 years, the domains include communication (receptive, expressive language), daily living skills (self-care/personal), socialization (interpersonal relations and play), and motor skills (gross and fine). The VABS-2 has been used in children with preschool developmental disabilities, including autism spectrum disorders. Used with children older than the chronological and developmental age of 6 years, the VABS-2 contains additional daily living skills, socialization, and communication items, comprising 297 items on the survey form and 577 items on the expanded form. The additional daily living skills items reflect meal preparation, chores, knowledge of time and money, and maintaining a budget. The socialization items include greetings, friendships, athletic participation, hobbies, and dating. The additional communication items involve reading, writing, and elaboration of ideas and long-term goals. For children older than 5 years, there is also a maladaptive behavior domain that includes internalizing, externalizing, and stereotypical and peculiar behaviors. The VABS-2 was concurrently used with the Kaufman Assessment Battery for Children, Second Edition (KABC-II; Kaufman & Kaufman, 2004). There are specific supplemental norm groups for individuals with disabilities.

Scales of
Independent Behavior–Revised

The Scales of Independent Behavior–Revised (SIB-R; Bruininks, Woodcock, Weatherman, & Hill, 1996) has an early development form of 40 items for ages birth to 5 years. For children of all ages there is a Short Form that includes 40 items. These have ratings of 0 (rarely or never performs), 1 (performs about 25% of the time), 2 (does fairly well or about 75% of the time), and 3 (does very well without being asked almost all the time). In the SIB-R, scores are categorized as

- *Pervasive*—reflecting developmental performance up to an 8-month level

- *Extensive*—reflecting developmental performance between a 9- and 12-month level

- *Frequent*—reflecting developmental performance between a 13- and 18-month level

- *Limited*—reflecting developmental performance between a 19- and 27-month level

- *Intermittent*—reflecting developmental performance between a 28- and 40-month level

- *Infrequent*—reflecting developmental performance between a 41- and 71-month level

A child scoring in the "limited" range is able to ambulate, feed him- or herself using a spoon and a cup, point, consistently indicate yes or no to basic need questions, and say 10 words. A child scoring in the intermittent range is able to ask questions and negotiate stairs and is toilet trained with supervision.

In the SIB-R, a child at 50 months is able to perform outerwear dressing such as putting on coats and gloves, obtain appropriate portions of food, follow two-part directions, and say his or her last name. In middle childhood, adolescence, and adulthood, emphasis is on social interaction and communication skills; personal living skills, including basic and extended activities of daily living; and community living skills of time and punctuality, money and value, work skills, and home and community orientations. Children age 8 and older are ex-pected to be able to change clothing if it is dirty, use a tissue for sneezing and coughing, tie shoelaces, adjust faucets before bathing, travel four blocks in a familiar environment with peers, read and understand books or magazines, write their complete address with zip code, and find a telephone number in a directory. In addition, the SIB-R contains eight domains of problem behavior: hurtful to self, hurtful to others, destruction of property, disruptive behavior, unusual or repetitive habits, socially offensive behaviors, withdrawn or inattentive behaviors, and uncooperative behaviors. Both frequency ratings (0 = never, to 3 = one or more times per week, to 5 = one or more times per hour) and severity ratings (0 = not serious to 3 = very serious) occur in the problem behavior domain.

The strength of the SIB-R is that it has application for basic and extended adaptive skills and problem behaviors for children with significant cognitive or autism spectrum disorders and can map to the American Association on Intellectual and Developmental Disabilities (AAIDD; formerly American Association on Mental Retardation) levels of support (Luccasson et al., 2002). The weaknesses are that there is a complex scoring system and that wide use of AAIDD classification levels in preschoolers with developmental challenges has not yet occurred.

Domain-Specific
Functional Assessment Instruments

The Alberta Infant Motor Scale (Darrah, Piper, & Watt, 1998), the GMFM, the MacArthur-Bates CDI, the Communication and Symbolic Behavior Scales Developmental Profile, the Infant-Toddler Social and Emotional Assessment (ITSEA; Carter & Briggs-Gowan, 2000; Carter, Briggs-Gowan, Jones, & Little, 2003), and the Vineland Social-Emotional Early Childhood (SEEC) Scale (Sparrow et al., 1997) are domain-specific functional assessments summarized in Table 22.3.

The Alberta Infant Motor Scale measures postural skills in both normal and at-risk infants from birth through the toddler age. The GMFM measures gross motor functional performance in rolling, sitting, crawling, standing,

Table 22.3. Domain-specific functional scales for childhood disabilities

Motor	**Alberta Infant Motor Scale** (AIMS; Darrah, Piper, & Watt, 1998)	**Gross Motor Function Measure** (GMFM; Russell, Rosenbaum, Avery, & Lane, 2002)
Domains	Prone, supine, sit, stand	Roll, sit, crawl, kneel, stand, walk, run, jump
Concurrent validity	Peabody Developmental Gross Motor Scale (Folio & Fewell, 2000)	Responsive to change in cerebral palsy, Down syndrome, and brain injury
	Bayley Scales 2 Performance Development Index (Bayley, 1993)	
Disability samples	Very low birth weight	Ontario Cerebral Palsy Treatment Centers
	Early intervention	Motor Curves Basis of Gross Motor Functional Classification System (GMFCS)
Communicative	**MacArthur-Bates Communicative Development Inventory** (CDI; Fenson et al., 2007)	**Communication and Symbolic Behavior Scales Developmental Profile** (CSBS-DP; Wetherby & Prizant, 2002)
Domains	Words and gestures, words and sentences	Social (emotion/gesture), speech (sounds/words), symbolic (understanding/toys)
Concurrent validity	Expressive One Word Picture Vocabulary Test (Gardner, 1981)	Mullen Scales of Early Learning (Mullen, 1995)
	Preschool Language Scale (Zimmerman, Steiner, & Pond, 2002)	
Disability samples	Preterm, twins, Down syndrome, prenatal drug exposure	Children with two of five Mullen domains (gross/fine motor, visual recognition, receptive/expressive language) scoring < 10%
Behavioral	**Infant Toddler Social & Emotional Assessment** (ITSEA; Carter & Briggs-Gowan, 2000)	**Vineland Social-Emotional Early Childhood Scales** (SEEC; Sparrow, Balla, & Cicchetti, 1997)
Domains	Externalizing, internalizing, dysregulation competencies	Interpersonal relationships, play and leisure time, coping skills
Concurrent validity	Mullen Scales of Early Learning Vineland SEEC MacArthur-Bates CDI	Battelle Personal Social Domain (Newborg, Stock, Wnek, Guidubaldi, & Svinicki, 1988)
		SIB Early Developmental Scale (Bruininks, Woodcock, Weatherman, & Hill, 1996)
Disability samples	78 children ages 1–2 years rated as difficult	Down syndrome, cerebral palsy, developmental delay, autism spectrum disorders

walking, running, and jumping, and its most difficult areas reflect gross motor skills done by 5-year-olds. It contains 88 items and is an evaluative measure for children with cerebral palsy. It is the basis for the Gross Motor Function Classification System (GMFCS; Wood & Rosenbaum, 2000), an ordinal ranking system of meaningful levels of functional performance

so that children receiving orthopedic, neurosurgical, pharmacological, orthotic, and rehabilitation interventions can be described over time. The MacArthur-Bates CDI assesses infants and toddlers ages 8–16 months for gestures and words, and children ages 16–30 months for words and sentences. The strength of this measure is that it captures 19 semantic categories of a child's initial words as well as a child's morphological and syntactic development. The ITSEA assesses attention, compliance, imitation, mastery and motivation, empathy, and prosocial functional behaviors in children ages birth to 3 years. It has both sound item construction from laboratory observations, as well as excellent psychometric properties. The SEEC Scale uses the VABS socialization domain for children birth to 6 years (Sparrow et al., 1997). The scale includes 44 items on interpersonal relationships, 44 on play and leisure time, and 34 on coping skills. There is excellent concurrent validity with the Personal Social Domain of the Battelle Developmental Screening Inventory as well as the Early Development Scale of the SIB-R.

A 42-item Brief Infant-Toddler Social and Emotional Assessment (BITSEA) has been validated against the ITSEA, the Child Behavior Check List for Ages 1.5–5 Years (Achenbach & Rescorla, 2000), the MacArthur-Bates CDI, and parental worry. In a cohort of 1,237 children ages 12–36 months, the BITSEA demonstrated appropriate sensitivity and specificity as a screening tool for delays in social-emotional competence (Briggs-Gowan et al., 2004). Almost 50% of children with low MacArthur-Bates CDI scores had low BITSEA scores, and almost 25% of children with abnormal BITSEA scores had low-score vocabulary. This discriminant validity reflects the comorbidity of social-emotional behavior problems and lower social competence among toddlers with language delays.

Measures of Family Context and Impact

Several measures are available to further assess family context and family impact on children with disabilities. The third edition of the Parenting Stress Index (PSI-3; Abidin, 1995) is a screening tool that examines the relationship between a parent's level of stress and the impact that stress has on the child. The PSI-3 is a 101-item scale divided into three domains: child domain (47 items), parent domain (54 items), and the optional Life Stress Scale (19 items). The PSI-3 has demonstrated good to excellent concurrent and discriminate validity with respect to children who are at risk for

emotional or behavior problems as well as parents who may be in need of parenting education and supports. There is also a 36-item short form (PSI-SF) that can be used for outpatient care. Three important factors captured in this scale are maternal self-esteem, parent–child interaction, and child self-regulation.

The Impact on Family Scale (Stein & Jessop, 2003) includes 15 items for the assessment of the social and family impact of a child's disability. As a measure of parental perception of the impact of a child's illness on family life, it measures psychological outcomes, social outcomes, and health service use. The scale also includes changes in family life and parental attributions of the impact of the child's illness on those changes.

The Family Resource Scale (Dunst & Leet, 1987) measures the adequacy of various resources in households with young children. It includes 31 items rated on a 5-point scale ranging from not at all adequate to almost always adequate. The hierarchy is derived from a conceptual framework that predicts that inadequacy of resources necessary to meet individually identified needs will negatively affect both personal well-being and parental commitment to carrying out professionally prescribed regimens unrelated to identified needs.

The Home Observation for Measurement of the Environment (HOME) was developed by Caldwell and Bradley (1984) to link environmental components of social disadvantage to practices that promote early childhood development. The HOME Inventory for Families of Infants and Toddlers has six subscales for ages birth to 3 years: responsibility, acceptance, organization, learning material, involvement, and enrichment. The domains of appropriate play material and maternal involvement are highly predictive of cognitive performance and identified children with developmental cognitive disability at age 3 more than two thirds of the time and those with IQ scores greater than 90 at age 3 more than 60% of the time. It can be a useful tool for support within high-risk environments for developmental cognitive disability (Bradley, 1995). It was also recently used in the Maternal Lifestyle Study of prospectively followed infants who were prenatally exposed to licit and illicit drugs (Messinger et al., 2004).

MEASURING HEALTH-RELATED QUALITY OF LIFE AND FUNCTIONAL STATUS

Several tools are available to health professionals for the assessment of the child's developmental and neurobehavioral status. These have been described in detail by Aylward (1994, 2002); Bracken (2000); Lidz (2003); Meisels and Fenichel (1996); Overton (1992); Sattler (2001, 2002); and Vohr, Wright, Hack, Aylward, and Hirtz (2004). Within the construct of health-related quality of life (HRQOL) are both explicit and implicit measures of physical, developmental, and behavioral functioning (Drottar, 1998; McDowell & Newell, 1996; Schalock, 1999). For this reason, HRQOL instruments that are applicable to children with neurodevelopmental impairments are reviewed in this section; a sample of three such instruments is provided in Table 22.4.

Health Utilities Index and Health Status Classification System–Preschool Version

The Health Utilities Index (HUI) is a set of multi-attribute health status classification systems (Torrance et al., 1996). Each HUI measurement system has two core components: 1) a generic multi-attribute health status ordinal rating and 2) a preference-based scoring function for assessing the outcomes of treatments. The HUI has been applied to children with cancer, spina bifida, asthma, and several other pediatric populations. In 1996, Saigal and colleagues had adolescents who were born extremely preterm evaluate their own health status at age 12–16 years. Adolescents from a normative community sample also evaluated their health status. Both groups had similar proportions rating their health status as optimal: 71% of ELBW teens and 73% of peers gave themselves a utility rating greater than .95 for health status (0 = imminent death, 1 = perfect health). Thus, these measures are an important component of long-term assessments and indicate that, although there are higher rates of neurodevelopmental impairments in ELBW infants, severe disability with perceived very low quality of life is rare.

In order to develop a health status–HRQOL tool for preschoolers and toddlers, Saigal and colleagues (2005) developed the Health Classification System–Preschool Version, a multi-attribute assessment of hearing, speaking, mobility, use of hands and fingers, self-care, feelings, learning and remembering, thinking and solving problems, pain and discomfort, general health, and behavior. Robust psychometric properties have been described for both Canadian and Australian ELBW survivors, a small group of children without prema-

Table 22.4. Health-related quality-of-life scales

	Health Utilities Index (HUI)	Child Health Questionnaire Parent Form 28 (CHQ-PF28)	Peds Quality of Life (PedsQL 4.0)
Domains	Multi-attribute health status classification: cognition, emotion, mobility, self-care, vision, hearing and communication, pain, fertility	Physical functioning, social emotional role, self-esteem, general health, bodily pain, mental health, behavior, parental impact, family activities and cohesion	Physical, emotional, social, and school functioning
Concurrent validity	Feeling Thermometer–Utilities	Disorder severity	Distinguishes between healthy children and children with special needs
Disability samples	Spina bifida, leukemia, epilepsy, extremely low birth weight	Epilepsy, cerebral palsy, attention-deficit/hyperactivity disorder, very low birth weight, juvenile rheumatoid arthritis, asthma	Cardiac disease, asthma, oncology, arthritis

turity or developmental challenges, and a large community.

Child Health and Illness Profile

Riley and colleagues (2004) developed the Child Report Form (CRF) and the Parent Report Form (PRF) of the Child Health and Illness Profile–Child Edition (CHIP-CE) for children ages 6–11 years. This 45-item questionnaire includes five domains: child health and self-esteem (8 items); comfort, or the degree to which a child experiences physical and emotional symptoms and their impact on activity limitations (12 items); resilience, which is a child's interpersonal, family support, and intrapersonal factors that enhance future health, such as regular physical activity (8 items); risk avoidance, which is the child's perception of how often there is engagement in behaviors that jeopardize future health or development (8 items); and academic and social achievement (9 items). Standardization involved more than 1,700 children in four geographic regions. There was adequate criterion validity with the physical functioning scale. The social competency measures correlated with friendships, academic achievement, and self-esteem. Both the CRF and PRF versions of the CHIP-CE assessments take approximately 20 minutes. More than 90% of the children and more than 80% of parents liked the format. Because the PRF requires a fifth-grade reading level, this tool has not yet been used directly in children with severe neurodevelopmental disorders but has been used in children with asthma and attention-deficit/hyperactivity disorder.

In 1993, Starfield and colleagues developed the Child Health and Illness Profile–Adolescent Edition (CHIP-AE), which covers health, discomfort, satisfaction with health, disorders, achievement of social expectations, risks, and resiliency in teenagers. The Spanish version has excellent validity (Rajmil, Serra-Sutton, Alonso, Herdman, et al., 2003; Rajmil, Serra-Sutton, Alonso, Starfield, et al., 2003). Validation has occurred for both children with chronic illness and children who were acutely ill (Starfield et al., 1996). Teens with chronic illness reported more activity limitations, greater dissatisfaction with their health, more chronic disorders, and less optimal physical fitness compared with school-age peers (Starfield

et al., 1995). Teens with acute illness reported more physical discomfort, minor illnesses, and lower physical fitness. Age, sex, and social class did not explain the differences, and there were substantial ranges of health status within teens with chronic illness and teens with acute illness. Overall, the CHIP-AE provides a means of documenting adolescent health needs and outcomes in populations of teenagers with acute or chronic illness and supports a person-focused (rather than a disease-focused) approach to assessing both needs for care and the impact of care on promoting health.

Child Health Questionnaires and Infant and Toddler Quality of Life Questionnaire

The Child Health Questionnaires (CHQ; Landgraf, Abetz, & Ware, 1996) measure physical functioning, role and social limitations, general health perception, bodily pain, self-esteem, parental impact of time and emotions, mental health, general behavior, family activities, family cohesion, and change in health among children 5 and older. There are three parent-completed versions of the CHQ, each with varying numbers of questions (28, 50, and 98 questions). There is also a child-completed version consisting of 87 questions for use with children 10 years and older. Administration time varies depending on the version. The instrument has been used to evaluate 199 children with cerebral palsy in the North American Growth and Cerebral Palsy Network (Liptak et al., 2001). These children were rated as having moderate to severe functional consequences using the GMFCS. Caregivers were administered the CHQ and a questionnaire designed to assess demographics, health, and functional status. Children with cerebral palsy had more significantly impaired physical health as measured by the CHQ physical summary score. In addition, the children's general health index was significantly associated with the GMFCS. The authors concluded that these children with cerebral palsy had overall poorer health status compared with the norm, and they have required more health-related treatments and resources than their peers.

The strength of the CHQ is that it measures physical, behavioral, and developmental status in middle childhood and adolescence, as well as a child's school and social functioning and family impact. The additional strength of this assessment tool is its uniformity for use with populations. This is facilitated by inclusion of explicit parental interview formats as well as a checklist for identifying ongoing conditions such as anxiety, asthma, inattention, behavioral problems, chronic allergies and sinus disorders, chronic musculoskeletal problems, chronic respiratory disorders, chronic rheumatic disease, depression, developmental delay or intellectual disabilities, diabetes, epilepsy, hearing or visual impairments, learning problems, speech problems, and sleep disturbances.

Building on the CHQ, Klassen and colleagues (2003) developed and validated a 103-item Infant and Toddler Quality of Life Questionnaire (ITQOL) for children ages 2 months to 5 years. Domains include physical abilities, growth and development, pain and discomfort, temperament and mood, general behavior, getting along with others, general health perception, and change in health. There are also five parental categories, including anxiety and worry about the child's health, limitations in time to meet parental needs because of the child's health, general health perception, and family cohesion. This instrument was used to assess more than 1,000 neonatal intensive care unit (NICU) survivors and almost 400 healthy term infants. Children who were in the NICU differed from healthy children in physical abilities, growth, development, temperament, mood, behavior, general health perceptions, and caregivers' burden (Klassen et al., 2004).

Child Health, Functional Status, Supports, and Participation Survey

Msall and Hogan developed the Child Health, Functional Status, Supports, and Participation Survey in 2000 (Hogan & Msall, 2007). Domains include descriptions of medical impairments, activity limitations, functional strengths and limitations, and ratings of physical, mental, and developmental health status. In addition, parents rated their physical and mental health status. For children ages 2 years and older, there are descriptions of health services, habilitative services, safety, and health status change. The overall goal of this effort was to capture key dimensions of child well-being and noncategorical components of child disability and to serve as a bridge between survey methodologies and more detailed clinical assessments. The Child Health, Functional Status, Supports, and Participation Survey domains are listed in Table 22.5.

Preliminary presentation of the domains occurred at the National Institutes of Health (NIH)–Casey Foundation Consensus Conference (Hogan & Msall, 2007; Msall & Tremont, 2002). This approach has also been used by Hogan and Park (2000) to link survey populations, family factors, and social support on developmental outcomes across very low, low, and normal birth weight survivors. It has also been used in the 8-year CRYO-ROP follow-up study (Msall et al., 2004).

Preschool Children Quality of Life Instrument

In the Netherlands, Fekkes and colleagues developed the Preschool Children Quality of Life Instrument (TAPQOL; Bunge et al., 2005; Fekkes, Theunissen, & Brugman, 2000). Domains include physical functioning, social functioning, cognitive functioning, and emotional functioning. The physical functioning domain includes motor skills such as walking, running, and coordination, as well as feeding and appetite, sleep, and health problems with breathing, digestion, and skin. Social functioning includes self-esteem, peer play, and social comfort, as well as problem behaviors of anger, irritability, short temper, aggression, restlessness, and making demands on caregivers. Cognitive functioning includes understanding what others say, speech, and elaboration in expressive language. Emotional functioning includes mood, anxiety, energy, and activity level. The TAPQOL was used to assess a cohort of preterm children born at 32–36 weeks' gestation as well as very preterm children born earlier than 32 weeks' gestation (Theunissen et al., 2001). Very preterm children, children with chronic medical impairments, children with lower parental rating of health status, and less happy children had significantly lower scores than comparison peers who were seen in primary well-child care (Fekkes et al., 2000).

Table 22.5. Child Health, Functional Status, Supports, and Participation Survey

Medical impairments

- Does your child currently require a tracheostomy, ventilator, feeding tube, dialysis, home intravenous infusion, or ear tubes?
- Has your child had any of the following: asthma, bronchopulmonary dysplasia, heart disease requiring medication or surgery, cerebral palsy, hydrocephalus, intellectual disabilities, autism, genetic disability, seizure disorder, sleep disorder, sickle cell anemia, anemia requiring ongoing transfusions, cystic fibrosis, diabetes, phenylketonuria, genetic metabolic disorder, Down syndrome, chromosomal disorder, gastroesophageal reflux disease, inflammatory bowel disease, systemic lupus erythematosis, juvenile rheumatoid arthritis, congenital immune deficiency, human immunodeficiency virus–acquired immunodeficiency syndrome, leukemia, cancer, or genetic disorder requiring surgery (cleft lip or palate, spina bifida)?

Participation and supports

- Compared with children of the same age, how well does your child (rated as *cannot do, below average, average, above average,* or *very talented*) play, make friends, and participate in sports, music, art, hobbies, scouts, or church?
- Does your child receive home nursing?
- Does your child have a personal care assistant at home?
- Is your child enrolled in early intervention?
- Does your child receive special education services?
- Does your child receive tutoring to keep up with homework?
- Does your child have an aide on the school bus or at school?

Functioning: Self-care and motor

- Does your child need more help than other children his or her age or have difficulty in completing the following activities due to an impairment or condition: eating, grasping objects, dressing, reaching overhead, bathing, lifting, toileting, bending, changing positions, walking, stooping, climbing stairs, or standing indefinitely?

Multi-attribute status: Sensory, communication, development, and behavior

- Describe your child's vision: 1) is blind; 2) has difficulty seeing even with glasses; 3) sees adequately with glasses; or 4) does not require correction.
- Describe your child's hearing ability: 1) is deaf; 2) has difficulty hearing even with hearing aid; 3) hears adequately with hearing aid; or 4) has no hearing problem.
- Describe your child's ability to communicate: 1) unable to communicate in words, gestures or sign language; 2) unable to communicate in conversations requiring sentences; 3) has difficulty being understood by others when speaking or signing; or 4) has no problem communicating.
- Describe your child's reading, mathematics, and writing skills at school: 1) is very far behind other children; 2) is behind other children; 3) is average; or 4) is above average.
- Describe your child's behavior with children of the same age: 1) very difficult; 2) sometimes difficult; 3) average; 4) somewhat easy; or 5) very easy.
- Describe your child's behavior with adults: 1) very difficult; 2) sometimes difficult; 3) average; 4) somewhat easy; or 5) very easy.
- Describe your child's judgment and maturity: 1) very far behind; 2) somewhat behind; 3) average; 4) above average; or 5) very advanced compared with peers.
- Does your child need physical therapy (for motor skills)?
- Does your child need occupational therapy (for fine motor–perceptual skills)?
- Does your child need speech therapy (for language)?
- Does your child need counseling/therapy (for behavior)?
- Does your child need tutoring for school subjects?
- Has your child missed more than 10 days of school in the past 12 months?
- Describe your child's experience with doctors or counselors for an emotional, developmental, or behavioral problem: 1) has not been seen; 2) has been seen; or 3) needs to be seen.
- If your child has been seen by a doctor or counselor for an emotional, developmental, or behavioral problem, when was the last time? Is your child receiving services? Is he or she receiving medication? Do you feel that it is helping and working?

Health status: Child and parent

Rate each as *excellent, very good, good, fair,* or *poor.*

- How would you rate your child's physical health?
- How would you rate your child's mental health?
- How would you rate your child's development?
- How would you as a parent rate your physical health?
- How would you as a parent rate your mental health?
- How would you as a parent rate your ability to work outside home?

Comparisons

- Compared with 12 months ago, is your child's health better, worse, or the same?
- Compared with other children his or her age, does your child require or use more medical care?
- Compared with other children his or her age, does your child require or use more mental health services?
- Compared with other children his or her age, does your child require or use more educational services?
- Compared with other children, how would you rate your child's height on a scale of short, somewhat average, average, tall, or very tall?
- Compared with other children, how would you rate your child's weight on a scale of very thin, thin, average, heavy, or very heavy?

Source: Hogan and Msall (2007).

Pediatric Quality of Life Inventory

Pediatric Quality of Life Inventory Version 4 (PedsQL 4.0) was designed to measure HRQOL in children and adolescents (Varni, Burwinkle, Seid, & Skarr, 2003). There are developmentally appropriate forms for ages 2–4, 5–7, 8–12, and 13–18 years. Pediatric self-report is measured in children and adolescents ages 5–18 years, and parent proxy-report is measured for children and adolescents ages 2–18 years. The generic core scale consists of 23 items covering physical functioning (8 items), emotional functioning (5 items), social functioning (5 items), and school functioning (5 items). This instrument distinguishes between healthy children and children with special needs. It has been translated into multiple languages, including Spanish. There are disease-specific versions for specific pediatric impairments, including cardiac disease, asthma, oncology, cerebral palsy, and arthritis. Initial studies demonstrate that the instrument is responsive to clinical change over time and can distinguish disease severity within a chronic health condition.

Domain-Specific HRQOL Measures

Two domain-specific HRQOL measures deserve comment. Camfield, Breau, and Camfield (2003) developed the Impact of Childhood Neurological Disability (ICND) Scale to assess the consequences of pediatric epilepsy on a child's functioning. Domains include behavior (inattentiveness, impulsiveness, or mood), cognitive (thinking and remembering), physical (movement, coordination, vision, or other sensory) and social consequences (with respect to seizure control, treatment, and side effects). There was excellent reliability, as well as concurrent validity with measures of parent stress, coping, and quality of life; children's self-esteem, isolation, and relation with siblings; and teacher's rating of academic performance. The ICND total score as well as scores for each domain were significantly related to quality-of-life ratings. In addition, families rated the negative impact of epilepsy on quality of life to be the largest for behavior, followed by cognition, physical/neurological disability, and finally epilepsy. Outside activity participation, social well-being, and home life were principal components that accounted for approximately half of the total variance of the ICND. Children with high ICND total scores had more parenting stress, lower self-esteem, and more emotional problems. Finally, children with "epilepsy plus" (i.e., children with epilepsy and cerebral palsy/intellectual disability/visual disability) had significantly higher total ICND scores as well as markedly elevated domain scores compared with those with epilepsy as their only neurological impairment.

Mackie, Jessen, and Jarvis (1998) developed the Lifestyle Assessment Questionnaire to measure the impact of cerebral palsy on children and their families. Sixty-six items encompass domains of communication, mobility, self-care, domestic life, interpersonal interactions, and relationship. Validation of the parent report form of this instrument shows that it can give a unique profile across neurodevelopmental disorders of mobility, communication, and cognition (Jessen, Colver, Mackie, & Jarvis, 2003; Mackie, Jessen, & Jarvis, 2002).

APPLICATIONS OF ADAPTIVE BEHAVIOR ASSESSMENT TOOLS

Use of the PEDI in the Midwest Newborn Lung Project

Palta, Sadek-Badawi, Evans, Weinstein, and McGuinness (2000) assessed 425 VLBW children at 5 years who were part of a neonatal regional study of respiratory complications after prematurity. Both the presence of severe intraventricular hemorrhage (IVH) and bronchopulmonary dysplasia independently predicted the presence of cerebral palsy, which occurred in almost 1 in 7 of those followed at age 5 years. Using the PEDI, children without IVH or with grade 1 IVH had self-care, mobility, and social function mean scores within the broad range of normal. Children with grade 3 or 4 IVH had scores between 1 and 1.8 standard deviation units (z) below the mean. This reflected functional challenges in self-care, mobility, and social function compared with typically developing kindergarten peers. Using scores more than 2 z below the mean as a criterion for functional limitations, children without cerebral palsy had 5% self-care functional limitations, 21% motor functional limitations, and 8% social functional limitations. In contrast, among children with cerebral palsy, self-care functional limitations occurred in 57%, mobility functional limitations in 89%, and social functional limitations in 32%. This effort helped highlight the wider spectrum of motor and social functional challenges in children

without cerebral palsy who were born with VLBW status.

Use of the VABS in Preschool Children with Communicative and Neurobehavioral Challenges

Rapin (1996) found that functional and adaptive assessment were important tools for preschool children with communicative disorders. This cohort included children with developmental language disorders, children with high-functioning (nonverbal IQ score 80+) and low-functioning (nonverbal IQ score < 80) autism spectrum disorders, and children with cognitive disability (IQ score < 70) but no features of autism spectrum disorder. Using the VABS, Rapin's team found the following mean daily living scores for each group of children: developmental language disorders = 85; high-functioning autism = 70; cognitive disability = 64; and low-functioning autism = 51. Among children with high-functioning autism spectrum disorder, picture vocabulary recognition predicted the VABS communication score. Among children with developmental language disorders, nonverbal IQ score predicted the VABS social score. Among children with low-functioning autism spectrum disorders, IQ score predicted the VABS communication score as well as the social score. Among children with cognitive disabilities, the verbal IQ score predicted the VABS communication and social scores. Thus, adaptive behavior can help inform the impact of a child's communicative or cognitive disability not only on communicative functioning but also on self-care and social skills.

HRQOL and Functional Outcome Measures for Children with Cerebral Palsy

Schneider, Gurucharri, Guiterrez, and Gaebler-Spira (2001) assessed 30 children ages 5–15 years (mean 8.5 years) using the GMFCS, the CHQ, the WeeFIM, and a Caregiver Questionnaire. The latter was a linear analogue scale of personal care, positioning, comfort, and interaction. Significant correlations were found between the Caregiver Questionnaire and the WeeFIM across total scores and subscale scores. Significant correlations were also found between CHQ subscales of parent time and family cohesion and Caregiver Questionnaire scores. There was a lack of correlation between the CHQ and the WeeFIM that was interpreted as indicating that functional status and HRQOL are different constructs. Both the WeeFIM and the Caregiver Questionnaire, however, reflected the impact of the child's condition on the caregiver.

McCarthy, Atkins, Harryman, Sponseller, and Hadley-Miller (2002) compared the GMFM, the PEDI, the CHQ, and the Pediatric Orthopedic Society of North America's Pediatric Outcomes Data Collection Instrument (POSNA-PODCI) in 115 children ages 3–10 years with spastic cerebral palsy. The POSNA-PODCI includes dimensions of upper extremity function, transfer and mobility, sports and physical function, comfort-pain free, happiness and satisfaction, expectation of treatment, and global function and comfort. The children's typology of cerebral palsy ranged from hemiplegia in 28 to diplegia in 49 and quadriplegia in 38. The mean GMFM scores were 89, 77, and 24, respectively. PEDI self-care scores were 66, 61, and 43, while social functioning scores were 65, 63, and 52. General health perception scores were 61, 57, and 56, and behavior scores were 65, 71, and 79. The POSNA-PODCI transfer and mobility scale and the PEDI mobility scale detected the most significant differences across typologies. The PEDI social function scale detected the largest difference in cognitive function between those with any degree of intellectual disability compared with those with IQ scores greater than 70.

Wake, Salmon, and Reddihough (2003) compare the GMFCS, the CHQ, and impact of intellectual disability and epilepsy in 80 children ages 5–18 years with cerebral palsy in Melbourne. Children with severe functional disability and cerebral palsy had poorer physical health, but psychosocial health and emotional impact on parents were similar for mild and severe cerebral palsy. Health status on the CHQ did not vary by the presence of intellectual/developmental disability or epilepsy.

Østensjø, Carlberg, and Vøllestad (2004) assessed 95 Norwegian children with cerebral palsy using the GMFCS and the PEDI. There were 44 children with diplegia, 19 with hemiplegia, and 32 with quadriplegia. Thirty-four percent were at a GMFCS of level 1/2, 10% at level 3, and 46% at level 4/5. As GMFCS level increased, caregiver assistance, modifications, and limitations in activity performance increased. Stepwise regression showed that the GMFCS level was a good predictor of everyday functioning, with both chronological age and cognition as contributing factors.

Overall, these studies demonstrate that, in assessing the functional status of children with cerebral palsy, generic HRQOL measures do not fully capture what can be assessed from both adaptive measures and functional status measures. These studies also illustrated that there is wide diversity in self-care, communicative, and learning competencies across types and severity of motor performance in children with cerebral palsy.

Spectrum of Gross Motor Function in ELBW Children with Cerebral Palsy at 18 Months of Age

A multicenter longitudinal cohort study was conducted of 1,868 ELBW infants born between 1995 and 1998 and evaluated at 18–22 months' corrected age (Vohr et al., 2005). Children were categorized into impairment groups based on the typology and physiology of neurological findings: spastic quadriplegia, triplegia, diplegia, hemiplegia, and monoplegia; hypotonic or athetotic cerebral palsy or both; other abnormal neurological findings; and normal. The abnormal neurological findings category was then compared with GMFCS level and Bayley motor scores. Two hundred eighty-two (15.2%) of the 1,860 children evaluated had cerebral palsy. Children with more limbs involved had more abnormal GMFCS levels and lower Bayley scores reflecting more severe functional limitations; however, for each cerebral palsy diagnostic category, there was a spectrum of gross motor functional levels and Bayley scores. More than 1 in 4 (26.6%) of the children with cerebral palsy had moderate to severe gross motor functional impairment, but almost 3 in 4 (73.4%) had motor functional skills that allowed for ambulation and self-mobility.

Kindergarten Functional Status, School Function, and 10-Year HRQOL

Children with severe neonatal retinopathy of prematurity (ROP) are the sickest, tiniest, and most medically fragile of VLBW and ELBW infants. The WeeFIM instrument was used at age 5.5 years with more than 1,000 children of less than 1,250 g birth weight enrolled in the NIH-sponsored Multi-center Randomized Trial of Cryosurgery for Retinopathy of Prematurity (CRYO-ROP; Msall, Phelps, et al., 2000). Overall, 88% of these children were followed across 23 centers. As severity of retinopathy increased, functional status declined and severe disability in social roles increased.

The complexity and severity of disability was worse in the 134 children with severe ROP and unfavorable visual acuity compared with that of the 81 children with severe ROP and favorable visual acuity. The former group had a rate of motor limitations of 43% compared with 5.2% for the latter group; a rate of self-care limitations of 78% compared with 25%; a rate of continency limitations of 51% versus 4.5%; and a rate of communicative/cognitive limitations of 67% versus 22%. Functional limitations in children without ROP were low: motor = 4%, self-care = 7%, continency = 4%, and communicative/cognitive limitations = 8%. Multiple logistic regression analysis revealed that favorable visual status and favorable 2-year neurological score predicted Wee-FIM functional status at age 5.5 years. The favorable 2-year neurological score included the absence of microcephaly, seizures, and/or hydrocephalus. Access to health insurance and African American race also contributed to better WeeFIM functional status at age 5.5 years.

Overall, this project demonstrated that functional assessment was a very useful measure of outcomes for children receiving new technologies and helped professionals and families understand developmental risk and resiliency. At age 8 years, outcome of the group that had the most severe ROP was examined with respect to developmental and educational outcome (Msall et al., 2004). Of 255 survivors, 85% were available for follow-up at age 8 years. Favorable visual and functional status at kindergarten entry and higher socioeconomic status were associated with significantly lower rates of special education services and below-grade-level educational achievement. Factors that were significantly associated with an increased risk for special education services included minority status, poverty, lack of access to a car, and Supplemental Social Security income because of disability and poverty. In multivariate regression analysis, the key predictors of special educational services at age 8 years were unfavorable visual status and unfavorable functional status at 5.5 years.

Additional studies by the CRYO-ROP Cooperative Group at age 10 years involved parental assessments with the HUI for HRQOL. The proportion of sighted children with limitations in four or more HUI attributes of mobility, speech, dexterity, cognition, emotion, pain, or hearing was 6.4% compared with 47% in children with blindness or low vision. The HRQOL score consists of a utility scale ranging from 1, indicating perfect health, to 0, reflecting death. The median HRQOL score was .87 for sighted children compared with .27 for blind/low vision children ($p < 0.001$) (Quinn et al., 2004). Thus this series of outcomes at ages 5.5 years, 8 years, and 10 years revealed the value of both functional assessment and HRQOL for children receiving new technologies. Because severe ROP occurred in just 6% of survivors with birth weights less than 1,251 g in this 1986–87 cohort, these efforts in linking functional status, educational status, and HRQOL reflect a very small subset of neonatal practices in the presurfactant era.

Use of the VABS or the WeeFIM in Children with Congenital Heart Disease

Limperopoulos et al. (2001) in Montreal examined functional assessment in children with congenital heart disease receiving open heart surgery in infancy (Limperopoulos et al., 2001). Children with hypoplastic heart syndrome were excluded. In a cohort of 118 survivors, 83% were followed at 18 months using either the WeeFIM or VABS ratings. For the

WeeFIM, mean quotients were 84 in self-care, 77 in mobility, and 92 in social cognition (normal = 100 ± 15). The WeeFIM total quotient was 84. Only 21% of the cohort was functioning similar to peers in basic skills. Moderate functional disability was noted in 37%, and severe functional disability in 6%. For the VABS, mean score for daily living skills was 84 and for socialization skills was 80 (normal = 100 ± 15). Functional difficulties in daily living skills were documented in 40%, with more than half of the children having poor socialization skills. Factors enhancing the risk for functional disabilities included perioperative neurodevelopmental status, microcephaly, length of deep hypothermic circulatory arrest, length of stay in the intensive care unit, age at surgery, and maternal education. This study demonstrates that there were high prevalence rates of functional limitations even as early as 18 months that have a significant impact on development and community care. In addition, there are opportunities for prospectively examining supports that enhance parent management skills involving some of these functional challenges.

Use of Functional Indicators in Population Surveys

One of the advantages of using functional measures is the ability to apply the construct to population surveys. For example, Hogan et al. (2000) examined functional limitations in mobility, self-care, communication, and learning in school-age children using the 1994–1995 National Health Interview Survey Disability Supplement. This was a representative, diverse sample of school-age children and allowed for population estimates. Among the 50 million schoolchildren ages 5–17 years, the prevalence of motor functional disability was 2.5 per 1,000; self-care disability was 5 per 1,000; communication-sensory disability was 30 per 1,000; and developmental disability in learning, attention, and behavior was 100 per 1,000. Overall there were 125,000 American schoolchildren with severe motor disability, 250,000 with self-care disability, 1,500,000 with communication-sensory disability, and 5,000,000 with learning/attention/behavior disability. Of children with multiple limitations in function-

ing, almost 3 in 5 had either a neurodevelopmental or learning-behavior disorder, approximately 1 in 5 had a physical disorder, and 1 in 5 did not have an identified impairment because they had not received medical services in the past year (Msall et al., 2003). Of additional concern was that more than half of the children needing or receiving special education services had had no recent contact with medical professionals.

CONCLUSION

In an era of fragmented and often scarce resources for supports to children with neurodevelopmental impairments, assessment strategies need to be developed that capture communicative, mobility, dexterity, self-care, peer interaction, and regulatory behaviors (joint attention, sleep, play) because they occur in usual activities. The advantage of functional assessment is that consideration of special equipment or assistive devices can occur in completing a task. In functional assessment, task performance, not the process used to achieve the outcome, is measured. In addition, functional assessment allows for a focus on the supports necessary for success in the classroom and in the community. Additional advantages of functional assessment are that it is criterion referenced, assesses typical performance, and can be linked to population surveys. As a tool, it can facilitate a common language for describing child disability. In this era of tremendous genetic, developmental, and neuroscience advances, our task is not only to prevent disability whenever possible but also to optimize outcomes of functional independence, family supports, and community participation.

REFERENCES

Abidin, R.R. (1995). *Parenting stress index* (3rd ed.). Odessa, FL: Psychological Assessment Resources.

Accardo, P.J., & Capute, A.J. (2005). *The Capute Scales: Cognitive Adaptive Test and Clinical Linguistic and Auditory Milestone Scale (CAT/CLAMS).* Baltimore: Paul H. Brookes Publishing Co.

Achenbach, T.M., & Rescorla, M.A. (Eds.). (2000). *Manual for the ASEBA Preschool Forms and Profiles.* Burlington: University of Vermont, Department of Psychiatry.

Aylward, G.P. (1994). *Practitioner's guide to developmental and psychological testing.* New York: Plenum Medical.

Aylward, G.P. (2002). Cognitive and neuropsychological outcomes: More than IQ scores. *Mental Retardation and Developmental Disabilities Research Reviews, 8*(4), 234–240.

Bayley, N. (1933). Mental growth during the first three years. *Genetic Psychology, 14,* 1.

Bayley, N. (1993). *Bayley Scales of Infant Development* (2nd ed.). San Antonio, TX: The Psychological Coporation.

Bayley, N. (2005). *Bayley Scales of Infant Development–Third Edition (BAYLEY-III).* San Antonio, TX: Harcourt Assessment.

Bracken, B.A. (Ed.). (2000). *The psychoeducational assessment of preschool children* (3rd ed.). Boston: Allyn & Bacon.

Bradley, R.H. (1995). Home environment and adaptive social behavior among premature, low birth weight children: Alternative models of environmental action. *Journal of Pediatric Psychology, 20*(3), 347–362.

Briggs-Gowan, M.J., Carter, A.S., Irwin, J.R., Wachtel, K., & Cicchetti, D.V. (2004). The Brief Infant-Toddler Social and Emotional Assessment: Screening for social-emotional problems and delays in competence. *Journal of Pediatric Psychology, 29,* 143–155.

Bruininks, R.H., Woodcock, R., Weatherman, R., & Hill B. (1996). *Scales of Independent Behavior–Revised.* Chicago: Riverside Publishing.

Bunge, E.M., Essink-Bot, M.-L., Kobussen, M.P.H.M., van Suijlekom-Smit, L.W.A., Moll, H.A., & Raat, H. (2005). Reliability and validity of health status measurement by the TAPQOL. *Archives of Disease in Childhood, 90,* 351–358.

Caldwell, B., & Bradley, R. (1984). *Home Observation for Measurement of the Environment (HOME) Inventory.* Little Rock: University of Arkansas at Little Rock.

Camfield, C., Breau, L., & Camfield, P. (2003). Assessing the impact of pediatric epilepsy and concomitant behavioral, cognitive, and physical neurologic disability: Impact of childhood neurologic disability scale. *Developmental Medicine and Child Neurology, 45,* 152–159.

Capute, A.J., & Accardo, P.J. (Eds.). (1996a). *Developmental disabilities in infancy and childhood* (2nd ed.). Baltimore: Paul H. Brookes Publishing Co.

Capute, A.J., & Accardo, P.J. (1996b). The infant neurodevelopmental assessment: A clinical interpretive manual for CAT-CLAMS in the first two years of life. *Current Problems in Pediatrics, 26,* 238–257 (Pt. 1); 279–306 (Pt. 2).

Capute, A.J., & Biehl, R.F. (1973). Functional developmental evaluation: Prerequisite to habilitation. *Pediatric Clinics of North America, 20,* 3–26.

Capute, A.J., & Shapiro (1985). The motor quotient: A method for the early detection of motor delay.

American Journal of Diseases of Children, 139(9), 940–942.

Carter, A.S., & Briggs-Gowan, M.J. (2000). *Manual of the Infant-Toddler Social and Emotional Assessment.* New Haven, CT: Yale University.

Carter, A.S., Briggs-Gowan, M.J., Jones, S.M., & Little, T.D. (2003). The Infant-Toddler Social and Emotional Assessment (ITSEA): Factor structure, reliability, and validity. *Journal of Abnormal Child Psychology, 31,* 495–514.

Chung, B.H., Wong, V.C., & Ip, P. (2004). Spinal muscular atrophy: Survival pattern and functional status. *Pediatrics, 114,* e548–e553.

Colvin, L., Fyfe, S., Leonard, S., Schiavello, T., Ellaway, C., De Klerk, N., et al. (2003). Describing the phenotype in Rett syndrome using a population database. *Archives of Disease in Childhood, 88,* 38–43.

Darrah, J., Piper, M., & Watt, M.J. (1998). Assessment of gross motor skills of at-risk infants: Predictive validity of the Alberta Infant Motor Scale. *Developmental Medicine and Child Neurology, 40,* 485–491.

Drotar, D. (Ed.). (1998). *Measuring health-related quality of life in children and adolescents: Implications for research and practice.* Mahwah, NJ: Lawrence Erlbaum Associates.

Dunn, L.M., & Dunn, L.M. (1997). *Peabody Picture Vocabulary Test–Third Edition (PPVT-III).* Circle Pines, MN: American Guidance Service.

Dunst, C.J., & Leet, H.E. (1987). Measuring the adequacy of resources in households with young children. *Child: Care, Health and Development, 13,* 111–125.

Fekkes, M., Theunissen, N.C., & Brugman, E. (2000). Developmental and psychological evaluation of the TAPQOL: A health related quality of life instrument for 1–5 year old children. *Quality of Life Research, 9,* 961–972.

Feldman, A.B., Haley, S.M., & Coryell, J. (1990). Concurrent and construct validity of the Pediatric Evaluation of Disability Inventory. *Physical Therapy, 70,* 602–610.

Fenson, L., Dale, P.S., Reznick, J.S., Thal, D.J., Hartung, J.P., Pethick, S., et al. (Eds.). (2007). *MacArthur-Bates Communicative Development Inventories: User's guide and technical manual* (2nd ed.). Baltimore: Paul H. Brookes Publishing Co.

Folio, M.R., & Fewell, R.R. (2000). *Peabody Developmental Motor Scales, Second Edition (PDMS–2).* Austin, TX: PRO-ED.

Gardner, M.F. (1981). *Expressive One-Word Picture Vocabulary Test.* Novato, CA: Academic Therapy Publications.

Gesell, A., Halverson, H.M., Thompson, H., Ilg, F.L., Castner, B.M., Ames, L.B., et al. (1940). *The first five years of life: A guide to the study of the preschool child.* New York: Harper & Row.

Gray, L.A., Lyon, N., Roistacher, J., Mariano, K., Baker, C.P., McKearnan, K., et al. (2006). Normative sample of the Warner Initial Developmental Evaluation of Adaptive and Functional Skills: Personal digital assistant network application in early childhood and in child disability. *Developmental Medicine and Child Neurology, 48* (Suppl. 106), 42(Abstract SP 33).

Griffiths, R. (1954). *The abilities of babies.* London: University of London Press.

Guyatt, G., Walter, S., & Norman, G. (1987). Measuring change over time: Assessing the usefulness of evaluative instruments. *Journal of Chronic Diseases, 40*(2), 171–178.

Haley, S.M., Coster, W.J., Ludlow, L.H., Haltiwanger, J.T., & Andrellos, P.J. (1992). *Pediatric Evaluation of Disability Inventory (PEDI) Version 1.* Boston: New England Medical Center–PEDI Research Group.

Haley, S.M., Fragala-Pinkham, M.A., Ni, P.S., Skrinar, A.M., & Kaye, E.M. (2004). Pediatric physical functioning reference curves. *Pediatric Neurology, 31,* 333–341.

Hayley, S.M., Ni, P., Ludlow, L.H., & Fragala-Pinkham, M.A. (2006). Measurement precision and efficiency of multidimensional computer adaptive testing of physical functioning using the pediatric evaluation of disability inventory. *Archives of Physical Medicine and Rehabilitation, 87*(9), 1223–1229.

Hogan, D.P., & Msall, M.E. (2007). Health and disability indicators for preschool and school age children. In B. Brown (Ed.), *Indicators of child and youth well-being: Completing the picture.* Mahwah, NJ: Lawrence Erlbaum Associates.

Hogan, D.P., & Park, J.M. (2000). Family factors and social support in the developmental outcomes of very low-birth weight children. *Clinics in Perinatology, 27,* 433–459.

Hogan, D.P., Rogers, M.L., & Msall, M.E. (2000). Functional limitations and key indicators of well-being in children with disability. *Archives of Pediatric and Adolescent Medicine, 154,* 1042–1048.

Illingworth, R.S. (1984). *The development of the infant and young child: Normal and abnormal* (8th ed.). London: Churchill Livingstone.

Jessen, E.C., Colver, A.F., Mackie, P.C., & Jarvis, S.N. (2003). Development and validation of a tool to measure the impact of childhood disabilities on the lives of children and their families. *Child: Care, Health and Development, 29,* 21–34.

Jongjit, J., Komsopapong, L., & Chira-Adisai, W. (2002). Measuring functional status in Thai children with disabilities. *Journal of the Medical Association of Thailand, 85,* 446–454.

Kaufman, A.S., & Kaufman, N.L. (2004). *Kaufman Assessment Battery for Children, Second Edition (KABC-II).* San Antonio, TX: Pearson Assessment.

Kirby, R.S., Brewster, M.A., Canino, C.U., & Pavin, M. (1995). Early childhood surveillance of developmental disorders by a birth defects surveillance system: Methods, prevalence comparisons, and mortality patterns. *Journal of Developmental and Behavioral Pediatrics, 16,* 318–326.

Kirschner, B., & Guyatt, G. (1985). A methodological framework for assessing health indices. *Journal of Chronic Diseases, 38*(1), 27–36.

Klassen, A.F., Landgraf, J.M., Lee, S.K., Barer, M., Raina, P., Chan, H.P., et al. (2003). Health related quality of life in 3 and 4 year old children and their parents: Preliminary findings about a new questionnaire. *Health and Quality of Life Outcomes, 1,* 1–12.

Klassen, A.F., Lee, S.K., Raina, P., Chan, H.W.P., Matthew, D., & Brabyn, D. (2004). Health status and health-related quality of life in a population-based sample of neonatal intensive care unit graduates. *Pediatrics, 113,* 594–600.

Koot, H.M., & Wallander, J.L. (Eds.). (2001). *Quality of life in child and adolescent illness: Concepts, methods, and findings.* New York: Taylor & Francis.

Kothari, D.H., Haley, S.M., Gill-Body, K.M., & Dumas, H.M. (2003). Measuring functional change in children with acquired brain injury (ABI): Comparison of generic and ABI-specific scales using the Pediatric Evaluation of Disability Inventory (PEDI). *Physical Therapy, 83,* 776–785.

Landgraf, J.M., Abetz, L., & Ware, J.E. (Eds.). (1996). *Child Health Questionnaire (CHR): A user's manual.* Boston: The Health Institute, New England Medical Center.

Leonard, S., Msall, M., Bower, C., Tremont, M., & Leonard, H. (2002). Functional status of school-aged children with Down syndrome. *Journal of Paediatrics and Child Health, 38,* 160–165.

Lidz, C.S. (2003). *Early childhood assessment.* New York: John Wiley & Sons.

Limperopoulos, C., Majnemer, A., Shevell, M.I., Rosenblatt, B., Rohlicek, C., Tchervenkov, C., et al. (2001). Functional limitations in young children with congenital heart defects after cardiac surgery. *Pediatrics, 108,* 1325–1331.

Liptak, G.S., O'Donnell, M., Conaway, M., Chumlea, W.C., Wolrey, G., Henderson, R.C., et al. (2001). Health status of children with moderate to severe cerebral palsy. *Developmental Medicine and Child Neurology, 43,* 364–370.

Lowen, D.E., Msall, M.E., Jenny, C., Tremont M, Showers J et al. (2000). Functional limitations in self-care, mobility, communication and learning after surviving inflicted head trauma. *Pediatric Research, 47*(4 Pt. 2), 206A, 1217.

Luckasson, R., Coulter, D.L., Polloway, S., Reiss, S., Schalock, R.L., Snell, M.E., et al. (2002). *Mental retardation: Definition, classification, and systems of supports* (10th ed.). Washington, DC: American Association on Mental Retardation.

Mackie, P.C., Jessen, E.C., & Jarvis, S. (1998). The Lifestyle Assessment Questionnaire: An instrument to measure the impact of disability on the lives of children with cerebral palsy and their families. *Child: Care, Health and Development, 24,* 473–486.

Mackie, P.C., Jessen, E.C., & Jarvis, S.N. (2002). Creating a measure of impact of childhood disability: Statistical methodology. *Public Health, 116,* 95–101.

McCarthy, M.L., Atkins, E.A., Harryman, S.E., Sponseller, P.D., & Hadley-Miller, N.A. (2002). Comparing reliability and validity of pediatric instruments for measuring health and well-being of children with spastic cerebral palsy. *Developmental Medicine and Child Neurology, 44,* 468–476.

McDowell, I., & Newell, C. (1996). *Measuring health: A guide to rating scales and questionnaires* (2nd ed.). New York: Oxford University Press.

Meisels, S.J., & Fenichel, E.S. (Eds.). (1996). *New visions for the developmental assessment of infants and young children.* Washington, DC: Zero to Three/National Center for Infants, Toddlers, and Families.

Messinger, D.S., Bauer, C.R., Das, A., Seifer, R., Lester, B.M., Lagasse, L.L., et al. (2004). The maternal lifestyle study: Cognitive, motor, and behavioral outcomes of cocaine-exposed and opiate-exposed infants through three years of age. *Pediatrics, 113*(6), 1677–1685.

Montgomery, T.R. (1988). Clinical aspects of mental retardation: The chief complaint. *Clinical Pediatrics, 27,* 529–531.

Msall, M.E., Avery, R.C., Tremont, M.R., Lima, J.C., Rogers, M.L., & Hogan, D.P. (2003). Functional disability and school activity limitations in 41,300 school age children: Relationship to medical impairments. *Pediatrics, 111,* 548–553.

Msall, M.E., DiGaudio, K., Duffy, L.C., LaForest, S., Braun, S., & Granger, C.V. (1994). WeeFIM: Normative sample of an instrument for tracking functional independence in children. *Clinical Pediatrics, 33,* 431–438.

Msall, M.E., DiGaudio, K., Rogers, B.T., LaForest, S., Lyon, N., Campbell, J., et al. (1994). The Functional Independence Measure for Children (WeeFIM): Conceptual basis and pilot use in children with developmental disabilities. *Clinical Pediatrics, 33,* 421–430.

Msall, M.E., Phelps, D.L., DiGaudio, K.M., Dobson, V., Tung, B., McClead, R.E., et al. (2000). Severity of neonatal retinopathy of prematurity is predictive of neurodevelopmental functional outcome at age 5.5 years. *Pediatrics, 106,* 998–1005.

Msall, M.E., Phelps, D.L., Hardy, R.J., Dobson, V., Quinn, G.E., Summers, C.G., et al., for the Cryotherapy for Retinopathy of Prematurity Cooperative Group. (2004). Educational and social competencies at 8 years in children with threshold retinopathy of prematurity in the CRYO-ROP multicenter study. *Pediatrics, 113,* 790–799.

Msall, M.E., & Tremont, M.R. (2002). Measuring functional outcomes after prematurity: Developmental impact of very low birth weight and extremely low birth weight status on childhood disability. *Mental Retardation and Developmental Disabilities Research Review, 8,* 258–272.

Msall, M.E., Tremont, M.R., & Ottenbacher, K.J. (2001). Functional assessment of preschool children: Optimizing developmental and family supports in early intervention. *Infants and Young Children, 14,* 46–66.

Mullen, E.M. (1995). *Mullen Scales of Early Learning.* Circle Pines, MN: American Guidance Service.

National Research Council and Institute of Medicine. (2004). *Children's health, the nation's wealth: Assessing and improving child health.* Committee on Evaluation of Children's Health, Board on Children, Youth, and Families, Division of Behavioral and Social Sciences and Education. Washington, DC: The National Academies Press.

Neligan, G., & Prudham, D. (1969). Norms for four standard developmental milestones by sex, social class and place in family. *Developmental Medicine and Child Neurology, 11,* 413–422.

Newacheck, P.W., Strickland, B., Shonkoff, J.P., Perrin, J.M., McPherson, M., McManus, M., et al. (1998). An epidemiologic profile of children with special health care needs. *Pediatrics, 102*(1 Pt 1), 117–123.

Newborg, J., Stock, J.R., Wnek, L., Guidubaldi, J., & Svinicki, J. (1988). *Battelle Developmental Inventory (BDI).* Chicago: Riverside Publishing.

Østensjø, S., Carlberg, E.B., & Vøllestad, N.K. (2004). Motor impairments in young children with cerebral palsy: Relationship to gross motor function and everyday activities. *Developmental Medicine and Child Neurology, 46,* 580–589.

Ottenbacher, K.J., Msall, M.E., Lyon, N.R., Duffy, L.C., Granger, C.V., & Braun, S. (1997). Interrater agreement and stability of the Functional Independence Measure for Children (WeeFIM): Use in children with developmental disabilities. *Archives of Physical Medicine and Rehabilitation, 78,* 1309–1315.

Ottenbacher, K.J., Msall, M.E., Lyon, N., Duffy, L.C., Granger, C.V., & Braun, S. (1999). Measuring developmental and functional status in children with disabilities. *Developmental Medicine & Child Neurology, 41,* 186–194.

Ottenbacher, K.J., Msall, M.E., Lyon, N., Duffy, L.C., Ziviani, J., Granger, C.V., et al. (2000a). Functional assessment and care of children with neurodevelopmental disabilities. *American Journal of Physical Medicine and Rehabilitation, 79,* 114–123.

Ottenbacher, K.J., Msall, M.E., Lyon, N.R., Duffy, L.C., Ziviani, J., Granger, C.V., et al. (2000b). The WeeFIM instrument: Its utility in detecting change in children with developmental disabilities. *Archives of Physical Medicine and Rehabilitation, 81,* 1317–1326.

Ottenbacher, K.J., Taylor, E.T., Msall, M.E., Braun, S., Lane, S.J., Granger, C.V., et al. (1996). The stability and equivalence reliability of the Functional Independence Measure for Children (WeeFIM). *Developmental Medicine and Child Neurology, 38,* 907–916.

Overton, T. (1992). *Assessment in special education: An applied approach.* New York: Maxwell Macmillan International.

Palta, M., Sadek-Badawi, M., Evans, M., Weinstein, M.R., & McGuinness, G. (2000). Functional assessment of a multicenter very low-birth-weight cohort at age 5 years. *Archives of Pediatrics and Adolescent Medicine, 154,* 23–30.

PRB/KIDS COUNT Special Report. (2002). *Children at risk: State trends 1990–2000.* Baltimore: Annie E. Casey Foundation.

Quinn, G.E., Dobson, V., Saigal, S., Phelps, D.L., Hardy, R.J., Tung, B., et al., for the CRYO-ROP Cooperative Group. (2004). Health-related quality of life at age 10 years in very low-birth-weight children with and without threshold retinopathy of prematurity. *Archives of Ophthalmology, 122,* 1659–1666.

Rajmil, L., Serra-Sutton, V., Alonso, J., Herdman, M., Riley, A., & Starfield, B. (2003). Validity of the Spanish version of the Child Health and Illness Profile–Adolescent Edition (CHIP-AE). *Medical Care, 41,* 1153–1163.

Rajmil, L., Serra-Sutton, V., Alonso, J., Starfield, B., Riley, A.W., & Vazquez, J.R., for the Research Group for the Spanish Version of the CHIP-AE. (2003). The Spanish version of the Child Health and Illness Profile–Adolescent Edition (CHIP-AE). *Quality of Life Research, 12,* 303–313.

Rapin, I. (1996). *Preschool children with inadequate communication: Developmental language disorder, autism, low IQ.* London: MacKeith Press.

Riley, A.W., Forrest, C.B., Starfield, B., Rebok, G.W., Robertson, J.A., & Green, B.F. (2004). The Parent Report Form of the CHIP–Child Edition: Reliability and validity. *Medical Care, 42,* 210–220.

Roid, G.H. (2003). *Stanford-Binet Intelligence Scales, Fifth Edition (SB5).* Chicago: Riverside Publishing.

Rosenbaum, P.L., Walter, S.D., Hanna, S.E., Palisano, R.J., Russell, D.J., Raina, P., et al. (2002). Prognosis for gross motor function in cerebral palsy: creation of motor development curves. *JAMA, 288*(11), 1357–1363.

Russell, D.J., Rosenbaum, P.L., Avery, L.M., & Lane, M. (Eds.). (2002). *Gross Motor Function Measure (GMFM-66 & GMFM-88) users manual.* London: MacKeith Press.

Saigal, S., Feeny, D., Rosenbaum, P., Furlong, W., Burrows, E., & Stoskopf, B. (1996). Self-perceived health status and health-related quality of life of extremely low-birth-weight infants at adolescence. *JAMA, 276*(6), 453–459.

Saigal, S., Rosenbaum, P.L., Stoskopf, B.L., Hoult, L., Furlong, W., Feeny, D., et al. (2005). Development, reliability and validity of a new measure of overall health for pre-school children. *Quality of Life Research, 14,* 243–257.

Sattler, J.M. (2001). *Assessment of children: Cognitive applications* (4th ed.). San Diego: Jerome M. Sattler.

Sattler, J.M. (2002). *Assessment of children: Behavioral and clinical applications* (4th ed.). San Diego: Jerome M. Sattler.

Schalock, R.L. (1999). *Adaptive behavior and its measurement: Implications for the field of mental retardation.* Washington, DC: American Association on Mental Retardation.

Schneider, J.W., Gurucharri, L.M., Guiterrez, A.L., & Gaebler-Spira, D.J. (2001). Health Related Quality of Life and Functional Outcome Measures for Children with Cerebral Palsy. *Developmental Medicine and Child Neurology, 43,* 601–608.

Shapiro, B.K. (2001). Specific reading disability: A multiplanar view. *Mental Retardation and Developmental Disabilities Research Review, 7,* 13–20.

Semel, E., Wiig, E.H., & Secord, W.A. (2003). *Clinical Evaluation of Language Fundamentals-Fourth Edition (CELF-4).* San Antonio, TX: Harcourt Assessment.

Simeonsson, R.J., Lollar, D., Hollowell, J., & Adams, M. (2000). Revision of the International Classification of Impairments, Disabilities and Handicaps: Developmental issues. *Journal of Clinical Epidemiology, 53,* 113–124.

Sparrow, S., Balla, D.A., & Cicchetti, D.V. (1984). *Vineland Adaptive Behavior Scales, Interview Edition, survey form manual.* Circle Pines, MN: American Guidance Service.

Sparrow, S.S., Balla, D.A., & Cicchetti, D.V. (1997). *Vineland Social-Emotional Early Childhood Scales (SEEC) manual.* Circle Pines, MN: American Guidance Service.

Sparrow, S.S., Balla, D.A., & Cicchetti, D.V. (2005). *Vineland Adaptive Behavior Scales-2 manual.* Circle Pines, MN: American Guidance Service.

Starfield, B., Bergner, M., Ensminger, M., Riley, A., Ryan, S., Green, B., et al. (1993). Adolescent health status measurement: Development of the Child Health and Illness Profile. *Pediatrics, 91,* 430–435.

Starfield, B., Forrest, C.B., Ryan, S.A., Riley, A.W., Ensminger, M.E., & Green, B.F. (1996). Health status of well vs. ill adolescents. *Archives of Pediatrics and Adolescent Medicine, 150,* 1249–1256.

Starfield, B., Riley, A.W., Green, B.F., Ensminger, M.E., Ryan, S.A., Kelleher, K., et al. (1995). The Adolescent Child Health and Illness Profile: A population-based measure of health. *Medical Care, 33,* 553–566.

Stein, R.E., & Jessop, D.J. (2003). The Impact on Family Scale revisited: Further psychometric data. *Journal of Developmental and Behavioral Pediatrics, 24,* 9–16.

Stein, R.E., & Silver, E.J. (1999). Operationalizing a conceptually based noncategorical definition: A first look at U.S. children with chronic conditions. *Archives of Pediatrics and Adolescent Medicine, 153,* 68–74.

Theunissen, N.C., Veen, S., Fekkes, M., Koopman, H.M., Zwinderman, K.A., Brugman, E., et al. (2001). Quality of life in preschool children born preterm. *Developmental Medicine and Child Neurology, 43,* 460–465.

Torrance, G.W., Feeny, D.H., Furlong, W.J., Barr, R.D., Zhang, Y., & Wang, Q. (1996). Multiattribute utility function for a comprehensive health status classification system: Health Utilities Index Mark 2. *Medical Care, 34,* 702–722.

Tsuji, T., Liu, M., Toikawa, H., Hanayama, K., Sonoda, S., & Chino, N. (1999). ADL structure for nondisabled Japanese children based on the Functional Independence Measure for Children (Wee-FIM). *American Journal of Physical Medicine and Rehabilitation, 78,* 208–212.

Varni, J.W., Burwinkle, T.M., Seid, M., & Skarr, D. (2003). The PedsQL 4.0 as a pediatric population health measure: Feasibility, reliability, and validity. *Ambulatory Pediatrics, 3,* 329–341.

Vohr, B.R., Msall, M.E., Wilson, D., Wright, L.L., McDonald, S., & Poole, W.K. (2005). Spectrum of gross motor function in extremely low birth weight children with cerebral palsy at 18 months of age. *Pediatrics, 116*(1), 123–129.

Vohr, B., Wright, L.L., Hack, M., Aylward, G., & Hirtz, D. (2004). Follow-up care of high-risk infants. *Pediatrics, 114,* 1377–1397.

Wake, M., Salmon, L., & Reddihough, D. (2003). Health status of Australian children with mild to severe cerebral palsy: Cross-sectional survey using the Child Health Questionnaire. *Developmental Medicine and Child Neurology, 45,* 194–199.

Wechsler, D. (2003). *Wechsler Intelligence Scale for Children–Fourth Edition (WISC–IV).* San Antonio, TX: Harcourt Assessment.

Wetherby, A.M., & Prizant, B.M. (Eds.). (2002). *Communication and Symbolic Behavior Scales Developmental Profile (CSBS DP).* Baltimore: Paul H. Brookes Publishing Co.

Wong, V., Wong, S., Chan, K., & Wong, W. (2002). Functional Independence Measure (WeeFIM) for Chinese children: Hong Kong cohort. *Pediatrics, 109,* E36.

Wood, E., & Rosenbaum, P. (2000). The gross motor function classification system for cerebral palsy: A study of reliability and stability over time. *Developmental Medicine and Child Neurology, 42*(5), 292–296.

World Health Organization. (Ed.). (2001). *International Classification of Functioning, Disability and Health.* Geneva: Author.

Zimmerman, I.L., Steiner, V.G., & Pond, N.E. (Eds.). (2002). *Preschool Language Scale–4.* San Antonio, TX: Psychological Corp.

Ziviani, J., Ottenbacher, K.J., Shephard, K., Foreman, S., Astbury, W., Ireland, P., et al. (2001). Concurrent validity of the Functional Independence Measure for Children (WeeFIM) and the Pediatric Evaluation of Disabilities Inventory in children with developmental disabilities and acquired brain injuries. *Physical and Occupational Therapy in Pediatrics, 21,* 91–101.

23

Family Functioning

BARBARA Y. WHITMAN

One needs only to stand in front of the "parenting and child-rearing" shelf of a local bookstore to conclude that parenting can be stressful and challenging. Book titles such as *Children: The Challenge* (Dreikurs, 1964/1990), *Raising Your Spirited Child* (Kurcinka, 2006), and *How to Talk So Kids Will Listen and How to Listen So Kids Will Talk* (Faber & Mazlish, 1999) bear witness to the fact that children bring unanticipated issues, challenges, and uncertainties. Further, despite several decades of "inclusion," most parents' introduction to intellectual or developmental disabilities is abrupt and emotional, occurring when they discover their child has, or is biologically at risk for, a developmental disorder. The impact of this discovery is pervasive, for these parents not only face the ordinary issues that every family faces, but they must also face, adjust to, and cope with challenges idiosyncratic to their child's developmental condition. For many, this follows a period during which their child required the immediate, combined expertise of numerous medical specialists, often in multiple medical settings. Thus, while trying to absorb the reality of their child's condition, these families may continue to face complex medical issues and financial demands that require extraordinary adjustments, accommodations, and complex coordination.

It has been long recognized that 1) the family is the principal context in which child development takes place, and 2) a child's development is not biologically fixed but is an ongoing interactional process mediated by the environment (Kelly, Booth-LaForce, & Spieker, 2005). In addition, care providers for those with developmental disabilities have long accepted that understanding each family and providing adequate and appropriate family support are central to the care process. The critical centrality of family support for maximizing their child's long-term developmental outcomes is reflected in the Education of the Handicapped Act Amendments of 1986 (PL 99–457). This federal legislation mandates early intervention and preschool programs in the United States to meet the dual goals of serving children with disabilities *and* providing support for their families. Often termed *family-centered care,* these mandates include 1) developing an individualized family service plan (IFSP) to assist each family in developing its ability to cope adaptively with the impact of the developmental concern; 2) including the family as part of the team that develops the IFSP; 3) using a family-directed assessment of family resources, priorities, and concerns; 4) developing and providing ways to address both child and family needs according to family preferences; 5) fully explaining the IFSP, family rights, and procedural safeguards; and 6) assigning a service coordinator to be responsible for implementing and coordinating the components of the plan (Ostfeld & Gibbs, 1990; Warfield, Krauss, Hauser-Cram, Upshur, & Shonkoff, 1999). Although not as intensive as that advocated in early intervention programs, family involvement at some level is mandated throughout the educational career of a child with a disability. While federally mandated family supports are tied to a child's enrollment in the educational system, family support needs extend beyond the completion of a child's education. Support needs for many families increase at this time as a result of increased isolation, fewer services, and uncertainty about the future.

Family-centered support and care encompass a wide range of activities guided by assumptions and models of family dynamics and both explicit and implied goals for intervention (Bailey & Powell, 2005). Several key principles frame best practices in a family-centered model. These include recognizing the family as a constant in the child's life, using a strengths perspective, attending to cultural diversity, thinking about children with disabilities as children first, working collaboratively with families in a way that is responsive to their needs and the needs of their children, enabling and empowering families, developing new skills and resources, supporting parent–child interactions and relationships, reducing stress, and linking with parent-to-parent and community resources (Leal, 1999; Yoder & DiVenere, 2004). Empowerment, the sine qua non of family-centered care, is defined as having the knowledge and confidence needed to take responsibility for, and control of, decision making (Dunst, 1985; Dunst, Trivette, & Johanson, 1994). Utilizing family systems and family life course theory as a framework for discussion, this chapter reviews the issues surrounding *family-centered care* for families in which one or more members have a developmental disorder (Aldous, 1996). For each stage of the family life course, the text examines the domains of tasks and needs, family relationships, and support and coping. Following that, the discussion deals separately with the issues of sexuality, siblings, and formal supports and finally revisits the parent–professional partnership.

UNIQUENESS OF FAMILIES

Families are complicated, dynamic, self-correcting systems including many individuals from several generations with varying relationships, experiences, and perceptions. These relationships, experiences, and perceptions form and are reformed through ongoing, culturally constrained interactions during which each participant continually responds to and shapes the behavior of the others. A family has an organized power structure, a specific set of rules, and assigned and ascribed roles for its members. The rules, while usually unstated and unwritten, are nonetheless known and mutually adhered to; in *healthy* families the rules change developmentally (Goldenberg & Goldenberg, 2000).

Furthermore, families, like individuals, follow a predictable life cycle. Common to most family life cycle models are the stages of marriage, birth and rearing of young children, raising school-age children, launching or departure of family members from the household, and retirement from the work force (Seltzer & Krauss, 2001). As a self-correcting system, a family can maintain complex patterns of balance within certain limits of variability. A family stressed beyond these variability limits may not be able to restore balance. When a family is stressed beyond its ability to recover, functioning may be permanently impaired. Changing demands, such as the birth of a child, introduce stress into the family and alter, at least temporarily, the ongoing balance. Across the family life cycle, both family environment factors and the quality of specific family relationships influence the range and variability of this balance and the family's ability to effectively weather expected and unexpected life events.

CULTURAL AND SOCIAL DIVERSITY OF FAMILIES

When viewed as a dynamic, relational system, family composition can assume many forms, including a traditional two-parent family, single parents, divorced and blended families, multigenerational families, grandparents as parents, and same-sex parents. Statistics indicate that, in 1998, 68% of U.S. children lived with two parents, compared with 77% living with two parents in 1980. At the same time, approximately 25% lived only with their mothers, 4% only with their fathers, and 4% with neither parent. In addition, although cultural, ethnic, and socioeconomic diversity varies by country, in all countries minority populations generally have fewer economic advantages. In the United States, the Latino population grew by 58% between the years 1990 and 2000. In the year 1999, the median income for U.S. white non-Latinos was $44,366, that for Latinos was $30,735, and that for African Americans, $27,910 (Hanson & Lynch, 2004). Many minority families have incomes below the official poverty level. Poverty is frequently associated with developmental risk (Hanson & Carta, 1996). According to Hanson and Lynch (2004), in 1986, the odds of children in poverty having a disability were 86% higher than they were for those children whose family income was above the poverty line. At the same time, having a child with a disability frequently limits parental employment opportunities, resulting in decreased financial resources. In a comparative survey of 245 mothers of children with developmental disabilities and 9,481 mothers of children without disabilities, Emerson (2003) found that families supporting a child with a disability were at significant economic disadvantage compared with those families whose children had no disability.

Separate from cultural beliefs regarding the meaning of a child's disability, the joint impact of poverty and the stress associated with having a child with a disability cannot be underestimated. Despite this, children from minority families are underrepresented in early childhood programs that are predominately staffed by professional-level service providers who are European American (Hanson, 1998). Furthermore, most service systems were not designed to accommodate the diversity common among today's families. The need for medical translators has become a daily occurrence in hospital clinics and emergency rooms. These families are also underrepresented in parent–professional partnerships because lack of transportation, employment demands, lack of translator services, and basic misunderstanding continue as barriers (McCallion, Janicki, & Grant-Griffin, 1997). Finally, these families are underrepresented in research on family stress and adjustment associated with a child's disability. Thus, those families who may benefit most from current family-centered, parent–professional partnership models for caregiving remain those least likely to participate.

PARENT–PROFESSIONAL PARTNERSHIPS

The family support movements that began in the 1960s and various family initiatives have raised awareness of the family as the primary context for child development and the primary decision maker for, and provider of, care. Furthermore, these efforts have spawned a new recognition of the need for parent–professional partnerships in caring for children and adults with disabilities. Thus, family-centered models hinge on collaborative, relationship-based decision making in the context of a multidisciplinary team. Advocates of the family-centered model make distinctions (often artificial) between older models that emphasized the provision of services to the child and current model assumptions that the relationships among family members and between family members and professionals, and the utilization of family strengths and resources, are primary to intervention and support processes (Dunst, Trivette, & Deal, 1988; Singer & Powers, 1993).

Although clearly family-centered care is an ideal, perhaps even *the* ideal, common sense and the true spirit of partnership often get lost in the rush to embrace these concepts. Thus, in many instances, there has been an open and disdainful diminishing and devaluation of role of the professional as a team member and of the role of formal supports, combined with an assertion that only family concerns are important (Hanson & Lynch, 2004). This imbalance is no more facilitative of care than the perceived imbalance of earlier decades, an imbalance that family-centered care aims at addressing.

As Guralnick noted,

This principle implies that the family's perspective be accorded considerable, if not absolute, weight. In practice, however, there are circumstances that make this principle difficult to implement in its most complete sense. Occasionally the team may perceive that the child's best interests and those of the family diverge, and there are instances in which the values of the team may not be concordant with the family's values. . . . [N]o easy solution is likely in these instances, but a vigorous negotiation process should be initiated in which the team states its case in a context of open communication. (2000, p. 11–12)

FAMILY LIFE CYCLE ISSUES

Birth and Early Childhood: Rearing Young Children

The stress associated with becoming a parent is well documented (Bailey & Powell, 2005;

Turnbull, Brotherson, & Summers, 1986). Major personal adjustments include changes in the spousal relationship, with marital roles tending to become more traditional; economic adjustments; increased fatigue; need for better time management; and decreased time for social activities. If, in addition, a child has, or is at risk for, a developmental disability, a wide range of emotional responses may be triggered. The impact is not limited to parents alone; grandparents and other extended family members are often profoundly affected by the discovery that a family member has a problem.

Early writers focused on this impact as a family crisis of such proportions that pathological outcomes were the norm, and recovery and normal family functioning the exception. By contrast, recent research suggests that, following an initial period of disruption, most families eventually recover normal functioning. Although episodic elevations of stress are common, chronic high levels of distress and pathological functioning are not typical for most families (Warfield et al., 1999). These contradictory findings may, in part, reflect a change in culture. Prior to 1970, people with developmental disabilities who lived with their families received little or no service support. With the thrust toward "normalization" and community integration, legislatively mandated family support services have created a radically different environment and culture for those children/adults with a disability and their families. Families today can expect to receive developmental services for children with a disability and support for the family immediately following a diagnosis.

Early childhood intervention services have been the norm only for the past two decades. Nonetheless, whereas earlier research may have overemphasized the negative family impact of a developmental disability, current literature tends to overemphasize those factors that promote positive family functioning in the context of family-centered early intervention, while ignoring the significant emotional impact and multiple life-altering challenges experienced by parents discovering that their child has, or is at risk for, a disability. Independent of a family's long-term adjustment, at the time of recognition of risk for or confirmation of a

developmental disorder, most parents, along with their extended families, describe a period of being stunned, shattered, or overwhelmed (Hanson & Lynch, 2004, p. 91; Roberts, 1984). These feelings often are followed by a sense of profound sadness and increased anxiety resulting from uncertainty over both the immediate and long-term implications of the child's disability for the child and for the family.

For many parents, the discovery can raise feelings of distress, guilt, or depression about having caused the condition and concern regarding their ability to effectively parent this child, particularly if, in addition to coping with the diagnosis, families are also having to deal with multiple medical issues. Ethnic, cultural, and religious beliefs about disability may further shape a family's response and adaptation to the probability that their child is facing atypical patterns of development, as well as affecting their use of professional and treatment services. The process of accepting the diagnosis, establishing some comfort regarding their ability to meet their child's needs, parent, and advocate for their child, and achieving a sense of family balance and stability can take several years.

Tasks and Needs in Early Childhood

The primary tasks for the family at this point, assuming a stable medical status, are to confirm and understand the implications of their child's diagnosis, to obtain a complete assessment and understanding of developmental status and needs, and to develop and participate in a comprehensive program of intervention. Often, this requires the coordination of multiple medical and therapeutic appointments, learning to communicate and deal with a variety of specialists—for some learning to handle complex medical situations and equipment—and becoming competent in navigating the service system and advocating for their child. Family financial resources may be stressed beyond capacity. At the same time, the family must regain a sense of emotional balance and learn to accommodate their child's special needs within the broader context of the family. Not infrequently these demands occur at a time when the marital relationship is young and the underlying capacity to trust that the spouse will be there when needed has yet to be established.

McWilliam (2005) highlighted three broad categories of family needs that affect parents' ability to complete these tasks: informational support, material support, and emotional support. Informational support includes specific information on the child's disorder, genetic information, an understanding of how typical children grow and develop, support and guidance for fostering their child's development (including how to play, talk with, and teach the child and handle the child's behavior), information about currently needed services and those that their child might need in the future, and a clear understanding of state and federal laws regarding their rights and responsibilities in the service system. Material support includes facilitating access to affordable necessary equipment, specialty diets, transportation, needed financial resources, and supportive or respite care services. Emotional support includes being sensitive and responsive to the family, showing interest in the whole family, being positive with and about the child and family, and supporting family functioning.

Currently, many of these tasks and needs can be obtained, coordinated, and accomplished in the context of an early childhood intervention program. Although there is wide variability among states in the availability, comprehensiveness, and effectiveness of these programs, the need to access and integrate their child and family into the available service system is common to all families. For many families, while ultimately seeking a source of help and hope, the process of seeking, qualifying for, and obtaining services is new, overwhelming, intrusive, and difficult. Recognizing this, inherent in the mandated early intervention process is the assignment of a service coordinator to facilitate moving the family through the assessment, assist with development of the IFSP, and support them during the intervention process.

Despite the strong family-centered focus undergirding early intervention programming, many families still experience the initial access and assessment process as one wherein they and their child are being examined, probed, calibrated, calculated, and labeled by multiple, often unfamiliar, professional specialists. Families are again brought face to face with the need to accept their child's condition while concurrently learning to understand and sort out advice from multiple sources of information. They are also learning to effectively advocate for their child in the midst of differences of opinion both among professionals and between professionals and themselves regarding the need for specific services, the extent of those services, and the ongoing effectiveness of those services. Nonetheless, having been thrust into unfamiliar, often unpleasant experiences, neither anticipated nor wanted, most families survive and eventually learn a new set of information, terminology, and skills. Still, the stress associated with these experiences cannot be understated.

Family Relationships in Early Childhood For young children, socioemotional and cognitive growth along with successful adaptation is primarily influenced by the physical and social environment; at that age the family is generally the most extensive and most powerful environmental influence on development (Glasser & Glasser, 1970). For those children with or at risk for a developmental disorder, the association between family functioning and outcome is particularly critical (Beckman, 1984; Bristol, 1987). Research documents that adaptive family functioning is more likely to provide the necessary substrate for maximizing developmental trajectories, for promoting the social competence and adaptive behavior necessary for participation in the least restrictive environment, and for preventing or reducing the likelihood of secondary, disability-related behavior and health problems (Bailey & Wolery, 1992; Hauser-Cram, Warfield, Shondoff, & Krauss, 2001). By contrast, high levels of stress can contribute to poor mother–child interactions and adversely affect a child's developmental outcomes (Orsmond, 2005).

Despite the clear recognition of the central role of the family in determining developmental outcomes, clearly there are differences between families and within any given family over time in their emotional and material resources and in the needed supports for enhancing optimal family functioning. In the context of maximizing a child's developmental outcomes through early intervention programming, a great deal of research has been conducted since the 1980s regarding 1) the key areas of family functioning associated with a child's development, 2) the level and kind of stress typically experienced by these families, and 3) how best to assess these characteristics. The collective research indicates that parents of young children with disabilities, including cerebral palsy, Down syndrome, and autism, report greater parent-related stress and experience greater caregiving demands than parents of more typically developing children (Britner, Morog, Pianta, & Marvin, 2003; Nachsen, Woodford, & Minnes, 2003; Tobing & Glenwick, 2002). Even greater stress has been associated with specific disabilities, including severe physical disabilities, autism, behavior problems, and neurological disorders. Because it remains the case that, independent of a child's disability status, mothers continue to assume the primary burden of child rearing, much of this research focuses on mothers. Some studies indicate different types of stress for mothers (social isolation, caregiving burden) than for fathers (financial); other studies document the stress associated with varying family structures (two-parent family versus single parent; size and quality of social network).

Having a child with disabilities often requires different accommodations than would be needed for a child who is developing typically. For instance, one study found that parents of children with Down syndrome had different patterns of time use, spending more time in child care, less time in social activities, and, for mothers, less time in employment than parents of typically developing children (Barnett & Boyce, 1995). Studies have found elevated parental stress associated with decreased income, so the impact of having a child with a disability on family income and ultimately on stress clearly is not trivial.

In addition, a child's behavior and temperamental characteristics have been demonstrated in multiple studies to affect parents' emotional status and ability to effectively parent during the earliest years of life. Parents of

young children with disabilities report greater stress related to their child's characteristics than do parents of children who are developing typically, especially with respect to feeling that their child is less adaptable and more demanding and active (Orsmond, 2005). Parenting a child with autism may produce greater stress than parenting children with other disabilities (Dumas, Wold, Fisman, & Culligan, 1991; Kasari & Sigman, 1997). Nor is this stress static. Using a longitudinal design with an early intervention population of children with Down syndrome, motor impairments, and other mild delays, Warfield et al. (1999) found increases over time in child-related stress such as that derived from demandingness and mood regulation; about one third of the sample parents scored in clinical ranges of stress by the time their child was 5 years old. Parent-related stress (e.g., derived from spousal relations and social isolation), however, appeared to remain relatively stable through the early years, although elevated compared with stress in parents of children without disabilities (Dyson, 1993).

Apparently, stress is not equally shared by mothers and fathers. Several studies document that, whereas mothers of children with autism or Down syndrome report greater parenting stress than mothers of typically developing children, fathers do not (Freeman, Perry, & Factor, 1991). Similarly, some authors report that mothers of children with a disability, particularly mothers of children with autism, have higher levels of depression and anxiety than parents of typically developing children, whereas fathers are less affected (Dumas et al., 1991; Hastings & Brown, 2002); other authors report no differences (Bristol, Schopler, & Gallagher, 1988). As would be predicted, single mothers are at highest risk for elevated stress and depression (Gottlieb, 1997).

The negative impact of marital discord on parenting behavior and child development is well documented (see Cummings & Davies, 2002, for review). In the general population, marital discord is negatively related to children's cognitive and social development, academic performance, behavior, physical health, mental health, and the development of positive coping abilities. Furthermore, marital discord has a negative impact on parenting and sibling relationships. As in the general population, research supports that the quality of the marital relationship is equally important in family adjustment to childhood developmental disabilities, as well as short-term parenting stress and mother's long-term parenting stress (Britner et al., 2003; Nihira, Myers, & Mink, 1980; Trute & Hiebert-Murphy, 2002). A number of studies have looked at the reciprocal relationship: the impact of having a child with a disability on the quality of the marital relationship. Both mothers and fathers of children with developmental disorders reported a greater negative impact of the child on the marriage than that reported by parents of children developing typically (Baker, Blatcher, Crnic, & Edelbrock, 2002; Freeman et al., 1991).

Support and Coping   As previously indicated, adapting to a having a child with a disability is a process that occurs over time. A number of variables have been found to mediate the process for young families adapting to a child with a disability. These include cognitive assessment of the child's disability, usual style of coping, a supportive social network, spousal support, and family cohesion.

Whereas the experience of being stunned and the accompanying sadness on learning that a child has a developmental disorder is almost universal, the subsequent emotions and adjustment depend in part on the subjective interpretation or meaning that parents place on the disability and its meaning in their family's life. For some parents, it will constitute a crisis carrying elements of harm, loss, and weakness. For others, the birth will be viewed as an unfortunate event, yet one that has positive implications. If the parents' interpretation is that of harm and loss, a positive long-term adaptation is clearly more difficult to accomplish.

Parents' interpretation of a child's disability is highlighted in a longitudinal study by Trute and Hiebert-Murphy (2002). The authors initially assessed 88 families with children age 5 years and younger for their subjective assessment of the impact of disability on the family. A reassessment 7 years later examined both the current subjective assessment of the impact of disability on the family and levels of parental and family stress. The findings suggested that parents develop co-occurring positive and negative assessments of family impact; the proportions of each were predictive of later psychological well-being, particularly for mothers. To the extent that negative assessments predominated, later well-being was compromised. Furthermore, these initial negative appraisals were essentially unchanged 7 years later. Interestingly, although both mothers and fathers held similar appraisals of negative impact, each sex independently, and often quite differently assessed positive impact.

In a separate study, Button, Pianta, and Marvin (2001) assessed subjective appraisals of the parent–child relationship among mothers of children with cerebral palsy or epilepsy and mothers of typically developing children. Measuring the mother's perception of child compliance, worry about the child's future, and emotional pain from the burden of caregiving, Button et al. found that mothers of children with cerebral palsy reported more feelings of worry and emotional pain and were less concerned with appropriate compliance than mothers in the other two groups. The authors suggested that negative interpretations regarding the child's future, coupled with the felt pain and burden of caregiving, are related to insensitive and unsupportive maternal behavior.

A parent's usual coping style or strategy for stress-related problem solving is also a factor affecting family adjustment. Contrasts are made between active, problem-focused coping strategies (seeking social support, making active efforts to alter the situation) and passive, emotion-focused coping strategies (wishful thinking, denial, avoidance). Research suggests that, particularly in mothers, problem-focused coping (e.g., seeking social support) generally results in reduced stress, whereas emotion-focused efforts (e.g., self-blame, bottled-up feelings, wishful thinking) were related to greater psychological distress and depressed mood (Kelly et al., 2005). Again defining seeking social support as an active problem-solving strategy and self-blame, bottled-up feelings, and wishful thinking as passive strategies, Judge (1998) found that active coping was associated with more confidence and sense of family strength, whereas passive strategies were related to lower perceived family strengths.

Having a social network of supportive relationships is well documented as a positive factor in family adjustment. Social support, especially informal social support, has been shown to be a positive influence on how mothers interact with their children, maternal life satisfaction, and maternal parenting satisfaction (Crnic & Stormshak, 1997). Several types of support accrue from these relationships. Among them are material support such as babysitting, respite care, and financial help; emotional support and a sense of being cared for even while caregiving; and facilitating, teaching, and modeling of active coping strategies. The role of social support has been extensively studied in families with a child with a disability. The ability to depend on these relationships for support is related to greater *personal* functioning for parents, more positive perceptions of their child's behavior, better *family* function, more positive parenting behavior, and more positive with less negative child affect (Dunst, Trivette, & Jodry, 1997).

It appears, however, that both a general ability to cope and the capacity to develop and utilize a supportive social network are highly dependent on the same variables: parental education, income, occupation, marital relationship, culture, and race. Some authors postulate that it is the quality rather than the size of the social network that is important. Among studies of those parents with smaller support networks, findings converge in suggesting that the quality of the network and the perception of satisfactory support from that network are positively related to parental adjustment (Kazak & Wilcox, 1984; Margalit, Raviv, & Ankonina, 1992).

In addition to a larger social support network, greater emotional connectedness and cohesiveness within families—in contrast to families characterized by isolation and disengagement—have a positive adaptive effect for young families of a child with a disability and a specific positive effect on maternal depression. Furthermore, the perception of spousal support predicts a more positive adaptation. For example, Simmerman and Blacher (2001) assessed the perceived and actual extent of, and satisfaction with, fathers' involvement in the lives of their young children with severe intellectual disability. Among the 60 families assessed, there was high agreement between mothers and fathers concerning the extent of fathers' help, which was highest in the areas of playing, nurturing, discipline, and deciding on services. Mothers' satisfaction with fathers' help related more strongly to family well-being and marital adjustment than the actual extent of fathers' help. Similar results were reported by Heller, Hsieh, and Rowitz (1997).

Families who successfully negotiate this early childhood stage emerge with an increased sense of competence and mastery. This sense of competence seems to improve a family's well-being, making family members better equipped to face the tasks of the next stage of the family life cycle, and they become more involved in the life of the child with a disability (Heller, 1993).

The School Years: Raising School-Age Children

The entry into and exit from the child's school years are marked by transitions that have significant impact for both the child and his or her family. As the child progresses through this stage, parents must help the child maximize his or her cognitive and intellectual development, encourage the development of self-help skills, facilitate socioemotional development and integration into the community, and negotiate the many changes that accompany adolescence and sexual development.

Tasks and Needs in the Early School Years At the entry to this stage, families must effectively negotiate the transition from early childhood services to the school environment. For children with a disability, transitions often involve multiple services and delivery systems and multiple adjustments for children and families. These adjustments may include physical and practical changes such as learning how to get to new places, learning new sets of rules, learning to work with new people, and adjustments to family schedules, as well as more difficult adjustments such as altering expectations and social ties. In addition to the process of making the transition from one service system to another, parents now have to adjust to the differences between the comprehensive special services by trained professionals characteristic of early childhood programs and the environment provided by those trained in general education. Furthermore, parents will have to educate themselves regarding differences in eligibility requirements for services, new demands for child participation, differing expectations for behavior, differences in staff and teacher commitment to accommodating special needs, and a different set of legislative and legal supports undergirding the intervention process and parent–professional partnership.

Ideally, the transition process should provide service continuity, reduce family disruption, prepare the child for the new educational setting, and meet legal requirements (Hanson, 2005). Nonetheless, for families who have come to terms with their child's diagnosis in the context of family-focused services central to early intervention programs, the move to school-based, child-focused services frequently reactivates parents' anxieties and concerns. Thus, for most families, the magnitude and meaning of the many adjustments required when a child moves from one service setting to another often render these transitions a protracted and emotional experience.

Accompanying the transition from early intervention to school-based services is another, often difficult realization. Although delays, or risk thereof, prompted entry into early intervention services, for those children now integrating into a setting where typically developing children predominate, the extent and severity of a child's delays and differences, by comparison, become more obvious. Furthermore, the type and severity of the child's disability, as well as any accompanying behavior concerns, will determine the services needed and may negatively influence available placement options. A child's ability to communicate, self-help skills, and ability to function independently factor into placement options and educational planning, and for some children preclude an inclusive setting. Current data suggest that, for those students with intellectual disabilities, as many as half continue to be educated in noninclusive settings (Katsiyannis, Zhang, & Archwamety, 2002); for students with significant disabilities, many school districts still have no clear plan for ensuring access to the general education curriculum (Agran, Alper, & Wehmeyer, 2002). For many parents, even those whose children integrate into inclusive classrooms, this transition may signal the first erosion of the previously held hope for eventual normalcy.

Family Relationships in the Early School Years Whereas the tasks of maximizing cognitive/intellectual development and self-help skills are addressed primarily in the context of the school environment, the family remains the central and core social context for nurturance, health and daily care, self-esteem development, socialization, recreation, community integration, and spiritual development. Just as the transition into school-based services marks a shift in school setting and educational focus, family transitions are also demanded, many with significant impact on family relations and day-to-day functioning. Few would question that family life today is extremely complex, requiring extraordinary coordination and organization to keep households running smoothly. These complexities and the time they require may be even greater in families in which a member has a developmental disability. Children with even mild disabilities frequently have more prolonged dependency needs than more typically developing children, requiring considerable parental planning, time, structure, and support to maintain behavior and accomplish even the most routine tasks. Even for these children, and certainly for those with greater physical or medical involvement, the most routine daily tasks such as bathing, dressing, and eating may require extra time. In addition, children with developmental delays or decreased social abilities (e.g., as seen in autism spectrum disorders) may require greater assistance from parents in initiating and maintaining peer friendships in the home and neighborhood than that demanded by similarly aged children without disabilities (Turnbull, Pereira, & Blue-Banning, 1999).

Friendships and relationships with peers in childhood serve many functions that contribute to long-term adjustment and quality of life. When positive, they can support efforts toward intellectual growth, social development, social support, and self-esteem. Without social interactions and friendships, people may experience isolation and loneliness (Geisthardt, Brotherson, & Cook, 2002). It is well documented that parents of both children and teens with disabilities believe it is important to help their children develop friendships, and they worry about the effect of lack of friendships on the quality of the children's lives. Also, at least one real, if unstated, goal of inclusive classroom environments is to increase the exposure to, and improve the quality of, peer social relationships for children with disabilities; yet, research suggests that, although inclusive environments do facilitate more peer interaction than specialized programs, 1) interaction with typically developing children still occurs less frequently that would be expected in terms of availability, 2) there is less acceptance and more rejection by peers, and 3) children with disabilities have more difficulty establishing reciprocal friendships than do developmentally matched typically developing children.

Similarly, in the home environment, and with clear effort on parents' part to facilitate neighborhood peer interactions for their child with disabilities, there is differential acceptance of children based on their disability. In both school and home environments, children whose disabilities were predominantly physical in nature were most actively involved with other children, whereas children with moderate to severe cognitive limitations or behavior problems were among those with the most limited peer contact (Geisthardt et al., 2002; Green & Stoneman, 1989). Thus, even in the younger grades, despite concerted remedial efforts and even in the absence of significant behavioral concerns, a pattern of increased social isolation for those with cognitive limitations is evident. The impact of these concerns on the family is reflected in higher rates of maternal distress (Emerson, 2003).

Furthermore, if they were not previously present, the early school years often herald the emergence of disruptive behavior problems. Children with developmental disabilities exhibit significantly more behavior problems when compared with typically developing children (Gortmaker, Walker, Weitzman, & Sobol, 1990). There is also evidence that the severity of behavior problems for children with disabilities is predictive of increased parent and family problems and greater service utilization, particularly mental health services (Floyd & Gallagher, 1997; Wallander, Varni, Babani, & Wilcox, 1990). The presence of behavior problems appears to be more important than the type of disability in determining family stress. Behavior problems limit access to normalized experiences for children with disabilities by keeping children in more restrictive school placements and by limiting joint family activities and family recreation, further exacerbating family stress (Turnbull & Ruef, 1996). As in all families, the advent of adolescence brings new challenges.

Coping with Adolescence The transitions from elementary school to middle school and again to high school presage dramatic changes for any student. For students with disabilities, these changes may have a significant impact. This transition will involve the same issues previously noted with the entry into grade school while adding many others. The safety and security of a single classroom in a familiar building is suddenly taken away. Classmates who have been together for several years may be dispersed. Students placed in an inclusive environment may need to adjust to several teachers and new groups of students in each class. Each teacher has his or her own style, expectations, and beliefs regarding his or her role vis-à-vis students with disabilities.

For most parents of a child with a disability, if they have not already accepted the permanent nature of their child's delays and differences, the entry into adolescence signals this permanency in an undeniable and often painful manner. Both the academic and the social gaps between the student with a disability and his or her classmates have continued to widen. For many parents, the issue of inclusion encompasses multiple concerns and anxieties, including the role of academics for their child and the impact of the school social environment for their child, and presages the life course of their child as an adult. Curriculum planning often shifts in emphasis from academics to functional life skills. In addition, a change in administrative, teaching, and support staff requires establishing multiple new relationships. The research literature does not provide clear answers for parents struggling with this issue.

Early studies suggested that interaction between high school students with disabilities and their typically developing peers may result in beneficial educational and social outcomes, such as an improvement in work skills for the student with a disability; enhanced learning, particularly with regard to standards-based learning, improved independence, and higher quality of life; and increased social interaction skills, such as initiating and responding to social interaction and better social acceptance from their peers without disabilities (Center & Curry, 1993; Hughes, Harmer, Killian, & Niarhos, 1995; Kennedy & Itkonen, 1994; Knowlton, 1998). More recent literature fails to support these benefits (Doré, Dion, Wagner, & Brunet, 2002; Hughes, Carter, Hughes, Bradford, & Copeland, 2002). Survey data suggest that most teachers do not support access to the general curriculum for students with disabilities, have such access as a low priority, are not actively involved in planning or teaching relating to access and curriculum, and view challenging behaviors as obstacles to full inclusion (Agran et al., 2002). For many students receiving instruction in an inclusive classroom, the instruction is student specific and given by an aide; true inclusion is illusory.

Social goals are not being met, as well. Anything more than obligatory social contact between high-school students with disabilities and their typically developing peers remains the exception rather than the rule (Hughes et al., 1999; Kraemer, Blacher, & Marshall, 1997). Even when structured settings specifically provide for social interactions, there is little generalization to nonstructured settings such as the cafeteria (Hughes et al., 2002). If inclusion has not yet provided a direct effect on social acceptance and education, there has been an indirect effect in terms of more positive attitudes toward and understanding of those with disabilities. A study by Krajewski, Hyde, and O'Keeffe (2002) examined high-school student attitudes toward students with a disability at two points in time, 1987 and 1999, in two separate

schools. In the 1987 survey, typically developing female students were significantly more positive toward inclusion than typically developing male students. By 1997, these differences had essentially disappeared as male students showed a trend toward more positive attitudes, but the differences were not statistically significant, nor did female students show an increase in positive attitudes. Furthermore, in 1997, both male and female students showed decreased acceptance of civil rights and less tolerance of social integration for students with disabilities. On the positive side of the ledger, there was a slightly decreased endorsement of subtle derogatory beliefs, but the overall findings are disheartening with regard to the positive educational or social impact of inclusion on either the student with a disability or his or her more typically developing peers.

Some would argue that attitudes are of little import if inclusion is resulting in better educational outcomes for the students with disabilities. In a national study of placement and educational outcomes, defined as "exit mode" (diploma, certificate, dropout), for students 14 and older at two separate points in time (1989 and 1998), Katsiyannis et al. (2002) found clear differences between disabilities. Comparing students with a variety of disabilities in 1989 with those in 1998, there was a 34.5% increase of students being placed and educated in an inclusive environment. Approximately half were receiving educational services in inclusive environments; however, for those with intellectual disabilities, there was only a slight upward trend toward educating students in general education classrooms, with more than half continuing to receive services in separate classrooms.

The positive educational impact of inclusive placement has not been realized. For all students with disabilities, there was a *decrease* in graduation rates with a diploma or certificate and no significant decrease in dropout rates. Furthermore, 3–5 years after leaving school, fewer than 8% of young adults with disabilities in the United States are reported to be fully employed or enrolled in postsecondary education, active socially, and living independently in the community (Hughes, 2001). Thus, it appears that the goals of improved educational outcomes have yet to be achieved. The negative impact of these findings on family functioning cannot be minimized (Emerson, 2003; Lam, Giles, & Lavander, 2003; Maes, Broekman, Dosen, & Nauts, 2003).

Support and Coping in the School Years   In contrast to the negative educational outcomes, families appear to fare better during the school years. Many families develop additional coping strategies such as depending or their faith and using tailored recreational experiences. In addition, many families that have adapted successfully to their child with a disability come to perceive that, despite the chronically elevated levels of stress associated with this child, the experience of this child is a positive one for their family. In a two-stage study of 43 families with children ranging in age from 3 to 19 years of age who had a variety of disabilities, Taunt and Hastings (2002) asked parents a series of questions, including questions about 1) the positive aspects of caring for their child with a disability, 2) what has been particularly rewarding, 3) the benefits of caring for their child, 4) whether the presence of this child has had any positive effects on the other children in the extended family, and 5) the family's hopes and fears regarding the future for their child with a disability and their family. Parents reported a number of positive effects, both for themselves and for their children without disabilities (Table 23.1). In addition, a significant proportion of the sample was generally positive about the future, with only a small minority expressing anxiety or fear in this regard. Similar positive findings emerged in a study of quality of life (Poston et al., 2003).

Many families get support from a religious faith. In a study specifically examining the role of spirituality and religion in the family quality of life for 78 families of children with a disability and 33 families without children with a disability, all families reported finding meaning from their religious beliefs, but those families with children with a disability specifically endorsed the importance of having faith, using prayer, and finding meaning in the disability as key contributors to the overall family quality of life (Poston & Turnbull, 2004). For many families of children with disabilities, faith and

prayer took on an additional role. At the same time, many of these families reported difficulty with church attendance, indicating that they felt their children were not accepted or that they had insufficient support to fully participate in church activities. Many families would choose to attend their local church, temple, synagogue, or mosque if their children had the appropriate supports. Without these supports, parents are reluctant to attend or are unable to benefit from attendance because they spend their time providing direct support to their child with a disability.

Among families with typically developing children, family recreational activities are thought to contribute positively to family relationships and the overall quality of family life. In a child's younger years, these activities often take the form of watching television or interactive play, activities that encourage family cohesion, facilitate communication, and encourage child socialization. For many families, once a child enters school, the focus of these efforts may shift to supporting a child's school- and community-based activities such as sports and scouting. Regardless of the family life stage, mothers are the primary organizers of family recreation and are more involved than other adult family members. Despite inclusion efforts, recent data suggest that individuals with developmental disabilities participate in recreation less frequently than others. Many families attempt to fill this void by organizing family activities for their child with a disability.

Mactavish and Schleien (2004) studied the nature of family recreational activities in 65 families that included children with mixed disabilities and a full range of functional abilities. The sample included 47 boys and 27 girls ranging in age from 2 to 22 years. Like families of their peers without disabilities, these families described a range of recreational activities, including passive (31 children), play (38), social (40), and entertainment/special events (35). In addition, many described regular participation in physical activities, including swimming (26 children), roughhousing or physical games such as playing catch or basketball (24), walking (18), and riding bikes (12); however, what clearly emerged was the concerted effort required by parents to provide

Table 23.1. Positive effects of a child with a disability on the family

Effects on parents	Effects on siblings and extended family	Feelings about the future
Changed perspective on life	**Changed perspective on life**	**Generally hopeful**
Don't take things for granted	Are content with what they have	
Have new goals	Have learned not to take life for granted	
Value other people more		
Have experienced changes in priorities		
Have increased appreciation of life		
Have increased sense of meaning/ purpose		
Have experienced changes in life/ career expectations		
Increased sensitivity	**Increased sensitivity**	**Generally anxious**
Have increased tolerance	Have increased understanding of disability	Worry about who will look after child
Have increased awareness of others	Have increased tolerance and patience	Worry about abuse in alternative living settings
Have improved sensitivity to child as a parent	Are more caring and willing to help others	
Have increased patience		
Are thoughtful and compassionate		
Support from other families	**Greater sense of responsibility**	**Hopes and fears**
Have an expanding social network	Have increased maturity	Feel that over time child will become more typical
Receive help from other families who have "been there"	Have pride in sibling with disability	Worry how child will be accepted
Share information	Are willing to stand up for people with a disability	
Have the chance to work with others to influence policies		
Opportunities to learn	**Positive attitude toward others**	**Not looking to future**
Have the opportunity to learn about disability, psychology, special education	Demonstrate caring and compassion	Don't worry ahead but live for the moment
Have the opportunity to learn about oneself	Are tender and warm	
Have the opportunity to learn from child	Are thoughtful and sensitive	
Have the opportunity to learn from many other professionals		
Increased confidence or assertiveness	**Opportunities to learn**	
Have increased confidence in dealing with others	Have the opportunity to learn about disabilities and other life difficulties	
Are involved in advocacy		
Improved family dynamics	**Improved family dynamics**	
Experience closer family relationships	Experience closer extended family relationships	
Rely on each other more	Are willing to help other family members	
Have a strengthened marriage		

From Taunt, H., & Hastings, R. (2002). Positive impact of children with developmental disabilities on their families: A preliminary study. *Education and Training in Mental Retardation and Developmental Disabilities, 37,* 410–420; adapted by permission of the Division on Developmental Disabilities.

these recreational activities for their child with a disability. Many indicated that these activities were pursued when the family's typically developing children were engaged in similar activities with their peers and were most often directed and attended by the mother. Generally, these efforts and interactions were informal and family initiated and occurred with equal frequency in home and community settings. For many parents, an educational as well as a social component prompted these efforts, providing a means for the child with a disability to connect with other family members, to develop skills, and to set foundations for the future. Furthermore, unlike their siblings without disabilities, who by adolescence generally seek individualized patterns of recreation, children with developmental disabilities appear to rely heavily on family recreation well into early adulthood and often beyond (Horna, 1994).

Adulthood:
The Launching or Departure of Family Members from the Household

Making the transition to adulthood is no easy process for families, for their child with a disability, and often for service providers as well. In a family, the completion of a child's educational career serves as the springboard for launching these children into the world as functional, financially and socially independent adults. By contrast, for most families whose adult child has a developmental disability, this launching does not occur; the adult child continues to live in the family home.

Tasks and Needs in Adulthood According to Braddock, Emerson, Felce, and Stancliffe (2001), in 1998 there were approximately 3.24 million adults with intellectual and other developmental disabilities living in the United States (1.2% of the population). Sixty percent lived with family caregivers, 13% in their own homes, and 15% with a spouse. Although independent supported community living for these adults is advocated as optimal, the need for residential spaces exceeds the capacity and continues to do so at an accelerating rate. Waiting lists for residential and community services are growing rapidly, as a large cohort of adults continue to live with aging parents who are in their 70s and 80s. Many observers predict a residential crisis for these adults within the next decade as elderly parents can no longer provide care due to their own disability or death. Also, as previously indicated, unemployment, financial dependence, and a lack of social relationships are the outcomes faced by many American adults with a disability after they leave high school. American students

with disabilities from high-poverty backgrounds and those of color are more likely to drop out of or be expelled from school, with even poorer social, employment, and community integration outcomes (Lewit, Terman, & Behrman, 1997). Although legislation has recently been enacted to improve the outcomes of secondary students making the transition into adulthood, the benefits of this legislation have yet to be realized.

Thus, for these families, there are material stresses as well as stresses associated with alterations in the stages of the family life course. Parents remain parents, albeit there may be an alteration with respect to the role and relationship that parents and other adult siblings have with the adult with a disability. Because parents remain parents, with a partly dependent adult child in residence, the life cycle process gets "stuck." Thus, the task for families at this point is to help the adult with a disability to develop as independent a life as possible within the family home, while continuing to prepare him or her for eventually living in an alternative setting. Similarly, the parents are faced with the task of struggling with the intermingling of their life needs with those of a deeply bonded dependent adult child (Boose, 2002). These tasks are faced with little guidance from the formal service system and virtually no financial resources because public expenditures for services are overwhelmingly targeted to adults who live in out-of-home settings, as are formal services and supports (Gordon, Seltzer, & Krauss, 1997; Parish, Pomeranz-Essley, & Braddock, 2003).

Although many states have a range of services for adults with disabilities, one of the first tasks for families whose child with a disability has just completed 18–21 years of early intervention and educational supports is to face the fact that there are no mandated services on which they can depend. Fuijura, Roccoforte, and Braddock (1994) estimated that, on average, parents spend more than $6,000 per year in out-of-pocket expenses for each adult child with a disability, a figure that has no doubt risen considerably in the years since this study. Furthermore, parents often must seek and advocate for services without the aid of an interdisciplinary team that has previously provided support. In a study of the experience of 30 Massachusetts families negotiating this transition with their young adult child with a disability, parents described the service-delivery systems as inconsistent, difficult to negotiate, lacking coordination, and unresponsive to parents' or their young adult children's needs (Timmons, McIntyre, Whitney-Thomas, Butterworth, & Allen, 1998). Against this background, the next section examines family relationships during this period.

Family Relationships in Adulthood Earlier literature converged in suggesting that families caring for adult children begin to experience reciprocity with their adult child, giving rise to more caregiving enrichment and lessened stress (Heller et al., 1997; Nachshen et al., 2003; Williams & Robinson, 2001); however, such positive outcomes are specific to families with little caregiving burden from behavior problems and for whom a clear and satisfactory long-term caregiving plan following parental death is in place. In an extensive review of the literature, Seltzer and Krauss (2001) concluded that adults with developmental disabilities who live with their parents tend to have close family relationships, characterized by the exchange of support and emotional involvement. In addition, parents' close relationship with their adult children without disabilities can provide an impetus for these siblings to also be involved with the individual with a disability. Thus, close family relationships for the child with a disability encompass intergenerational patterns extending to adult siblings as well as mothers and fathers and are particularly notable among sisters of people with disabilities.

These findings, however, must be placed in context. For decades, behavior problems were the most significant predictor of an out-of-home placement of adults with disabilities (Borthwick-Duffy, Eyman, & White, 1987; Bromley & Blacher, 1991). Less brittle adults often remained in the parental home. With the current trend toward continued home placement throughout the life span, a very different picture emerges (Larson, Lakin, Anderson, & Kwak, 2001). At least two factors influence these findings: 1) the burden for caregivers of

significant behavior difficulties and 2) the age of the caregiving parents.

A number of studies document that caring for an adult with significant behavior problems as part of their disability increases the caregiving burden and is reflected in increased maternal pessimism, depressive symptoms, and dissatisfaction with the quality of the parent–child relationship, especially for mothers (Greenberg, Seltzer, Krauss, & Kim, 1997; Heller et al., 1997). In a complex longitudinal study, Orsmond, Seltzer, Krauss, and Hong (2003) followed 193 families of adults with disabilities living at home for 12 years, encompassing eight data collection points each 18 months apart. Only about 25% of the adults had no behavior difficulties during that time, with the remaining adults presenting behavior challenges throughout the study period; at least one fourth had clinically significant behavior difficulties. Furthermore, the findings indicated that the adult child's behavior problems were a chronic stressor, particularly for the mother, eventually taking their toll on maternal well-being and resulting in increased feelings of caregiving burden, depressive symptoms, and pessimism about the child's future and a less positive mother–adult child relationship. In addition, the findings indicated that, as mothers became less functional, the behavioral and functional status of the adult child was affected as well, resulting in a downward spiral of behavioral and emotional functioning. Clearly, the emotional toll on all family members is considerable.

Seltzer and Krauss (2001) pointed out that one unique aspect of family relationships among adults who live at home with their parents, even those who have done so for many years, is the impermanence of this caregiving arrangement. With the increased life span for adults with disabilities, it is the norm for their parents to predecease them. The probability of this event is a source of considerable and chronic stress for many families in the context of the limited and insufficient availability of alternative living settings. As previously noted, among those families who have actively and successfully engaged in future planning, close and positive family relationships remain stable; failure to have or be able to effectively develop such a plan can erode a previously positive adjustment for the family and the adult with disabilities.

Support and Coping   Although parents and families in this life stage use an array of coping strategies similar to those found in younger parents, there are some data to suggest that older family caregivers more frequently use cognitive coping strategies such as making favorable comparisons and reliance on faith. By the same token, some families simply become resigned (Grant & Whittell, 2001). For many families in this life cycle stage, the social network of support on which many have relied begins to shrink, both because of an inability of the caregiving family to participate in many activities and, as the caregiving parents age, because of death of network members (Bigby, 1997). As a result, many families report increased isolation and stress with decreased ability to cope. With the substantial increase in adults with disabilities remaining in their parental home, and the lengthened life span of these adults, directed efforts toward extending the benefits of family-centered care to these vulnerable families are needed.

SEXUALITY

Perhaps no area of child rearing is more challenging for parents than the young adolescent's emerging expressions of sexuality and sexual behavior. For many parents whose child has a disability, the emergence of sexuality and sexual behavior evokes a myriad of emotions and reactions. In addition, among all of the decision-making areas within which parents and professionals must relate, sexuality is the one most likely to bring parents into direct conflict with professionals. Much of this conflict results from historical forces that have shaped the current medical, legal, and professional caregiving environment. At the heart of conflict is the legacy of eugenics, historically exemplified by the Kallikak family, that has played out across multiple decades of social control through unrestrained, nonconsensual sterilization of those deemed "different" or "inferior." As a result, the legal, professional, and caregiving position is that sexuality and "sexual expression" (i.e.,

sexual intercourse) are rights for those with developmental disabilities (Ailey, Marks, Crisp, & Hahn, 2003). Thus, for many parents of adolescents and adults with disabilities, the emergence of sexuality and sexual behavior not only raises appropriate concerns regarding the best approach for helping their offspring understand and manage this area of their lives, but also raises the specter of total loss of ability to influence and guide their children in this area as others encourage these children to "exercise their rights." In no other area is the concept of family-centered care more ignored, with the justification of assertively protecting the unbridled "rights" of the individual with disabilities.

Are parents simply being overprotective, or unconsciously sabotaging appropriate independence for their child with a disability (Greydanus, Rimsza, & Newhouse, 2002)? Although this may be true for some children, in most instances parental concerns are not without a sound basis. It is well documented that individuals with developmental disabilities are more susceptible to sexual abuse and exploitation than the general population (Tharinger, Horton, & Millea, 1990). Also, once sexually active, those with developmental disabilities have a higher rate of pregnancy than their peers without disabilities (McCabe & Cummins, 1996). Thus, families need to be helped in finding appropriate and ongoing sexual education for their children and for themselves in terms of how to handle this issue with their young adults. Furthermore, parents may need help in finding sensitive, responsive, and comprehensive medical care for their young adult in a setting that can understand and address parental concerns as well. Finally, families helping their young adults make the transition into supported living settings need encouragement and support in openly discussing their wishes and family values regarding this issue with prospective caregivers.

SIBLINGS

Siblings have an important but often neglected role in the family. A passive "neglect" of typically developing siblings is reflected in the activities and physical structure of hospital clinics as well as other family-centered service providers; yet, it is clear that, in families in which a child has a disability, the daily life and experiences of siblings may be different from those of their peers in a number of ways. Findings concerning the effects on children of having a sibling with a disability are inconsistent. Some studies have found negative outcomes for typically developing siblings, including loneliness, embarrassment regarding their sibling with a disability, difficulty handling and dealing with concomitant behavior problems, and an increased risk for internalizing disorders and adjustment problems. Others have found no differences among siblings on a number of dimensions, including self-esteem, social competence, adjustment, and emotional difficulties. A study of siblings of a child with autism found that siblings reported both more acceptance and more embarrassment than siblings of children without disabilities (Roeyers & Mycke, 1995). Collectively, available research and personal testimonies reveal complex and multifaceted sibling relationships and experiences that vary across time and are mediated by the quality of family dynamics (Seltzer, Greenberg, Krauss, Gordon, & Judge, 1997; Stoneman & Berman, 1993). The quality of the relationship between siblings with and without disabilities, and the long-term adjustment of siblings without a disability, is clearly influenced by the family's subjective assessment of the nature and burden of the disability, the assessment by parents of their personal adequacy in meeting the needs of their children without a disability, and the overall pattern of family adaptation (Guite, Labato, Kao, & Plante, 2004; Swados, 1991; Trevino, 1983; Zetlin, 1986).

Collective interview data reveal a number of common concerns among siblings of a child with a disability. These include (survivor-type) guilt, embarrassment at the appearance of the sibling with a disability, fear that they themselves will develop the disability or have a child with the disability, anger and jealousy at the time and care provided to the sibling with a disability, resentment at having to spend time with this sibling, confusion about both the disability and their role in that sibling's care, isolation, being alone in their feelings, pressure particularly to achieve and make up for their sibling's disability, being burdened by their part in care provision, and concern over the future of their sibling with a disability (South Carolina Department of Disabilities and Special Needs, 1994).

As adults, however, when contrasted with siblings of adults with serious mental illness, siblings of adults with intellectual disabilities had a closer relationship with their siblings than the comparison group; were more likely to perceive that having a brother or sister with a developmental disability had a pervasive influence on their life decisions and to evaluate their sibling experience as mostly positive; and had better psychological well-being when they had a close relationship with their sibling with a disability. By contrast, adult siblings of those with mental illness had more favorable psychological well-being when they perceived a less pervasive impact of their brother or sister on their life (Seltzer et al., 1997). Common between the two groups was the impact of behavior problems of a sibling with a disability on the psychological outcome of the sibling without a disability.

The implication of both the collective interview data and the study of adults is clear. Family-centered services must be more systematic and purposeful in assessing and supporting siblings of those with disabilities. Because many will, as adults, assume some portion of responsibility for their sibling with a disability, including siblings without a disability from the time of system entry and throughout the life span is clearly indicated.

FORMAL SUPPORT SYSTEMS

In addition to the social network and support systems of individual families, service providers need to be aware of the continuum of formal psychosocial support services. These include support groups that are often disability specific, educational programs and courses, psychotherapeutic groups, self-help groups, events and activities, and Internet-based support services.

Support groups are those programs that bring together individuals with similar diagnoses and problems for the purpose of learning, sharing, and mutual support (Johnson, 2000).

Support groups are ongoing; have relatively open agendas; provide mutual support rather than therapy; and can have a very formal structure, with officers, dues, and guidelines, or an informal structure with only a designated meeting time and place (Johnson & Johnson, 1998). Although many disabilities have national organizations (e.g., Down syndrome), state-based chapters often work in conjunction with an interested professional providing backup. One study, however, reported that half of the parents surveyed had no access to parent support groups or other self-help groups (Herman & Thompson, 1995).

Educational programs are structured educational efforts provided in a supportive environment. These programs are usually conducted by a professional, meet for a specified number of sessions, and are specifically focused on increased knowledge, which can empower attendees.

Events and activities such as camps, retreats, walk-a-thons, picnics, and other such efforts usually have as their focus fun and family-to-family support in the context of recreational activities. Both families and their children with disabilities can develop friendships and broaden their peer support network through events and activities.

Self-help groups, both face to face and on-line, are peer-directed efforts that serve the goals of increased peer support, education, empowerment and advocacy, and information sharing. In particular, Internet self-help groups can reach populations that are rural or have physical disabilities more effectively than face-to-face groups because they eliminate transportation and access issues. Research documents the effectiveness of these "virtual" groups (Houston, Cooper, & Ford, 2002). Furthermore, earlier studies indicated that parents who had access to other parents whom they perceived as helpful were more likely to see their basic and child-related resources as adequate (Herman & Thompson, 1995).

Some families may need the more intensive services of a psychotherapeutic group. Psychotherapeutic groups are directed by trained professionals and have a more intense focus than other support efforts.

CONCLUSION

The capacity to effectively listen and sensitively communicate is the substrate of all relationships, including the parent–professional collaborative partnership at the basis of family-centered care. Nonetheless, even in the best of circumstances, misunderstandings and disagreements will occur. At that point, it is often useful to ask parents for their perceptions of how the communication got off track. Parents who are themselves professionals in the field of developmental disabilities can often be quite instructive. The following list of points was developed by a pediatric audiologist whose son has a rare, degenerative metabolic disease. At age 4, "C.J." has profound hearing impairment, little to no vision, and very little motor functioning, and is frequently hospitalized. Having been told that C.J. would not live to see his first birthday and having made a very conscious decision regarding end-of-life procedures for C.J., his parents are frequently at odds with providers in all sectors. Their list of do's and don'ts should serve as cautions to all who seek to develop a good parent–professional partnership. Using their title, this chapter will close with "The Top 10 Things Parents of a Developmentally Delayed Child Want You to Know" (K. Geier, personal communication, 2005):

1. Never use the word *fine* (i.e., "Suzy will be fine."). This is far too ambiguous and can lead to misinterpretation. What parents hear is "Suzy will be normal." Don't say it unless you mean it. Be specific and don't dance around a situation. Use phrases such as the following: "Suzy is medically stable." "Suzy can go home soon." "The goal is for Suzy is to eventually (insert word here, e.g., walk, talk, communicate), but we don't know if she ever will."

2. It's okay to say, "I don't know." The best thing to do in this situation is to acknowledge the parents' frustration and disappointment at the uncertainty. "Only time will tell. I know that really stinks, but in the meantime we are going to do every-

thing we can to help her along (e.g., physical and occupational therapy)."

3. Try never to give timelines for ANYTHING (especially when discussing end-of-life issues) unless you are absolutely certain (which you can't be)! For example, don't say, "She won't make it to 12 months old." "In 6 months, Suzy should be sitting." "Based on his diagnosis, he should walk by the time he is 4." When you say things like this, parents practically mark it on the calendar. When the event doesn't happen in the time allotted, they often feel it's their fault, and they didn't do enough to make it happen. When the event happens prior to the time stated, they will lose trust in you ("HA! It happened before they said it would. What do they know?").

4. Never ask for a list of developmental milestone questions based on the child's age. It is humiliating answering "no" to every question, and parents can often become sarcastic in their answers (e.g., "Does it look like she cans sit independently? She can't even hold her head up!"). Instead, ask what the current therapy goals are, or ask when the child achieved a milestone that you are observing ("So, when did she start sitting?"). Just be sensitive when you ask these questions.

5. When giving treatment options, give ALL of the options that are appropriate, not just the ones that YOU find appropriate. Sometimes not doing a surgery or particular therapy is an option (not all the time). When appropriate, parents need to be given the option to do nothing and feel that this is an acceptable option and no one will think they are bad parents or being neglectful. This is especially true in end-of-life situations.

6. More therapy does not always mean a better outcome. Just because a child can get more therapy (physical therapy three times per week instead of two times per week) doesn't mean they should. Parents still need to be parents first, not therapists. That is not to say they should not be involved in the therapy process, and carryover in the home is necessary. But often parents feel guilty if they do not do their child's "therapy homework" every day, or they can become so controlling and overdemanding, their child becomes overprogrammed. Children with special needs often become their parents' (usually mother's) project. There is a happy medium in there somewhere.

7. Never ignore the power of a genetics consult. For many parents, a genetic diagnosis is the answer to "why me?" Knowing what the chances are that you will have another child like this, and knowing the disorder has a name, can often be extremely helpful through the denial stage, even if it is a fluke. Even if a child has autism, a genetics consult could be revealing. Many genetic diagnoses, such as unbalanced chromosomal translocations, appear as autism at first glance, when in actuality the chromosomal abnormality is causing the child to have autistic behaviors. Again, it is extremely helpful for a parent to know "why" (e.g., "It's not because I didn't get enough folic acid during pregnancy, or all those Diet Cokes I drank").

8. Do not forget this child is part of a family. Children with developmental delays are often the focus or center of attention for the family. Siblings within a family can easily be left out. Suggest a local SibShop program for siblings, and try to get the family connected with a support group, even if the group is not specifically for the child's diagnosis. Gently remind parents that their child with special needs is just one aspect of their lives, not their entire lives. It's easy for the child to become the parent's identity.

9. Teach parents that they are their child's advocate. No one is going to do the work for them or in the time frame they feel is appropriate. Teach them that social workers, case managers, and therapists are there for suggestions and to lead fami-

lies in the right direction, not to do all the work for them. The parent is the child's primary case manager.

10. Reassure the family that it does get easier over time. The first year is hell, and the first several years (until a child begins an early childhood program) are difficult and can be isolating. The problems and behaviors don't necessarily become easier, but the parent's ability to handle difficulties seems to become better over time, or they are less hesitant to reach out and ask for advice.

REFERENCES

Agran, M., Alper, S., & Wehmeyer, M. (2002). Access to the general curriculum for students with significant disabilities: What it means to teachers. *Education and Training in Mental Retardation and Developmental Disabilities, 37,* 123–133.

Ailey, S.H., Marks, B., Crisp, C., & Hahn, J.E. (2003). Promoting sexuality across the life span for individuals with intellectual and developmental disabilities. *Nursing Clinics of North America, 38,* 229–252.

Aldous, J. (1996). *Family careers: Rethinking the developmental perspective.* Thousand Oaks, CA: Sage Publications.

Bailey, D.B., & Powell, T. (2005). Assessing the information needs of families in early intervention. In M. Guralnick (Ed.), *The developmental systems approach to early intervention* (pp. 151–184). Baltimore: Paul H. Brookes Publishing Co.

Bailey, D.B., & Wolery, M. (1992). *Teaching infants and preschoolers with disabilities* (2nd ed.). Upper Saddle River, NJ: Prentice Hall.

Baker, B.L., Blatcher, J., Crnic, K.A., & Edelbrock, C. (2002). Behavior problems and parenting stress in families of three-year old children with and without developmental delays. *American Journal on Mental Retardation, 107,* 433–444.

Barnett, W.S., & Boyce, G. (1995). Effects of children with Down syndrome on parents' activities. *American Journal on Mental Retardation, 100,* 115–127.

Beckman, P. (1984). A transactional view of stress in families of handicapped children. In M. Lewis (Ed.), *Beyond the dyad* (pp. 45–53). New York: Plenum Press.

Bigby, C. (1997). When parents relinquish care: Informal support networks of older people with intellectual disability. *Journal of Applied Research in Intellectual Disabilities, 10,* 333–344.

Boose, L. (2002). *Parents living with an adult dependent child with a disability.* Portland, OR: Author.

Borthwick-Duffy, S.A., Eyman, R.K., & White, J.F. (1987). Client characteristics and residential placement patterns. *American Journal of Mental Deficiency, 92,* 24–30.

Braddock, D., Emerson, E., Felce, D., & Stancliffe, R.J. (2001). Living circumstances of children and adults with mental retardation or developmental disabilities in the United States, Canada, England and Wales, and Australia. *Mental Retardation and Developmental Disabilities Research Reviews, 7,* 115–121.

Bristol, M.M. (1987). Mothers of children with autism or communication disorders: Successful adaptation and the double ABCX model. *Journal of Autism and Developmental Disorders, 17,* 469–486.

Bristol, M.M., Schopler, E., & Gallagher, J.J. (1988). Mothers and fathers of young developmentally disabled and nondisabled boys: Adaptation and spousal support. *Developmental Psychology, 24,* 441–451.

Britner, P.A., Morog, M., Pianta, R.C., & Marvin, R.S. (2003). Stress and coping: A comparison of self-report measures of functioning in families of young children with cerebral palsy or no medical diagnosis. *Journal of Child and Family Studies, 12,* 335–348.

Bromley, B.E., & Blacher, J. (1991). Parental reasons for out-of-home placement of children with severe handicaps. *Mental Retardation, 29,* 275–280.

Button, S., Pianta, R., & Marvin, R.S. (2001). Mothers' representations of relationships with their children: Relations with parenting behavior, mother characteristics, and child disability status. *Social Development, 10,* 455–472.

Center, Y., & Curry, C. (1993). A feasibility study of a full integration model developed for a group of students classified as mildly intellectually disabled. *International Journal of Disability, Development, and Education, 40,* 217–235.

Crnic, K., & Stormshak, E. (1997). The effectiveness of providing social support for families of children at risk. In M. Guralnick (Ed.), *The effectiveness of early intervention* (pp. 209–225). Baltimore: Paul H. Brookes Publishing Co.

Cummings, E.M., & Davies, P. (2002). Effects of marital conflict on children: Recent advances and emerging themes in process-oriented research. *Journal of Child Psychology and Psychiatry, 43,* 31–63.

Doré, R., Dion, E., Wagner, S., & Brunet, J.P. (2002). High school inclusion of adolescents with mental retardation: A multiple case study. *Education and Training in Mental Retardation and Developmental Disabilities, 37,* 253–261.

Dreikurs, R., with Soltz, V. (1990). *Children: The challenge.* New York: Plume. (Original work published 1964)

Dumas, J.E., Wold, L., Fisman, S.N., & Culligan, A. (1991). Parenting stress, child behavior problems and dysphoria in parents of children with autism, Down syndrome, behavior disorders, and normal development. *Exceptionality, 2,* 97–110.

Dunst, C.J. (1985). Rethinking early intervention. *Analysis and Intervention in Developmental Disabilities, 5,* 165–201.

Dunst, C.J., Trivette, C., & Deal, A.B. (1988). *Enabling and empowering families: Principles and guidelines for practice.* Cambridge, MA: Brookline Books.

Dunst, C.J., Trivette, C., & Jodry, W. (1997). Influences of social support on children with disabilities and their families. In M. Guralnick (Ed.), *The effectiveness of early intervention* (pp. 499–522). Baltimore: Paul H. Brookes Publishing Co.

Dunst, C.J., Trivette, C., & Johanson, C. (1994). Parent–professional collaboration and partnerships. In C.J. Dunst, A.G. Deal, & C.M. Trivette (Eds.), *Supporting and strengthening families: Vol. 1. Methods, strategies and practices* (pp. 197–211). Cambridge, MA: Brookline Books.

Dyson, L.L. (1993). Response to the presence of a child with disabilities: Parental stress and family functioning over time. *American Journal on Mental Retardation, 98,* 207–218.

Education of the Handicapped Act Amendments of 1986, PL 99–457, 20 U.S.C. §§ 1400 *et seq.*

Emerson, E. (2003). Mothers of children and adolescents with intellectual disability: Social and economic situation, mental health status, and the self-assessed social and psychological impact of the child's difficulties. *Journal of Intellectual Disability Research, 47,* 385–399.

Faber, A., & Mazlish, E. (1999). *How to talk so kids will listen and how to listen so kids will talk* (20th anniversary ed.). New York: Avon Books.

Floyd, F.J., & Gallagher, E. (1997). Parental stress, care demands, and use of support services for school-age children with disabilities and behavior problems. *Family Relations, 46,* 359–371.

Freeman, N.L., Perry, A., & Factor, D.C. (1991). Child behaviors as stressors: Replicating and extending the use of the CARS as a measure of stress. A research note. *Journal of Child Psychology and Psychiatry, 32,* 1025–1030.

Fuijura, G.T., Roccoforte, J., & Braddock, D. (1994). Costs of family care for adults with mental retardation and related developmental disabilities. *American Journal on Mental Retardation, 99,* 250–261.

Geisthardt, C., Brotherson, M., & Cook, C.C. (2002). Friendships of children with disabilities in the home environment. *Education and Training in Mental Retardation and Developmental Disabilities, 37,* 235–252.

Glasser, P.H., & Glasser, L. (1970). *Families in crisis.* New York: Harper & Row.

Goldenberg, I., & Goldenberg, H. (2000). *Family therapy: An overview* (5th ed.). Pacific Grove, CA: Brooks/Cole Thomson Learning.

Gordon, R.M., Seltzer, M., & Krauss, M.W. (1997). The aftermath of parental death: Changes in the context and quality of life. In R.L. Schalock (Ed.), *Quality of life: Vol. 2. Applications to persons with disabilities* (pp. 25–42). Washington, DC: American Association on Mental Retardation.

Gortmaker, S.L., Walker, D., Weitzman, M., & Sobol, A.M. (1990). Chronic conditions, socioeconomic risks, and behavioral problems in children and adolescents. *Pediatrics, 85,* 267–276.

Gottlieb, A.S. (1997). Single mothers of children with developmental disabilities: The impact of multiple roles. *Family Relations, 46,* 5–12.

Grant, G., & Whittell, B. (2001). Do families and care managers have a similar view of family coping? *Journal of Learning Disabilities, 5,* 111–120.

Green, A.L., & Stoneman, Z. (1989). Attitudes of mothers and fathers of nonhandicapped children. *Journal of Early Intervention, 13,* 292–304.

Greenberg, J., Seltzer, M., Krauss, M.W., & Kim, H.W. (1997). The differential effects of social support on the psychological well-being of aging mothers of adults with mental illness or mental retardation. *Family Relations, 46,* 383–394.

Greydanus, D.E., Rimsza, M., & Newhouse, P.A. (2002). Adolescent sexuality and disability. *Adolescent Medicine: State of the Art Reviews, 13,* 223–247.

Guite, J., Labato, D., Kao, B., & Plante, W. (2004). Discordance between sibling and parent reports of the impact of chronic illness and disability on siblings. *Children's Health Care, 33*(1), 77–92.

Guralnick, M. (2000). Interdisciplinary team assessment for young children: Purposes and processes. In M. Guralnick (Ed.), *Interdisciplinary clinical assessment of young children with developmental disabilities* (pp. 3–15). Baltimore: Paul H. Brookes Publishing Co.

Hanson, M.J. (1998). Ethnic, culture and language diversity in intervention settings. In M. Hanson & E.W. Lynch (Eds.), *Developing cross-cultural competence: A guide for working with children and their families* (2nd ed., pp. 3–22). Baltimore: Paul H. Brookes Publishing Co.

Hanson, M.J. (2005). Ensuring effective transitions in early intervention. In M. Guralnick (Ed.), *The developmental systems approach to early intervention* (pp. 373–400). Baltimore: Paul H. Brookes Publishing Co.

Hanson, M.J., & Carta, J.J. (1996). Addressing the challenges of families with multiple risks. *Exceptional Children, 62,* 201–212.

Hanson, M.J., & Lynch, E. (2004). *Understanding families: Approaches to diversity, disability, and risk.* Baltimore: Paul H. Brookes Publishing Co.

Hastings, R.P., & Brown, T. (2002). Behavior problems of children with autism, parental self-efficacy, and mental health. *American Journal on Mental Retardation, 107,* 222–232.

Hauser-Cram, P., Warfield, M.E., Shondoff, J.P., & Krauss, M.W. (2001). Children with disabilities: A longitudinal study of child development and parental well-being. *Monographs of the Society for Research in Child Development, 66*(3, Serial No. 266).

Heller, T. (1993). Self-efficacy coping, active involvement, and caregiver well-being throughout the life course among families of persons with mental retardation. In A.P. Turnbull, S.K. Behr, D.L. Murphy, J.G. Marquis, & M.J. Blue-Banning (Eds.), *Cognitive coping, families, and disability* (pp.

195–206). Baltimore: Paul H. Brookes Publishing Co.

Heller, T., Hsieh, K., & Rowitz, L. (1997). Maternal and paternal caregiving of persons with mental retardation across the lifespan. *Family Relations, 46,* 407–415.

Herman, S.E., & Thompson, L. (1995). Families perceptions of their resources for caring for children with developmental disabilities. *Mental Retardation, 33,* 73–84.

Horna, J. (1994). *The study of leisure: An introduction.* Toronto, Ontario: Oxford University Press.

Houston, T.K., Cooper, L.A., & Ford, D.E. (2002). Internet support groups for depression: A 1-year prospective cohort study. *American Journal of Psychiatry, 159,* 2062–2068.

Hughes, C. (2001). Transition to adulthood: Supporting young adults to access social, employment, and civic pursuits. *Mental Retardation and Developmental Disabilities Research Reviews, 7,* 84–90.

Hughes, C., Carter, E.W., Hughes, T., Bradford, E., & Copeland, S.R. (2002). Effects of instructional versus non-instructional roles on the social interactions of high school students. *Education and Training in Mental Retardation and Developmental Disabilities, 37,* 146–162.

Hughes, C., Harmer, M., Killian, D.J., & Niarhos, F. (1995). The effects of multiple-exemplar self-instructional training on high school students' generalized conversational interactions. *Journal of Applied Behavior Analysis, 28,* 201–218.

Hughes, C., Rodi, M., Lorden, S.W., Pitkin, S.E., Derer, K.R., Hwang, B., et al. (1999). Social interactions of high school students with mental retardation and their general education peers. *American Journal on Mental Retardation, 104,* 533–544.

Johnson, J. (2000). An overview of psychosocial support services: Resources for healing. *Cancer Nursing, 23,* 310–333.

Johnson, J., & Johnson, M. (1998). Programmatic approaches to psychosocial support. In R.M. Carroll-Johnson, L.M. Gorman, & N.J. Bush (Eds.), *Psychosocial nursing care along the cancer continuum.* Pittsburgh: Oncology Nursing Press.

Judge, S.L. (1998). Parental coping strategies and strengths in families of young children with disabilities. *Family Relations, 47,* 263–268.

Kasari, C., & Sigman, M. (1997). Linking parental perceptions to interactions in young children with autism. *Journal of Autism and Developmental Disorders, 27,* 39–57.

Katsiyannis, A., Zhang, D., & Archwamety, T. (2002). Placement and exit patterns for students with mental retardation: An analysis of national trends. *Education and Training in Mental Retardation and Developmental Disabilities, 37,* 134–145.

Kazak, A.E., & Wilcox, B. (1984). The structure and function of social support networks in families with handicapped children. *American Journal of Community Psychology, 12,* 645–661.

Kelly, J., Booth-LaForce, C., & Spieker, S. (2005). Assessing family characteristics relevant to early intervention. In M. Guralnick (Ed.), *The developmental systems approach to early intervention* (pp. 235–265). Baltimore: Paul H. Brookes Publishing Co.

Kennedy, C.H., & Itkonen, T. (1994). Some effects of regular class participation on the social contacts and social networks of high shool students with severe disabilities. *Journal of The Association for Persons with Severe Handicaps, 19,* 1–10.

Knowlton, E. (1998). Considerations in the design of personalized curricular supports for students with developmental disabilities. *Education and Training in Mental Retardation and Developmental Disabilities, 33,* 95–107.

Kraemer, B.R., Blacher, J., & Marshal, M.P. (1997). Adolescents with severe disabilities: Families, school, and community intergration. *Journal of The Association for Persons with Severe Handicaps, 22,* 224–234.

Krajewski, J.J., Hyde, M.S., & O'Keeffe, M.K. (2002). Teen attitudes toward individuals with mental retardation from 1987 to 1998: Impact of respondent gender and school variables. *Education and Training in Mental Retardation and Developmental Disabilities, 37,* 27–39.

Kurcinka, M.S. (2006). *Raising your spirited child: A guide for parents whose child is more intense, sensitive, perceptive, persistent, energetic* (Rev. ed.). New York: Harper.

Lam, D., Giles, A., & Lavander, A. (2003). Carers' expressed emotion, appraisal of behavioural problems and stress in children attending schools for learning disabilities. *Journal of Intellectual Disability Research, 47,* 456–463.

Larson, S., Lakin, C., Anderson, L., & Kwak, N. (2001). Characteristics of and service use by persons with MR/DD living in their own homes or with family members: NHIS-D analysis. *MR/DD Data Brief, 3,* 1–12.

Leal, L. (1999). *A family centered approach to people with mental retardation.* Washington, DC: American Association on Mental Retardation.

Lewit, E.M., Terman, D., & Behrman, R.E. (1997). Children and poverty: Analysis and recommendations. *Child Poverty, 7,* 4–24.

Lustig, D. (2002). Family coping in families with a child with a disability. *Education and Training in Mental Retardation and Developmental Disabilities, 37,* 14–22.

Mactavish, J.B., & Schleien, S. (2004). Re-injecting spontaneity and balance in family life: Parents' perspective on recreation in families that include children with developmental disability. *Journal of Intellectual Disability Research, 48,* 123–141.

Maes, B., Broekman, T.G., Dosen, A., & Nauts, J. (2003). Caregiving burden of families looking after persons with intellectual disability and behavioural or psychiatric problems. *Journal of Intellectual Disability Research, 47,* 447–455.

Margalit, M., Raviv, A., & Ankonina, D.B. (1992). Coping and coherence among parents with disabled children. *Journal of Clinical Child Psychology, 21*, 202–209.

McCabe, M.P., & Cummins, R. (1996). The sexual knowledge, experience, feelings and needs of people with mild intellectual disability. *Education and Training in Mental Retardation and Developmental Disabilities, 31*, 13–21.

McCallion, P., Janicki, M., & Grant-Griffin, L. (1997). Exploring the impact of culture and acculturation on older families caregiving for persons with developmental disabilities. *Family Relations, 46*, 347–357.

McWilliam, R. (2005). Assessing the resource needs of families in the context of early intervention. In M. Guralnick (Ed.), *The developmental systems approach to early intervention* (pp. 215–234). Baltimore: Paul H. Brookes Publishing Co.

Nachsen, J.S., Woodford, L., & Minnes, P. (2003). The family stress and coping interview for families of individuals with developmental disabilities: A lifespan perspective on family adjustment. *Journal of Intellectual Disability Research, 47*, 285–290.

Nihira, K., Myers, C., & Mink, I.T. (1980). Home environment, family adjustment, and the development of mentally retarded children. *Applied Research in Mental Retardation, 1*(1–2), 15–24.

Orsmond, G. (2005). Assessing interpersonal and family distress and threat to confident parenting in the context of early intervention. In M. Guralnick (Ed.), *The developmental systems approach to early intervention* (pp. 185–214). Baltimore: Paul H. Brookes Publishing Co.

Orsmond, G., Seltzer, M., Krauss, M.W., & Hong, J. (2003). Behavior problems in adults with mental retardation and maternal well-being: Examination of the direction of effects. *American Journal on Mental Retardation, 108*, 257–271.

Ostfeld, B.M., & Gibbs, E. (1990). Use of family assessment in early intervention. In E.D. Gibbs & D.M. Teti (Eds.), *Interdisciplinary assessment of infants: A guide for early intervention professionals* (pp. 249–267). Baltimore: Paul H. Brookes Publishing Co.

Parish, S., Pomeranz-Essley, A., & Braddock, D. (2003). Family support in the United States: Financing trends and emerging initiative. *Mental Retardation, 41*, 174–187.

Poston, D., & Turnbull, A. (2004). Role of spirituality and religion in family quality of life for families of children with disabilities. *Education and Training in Mental Retardation and Developmental Disabilities, 39*, 95–108.

Poston, D., Turnbull, A., Park, J., Mannan, H., Marquis, J., & Wang, M. (2003). Family quality of life: A qualitative inquiry. *Mental Retardation, 41*, 313–328.

Roberts, J. (1984). Families with infants and young children who have special needs. In J.C. Hansen (Ed.), *Families with handicapped members* (pp. 1–17). Rockville, MD: Aspen Publications.

Rodrigue J.R., Morgan, S., & Geffken, G.R. (1992). Psychosocial adaptation of fathers of children with autism, Down syndrome, and normal development. *Journal of Autism and Developmental Disorders, 22*, 249–263.

Roeyers, H., & Mycke, K. (1995). Siblings of children with autism, with mental retardation and with normal development. *Child Care, Health, and Development, 21*, 305–319.

Seltzer, M.M., Greenberg, J., Krauss, M.W., Gordon, R.M., & Judge, K. (1997). Siblings of adults with mental retardation or mental illness: Effects on lifestyle and psychological well-being. *Family Relations, 46*, 395–405.

Seltzer, M.M., & Krauss, M. (2001). Quality of life of adults with mental retardation/developmental disabilities who live with family. *Mental Retardation and Developmental Disabilities Research Reviews, 7*, 105–114.

Simmerman, S., & Blacher, J. (2001). Fathers' and mothers' perceptions of father involvement in families with young children with a disability. *Journal of Intellectual and Developmental Disability, 26*, 325–338.

Singer, G.H.S., & Powers, L. (1993). *Families, disability, and empowerment: Active coping skills and strategies for family intervention.* Baltimore: Paul H. Brookes Publishing Co.

South Carolina Department of Disabilities and Special Needs. (1994). *Family matters: A guide for adult brothers and sisters of people with developmental disabilities.* Columbia, SC: Author.

Stoneman, Z., & Berman, P. (1993). *The effects of mental retardation, disability, and illness on sibling relationships: Research issues and challenges.* Baltimore: Paul H. Brookes Publishing Co.

Swados, E. (1991). *The four of us: The story of a family.* New York: Farrar, Strauss, and Giroux.

Taunt, H., & Hastings, R. (2002). Positive impact of children with developmental disabilities on their families: A preliminary study. *Education and Training in Mental Retardation and Developmental Disabilities, 37*, 410–420.

Tharinger, C., Horton, B., & Millea, S. (1990). Sexual abuse and exploitation of children and adults with mental retardation and other handicaps. *Child Abuse and Neglect, 14*, 301–312.

Timmons, J.C., McIntyre, J., Whitney-Thomas, J., Butterworth, J., & Allen, D. (1998). Barriers to transition planning for parents of adolescents with special health care needs. *Research to Practice, 4*(7), 3–4.

Tobing, L.E., & Glenwick, D. (2002). Relation of the Childhood Autism Rating Scale–Parent version to diagnosis, stress, and age. *Research in Developmental Disabilities, 23*, 211–223.

Trevino, F. (1983). Siblings of handicapped children: Identifying those at risk. In L. Wikler & M.P.

Keenan (Eds.), *Developmental disabilities: No longer a private tragedy.* Washington, DC: National Association of Social Workers/American Association on Mental Deficiency.

Trute, B., & Hiebert-Murphy, D. (2002). Family adjustment to childhood developmental disability: A measure of parent appraisal of family impacts. *Journal of Pediatric Psychology, 27,* 271–280.

Turnbull, A., Brotherson, M., & Summers, J.A. (1986). Family life cycle: Theoretical and empirical implications and future directions for families with mentally retarded members. In J.J. Gallagher & P. Vietz (Eds.), *Families of handicapped persons: Research, programs, and policy issues* (pp. 45–66). Baltimore: Paul H. Brookes Publishing Co.

Turnbull, A., Pereira, J., & Blue-Banning, M.J. (1999). Parents' facilitation of friendships between their children with a disability and friends without a disability. *Journal of The Association for Persons with Severe Handicaps, 24,* 85–99.

Turnbull, A., & Ruef, M. (1996). Family perspectives on problem behavior. *Mental Retardation, 34,* 280–293.

Wallander, J.L., Varni, J., Babani, L., Banis, H.T., & Wilcox, K.T. (1989). Family resources as resistance factors for psychological maladjustment in chronically ill and handicapped children. *Journal of Pediatric Psychology, 14,* 157–173.

Warfield, M.E., Krauss, M.W., Hauser-Cram, P., Upshur, C.C., & Shonkoff, J.P. (1999). Adaptation during early childhood among mothers of children with disabilities. *Journal of Developmental and Behavioral Pediatrics, 20,* 9–16.

Williams, V., & Robinson, C. (2001). He will finish up caring for me: People with learning disabilities and mutual care. *British Journal of Learning Disabilities, 29,* 56–62.

Yoder, J., & DiVenere, N. (2004). Family-centered care and the family's perspective: Traumatic brain injury, cancer, and co-morbid learning challenges. In C.M. Vargas & P.A. Prelock (Eds.), *Caring for children with neurodevelopmental disabilities and their families* (pp. 35–68). Mahwah, NJ: Lawrence Erlbaum Associates.

Zetlin, A.G. (1986). Mentally retarded adults and their siblings. *American Journal of Mental Deficiency, 91,* 217–225.

24

Neuroradiology

ERROL J. CANDY,
ALEXANDER H. HOON, JR., AND DORIS D.M. LIN

Neuroimaging modalities, including computed tomography (CT) and magnetic resonance imaging (MRI), are important components in the etiological workup of children with developmental delay or neurological impairment. In children with static encephalopathies, findings can also be used to establish etiological associations and the timing of insults, as well as to determine the need for neurosurgical intervention. In those children with metabolic diseases or progressive encephalopathies, abnormalities can provide important clues as to likely diagnoses and direct further metabolic testing.

In the acute setting, CT has great utility. There is ready access to the patient during scanning in the event of patient decompensation. Diagnostically, CT is very sensitive for detection of hemorrhage or calcium, both of which are often difficult to appreciate with MRI. CT should be performed in most emergency situations, including head trauma; acute neurological deficit where hemorrhage or ischemia is suspected; and asphyxia. Other indications for CT are unstable newborns for whom bedside ultrasonography does not provide the necessary information and cases of suspected congenital infection or other conditions in which calcium might be present.

MRI, because of its unique soft tissue discrimination and clear distinction between gray and white matter, plus its ability to generate images in multiple planes, allows visualization of the brain in a way previously unavailable before autopsy. Therefore, in most commonly encountered clinical situations, MRI should be the brain imaging modality of choice in an etiological workup.

To maximize benefit to the patient and maintain cost-effectiveness, clinicians should become familiar with the uses and limitations of both MRI and CT. Radiological consultation should be obtained if there is uncertainty whether imaging is likely to be useful or if there is a need to determine the study of choice. Consultation between the clinician and radiologist is an integral part of modern-day radiology and is important for utilization of imaging resources most efficiently and maximizing benefit to the patient. Emergency imaging is not covered in this chapter; the discussion is limited primarily to those conditions more likely to be encountered by developmental pediatricians and pediatric neurologists.

SEDATION

With a few exceptions, children 6 years and younger will require sedation during MRI and CT studies. Sedation should be administered by trained personnel in the radiology department, hospital, or imaging center. The American Academy of Pediatrics recommended close monitoring with pulse oximetry, cardiorespiratory monitoring, or both for all patients undergoing conscious sedation (American Academy of Pediatrics, 1992). It is important for clinicians to coordinate plans with the radiologist when arranging scans of children who are outpatients so that the parents can be given

We thank Professor Peter Barker for supplying Figures 24.36 and 24.39 and for reading the manuscript.

instructions regarding withholding oral intake and possible sleep deprivation prior to the child's appointment.

Oral chloral hydrate (75–100 mg/kg) has been shown to be safe and effective up to a maximum dose of 2.5 g, or on average, in children from birth to 2 years of age (Greenberg, Faerber, & Aspinall, 1991). Because of maximal dosage restraints, chloral hydrate yields adequate sedation only in children up to 25 kg in weight. At times, its effect can be augmented by administration of diphenhydramine (Benadryl) once the maximal dosage has reached. Most inpatients who are sedated on the ward prior to arriving in the radiology department are given too little medication. This results in a nondiagnostic or suboptimal study in many cases (50% failure rate if < 65 mg/kg is given) because of patient motion. Improper sedation is time consuming, expensive, and stressful to the patient. In addition, such a situation can be frustrating for the radiology and nursing staff who are closely involved with the patient during imaging (Bluemke & Breiter, 2000).

Intravenous pentobarbital sodium (Nembutal) at a dosage of 2–4 mg/kg, not exceeding 150 mg total dose, has been shown to be safe and effective in experienced hands for pediatric sedation (Strain, Campbell, Harvey, & Foley, 1988) and can be used in older children (usually 2 to 6 years of age) or when intravenous access is available in younger patients older than 6 months of age.

Beyond the dose limit that can be safely delivered using Nembutal, for some older children (6–18 years) the use of anxiolytics such as Diazepam (Valium) can be effective. General anesthesia may be necessary 1) if these are not effective, 2) for those children who require airway protection, and 3) for some with underlying metabolic abnormality.

The sedation of premature or severely ill infants is performed with caution, with specific input from the neonatologist on the recommended dose and whether sedation is indeed required.

BASIC PRINCIPLES OF MAGNETIC RESONANCE IMAGING

There are two ways in which brain lesions can be identified by CT or MRI. The first, when there is a change in the brain geometry, is commonly referred to as mass effect. CT and MRI are approximately equal in their detection of mass lesions. The second method of identifying lesions is by their inherent tissue contrast. When compared with CT, MRI provides markedly greater inherent tissue contrast.

CT imaging relies on transmission of X-rays, the absorption of which is related to electron density (ED) of the tissue. High-ED tissue, such as bone, absorbs (blocks) X-rays and therefore appears bright, whereas low-ED tissue, such as cerebrospinal fluid (CSF), transmits X-rays (more transparent) and appears dark.

MRI is not a technique based on X-ray transmission. It relies on receiving radiofrequency signals emitted from protons in the body tissues. In a CT scan of the brain, the gray matter–white matter difference in tissue contrast is approximately 2%, whereas MRI can readily produce a 20% difference, depending on the scanning parameters used. Brain pathology such as demyelination, brain neoplasms, and edema has even greater tissue contrast, approaching several hundred percent.

This chapter is not intended to provide a complete discussion of the physics of MRI; only a simplified summary is given. Clinical MRI relies primarily on what are known as spin echo techniques. When a patient is placed within the extremely strong magnetic field of the MRI machine, protons in the body tissues align themselves parallel to the magnetic field. Protons in the tissue being scanned are then momentarily deflected from their alignment via a specific radiofrequency pulse sent from a transmitter coil. When the pulse is turned off, the protons begin to return to their original alignment within the magnetic field. In so doing, they emit a small radiofrequency signal of their own, which is detected by a receiver coil. A computer registers the intensity of this signal and identifies its location within the brain or body part being imaged using gradients of the magnetic field strength. This entire process is repeated multiple times to obtain the final image.

For morphological delineation, the three most frequent types of images obtained are T1-weighted spin echo, T2-weighted fast spin

Table 24.1. Tissue appearances on computed tomography (CT) and magnetic resonance imaging (MRI)

Tissue	CT	MRI			
		T1	PD	FLAIR	T2
Gray matter	Light gray	Gray	Light gray	Light gray	Gray
White matter	Dark gray	Light gray	Dark gray	Dark gray	Darker gray
CSF	Dark	Dark	Gray	Dark	Bright
Fat	Very dark	Bright	Gray[a]	Bright[a]	Bright[a]
Bone/calcium	Bright	Dark[b]	Dark	Dark	Dark
Edema	Dark	Dark	Bright	Bright	Bright
Protein	Gray	Bright	Bright	Bright	Bright
Air	Black	Black	Black	Black	Black
Acute blood	Bright	Gray	Gray	Gray	Dark
Subacute blood	Gray	Bright	Bright	Bright	Bright
Chronic blood	Dark	Variable	Gray	Dark	Dark

Key: CSF, cerebrospinal fluid; FLAIR, fluid-attenuated inversion recovery image; PD, proton density image; T1, T1-weighted image; T2, T2-weighted image (features described are for fast spin echo T2-weighted image).

[a]Fat can be dark on PD, T2, and FLAIR images if fat suppression is applied.

[b]Calcium can be bright on T1-weighted image depending on the degree of calcification.

echo, and fluid-attenuated inversion recovery (FLAIR) images. In the past, proton (spin) density images were often acquired simultaneously with T2-weighted images, and these two are referred to as a *double echo sequence*. For nearly all applications, FLAIR imaging has now replaced proton density, although proton density can be useful in neonates when myelination is incomplete. The various tissue appearances are summarized in Table 24.1, with an example of the appearance of a normal brain in Figure 24.1. More advanced magnetic resonance (MR) sequences, including diffusion-weighted imaging, perfusion imaging, MR spectroscopic imaging, and functional MRI, are now increasingly utilized to provide physiological or functional information. The use of these sequences is discussed further at the end of this chapter.

NORMAL BRAIN DEVELOPMENT

Because brain development has been discussed in detail elsewhere (see Chapter 2, this volume), only aspects pertinent to imaging are covered here.

Myelination

Myelination is a marker of maturation in the developing infant brain. Until recently, myelination could be studied only in postmortem specimens (Yakovlev & Lecours, 1967). With the advent of MRI, myelination can now be studied in vivo (Barkovich, Kjos, Jackson, & Norman, 1988), with important clinical ramifications.

With central nervous system (CNS) maturation, the white matter becomes myelinated in an orderly sequence. The overall pattern is caudal to rostral, and sensory to motor (Table 24.2). Myelination begins during the fifth week of intrauterine life and progresses rapidly until 2 years of age, although a few tracts continue to myelinate into adulthood. Although myelination progresses as a continuum, it appears to evolve in two separate stages on MRI. Initially, myelin demonstrates increased signal (bright) relative to gray matter on T1-weighted images. This is presumably the result of laying down of precursor myelin tubules, which are high in cholesterol. This correlates best with degree 1 or 2 (out of a maximum of 4) on the myelin staining techniques and has been referred to as immature myelin (or premyelin).

During the second stage, immature myelin undergoes dehydration and demonstrates decreased signal (dark) relative to gray matter on T2-weighted images. This correlates fairly closely with mature myelin (degree 3 or 4). The decreased signal is probably related to dehydration (fewer protons) and organization (proton immobility), when the myelin becomes more densely packed.

When assessing myelination with MRI, the T1-weighted images are the most useful in the first 6 postnatal months, and the T2-weighted images are the most useful there-

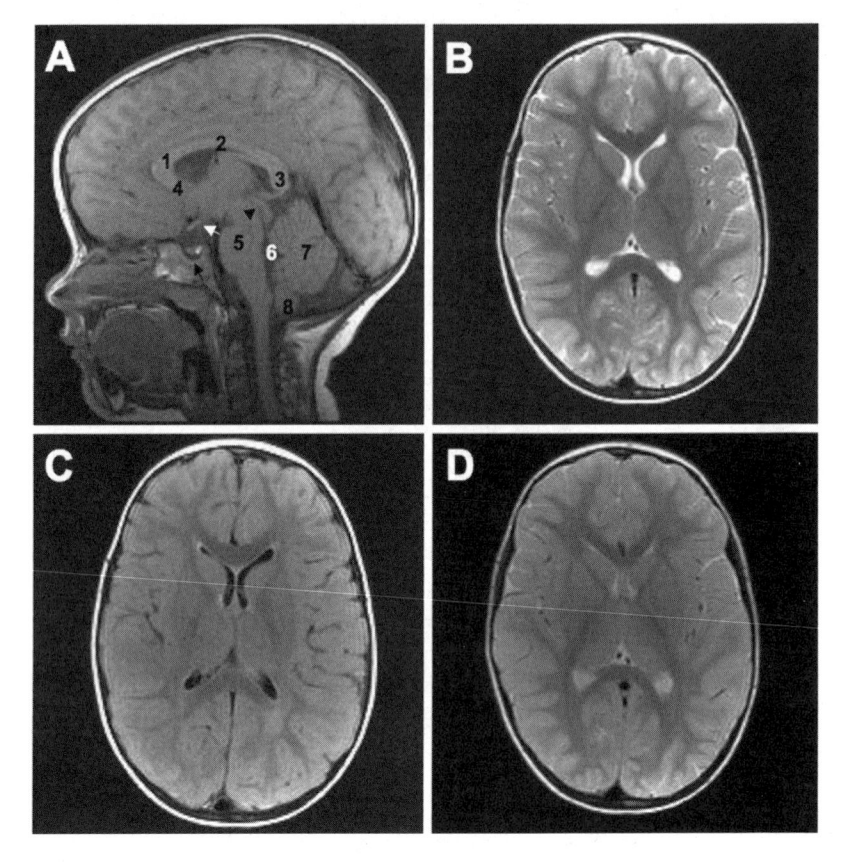

Figure 24.1. Normal 3-year-old brain. *A,* Sagittal T1-weighted image demonstrating good midline detail of the corpus callosum comprising, in order of embryological development: 1) genu, 2) body, 3) splenium, and 4) rostrum. (*Key:* White arrow, optic chiasm; black arrow, pituitary gland; arrowhead, cerebral acqueduct; 5, brainstem; 6, fourth ventricle; 7, cerebellar vermis; 8, cerebellar tonsils.) Note that cerebrospinal fluid (CSF) is black, white matter of the corpus callosum is light gray, and gray matter is darker gray. *B,* Axial T2-weighted image at the level of the foramen of Monro shows characteristic bright CSF within the lateral ventricles. The gray matter is gray, and the mature white matter is dark. *C,* Axial FLAIR image shows suppressed CSF signal, which is black. The gray matter is gray (similar to T2-weighted image) and the white matter is dark gray. *D,* Axial proton density image shows that the gray matter is gray, the white matter is dark gray, and CSF is lighter gray.

after. In a given anatomic site, if tissue with increased signal on the T1-weighted image also appears bright on the T2-weighted image, then this is immature myelin. Conversely, if those regions of increased signal on the T1-weighted image demonstrate decreased signal on the T2-weighted image, this is mature myelin (note that both immature and mature myelin are bright on T1-weighted images).

Attainment of gross cognitive and motor skills is the end result of complex neurological development. Mature myelination is a major factor in this development, but it remains uncertain whether this is the rate-limiting step. Therefore, delays in myelination should be interpreted in the context of other clinical findings.

CONGENITAL BRAIN ANOMALIES

Congenital brain anomalies are found in approximately 20% of children with cerebral palsy (Candy, Hoon, Capute, & Bryan, 1993; Schouman-Claeys et al., 1989; Truwit, Barkovich, Koch, & Ferriero, 1992). Table 24.3 shows the intrauterine timing of the brain insults.

Dysgenesis of the Corpus Callosum

At approximately 8 weeks of gestation, the corpus callosum begins to develop from the lamina reuniens in a specific order: genu, body, splenium, and then the rostrum (Jinkins, Whittemore, & Bradley, 1989). When there is dysgenesis, the rostrum is always absent, followed by the splenium, body, and so forth de-

Table 24.2. Brain myelination sequence and timing on magnetic resonance imaging

Anatomic region	Immature myelin: T1 bright (months)	Mature myelin: T2 dark (months)
Posterior fossa		
Middle cerebellar peduncle	Birth to 1	3–6
Cerebellar white matter	1–3	8–18
Supratentorial		
PLIC		
Posterior	Birth	Birth to 2
Anterior	Birth	4–7
Splenium	3–4	4–6
Genu	4–6	5–8
ALIC	2–3	7–11
Centrum semiovale	2–4	7–11
Occipital white matter		
Central	3–5	9–14
Peripheral	4–7	11–15
Frontal white matter		
Central	3–6	11–16
Peripheral	7–11	14–18

From Barkovich, A.J., Kjos, B.O., Jackson D.E., and Norman, D. (1988). Normal maturation of the neonatal and infant brain: MR imaging at 1.5T. *Radiology, 166,* 173–180; adapted by permission of Radiological Society of North America. *Key:* ALIC, anterior limb internal capsule; PLIC, posterior limb internal capsule.

pending on the severity. When the corpus callosum is secondarily destroyed, however, the rostrum is always present, making it possible to distinguish dysgenesis from destructive lesions. Partial or total absence of the corpus callosum can occur as an isolated anomaly (Figure 24.2) or, more frequently, in association with a variety of other midline anomalies, including in-

Table 24.3. Timing of congenital central nervous system anomalies

Anomaly	Age (gestational weeks)
Chiari malformations	4
Encephaloceles	4
Holoprosencephaly	5–6
Septo-optic dysplasia	6–7
Dandy-Walker malformation	7–10
Dysgenesis of corpus callosum	10–24
Schizencephaly	8
Agyria	11–13
Pachygyria	13–22
Gray matter heterotopia	18–22
Polymicrogyria	22
Primary hydranencephaly	14–28

terhemispheric cyst or lipoma (Figure 24.3), Chiari II malformation, Dandy-Walker malformation, encephaloceles, midline facial anomalies, and septo-optic dysplasia.

POSTERIOR FOSSA ABNORMALITIES

Most posterior fossa anomalies occur secondary to associated supratentorial or spinal malformations.

Chiari Malformations

In 1891, Chiari described a malformation that was characterized by herniation of the posterior fossa contents below the level of the foramen magnum. With modern imaging techniques, the Chiari malformation has been categorized into types I, II, and III.

Chiari malformations are treated with posterior fossa decompression by a number of neurosurgical techniques, all employing a suboccipital craniectomy in conjunction with an upper cervical laminectomy (Dyste, Menezes, & VanGilder, 1989). If there is an associ-

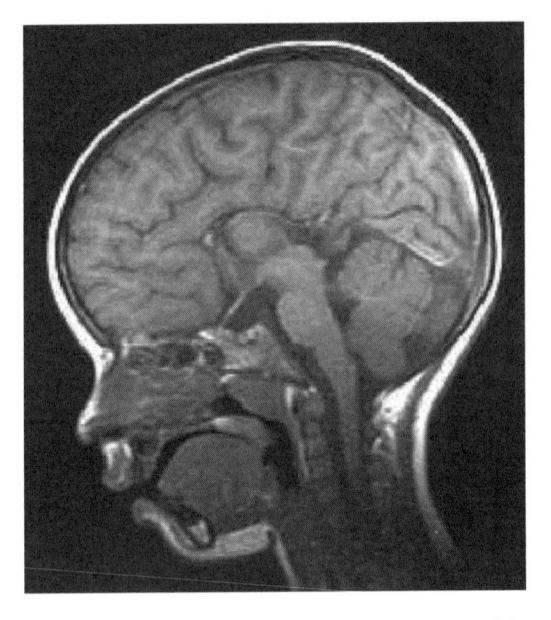

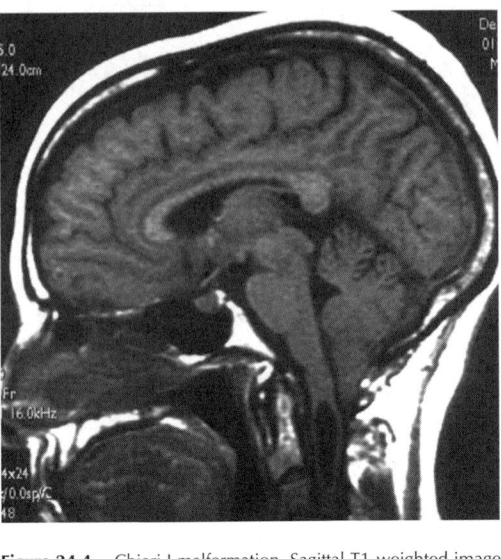

Figure 24.4. Chiari I malformation. Sagittal T1-weighted image shows inferior descent of the cerebellar tonsils below the foramen magnum to the level of the C1 arch. Note also a cystic cavity, reflecting syringohydromyelia, within the C2–3 cord.

Figure 24.2. Sagittal T1-weighted image showing agenesis of the corpus callosum.

ated cervical cord syrinx, it can sometimes be alleviated by posterior fossa decompression. If not, a syrinx is treated by drainage using a variety of methods, including syringosubarachnoid shunts, syringoperitoneal shunts, combinations of these, or a syringopleural shunt.

Chiari I Malformation   Although originally described as tonsillar ectopia through the

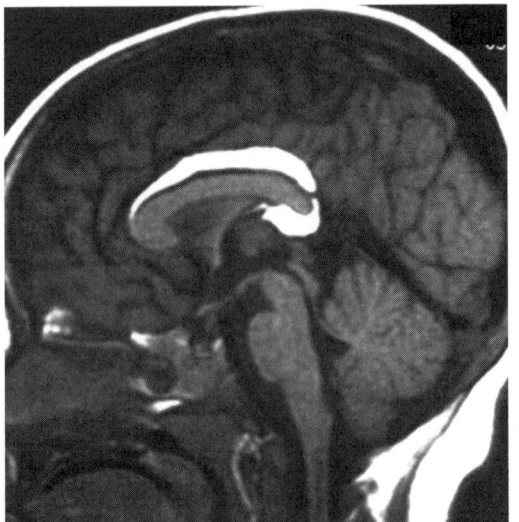

Figure 24.3. Sagittal T1-weighted image showing a callosal lipoma associated with a slightly foreshortened splenium of the corpus callosum.

foramen magnum of greater than 3 mm, this anomaly has been redefined with the advent of MRI as herniation of 5 mm or more (Figure 24.4). The herniated cerebellar tonsils are typically wedge shaped, and there may be associated craniocervical osseous anomalies such as segmentation defects (Klippel-Feil), platybasia, and basilar impression. Herniation can be caused by craniocervical anomalies, can be a sequela of intrauterine hydrocephalus, or can be idiopathic. Hydrocephalus appears in fewer than 20% of Chiari I cases, and syringohydromyelia in 20%. With Chiari I malformation, there is no meningomyelocele. Children can present with symptoms and signs related to hydrocephalus or a syrinx, if either is present. Treatment of hydrocephalus is with a standard ventriculoperitoneal shunt.

If only tonsillar ectopia is present, there may be symptoms and signs suggestive of cerebellar, bulbar, or cervical cord dysfunction; however, Chiari I malformation may be an incidental finding. Therefore, in order to avoid unnecessary surgery, attempts should be made to correlate the clinical findings with the degree of tonsillar ectopia (Barkovich, Wippold, Sherman, & Citrin, 1986); clinical findings generally increase with greater ectopia, although this topic remains somewhat controversial

(Milhorat et al., 1999). Headaches occur in about 50% of all children with Chiari I malformation. In one series, however, only half of the children with headaches had a characteristic headache pattern that was temporarily aggravated by either a sustained Valsalva maneuver, physical effort, cough, or significant body or head postural changes (Pascual, Oterino, & Berciano, 1992).

Chiari II Malformation The Chiari II malformation is a complex anomaly involving the hindbrain, spine, and mesoderm that is ideally imaged with MRI (Wolpert, Anderson, Scott, Kwan, & Runge, 1987). The key imaging finding is a small posterior fossa. Chiari II malformation consists of four consistent features (Figure 24.5): 1) deformity of the quadrigeminal (tectal) plate, 2) inferior displacement of the pons, 3) inferior displacement and elongation of the fourth ventricle, and 4) cerebellar vermis with or without tonsillar ectopia. Virtually all children with Chiari II malformation have a meningomyelocele, which, when repaired, will result in hydrocephalus requiring shunting within a few days. Apart from hydrocephalus in about 95% of Chiari II malformation cases, other abnormalities include an enlarged massa intermedia (75%–95%), corpus callosum dysgenesis (85%; see Figure 24.5A), fenestrated falx with interdigitation of the cerebral hemispheres, cervicomedullary kink (70%), and syrinx (40%–95%). Surgical management is a ventriculoperitoneal shunt for the hydrocephalus. Interestingly, the posterior fossa abnormalities are symptomatic in fewer than 20% of children (Park, Hoffman, Hendrick, & Humphreys, 1983).

In older children, symptoms usually present gradually, with upper extremity weakness and long tract signs. Posterior fossa decompression provides good results in these children (Park et al., 1983). The clinical picture is more severe in neonates, with dysfunction of the lower cranial nerves, caudal brainstem, and cerebellum that results in apneic spells, vocal cord paralysis, and frequently death. Early recognition and prompt decompression, however, usually provide good results (Vandertop et al., 1992); MRI has made a great impact on early and accurate diagnosis of Chiari II malformation in neonates. It should be stressed that any child with apneic attacks or signs of brainstem compression or both should undergo MRI under general anesthesia for complete airway control and ventilation.

Chiari III Malformation The Chiari III malformation is an extremely rare anomaly that is associated with an occipital or upper cervical cephalocele or both. It is not covered in this chapter.

POSTERIOR FOSSA CYSTIC MALFORMATIONS

There is much confusion in the current literature regarding the classification and terminology of posterior fossa cystic malformations. The terminology used in this chapter is based on contributions made by MRI, in conjunction with an understanding of neuroembryology. In the developing brain, the cerebellum is formed between 6 and 15 gestational weeks, with the vermis antedating the cerebellar hemispheres by 4–8 weeks.

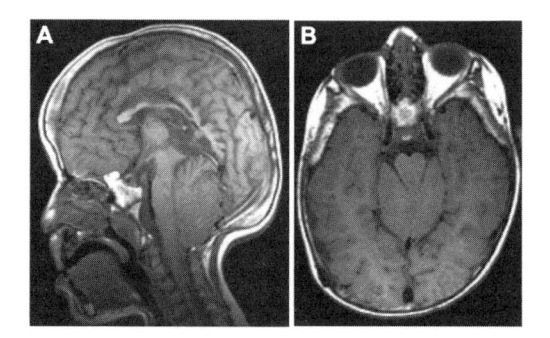

Figure 24.5. Chiari II malformation in a 4-year-old girl with myelomeningocele and hydrocephalus for which she is shunted. *A,* Sagittal T1-weighted image shows a small posterior fossa cranium, resulting in inferior displacement of the cerebellum and brainstem, crowding of the foramen magnum, tectal beaking, enlarged massa intermedia, and associated partial agenesis of the corpus callosum. Note that the corpus callosum is diffusely thinned; in addition, the splenium and rostrum are not formed. *B,* Axial T1-weighted image shows a towering cerebellum through the incisura, appearing heart-shaped and wrapping around the brainstem.

Dandy-Walker Complex

The Dandy-Walker complex is a spectrum of related anomalies ranging from the Dandy-Walker malformation (the most severe), to the less severe Dandy-Walker variant, and finally to the least severe mega cisterna magna (Altman, Nadich, & Braffman, 1992). The Dandy-Walker anomalies most likely represent a continuum of developmental anomalies (Barkovich, Kjos, Norman, & Edwards, 1989).

Dandy-Walker Malformation   Dandy-Walker malformations are caused when the roof of the fourth ventricle, which normally closes at about 8 weeks of gestation, fails to close. As a result, the membranous fourth ventricle ''balloons'' out to expand and occupy a large portion of the posterior fossa. The key imaging finding for this diagnosis is an enlarged posterior fossa. The disorder is characterized by three associated features: 1) cystic dilation of the fourth ventricle; 2) complete or partial agenesis of the cerebellar vermis; and 3) enlarged posterior fossa, including elevation of the cerebellar tentorium, the torcula, and the straight and transverse sinuses (Figure 24.6). In addition, there is usually associated hydrocephalus (> 80%), which should be considered a complication and not part of the malformation. Hydrocephalus is often not present at

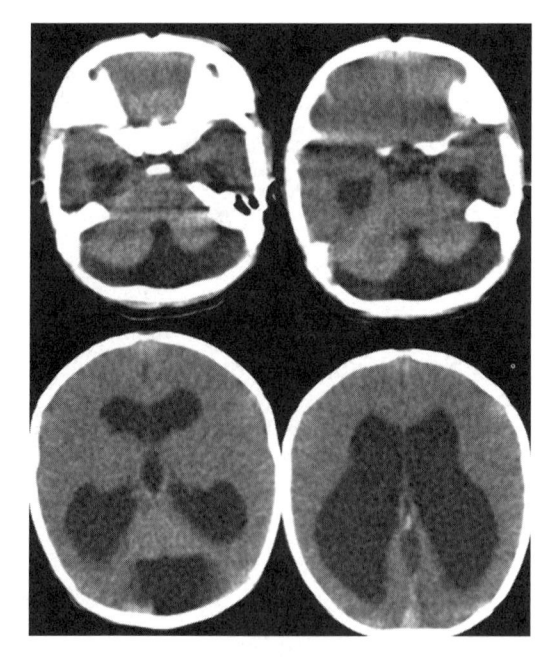

Figure 24.6.   Dandy-Walker malformation in a 4-day-old boy. Axial computed tomography shows a dorsal posterior fossa cyst communicating with the fourth ventricle, hypoplastic cerebellar vermis, and enlarged third and lateral ventricles resulting from hydrocephalus.

birth but develops by 3 months of age. Associated CNS anomalies occur in 68% of cases; many patients have brainstem dysplasias. The most common supratentorial anomalies are corpus callosum dysgenesis (20%–25%) and gray matter heterotopias (5%–10%).

Other Dandy-Walker malformations include agyria, polymicrogyria, schizencephaly, lipomas, and cephaloceles. Associated peripheral malformations occur in 20%–33% of cases and include cleft lip and palate, cardiac malformations, and urinary tract abnormalities.

Clinically, the Dandy-Walker malformation accounts for 14% of posterior fossa cystic malformations (Raybaud, 1982). It is usually a sporadic disorder with low risk of occurrence in siblings (1%–5%), unless associated with chromosomal anomalies (Murray, Johnson, & Bird, 1985). The prognosis depends primarily on the type and extent of the supratentorial abnormalities, but the severity of impairments has probably been overestimated in the past. In a study of 19 patients, 47% had normal intellect with little or no motor deficit; 26% had learning disabilities with little or no motor deficit; 11% had moderate developmental delay with little or no motor deficit; and 16% had severe delay with spastic cerebral palsy (Maria, Zinreich, Carson, Rosenbaum, & Freeman, 1987).

As with the Chiari malformations, there are also various surgical treatment approaches. Although it would seem logical to shunt only the posterior fossa cyst, this can cause downward transtentorial herniation if the cerebral aqueduct is obstructed and is only successful in a minority of patients. Similarly, ventricular shunting alone can produce upward herniation of the cerebellum and is not always successful. Most patients, therefore, require a combined cystoperitoneal-ventriculoperitoneal shunt (Bindal, Storrs, & McLone, 1990–1991).

Dandy-Walker Variant   There is some controversy about the definition of the Dandy-Walker variant, but, simply stated, it has two of the three features of a Dandy-Walker malformation: 1) cystic dilation of the fourth ventricle and 2) hypoplasia of the cerebellar vermis. The posterior fossa, however, is normal in size, with the tentorium in the normal position.

It has therefore been suggested that Dandy-Walker variant be renamed vermian-cerebellar hypoplasia (Kollias, Ball, & Prenger, 1993).

The Dandy-Walker variant accounts for 30% of posterior fossa malformations. Children can present with an enlarging head circumference or developmental delay. As with the Dandy-Walker malformation, there are associated supratentorial anomalies, which suggests a similar etiology and timing. These anomalies include dysgenesis of the corpus callosum (21%) and neuronal migration anomalies (21%), and cognitive impairment is related to them. Shunting is performed only if hydrocephalus (occurring in approximately 30% of cases) is present.

Associated Syndromes Although associated supratentorial abnormalities often occur with Dandy-Walker variant, these usually cannot be classified as defined syndromes. Nevertheless, some syndromes can be identified that are important for prognosis and genetic counseling.

Joubert Syndrome Described by Joubert, Eisenring, Robb, and Andermann in 1969, this extremely rare syndrome usually presents in infancy with hyperpnea and nystagmus but can present in older children with ataxia, psychomotor retardation, and facial asymmetry. It is inherited as an autosomal recessive trait, and the genetic loci have been mapped with identification of mutations in two genes (Louie & Gleeson, 2005). There can be either complete or partial vermian agenesis, which is well demonstrated by MRI. The fourth ventricle has a characteristic "bat wing" or "molar tooth" shape secondary to the hypoplasia of the cerebellar peduncles. The fourth ventricle balloons posteriorly to various degrees as a result of vermian dysgenesis (Figure 24.7).

Walker-Warburg Syndrome Walker-Warburg syndrome is characterized by type II lissencephaly, as well as retinal and cerebellar malformations (Dobyns, Pagon, & Armstrong, 1989). The cerebellar abnormalities include polymicrogyria of the hemispheres and inferior vermian hypoplasia, with enlargement of the fourth ventricle but without expansion of the

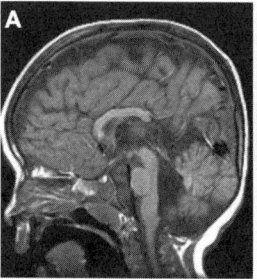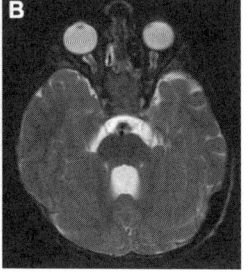

Figure 24.7. Joubert syndrome in a 3-year-old boy with oculomotor apraxia and developmental delay. Sagittal T1-weighted image (A) and axial T2-weighted image (B) demonstrate hypoplasia of the cerebellar vermis with an enlarged fourth ventricle, elongated cerebellar peduncles, and a suggestion of a molar tooth sign. In addition, the corpus callosum is hypogenetic posteriorly.

posterior fossa. Walker-Warburg syndrome is inherited as an autosomal recessive trait and has a poor prognosis, with most affected children dying early.

Other Syndromes Other syndromes that have vermian hypoplasia are Meckel-Gruber syndrome, Coffin-Siris syndrome, Ellis-van Creveld syndrome, and Fraser cryptophthalmos. Syndromes that may be associated with vermian hypoplasia, but not invariably, are dominant X-linked Aicardi syndrome and Cornelia de Lange syndrome.

Mega Cisterna Magna Mega cisterna magna is a fairly common malformation, accounting for 54% of cyst-like posterior fossa anomalies. It describes expansion of the cisterna magna, which freely communicates with the ventricles and subarachnoid spaces. In this malformation, the vermis and cerebellar hemispheres are usually normal. Mega cisterna magna is thought to be caused by cystic dilation of the tela choroidea at approximately 18 weeks of intrauterine life (Blake, 1900). This is considered a normal phase of embryological development, but in the malformation these outpouchings fail to regress. The result is a posterior fossa that appears to have an enlarged subarachnoid (CSF) space along the inferior aspect of the cerebellar vermis. Cysts can be large, extending beyond the normal limits of the cisterna magna and supratentorially through a posterior dehiscence of the tentorium. The falx cerebelli is seen in about 60% of cases. Occa-

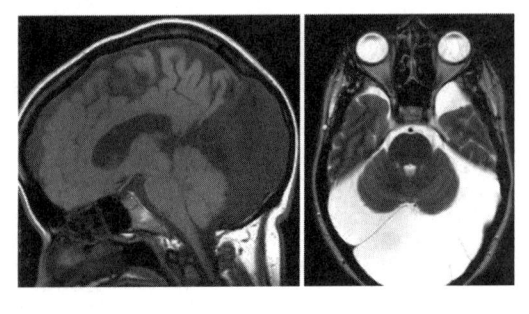

Figure 24.8. Large posterior fossa and small left middle cranial fossa arachnoid cysts. Note smooth erosion and scalloping of the inner table of the occipital skull and apparent mass effect on the cerebellum, which is displaced anteriorly, characteristic of arachnoid cysts.

sionally, mild compression of the vermis is present, but differentiation from Dandy-Walker variant is made by identifying all nine vermian lobules and noting no brainstem hypoplasia with mega cisterna magna. This anomaly is usually asymptomatic and, if so, should be considered an incidental finding.

Posterior Fossa Arachnoid Cyst

As with supratentorial arachnoid cysts, a posterior fossa arachnoid cyst arises from a developmental split in the arachnoid membrane. If it occurs in the midline, it can often be difficult, if not impossible, to distinguish from mega cisterna magna (Figure 24.8). Arachnoid cysts are unilocular, however, and often cause scalloping of the inner table of the skull. Unlike the mega cisterna magna, they do not communicate freely with the subarachnoid space and can be demonstrated by cisternography and, more recently, with CSF flow studies using MRI.

Occasionally arachnoid cysts are large and produce significant mass effect, but they are usually found incidentally when the child undergoes imaging for other reasons. Arachnoid cysts are seldom symptomatic. If hydrocephalus or posterior fossa symptoms are absent, it is reasonable to group the midline cysts with mega cisterna magna. To alleviate parental anxiety, arachnoid cysts should be referred to as incidental findings.

HOLOPROSENCEPHALY

Holoprosencephaly results from failure of cleavage of the prosencephalon (forebrain)

into two cerebral hemispheres and differentiation of the telencephalon from the diencephalon during early embryonic development, at about the fifth week of gestation (Simon & Barkovich, 2001). The etiology for this complex brain malformation is diverse, including environmental, metabolic, toxic, and infectious factors, as well as several chromosomal abnormalities (Dubourg et al., 2004). There are a number of associated midline facial deformities, commonly including dysmorphic features and hypotelorism, midline cleft, and, in the extreme case, a single fused eye at midline (cyclopia) and proboscis. Holoprosencephalies present as a spectrum of anomalies, classified by De Meyer (1971) into alobar, semilobar, and lobar types, ranging from the most severe form to the mildest. Depending on the severity of involvement, clinical manifestations range from stillborn and very short-lived infants affected by alobar holoprosencephaly, to children with variable degrees of seizures, developmental delay, intellectual disabilities, and endocrine and visual abnormalities (Hahn & Plawner, 2004).

Alobar Holoprosencephaly

In the alobar type, which has severe malformations, the brain is undivided (Hahn & Pinter, 2002). The interhemispheric fissure and cerebral falx are absent and there is a monoventricle, fusion of the thalami, and lack of formation of the third ventricle and corpus callosum, as well as absent olfactory bulbs, olfactory tracts, and optic tracts (Figure 24.9). There is frequently a large dorsal cyst contiguous with the monoventricle.

Semilobar Holoprosencephaly

In the semilobar type, there is partial division of the brain and moderate deformity of structures; the posterior portion of the brain is segmented into two hemispheres but not the frontal portion (Figure 24.10). The splenium of the corpus callosum is formed, but the anterior portion of the corpus callosum is absent. A variant type described by Barkovich, called holoprosencephaly with middle interhemispheric fusion or syntelencephaly, was considered a

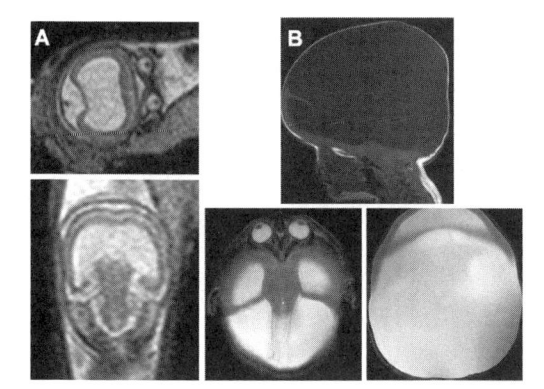

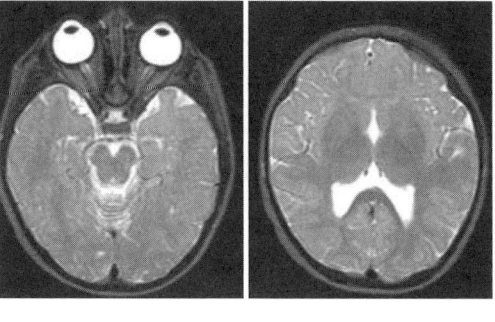

Figure 24.9. Alobar holoprosencephaly. *A,* Fetal magnetic resonance imaging shows a dilated monoventricle, thin cortical mantle, and hypotelorism. *B,* Sagittal T1-weighted and axial T2-weighted images of a stillborn show a single ventricle and markedly large dorsal cyst, compressed and thinned cortical mantle, and close-set eyes.

Figure 24.11. Lobar holoprosencephaly in a 19-month-old girl with microcephaly and diabetes insipidus. The posterior cerebral hemispheres are well formed but the anterior interhemispheric fissure is hypoplastic. There remains partial fusion of the superior frontal gyri, the cingulate gyri, and the anterior portion of the caudate nuclei. The septum pellucidum is absent.

form of semilobar holoprosencephaly (Barkovich & Quint, 1993). In this variant, the middle portion of the brain, including the posterior frontal and parietal regions, is fused while the interhemispheric fissures are normally formed anteriorly and posteriorly.

Lobar Holoprosencephaly

In the lobar type, the deformity is mild; although the septum pellucidum is absent and there is partial fusion of some structures, the interhemispheric fissure is well formed (Figure

24.11). Septo-optic dysplasia (Figure 24.12) may represent the mildest form of holoprosencephaly spectrum or an overlapping syndrome and is characterized by absence or hypoplasia of the septum pellucidum and hypoplasia of the optic nerves, with frequently associated pituitary dysfunction.

NEURONAL MIGRATION ANOMALIES

Insults to the fetal brain, whether genetic, infectious, ischemic, metabolic, or toxic, can result in arrest of cortical development or damage to the developing cortex. An understanding of the embryology of the cortex is required for discussion of the pathology and imaging of these anomalies (Gressens, 2006).

At 12–24 weeks of intrauterine life, neurons migrate from the germinal matrix along glioependymal processes through the cerebral hemispheres to the pial surface. This migration proceeds in consecutive "waves," thereby forming the six cortical layers. Cortical organization, occurring between 22 weeks' gestation

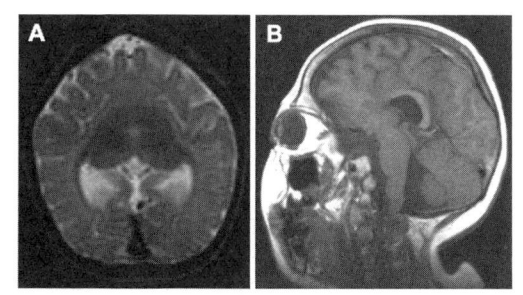

Figure 24.10. Semilobar holoproscencephaly. *A,* Axial T2-weighted image in an infant with seizures shows developed posterior interhemispheric fissure and division of cerebral hemispheres posteriorly. The lateral ventricles, however, are only partially divided, and the anterior cerebrum, thalami, and basal ganglia are fused at midline and poorly differentiated. *B,* Sagittal T1-weighted image of a 7-year-old girl with seizures and marked developmental delay. In holoprosencephaly, the posterior portion of the corpus callosum is formed but the anterior portion is not because there is incomplete ventral induction and cleavage of anterior cerebral structures.

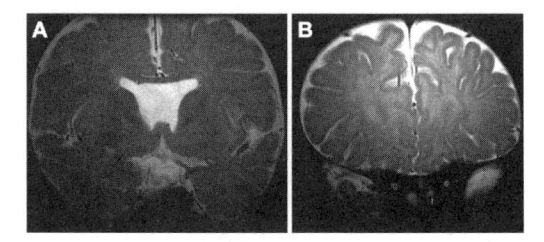

Figure 24.12. Septo-optic dysplasia, or de Morsier syndrome. Coronal T2-weighted images show absent septum pellucidum (*A*) and hypoplastic, pinpoint optic nerves (*B*).

and 2 years of age, depends on normal neuronal migration. Any insult that inhibits this chemotaxis of neurons can cause a migration anomaly.

The timing of such an event is thought to determine the type of anomaly that occurs (Smith & Blaser, 1989). These anomalies include schizencephaly, lissencephaly (agyria and pachygyria), polymicrogyria, gray matter heterotopias, and unilateral hemimegalencephaly. Because of its exquisite gray matter–white matter differentiation, MRI is ideally suited to the study of these migration anomalies.

Schizencephaly

Schizencephaly is thought to develop at approximately 8 weeks of intrauterine life because of injury to the migrating neurons in the region of the germinal matrix. The result is a full-thickness cleft (schism) in the cerebral hemisphere connecting the ventricular ependymal lining and the outer pial membrane. Neurons are detoured from their normal migrational route and settle along the edges of the cleft, thereby producing a gray matter lining. The appearance of this lining distinguishes schizencephaly from infarction, in which there is destruction of brain parenchyma and no gray matter lining. Clefts can be unilateral or bilateral and are usually in the peri-sylvian regions. They can be closed (little or no CSF seen extending along the cleft) or open (CSF easily seen). Schizencephaly is often bilateral or occurs in association with contralateral cortical dysplasia (focal heterotopia).

In general, presenting symptoms depend on the severity of the lesion (Granata et al., 2005). Patients with closed-lipped, unilateral schizencephaly (Figure 24.13A) usually have seizures and mild hemiparesis or visual disturbances. Progressively larger clefts and bilateral clefts present with more severe motor and cognitive impairments as more brain parenchyma is involved, the most severe being bilateral open-lipped schizencephaly (Figure 24.13B).

Lissencephaly (Agyria/Pachygyria)

Lissencephaly (smooth brain) is sometimes used as a synonym for agyria and at other times

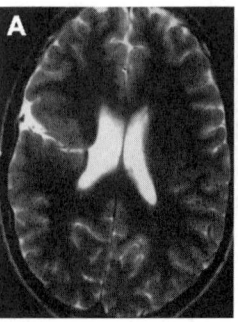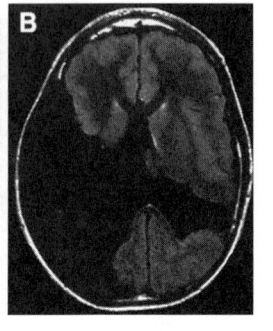

Figure 24.13. Schizencephaly. *A,* Axial T2-weighted image shows closed-lipped schizencephaly in a child with seizures, developmental delay, and visual impairment. Note that gray matter lines the cerebrospinal fluid cleft extending to the right lateral ventricle, associated with mild tenting of the ventricular margin. *B,* Axial FLAIR image in a different child shows bilateral open-lipped schizencephaly, larger on the right side.

as a more general term meaning the agyria/pachygyria complex (Kato & Dobyns, 2003). The latter term is gaining acceptance and is used in this discussion. Agyria/pachygyria represents a continuum from mild to severe and is a condition in which children have microcephaly, severe retardation, and seizures at an early age.

Agyria The most severe manifestation of the agyria/pachygyria spectrum, agyria is thought to result from an arrest of neuronal migration at 11–13 weeks' gestation. The initial layer of cortical neurons is theorized to be abnormal, thereby preventing the second and subsequent neuronal layers from migrating to their more superficial locations. This abnormal cortical layering alters the process of gyration, resulting in the smooth, thickened cortical mantle of agyria. There is "waisting" in the region where the sylvian fissures should be, thereby giving the brain a "figure-of-8" appearance (Figure 24.14). The brainstem is often hypoplastic because many of the corticospinal and corticobulbar tracts are absent.

Agyria has also been described as complete lissencephaly. If patients have the typical associated facial and somatic dysmorphism, they are classified as having Miller-Dieker syndrome, with an associated deletion on chromosome 17 in the majority of cases (Dobyns, Strutton, & Greenberg, 1984). If there are no typical dysmorphisms, the agyria is called isolated lissencephaly sequence.

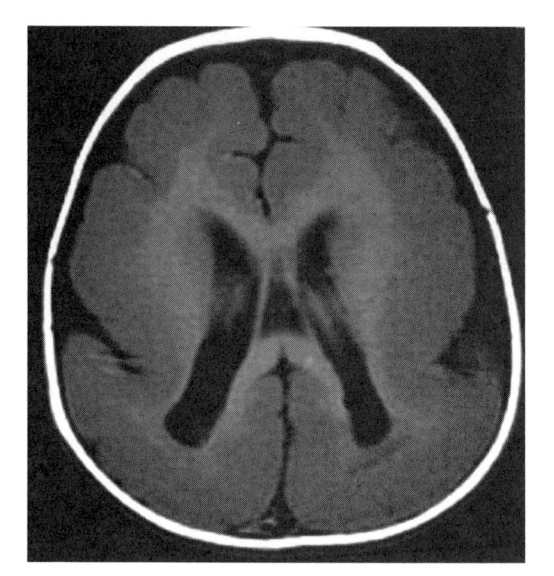

Figure 24.14. Lissencephaly, or agyria, in a 1-year-old boy presenting with developmental delay and hypotonia. Axial T1-weighted image shows diffusely thick and smooth cortex with lack of normal gyration and somewhat diminished white matter.

Pachygyria Also called incomplete lissencephaly, pachygyria appears on imaging as a thickened cortex, shallow sulci, broad flat gyri, and poor arborization of the thinned white matter (Figure 24.15). Pachygyria is presumed to result from a disturbance of neocortex formation after the 13th gestational week but before completion of neuronal migration. It often involves both cerebral hemispheres but can be more focal. Children with pachygyria tend to have less severe clinical presentations than do children with agyria (de Rijk-van Andel, Arts, Barth, & Loonen, 1990), although most are markedly affected.

Polymicrogyria

Polymicrogyria occurs from 22 weeks' gestational age up to 2 years after birth. The term describes a region of thickened cortex with an increased number of small sulci and gyri, grossly having the dimpled appearance of the surface of a basketball (Figure 24.16). The cortex consists of only four layers but is more organized than in agyria/pachygyria. The thickness of underlying white matter is usually normal, but on MRI it can demonstrate increased T2 signal (gliosis), probably resulting from the same insult causing the polymicrogyria (Barkovich, Chuang, & Norman, 1988). Polymicrogyria can also be associated with abnormally draining veins and should not be mistaken for an arteriovenous malformation. Recognition of the neuronal migration anomaly should prevent an unnecessary arteriogram.

Even using MRI, it can be extremely difficult to make a diagnosis of polymicrogyria. Generally, polymicrogyria is best recognized on high-spatial-resolution three-dimensional T1-weighted MRI sequences. Because this condition often occurs in association with the more easily recognized pachygyria and heterotopias, in many cases making a definitive diagnosis may not be essential.

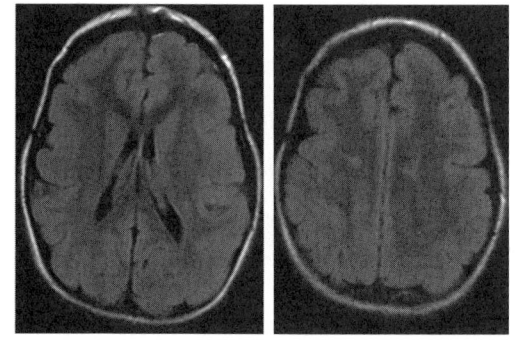

Figure 24.15. Diffuse pachygyria/polymicrogyria in a 6-year-old girl with microcephaly, craniosynostosis, and headaches. Axial FLAIR images show thickened cortex and shallow sulci, most notable in the frontal lobes bilaterally. Note also that, at the level of the centrum semiovale, bilateral linear FLAIR hyperintensity foci likely represent gliosis or migration lines.

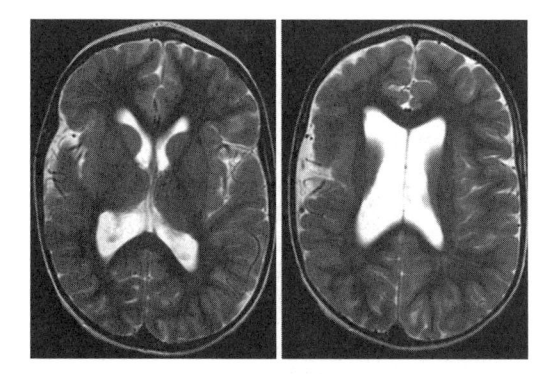

Figure 24.16. Imaging study of a 3-year-old girl with DiGeorge syndrome and right-sided polymicrogyria. Axial T2-weighted images show multiple shallow and small sulci with an undulated appearance of the cortex in the right frontoparietal, perisylvian, and temporal regions.

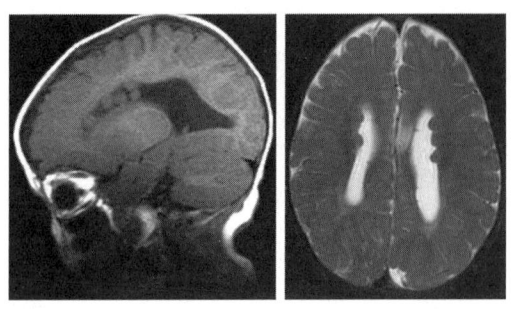

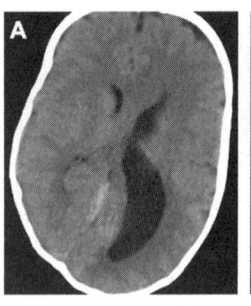
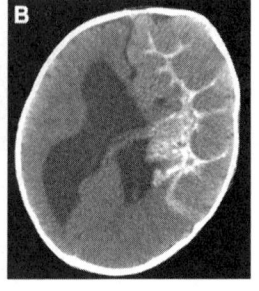

Figure 24.17. Periventricular nodular heterotopia in a child with developmental delay and seizures. Sagittal T1-weighted image and axial T2-weighted image show multiple nodules that are isointense to the gray matter along the ependymal surface of the lateral ventricles.

Figure 24.18. *A,* Hemimegalencephaly in a 2-year-old boy with macrocephaly and seizures. Axial computed tomography of the head shows asymmetrically larger left cerebral hemisphere and ipsilateral ventriculomegaly, characteristic of left hemimegalencephaly. *B,* Another patient with left-sided hemimegalencephaly showing herniation of the left cerebrum toward the right side, resulting in obstructive hydrocephalus. There is also extensive dystrophic calcification of the white matter in the left cerebral hemisphere likely related to in utero insult.

Gray Matter Heterotopias

Theoretically resulting from an insult late in the neuronal proliferation stage, gray matter heterotopias consist of collections of neurons in abnormal locations from the subependymal zone to the cortex (Figure 24.17). Heterotopias can be isolated or associated with other CNS anomalies such as Chiari II malformation or polymicrogyria. When patients present with seizures, surgical excision of the offending lesion frequently stops the seizures (Andermann, 2000).

Hemimegalencephaly

In hemimegalencephaly, a rare malformation, there is unilateral hypertrophy of the brain (Barkovich & Chuang, 1990, Tinkle, Schorry, Franz, Crone, & Saal, 2005). The affected hemisphere has a pachygyric cortex without cell layering, and frequently gliosis of the white matter (Figure 24.18). The imaging key to the diagnosis is enlargement of the lateral ventricle on the affected side on MRI or CT with less compression than typically is associated with a neoplasm.

Primary Hydranencephaly

Primary hydranencephaly, a severe CNS malformation, involves destruction of the cerebral hemispheres and is presumed to be caused by second-trimester infarction of the internal carotid artery territories; by infections such as cytomegalovirus (CMV), toxoplasmosis, or herpes; or by both (Raybaud, 1983). Morphologically, the cerebral hemispheres are replaced

by a thin membranous sac filled with CSF and necrotic debris, and the falx is present. The membrane of the sac is translucent, with its outer layer representing the relatively intact leptomeninges and its inner layer formed from remnants of nervous tissue with no ependyma. Some of the brain mantle may be preserved, usually the inferior frontal lobes and the inferior and medial aspects of the temporal plus occipital lobes. The basal ganglia, or at least the thalami, are typically preserved but atrophic. The brainstem is atrophic, and the cerebellum is usually normal (Figure 24.19A).

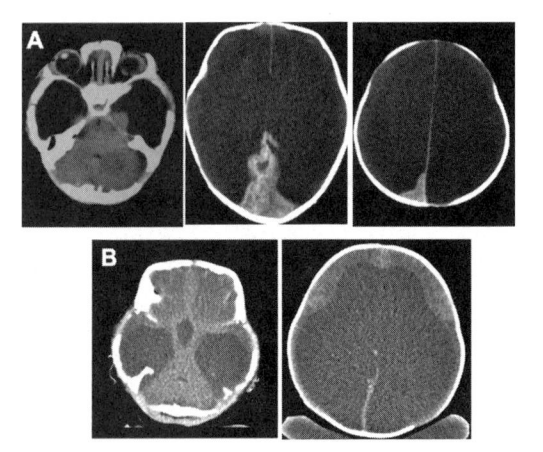

Figure 24.19. Hydranencephaly in a newborn. *A,* Axial computed tomography of the head shows complete destruction of the cerebrum with sparing of the posterior fossa and a small nubbin of residual mesial temporal tissues. Note that the superior falx is completely formed, the ventricular system cannot be distinguished, and no cortical mantle can be discerned. This pattern can be contrasted with that of massive congenital hydrocephalus resulting from aqueductal stenosis (*B*), in which there is marked enlargement of the lateral ventricles but a thinned cortical mantle can be identified.

Because primary hydranencephaly can be confused with treatable hydrocephalus, imaging is performed in these cases in an attempt to differentiate the two conditions (Mori, 2000). MRI is the study of choice, because differentiation of hydranencephaly from hydrocephalus may be difficult using CT. Even in severe hydrocephalus (Figure 24.19B) there is some cerebral mantle, including gray and white matter and ependyma. The most important feature is that these children have enlarged heads, whereas patients with hydranencephaly are normocephalic or microcephalic.

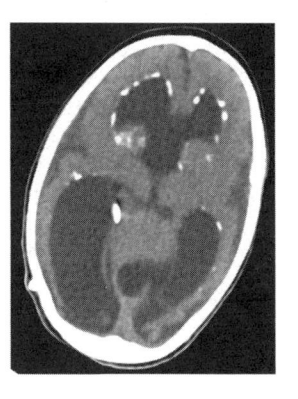

Figure 24.20.   Axial head computed tomography shows periventricular calcification and lissencephaly (diffuse pachygyria) resulting from in utero cytomegalovirus infection.

CONGENITAL INFECTIONS

The congenital infections of toxoplasmosis, syphilis, rubella, CMV, and herpes simplex have been grouped together as the TORCH infections (Stamos & Rowley, 1994; see Chapter 10, this volume). Recently, human immunodeficiency virus has become more common in the pediatric population. Congenital infection occurs in utero via direct transmission across the placenta (fortunately in a minority of maternal infections) or, less commonly, through the cervix. Perinatal exposure occurs during vaginal delivery. In general, the sequelae of intrauterine infection reflect the agent involved and the stage of fetal development when exposure occurred (Mendelson, Aboudy, Smetana, Tepperberg, & Grossman, 2006).

Cytomegalovirus

Cytomegalovirus is a DNA virus of the herpesvirus group and is the most common congenital infection (Ross & Boppana, 2005). It has been reported in 1% of neonates, 5% of whom are symptomatic. The more severe manifestations occur when the fetus is infected during the primary episode of maternal infection, the prevalence being 40%. Conversely, asymptomatic infection is more common if maternal viremia is due to reactivation of latent infection or if neonatal exposure occurs during delivery.

Clinical manifestations of congenital CMV infections include seizures, intellectual disabilities, chorioretinitis, cataracts, optic atrophy, sensorineural hearing loss, and hydrocephalus. In the brain, the virus has an affinity for the rapidly growing cells of the germinal matrix, thereby causing periventricular calcifications and neuronal migration anomalies (Bignami & Appicciutolo, 1964). Other imaging findings include cerebellar hypoplasia, cerebral atrophy, encephalomalacia, hydrocephalus, and delayed myelination (Bale, 1984; Haginoya et al., 2002). Whereas CT is the best modality to identify the periventricular calcifications (Figure 24.20), parenchymal disease is better evaluated using MRI (Holland et al., 1985).

Toxoplasmosis

Toxoplasma gondii, an obligate intracellular parasite, causes congenital infection through transplacental transmission. Pregnant women usually acquire the infection by ingestion of oocysts in poorly cooked meat. Toxoplasmosis affects 1% of all pregnancies, with the fetus being affected in 50%. CNS findings include chorioretinitis (leading to visual impairment in many cases), abnormal CSF, hydrocephalus, seizures, and intellectual disabilities (Eichenwald, 1956).

Findings on brain imaging are similar to and often indistinguishable from those with CMV. Calcifications are common in the periventricular regions (although usually less than in CMV), basal ganglia, and cortex. Encephalomalacia and hydrocephalus can also be seen in more severe cases. Unlike CMV, however, neuronal migration anomalies are not a feature of toxoplasmosis.

If infection occurs before 20 weeks' gestation, the clinical and imaging findings tend to be severe. With infection between 20 and 30 weeks, the picture is more variable, and after 30 weeks there are usually mild clinical manifestations with small periventricular and intracerebral calcifications seen on CT (Diebler, Dusser, & Dulac, 1985).

Herpes Simplex

Herpes simplex virus types 1 and 2 belong to the herpesvirus group. Type 2 accounts for nearly all of congenital herpes infections and 80%–90% of neonatal infections. Although infection is relatively rare, the sequelae are usually severe (Hutto, Arvin, & Jacobs, 1987). Intrapartum transmission is the usual mode of spread, rather than transplacental, and approximately 50% of cases have CNS involvement. All cells of the brain can be affected, but there is a predilection for endothelial cells, resulting in vascular thrombosis and hemorrhage.

Imaging features seen in the chronic stage of herpes simplex are a more accurate indicator of prognosis. These include encephalomalacia (Figure 24.21) plus dystrophic calcification involving the basal ganglia and, in a gyriform pattern, the cortex, thought to result from cortical laminar necrosis (Noorbehesht, Enzmann, Sullinder, Bradley, & Arvin, 1987).

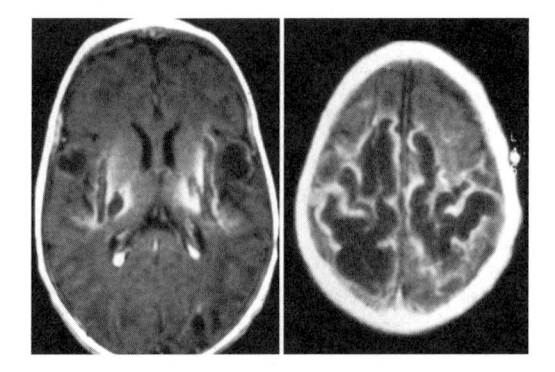

Figure 24.21. Sequelae of herpes simplex virus type 2 (HSV-2) infection in a child. Axial FLAIR images show tissue destruction with encephalomalacia involving the bilateral basal ganglia and frontoparietal cortices, which show cystic change and gliosis.

ISCHEMIC BRAIN INSULTS

The timing of ischemic brain injuries can be divided into two broad categories: those associated with prematurity and perinatal ischemic insults.

Prematurity-Related Ischemic Injury

Brain injury in the premature infant requires special mention (Volpe, 2005). More than 40,000 children are born each year in the United States with a birth weight of 1,500 g or less. Approximately 85% of these infants survive, of whom 5%–15% exhibit major spastic motor deficits ranging from spastic diplegia to quadriplegia. Some also have intellectual disabilities. Twenty-five percent to 50% of patients may have less prominent developmental disabilities, or primarily school failure (Volpe, 1989).

With the increase in survival rates of very low birth weight babies in recent years, the prevalence of cerebral palsy in this group is increasing, and prevention of brain injury has become an important focus of research and clinical care (Kuban & Leviton, 1994).

Periventricular Leukomalacia Most premature children with spastic diplegia have periventricular leukomalacia (PVL) (Truwit et al., 1992; Volpe, 2003). PVL is thought to be caused by an ischemic insult to the periventricular white matter and results in focal necrosis of the white matter dorsal and lateral to the external angles of the lateral ventricles (Banker & Larroche, 1962). The two most common sites are adjacent to the atria of the lateral ventricles and adjacent to the frontal horns, although studies also often report diffuse involvement of periventricular white matter (Counsell et al., 2003).

Pathogenesis may be related to a combination of factors including vulnerability of oligodendroglia precursor cells, neurocytotoxic activation of reactive oxygen free radical and nitrogen species by infectious agents or ischemia, and the presence of regional vascular border zones (Billiards et al., 2006; Volpe, 2003). Ischemic injury in the premature infant tends to occur in different regions when compared with term infants because the watershed areas change in location between 24 weeks and term. Nearly all of the blood supply to the cerebral white matter in the premature infant comes from vessels coursing inward from the surface of the brain, thereby producing watershed areas at the furthest points adjacent to the lateral ventricles (Takashima & Tanaka, 1978). As gestation progresses through the third trimester, vessels begin to course into the cerebral hemispheres from the lateral ventricles, moving the watershed area from the periventricular region to the brain surface (Figure 24.22). Research suggests that oligodendroglia may be vulnerable to injury on the basis of excess glutamate. This glutamate causes cell death by disrupting a cystine pump, leading to glutathione depletion and loss of free radical scavengers (Oka, Belliveau, Rosenberg, & Volpe, 1993).

The major long-term clinical correlates of PVL are spastic diplegia and, to a lesser extent, intellectual deficits. In spastic diplegia, the lower extremities are affected more than the upper extremities because PVL is located in the region of cerebral white matter more likely to

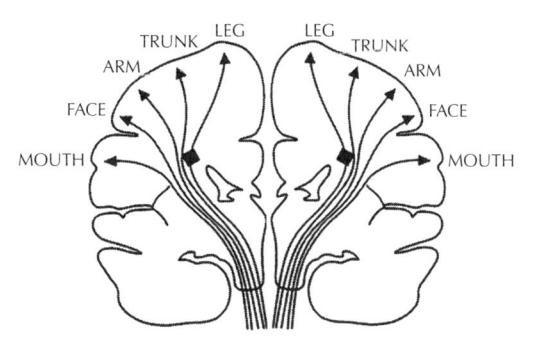

Figure 24.23. Diagram of the corticospinal tracts from their origin in the motor cortex, with descent through the periventricular region into the internal capsule. Loci of periventricular leukomalacia (black squares) are expected to affect descending fibers for the lower extremities more so than more laterally placed fibers for the upper extremities and face. (From Volpe, J.J. [1989]. Current concepts of brain injury in the premature infant. *AJR: American Journal of Roentgenology, 153,* 245. Reprinted with permission from the American Journal of Roentgenology).

injure the motor tracts innervating the legs than those of the arms (Figure 24.23). Research reports suggest that sensory pathway injury may be an important component of motor phenotypes (Fan, Yu, Quan, Sun, & Guo, 2006; Hoon et al., 2002).

In the neonatal period, cranial sonography is the imaging study of choice because the instrument is portable, and it provides relatively good resolution with lack of ionizing radiation at lower cost than CT or MRI. Nevertheless, only 28% of PVL is identified with sonography. In older children, MRI has become the study of choice in recent years (Baker, Stevenson, & Enzmann, 1988). There is a characteristic triad of findings with MRI: 1) abnormally increased proton density and T2 signal in the periventricular white matter, 2) loss of volume of periventricular white matter, and 3) compensatory enlargement of the lateral ventricles, greatest in the atria, often with angulation and irregularity (Figure 24.24) (Skranes et al., 2005). A spectrum of MRI findings in children with PVL correlates well with gestational age. Those infants born at less than 30 weeks demonstrate loss of periventricular white matter with little or no abnormal signal because the immature brain cannot mount a gliotic (scar) response. In those infants born between 30 and 33 weeks' gestational age, there is some loss of periventricular white matter that is associated with abnormal signal (gliosis) in this region. In infants

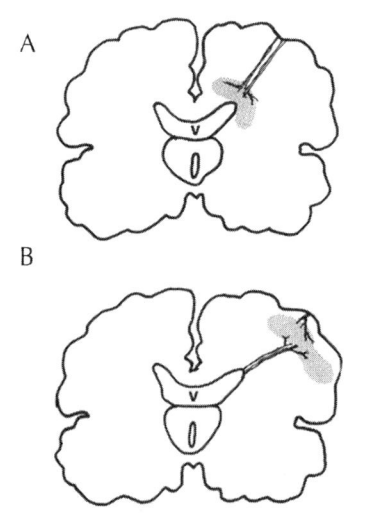

Figure 24.22. Diagram showing the change in blood supply to the cerebral hemispheres during the third trimester. *A,* The immature pattern, in which the periventricular white matter is supplied by penetrating arteries that extend from the surface of the brain. The periventricular region (shaded), therefore, is the watershed zone. (*Key:* V, lateral ventricles.) *B,* The mature pattern after 36 gestational weeks, wherein the vessels extend from the lateral ventricles, thereby moving the watershed zone to the cortical and subcortical areas (shaded).

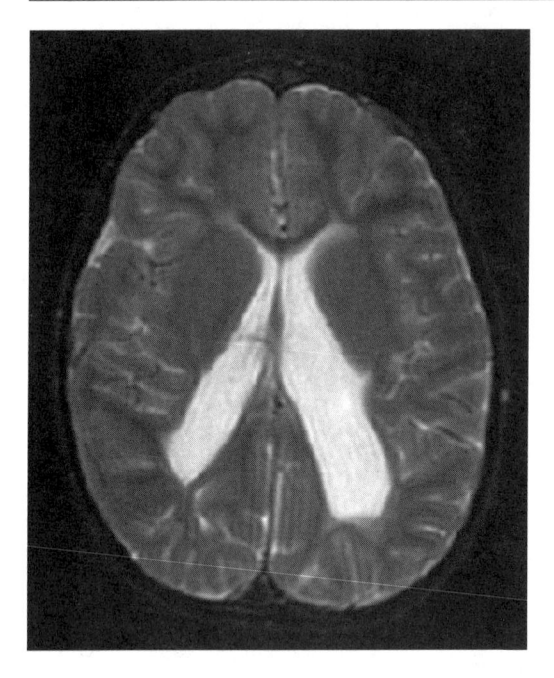

Figure 24.24. Periventricular leukomalacia (PVL) in a 4-year-old with seizure. Axial T2-weighted image shows dilated lateral ventricle predominantly in the mid- to posterior bodies and atria, with the ventricular margins having a faceted appearance. There is also paucity of adjacent white matter.

born after 33 weeks, there is usually minimal white matter volume loss and primarily abnormal signal. This should not be confused with the mildly increased signal in this region seen in children without periventricular abnormalities.

Periventricular-Intraventricular Hemorrhage Premature infants also suffer from periventricular-intraventricular hemorrhages, which are graded I to IV. Such hemorrhage is best visualized in the neonatal period with cranial ultrasound, on which the blood appears as a region of increased echogenicity. Grade I hemorrhage involves only the germinal matrix, grade II extends into the lateral ventricles, and grade III extends into the ventricles but also causes dilation of the ventricles. Initially, grade IV hemorrhage was described as extension of the hemorrhage from the lateral ventricles into the brain parenchyma, but it is now believed that the abnormality is caused by hemorrhagic venous infarction in the periatrial white matter. This occurs in 15% of infants with intraventricular hemorrhage. These areas of infarction evolve into encephalomalacia.

Isolated grade I hemorrhage is usually of little clinical significance, whereas the risk of developmental impairments increases from grade II to grade IV hemorrhage.

Perinatal Brain Injury

Perinatal brain injury in the term infant encompasses a variety of imaging findings (Rorke & Zimmerman, 1992), most often resulting from hypoxic-ischemic injury mediated by glutamate toxicity (Lipton & Epstein, 1994). All are well demonstrated by MRI imaging. Recognizable patterns include the following:

1. Global necrosis (multicystic encephalomalacia), which may cause microcephaly, cystic necrosis of brain tissue, and sclerosis (Figure 24.25)

2. Border zone infarction, which is limited to border zone regions between arterial distributions (Figure 24.26)

3. Hippocampal sclerosis; the subiculum and cornu ammonis field 1 of the hippocampus are particularly vulnerable to ischemia.

4. Involvement of the basal ganglia and thalamus (Figure 24.27). The deep gray nuclei have increased metabolic activity during the newborn period and, therefore, are particularly susceptible to injury, including perinatal insults of asphyxia and kernicterus, accounting for clinically recognizable extrapyramidal syndromes (Hoon, Belsito, & Nagae-Poetscher, 2003). Infants

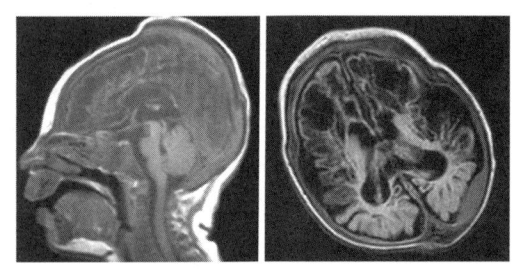

Figure 24.25. Sequelae of diffuse hypoxic/anoxic injury in a full-term baby boy who suffered from meconium aspiration with an episode of hypoxia resulting from respiratory decompensation. Sagittal T1-weighted image (left) and axial FLAIR image (right) show cystic encephalomalacia throughout the cerebral hemispheres, with some relative sparing of the occipital regions. A chronic subdural hematoma is present in the left parieto-occipital convexity.

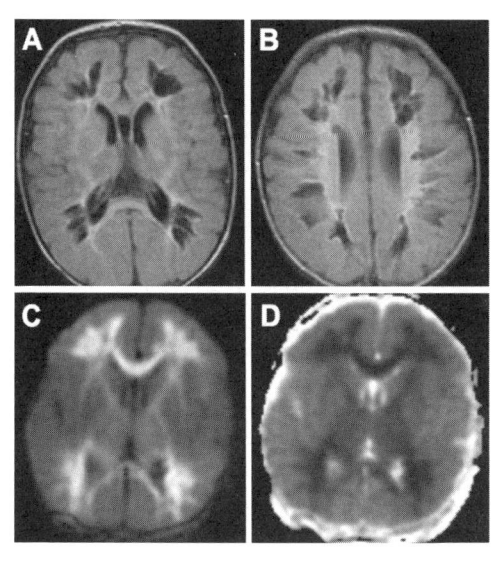

Figure 24.26. Watershed infarct in a 1-month-old infant. Axial FLAIR images show cystic encephalomalacic change in the white matter bordering the anterior-middle and middle-posterior cerebral artery territories (A) and in the corona radiata in a parasagittal distribution characteristic of border zone infarction (B). These areas can be most sensitively depicted by diffusion-weighted images in the acute setting (3 weeks before A and B) as seen in C, which shows hyperintensity in the border zone, including the corpus callosum, corresponding to dark signal on the apparent diffusion coefficient (ADC) maps in D.

nosis with advanced imaging modalities such as diffusion-weighted images and MR spectroscopy would potentially be useful in identifying those asphyxiated infants who might benefit from neuroprotective interventions to prevent later motor impairment. Currently, the American Academy of Neurology recommends early CT to exclude hemorrhage and conventional MRI later in the first week of life to determine location and extent of injury, and to establish prognosis (Ment et al., 2002). Kernicterus can cause a newborn encephalopathy similar to hypoxic-ischemic encephalopathy (HIE) with manifestation of seizures, coma, and decreased central respiratory drive, as well as choreoathetoid cerebral palsy later on in childhood. MRI shows selective involvement of the globus pallidus in kernicterus, in contradistinction to the putamen-thalamus in HIE (Yilmaz et al., 2001).

5. Vascular distribution that can involve the cortex of the motor-sensory strip (Figure 24.28); however, the middle cerebral ar-

who have suffered asphyxia may develop athetoid and dystonic cerebral palsy during childhood, and MRI commonly demonstrates a characteristic pattern of signal abnormalities in the putamen, thalamus, and motor strip corresponding to glutaminergic synapses (Johnston & Hoon, 2000; Menkes & Curran, 1994). Early diag-

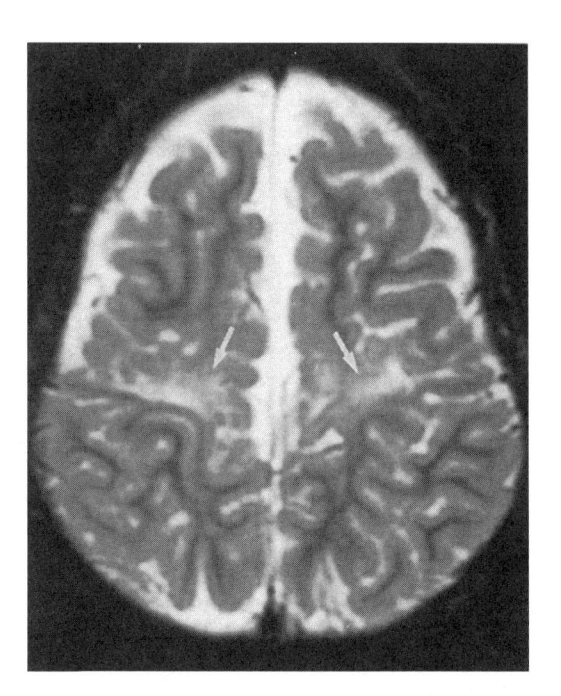

Figure 24.28. Imaging study in in a 5-year-old girl presenting with motor and cognitive impairment who suffered a perinatal hypoxic brain injury at term. Axial T2-weighted image showing infarction of the motor strip (arrows), which is a typical location of perinatal hypoxic injury.

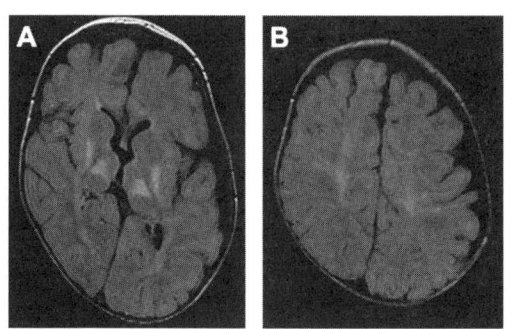

Figure 24.27. Imaging studies in a 2-year-old with cerebral palsy and seizures who was a full-term baby who suffered an anoxic event in the neonatal period. Axial FLAIR images show abnormal hyperintensity involving the ventrolateral thalami and dorsal putamina (A), as well as in bilateral peri-rolandic regions (B). These are characteristic regions sensitive to hypoxic/anoxic insult in a full-term infant.

tery distribution can be infarcted, which often appears to occur prenatally late in the third trimester and is of uncertain etiology. These children present as having congenital hemiplegia, and, for unknown reasons, isolated right hemiplegia occurs twice as often as isolated left hemiplegia.

NEUROCUTANEOUS SYNDROMES

The phakomatoses, which include neurofibromatosis, tuberous sclerosis, Sturge-Weber syndrome, and von Hippel-Lindau disease, are a diverse group of conditions that affect tissues of ectodermal origin, including the skin, eye, and CNS. Recently, it has become evident that MRI of the brain can sometimes be the first indication of disease because the skin manifestations may not be present early in life (Korf, 2004).

Neurofibromatosis

Neurofibromatosis type 1 (NF1), the classic form of von Recklinghausen disease, is characterized by multiple skin lesions (café-au-lait spots, neurofibromas), mesodermal dysplasias (dural ectasia), and CNS neoplasms (gliomas) (Yohay, 2006). NF1 is transmitted as an autosomal dominant trait in approximately 50% of cases, with the other half resulting from a spontaneous mutation on chromosome 17 (Riccardi & Eichner, 1986).

Plexiform neurofibromas are associated with peripheral nerves and can be problematic if they occur in the spine, where there may be progressive cord compression, or in the orbit, where vision may be threatened. CNS tumors are most often gliomas in the optic nerve or chiasm, occurring in 5%–15% of NF1 patients (Figure 24.29A and B). Fortunately, these gliomas tend to be slow growing and, if small, may not affect vision drastically. Other tumors include lower grade astrocytomas, ependymomas, and glioblastomas.

NF1 patients may also exhibit multiple foci of increased T2 signal in the basal ganglia, optic radiations, cerebellar peduncles, and brainstem (Figure 24.29C and D). These lesions may be the first manifestation of NF1 before the diag-

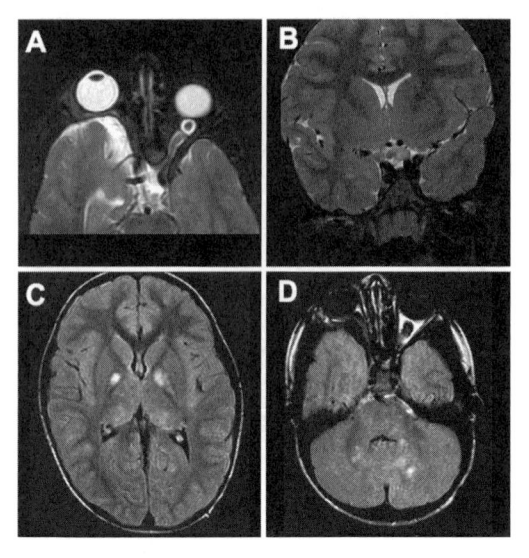

Figure 24.29. Neurofibromatosis type 1 in a 10-year-old boy. *A*, Axial T2-weighted image of the orbits shows right sphenoid wing dysplasia causing asymmetrical right exophthalmos. Mild fusiform enlargement of the intraorbital left optic nerve reflects optic glioma. *B*, Coronal T2-weighted image in the same patient shows more prominent involvement of the prechiasmatic left optic nerve and optic chiasm, which show expansion and T2 hyperintensity. *C* and *D*, Axial FLAIR images demonstrate hyperintense lesions involving the bilateral globus pallidi and thalami (*C*) and the brainstem, middle cerebellar peduncles, and dentate nuclei (*D*) resulting from characteristic spongiform changes in NF1.

nosis is clinically apparent and typically undergo evolution of shifting size, number, and location in the late teens (Kraut et al., 2004) but gradually resolve in adulthood. On pathology based on autopsy series, these lesions correspond to spongiform or vacuolar changes in the myelin sheath (DiPaolo et al., 1995; Itoh et al., 1994). They are not associated with any mass effect or enhancement. Although these lesions do not cause neurological symptoms, they have been correlated with learning disabilities (Cutting et al., 2000).

Neurofibromatosis type 2 (NF2) should be separated from NF1 because its genetic basis and presentation are unique. NF2 is transmitted as an autosomal dominant trait with nearly 100% penetrance and is caused by a defect on the long arm of chromosome 22. Typically, children with NF2 have bilateral vestibular schwannomas (Figure 24.30A), and they also can have schwannomas of cranial or spinal nerves (Figure 24.30B); meningiomas, which are frequently multiple; and intramedullary ependymomas (Figure 24.30C).

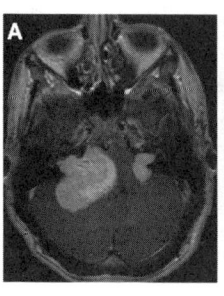
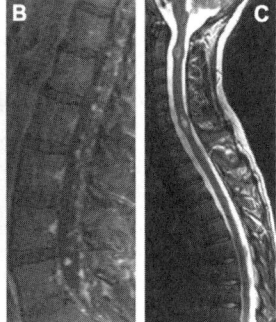

Figure 24.30. Neurofibromatosis type 2. *A*, NF2 in a 23-year-old man. Axial T1-weighted image after contrast infusion shows bilateral large, avidly enhancing extra-axial masses in the cerebellopontine angles with extension into and expansion of the internal auditory canals, reflecting bilateral vestibular schwannomas. Note that there is moderate compression of the pons at this level and partial effacement of the fourth ventricle. *B*, NF2 in an 18-year-old woman. Postcontrast sagittal T1-weighted image of the lumbar spine showing multiple small enhancing nodes in the intradural extramedullary compartment coating the surface of the conus medullaris and cauda equina fibers. These most likely reflect schwannomas in an individual with NF2, but may also reflect a combination of schwannomas, meningiomas, and gliomas. *C*, Sagittal T2-weighted image of the cervical and thoracic spine in the same patient as *B* shows two ovoid hyperintense intramedullary lesions expanding the cord at the level of C2 and C6. Both lesions enhance avidly (not shown) and represent ependymomas.

Tuberous Sclerosis

Tuberous sclerosis is an autosomal dominant disorder with a classic clinical triad of adenoma sebaceum, seizures (80%–100%), and intellectual disabilities (50%) (Quigg & Miller, 2005). Although fewer than one third of children with tuberous sclerosis will have all these features, at least 95% will demonstrate some cutaneous manifestations, including facial angiofibromata (adenoma sebaceum being a misnomer), fibromas, hypopigmented macules, or shagreen patches. The chromosomal abnormality has been localized to 9q34, encoding *TSC1* or hamartin (van Slegtenhorst et al., 1997), and to 16p13.3, encoding *TSC2* or tuberin (European Chromosome 16 Tuberous Sclerosis Consortium, 1993). Both gene products form a cytoplasmic protein heteromeric complex and act as tumor suppressors affecting the regulation of cellular growth, adhesion, and migration (Narayanan, 2003; van Slegtenhorst et al., 1998).

Cortical and subcortical tubers occur in 95% of affected children, and the number of tubers is directly related to the degree of intellectual disability (Roach, Williams, & Laster,

1987). They are hamartomatous lesions composed of variable amounts of disordered glial tissue, heterotopic neurons, giant cells, and dystrophic calcifications. Calcified tubers are well seen on CT, but, if noncalcified, they are far better visualized by MRI, particularly on the FLAIR sequence, which demonstrates hyperintense foci (Figure 24.31A).

White matter lesions are seen in approximately 90% of children with tuberous sclerosis and are usually linear bands, 10% of which enhance with gadolinium. The distribution of abnormal giant cells along the usual migratory pathway of neurons within the white matter, and their common association with overlying cortical tubers, imply a shared dysgenetic migrational origin.

Subependymal nodules occur in 95% of children with tuberous sclerosis and are usually bilateral. They tend to calcify progressively with time so that they are dark on a T2-

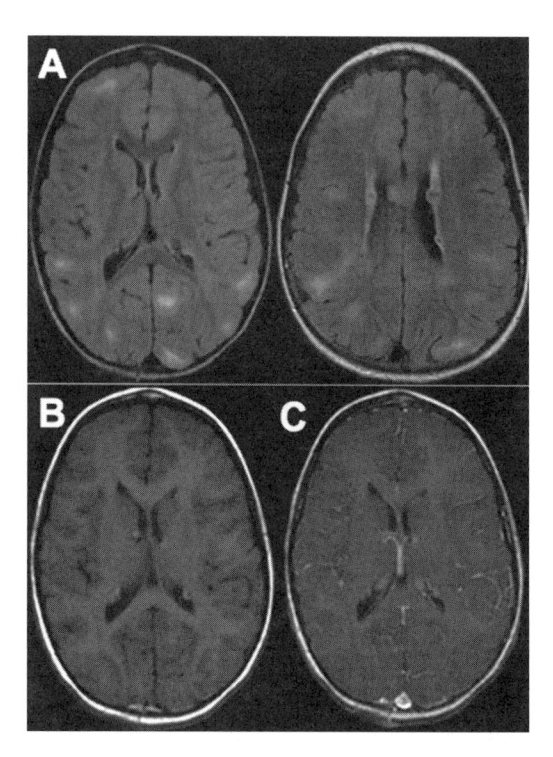

Figure 24.31. Tuberous sclerosis in a 7-year-old girl. *A*, FLAIR images show multiple hyperintense cortical and subcortical tubers. In addition, several small subependymal hamartomas are present, showing slight FLAIR and T2 hypointensity likely reflecting calcification. T1-weighted pre- (*B*) and postcontrast (*C*) images show that the subependymal hamartomas are T1 hyperintense without additional enhancement, also consistent with calcific deposits.

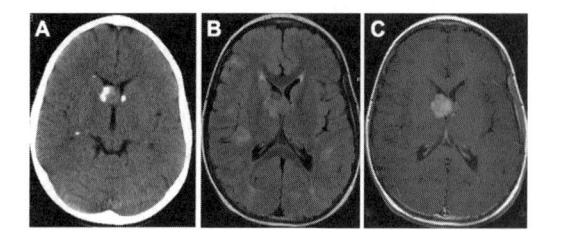

Figure 24.32. Tuberous sclerosis. *A,* Non–contrast enhanced head computed tomography shows a partially calcified intraventricular mass near the foramen of Monro representing a subependymal giant cell astrocytoma. Additional punctate calcifications reflect calcified subependymal nodules. *B,* FLAIR image shows multiple cortical and subcortical tubers to best advantage. *C,* Postcontrast (gadolinium-DTPA) T1-weighted axial image shows avid contrast enhancement in the foramen of Monro giant cell astrocytoma. There was no hydrocephalus in this case.

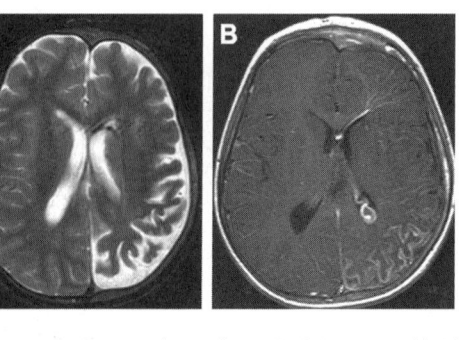

Figure 24.33. Sturge-Weber syndrome (SWS) in a 4-year-old girl with left facial port-wine stain, seizures, and developmental delay. *A,* Axial T2-weighted image shows left cerebral hemiatrophy, most prominent in the left parietal and occipital lobes. *B,* Postcontrast axial T1-weighted image shows leptomeningeal enhancement in the similar affected region. Note also left frontal white matter venous angiomas and a prominent choroid glomus within the atrium of the left lateral ventricle, often seen in SWS as a collateral pathway for ineffective cortical venous drainage.

weighted image and FLAIR (Figure 24.31A) and may show slight hyperintensity on T1-weighted images (Figure 24.31B), and they are well seen on CT (Figure 24.32A). Noncalcified nodules are better visualized using MRI, however, and 30% of these enhance with gadolinium (Figure 24.31C). In approximately 15% of children with tuberous sclerosis, a subependymal nodule will undergo neoplastic change by transforming into a giant cell astrocytoma. These usually occur close to the foramen of Monro and should be suspected if a subependymal nodule enlarges or produces hydrocephalus (Figure 24.32).

Sturge-Weber Syndrome

Sturge-Weber syndrome is a noninherited abnormality consisting of a port-wine facial nevus in the distribution of the trigeminal nerve (usually V1), choroid plexus glomus, and angiomas of the ocular choroid and the pia, the latter of which are associated with abnormal cortical venous drainage (Figure 24.33). The abnormal venous drainage leads to atrophy of the underlying cerebral hemisphere and shunting of blood through deep medullary veins into the deep venous system, which should not be misinterpreted as an arteriovenous malformation. The cortex may be normal in young infants but undergoes progressive dystrophic calcification (Benedikt & Voyl, 1993).

   Clinically, children with Sturge-Weber syndrome usually develop normally until they begin to have seizures, often in the first few years of life. The seizures become progressively refractory to treatment and are accompanied by hemiplegia and homonymous hemianopia in approximately 30% of children. The majority of these children have intellectual disabilities.

Von Hippel-Lindau Disease

Von Hippel-Lindau disease is an autosomal dominant disorder with incomplete penetrance caused by a gene abnormality on chromosome 3 (Maher, 2004). It is characterized by retinal angiomas; cerebellar and spinal cord hemangioblastomas; renal cell carcinomas; pheochromocytomas; and cysts of the pancreas, kidney, liver, and epididymis. Individuals with von Hippel-Lindau disease tend to present in their mid-20s to mid-30s with retinal detachments, symptoms of a posterior fossa mass, or both.

METABOLIC DISORDERS

In inborn errors of metabolism, metabolic pathways are blocked, resulting in accumulation of intermediate products that can cause neurological symptoms. Metabolic diseases are now recognized more frequently because their biochemical bases are better understood (see Chapter 5, this volume). Neuroimaging has become an indispensable tool in identifying affected regions, progression of disease, and therapeutic effectiveness (Naidu & Moser, 1991). In some cases, especially if a child with developmental delay has an atypical presentation, MRI may provide the first indication of a possible metabolic disorder (Lyon, Adams, & Kolodny, 1996). Although the following disease entities are rare, the clinician should not overlook the possibility of their occurrence during the patient's evaluation.

White Matter Diseases

A number of childhood white matter diseases have important findings on MRI. *X-linked adrenoleukodystrophy* (XALD) is a demyelinating disease that has several different forms, approximately 50% of which are rapidly progressive childhood cerebral forms predominantly affecting young and adolescent boys (Moser, 2006). It is an X-linked recessive disorder resulting from impaired capacity of degradation of very-long-chain fatty acids that takes place in peroxisomes. Accumulation of very-long-chain fatty acids occurs in plasma and tissues, including the brain and adrenal glands, and serum diagnosis can be made using chromatography. The defective gene has been mapped to Xq28, which encodes a peroxisomal membrane protein called adrenoleukodystrophy protein, or ALDP, a member of the ATP-binding cassette transporter superfamily (Mosser et al., 1993). Acoustic pathways, optic pathways, and the pyramidal tracts are often involved. MRI of adrenoleukodystrophy patients most commonly demonstrates inflammatory demyelination in the parieto-occipital white matter and splenium of the corpus callosum, with sparing of the subcortical U fibers, although frontal pathways may also be involved (Kumar et al., 1987) (Figure 24.34). Contrast enhancement with gadolinium often can be seen along the leading edge of the abnormal white matter. It is now recognized that there is a wide range of phenotypic variation in XALD (Moser, Raymond, & Dubey, 2005). Adrenomyeloneuropathy is an adult form that presents as a slowly progressive paraparesis resulting from noninflammatory distal axonopathy affecting the long tracts of the spinal cord, without radiological evidence of diffuse cerebral involvement. Women heterozygous for

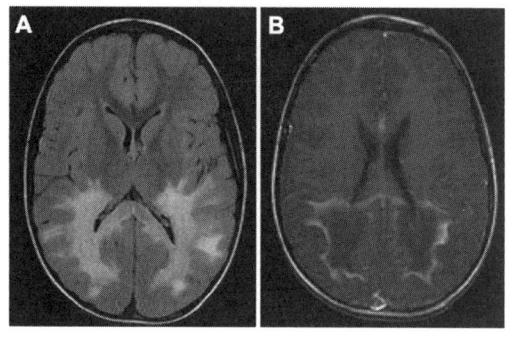

Figure 24.34. Adrenoleukodystrophy in a 6-year-old boy. *A,* Axial FLAIR image shows bilateral symmetrical hyperintense signal abnormality involving the parieto-occipital white matter and the splenium of the corpus callosum. *B,* Postcontrast axial T1-weighted image shows enhancement in the margin of the white matter signal abnormality (so-called advancing front), representing areas of active demyelination.

XALD may also manifest adrenomyeloneuropathy-like symptoms even while adrenal insufficiency and cerebral involvement are rare, and diagnosis in these carriers is more reliably established by DNA analysis than by imaging or serum assay.

Two white matter diseases, Alexander disease and Canavan disease, both present with macrocephaly (Maria, Deidrick, Moser, & Naidu, 2003). The cause of *Alexander disease* is unknown, but it presents with both infantile (birth to 2 years) and juvenile (7–14 years) forms. Abnormal astrocytes containing Rosenthal fibers constitute the diagnosis on brain biopsy. MRI of Alexander disease demonstrates frontal lobe predilection for demyelination (Figure 24.35). After contrast injection, enhancement adjacent to the frontal horns can be seen early in the disease.

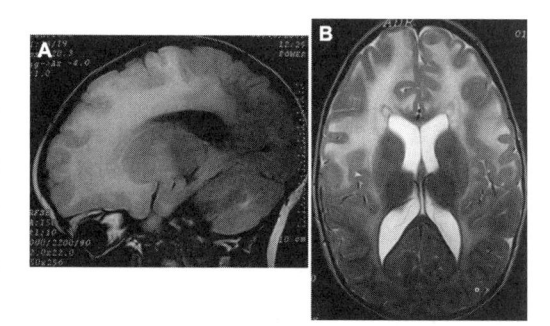

Figure 24.35. Alexander disease in a child with macrocephaly. Sagittal FLAIR (*A*) and axial T2-weighted (*B*) images show extensive hyperintense signal abnormality preferentially involving the anterior cerebral white matter.

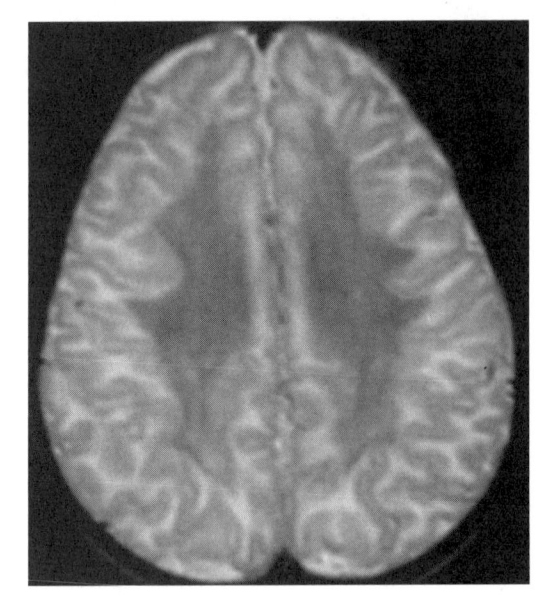

Figure 24.36. Canavan disease. Axial T2–weighted image shows diffuse white matter hyperintensity extending to the subcortical U fibers. This case is somewhat unusual in that there is some sparing of the centrum semiovale.

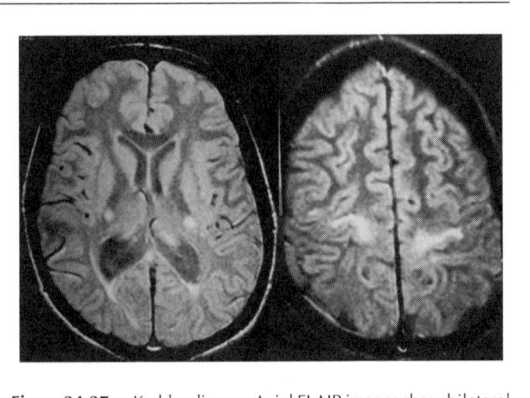

Figure 24.37. Krabbe disease. Axial FLAIR images show bilateral hyperintense signal abnormalities involving the corticospinal tracts at the level of the precentral gyri and posterior limbs of the internal capsules.

Canavan disease is an autosomal recessive disorder caused by an aspartocyclase deficiency that results in an accumulation of *N*-acetyl aspartic acid in the brain and urine. MRI shows diffuse involvement of the white matter, including the subcortical U fibers (Figure 24.36).

Another autosomal recessive disorder, *metachromatic leukodystrophy,* also has infantile and juvenile forms. It is caused by arylsulfatase A deficiency, producing an accumulation of sulfatides in the brain. Diagnosis of metachromatic leukodystrophy is obtained through tissue fibroblast analysis. MRI demonstrates frontal white matter involvement more so than parieto-occipital.

Pelizaeus-Merzbacher disease is an X-linked recessive white matter disease causing proteolipid protein deficiency and is characterized by pendular nystagmus. MRI shows symmetrical involvement of the supra- and infratentorial white matter with diffuse hypomyelination.

Krabbe disease is inherited as an autosomal recessive disorder and presents early in life with optic atrophy and spasticity. CT demonstrates increased density in the basal ganglia and thalami. Diffusely abnormal white matter can be seen on MRI, which often demonstrates involvement of the corticospinal tract, splenium of the corpus callosum, and cerebellum (Figure 24.37).

To summarize and simplify this discussion, in a child with white matter disease who is macrocephalic, Alexander or Canavan disease is a diagnostic consideration. Alexander disease affects the frontal white matter, whereas Canavan disease is more diffuse. Adrenoleukodystrophy affects boys and usually involves the occipitoparietal white matter. Pelizaeus-Merzbacher disease presents clinically with nystagmus and often can be seen throughout a family history. Metachromatic leukodystrophy has nonspecific features but can be diagnosed with fibroblast analysis for deficiency of arylsulfatase A in suspected children. On CT scans, Krabbe disease demonstrates increased density in the region of the basal ganglia.

ORGANIC ACIDEMIAS

In children with abnormal basal ganglia on MRI and no history of hypoxia, the organic acidemias should be considered. The following examples describe the neuroimaging correlates of basal ganglia abnormalities and other associated findings that may suggest the diagnosis.

Glutaric acidemia type 1, an autosomal recessive organic acidemia, results in a deficiency of the mitochondrial protein glutaryl-coenzyme A (CoA) dehydrogenase, thereby causing a buildup of glutaric acid (Strauss & Morton, 2003). Megalencephaly presents in infancy, and children present with neurological deterioration that is primarily extrapyramidal, with acute episodic vomiting and lethargy.

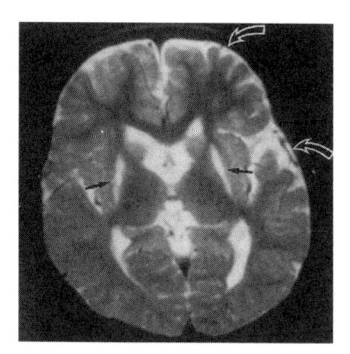

Figure 24.38. Glutaric acidemia type 1. Axial T2-weighted image showing typical involvement of the basal ganglia (solid arrows), with early frontal and temporal atrophy (open arrows).

MRI shows progressive frontotemporal atrophy, and abnormal signal is often seen in the basal ganglia (Figure 24.38). Arachnoid cysts have been reported to be more frequent in these patients than in the general population. Although the diagnosis can be made by analysis of urinary organic acids, there are some patients in whom the results are negative. Therefore, if a child presents with choreoathetosis and has basal ganglia lesions, arachnoid cysts, or both on MRI, skin fibroblast analysis for glutaryl-CoA dehydrogenase is warranted.

A major metabolic pathway passes via propionyl-CoA through methylmalonyl-CoA to the tricarboxylic acid cycle. Different metabolic defects may block the breakdown of propionyl-CoA, causing *propionic acidemia,* or the breakdown of methylmalonyl-CoA, causing *methylmalonic acidemia* (Figure 24.39). These two disorders, although rare, are among the more common of the organic acidemias (Brismar &

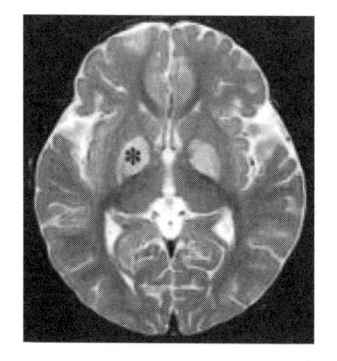

Figure 24.39. Methylmalonic acidemia. Axial T2-weighted image shows bilateral symmetrical hyperintensity involving the globus pallidi (*).

Ozand, 1994). Both diseases are inherited as autosomal recessive disorders and are characterized by failure to feed, frequent vomiting, metabolic acidosis, frequent infections, hypotonia, and seizures. MRI usually demonstrates prominence of the subarachnoid spaces, plus abnormal signal in the basal ganglia and white matter. Basal ganglia lesions in methylmalonic acidemia are limited to severe involvement of the globus pallidus, however, and not the putamen or caudate. Propionic acidemia tends to involve the entire basal ganglia, including the globus pallidus, putamen, and caudate.

TRAUMA

Unfortunately, accidental and nonaccidental brain trauma accounts for a large proportion of morbidity in children. CT is the study of choice in the acute stage, but MRI is more sensitive for all types of parenchymal injury in the subacute and chronic stages. Only the chronic imaging findings, which are more relevant to developmental pediatrics, are discussed here.

Because of its lack of rigidity, the brain has little protection against shear-strain deformation, and most intra-axial brain injury (involving the parenchyma) is considered to be caused by this type of force (Holbourn, 1945). Parenchymal brain injury can be divided into four types (Gentry, Godersky, & Thompson, 1988):

1. *Diffuse axonal injury (DAI)*—This is the most common type of injury and is produced by acceleration and rotational forces. The MRI era has enabled visualization of shearing injuries of axons, 50% of which usually occur at the gray matter–white matter junction (Figure 24.40) because the gray and white matter have different rigidity. The remainder of the lesions occur in the large white matter fiber bundles of the corpus callosum (22%), corona radiata (19%), and internal capsule (8%). These lesions are usually small, may contain a small amount of hemorrhage, and tend to increase with more severe head trauma and prolonged loss of consciousness.

2. *Cortical contusions*—These are the second most frequent injuries and are less likely to be associated with severe initial impair-

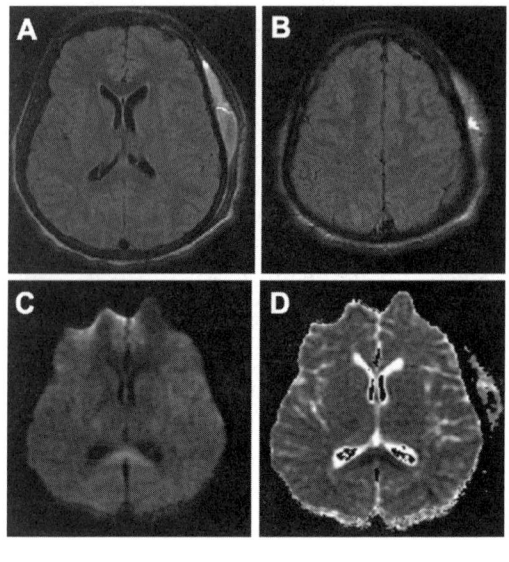

Figure 24.40. Diffuse axonal injury in a 5-year-old girl involved in a motor vehicle accident. *A,* Axial FLAIR image shows left frontal scalp swelling. Intracranially, there are a few punctate foci of hyperintensity in the right frontal and right parietal white matter reflecting edema. *B,* Additional punctate hyperintense foci in the centrum semiovale on the right near the corticomedullary junction. *C,* Diffusion-weighted image shows hyperintense signal in the splenium of the corpus callosum that corresponds to restricted (decreased) diffusion the calculated apparent diffusion coefficient maps in *D,* indicative of traumatic shearing injury.

ment of consciousness. They are often hemorrhagic and frequently involve the temporal or inferior frontal lobe. In the chronic stage, the contusions may progress to encephalomalacia.

3. *Deep gray matter lesions*—Although uncommon, these lesions are associated with severe head injuries, and most are hemorrhagic. They may be caused by disruption of multiple small perforating vessels and in the chronic stage have the appearance of infarction (Adams, 1984).

4. *Primary and secondary brainstem lesions*—Associated with the most severe head injuries, these lesions are most likely the result of DAI (Adams, 1984; Gentry, Godersky, & Thompson, 1989). They may be classified as those occurring at the time of trauma (primary brainstem injury) and those that develop later (secondary brainstem injury). Most primary brainstem injuries tend to occur in the dorsolateral aspect of the upper brainstem as a result of indirect DAI and typically are accompanied by su-

pratentorial DAI lesions. A small percentage of primary brainstem lesions result from direct trauma from the adjacent rigid tentorial incisura. Secondary brainstem injury can be caused by transtentorial herniation or hypoxia. Most of these brainstem lesions cannot be identified on CT; therefore, MRI is the study of choice. In the acute phase, MRI demonstrates foci of increased FLAIR and T2 signal, and the brainstem becomes progressively atrophic with time.

EVOLVING IMAGING MODALITIES

A number of other imaging modalities being developed may have diagnostic applicability in children with static and progressive encephalopathies. Until recently, only morphological imaging of the brain could be performed; however, with MRI hardware advances and the development of newer techniques, it is now possible to perform "functional imaging" of the brain. The underlying physical principles and clinical applications of these techniques are thoroughly covered in the book *Clinical MR Neuroimaging: Diffusion, Perfusion and Spectroscopy* (Gillard, Waldman, & Barker, 2005).

Magnetic Resonance Spectroscopy

MR spectroscopy is a noninvasive technique for obtaining information concerning tissue metabolism (Cecil, 2006). Phosphorus-31 MR spectroscopy allows detection of compounds involved in energy metabolism, including phosphocreatine, inorganic phosphate, and adenosine triphosphate, as well as measurement of tissue pH. Proton (^{1}H) MR spectroscopy can be used to measure *N*-acetyl aspartate (NAA), choline, creatine, glutamate, glutamine, *myo*-inositol, and lactic acid.

Localized image-guided MR spectra have been obtained in human brains in a variety of conditions, including adrenoleukodystrophy, brain neoplasms, epilepsy, and infarction. From information gathered to date, it appears that, in many diseases affecting the brain, MR spectroscopy is more sensitive than routine MRI (Barker & Horska, 2004). For instance, choline is often observed to be elevated in demyelinating diseases, whereas NAA is reduced in most etiologies associated with neuronal loss or dysfunction. Only in the case of Canavan disease is NAA higher than normal. This technique holds promise for diagnosis and monitoring of diseases and of response to therapy, especially in neurodegenerative disorders.

Echo-Planar Magnetic Resonance Imaging

Echo-planar MRI is an extremely fast imaging technique that collects all of the data to reconstruct an image in less than 0.1 second. This technique has allowed development of functional brain imaging, including imaging of perfusion, diffusion, and cortical activation (Edelman, Wielopolski, & Schmitt, 1994).

Magnetic Resonance Diffusion Imaging

Diffusion is the process of random thermal motion of molecules. When this occurs in a magnetic field gradient, there is loss of signal on spin echo–based MRI scans. Because diffusion occurs at a scale on the order of tenths or hundredths of a millimeter per second, it requires a large gradient strength or duration, or both, to produce observable signal loss. With the advent of rapid echo-planar imaging, it is possible to demonstrate diffusion of water within the brain. This technique may provide useful information about tissue structure and function because diffusion coefficients are related to the temperature and physical characteristics of the molecules. For example, water diffusion imaging provides information about white matter orientation and maturity, and this technique may prove to be a more sensitive assessment of development of myelination than conventional spin echo images. Diffusion imaging is particularly sensitive to the detection of acute ischemic injury to the brain, which results in decreased water diffusion (Sagar & Grant, 2006).

Magnetic Resonance Perfusion Imaging

With MR perfusion imaging, blood perfusion of the brain can be mapped either by administering an intravenous paramagnetic contrast agent or by "tagging" incoming blood (called *arterial spin labeling* [ASL]). This method is particularly useful in detecting areas of hypoperfusion (e.g., cerebral ischemia) or hyperperfusion (as in an epileptic focus).

Perfusion imaging can also be used for localization of cortical activity. It is thought that cortical activity increases blood flow, which can be visualized by perfusion imaging. Previously, this was mostly the domain of positron emission tomography (PET), which is expensive, has limited availability, requires administration of radioactive isotope, and may require averaging of studies across subjects. Perfusion imaging provides better spatial resolution than does PET, and it allows localization of cortical activity in an individual. In addition, because ASL-based MR perfusion imaging is noninvasive, activation studies can be performed repeatedly.

CONCLUSION

In the past decade, cranial neuroimaging has become an invaluable tool in the workup of children with neurological diseases, developmental delay, or both. Not only can it confirm suspected clinical diagnoses, but in many instances it can provide the earliest diagnosis of an unsuspected condition as well as provide insight into the timing of insults. Nevertheless, even though conventional MRI provides exquisite anatomic detail, there are some children who have neurological abnormalities, but whose brains have a normal appearance. It is for this group that functional imaging holds the most promise. Examples are children who have cerebral palsy but whose brain MRIs are normal, including those with choreoathetoid cerebral palsy, in whom the basal ganglia are anatomically normal. Another group includes children with intellectual disabilities whose brains demonstrate no conventional MRI abnormality. In the future, functional imaging offers great promise and may further advance our understanding of neurological diseases in children.

REFERENCES

Adams, J.H. (1984). Head injury. In J.H. Adams, J.A.N. Corsellis, & L.W. Duchen (Eds.), *Greenfield's neuropathology* (4th ed., pp. 85–124). New York: John Wiley & Sons.

Altman, N.R., Nadich, T.P., & Braffman, B.H. (1992). Posterior fossa malformations. *AJNR: American Journal of Neuroradiology, 13,* 691–724.

American Academy of Pediatrics, Committee on Drugs. (1992). Guidelines for monitoring and management of pediatric patients during and after sedation for diagnostic and therapeutic procedures. *Pediatrics, 90,* 1110–1115.

Andermann, F. (2000). Cortical dysplasias and epilepsy: A review of the architectonic, clinical, and seizure patterns. *Advances in Neurology, 84,* 479–496.

Baker, L.L., Stevenson, D.K., & Enzmann, D.R. (1988). End-stage periventricular leukomalacia: MR evaluation. *Radiology, 168,* 809–815.

Bale, J.F., Jr. (1984). Human cytomegalovirus infection and disorders of the nervous system. *Archives of Neurology, 41,* 310–320.

Banker, B.Q., & Larroche, J.C. (1962). Periventricular leukomalacia of infancy. *Archives of Neurology, 7,* 32–50.

Barker, P.B., & Horska, A. (2004). Neuroimaging in leukodystrophies. *Journal of Child Neurology, 19,* 559–570.

Barkovich, A.J. (1990). *Pediatric neuroimaging: Metabolic and destructive brain disorders* (pp. 35–42). New York: Raven Press.

Barkovich, A.J., & Chuang, S.H. (1990). Unilateral megalencephaly: Correlation of MR and pathologic characteristics. *AJNR: American Journal of Neuroradiology, 11,* 523–531.

Barkovich, A.J., Chuang, S.H., & Norman, D. (1988). MR of neuronal migration anomalies. *AJR: American Journal of Roentgenology, 150,* 179–187.

Barkovich, A.J., Kjos, B.O., Jackson, D.E., & Norman, D. (1988). Normal maturation of the neonatal and infant brain: MR imaging at 1.5T. *Radiology, 166,* 173–180.

Barkovich, A.J., Kjos, B.O., Norman, D., & Edwards, M.S. (1989). Revised classification of posterior fossa cysts and cystlike malformations based on the results of multiplanar MR imaging. *AJR: American Journal of Neuroradiology, 10,* 977–988.

Barkovich, A.J., & Quint, D.J. (1993). Middle interhemispheric fusion: An unusual variant of holoprosencephaly. *AJNR: American Journal of Neuroradiology, 14,* 431–440.

Barkovich, A.J., Wippold, F.J., Sherman, J.L., & Citrin, C.M. (1986). Significance of cerebellar tonsillar ectopia on MR. *AJNR: American Journal of Neuroradiology, 7,* 795–799.

Benedikt, R.A., & Voyl, T.J. (1993). MR imaging of Sturge-Weber syndrome. *AJNR: American Journal of Neuroradiology, 14,* 409–417.

Bignami, A., & Appicciutolo, L. (1964). Micropolygyria and cerebral calcification in cytomegalic inclusion disease. *Acta Neuropathologica, 4,* 127–137.

Billiards, S.S., Haynes, R.L, Folkerth, R.D., Trachtenberg, F.L., Liu, L.G., Volpe, J.J., et al. (2006). Development of microglia in the cerebral white matter of the human fetus and infant. *Journal of Comparative Neurology, 497,* 199–208.

Bindal, A.K., Storrs, B.B., & McLone, D.G. (1990–1991). Management of the Dandy-Walker syndrome. *Pediatric Neurosurgery, 16,* 163–169.

Blake, J.A. (1900). The roof of the lateral recesses of the fourth ventricle, considered morphologically and embryologically. *Journal of Comparative Neurology, 10,* 79–108.

Bluemke, D.A., & Breiter, S.N. (2000). Sedation procedures in MR imaging: Safety, effectiveness, and nursing effect on examinations. *Radiology, 216,* 645–652.

Brismar, J., & Ozand, P.T. (1994). CT and MR of the brain in disorders of propionate and methylmalonate metabolism. *AJNR: American Journal of Neuroradiology, 15,* 1459–1473.

Candy, E.J., Hoon, A.H., Capute, A.J., & Bryan, R.N. (1993). MRI in motor delay: Important adjunct to classification of cerebral palsy. *Pediatric Neurology, 9,* 421–429.

Cecil, K.M. (2006). MR spectroscopy of metabolic disorders. *Neuroimaging Clinics of North America, 16,* 87–116.

Chiari, H. (1891). Ueber Veranderungen des Kleinhirns infolg von hydrocephalie des grosshims. *Deutsche Medizinische Wochenschrift, 17,* 1172–1175.

Counsell, S.J., Allsop, J.M., Harrison, M.C., Larkman, D.J., Kennea, N.L., Kapellou, O., et al. (2003). Diffusion-weighted imaging of the brain in preterm infants with focal and diffuse white matter abnormality. *Pediatrics, 112,* 1–7.

Cutting, L.E., Koth, C.W., Burnette, C.P., Abrams, M.T., Kaufmann, W.E., & Denckla, M.B. (2000). Relationship of cognitive functioning, whole brain volumes, and T2-weighted hyperintensities in neurofibromatosis-1. *Journal of Child Neurology, 15,* 157–160.

De Meyer, W. (1971). Classification of cerebral malformations. *Birth Defects Original Article Series, 7,* 78–93.

de Rijk-van Andel, J.F., Arts, W.F.M., Barth, PG., & Loonen, M.C.B. (1990). Diagnostic features and clinical signs of 21 patients with lissencephaly type 1. *Developmental Medicine and Child Neurology, 32,* 707–717.

Diebler, C., Dusser, A., & Dulac, O. (1985). Congenital toxoplasmosis: Clinical and neuroradiological evaluation of the cerebral lesions. *Neuroradiology, 27,* 125–130.

DiPaolo, D.P., Zimmerman, R.A., Rorke, L.B., Zackai, E.H., Bilaniuk, L.T., & Yachnis, A.T. (1995). Neurofibromatosis type 1: Pathologic substrate of high-signal-intensity foci in the brain. *Radiology, 195,* 721–724.

Dobyns, W.B., Pagon, R.A., & Armstrong, D. (1989). Diagnostic criteria for the Walker-Warburg syndrome. *American Journal of Medical Genetics, 32,* 195–210.

Dobyns, W.B., Strutton, R.F., & Greenberg, F. (1984). Syndromes with lissencephaly. *American Journal of Medical Genetics, 18,* 509–526.

Dubourg, C., Lazaro, L., Pasquier, L., Bendavid, C., Blayau, M., Le Duff, F., et al. (2004). Molecular screening of SHH, ZIC2, SIX3, and TGIF genes in patients with features of holoprosencephaly spectrum: Mutation review and genotype-phenotype correlations. *Human Mutation, 24,* 43–51.

Dyste, G.N., Menezes, A.H., & VanGilder, J.C. (1989). Symptomatic Chiari malformations. *Journal of Neurosurgery, 71,* 159–168.

Edelman, R.E., Wielopolski, P., & Schmitt, F. (1994). Echo-planar MR imaging. *Radiology, 192,* 600–612.

Eichenwald, H.F. (1956). Human toxoplasmosis. In *Proceedings of the conference on clinical aspects and diagnostic problems of toxoplasmosis in pediatrics.* Baltimore: Williams & Wilkins.

European Chromosome 16 Tuberous Sclerosis Consortium. (1993). Identification and characterization of the tuberous sclerosis gene on chromosome 16. *Cell, 75,* 1305–1315.

Fan, G.G., Yu, B., Quan, S.M., Sun, B.H., & Guo, Q.Y. (2006). Potential of diffusion tensor MRI in the assessment of periventricular leukomalacia. *Clinical Radiology, 61,* 358–364.

Gentry, L.R., Godersky, J.C., & Thompson, B. (1988). MR imaging of head trauma: A review of the distribution and radiopathologic features of traumatic lesions. *AJR: American Journal of Roentgenology, 150,* 663–672.

Gentry, L.R., Godersky, J.C., & Thompson, B.H. (1989). Traumatic brainstem injury: MR imaging. *Radiology, 171,* 177–187.

Gillard, J., Waldman, A., & Barker, P. (Eds.). (2005). *Clinical MR neuroimaging: Diffusion, perfusion and spectroscopy.* Cambridge, England: Cambridge University Press.

Granata, T., Freri, E., Caccia, C., Setola, V., Taroni, F., & Battaglia, G. (2005). Schizencephaly: Clinical spectrum, epilepsy, and pathogenesis. *Journal of Child Neurology, 20,* 313–318.

Greenberg, S.B., Faerber, E.N., & Aspinall, C.L. (1991). High dose chloral hydrate sedation for children undergoing CT. *Journal of Computer Assisted Tomography, 15,* 467–469.

Gressens, P. (2006). Pathogenesis of migration disorders. *Current Opinion in Neurology, 19,* 135–140.

Haginoya, K., Ohura, T., Kon, K., Yagi, T., Sawaishi, Y., Ishii, K.K., et al. (2002). Abnormal white matter lesions with sensorineural hearing loss caused by congenital cytomegalovirus infection: Retrospective diagnosis by PCR using Guthrie cards. *Brain Development, 24,* 710–714.

Hahn, J.S., & Pinter, J.D. (2002). Holoprosencephaly: Genetic, neuroradiological, and clinical advances. *Seminars in Pediatric Neurology, 9,* 309–319.

Hahn, J.S., & Plawner, L.L. (2004). Evaluation and management of children with holoprosencephaly. *Pediatric Neurology, 31,* 79–88.

Holbourn, A.H.S. (1945). The mechanics of brain injuries. *British Medical Bulletin, 3,* 147–149.

Holland, B.A., Kucharcyzk, W., Brant-Zawadski, M., Norman, D., Haas, D.K., & Harper, P.S. (1985). MR imaging of calcified intracranial lesions. *Radiology, 157,* 353–356.

Hoon, A.H., Jr., Belsito, K.M., & Nagae-Poetscher, L.M. (2003). Neuroimaging in spasticity and movement disorders. *Journal of Child Neurology, 18*(Suppl. 1), S25–S39.

Hoon, A.H., Jr., Lawrie, W.T., Jr., Melhem, E.R., Reinhardt, E.M., Van Zijl, P.C., Solaiyappan, M., et al. (2002). Diffusion tensor imaging of periventricular leukomalacia shows affected sensory cortex white matter pathways. *Neurology, 59,* 752–756.

Hutto, C., Arvin, A., & Jacobs, R. (1987). Intrauterine herpes simplex virus infections. *Journal of Pediatrics, 110,* 97–101.

Itoh, T., Magnaldi, S., White, R.M., Denckla, M.B., Hofman, K., Naidu, S., et al. (1994). Neurofibromatosis type 1: The evolution of deep gray and white matter MR abnormalities. *AJNR: American Journal of Neuroradiology, 15,* 1513–1519

Jinkins, J.R., Whittemore, A.R., & Bradley, W.G. (1989). MR imaging of callosal and corticocallosal dysgenesis. *AJNR: American Journal of Neuroradiology, 10,* 339–344.

Johnston, M.V., & Hoon, A.H., Jr. (2000). Possible mechanisms in infants for selective basal ganglia damage from asphyxia, kernicterus, or mitochondrial encephalopathies. *Journal of Child Neurology, 15,* 588–591.

Joubert, M., Eisenring, J., Robb, J.P., & Andermann, F. (1969). Familial agenesis of the cerebellar vermis. *Neurology, 19,* 813–825.

Kato, M., & Dobyns, W.B. (2003). Lissencephaly and the molecular basis of neuronal migration. *Human Molecular Genetics, 12*(Spec. No. 1), R89–R96.

Kollias, S.S., Ball, W.S., & Prenger, E.C. (1993). Cystic malformations of the posterior fossa: Differential diagnosis clarified through embryologic analysis. *RadioGraphics, 13,* 1211–1231.

Korf, B.R. (2004). The phakomatoses. *Neuroimaging Clinics of North America, 14,* 139–148.

Kraut, M.A., Gerring, J.P., Cooper, K.L., Thompson, R.E., Denckla, M.B., & Kaufmann, W.E. (2004). Longitudinal evolution of unidentified bright objects in children with neurofibromatosis-1. *American Journal of Medical Genetics Part A, 129,* 113–119.

Kuban, K.C.K., & Leviton, A. (1994). Cerebral palsy. *New England Journal of Medicine, 330,* 188–193.

Kumar, A.J., Rosenbaum, A.E., Naidu, S., Wener, L., Citrin, C.M., Lindenberg, R., et al. (1987). Adrenoleukodystrophy: Correlating MR imaging with CT. *Radiology, 165,* 497–504.

Lipton, S.A., & Epstein, F.H. (1994). Excitatory amino acids as a final common pathway for neurological disorders. *New England Journal of Medicine, 330,* 613–621.

Louie, C.M., & Gleeson, J.G. (2005). Genetic basis of Joubert syndrome and related disorders of cerebellar development. *Human Molecular Genetics, 24*, 235–242.

Lyon, G., Adams, R.D., & Kolodny, E.H. (1996). *Neurobiology of hereditary metabolic diseases of children.* New York: McGraw-Hill.

Maher, E.R. (2004). Von Hippel-Lindau disease. *Current Molecular Medicine, 4*, 833–842.

Maria, B.L., Deidrick, K.M., Moser, H., & Naidu, S. (2003). Leukodystrophies: Pathogenesis, diagnosis, strategy, therapies, and future research directions. *Journal of Child Neurology, 18*, 578–590.

Maria, B.L., Zinreich, S.J., Carson, B.C., Rosenbaum, A.E., & Freeman, J.M. (1987). Dandy-Walker syndrome revisited. *Pediatric Neuroscience, 13*, 45–51.

Mendelson, E., Aboudy, Y., Smetana, Z., Tepperberg, M., & Grossman, Z. (2006). Laboratory assessment and diagnosis of congenital viral infections: Rubella, cytomegalovirus (CMV), varicella-zoster virus (VZV), herpes simplex virus (HSV), parvovirus B19 and human immunodeficiency virus (HIV). *Reproductive Toxicology, 21*, 350–382.

Menkes, J.H., & Curran, J. (1994). Clinical and MR correlates in children with extrapyramidal cerebral palsy. *AJNR: American Journal of Neuroradiology, 15*, 451–457.

Ment, L.R., Bada, H.S., Barnes, P., Grant, P.E., Hirtz, D., Papile, L.A., et al. (2002). Practice parameter. Neuroimaging of the neonate: Report of the Quality Standards Subcommittee of the American Academy of Neurology and the Practice Committee of the Child Neurology Society. *Neurology, 58*, 1726–1738.

Milhorat, T.H., Chou, M.W., Trinidad, E.M., Kula, R.W., Mandell, M., Wolpert, C., et al. (1999). Chiari I malformation redefined: Clinical and radiographic findings for 364 symptomatic patients. *Neurosurgery, 44*, 1005–1017.

Mori, K. (2000). Actualities in hydrocephalus classification and management possibilities. *Neurological Research, 22*, 127–130.

Moser, H.W. (2006). Therapy of X-linked adrenoleukodystrophy. *NeuroRx, 3*, 246–253.

Moser, H.W., Raymond, G.V., & Dubey, P. (2005). Adrenoleukodystrophy: New approaches to a neurodegenerative disease. *JAMA, 294*, 3131–3134.

Mosser, J., Douar, A.M., Sarde, C.O., Kioschis, P., Feil, R., Moser, H., et al. (1993). Putative X-linked adrenoleukodystrophy gene shares unexpected homology with ABC transporters. *Nature, 361*, 726–730.

Murray, J.C., Johnson, J.A., & Bird, T.D. (1985). Dandy-Walker malformation: Etiologic heterogeneity and empiric recurrence risks. *Clinical Genetics, 28*, 272–283.

Naidu, S., & Moser, H.W. (1991). Value of neuroimaging in metabolic diseases affecting the CNS. *AJNR: American Journal of Neuroradiology, 12*, 413–416.

Narayanan, V. (2003). Tuberous sclerosis complex: Genetics to pathogenesis. *Pediatric Neurology 29*, 404–409.

Noorbehesht, B., Enzmann, D.R., Sullinder, W., Bradley, J.S., & Arvin, A.M. (1987). Neonatal herpes simplex encephalitis: Correlation of clinical and CT findings. *Radiology, 162*, 813–819.

Oka, A., Belliveau, M.J., Rosenberg, P.A., & Volpe, J. (1993). Vulnerability of oligodendroglia to glutamate: Pharmacology, mechanisms, and prevention. *Journal of Neuroscience, 13*, 1441–1453.

Park, T.S., Hoffman, H.J., Hendrick, E.B., & Humphreys, R.P. (1983). Experience with surgical decompression of the Arnold-Chiari malformation in young infants with myelomeningocele. *Neurosurgery, 13*, 147–153.

Pascual, J., Oterino, A., & Berciano, J. (1992). Headache in type I Chiari malformation. *Neurology, 42*, 1519–1521.

Quigg, M., & Miller, J.Q. (2005). Clinical findings of the phakomatoses: Tuberous sclerosis. *Neurology, 65*, E22–E23.

Raybaud, C. (1982). Cystic malformations of the posterior fossa. *Journal of Neuroradiology, 9*, 103–133.

Raybaud, C. (1983). Destructive lesions of the brain. *Neuroradiology, 25*, 265–291.

Riccardi, V.M., & Eichner, J.E. (1986). *Neurofibromatosis: Phenotype, natural history and pathogenesis.* Baltimore: The Johns Hopkins University Press.

Roach, E.S., Williams, D.P., & Laster, D.W. (1987). Magnetic resonance imaging in tuberous sclerosis. *Archives of Neurology, 44*, 301–303.

Rorke, L.B., & Zimmerman, R.A. (1992). Prematurity, postmaturity, and destructive lesions in utero. *AJNR: American Journal of Neuroradiology, 13*, 517–536.

Ross, S.A., & Boppana, S.B. (2005). Congenital cytomegalovirus infection: Outcome and diagnosis. *Seminars in Pediatric Infectious Diseases, 16*, 44–49.

Sagar, P., & Grant, P.E. (2006). Diffusion-weighted MR imaging: Pediatric clinical applications. *Neuroimaging Clinics of North America, 16*, 45–74.

Schouman-Claeys, E., Picard, A., Laland, G., Kalifa, G., Lacert, P., Brentanos, E., et al. (1989). Contribution of computed tomography in the etiology and prognosis of cerebral palsy in children. *British Journal of Radiology, 62*, 248–252.

Simon, E.R., & Barkovich, A.J. (2001). Holoprosencephaly: New concepts. *Magnetic Resonance Imaging Clinics of North America, 9*, 149–164.

Skranes, J.S., Martinussen, M., Smevik, O., Myhr, G., Indredavik, M., Vik, T., et al. (2005). Cerebral MRI findings in very-low-birth-weight and small-for-gestational-age children at 15 years of age. *Pediatric Radiology, 35*, 758–765.

Smith, A.S., & Blaser, S.I. (1989). Magnetic resonance imaging of disturbances in neuronal migration: Illustration of an embryological process. *RadioGraphics, 9*, 509–522.

Stamos, J.K., & Rowley, A.H. (1994). Timely diagnosis of congenital infections. *Pediatrics Clinic of North America, 41,* 1017–1033.

Strain, J.D., Campbell, J.B., Harvey, L.A., & Foley, L.C. (1988). IV Nembutal: Safe sedation for children undergoing CT. *AJR: American Journal of Roentgenology, 151,* 975–979.

Strauss, K.A., & Morton, D.H. (2003). Type I glutaric aciduria, part 2: A model of acute striatal necrosis. *American Journal of Medical Genetics Part C: Seminars in Medical Genetics, 121,* 53–70.

Takashima, S., & Tanaka, K. (1978). Development of cerebrovascular architecture and its relationship to periventricular leukomalacia. *Archives of Neurology, 35,* 11–16.

Tinkle, B.T., Schorry, E.K., Franz, D.N., Crone, K.R. & Saal, H.M. (2005). Epidemiology of hemimegalencephaly: A case series and review. *American Journal of Medical Genetics Part A, 139,* 204–211.

Truwit, C.L., Barkovich, A.J., Koch, T.K., & Ferriero, D.M. (1992). Cerebral palsy: MR findings in 40 patients. *AJNR: American Journal of Neuroradiology, 13,* 67–78.

van Slegtenhorst, M., de Hoogt, R., Hermans, C., Nellist, M., Janssen, B., Verhoef, S., et al. (1997). Identification of the tuberous sclerosis gene TSC1 on chromosome 9q34. *Science, 277,* 805–808.

van Slegtenhorst, M., Nellist, M., Nagelkerken, B., Cheadle, J., Snell, R., van den Ouweland, A., et al. (1998). Interaction between hamartin and tuberin, the TSC1 and TSC2 gene products. *Human Molecular Genetics, 7,* 1053–1057.

Vandertop, W.P., Asai, A., Hoffman, H.J., Drake, J.M., Humphreys, R.P., Rutka, J.T., et al. (1992). Surgical decompression for symptomatic Chiari II malformation in neonates with meningomyelocele. *Journal of Neurosurgery, 77,* 541–544.

Volpe, J.J. (1989). Current concepts of brain injury in the premature infant. *AJR: American Journal of Roentgenology, 153,* 243–251.

Volpe, J.J. (2003). Cerebral white matter injury of the premature infant—more common than you think. *Pediatrics, 112,* 176–180.

Volpe, J.J. (2005). Encephalopathy of prematurity includes neuronal abnormalities [Commentaries]. *Pediatrics, 116,* 221–224.

Wolpert, S.M., Anderson, M., Scott, R.M., Kwan, E.S.K., & Runge, V.M. (1987). Chiari 2 malformation: MR imaging evaluation. *AJR: American Journal of Roentgenology, 149,* 1033–1042.

Yakovlev, P.I., & Lecours, A.R. (1967). The myelogenetic cycles of regional maturation of the brain. In A. Mankowski (Ed.), *Regional development of the brain in early life* (pp. 3–70). Oxford, UK: Blackwell.

Yilmaz, Y., Alper, G., Kilicoglu, G., Celik, L., Karadeniz, L., & Yilmaz-Degirmenci, S. (2001). Magnetic resonance imaging findings in patients with severe neonatal indirect hyperbilirubinemia. *Journal of Child Neurology, 16,* 452–455.

Yohay, K. (2006). Neurofibromatosis types 1 and 2. *Neurologist, 12,* 86–93.

▲
25

Visual Impairment

CHRISTOPHER T. LEFFLER

If the visual system does not receive clear images from well-aligned eyes during childhood, the ability to develop normal binocular vision is lost permanently. Therefore, proper assessment and treatment of visual disorders in childhood can have a profound influence on lifelong visual function. For instance, childhood refractive correction, optical treatment of visual deprivation or suppression (amblyopia), removal of media opacities such as congenital cataracts, and laser treatment to prevent retinal detachments in premature babies are some of the most effective treatments in all of medicine.

Although the fundamentals of visual assessment and treatment are the same for all children, those with developmental disabilities present particular challenges. The assessment relies more heavily on objective tests when verbal feedback is limited or delayed. It may not be clear to caregivers whether functional problems are due to disorders in the visual, neurological, other, or multiple systems. Some procedures, including eye examinations, must be done under general anesthesia, and additional precautions must be taken after surgery to protect the eyes. This chapter describes the assessment, criteria for ophthalmological referral, and overview of treatment options for visual disorders in children while highlighting aspects relevant to those with developmental disabilities.

VISUAL ANATOMY AND PHYSIOLOGY

The primary refractive element of the eye is the air–tear interface, the power of which is determined by the corneal curvature. While traversing the aqueous-filled anterior segment, light passes through the pupillary aperture, the size of which is determined largely by the ambient light level. Light is then refracted by the crystalline lens. The power of the lens is adjusted by the accommodative mechanism so that the target image is focused on the retina. After passing through the clear vitreous and inner layers of the retina, the light is absorbed by the outer retinal photoreceptor elements, consisting of rods and cones. Rods are relatively more sensitive in low-light, or scotopic, conditions and are more numerous in the retinal periphery. Cones are concentrated in the center of the retina where the image is focused. There are three types of cones that have different absorption spectra to permit color perception. The photoreceptor signals are then transduced by intervening bipolar cells to activate ganglion cells, which have their cell bodies in the inner retina. The ganglion cell axons constitute the optic nerve and the optic tracts, which conduct the visual stimuli to the lateral geniculate body of the thalamus. Nasal optic nerve fibers, carrying information on the temporal visual field, cross at the optic chiasm. The postchiasmal optic segments, termed the *optic tracts*, carry information on the contralateral visual field. The lateral geniculate nucleus sends information via the optic radiations to the primary visual cortex.

ASSESSMENT OF THE EYE

Pediatric eye examination requires principles generally relevant to childhood medical assessment. Examination must be opportunistic and must progress from the least disturbing (observation at a distance, determination of ability to fix and follow interesting targets) to the most noxious (indirect ophthalmoscopy, dilating drops) so that the maximum amount of information can be gleaned before the child stops cooperating. Observing the child while discussing the history with the family provides significant information about the level of attention, visual acuity, and intermittent ocular misalignment.

Timing of Examinations

Pediatricians begin evaluating the eye at birth (Table 25.1). Visual acuity testing with vision charts begins in the pediatrician's office at least by age 3. Friedman and Kaufman (2003) have recommended routine comprehensive dilated eye examinations by a pediatric ophthalmologist at age 4. The rationale is to detect subtle

Table 25.1. Development and assessment of the eye

Age	Development and assessment
Gestational age	
22 days	Optic primordia appears.
At birth, any age	*Fundus checked for red reflex.
	*Corneal light reflex tested.
	*Cover test performed.
30 weeks	*Screening for retinopathy of prematurity by ophthalmologist required for gestational age < 30 weeks or birth weight < 1500 g (AAP, 2006).
	Pupillary light reflexes may be present.
	Lid closure in response to light.
34 weeks	Vestibular eye rotations (doll's eye reflex) well developed.
Term age	
Birth	Visual fixation present. Optokinetic nystagmus and conjugate horizontal gaze well developed. Visual acuity 20/400.
1 month	Pupillary light reflex well developed.
2 months	Fixation and conjugate vertical gaze well developed. Color vision present.
2–5 months	Blink response to visual threat.
3 months	Visual following well developed.
4 months	Accommodation well developed. Eyes should be well aligned in the absence of pathology.
6 months	Color vision at adult level. Fusional convergence and iris stromal pigmentation well developed. Stereopsis developed.
1 year	Visual acuity 20/50.
2 years	*Check acuity by grading preferential looking or Snellen chart at adult level (20/20).
	*Check fundus with direct ophthalmoscope.
3 years	*Check visual acuity.
	Refer if < 4 of 6 correct on 20-ft line with either eye tested at 10 ft (< 10/20 or < 20/40) (AAP, 1996).
	Refer if two-line difference between eyes (i.e., 10/12.5 and 10/20, or 20/25 and 20/40) (AAP, 1996).
	*Cover test at 10 ft. Refer for any eye movement (AAP, 1996).
	*Random-dot–E stereo test at 40 cm (630 seconds of arc). Refer if < 4 of 6 correct (AAP, 1996).
6 years	*Check visual acuity.
	Refer if < 4 of 6 correct on 15-ft line with either eye tested at 10 ft (i.e., < 10/15 or < 20/30) (AAP, 1996).
	Refer if two-line difference between eyes (i.e., 10/10 and 10/15, or 20/20 and 20/30) (AAP, 1996).
7 years	Stereoacuity at adult level.
10 years	End of critical period for monocular visual deprivation.

Sources: American Academy of Pediatrics (AAP, 1996); Edward and Kaufman (2003).
*Denotes required tests that may result in ophthalmology referral. An older child failing a test that results in referral at a younger age should also be referred.

disease that can be missed by non-ophthalmologists at a time when visual deficits are still amenable to treatment. These authors also recommended routine follow-up ophthalmology evaluations at least every 4–5 years. There is a consensus that examinations by a pediatric ophthalmologist are indicated in children with developmental disabilities such as cerebral palsy (Ashwal et al., 2004).

Visual Acuity

Visual acuity refers to the ability to resolve two closely spaced points. Visual acuity is denoted by a fraction in which the numerator is the distance to the target and the denominator is the distance at which a normal adult can distinguish the target features. For instance, 20/40 indicates that, from 20 ft, the patient can distinguish a target that a normal adult can discern from 40 ft. If the patient cannot see the largest target, which often corresponds with 20/400 vision, the target can be moved closer, or it can be noted whether the patient can count outstretched fingers ("count fingers vision"), can identify hand movement ("hand motions vision"), or can see light but not form ("light perception vision").

Young children and some patients with disabilities cannot verbalize the identity of a visual target. Therefore, objective examination techniques are used to assess the level of vision. As noted earlier, observation while discussing the history often clarifies whether the child spontaneously fixates on faces or other targets of interest. A toy, a brightly colored object, or a penlight can be passed in front of the child to see if the child can fixate on and follow the target. If the child succeeds with both eyes open, each eye should be tested individually. The child may object more strenuously when one eye is covered compared with the other. This fixation preference suggests a difference in visual acuity between the eyes.

Optokinetic nystagmus is elicited by spinning a drum with vertical stripes to elicit slow horizontal ocular pursuit followed by rapid return saccades. Optokinetic nystagmus is tested at near and corresponds with a vision of at least 20/200 to 20/400.

Babies and nonverbal patients can be tested by preferential looking techniques. Older children can be tested with a number of visual acuity charts that require progressively more sophisticated responses. The "tumbling E" chart has a series of letter Es that the child identifies as being oriented "up," "down," or "to the side." It is not useful to ask the child to distinguish orientation to the right or the left. Some children will not correctly describe the distant target but can match it with an image on a near-vision card. Some children will not be able to determine the orientation of the letter E but can match the orientation of a picture of a hand with their own hand. Visual acuity charts with standardized shapes can be used. The child may need to be familiarized with the shape names at near. Older children and adults can be tested with the standard Snellen or other alphabetical charts. In general, it is helpful to use the method that requires the most sophisticated response that the child can muster. Because children of the same age may vary in their verbal abilities, several charts may need to be tried. Although children are known to test better on average on the simpler tests, there is wide interindividual and intraindividual variation. In practice, the best reproducible response is used for clinical decisions, although all results are documented.

Referral to an ophthalmologist should be made if there is a two-line intereye difference in visual acuity, or if visual acuity is worse than 20/40 at ages 3–5 or worse than 20/30 at age 6 (see Table 25.1).

Visual Fields

The peripheral visual field can be tested by confrontation, using the examiner's visual field as a control. In current clinical practice, management decisions about glaucoma and other optic neuropathies are usually based on automated perimetry of the central 24 or 30 degrees. Automated perimetry of the more peripheral visual field is not reliable enough to be routinely useful. Testing of the more peripheral visual field is typically done with Goldmann kinetic perimetry, or using a manual wall-mounted tangent screen.

Visual Impairment Categories

Visual impairment grading is important for determining qualification for social services and occupations, as well as the best low-vision aids. Most schemes for categorizing visual impairment are based on visual acuity as well as the horizontal peripheral visual field. For instance, in the United States, legal blindness is defined as a corrected visual acuity of 20/200 or less, or a visual field of 20 degrees or less. Driving requirements vary from state to state and for whether driving is commercial or noncommercial. In the United States, corrected visual acuity of 20/40 or better is required in both eyes for interstate commercial driving. A low-vision specialist should be consulted when long-term severe visual impairment is expected. Of course, this assessment will consider aspects of visual function besides visual acuity and fields, such as accommodation, contrast sensitivity, and occupational or other visual needs.

Eye Alignment

Assessment of eye alignment begins simply by watching the child while interviewing the parents. Some ocular deviations will vary based on the direction of gaze, target distance, level of fatigue, or other factors. The child may not cooperate with attempts to elicit different gaze directions during the examination. Therefore, the more time spent watching the child, the better.

The examiner attempts to determine if both eyes are aligned on the same target. Ocular deviation may be medial (esotropia), lateral (exotropia), upward (hypertropia), or downward (hypotropia). At all ages, ocular alignment can be assessed by holding a penlight in front of the eyes and examining the reflection in the cornea, termed the *corneal light reflex*. Fixation on the penlight with either eye should result in a well-centered corneal light reflection in both eyes.

If the patient can fixate with both eyes, one can perform the cover test for a manifest deviation, termed a *tropia*. Here, the examiner simply covers the eye that appears to be fixating. If the other eye moves in any direction to fixate on the target, then that eye was indeed not previously fixating on the target and a tropia is present. One must test both eyes several times to be certain.

Sometimes no manifest deviation is present, but the patient has an underlying tendency for deviation, termed a *phoria*. The total deviation (phoria plus tropia) is elicited by the alternate cover test. One eye is covered to eliminate fusion, and the uncovered eye fixates on a target. Then, the occluder is rapidly moved to the other eye. If the previously covered eye moves to fixate on the target, then a phoria, apparent only in the absence of fusion, is present. A small phoria may be a normal finding; however, if the family describes a tropia outside the office, then a phoria on alternate cover testing may represent an intermittent tropia, and referral decisions should be made as if a tropia were seen in the office.

Nystagmus

Nystagmus, or rhythmic extraocular movements, may be either sensory or motor in origin. Severe visual deprivation will result in nystagmus. Multiple inherited conditions are associated with nystagmus (see Table 25.2 later). Severe congenital nystagmus decreases foveation time, which lowers visual acuity. Medical, optical, or surgical treatments that reduce eye movement can improve visual acuity (Maybodi, 2003). Retrobulbar or intramuscular botulinum toxin injection can reduce nystagmus amplitude, but for children or any person with developmental disability who cannot tolerate in-office procedures, the necessity for periodic re-injections makes this impractical. Horizontal rectus muscle recessions have been used successfully in children with no null point (Alio, Chipont, Mulet, & De La Hoz, 2003), and recession/resection procedures are used if a null point is observed (Maybodi, 2003; Pratt-Johnson, 1991).

Spasmus nutans is a benign high-frequency oscillation seen in young children in association with torticollis and head bobbing. The condition resolves spontaneously, but a magnetic resonance imaging (MRI) scan should be obtained to rule out chiasmal tumors.

Ophthalmoscopy

Clarity of the ocular media is assessed at all ages with the red reflex test, in which an ophthalmoscope is used from a distance of a few feet and a red retinal reflection should be seen through the pupil. A dark red reflex may represent a severe refractive error, a very small pupil, strabismus, or cataract or other media opacity. A white red reflex may represent retinoblastoma or exudative retinal processes such as Coats' disease. An abnormal red reflex requires a referral.

The direct ophthalmoscope can also be used in cooperative children to examine the fundus, including the optic nerve. The high magnification of the direct ophthalmoscope is associated with a narrow field that does not permit viewing in the presence of substantial eye movement. Therefore, ophthalmologists typically use the indirect ophthalmoscope to obtain a wide-field view of the fundus even with uncooperative patients. Scleral depression with topical anesthesia is used to stabilize the eye and see the peripheral retina.

Pupils

Constriction of the pupils in response to light occurs by a reflex arc that is present to some degree at 30 weeks' gestational age and reliably at 34 weeks. Pupillary fibers leave the posterior portion of the optic tract to reach the midbrain at the level of the superior colliculus, where they synapse in the pretectal nuclei. Efferent fibers from each pretectal nucleus pass to both the right and left Edinger-Westphal nuclei, with decussating fibers running both anterior and posterior (in the posterior commissure) to the cerebral aqueduct. Preganglionic parasympathetic fibers pass from the Edinger-Westphal nucleus via the inferior division of the third cranial (oculomotor) nerve to synapse in the ciliary ganglion of the orbit. The postganglionic short ciliary nerves include fibers for both iris constriction and ciliary muscle action (accommodation).

Of note, partial decussation of fibers in the optic chiasm and of fibers leading to the Edinger-Westphal nuclei results in equal efferent pupillomotor output to both eyes. There-fore, if a flashlight is passed quickly from one eye to the other, the direction of pupillary movement will be the same in both eyes. In other words, the pupils of both eyes will either constrict, dilate, or remain unchanged. Only the last response is normal. Constriction of the pupils of both eyes means that the afferent system of the second eye transmits a stronger impulse, and the first eye has a relative afferent pupillary defect. Dilation of the pupils of both eyes means that the second eye has an afferent pupillary defect. An afferent pupillary defect always requires an ophthalmology referral. The most common cause of an afferent pupillary defect is optic nerve disease. Sometimes a high degree of retinal disease, dense media opacities (vitreous hemorrhage, but not cataract), or amblyopia can cause an afferent pupillary defect. When performing the swinging flashlight test, it is important to test in the dark and to hold the light in front of each eye long enough to permit system equilibration before rapidly swinging the light to the other eye.

Intraocular Pressure

The intraocular pressure is a universal measurement during adult ophthalmology visits, but the difficulty in obtaining the pressure in uncooperative patients means that it is obtained less often in children. Pediatricians are not expected to routinely check the pressure, but it is reasonable to palpate the eye gently if there is a clinical question. Applanation tonometry at the slit lamp, the standard in adults, cannot be done in uncooperative patients. Therefore, the Tono-Pen is routinely used in the office in children, although lid squeezing, crying, and moving may cause errors. During examination under anesthesia, the weighted Schiötz tonometer, the Perkins applanation tonometer, or the Tono-Pen can be used.

Congenital glaucoma produces symptoms of epiphora, photophobia, and blepharospasm. Any of these findings should prompt ophthalmological referral if another cause is not obvious. Congenital glaucoma produces corneal edema, an enlarged eye (buphthalmos), elevated intraocular pressure, and optic disc cupping. The normal horizontal corneal diameter is 9.5–10.5 mm at birth and 10–11.5 mm at age

1 year. Glaucoma is suggested by a horizontal corneal diameter more than 1 mm above these limits or in excess of 13 mm at any age (American Academy of Ophthalmology, 2004).

Electrophysiology

Visual electrophysiology may be used to help determine the site and severity of visual disturbance. The electroretinogram records the electrical response of the retina to a bright flash of light or to an alternating checkerboard pattern. The size of the checkerboard producing a response can help assess the visual acuity. The visual evoked potential records the electroencephalographic response to visual stimulation. Visual electrophysiologic responses mature substantially during the first year and especially the first 6 months of life (Brecelj, 2003; Edward & Kaufman, 2003). Therefore, the laboratory must have experience with and knowledge of the expected responses with their protocol if infants are tested.

PEDIATRIC OPHTHALMOLOGY FINDINGS

A number of childhood eye disturbances are routine in pediatric ophthalmology. Because multiple pediatric disorders have both ophthalmological and neurological effects (Table 25.2), visual disorders are even more common in multiple types of developmental disability.

Prematurity

Prematurity is associated with both visual and neurological impairment. The most devastating ophthalmological complication is retinopathy of prematurity (ROP). The child is born before the retina is completely vascularized. The peripheral avascularized retina is presumably ischemic and secretes neovascular growth factors. Fibrovascular proliferation into the vitreous at the border between the vascularized and avascular retina leads to retinal detachment and, therefore, blindness. All infants under 1,500 g or of gestational age of 30 weeks or less must be screened by an ophthalmologist for ROP. The first examination is performed at 31–33 weeks' postgestational age (American

Academy of Pediatrics, 2006). Retinal detachment can be prevented in many infants by ablation of the peripheral avascular retina with cryotherapy. More recently, peripheral retinal laser photocoagulation has been found to be effective and better tolerated. One major sign that ocular stress is severe enough to lead to retinal detachment is the presence of significant vascular tortuosity and dilation, termed *"plus" disease*. The current criteria for laser treatment from the Early Treatment for Retinopathy of Prematurity (ETROP) study rely heavily on the presence of plus disease, although fibrovascular proliferation and posterior location of the avascular retinal border also play a role (Good, 2004).

Lowering ambient light levels has been found not to affect the likelihood of retinopathy. The presence of retinopathy in children who are sick enough to require high levels of inspired oxygen, the higher peripheral oxygen tensions potentially present after birth, and the theoretical role of oxidative damage have led to the commonly held notion that oxygen causes ROP. Clearly, inspired oxygen tensions over one-half atmosphere cause pulmonary damage in people of any age. As a practical matter, one needs to provide enough oxygen to avoid peripheral ischemia but not enough to cause pulmonary and possibly ocular damage. This issue was addressed empirically in the Supplemental Therapeutic Oxygen for Prethreshold Retinopathy of Prematurity (STOP-ROP) study, which compared conventional oxygen saturation (89%–94%) with higher target saturation levels (96%–99%) in premature infants with prethreshold retinopathy (Supplemental Therapeutic Oxygen, 2005). As one might expect, it was found that higher levels of oxygenation resulted in more cases of pulmonary complications, longer hospitalizations, and a higher mortality rate. There was no difference, however, between the two groups in terms of the progression of retinopathy.

Premature babies are also more likely to have refractive errors, strabismus, and glaucoma. Therefore, they need to have regular eye examinations throughout childhood. Infant formulas containing two long-chain polyunsaturated fatty acids, arachidonic acid and docosahexaenoic acid, are now commercially

Table 25.2. Disorders causing both ocular and neurological impairment

Disorder	Eye findings	Other findings	Inheritance/etiology
Associated with pigmentary retinopathy			
Refsum disease	Retinitis pigmentosa, optic atrophy	Ataxia, polyneuropathy, deafness, anosmia, distal extremity weakness, cardiac arrhythmias	AR/phytanic acid accumulation due to phytanoyl-CoA hydroxylase deficiency
Laurence-Moon-Bardet-Biedl syndrome	Retinitis pigmentosa	ID, polydactyly, obesity, hypogenitalism, paraplegia	AR/multiple loci
Usher syndrome	Retinitis pigmentosa	SNHL: type 1 (ataxia), type 2 (no ataxia, less severe SNHL)	AR
Bassen-Kornzweig syndrome (abetalipoproteinemia)	Retinitis pigmentosa, restrictive ocular motility	Spinocerebellar ataxia, acanthocytosis, celiac disease, diarrhea	Abetalipoproteinemia, mutation in microsomal triglyceride transfer protein gene
Kearns-Sayre syndrome	Progressive external ophthalmoplegia after age 5, "salt and pepper" pigmentary retinopathy with normal arterioles, rarely bone spicules, nyctalopia, ptosis Onset younger than age 20, possibly in infancy	Heart block, SNHL, vestibular dysfunction, cerebellar ataxia, corticospinal dysfunction, muscular dystrophy, ID, spongiform CNS degeneration, short stature, diabetes mellitus Treat with coenzyme Q10	Usually sporadic/mitochondrial DNA deletion
Cockayne syndrome	Pigmentary retinal degeneration, cataracts, optic atrophy	ID, dwarfism, deafness, progeria, photosensitive rashes	AR/chromosome 5 (Cockayne syndrome type A gene) or chromosome 10 (helicase)
Alstrom syndrome	Cone–rod retinal dystrophy	SNHL, diabetes mellitus, obesity, dilated cardiomyopathy	AR/chromosome 2p13 (Hearn et al., 2002)
Olivopontocerebellar atrophy (a spinocerebellar ataxia)	Pigmentary retinal degeneration, nystagmus, slow saccades, optic atrophy	Cerebellar and brain stem atrophy, dementia, dysphagia, dysarthria	AD/*SCA1* and *SCA2* genes on chromosomes 6 and 12, respectively (Koeppen, 1998)
Neuronal ceroid lipofuscinosis (Batten disease)	Pigmentary retinal degeneration, optic atrophy, ERG extinction	Cerebral atrophy, ataxia, seizures, dementia	AR/multiple lysosomal gene mutations (Mole, Mitchison, & Munroe, 1999)
Zellweger (hepatocerebrorenal) syndrome	Infantile pigmentary retinal degeneration, nystagmus, hypertelorism, cataract, microphthalmia	Psychomotor retardation, hypotonia, seizures, dysmorphic features, renal cortical cysts, hepatosplenomegaly	AR/abnormality in peroxisomal enzymes on chromosomes 8, 1, or 7
Neonatal adrenoleukodystrophy	Cataract, optic atrophy, pigmentary retinopathy	Psychomotor retardation, ID, seizures, adrenal insufficiency	AR
Metabolic storage diseases			
Tay-Sachs disease (GM_2 gangliosidosis type I)	Foveal cherry-red spot, optic atrophy, abnormal visual evoked responses	ID, muscle weakness, seizures	AR/hexosaminidase A deficiency (chromosome 15) (Kaback & Desnick, 2001)

(continued)

Table 25.2.   *(continued)*

Disorder	Eye findings	Other findings	Inheritance/etiology
Sandhoff disease (GM$_2$ gangliosidosis type II)	Foveal cherry-red spot	ID, muscle weakness, hepatosplenomegaly	AR/hexosaminidase A and B deficiency (chromosome 5)
Generalized gangliosidosis (GM$_1$ gangliosidosis type I)	Foveal cherry-red spot, optic atrophy, corneal clouding	Developmental delay/ arrest, neurological deterioration, hepatosplenomegaly, skeletal dysplasia	AR/β-galactosidase deficiency (chromosome 3) (Suzuki et al., 1991)
Mucolipidosis type I (cherry-red spot–myoclonus syndrome)	Foveal cherry-red spot, optic atrophy, corneal opacities, lamellar cataracts	Ataxia, myoclonic epilepsy, hepatosplenomegaly	AR/neuraminidase (sialidase) deficiency (chromosome 6) (Bonten et al., 2000)
Mucopolysaccharidosis I H (Hurler syndrome) and I S (Scheie syndrome)	Retinal pigmentary degeneration with spiculated appearance, optic atrophy, progressive corneal opacity without edema, ERG abnormalities	ID, coarse facies, short stature, joint stiffness, dysostosis multiplex, rhinitis, enlarged tongue. Type I S is less severe than type I H.	AR/deficiency of lysosomal α-L-iduronidase with accumulation of dermatan sulfate and heparan sulfate (chromosome 4) (Scott et al., 1990)
Mucopolysaccharidosis II (Hunter syndrome)	Retinal pigmentary degeneration with arteriolar narrowing, optic atrophy, corneal clouding, ERG abnormalities	ID, coarse facies, short stature	XR
Mucopolysaccharidosis III (Sanfilippo syndrome)	Retinal pigmentary degeneration with spiculated appearance, optic atrophy, corneal clouding, ERG abnormalities	ID, coarse facies, short stature	AR
Niemann-Pick disease	Foveal cherry-red spot (primarily in type A), anterior capsular brownish opacification and posterior capsular cataract	ID in infantile (type A), lung disease, hepatosplenomegaly, short stature, pancytopenia	AR/sphingomyelinase deficiency (chromosome 11p15): sphingomyelin accumulation in lysosomes of macrophages
Angiokeratoma corporis diffusum (Fabry disease)	Cream-colored corneal verticillata; posterior spoke-like subcapsular, punctate, or wedge-shaped cataracts; conjunctival or retinal vascular abnormalities; normal vision	Cutaneous angiokeratomas, hypohydrosis, acral pain and paresthesias, renal cysts and failure, myocardial ischemia, febrile crises, cerebral ischemia or hemorrhage, seizures	XR/α-galactosidase-A deficiency (chromosome Xq22): accumulation of glycosphingolipids, including globotriaosylceramide
Phakomatoses			
Neurofibromatosis type 1 (von Recklinghausen disease)	Lisch nodules (iris hamartomas) in almost 100% of type 1 by age 21. Relatives should be examined for Lisch nodules. Optic nerve glioma, glaucoma, conjunctival neurofibromas, enlarged corneal nerves, pulsatile proptosis	ID, learning disabilities, seizures, neurofibromas, axillary and inguinal freckling, sphenoid hypoplasia, glioma, pheochromocytoma	AD/chromosome 17

Neurofibromatosis type 2	Posterior subcapsular cataracts, optic nerve gliomas and meningiomas	Vertigo, seizures, ID, acoustic neuromas, hearing loss, CNS glioma, meningioma, pheochromocytoma	AD/chromosome 22
Tuberous sclerosis (Bourneville disease)	Retinal or optic nerve astrocytic hamartoma	Seizures, ID possible, CNS astrocytic hamartomas, achromic nevi (ash-leaf spots), café-au-lait spots, shagreen patches; visceral hamartomas in kidneys, bone, and heart	AD/chromosome 9
Ataxia-telangiectasia (Louis-Bar syndrome)	Oculomotor apraxia, bulbar conjunctival telangiectasias	ID, progressive cerebellar ataxia in second year of life, skin telangiectasias, thymus hypoplasia, poor immune function, increased incidence of leukemia and lymphoma	AR/chromosome 11
Angiomatosis retinae (von Hippel–Lindau disease)	Retinal capillary hemangiomas with dilated feeder vessels and associated hemorrhage or exudates	Cerebellar hemangioblastomas, renal cell carcinomas; cysts in pancreas, liver, epididymis, or ovaries; pheochromocytoma	AD/chromosome 3
Encephalofacial angiomatosis (Sturge-Weber syndrome)	Choroidal hemangiomas, glaucoma ipsilateral to eyelid or conjunctival hemangiomas	Seizure, ID, CNS and meningeal hemangiomas, facial hemangioma, nevus flammeus present at birth	Sporadic occurrence
Racemose angioma (Wyburn-Mason syndrome)	Retinal arteriovenous anastomoses	ID; intracranial, especially midbrain, arteriovenous malformations with calcification	Sporadic occurrence
Other genetic conditions			
Joubert syndrome	Congenital retinal dystrophy, oculomotor abnormalities	Cerebellar hypoplasia, ataxia, ID, episodic hyperventilation	AR
Leber congenital amaurosis	Poor vision, sluggish pupillary responses, large-amplitude nystagmus within first few months, eye pressing (ocular digital sign)	ID, seizures, SNHL in 5%	AR/rod–cone dystrophy
	Retina normal initially, then with vessel attenuation, optic disc pallor, retinal pigment changes		
	Hyperopia, keratoconus, abnormal or absent ERG		

(continued)

Table 25.2. *(continued)*

Disorder	Eye findings	Other findings	Inheritance/etiology
Aicardi syndrome	Optic nerve hypoplasia, clear retinal lacunae	Seizures, infantile spasms, ID; lethal in boys, seen only in girls; absence of corpus callosum, gray matter abnormalities on MRI	
Down syndrome	Strabismus, nystagmus, keratoconus, total or punctate "snowflake" cataracts, myopia, astigmatism, glaucoma, ptosis, Brushfield spots (yellow iris spots), epicanthal folds, eyelid laxity	ID, large tongue, facial hypoplasia, short and webbed neck, short digits, palmar crease, congenital heart disease	Trisomy 21
Friedreich's ataxia	Optic atrophy, nystagmus	Spinocerebellar degeneration, ataxia, SNHL	AR/*FRDA* gene on chromosome 9, which encodes frataxin (Bradley et al., 2000)
Septo-optic dysplasia (de Morsier syndrome)	Optic nerve hypoplasia	Absence of septum pellucidum and agenesis or thinning of the corpus callosum, pituitary abnormalities, encephalocele. Brain MRI and endocrine evaluation warranted	Usually sporadic, can be AR/*HESX1* gene mutations (Bennett, 2002)
Albinism	Foveal and optic nerve hypoplasia, nystagmus, reduced visual acuity, iris transillumination defects, refractive errors, strabismus, decreased proportion of uncrossed fibers at optic chiasm	ID and immune defects (in Chédiak-Higashi syndrome)	AR (Chédiak-Higashi syndrome)/Tyrosinase negative in complete oculocutaneous form
Galactosemia	Oil droplet, lamellar, nuclear, or total cataract shortly after birth in 75%	Lethargy, hypotonia, hepatomegaly, sepsis, poor growth, language deficits. Treat with galactose restriction	AR/defect of galactose-1-phosphate uridyltransferase at chromosome 9p13
Aniridia	Iris hypoplasia or absence, nystagmus, anterior polar or disk-like cataracts, foveal hypoplasia, glaucoma	ID, Wilms' tumor in sporadic patients	⅔ AD, ⅓ sporadic/chromosome 11 deletion
Homocystinuria	Myopia, lens subluxation, cataracts, glaucoma, pigmentary retinal degeneration	ID, marfanoid appearance, thromboembolism, leg weakness	AR/deficiency of cystathionine synthase with accumulation of homocysteine (chromosome 21q22.3) (Kraus, 1994)

Lowe's (oculocerebrorenal) syndrome	Cataracts, glaucoma Carriers have punctate cortical opacities	Hypotonia, ID, rickets, aminoaciduria	AR or XR/decreased renal ammonia production
Cornelia de Lange syndrome	Common: myopia, ptosis, nystagmus Also: optic atrophy, optic nerve colobomas, microcornea, astigmatism, strabismus	Prematurity, intrauterine growth retardation, low-pitched weak cry, initial hypertonicity, ID	Usually sporadic, rarely AD or AR
Myotonic dystrophy (Steinert disease)	"Christmas tree" or posterior subcapsular cataract	Swallowing and speech disability, muscle wasting	AD
Congenital infections and toxins			
Congenital cytomegalovirus (CMV) infection	Chorioretinal inflammation, retinal hemorrhage	ID, intrauterine growth retardation, hepatosplenomegaly, petechiae, cerebral atrophy, cerebral calcifications, SNHL in 1% of newborns with congenital CMV infection	Maternal infection with CMV
Congenital toxoplasmosis	Retinochoroiditis, focal atrophic and pigmented scars, focal vitritis	Cerebral calcifications, convulsions, fever, hydrocephalus, microcephaly	Maternal infection with *Toxoplasma gondii*
Congenital rubella	"Salt and pepper" retinopathy, nuclear or total cataract, glaucoma, microphthalmos	Cardiac defects, deafness	Maternal infection during first trimester
Herpes simplex, intrauterine	Chorioretinitis, microphthalmos	Encephalitis	Intrauterine disease less likely than transplacental acquisition
Congenital syphilis	Choroiditis	Hepatosplenomegaly, pneumonia, rhinitis, neurosyphilis, skin lesions	Transplacental passage of *Treponema pallidum*
Fetal alcohol syndrome	Small palpebral fissures (blepharophimosis), ptosis, telecanthus, anterior segment dysgenesis, strabismus, corneal opacities, optic nerve hypoplasia, retinal vascular tortuosity	Cognitive impairment, congenital heart disease, facial abnormalities with absence of philtrum and a broad upper lip	Maternal ethanol ingestion
Cerebral palsy	Strabismus, optic atrophy, nystagmus, refractive errors (Ashwal et al., 2004)	Posture or movement disorder caused by lesion of the developing brain	Multiple etiologies: genetic, toxic, infectious, vascular insufficiency

Key: AD, autosomal dominant; AR, autosomal recessive; CNS, central nervous system; CoA, coenzyme A; ERG, electroretinography; ID, intellectual disabilities; MRI, magnetic resonance imaging; SNHL, sensorineural hearing loss; XR, X-linked recessive.

available. The latter has been shown to result in better visual acuity, particularly in preterm infants (Carver, 2003).

Refractive Errors

Significant refractive errors are quite common in the general pediatric population and are found in more than 40% of patients with intellectual disabilities (van Splunder, Stilma, Bernsen, Arentz, & Evenhuis, 2003; Warburg, 2001). Correction of refractive errors can have lifelong visual benefits. The pediatrician is not expected to perform refraction testing. Refraction testing can be performed even in nonverbal or young patients by retinoscopy with a skiascopy rack. In verbal patients, this refraction test can be subjectively refined.

Amblyopia

Amblyopia is a unilateral or bilateral decrease in visual acuity caused by an absolute or relative absence of a clear image, or by strabismus, during the visual development period. Amblyopia is not associated with any anatomic findings on clinical examination. Amblyopia is found in approximately 2%–4% of the North American population and is highly treatable during the visual development period (American Academy of Ophthalmology, 2004). This period was historically regarded as ending at age 8, although Scheiman et al. (2005) have shown that some visual acuity improvement can be attained at least through age 12 and possibly through age 17. Younger children have a higher probability of successful treatment. For instance, in a trial of patching for amblyopia, children age 5 or 6 improved 3.8 lines, while children age 3 or 4 improved 5.5 lines, a 50% difference (Holmes et al., 2003).

Initial treatment consists of refractive correction. If some degree of amblyopia persists, vision in the better eye is reduced by patching, by eliminating accommodation with atropine, or by optical blurring. By forcing the patient to use the amblyopic eye, treatment improves the ability to process visual input from this eye. Randomized studies have demonstrated that both atropine and patching are effective and that patching regimens involving fewer hours

during the day are effective (Holmes et al., 2003). Finally, strabismus is corrected if present.

Strabismus

Strabismus represents a misalignment of the eyes and can result in permanent loss of visual acuity or stereopsis. Most childhood strabismus is comitant, that is, the deviation is the same in all directions of gaze. A small exotropia is present in many newborns and usually disappears spontaneously as fusional mechanisms develop.

Concomitant esotropia in childhood is typically divided into two major types: infantile and accommodative. Onset of infantile esotropia is at several months of age. The deviation may be large-angle and is not typically associated with hyperopia. Correction requires strabismus surgery or botulinum toxin injection (McNeer, Tucker, & Spencer, 1997). Patients older than age 4 months with constant large-angle (> 40 prism diopters) esotropia without significant hyperopia can be considered for early surgery (Hutcheson, 2004).

Accommodative esotropia occurs after 1 year of age and is associated with an intermittent angle, usually worse at near, and hyperopia. The accommodation required to obtain a clear image in the setting of hyperopia is associated with convergence. In some cases, the child is not unusually hyperopic, but accommodation is associated with an unusually high degree of near convergence. Accommodative esotropia is treated with refractive correction.

These types of esotropia are not mutually exclusive. Some early-onset esotropia is associated with hyperopia, and refractive correction is a reasonable first step even though strabismus surgery may be necessary later. Likewise, surgery may be necessary to treat residual deviation after refractive correction of late-onset accommodative esotropia.

Cataract

Congenital cataract is detected with the red reflex examination and requires immediate ophthalmological referral. Cataracts are found in 8%–54% of patients with intellectual disabilities (Wu, Amini, Leffler, & Schwartz, 2005) and are seen in many developmental conditions (see Table 25.2). Childhood cataract morphology is related to the associated systemic condition (Amaya, Taylor, Russell-Eggitt, Nischal, & Lengyel, 2003). Associated systemic disorders are usually apparent at the time of cataract evaluation. A TORCH titer (toxoplasmosis, other infections, rubella, cytomegalovirus, and herpes simplex virus), red blood cell transferase level, and galactokinase level constitute the basic metabolic workup to rule out galactosemia and congenital infections. More extensive metabolic evaluation may be warranted in selected cases (Buckley, Tesser, & Hess, 2005).

Surgical removal of severe congenital cataracts is indicated. Aphakic spectacles can be worn if cataracts are removed bilaterally. Comparison of optical correction with a contact lens versus intraocular lens implantation in cases of unilateral infantile cataract is an area of ongoing investigation (Lambert et al., 2003). Congenital cataract surgery may be associated with late-onset glaucoma.

Delayed Visual Maturation

An apparently delayed ability to see despite the absence of other developmental delays is termed *delayed visual maturation* (Mercuri et al., 1997). The family notices an inability to fixate on targets. A complete eye examination is indicated. Sometimes correction of hyperopia is associated with resolution. An MRI scan may be indicated to search for neurological abnormalities. Visual electrophysiology can document the degree of function of the retina and optic nerve.

Retinal Disorders

A number of disorders associated with developmental delay or disability can produce retinal disease. Metabolic storage diseases result in accumulation of light-colored metabolic precursors in retinal ganglion cells surrounding the fovea, resulting in the appearance of a "cherry-red spot" in the macula (see Table 25.2). Retinitis pigmentosa describes a group of inherited conditions that diffusely affect photoreceptor and pigment epithelial function, resulting in visual field constriction and abnormal electroretinogram responses. Many causes of pigmentary retinopathy are associated with neurological findings. It is particularly important to diagnose treatable causes. Refsum disease, associated with high serum phytanic acid levels, is treated with a low–phytanic acid and low-phytol diet. Hereditary abetalipoproteinemia (Bassen-Kornzweig syndrome) is associated with decreased serum apolipoprotein B levels and is treated with supplementation of vitamins A, E, and K and dietary fat restriction. Kearns-Sayre syndrome, associated with ptosis and ophthalmoplegia, may require a pacemaker to prevent atrioventricular block and may benefit to some degree from coenzyme Q10 administration. Congenital syphilis can be identified with standard treponemal serology.

Optic Nerve Disorders

Optic atrophy is noted as optic nerve pallor, loss of the disc capillary net, or nerve fiber layer dropout. Any congenital or acquired process that damages the retinal ganglion cells or their axons can produce optic nerve atrophy. Compressive lesions, trauma, hydrocephalus, and hereditary conditions can cause optic atrophy. Associated disorders include cerebral palsy, retinitis pigmentosa, and metabolic storage diseases (see Table 25.2).

Optic nerve hypoplasia consists of a unilateral or bilateral congenitally small optic nerve with a surrounding halo of scleral tissue. This yellow outer ring produces the so-called double-ring sign. The border of the inner ring represents the termination of the retinal pigment epithelium. The total size of the optic nerve plus the peripapillary halo is equal to the size of the normal optic disc. A poor foveal light reflex or vessel tortuosity may also be seen. Optic nerve hypoplasia is seen in multiple conditions, including septo-optic dysplasia (de Morsier syndrome), albinism, aniridia, and Aicardi syndrome (see Table 25.2). Maternal gestational diabetes and maternal exposure to alcohol, phenytoin, and corticosteroids are also associated with optic nerve hypoplasia (Sergott & Hug, 2005). Visual acuity is variable. In asymmetrical cases, a portion of the vision drop may be amenable to amblyopia therapy. An MRI scan to evaluate for the midline brain structure of de Morsier syndrome is indicated. An endocrinological evaluation is critical because patients with de Morsier syndrome may have life-threatening pituitary abnormalities, as well as treatable growth hormone deficiency.

CONCLUSION

The fundamentals of visual assessment and treatment in children with developmental disabilities are the same as for all children. Proper assessment of the red reflex, eye alignment, ocular motility, visual acuity, stereopsis, and pupils will result in appropriate ophthalmologic referrals. Timely treatment of retinopathy of prematurity, refractive errors, cataracts, amblyopia, and strabismus can have a lifelong impact on ultimate visual outcome. Numerous developmental disorders affect both the neurologic and visual systems. Therefore, ophthalmologic disorders are more common in individuals with developmental disabilities, and a baseline assessment by an ophthalmologist is essential. Whenever there is doubt about the proper functioning of the visual system, an ophthalmologic evaluation is warranted.

REFERENCES

Alio, J.L., Chipont, E., & De La Hoz, F. (2003). Visual performance after congenital nystagmus surgery using extended hang back recession of the four horizontal rectus muscles. *European Journal of Ophthalmology, 13,* 415–423.

Amaya, L., Taylor, D., Russell-Eggitt, I., Nischal, K.K., & Lengyel, D. (2003). The morphology and natural history of childhood cataracts. *Survey of Ophthalmology, 48,* 125–144.

American Academy of Ophthalmology. (Ed.). (2004). *Basic and clinical science course: Section 6. Pediatric ophthalmology and strabismus.* San Francisco: Author.

American Academy of Pediatrics, Committee on Practice and Ambulatory Medicine, Section on Ophthalmology. (1996). Vision screening guidelines. *Pediatrics, 98,* 156.

American Academy of Pediatrics, Section on Ophthalmology; American Academy of Ophthalmology; & American Association for Pediatric Ophthalmology and Strabismus. (2006). Screening examination of premature infants for retinopathy

of prematurity. *Pediatrics, 117*(2), 572–576. (Erratum in *Pediatrics, 188*[3], 1324)

Ashwal, S., Russman, B.S., Blasco, P.A., Miller, G., Sandler, A., Shevell, M., et al. (2004). Practice parameter. Diagnostic assessment of the child with cerebral palsy: Report of the Quality Standards Subcommittee of the American Academy of Neurology and the Practice Committee of the Child Neurology Society. *Neurology, 62,* 851–863.

Bennett, J.L. (2002). Developmental neurogenetics and neuro-ophthalmology. *Journal of Neuroophthalmology, 22,* 286–296.

Bonten, E.J., Arts, W.F., Beck, M., Covanis, A., Donati, M.A., Parini, R., et al. (2000). Novel mutations in lysosomal neuraminidase identify functional domains and determine clinical severity in sialosis. *Human Molecular Genetics, 9,* 2715–2725.

Bradley, J.L., Blake, J.C., Chamberlain, S., Thomas, P.K., Cooper, J.M., & Schapira, A.H. (2000). Clinical, biochemical, and molecular genetic correlations in Friedreich's ataxia. *Human Molecular Genetics, 9,* 275–282.

Brecelj, J. (2003). From immature to mature pattern ERG and VEP. *Documenta Ophthalmologica, 107,* 215–224.

Buckley, E.G., Tesser, R.S., & Hess, D.B. (2005). Pediatric cataracts and lens anomalies. In L.B. Nelson & S.E. Olitsky (Eds.), *Harley's pediatric ophthalmology* (5th ed., pp. 255–284). Baltimore: Lippincott, Williams & Wilkins.

Carver, J.D. (2003). Advances in nutritional modifications of infant formulas. *American Journal of Clinical Nutrition, 77*(Suppl), 1550S–1554S.

Edward, D.P., & Kaufman, L.M. (2003). Anatomy, development and physiology of the visual system. *Pediatric Clinics of North America, 50,* 1–23.

Friedman, L.S., & Kaufman, L.M. (2003). Guidelines for pediatrician referrals to the ophthalmologist. *Pediatric Clinics of North America, 50,* 41–53.

Good, W.V., for the Early Treatment for Retinopathy of Prematurity Cooperative Group. (2004). Final results of the Early Treatment for Retinopathy of Prematurity (ETROP) randomized trial. *Transactions of the American Ophthalmological Society, 102,* 233–248.

Hearn, T., Renforth, G.L., Spalluto, C., Hanley, N.A., Piper, K., Brickwood, S., et al. (2002). Mutation of *ALMS1,* a large gene with a tandem repeat encoding 47 amino acids, causes Alstrom syndrome. *Nature Genetics, 31,* 79–83.

Holmes, J.M., Kraker, R.T., Beck, R.W., Birch, E.E., Cotter, S.A., Everett, D.F., et al. (2003). A randomized trial of prescribed patching regimens for treatment of severe amblyopia in children. *Ophthalmology, 110,* 2075–2087.

Hutcheson, K.A. (2004). Childhood esotropia. *Current Opinion in Ophthalmology, 15,* 444–448.

Kaback, M.M., & Desnick, R.J. (2001) Tay-Sachs disease: From clinical description to molecular defect. *Advances in Genetics, 44,* 1–9.

Koeppen, A.H. (1998). The hereditary ataxias. *Journal of Neuropathology and Experimental Neurology, 57,* 531–543.

Kraus, J.P. (1994). Komrower Lecture. Molecular basis of phenotype expression in homocystinuria. *Journal of Inherited Metabolic Disease, 17,* 383–390.

Lambert, S.R., Lynn, M., Drews-Botsch, C., DuBois, L., Wilson, M.E., Plager, D.A., et al. (2003). Intraocular lens implantation during infancy. *Journal of the AAPOS, 7,* 400–405.

Maybodi, M. (2003). Infantile-onset nystagmus. *Current Opinion in Ophthalmology, 14,* 276–285.

McNeer, K.W., Tucker, M.G., & Spencer, R.F. (1997). Botulinum toxin management of essential infantile esotropia in children. *Archives of Ophthalmology, 115,* 1411–1418.

Mercuri, E., Atkinson, J., Braddick, O., Anker, S., Cowan, F., Pennock, J., et al. (1997). The aetiology of delayed visual maturation: Short review and personal findings in relation to magnetic resonance imaging. *European Journal of Paediatric Neurology, 1,* 31–34.

Mole, S.E., Mitchison, H.M., & Munroe, P.B. (1999). Molecular basis of the neuronal ceroid lipofuscinoses: Mutations in *CLN1, CLN2, CLN3,* and *CLN5. Human Mutation, 14,* 199–215.

Pratt-Johnson, J.A. (1991). Results of surgery to modify the null-zone position in congenital nystagmus. *Canadian Journal of Ophthalmology, 26,* 219–223.

Scheiman, M.M., Hertle, R.W., Beck, R.W., Edwards, A.R., Birch, E., Cotter, S.A., et al. (2005). Randomized trial of treatment of amblyopia in children aged 7 to 17 years. *Archives of Ophthalmology, 123,* 437–447.

Scott, H.S., Ashton, L.J., Eyre, H.J., Baker, E., Brooks, D.A., Callen, D.F., et al. (1990). Chromosomal localization of the human alpha-L-iduronidase gene (IDUA) to 4p16.3. *American Journal of Human Genetics, 47,* 802–807.

Sergott, R.C., & Hug, D. (2005). Pediatric neuro-ophthalmology. In L.B. Nelson & S.E. Olitsky (Eds.), *Harley's pediatric ophthalmology* (5th ed.). Baltimore: Lippincott, Williams & Wilkins.

Supplemental Therapeutic Oxygen for Prethreshold Retinopathy of Prematurity (STOP-ROP), a randomized, controlled trial. I: Primary outcomes. (2005). *Pediatrics, 105,* 295–310.

Suzuki, Y., Sakuraba, H., Oshima, A., Yoshida, K., Shimmoto, M., Takano, T., et al. (1991). Clinical and molecular heterogeneity in hereditary beta-galactosidase deficiency. *Developmental Neuroscience, 13,* 299–303.

Van Splunder, J., Stilma, J.S., Bernsen, R.M., Arentz, T.G., & Evenhuis, H.M. (2003). Refractive errors and visual impairment in 900 adults with intellectual disabilities in the Netherlands. *Acta Opthalmologica Scandinavica, 81,* 123–129.

Warburg, M. (2001). Visual impairment in adult people with moderate, severe, and profound intellectual disability. *Acta Ophthalmologica Scandinavica, 79,* 4504.

Wu, T.T., Amini, L., Leffler, C.T., & Schwartz, S.G. (2005). Cataracts and cataract surgery in mentally retarded adults. *Eye & Contact Lens, 31,* 50–53.

Practice Issues

V

26

Early Intervention and Its Efficacy

PAUL H. LIPKIN AND MITCHELL SCHERTZ

Early therapeutic intervention for the child with developmental disabilities is universally available in the United States for any infant or preschool child upon identification of a disability. The term *early intervention* (EI) has come to be used generically by professionals in the field of developmental disabilities to represent a wide array of developmentally based therapies or programs being used with children with developmental problems, or at "high risk" for such problems, during the infancy and preschool periods, with the intent of improving performance in one of the developmental spheres.

Although EI services are federally mandated and readily accessible, many issues regarding program efficacy remain unresolved. It is difficult to determine whether EI is effective without addressing such issues as what the intervention is, to whom it is being applied, and how one defines "efficacy." The following questions must be answered in any study of the efficacy of EI:

1. What is the population being treated? Is this a homogeneous treatment group, based on disability, age, or other demographic characteristics?

2. What is the intervention being applied? Is this treatment well defined?

3. How is "early" defined? At what age is the treatment being applied?

4. How is "efficacy" defined?

5. What is the outcome being measured?

6. When is the outcome being measured?

Because the studies of efficacy have differed in their answers to these questions, no single answer regarding program efficacy has emerged. Public consensus, however, has developed favoring such intervention based on some of the positive effects reported (Majnemer, 1998). Before reviewing the results of these studies, we present a brief history of EI and the federal mandates supporting it.

HISTORY OF EARLY INTERVENTION

The history of EI reveals the emergence of pilot programs geared toward improving the development of children with intellectual disabilities early in this century (Skeels & Dye, 1939). These "infant stimulation" programs, as they were called until only recently, grew in number during the 1950s and expanded to cover children with other disabilities, such as cerebral palsy (CP) (Denhoff, 1981). These programs emerged at a time when affected children were commonly placed in institutional settings for their long-term care. These new alternative programs instead emphasized individualized attention, family involvement, and parent support in the care of the children. As these programs evolved, the scope of services expanded from, initially, provision of isolated therapies focusing on a single disability, such as physical therapy for CP, to more comprehensive programming addressing multiple spheres of development, such as socialization, cognition, and communication. By the 1970s, many programs had emerged, but without clear guidelines, so the United Cerebral Palsy Associations and the Bureau of the Handicapped of the U.S. Department of Health, Education and Welfare developed a five-center study of infant stimulation program efficacy (Schilling, Siepp, Patterson, et al., 1974, cited in Denhoff, 1981). These centers adopted a set of principles that continue to guide services at the present time: 1) parents should be primary care providers, with most care provided in the home; 2) specially trained educators of infants and children with developmental disabilities will instruct parents in the care of the children; and 3) a multidisciplinary team and support services will assist the family and the educators as needed. Because of the heterogeneous nature of the population studied, conclusions regarding efficacy were unclear; however, a model of care for infants with disabilities emerged that has been carried into the federal mandates for EI services (see later).

At the same time that EI services for children with disabilities were increasing in availability, similar services were emerging for children believed to be at increased risk for disability. The terms *high risk* and *at risk* emerged, based on research indicating that some infant populations were more likely than others to develop disabilities. These populations have often been separated into those at "biological risk" and those at "environmental risk." Biological risk factors included perinatal factors, such as prematurity or perinatal asphyxia; specific medical disorders, such as congenital malformations, genetic disorders, or syndromes; and abnormal neurodevelopmental findings, such as tone abnormalities or hearing loss. Increased environmental risk was thought to be present in homes where there was limited stimulation or increased stress. More specifically, this group included children of teenage mothers, children with lower socioeconomic status (SES), those with parents with cognitive or physical disabilities, and those who had experienced child abuse or neglect.

Although increased risk was identified in these children, the degree of risk appropriate to classification as "high risk" was never established, leading to such classification of large numbers of children, most of whom would have normal developmental outcomes. Nevertheless, programs were established to foster improved development in these children. For example, it was the notion of increased environmental risk that inspired the federal government's Head Start program, begun in 1965 during the Johnson administration as one of the Great Society programs. Other programs focusing on the child at environmental risk include the Abecederian Project (Ramey & Campbell, 1991); the Ypsilanti Perry Preschool Project (Schweinhart, Berrueta-Clement, Barnett, Epstein, & Weikart, 1985) and the Yale Child Welfare Program (Provence, 1985), while the Infant Health and Development Program (1990) is centered on low birth weight infants. These programs are among those best studied for efficacy because developmental "risk" was much greater in frequency than established disability, allowing for greater sample recruitment.

Federal Mandates for Early Intervention Services

Public Law 94-142 The most important events fostering dramatic expansion of EI services for children with disabilities began in 1975 with passage of the Education for All Handicapped Children Act (PL 94-142). With this act, Congress established that all children with disabilities, regardless of the severity of the disability, were entitled to a "free appropriate public education" from ages 3 to 21. Educational programs were mandated for children older than age 5, with incentive grants provided to those states initiating services at 3 years of age. Although services for children from birth to 3 years were not included, a precedent for EI was established when states were encouraged to establish programs for children with disabilities beginning in the preschool years at age 3. Several important concepts, in addition to that of a free appropriate public education for children with disabilities, were established with this law.

While special services were being implemented, Congress supported the concept of "mainstreaming" by requiring that these services be provided in "the least restrictive environment," allowing the child with disabilities every possible opportunity to be with children without disabilities. The range of services available were now to include physical education, home or hospital instruction, and "related services." The latter services were those required to allow the child to participate in the educational program and included transportation, speech and audiology services, psychological services, counseling services, physical and occupational therapy services, recreation, and medical services. The medical services were to be limited to diagnostic and evaluation services and could be provided only if these were necessary to identify and assess a disabling condition, in order that the child might benefit from special education. Although the law thus restricted the use of medical services, it nevertheless codified a link between the educational and medical community in serving the child with disabilities.

In order to determine a child's eligibility, a multidisciplinary team evaluation was required, thereby endorsing this model for care of children with disabilities. From the team evaluation, an individualized education program (IEP) was to be created, establishing a specific curriculum annually for each child that was designed to meet his or her particular developmental needs. The IEP had to include statements regarding current level of performance, annual goals, specific services to be provided, dates of initiation and duration of the services, and objective criteria and evaluation procedures and schedules for determining annually whether the objectives were being achieved. Finally, a set of procedural "due process" safeguards were put in place in order to guarantee the child and his or her family such a free and appropriate program.

Public Law 99-457 and the Individuals with Disabilities Education Act

Although PL 94-142 set a critical precedent in the establishment of special education, it additionally provided an important endorsement of the notion of EI by encouraging special services to children with disabilities early in childhood in order to optimize current and future development. This endorsement was translated into a new mandate in 1986 with the passage of the Education of the Handicapped Act Amendments (PL 99-457). This law now required that all states provide special services to children with disabilities beginning at age 3, thus replacing the preschool incentive grants of PL 94-142, and added a new incentive program for establishment of services for children from birth to 3 years of age.

The goals outlined by PL 99-457 were "to enhance the development of handicapped infants and toddlers and to minimize the potential for developmental delay" and, more specifically, "to reduce the educational costs to our society,...minimizing the need for special education and related services after handicapped infants and toddlers reach school age" (Section 671). Under the incentive grant program of this law, each state was given financial support for the establishment and later continuation of EI services for infants and toddlers with disabilities. These programs were specifically intended to be comprehensive, coordinated, and multidisciplinary in nature and were to include screening, identification, referral, and treatment services. In addition to serving those children with disabilities, there was also an option of providing services to children "at risk." Just as PL 94-142 imprinted new concepts of service and new terminology into the area of education, so did PL 99-457 for EI.

Perhaps the greatest change emerging from this legislation has been its focus on the family and the community, with particular emphasis on caring for the child with developmental disabilities in community settings, especially in his or her own home, with mandated family involvement, distinguishing it clearly from PL 94-142 and its focus only on the child in school. This is highlighted most clearly by the substitution of the individualized family service plan (IFSP) for the IEP of the previous law. The IFSP is a family-directed assessment of resources, priorities, and concerns relating to enhancing the development of the child. It is similar to the IEP in its inclusion of a statement regarding a child's current level of functioning, except that, rather than focusing strictly on educational levels, it broadens the description of functioning to include all of the defined areas of development: physical (including motor, hearing, and vision), cognitive, communicative, social or emotional, and adaptive. The IFSP must also include a statement of major outcomes expected for the child and family, with criteria, procedures, and time lines for achieving them. The specific services necessary to meet the child's and family's unique needs to achieve these outcomes must be stated, including their frequency, intensity, duration, location, method of service delivery, and dates of initiation.

Whereas the previous law discussed services in the least restrictive environment, PL 99-457 required that these services be provided in the child's "natural environment, including the home and community settings" as appropriate, where children without disabilities may participate. In order to further emphasize the family and community foci, other services necessary for the child but not required by this law can also be described in the IFSP, with a plan outlined for their implementation. Finally, the IFSP must designate a "service coordinator," a professional who will be responsible for its implementation, coordinating services for the child.

Since its original passage, this legislation has undergone several revisions. First, the Education of the Handicapped Act was renamed the Individuals with Disabilities Education Act (IDEA; PL 101-476) in 1990 and was modified further in the Individuals with Disabilities Education Act Amendments of 1991 (PL 102-119) and 1997 (PL 105-17). With these changes, the incentive program of PL 99-457 was replaced with mandated services for children from birth to 3 years of age (named Part C). In addition, coverage of disabilities was expanded to include autism and traumatic brain injury. The EI services to which the infant or toddler with disabilities is entitled in IDEA include those traditionally provided through PL 94-142 (e.g., psychological services, occupational therapy, physical therapy, speech and language services) but are further expanded to meet the broader needs of assisting the child and family in the community. Services added include family training, counseling, and home visits; expanded health services (diagnostic medical services, nursing services, nutrition services); vision services; and "special instruction," with the latter term de-emphasizing the educational focus of the services for older children.

Eligibility for services now is determined through a three-pronged approach: early identification, screening, and assessment. Assessment remains multidisciplinary in approach, but a child no longer must be classified into a specific disability category. Instead, children need only be defined as having "develop-mental delays" in one or more of the areas of development (physical, cognitive, communicative, social or emotional, and adaptive), with each state defining criteria for "delay," or have "a diagnosed physical or mental condition that has a high probability of resulting in developmental delay." Services for children "at risk" are at each state's discretion.

In 2004, IDEA was reauthorized as the Individuals with Disabilities Education Improvement Act (PL 108-446). The most significant change in this law affecting EI services is the allowance for extension of the infant and toddler services (Part C) until kindergarten, with a parent's permission. In contrast to the prior mandate for transition of these services into the preschool services at age 3, children can now continue with the family-centered, natural environment model for EI. In so doing, a child will continue to have an IFSP until kindergarten, with services provided identical to those provided for younger children, rather than the school-based model centered on an IEP. All such children must have an educational component provided, however. This new model will assure continuity of services for children who would benefit from such, with later transition into the educational model.

A new era in EI services began with the passage of IDEA. In effect, the federal government said that children with disabilities deserve early assistance in their development and in helping them and their families adapt to living with a disability; at the same time, society must accept entry of these children into the community just as children without disabilities are accepted. This does not imply that the question of program efficacy is resolved, however. Instead, we now must ask which services are appropriate for which children and how we should provide them. Bearing these questions in mind, one can delve into the question of efficacy. Studies have divided into those focusing on children with identified disabilities and those centered on children at risk for future disability.

EARLY INTERVENTION FOR CHILDREN WITH KNOWN DEVELOPMENTAL DISABILITIES

What does the literature say regarding the efficacy of EI in children with known specific developmental disabilities some 40 years after its introduction? Despite a large body of research, many questions remain, and our recommendations are currently tentative at best. In this section, we open with an overview of the context in which this research has been performed. We then examine the question of efficacy of EI from both an overall and a disability-specific approach as reflected in published reviews as well as summaries of relevant primary studies. Specific areas examined include CP, Down syndrome (DS), and autism.

Information is presented in great detail because it is now becoming quite clear that simple statements, if not meaningless, are of only minimal value. Beyond the obvious need for assistance for children with disabilities lies the task of deciding how best to provide that assistance. For the health care professional charged with caring for children with disabilities, an understanding of this literature is essential if one is to be able to draw valid conclusions and provide proper direction to parents seeking information about EI programs for their children.

With the widespread establishment in the 1960s of EI programs, studies providing efficacy data on particular programs started appearing in the literature in significant numbers in the 1970s and 1980s. Fewer studies have appeared in the 1990s (Farran, 2000). Whereas earlier studies had major methodological problems, more recent studies tend to have improved research designs, including increasing use of randomized controlled studies.

Initial research in this field focused on the general question of efficacy in the child with developmental disabilities. Since the late 1980s, concurrent with claims by multiple researchers that EI was or had the potential to be effective, there were calls to go beyond the general question and start delving into specifics (Guralnick, 1991; Shonkoff, Hauser-Cram, Krauss, & Upshur, 1988). In this next stage, termed *second-generation research* (Guralnick, 1997), focus was turned toward particulars of EI, including for which disability or age, using what interventions, and with what intensity is it effective.

The vast majority of the efficacy studies in children with disabilities have reported on children having as their major disability either intellectual disabilities (particularly DS), CP, or autism. Reviews of the literature have been either general critiques of study methodology and results or meta-analytical studies. The technique of meta-analysis, developed by Glass (1976), aggregates and synthesizes data from several studies, using summary statistics to calculate effect sizes. "Effect size" is defined as the mean difference on the outcome variable between treated and untreated subjects, divided by the within-group standard deviation. Stated differently, for each variable, mean effect size for the experimental group is calculated and compared with the mean effect size for the control group. This technique is very helpful for demonstrating significant patterns of findings across studies with small sample sizes, for which statistical significance is hard to obtain. Limitations of this technique relate to the limitations of the primary studies themselves. If certain data are not provided in the original studies, performing a meta-analysis on these studies will not provide answers as if such data were present. In addition, it is important that studies included in such an analysis have similar content. Both of these limitations are particularly relevant to the EI literature and have precluded in a number of studies the performance of meta-analyses. Many of the original studies lack very pertinent information, such as parental SES or type of disability, and are not very rigorous in their use of definitions.

General Reviews

Through 1990, a number of comprehensive global reviews, either using a methodological or meta-analytical approach, have examined the efficacy of EI for children with disabilities (Casto & Mastropieri, 1986; Dunst & Rheingrover, 1981; Farran, 1990; Shonkoff & Hauser-Cram, 1987; Simeonsson, Cooper, & Schemer, 1982). Since 1990, there has been only one general review (Farran, 2000).

In 1981, Dunst and Rheingrover examined 49 studies conducted from 1967 to 1980 that assessed EI efficacy in "organically impaired" infants. Of the 49 studies examined, only 4 were of true experimental design and adequately controlled for the seven threats to internal validity. Seventy-one percent of the studies had designs that were either pre-experimental or nonequivalent control group designs, which, according to the authors, made the results of those studies "fundamentally un-interpretable." Dunst and Rheingrover con-cluded that the large majority of the studies *did not* provide evidence of efficacy of EI in chil-dren with organic impairments. They did note that EI may be efficacious, but, given the meth-odological flaws of these studies, conclusions to that effect were impossible to draw.

Simeonsson et al. (1982) reviewed 27 studies conducted from 1975 to 1982 that ex-amined the efficacy of EI for infants and chil-dren with "biological disabilities." The nature of the intervention was a combination ap-proach in half of the studies and physical ther-apy and vestibular stimulation in one third of the studies. Seventy percent of the studies specified roles for the parents. Standardized evaluation instruments were used in 70% of the studies; however, no single instrument was used in the majority of the studies. Examina-tion of the methodology revealed that only 5 of the 27 studies had an experimental design that was prospective, with random assignment of control group. Simeonsson et al. (1982) stated that only a limited number of studies met common criteria for research. In 25 studies (93%), the authors of the primary studies re-ported efficacy of intervention; however, sta-tistical support was only presented in 13 (48%) of the studies. Simeonsson et al. concluded that, despite the methodological limitations, the "research does provide qualified support for the effectiveness of early intervention" (1982, p. 638).

In 1986, Casto and Mastropieri performed a meta-analysis of EI studies of preschoolers with disabilities. Studies were obtained from a data set of more than 200 published and un-published studies compiled at the Early Inter-vention Research Institute at Utah State Uni-versity. A total of 74 studies from 1937 to 1984 were included in the analysis. The authors de-scribed a detailed coding system, which in-cluded introduction, description of subjects, type of intervention, research design and out-come (including outcome measures used), and conclusions, that allowed integration of these varied studies. They reported on 216 effect

sizes calculated from the 74 studies. Of the sub-jects, 44% had intellectual disabilities, 28% had multiple disabilities, 10% had orthopedic impairments, 8% had speech-language impair-ment, 4% had emotional disturbances, 3% had general developmental delay, and 2% had hearing impairment. Intelligence quotient (IQ) score was the outcome measure used most fre-quently.

Casto and Mastropieri (1986) concluded that EI does result in moderately large immedi-ate benefits (effect size = 0.68) for preschool-ers with disabilities that are evidenced over a variety of outcome variables, including IQ score, motor skill, language skill, and aca-demics. Few conclusions could be drawn about effects on self-concept, social competency, and family or peer relationships. Similarly, few conclusions could be made specifically regard-ing preschoolers with severe disabilities, sen-sory impairment, behavior disorders, or speech-language impairment. Notable was their qualification that the effect size was sig-nificantly lower (0.40) when only good-quality studies were included in the analysis. Further analysis of program variables found that evi-dence was not supportive of the need for pa-rental involvement, earlier age of entrance, or increased degree of program structure, dura-tion, or intensity. Finally, no good studies ex-isted that examined whether short-term gains were maintained over the long term.

Shonkoff and Hauser-Cram (1987) fol-lowed with another meta-analysis of a subset of the same 230 studies that were considered by Casto and Mastropieri (1986) but excluded studies that had major methodological flaws. From 31 selected studies, they assessed 91 cal-culated effects. The mean effect size of EI ser-vices was 0.62 when measured for IQ/develop-mental quotient (DQ) (as compared with the 0.68 effect size reported by Casto and Mastro-pieri). Stated otherwise, this means that EI pro-vides children with approximately 0.5 standard deviation benefit. The investigators referred to this as a "moderate positive effect," generally considered clinically significant.

Closer examination of the "effects" showed that three fourths of the measured ef-fects were IQ/DQ related. Motor improvement had the least effect (0.43), and language improvement had the greatest effect (1.17). The population that appeared to have benefited the most was a "mixed" population (0.94), followed by those with "developmental delay" (0.70) and intellectual disabilities (0.42). The lowest effect size was for those children who had orthopedic impairments (0.11). Age of enrollment was found to be important in the children with mild disabilities. Program features that were noted to have an effect included a highly structured program and extensive parental involvement, especially if the parent and child were both enrolled in the program.

Shonkoff and Hauser-Cram (1987) pointed to the lack of important data on the child, family, and program in the studies they examined. Outcome was focused disproportionately on cognitive development and not on other items such as social competence or motivation. No outcome measures were included for family function. The reviewers concluded that the data clearly suggest that EI services are effective in promoting developmental progress for many children with disabilities who are younger than 3 years of age. They did note that not all children benefit. Type of disability was associated with different rates of improvement, with those children classified as "developmentally delayed" showing the most improvement and those classified as "orthopedically impaired" showing the least. Age of entry younger than 6 months was associated with better outcome than later ages of entry except in the children with more severe disabilities, in whom there appeared to be no difference.

Farran (1990) examined 42 studies that were published from 1977 to 1986 and reported on the efficacy of EI for children with disabilities. Thirteen of these studies dealt exclusively with children with DS and are discussed later. The remaining 29 studies dealt with a mixed population that had a large number of children with CP. Farran noted multiple concerns regarding the studies reviewed, including problems with methodology (especially outcome measures), minimal information regarding families, and wide variation between studies on crucial elements examined, including area of development examined, age of entry, and length of intervention. Only five of the studies had long-term follow-up. Farran

felt that conclusions regarding efficacy were difficult to determine due to outcome measures used and lack of a control group in many of the studies. There was no evidence supporting the use of any particular program. Because of mixed groups, it was possible that positive effects were lost in statistical analysis.

Farran (2000) performed a follow-up review of studies published since 1987. Results of second-generation research allowed her to draw conclusions regarding the "particulars," including effects with respect to age of child, severity of diagnosis, family characteristics, location where service was provided, and intervention approach used. In examination of this review, it is worthwhile focusing in on a number of selected studies she discussed.

Farran (2000) examined the studies that characterized how services were being provided to children ages birth to 3 enrolled in EI by surveying the parents, following the children, or both. Responses found that those with highest education, positive family characteristics, and few needs for support had received the most support, in contrast to families of low income, who received less. Consistent with this, children with similar diagnoses and needs got markedly different services. Children with more severe impairments, as compared with those with milder impairments, received more services but made less progress. The child's and family's characteristics were much stronger predictors for progress than particular aspects of EI (Shonkoff, Hauser-Cram, Krauss, & Upshur, 1992). One study reported sobering findings on parent interview done at the time children with disabilities were making the transition to regular school. Many parents reported being disillusioned. Instead of seeing EI as helping their child catch up, they saw preschool special education as solidifying their child's permanent placement into special education in the future.

One study examining effects of intensity and lag treatment compared progress in children birth to 3 years participating in a full-time versus part-time group (Dihoff et al., 1994). Initial evaluation at 6 months found the full-time group to be more advanced as compared to the part-time group. Follow-up at 12 months, however, found no difference between the groups.

Farran (2000) reviewed three examples of systematic investigations of intervention approaches. One example used a transactional approach to development (Sameroff & Fiese, 1990). This model sees developmental outcomes at any point in time to be the result of a three-part process that starts with child behavior that triggers family interpretation that produces a parental response. Implementation consisted of the mother interacting with her infant while receiving coaching that was followed by direct intervention with the child while the mother was in a parent support group. Findings of a later study using this model (Brinker, Seifer, & Sameroff, 1994) indicated that overall the child did *not* make significant progress in the intervention; however, further examination revealed surprising results, with maternal SES and stress level affecting how the child responded to the intervention. For example, children of mothers of low SES and high stress levels who participated in intervention did less well. These studies highlight the need to take into account family and child characteristics when planning interventions.

The second approach examined was the use of Milieu Teaching (MT) in children with disabilities (Kaiser, Yoder, & Keetz, 1992). MT is a naturalistic intervention strategy that incorporates following the child's lead or interest, use of explicit prompts for the child's language, rewards within naturally occurring consequences, and embedding the intervention in ongoing interaction between the clinician and child. In a number of well-performed studies comparing this technique with other interventions, it was found that MT was better for children who spoke little, who did not self-initiate, and whose speech was not intelligible at the outset. This technique was extended to use with prelinguistic functioning children by using a pre-MT intervention. This latter technique incorporated transactional effects and was found effective in increasing prelinguistic intentional requesting behaviors within the sessions that also generalized to the classroom and to teachers who had not been part of the intervention. It should be noted that Prelin-

guistic MT has recently been reported to be of value with preschoolers with autism (Yoder & Stone, 2006).

The third approach examined was the aptitude-by-treatment interactions approach (Cole & Dale, 1986; Cole, Mills, Dale, & Jenkins, 1991). In this approach, the child's characteristics or "aptitude" interacts with the type of treatment he or she receives so as to identify which type of child responds best to which type of treatment (a central second-generation research question). Over a number of studies, the authors examine the effect of different types of instruction and school settings (segregated vs. integrated) on children with mild disabilities at the preschool and kindergarten ages. At the end of the interventions, there were no differences between groups regarding the likelihood of going into special education. At age 9, two thirds of the group were learning in special education classes; however, further inspection revealed aptitude-by-treatment interactions. Higher functioning children benefited from one type of intervention and did better in integrated classes. In contrast, lower functioning children benefited from a second type of intervention and did better in segregated classes. These findings have held up in a recent follow-up study by this same group when these children were age 16 (Dale, Jenkins, Mills, & Cole, 2005).

Farran (2000), in conclusion, noted that, despite studies being so diverse, certain initial statements regarding EI could be made, including the following:

1. In children with disabilities identified in the preschool period, EI of all types and in all locations produces more gains on standardized testing for those with mild impairments than for those with more severe impairments.

2. EI for 3- to 5-year-olds who have language impairment appears to be generally effective and associated with participation in mainstream education.

3. In newborns to 3-year-olds, focused interventions appear to be less effective than general global infant interventions focused on positive family interactions.

From her review of systematic approaches to EI, Farran noted that, in EI, "one size does not fit all." These sets of studies, however, begin to identify a major second-generation research question, namely which children respond better to which interventions and at which time in their development. Significant issues remaining include the need for examination of long-term outcomes and for recognizing and addressing the complexity of interaction between family and child characteristics when planning services.

Currently underway and worth following is the National Early Intervention Longitudinal Study (NEILS). The goal of this study is to provide information about children and their families participating in Part C (serving ages birth to 3 years) EI programs. At this early stage, only limited information on child development and families' perception of the EI process has been published. Early 1-year results on child outcome are not interpretable as currently presented, given lack of any standardized outcome data; however, recently published family data are worthy of mention. The report (Bailey et al., 2005) summarized the investigators' findings on the 2,586 families that provided answers to eight questions posed to them by the investigators via a telephone interview. In their responses, parents reported a high degree of satisfaction with EI programs and services. Most parents noted that EI professionals made them feel optimistic and hopeful about their child's future. Parents perceived that EI had a positive impact on their child's development and that their family was better off as a result of help and information received from the programs. Most parents were hopeful about the future and expected both their child's and family's future life situation would be excellent to good. Echoing previous parent surveys, however, these findings were not as strong for families of low income or if the child was in poor health. These findings are complementary to those reported by Farran (2000) earlier.

Early reviews in the area of EI efficacy were replete with comments regarding the significant methodological shortcomings found in the primary studies. Most studies performed failed to meet basic research design criteria and lacked crucial data regarding child, family, and intervention that would allow meaningful conclusions to be drawn. Surprisingly, a number of these reviewers nevertheless concluded that EI was effective in children with disabilities. Findings by Farran (2000) reporting greater benefit of EI for those children with milder disabilities are consistent with those previous reports. Data from studies examining MT and aptitude-by-treatment interactions approaches should alert us to the need to match intervention approaches to the type and degree of disability of the child. Findings suggest that children with milder cognitive and language disabilities appear to benefit from a more direct and explicit teaching method in an integrated classroom, whereas those with more severe disabilities benefit from a teaching method that provides more support, teaches more learning strategies, and is located within a segregated classroom. Regarding families, EI seems to provide structure and support for families of children with disabilities; however, it is especially incumbent on the clinician to verify that families of lesser means receive these EI services and that the effects are closely monitored.

Early Intervention for Cerebral Palsy

In an early case review, Paine (1962) reported that many children with CP who were not treated with physical therapy developed motor skills at a rate equal to that of their treated peers; however, anecdotal evidence was reported on the treated group having an improved appearance of gait and on the possible prevention of contractures in some children. Since this publication, our ability to classify and assess function and change in children with CP has improved substantially. Most recent has been the development of the World Health Organization's International Classification of Functioning, Disability and Health. This tool provides a standardized language and system for classifying human function and disability (Simeonsson et al., 2003). A number of well-standardized and validated instruments to assess both impairment and function in this population of children with motor disabilities have been published. Examples include the Gross Motor Function Measure (GMFM; Russell et al., 1989) and the Pediatric Evaluation of Disability Inventory (PEDI; Feldman, Haley, & Coryell, 1990), which measure function, and the Gross Motor Function Classification System (GMFCS; Palisano et al., 1997), which classifies level of impairment.

Unfortunately, less progress has been made in identifying interventions that actually bring about such sought-after change. Such therapies as neurodevelopmental treatment (NDT), which were considered mainstays for much of the last century, are now being clearly shown to have deficiencies that warrant a reassessment of approach (Blauw-Hosper & Hadders-Algra, 2005; Butler & Darrah, 2001). In contrast, there are emerging signs that other approaches may be of value in the treatment of children with CP. These include interventions that use a functional approach and employ well-studied principles such as motor learning. It is important to review a number of relevant studies that have led to these conclusions.

In this section, a brief description of the different interventions that are currently being used in the treatment of children with CP is provided. This is followed by an examination of CP efficacy literature with focus on the reviews and relevant studies published over the past decade.

Interventions for Children with Cerebral Palsy

Harris (1997) reviewed the major forms of EI for infants and young children with motor disabilities. These included neurofacilitation approaches, neurobehavioral motor intervention, conductive education (CE), and specific environmental adaptations such as adaptive seating, powered mobility, and orthoses. Since that review, studies on a number of other nonpharmacological interventions have been published, including constraint-induced movement therapy, treadmill training, strengthening, and therapeutic riding or hippotherapy. Electrical stimulation, environmental adaptations, therapeutic riding, and use of medications such as botulinum toxin (Botox) and baclofen are not addressed in this review.

The neurofacilitation approaches (Harris, 1990) include most prominently NDT, developed by Bobath and Bobath (1984). Other authors refer to these approaches as neurophysiological or neuromaturational and include within them the Vojta approach (Ketelaar, Vermeer, Hart, van Petegem-van Beek, & Helders, 2001). Neurofacilitation is based on a hierarchical model of motor control (Harris, Atwater, & Crowe, 1988), which suggests that lesions in the central nervous system will result in a lack of higher-level control over movements and release of primitive and abnormal reflexes at lower levels. As such, goals of this approach are to inhibit abnormal muscle tone and primitive reflexes and facilitate normal movement patterns.

CE was conceived in the 1940s by Dr. Andreas Peto of Hungary to assist children with motor dysfunction to attain what he called "orthodysfunction," enabling them to attend school with the maximum degree of independence (Darrah, Watkins, Chen, & Bonin, 2004). The intervention model is educational and functional in nature. In addition to motor function, it addresses social and academic skills. Traditionally, CE is provided by teacher-therapists, termed *conductors,* to groups of children with CP. Activities are highly structured and accompanied by the use of rhyme and song termed *rhythmical intention.* Physical assistance from the conductor is minimal. Wooden slatted beds and ladder-back chairs to assist with movement are widely used, but adaptive equipment is not generally recommended.

Functional or neurobehavioral approaches to intervention have evolved as a result of alternative theories regarding motor development and motor control. Theories described as ecological (Gibson, 1979) or dynamic systems (Kelso, 1995; Thelen & Smith, 1994) differ notably from the neurofacilitation approaches in viewing motor development as emerging from the dynamic interaction of many subsystems in a task-specific context (Ketelaar et al., 2001). This approach combines a functional/behavioral approach with motor intervention techniques similar to those used in neurofacilitation. Variations on this intervention exist but involve a task-oriented model that focuses on function with emphasis on the role of the environment and the task in the performance of functional activities (Horak, 1991). This approach takes an active view of motor learning whereby people learn by actively attempting to solve problems inherent to a functional task by repetitive practice of goal-related tasks.

Constraint-induced movement therapy is a relatively new rehabilitation approach that is being employed in the treatment of children with CP. It involves intensive targeted practice with the involved extremity along with the use of a restraint of the unaffected arm. It is administered by a trained practitioner and combines principles from the fields of behavioral psychology and motor learning (Gordon, Charles, & Wolf, 2005). Similar to this approach is forced use therapy, which differs from constraint-induced movement therapy in that it is done with or without physical or occupational therapy (Willis, Morello, Davie, Rice, & Bennett, 2002). Initial work in this field originated with work on monkeys, where it was found that these animals could be induced to make use of a deafferented limb by restricting movement of the intact limb. Initial human studies were done in stroke victims, and only recently has this technique begun to be introduced in children with CP.

The use of muscle strengthening has been considered since the time at which physical therapy was first used in children with CP; however, only recently has it been reconsidered and reintroduced as a mode of therapy as a means to improve function in children with CP. This is a consequence of the growing evidence that muscle weakness represents a significant impairment in children with CP (Damiano, Dodd, & Taylor, 2002). Strengthening generally involves short-term exercises or interventions either to improve function of specific muscle groups or to improve overall function. No single approach currently exists. Related to this has been the recent introduction of treadmill training that is aimed at improving motor skills in children with CP. Additional research is being done on the metabolic effects of this intervention. Again, because of its preliminary nature, no single protocol is currently in use.

General Efficacy Reviews of Cerebral Palsy Interventions

Initial reviews in this area were more exploratory in nature and addressed the more global question as to the efficacy of therapy in CP; however, as the field matured, published studies as well as subsequent reviews have provided us with the ability to make more conclusive statements as to what does not work as well as to what indeed may work. Consistent with the previously noted call for second-generation research, more recent studies have begun examining which interventions work best for whom and under what conditions.

Early reviews of the literature evaluating the efficacy of physical therapy in CP included general overviews of the primary research studies (Campbell, 1990; Parette & Hourcade, 1984; Scherzer & Tscharnuter, 1990) and both quantitative (meta-analytical) (Turnbull, 1993) and qualitative (Piper, 1990; Tirosh & Rabino, 1989) approaches. All reported that significant deficiencies in the scientific method employed by the primary research studies limited their ability to draw clear conclusions regarding the efficacy of physical therapy.

Harris (1997), in her review of the effectiveness of EI for children with CP, examined the literature on children ages 6 and younger that was published after 1985. Results from two randomized controlled interventions (Law et al., 1991; Palmer et al., 1988) did not support efficacy of NDT. Regarding the value of a neuromotor behavioral approach, Harris reported on preliminary results from one published study that demonstrated benefit and suggested the need for follow-up on these promising findings. Based on poor data supporting the value of CE, Harris suggested "restraint in recommending this approach for young children with CP" (p. 337).

Blauw-Hosper and Hadders-Algra (2005) performed a focused systematic review of studies that reported on the effect of EI on motor development. The review focused on studies performed from 1964 to date on infants up to 18 months of age who were either at risk for or had developmental disabilities. Studies that met inclusion criteria were classified as to the type and size of the group, internal and external validity, and level of evidence. Levels of evidence were ranked from I to V, with level I designating studies that were randomized controlled trials, II nonrandomized controlled trials, III case studies with control participants,

level IV case series without control participants, and level V case reports. Given the great
heterogeneity of the studies, including types
of intervention, outcomes measures used, and
age at outcome, the authors noted that no
meta-analysis could be performed.

Of the 36 studies included, 10 were of children with developmental disabilities. These
studies varied considerably. Six studies examined the effects of intervention on children
with CP. The intervention approaches used
were NDT, Vojta, CE, developmental stimulation, or an unspecified physical therapy approach. Three studies examined the effects of
NDT (Mahoney, Robinson, & Fewell, 2001;
Mayo, 1991; Palmer et al., 1988), one examined the effect of Vojta treatment (Kanda, Pidcock, Hayakawa, Yamori, & Shikata, 2004),
and one examined the effect of a CE approach
(Reddihough, King, Coleman, & Catanese,
1998). All of the studies except one (Kanda
et al., 2004) had an evidence level of either I
(definitive) or II (tentative) and had fair to high
internal and external validity; the study by
Kanda et al. had an evidence level of III. Outcome results for these six studies included two
in which the intervention group performed
better than the control group, one in which
the control group performed better than the
intervention group, and three for which there
was no difference between the intervention
and control groups.

Blauw-Hosper and Hadders-Algra (2005)
concluded that NDT during the first years of
life does not have measurable effects on motor
development. Similar findings were noted for
Vojta treatment; however, it should be noted
that there were only two studies that examined
this intervention, one of which was a level III
study. In contrast, specific developmental
training and general developmental programs,
in which parents learn how to promote infant
development, were noted to have a positive
effect on motor development.

Efficacy for Specific
Interventions in Cerebral Palsy

Neurodevelopmental Treatment   Butler
and Darrah (2001) performed a systematic review of the evidence regarding the value of

NDT in the treatment of CP. Of 65 studies examined, 21 met inclusion criteria. Studies were
classified based on type of evidence (dimensions of disability) and level of evidence (type
of research design employed). Dimensions of
disability included pathophysiology, impairment, activity, participation, and societal limitation. Twenty-one studies were classified,
with 14 meeting level I or level II criteria. This
led the reviewers to decide that conclusions
drawn from these studies would be credible.
They also noted the limited (416 children) and
heterogeneous population that formed the
basis of these studies.

Findings were not supportive for the value
of NDT in regard to motor response or prevention of contractures and deformity. Findings
regarding its effect on gross motor development were not consistent, and all three studies
that examined its effect on fine motor development showed no advantage to this intervention. Studies that compared different intensities of NDT intervention showed differences
between groups after the intervention. Similar
to the lack of support for NDT in effecting
change in the level of impairment, there was
almost no support for its value in regard to its
improvement of function or for its effect on
mother–child interaction as compared with
other interventions. Finally, examination of
subgroups for which NDT might be more or less
effective did not yield any conclusive findings.
The authors concluded by suggesting the need
to investigate other therapeutic approaches despite the existence of gaps in the evidence regarding NDT.

Since Butler and Darrah's (2001) publication, two more studies evaluating NDT
(Knox & Evans, 2002; Tsorlakis, Evaggelinou,
Grouios, & Tsorbatzoudis, 2004) have been
published. The study by Knox and Evans,
which the authors described as preliminary,
consisted of 15 children with varied types of
CP. Ages ranged from 2 to 12 years. Using a
repeated-measures design with the GMFM and
PEDI, they examined the functional effects of
NDT delivered over the course of 6 weeks. At
the end of the intervention, they reported significant improvement on the GMFM total
score. Limitations in this study include the lack
of a control group and small sample size. Tsor-

lakis et al. (2004), using a randomized study design, compared the effect of twice-weekly versus five-times-weekly NDT on gross motor function of children with spastic CP. The intervention was administered over a period of 16 weeks to 34 children, ages 3–14 years, whose GMFCS level ranged from I to III. Outcome as measured using the GMFM found that both groups improved significantly at the end of the intervention. The group receiving the more intensive intervention showed somewhat greater improvement than the control group; however, it should be noted that, although changes were statistically significant, questions remain as to their clinical or functional relevance.

Functional Treatment Ketelaar et al. (2001) compared the effects of a functional therapy program to that of NDT or Vojta treatment on motor abilities in children with CP. The functional program had an emphasis on practicing functional activities important to the child and the parent and not on normalization of movement. This was a semirandomized controlled study that included 55 children with mild to moderate CP ages 2–7 years. Longest follow-up was at 18 months. Outcome measures included the GMFM and the PEDI. Both groups were reported to have improved after treatment, with no difference between groups on their ability to perform basic motor skills as measured by the GMFM. The group receiving the functional therapy program, however, performed significantly better than the NDT/Vojta group as measured by the PEDI.

Occupational Therapy Steultjens et al. (2004) performed a systematic review on the effects of occupational therapy in children with CP. Intervention categories examined included comprehensive occupational therapy, training of sensorimotor functions, training of skills, parent counseling, advice and instruction regarding use of assistive devices, and provision of splints. Steultjens et al. included 17 studies in the review. Seven were randomized controlled studies, but only one was of high methodological quality. Because of the poor methodological quality of the identified studies, the reviewers concluded that there was insufficient evidence to support or refute the efficacy of occupational therapy in children with CP.

Conductive Education Darrah et al. (2004) performed a systematic review of studies that used CE to treat children with CP. Fifteen studies met inclusion criteria; however, only four were of level I or II quality and, of these, only two controlled adequately for threats to internal validity. In examining the strongest studies in terms of both research design and conduct of the study, Darrah et al. found that the majority of the studies revealed no differences in outcome between groups receiving CE intervention and controls or between pre- and post-CE group results. The reviewers also noted that, of the 20 statistically significant findings, 10 favored CE and 10 favored controls, with no one outcome measure showing consistent improvement in the CE group.

Darrah et al. concluded that the literature at this time does not provide evidence either supporting or refuting the value of CE in the treatment of children with CP. The reviewers raised the need for standardization of the CE approach as well as the need for studies to report their results in greater detail. They further questioned whether the intervention as initially described, including not advocating for assistive equipment, is appropriate in today's environment where accessibility and use of assistive technology are commonplace.

Constraint-Induced Movement Therapy/ Forced Use Therapy Studies to date on both of these relatively new approaches have been limited to either case reports or studies with small samples (Boyd, Morris, & Graham, 2001; DeLuca, Echols, Ramey, & Taub, 2003; Eliasson, Bonnier, & Krumlinde-Sundholm, 2003; Eliasson, Krumlinde-Sundholm, Shaw, & Wang, 2005; Gordon et al., 2005; Naylor & Bower, 2005; Taub, Ramey, DeLuca, & Echols, 2004; Willis et al., 2002).

Taub et al. (2004) performed a randomized controlled trial with 18 children with hemiparesis resulting from CP. The children ranged in age from 7 to 96 months, and 16 of the 18 had spastic CP. Level of severity of affected limb was reported as ranging from mild to severe. The intervention consisted of two components: 1) casting of the less affected upper extremity for 6 hours/day for 21 consecutive days; and 2) training procedures using shaping performed by an occupational therapist, physical therapist, or physical therapy assistant for 6 hours/day for the 21 days. Children in the control group received conventional physical or occupational therapy for a mean 2.2 hours/week. At outcome, children receiving the intervention performed significantly better at acquiring more motor skills along with increased use of and improved quality of the affected upper limb. Benefits were noted to persist at 6-month follow-up. Limitations in this study include the significantly greater number of hours of intervention received by the experimental group versus the control group.

Eliasson et al. (2005) reported the results of a clinically controlled trial of 41 children with hemiplegic CP, ages 18 months to 4 years. Intervention consisted of wearing a restraining glove on the dominant hand for 2 hours/day over 2 months. In addition the parents and teachers received an introductory seminar prior to treatment and were responsible for employing the learning opportunities. During the 6-month study period, both the intervention and control groups continued to receive the same ongoing physical (2 times per month) and occupational (once per month) therapy. Outcome measured at 2 and 6 months found that those receiving CIMT improved their use of the affected hand more significantly than children in the control group did. Interestingly, both more affected and older children gained more from the intervention.

Sung et al. (2005) reported on a randomly controlled study that demonstrated the benefit of forced-use therapy *combined* with conventional rehabilitation over conventional rehabilitation alone on a young group (mean age 3–43 months) of 31 children with hemiplegic CP. The forced use therapy employed the use of a short arm cast that was worn for 6 weeks. The rehabilitation consisted of stretching exercise and functional occupational therapy for the upper extremity.

In a randomly controlled study, Gordon, Wolf, and Charles (2006) compared the use of CIMT on 20 children with hemiplegic CP and

found the intervention efficacious and not age dependent. Another study from that group (Charles, Wolf, Schneider, & Gordon, 2006) further noted that while the CIMT intervention improved movement efficiency it did *not* affect muscle strength, sensibility or tone.

Numerous issues remain to be clarified regarding this promising but still somewhat preliminary intervention for children with hemiplegia. These include but are not limited to inclusion criteria, type of personnel, type of restraint used, duration and intensity of intervention, location of the intervention, and assessment tools (Gordon et al., 2005). It should be stressed that this approach is in its early stages and needs to be applied with caution.

Strengthening and Treadmill Training

Darrah, Fran, Chen, Nunwieler, and Watkins (1997) performed a systematic review of the literature regarding the effects of resistive exercise in children with CP. Of seven articles reviewed, only one met level I evidence criteria, though all studies reported beneficial effects of exercise training. The reviewers concluded that such exercise increases muscle performance, though its effect on function was not yet clear.

Damiano et al. (2002), in a summary of existing research on this topic, found consistent evidence to state that strengthening programs predictably increase the ability to produce force and that training programs of short duration can improve gait, wheelchair propulsion, and other aspects of motor performance. Notably, they reported on a study by McCubbin and Shasby (1985) that determined that repetition alone (namely motor learning) was not sufficient to have a beneficial effect and that the use of a resistive component was necessary to achieve the beneficial effects of this exercise.

Dodd, Taylor, and Damiano (2002) performed a systematic review of the effectiveness of strength training programs for people with CP. Twenty-three articles were selected to be examined in detail and rated for methodological rigor, with 11 studies meeting inclusion criteria. Only one randomized controlled trial was identified. With respect to impairment, 8 of the 10 empirical studies reported strength increases as a result of a strength-training program (effect sizes, 1.16–5.27). Two studies reported improvements in activity, and one study reported improvement in self-perception. No negative effects, such as reduced range of motion or spasticity, were reported.

Five studies have been published since this review, with all reporting on benefits of strength training (Blundell, Shepherd, Dean, Adams, & Cahill, 2003; Dodd, Taylor, & Graham, 2003; Eagleton, Iams, McDowell, Morrison, & Evans, 2004; McBurney, Taylor, Dodd, & Graham, 2003; Morton, Brownlee, & McFadyen, 2005); however, only one was a randomized clinical trial (Dodd et al., 2003). Sample sizes for all these studies were small (maximum of 11). The interventions described lasted for up to 6 weeks. The youngest of the participants was 4 years old, with the majority being adolescents, thus limiting the applicability of these results to the EI population. The trials suggest that training can increase strength and may improve motor activity in people with CP, with no studies reporting adverse effects.

Two studies have examined the effects of treadmill training in children with CP on improving motor function. Richards et al. (1997) reported on the addition of treadmill training to a traditional physical therapy program for four nonambulatory children with CP, ages 1.7–2.3 years. Two children showed improvement in supported gait, and two achieved independent ambulation during the study. Schindl, Forstner, Kern, and Hesse (2000) demonstrated improved walking and other motor skills, such as transferring, independent standing, and stair climbing, in 8 of 10 children between 6 and 12 years of age with CP who received treadmill training. These studies are consistent with another study reporting on the effects of this intervention in children with DS that is discussed in the next section.

Conclusions   At the writing of our previous review in 1995, evidence supporting physical therapy as an efficacious treatment for children with CP was found to be lacking. Today that statement deserves modification. The literature now contains studies that do allow us to at least make preliminary recommendations. Researchers have clearly heeded the call for

performing studies that meet necessary methodological requirements. The data, while not totally conclusive, appear sufficient to state that neurofacilitation approaches should *not* be the major or initial approach used in children with CP. Rather, the data suggest that a functional/behavioral approach should be considered as the initial approach to treatment. Specific interventions such as CIMT appear promising and warrant careful consideration by therapists planning intervention for children with hemiplegia. Similarly, use of strengthening should be strongly considered as a component of treatment in this population. The use of treadmill training appears promising, though definitive recommendations await further clinical studies. Final conclusions regarding CE are not yet in; however, pending data that clearly support efficacy, caution is warranted.

Early Intervention for Down Syndrome

Children with DS, the most common cause of intellectual disabilities resulting from a chromosomal aberration, represent a unique group among the children receiving intervention services. They are readily diagnosed at birth and share a common biology explaining their disability. The relative homogeneity of this population removes questions pertaining to diagnostic definition that exist when studying other groups of children with disabilities who are receiving intervention services, thus making examination of the efficacy of such interventions more straightforward. A number of studies (e.g., Carr, 1988; Piper, Gosselin, Gendron, & Mazer, 1986) have reported that the child with DS will undergo a general decline in IQ score from infancy to late childhood, a finding that further differentiates this population and is of importance when assessing efficacy.

Review of Efficacy Studies   Gibson and Harris (1988) examined 21 studies of EI for infants and children with Down syndrome. Most of the programs assessed were comprehensive and parent and child centered, but significant methodological limitations were found. Only three had a control or comparison group, with the majority testing efficacy of treatment by comparing the intervention group with published developmental norms of children with DS raised at home who did not receive EI. Efficacy was assessed across a number of different domains, including gross motor, fine and visual motor, socialization and self-help skills, speech and language, mental age, cognition, and academic performance. Fine motor and visual-motor skills, socialization/self-help skills, and mental age were areas in which short-term benefits of significant magnitude were observed more consistently. There was a diversity of outcome across different studies despite the similar program content and means of delivery; however, there were differing lengths of treatment intervention, age of subjects, and sample size. Among the three studies that had controls, there was little agreement regarding the nature of the program benefit. This latter finding raises questions as to the overall claim of efficacy of EI, but it also focuses the reader on the need to consider that particular types of intervention may be suited to children with DS who have particular characteristics.

Gibson and Harris (1988), although concluding that there may be some evidence for short-term benefits, had significant questions regarding the persistence of such initial gains over the long term. There appears to be a tendency in children with DS to experience a decline in their initial gains from EI to the level of control subjects or population test norms for untreated children with DS at home. Long-term effects of EI appear to be limited to social acceptance in school. Gibson and Harris suggested the need for more methodologically sound studies and for the development of acceptable, agreed-on developmental markers for the child with DS, akin to a standardized growth chart of developmental milestones for these children. They maintained that continued research is needed into newer and more effective intervention technologies. In addition, currently available knowledge on how children with DS learn must be incorporated into EI programs; it is suggested that these children are unlikely to profit from formal cognitive and meta-cognitive training given prior to later childhood and early adult years.

Farran (1990), in her examination of efficacy studies as they relate to children with DS, raised concerns similar to those of Gibson and

Harris (1988). She was critical of studies that used developmental norms of children with DS raised at home, noting disagreement among studies that attempt to "plot" a normal developmental function for the population of children with DS. Similarly, studies that used untreated control groups were not properly matched, thus raising questions regarding the comparison made. She did note that two of three more rigorously designed studies reported on positive immediate effects without any long-term effects. Farran summarized her analysis by concluding, "in no prospective study has any particular intervention effect been established for children with Down syndrome" (1990, p. 526). She concluded by stating that deinstitutionalization has resulted in a change of the developmental pattern of children with DS whereby they have improved from the severe-to-profound to the mild-to-moderate levels of disability.

In a long-term follow-up study on children with DS, Connolly, Morgan, Russell, and Fulliton (1993) compared long-term motor, cognitive, and adaptive functioning in a sample of 10 adolescents with DS who had received EI services as infants and children with such functioning in an untreated age-matched group of adolescents with DS. Gross and fine motor skills in the EI group were below chronological age, though gross motor skills were better than fine motor skills. This group performed significantly better than the comparison group on both cognitive and adaptive functioning. Although the EI group did show the typical decline in cognitive abilities, they did not show a decline in adaptive functioning. Because of methodological concerns, Connolly et al. were hesitant to attribute the benefits seen in the treated population to the EI program they received. Although this study does not supply definitive evidence for efficacy of EI, it provides sufficient evidence to continue the search for it and shows the incredible practical and methodological difficulties in performing significant long-term studies from which definitive conclusions can be drawn.

Hines and Bennet (1996) reviewed evidence for efficacy of EI in children with DS. Studies reviewed were very similar to those mentioned in the review by Gibson and Harris

(1988), except for one additional study (Irwin, 1989). Hines and Bennet noted the significant methodological limitations inherent in the current literature and the lack of robust findings regarding long-term IQ improvement. They noted, however, that the overall findings of positive changes in children receiving EI were consistent, especially in terms of independence, community function, and improved quality of life. They suggested that children with DS and their families are likely to benefit from EI.

Spiker and Hopmann (1997), in their review of EI for children with DS, pointed out the incongruence between the evidence for efficacy of EI in DS and the conclusions being drawn. They noted that many in the field accept EI as being beneficial and efficacious, to the point that no-treatment conditions should be considered unethical in treatment protocols (Shonkoff et al., 1992). In contrast, Spiker and Hopmann quoted the previously mentioned opinions of Gibson and Harris (1988), who dispute that claim, stating that evidence as to efficacy has not yet been demonstrated.

Spiker and Hopmann (1997) reviewed the evolving literature that has begun to describe how children with DS develop, especially studies focusing on qualitative function. Although children with DS were initially thought to develop similarly to, albeit more slowly than, typically developing children, current research is now showing the existence of qualitative differences between these groups. These findings extend to almost all areas examined, including cognition, language and communication, play behavior and attention, attachment and temperament, and parent–child interactions. Some of these differences include taking longer to learn contingencies, having difficulties consolidating and generalizing newly learned skills (Wishart, 1993), being less engaged in motivation tasks, having poorer play when left alone with toys (Ruskin, Kasari, Mundy, & Sigman, 1994), and being less readable in terms of the social, emotional, and communicative cues they emit in social interaction situations. In line with this, children with DS are thought to be more difficult and less gratifying as social partners, to take less initiative, and to respond in a less predictable manner. Awareness of

these developmental characteristics in infants and children with DS is crucial in being able to construct effective intervention approaches.

A number of relevant studies mentioned in Spiker and Hopmann's review (1997), as well as some of the study conclusions, deserve mention. In one of the few studies utilizing recent research about the developmental characteristics of children with DS, Wishart (1986), in a study of 10 1- to 3-year-olds with DS, examined the effects of object concept training. Although the children registered statistically relatively few gains, Wishart reported on a marked improvement in the quality of the searches made by most of the children with DS over these training sessions. Studies like these, despite their limitations, are crucial if we are to begin to gain a basic understanding of how to work with this population.

In examining the literature on *alternative communication* that employed use of speech and manual signs, Spiker and Hopmann (1997) noted that preliminary work from a number of different investigators suggests that such an approach for young children with DS may be valuable both before and during the one-word stage. The literature regarding *motor interventions* in DS was also inconclusive. Harris et al. (1988) suggested benefits of NDT in children with DS, but conclusions were limited because of poor methodological rigor, a finding noted earlier in a review by Naganuma (1987). Other noted studies also reported benefits but again were plagued by poor methodology. Only a single study was found that examined effects of *inclusion* in integrated settings. That study reported on a group of 36 children (ages 3 years 8 months to 10 years) with DS, half of whom attended general nursery or primary school and half of whom attended segregated special schools. Placement was determined by the school district; thus there was no random assignment. Groups were matched for mental age. Outcomes were measured using standardized intelligence and academic tests. Over the 2-year study period, the mainstreamed group had a significantly greater mean mental age gain of 19 months compared with 14.2 months for the special school groups. (Compare these results with findings noted previously regarding the aptitude-by-treatment interactions approach in General Reviews.)

In examining the review by Spiker and Hopmann (1997), what stands out is the striking contrast between the advances that have been made in characterizing development in children with DS and the paucity of methodologically sound intervention studies. This is especially true regarding studies that based interventions on previously mentioned research about developmental characteristics in children with DS. Their review is clearly successful in its goal of moving our focus beyond the simplistic question of overall efficacy toward forcing the research and treatment community to grapple, however difficult and frustrating that may be, with the minutiae necessary to extract relevant data and plan future interventions.

Foreman and Crews (1998) reported on the use of augmentative communication in 19 children with DS, ages 2–4 years, who had been in an EI program for at least 6 months. The intervention consisted of teaching all of the children to communicate 12 single words via four different methods: verbal instruction alone, a symbol method (containing computerized pictographs), a sign method (Makaton), or a multimodal method (verbal + sign + symbol). The intervention lasted 4 days. Each day the child was taught 3 words over three teaching sessions, including an initial session, a post-teaching session 15 minutes later, and a follow-up session 24 hours later. Change was measured via a repeated-measures technique. The study found that the sign method (which incorporated use of verbal instruction) or the multimodal method resulted in significant improvement for all children. Of importance was the finding that none of the children were able to communicate the names of items taught solely with verbal instruction.

Ulrich, Ulrich, Angulo-Kinzler, and Yun (2001) reported on the value of treadmill training for infants with DS in reducing delay of time to walking. Subjects included 30 infants who began participation when they could sit alone for 30 seconds. The intervention consisted of practice stepping on a small, motorized treadmill 5 days per week for 8 minutes in their home. Both the intervention and control groups received traditional physical therapy at least every other week. The experimental group learned to walk significantly sooner than the control group (74 vs. 101 days). The authors noted that, in their view, the need for targeting a specific skill (in this case stepping) is key in performing a successful intervention.

Mahoney et al. (2001) reported on the effects of early motor intervention in children with DS or CP using either an NDT or a Developmental Skills model in sessions that were provided at nine different clinical sites over a period of 1 year. NDT was described previously in this chapter. The Developmental Skills program as reported by Mahoney et al. focused on learning and mastery of a set of normally sequenced motor milestones. Treatment strategies tended to be behavioral in nature, with children encouraged to engage in the activity and extrinsically reinforced when they demonstrated greater approximations of the desired behavior. Data were presented separately for children with DS or CP as well as for children who received the NDT or the Developmental Skills intervention. At entrance into the study, the 27 children with DS had a mean age of 13.9 months. Motor function, as measured by the Peabody gross motor scale, was 7.5 months, and gross motor classification as per the GMFCS ranged from I to IV. No significant differences were noted between the children with DS who received the NDT versus the Developmental Skills intervention. Significant changes were apparent at the end of the intervention as compared with at entrance; however, there was no evidence that the intervention accelerated development or improved movement quality beyond what could be expected from maturation. No differences were noted between the types of intervention received.

Conclusions Evidence for the efficacy of EI in the population of children with DS that is based on methodologically sound research studies remains limited, a conclusion not significantly different from our previous review a decade ago. Few new relevant studies have been published since. There do seem to be suggestions that EI may be beneficial in preventing declines in IQ score, but again the evidence is far from definitive. There have been a few studies centered around specific interventions that have provided preliminary evidence for efficacy, including treadmill training and augmentative communication. Although there have been significant advances in our understanding of development of children with DS, there are, as of today, few, if any, rigorously studied interventions that have been found valuable in this population.

Early Intervention for Autism

Of all the areas of major childhood disability, the search for effective comprehensive approaches for treating children with autism has shown the most progress and promise. Prior to the 1980s, studies with limited methodological rigor were the norm; therefore, it was difficult to draw conclusions and make recommendations regarding treatment interventions. Since then, however, increasing numbers of studies of at least preliminary methodological quality began appearing in the literature. It is instructive to examine salient studies and reviews of this literature in order to provide an understanding of the complex and sometimes conflicting issues that continue to direct further research in this field and that have implications regarding treatment recommendations.

In 1987, Lovaas published a landmark study reporting on an unprecedented improvement in the development of children with autism who had received early intensive behavioral intervention. The intervention consisted of 40 hours of one-to-one behavioral treatment per week, provided for a period of 2 years or more, to children with autism who were younger than 4 years of age at the time of enrollment. The intervention included extensive parent training and inclusion of the children in regular preschool environments. The treatment focused on developing language, increasing social behavior, and promoting cooperative play with peers and independent toy play. Efforts were also aimed at decreasing rituals, tantrums, and aggressive behaviors.

Nineteen children were treated, with another 19 acting as controls (internal control group). The treatment and control groups were similar in IQ score and severity of disturbance. The only significant bias was that assignment

to groups was not randomized. Treatment intervention for the internal control group consisted of 10 hours or less of one-to-one behavioral treatment and other treatments provided by community agencies, including parent intervention and special education services. In addition, an "outside control group" consisting of 21 children with autism and similar IQ levels was followed over time but not referred to the study. Reevaluation at a mean age of 7 years revealed that the experimental group had gained an average of 20 IQ points and made significant educational gains. Nine of the 19 children had IQ scores in the average range and had completed a regular first-grade class. In contrast, only 1 of the 40 total control subjects had achieved typical IQ or educational levels. It was, therefore, concluded that the behavioral treatment was effective in improving outcome. At follow-up 6 years later, McEachin, Smith, and Lovaas (1993) reported that the gains were maintained in all of the children, with 9 of 19 children (47%) in the experimental group attending general classes, whereas none of the 19 children in the internal control group were in a general class.

As can be seen in a review by Simeonsson, Olley, and Rosenthal (1987), the study by Lovaas was truly a breakthrough. In their review of EI for children with autism, they found that only 3 of 10 intervention studies published since 1975 (Fenske, Zalenski, Krantz, & McClannahan, 1985; Lovaas, 1987; Strain, Hoyson, & Jamieson, 1985) were comprehensive in nature and included structured behavioral treatment, parental involvement, treatment at an early age, intensive treatment, and generalization across settings.

One decade later, Dawson and Osterling (1997) reported on eight model EI programs for autism in the United States. Three of these were continuations of those reported previously by Simeonsson et al. (1987). All eight programs contained within them the comprehensive approach noted previously. Furthermore, these programs included, at a minimum, some form of standardized assessment of verbal and nonverbal abilities, autistic symptoms, and adaptive function. Program age at entrance ranged from 2 years 8 months in one program (Lovaas) to between 3 and 4 years in the others. At entrance, full-scale IQ scores ranged from 49 to 70, and half the programs included children diagnosed with pervasive developmental disorder not otherwise specified as well as autism.

Program outcome data were reported as post-preschool placements of the children, as specific developmental gains, or both. In four of the six programs reporting placement data, 50% of the children were integrated into a general classroom by the end of the intervention. Children gained an average of 20 IQ points as compared with their IQ scores when entering the intervention. This was very significant in light of the finding that, *prior* to entering the intervention, most children had an IQ score of 70 or below. Yet, Dawson and Osterling (1997) noted that, given the significant methodological limitations, including lack of randomization, these studies did not meet the requirements for "true experimental studies."

Rogers (1998) performed a similar but more systematic review of the autism EI literature. Overall, she noted that the studies all reported significant improvements in outcome for children enrolled in their respective treatment programs. In applying criteria for empirically supported treatments to the studies examined, Rogers found the Lovaas (1987) study to have the strongest design. This is despite certain deficiencies in methodologies, most significantly the lack of randomization. Two studies (Birnbrauer & Leach, 1993; Sheinkopf & Siegel, 1998) that were partial replications of the Lovaas approach were the only other studies to contain control groups. A third replication study of the Lovaas approach (Anderson, Avery, Dipietro, Edwards, & Christian, 1987), along with two other studies (Fenske et al., 1985; Harris, Handleman, Gordon, Kristoff, & Fuentes, 1991) that employed similar behavioral intervention approaches, all employed pre–post designs. Finally, two other studies using somewhat different treatment approaches, one a developmental/behavioral curriculum (Hoyson, Jamieson, & Strain, 1984) and another a developmentally oriented program (Rogers & DiLalla, 1991), also employed pre–post designs.

Rogers (1998) noted that, despite the positive outcomes reported by all of the programs, the studies reviewed did not meet criteria for determining empirically supported treatments. She likened the value of such studies to those of open trials of medication whose positive results await confirmation in more methodologically rigorous designs, including, among other design aspects, matching, randomization, and blind raters.

Kasari (2002), in a literature review of essentially the same studies, drew conclusions similar to those of Rogers (1998). Although she noted that the current corpus of studies, because of internal threats to validity, represent only directions, Kasari found suggestions that the active components of treatment programs may be specific treatment approaches and content, setting effects (home vs. center), and number of hours of intervention. Further elaborating on this is the suggestion that focusing on joint attention and symbolic play in a direct manner may lead to improved gains.

Diggle, McConachie, and Randle (2003) performed a systematic review of the literature for evidence of efficacy of parent-mediated EI for young children with autism. Only studies that were randomized or quasi-randomized controlled trials and were found to have low to moderate risk of bias were considered for review. Only 2 of the 68 available studies (Jocelyn, Casiro, Beattie, Bow, & Kneisz, 1998; Smith, Groen, & Wynn, 2000) met inclusion criteria, and they are summarized here.

The study by Jocelyn et al. (1998) was a randomized controlled study that compared parent training plus community child care with community child care alone. The experimental group was composed of 16 parents who were trained for 15 hours over 10 weeks in the areas of functional analysis, empathy skills, and coping with problem behavior. Parents participated in three case conferences, and two home visits were made by social workers. Children attended child care for an average of 21 hours/week over 12 weeks. Nineteen families in the control group had their child in child care for an average of 4 hours/day over 12 weeks and received social work support. At the conclusion of the 12 weeks, the experimental group showed significantly greater gains in the child's language abilities, as well as increases in caregivers' knowledge about autism.

Smith et al. (2000) carried out a randomized controlled study comparing intensive treatment based on a Lovaas behavioral approach with parent training. There were 15 families in the intensive treatment group versus 13 in the parent training group. In the intensive treatment group, children received 30 hours of intervention per week for up to 3 years by four to six student therapists. In the parent training group, parents were taught the Lovaas treatment method from the manual. Parents received two sessions per week (5 hours) for 3–9 months. Parents were asked to work with their child for 5 hours/week. Children in this group were in special education classes for up to 15 hours/week during this period. Follow-up was performed at an average of 4 years 10 months. Results favored the intensive treatment group in regard to child outcome measures, including an IQ gain of approximately 16 points; however, no differences were noted with respect to parent or teacher perspectives.

In attempting to summarize the findings of these two studies, Diggle et al. (2003) noted that short-term language improvements were greater for children of those parents receiving parent training as compared with children who received child care alone. In addition, it was noted that mothers and child care workers who received parent training gained knowledge about autism. They further noted that one could consider that parent-mediated behaviorally oriented EI is better than child care but not as effective as intensive home-based treatments as seen in the study by Smith et al. (2000). Diggle et al., however, raised numerous other possibilities that could explain the current findings, including the fact that the difference between the intensive intervention group and the parent training group was due to the difference of hours of intervention. Consequently, they do not see these two studies as allowing one to make conclusions regarding the added value of parent intervention for young children with autism.

Diggle et al. (2003) pointed to less reliable evidence from 13 nonrandomized but controlled studies that overall reported at least some positive results for parent training interventions. These include five studies suggesting improvements in child outcomes, five reporting improvements in parent outcomes, and two that found improvements in both child and parent outcomes. Diggle et al. also noted that only 1 of the 13 studies found no effect for intervention.

It is instructive to compare the behavioral versus developmental approaches noted previously. As described by Farran (2000), the behavioral approach, as developed by Lovaas, sees children with autism, given their abnormal central nervous system, as not being able to learn from their regular environment. This necessitates an intensive, highly structured and predetermined, all-encompassing intervention approach requiring extensive manipulation of the environment while employing laws of learning. In contrast, the developmental approach, also known as the play-based approach, sees the all-encompassing social impairment in children with autism not as a deficit but as a functional and communicative issue. The goal of intervention is to teach alternative modes of communication that serve as effectively as the odd/problem behaviors. This approach sees the child as an active participant in treatment. Skills should be modeled on naturally occurring patterns in typical situations and should employ a highly individualized approach that is based on family resources, values, and preferences. Thus, a behavioral approach is teacher-directed whereas a developmental approach is child-initiated.

In addition to the ongoing discussion as to the value of EI programs in general, Howlin (2003) raised questions regarding the specific effects of the EI programs. Among the many questions remaining are those regarding effects of particular curricula (behavioral vs. developmental), one-to-one versus group teaching, home-based versus school-based programs, and necessary number of hours of intervention (intensity). Despite the limitations of the current state of research, there do seem to be suggestions that programs of 20 hours produce results that are better than shorter ones. Also, there appears to be a consensus that earlier is better in terms of initiating treatment.

Although answers to many of these questions remain unclear, Howlin did list a number of effective components of intervention. These include consideration of social, communication, and behavioral deficits when planning an intervention; emphasis on skill development; employment of a structured, behavior-based approach; utilization of a functional analysis approach to behavior problems; focus on development of effective communication skills; modification of environment to enhance learning and reduce stress; use of naturally occurring opportunities for teaching and reinforcement; and understanding of the importance of predictability and routine in teaching new skills and reducing problem behaviors and in fostering integration with typically developing peers.

Following up on the now incessant call for more rigorously performed studies were two pilot studies that reported on the results of parent training interventions for children with autism as well as a replication study of Lovaas' early intensive behavioral intervention all using a randomized controlled design. Drew et al. (2002) reported on a parent training intervention that focused on joint attention and joint action routines. Twenty-four children with autism with a mean age of 23 months were randomized to a parent training group or to local services. Follow-up 1 year later showed very marginal improvement of the intervention group versus the control group; however, the authors noted multiple limitations, including the fact that three of the control group children received intensive home-based behavioral interventions during the study.

Aldred, Green, and Adams (2004) performed a study similar to that of Drew et al. with a focus on social communication. The study group consisted of 28 children with autism, ages 2–6 years, who in addition to receiving routine ongoing care were (after matching) randomized to receive a social communication intervention for children with autism. This intervention, recognizing the lack of joint attention skills and the pragmatic difficulties in working with children with autism, focused on improving parental adaptation and communication with children with autism. At 1 year, significant improvements as compared to controls were reported both on the Autism Diagnostic Observation Schedule (ADOS; Lord et al., 1989) total score, especially in the reciprocal social interaction, and on measures of ex-

pressive language, communicative initiation, and parent–child interaction.

Sallows and Graupner (2005) examined the 4-year outcome of 24 children who received either a clinic-directed early intensive behavior intervention or a parent-directed group that also received intensive intervention but with less clinic supervision. Findings were very similar to those of Lovaas with 48% of all children functioning in a general education class by age 7 years. Of further importance was the finding that treatment outcome was best predicted by pretreatment variables including imitation, language, and social responsiveness skills.

Tonge et al. (2006), in a randomized controlled study, reported of the benefit of parent education and behavior management program for parents of children with autism on parental mental health, suggesting a role for it alongside EI training directed at improving the child's function.

Finally, when reviewing the EI literature on autism, it is worthwhile mentioning the existence of an intervention referred to as the Developmental, Individual-Difference, Relationship-Based (DIR/Floortime) program (Greenspan & Wieder, 1997; Wieder & Greenspan, 2003), which has gained widespread use with much anecdotal reporting of its value. This model focuses on the building blocks of relating, communicating, and thinking and addresses the individual variations in sensory processing, sensory discrimination and modulation, and motor planning and sequencing as well as family interactive patterns. There is, however, extremely scant evidence for efficacy as published in peer-reviewed journals, with no controlled or replicated studies found. Consequently, it is not mentioned in any of the previously discussed reviews.

Conclusions Of the three areas examined in this chapter, evidence for the efficacy of EI in the population of children with autism is clearly the strongest. Although the literature still has limitations, there is at least good preliminary evidence suggesting that early intensive intervention, be it behaviorally or developmentally based, provided for at least 20 hours/week from as early an age as possible seems to be indicated. Further research will allow better delineation of the components that are most effective in treating this population.

Efficacy of Early Intervention with Known Developmental Disabilities: Conclusions and Implications

Evidence for EI in children with specific developmental disabilities is increasing, albeit at a slow rate. Whereas the early literature was plagued by studies with poor methodology, more recent studies in almost all areas are beginning to be of a quality that allows clinicians to draw some conclusions. A notable exception is in the field of DS, where, unfortunately, new data are limited. In the field of CP, we are beginning to see that the evidence for previously mainstay therapies such as NDT is limited, and thus such therapies should not be employed as the major approach to treatment. In their place, functionally based approaches should be considered. In children with DS, given that data do suggest short-term benefits for "intervention," some form of EI seems warranted, though parents and providers should be keenly aware that benefits of current programs are not certain. Knowledge of the learning characteristics of children with DS must be considered when planning these interventions. In the field of autism, where the most progress has been made, early intensive behavioral or developmental approaches should be considered standard pending further data.

Ethically there is no question that children with disabilities need assistance and intervention. Examination of efficacy is not meant to deny the need for such treatment or that treatment causes change. In fact, general systems theory and the theory of self-organization assert that any outside intervention obliges a system to reorganize its structure in response to its environment (Pretis, 2000); however, only through careful and systematic examination of all interventions will we gain the knowledge necessary to advise parents as to which interventions warrant their attention and their valuable and limited resources. Given that many of the answers are still not available, it will be incumbent on professionals serving children to closely follow this evolving literature.

What is very clear from review of this body of literature is the need to plan interventions with clearly delineated goals that are functional in nature and decided on in collaboration with parents. Periodic objective assessments should be mandatory. The practice of limiting enrollment of children with different developmental disabilities to different arms of clinical trials, akin to studies found in the oncology literature, should strongly be considered.

EARLY INTERVENTION IN CHILDREN AT RISK FOR DEVELOPMENTAL DISABILITIES

Two models of EI of children at risk for developmental disabilities have emerged: one for the child "at environmental risk" and the other for the child "at biological risk." Those children in the former category have primarily included children growing up in backgrounds of poverty, abuse, or neglect or with limited parental stimulation, as might be found for children of teenage parents. This group stimulated the development of the federal Head Start program, as the country sought to find early solutions to the problems of poverty and crime. Therefore, while intervening for developmental disabilities was not the original intent, it has come to be believed that these services might prevent cognitive problems, such as mild intellectual disabilities, borderline levels of intelligence, and learning disabilities, and hence improve school achievement. Contributing to this belief was the popular notion that mild intellectual disabilities and borderline intelligence are primarily of "sociocultural" etiology. It is also commonly suggested that such intervention may be able to prevent emotional and behavior disorders, such as attention-deficit/hyperactivity disorder or depression. Programs for children at biological risk focused their attention on children with medical conditions known to have high incidences of disabilities. The low birth weight or premature infant has been the primary model for these programs, with interventions beginning as early as the newborn period in the neonatal intensive care unit.

Intervention for
Children at Environmental Risk

Dozens of programs have intervened with populations of children considered to be at increased environmental risk, and attempts have been made to study their efficacy. In the review by Farran (1990), 32 projects with results published between 1977 and 1986 and centered on "disadvantaged" children receiving services as a result of their low SES were examined. A total of 5,000 children received services, and they were compared with 2,000 controls. Interventions focused primarily on cognitive remediation, some center-based and others home-based. Age at program enrollment varied from infancy to the prekindergarten years. Among the home-based programs, short-term improvements were seen in IQ performance of treated children compared with controls, but, with longitudinal follow-up, the improvement continued in only one of four studies. In center-based programs begun in infancy, improvements in test performance were noted among treated children through age 3; however, by ages 4–5, improvements were occurring in control subjects as well, limiting the differences between the groups and creating questions regarding long-term benefits of the interventions. Studies involving 2- and 3-year-old children had mixed results, with limited positive effects. Those programs for 4- to 6-year-old children included those enrolled in Head Start programs, and these too showed positive short-term effects, with absence of convincing long-term improvements unless similar services continued into the elementary school years.

In more recent reviews of the efficacy of early childhood education on children of poverty, longer-term benefits of such intervention have been reported. In the Carolina Abecederian Project (n.d.), follow-up of a cohort of 104 children to age 21 has revealed remarkable differences between those children who received early childhood education and those who did not. Treated children had higher cognitive scores, language skills, and reading and mathematics achievement than controls. They also reached significantly higher levels of education and enjoyed higher employment rates. The positive cognitive effects seen in children treated in this program as well as the related Project CARE were greatest for those children of lesser-educated mothers (Ramey & Ramey, 1998). Similar conclusions were reached in a review of 38 studies (Barnett, 1998) and in a study involving more than 1,500 low-income children (Reynolds, Temple, Robertson, & Mann, 2001). Both concluded that there are long-term cognitive and academic benefits from early childhood education for children in poverty. Although some studies reported a fading out of IQ advantage, gains in educational achievement generally appeared to remain robust. Cost–benefit analysis based on a single study also suggested an economic benefit to society of such programs.

It is now four decades since Head Start and related programs began providing early childhood education to children in low-income households and with lower educated parents. In this population there appears to be convincing evidence of both short- and long-term benefit from EI preschool services.

Intervention for
Children at Biological Risk

Intervention studies of children at biological risk have primarily focused their attention and efforts on the low birth weight premature infant population, given their large numbers, their relative homogeneity, and the ease of accessibility of this group. Services have ranged from those begun in the newborn period, with direct intervention to the hospitalized infant, to home- or center-based services begun later.

In the neonatal intensive care unit (NICU), interventions have ranged from traditional physical therapy to multimodal, varied, and often unconventional methods of infant stimulation, including modalities such as touch (e.g., massage, special positioning, stroking); movement (e.g., rocking for vestibular stimulation, waterbeds); sound (e.g., placental sounds, music, human voice); and sight (e.g., picture cues, ambient light adjustment). Some interventions have been implemented through the infant's parents, whereas others have involved primarily a therapist, including physical therapists, psychologists, infant educators, and nurses. Studies of the effectiveness of these services reveal varied results, with the majority of the results generally compromised by small numbers of infants studied, limited controls, and extreme program diversity and with each program's design being idiosyncratic to the investigators involved or the population studied. In their review of these services, Bennett and Guralnick (1991) noted conflicting results and difficulties in generalizability, precluding recommendation of such services.

Since this review, neonatal developmental intervention has increased in the NICU. In a more recent review of such care, Symington and Pinelli (2006) examined 36 randomized controlled trials involving 2,220 neonates. Study sample sizes ranged from 16 to 259 subjects, with 22 studies involving fewer than 50 infants. These interventions were grouped into four categories: positioning, clustering of nursery care activities, modification of external stimuli, and individualized developmental care. It was these authors' conclusion that these interventions demonstrated limited benefits, with decreased moderate-severe chronic lung disease, decreased necrotizing enterocolitis, and improved family outcome. There was limited evidence of long-term benefit, with the Newborn Individualized Developmental Care and Assessment Program (NIDCAP; Als, 1998) having very limited effect on behavior and movement and no effect on cognition at five year outcome.

Other individualized interventions showed some effect in enhancing outcomes, but the results often conflicted. There were significant design limitations seen, including half of the studies being flawed by absence of blinding of the assessors. The authors called for more consistent evidence of benefit in short- and long-term outcomes before recommendations could be made for a clear direction for practice. They also note that the costs of such interventions and their related economic impact have not been studied and considered. In meta-analyses of five randomized clinical trials and three prospective phase-lag cohort studies using the Newborn Individualized Developmental Care and Assessment Program (NIDCAP; Als, 1998) with 321 low birth weight infants, neither clear benefit nor adverse effect was seen in the short-term medical outcomes or the neurodevelopmental outcomes at 24 months of age (Jacobs, Sokol, & Ohlsson, 2002). Therefore, despite the widespread use and acceptance of developmental intervention in the NICU, there remain no clear scientific conclusions of a short-term benefit or improved long-term outcomes of treated low birth weight infants.

Studies of intervention begun with the low birth weight infant after discharge from the NICU have had similar weaknesses; however, the multicenter Infant Health and Development Program (1990) has overcome many of these obstacles through its creation of a randomized intervention trial involving eight sites and nearly 1,000 infants. In this study, infants were recruited from two birth-weight classes, those weighing between 2,000 and 2,500 g and those weighing 2,000 g or less, with 608 infants receiving no intervention and 377 infants receiving an intensive intervention program. The intervention began on discharge from the nursery and continued until 36 months of age (corrected for prematurity). It consisted of three components: home visits, center-based services, and parent group meetings. The home visits occurred weekly for the first year and biweekly for the following years and consisted of family support, provision of health and developmental information, and implementation of two developmental instructional curricula. From 12 to 36 months of age, children attended a center-based intervention program 5 days per week that utilized the same curricula. The parent groups were begun when the infants were 12 months of age, with meetings occurring bimonthly and giving information on child rearing, health and safety, and other parenting concerns, as well as providing a social support (Ramey et al., 1992).

Outcome now has been assessed through 8 years of age and has consisted of assessments of cognition, academic achievement, parental report of school performance behavior, and health status (McCormick, McCarton, Brooks-Gunn, Belt, & Gross, 1998). At 36 months of age, in both weight groups, children receiving intervention scored higher on IQ tests, with the greatest effect occurring among those weighing 2,000–2,500 g. Intervention with infants weighing less than 1,500 g appeared to have the least effect, although differences in IQ score were also noted among this group (McCormick, McCarton, Tonascia, & Brooks-Gunn, 1993). Equal numbers of intervention and control infants tested as having an IQ score less than 70 at 36 months of age, however (Infant Health and Development Program, 1990). Thus, the effect of the intervention was greatest among the heavier children. Behavioral outcome revealed better performance in the intervention group, although only for those infants with mothers having less than a college education. In general, children whose mothers had a high school education or less benefited most from the intervention (Brooks-Gunn, Gross, Kraemer, Spiker, & Shapiro, 1992). The intellectual performance of those children with greater family participation was significantly better than that of those with lower family participation, suggesting that greater intensity of service was linked to better cognitive outcome (Ramey et al., 1992).

With reassessment at age 5, 2 years after discontinuation of the intervention, and again at age 8, the beneficial effects of the intervention were significantly reduced (McCarton et al., 1997). Only children in the heavier group (2,001–2,500 g birth weight) showed improved cognitive performance, with a modest increase of 4.4 IQ points and improved mathematics achievement and receptive vocabulary performance (Brooks-Gunn et al., 1994). Those children in the lighter group showed no improvements over the controls on any measure of performance. Neither birthweight group differed from the control sample in behavioral outcome. While no change was observed in health status at age 5, at 8 years the children in the intervention group were rated lower in motor activities than the controls. The health outcomes of the children in the heavier group did not differ with intervention, whereas those in the lighter group who received intervention were rated lower by their mothers in social limitations caused by behavior.

The Infant Health and Development Program (1990) thus has given some support to the provision of EI services to low birth weight infants as a means of improving cognitive outcome, although the effect was modest and was seen only in children weighing between 2,000 and 2,500 g at birth and with mothers with a high school education or less. It must be borne in mind that these improvements in outcome were limited to cognitive performance, with no benefit found in behavioral, functional, or health outcomes. Presence or absence of frank developmental disability was not specifically assessed, although motor outcome of those in the intervention group may have been worse. In addition, the effect was least among those children at greatest risk for disability, the very low birth weight infants below 1,500 g at birth. McCormick et al. (1998) suggested that the lighter group may have a higher proportion of children with neurological impairments who would not benefit from this specific intervention. Children in the heavier group, in whom the only significant effect was seen, are at significantly lesser risk of disability and require significantly less neonatal medical care. Although the authors have concluded that intensive preschool intervention can improve the outcomes of low birth weight infants, these findings suggest an effect identical to that seen in those children at environmental risk, with the benefit seen in children at lower biological risk but higher risk based on social and educational factors.

Efficacy of Early Intervention in Children at Risk: Conclusions

Many studies of EI with children at risk, whether this is an environmental or a biological risk, have provided encouragement to those who seek to prevent future problems through special programs for infants, toddlers, and preschoolers; however, it appears that it is specifically those children at environmental risk who are benefiting most. In particular, children from low-income households and born to lower educated mothers appear to be deriving the greatest advantage from this intervention. In children at biological risk, as exemplified by low birth weight infants, these same social variables appear to mediate the intervention effects, rather than any biological factor. In those children at greatest biological risk with very low birth weight, the efficacy of early childhood intervention remains debatable and demands further investigation of the methods of treatment, long-term outcome, and risk–benefit analysis.

CONCLUSION

Since the 1900s, we have witnessed a major change in the public perception of children with disabilities and a similarly major change in the methods by which we care for them. No longer are we sending affected children into institutional settings focused on custodial care. Instead, the children have been afforded individual rights, now mandated by law, allowing them to experience the same opportunities that other children have for care by their families, for socialization, and for education. The availability of EI services, coupled with the enactment of PL 101-336, assures that people with disabilities can receive special assistance in accessing the services of their community and thus become integrated into it throughout their life span.

With the passage and subsequent revisions of the IDEA, EI has become a model both for integration of children with disabilities into the community and for prevention of developmental problems in high-risk populations. This differs from its original therapeutic intent of changing the child's developmental performance outcome. As reviewed in this chapter, current research suggests that the efficacy of EI in improving outcome is mixed. In populations at risk, the greatest support for its efficacy comes from studies of children at environmental or socioeconomic risk. In those with identified disabilities, the greatest benefits have been demonstrated in children with autism receiving early intensive interventions. While efficacy of neurodevelopmental therapy for children with CP and motor disorders has not been clearly seen, other techniques showing promise have emerged for children with these conditions. Therapeutic benefit from EI has been less clearly delineated for intellectual disabilities, as in the example of children with DS, although some gains have been suggested in more recent work.

It is now clear that investigation of the efficacy of EI requires varying techniques and methodologies, depending on the population being investigated. Infants with disabilities are far fewer in number than those at risk, making large, meaningful studies more difficult to design. The variety of disabling conditions is also wide, resulting in significant heterogeneity in designing programs and studies for affected children. In contrast, children at risk can be provided broader, less specific, and perhaps less costly services that focus on "development" in the most general sense, with fewer expectations for progress. We anticipate that the child with CP will develop walking skills, an accomplishment that may be significant if there is severe neurological damage, whereas we merely hope that the at-risk child does generally better in school, not knowing for sure if there are biological obstacles standing in his or her way.

We are now in the era of "second-generation research" (Guralnick, 1997) on EI, in which greater specificity and better methodology, such as randomized controlled trials, are being used in research design. More population specificity and uniformity are being used in research involving both high-risk children and children with specific disabilities, including critical elements such as entry criteria, disability definition, and demographic variables of age and socioeconomic status. Greater specificity of therapeutic techniques is also being employed, providing better answers as to what methods may offer the greatest benefit.

Professionals in the field of developmental disabilities should continue to seek answers to questions regarding efficacy of EI through appropriately designed studies, so that they can create programs and services with optimal benefit. The therapeutic model for a specific group of children may need to be revised, replaced, or supplemented with a family-social model for EI programming. Service providers can assist through ongoing review of the efficacy of treatments provided, accepting that some treatments may be ineffective in some circumstances, and the better course may be substitution of other techniques that have demonstrated efficacy. The providers should also help families by guiding them into appropriate services and expectations for their child. It is clear that EI will continue as the model for care of the infant and preschooler with disabilities. We must be sure that it achieves all it can in assisting these children and their families to integrate optimally into the community at large.

REFERENCES

Aldred, C., Green, J., & Adams, C. (2004). A new social communication intervention for children with autism: Pilot randomized controlled treatment study suggesting effectiveness. *Journal of Child Psychology and Psychiatry, 45,* 1420–1430.

Als, H. (1998). Developmental care in the newborn intensive care unit. *Current Opinion in Pediatrics, 10,* 138–142.

Americans with Disabilities Act of 1990, PL 101-336, 42 U.S.C. §§ 12101 *et seq.*

Anderson, S.R., Avery, D.L., DiPietro, E.K., Edwards, G.L., & Christian, W.P. (1987). Intensive home-based early intervention with autistic children. *Education and Treatment of Children, 10,* 352–366.

Bailey, D.B., Jr., Hebbeler, K., Spiker, D., Scarborough, A., Mallik, S., & Nelson, L. (2005). Thirty-six-month outcomes for families of children who have disabilities and participated in early intervention. *Pediatrics, 116*(6), 1346–1352.

Barnett, W.S. (1998). Long-term cognitive and academic effects of early childhood education on children in poverty. *Preventive Medicine, 27,* 204–207.

Bennett, F.C., & Guralnick, M.J. (1991). Effectiveness of developmental intervention in the first five years of life. *Pediatric Clinics of North America, 38,* 1513–1528.

Birnbrauer, J.S., & Leach, D.J. (1993). The Murdock Early Intervention Program after 2 years. *Behavior Change, 10,* 63–74.

Blauw-Hosper, C.H., & Hadders-Algra, M. (2005). A systematic review of the effects of early intervention on motor development. *Developmental Medicine and Child Neurology, 47,* 421–432.

Blundell, S.W., Shepherd, R.B., Dean, C.M., Adams, R.D., & Cahill, B.M. (2003). Functional strength training in cerebral palsy: A pilot study of a group circuit training class for children aged 4–8 years. *Clinical Rehabilitation, 17,* 48–57.

Bobath, K., & Bobath, B. (1984). The neurodevelopmental treatment. In D. Scrutton (Ed.), *Management of the motor disorders of children with cerebral palsy* (pp. 6–18). London: Spastics International Medical Publications.

Boyd, R.N., Morris, M.E., & Graham, H.K. (2001). Management of upper limb dysfunction in children with cerebral palsy: A systematic review. *European Journal of Neurology, 8*(Suppl. 5), 150–166.

Brinker, R.P., Seifer, R., & Sameroff, A.J. (1994). Relations among maternal stress, cognitive development, and early intervention in middle- and low-SES infants with developmental disabilities. *American Journal of Mental Retardation, 98,* 463–480.

Brooks-Gunn, J., Gross, R.T., Kraemer, H.C., Spiker, D., & Shapiro, S. (1992). Enhancing the cognitive outcomes of low birth weight, premature infants: For whom is the intervention most effective? *Pediatrics, 89,* 1209–1215.

Brooks-Gunn, J., McCarton, C.M., Casey, P.H., McCormick, M.C., Bauer, C.R., Bembaum, J.C., et al. (1994). Early intervention in low-birth-weight premature infants: Results through age 5 years from the Infant Health and Development Program. *JAMA, 272,* 1257–1262.

Butler, C., & Darrah, J. (2001). Effects of neurodevelopmental treatment (NDT) for cerebral palsy: An AACPDM evidence report. *Developmental Medicine and Child Neurology, 43,* 778–790.

Campbell, S.K. (1990). Efficacy of physical therapy in improving postural control in cerebral palsy. *Pediatric Physical Therapy, 2,* 135–140.

Carolina Abecedarian Project. (n.d.). *Early learning, later success: The Abecedarian Study. Early childhood educational intervention for poor children. Executive summary.* Retrieved June 30, 2005, from http://www.fpg.unc.edu/~abc/summary.cfm

Carr, J. (1988). Six weeks to twenty-one years old: A longitudinal study of children with Down's syndrome and their families. *Journal of Child Psychology and Psychiatry, 29,* 407–431.

Casto, G., & Mastropieri, M. (1986). The efficacy of early intervention programs: A meta-analysis. *Exceptional Children, 52,* 417–424.

Charles, J.R., Wolf, S.L., Schneider, J.A., & Gordon, A.M. (2006). Efficacy of a child-friendly form of constraint-induced movement therapy in hemiplegic cerebral palsy: A randomized control trial. *Developmental Medicine and Child Neurology, 48,* 635–642.

Cole, K.N., & Dale, P.S. (1986). Direct language instruction and interactive language instruction with language delayed preschool children: A comparison study. *Journal of Speech and Hearing Research, 29,* 206–217.

Cole, K.N., Mills, P.E., Dale, P.S., & Jenkins, J.R. (1991). Effect of preschool integration for children with disabilities. *Exceptional Children, 58,* 36–45.

Connolly, B.H., Morgan, S.B., Russell, F.F., & Fulliton, W.L. (1993). A longitudinal study of children with Down syndrome who experienced early intervention programming. *Physical Therapy, 73,* 170–179.

Dale P.S., Jenkins, J.R., Mills, P.E., & Cole, K.N. (2005). Follow-up of children from academic and cognitive preschool curricula at ages 12 and 16. *Exceptional Children, 16,* 861–865.

Damiano, D.L., Dodd, K., & Taylor, N.F. (2002). Should we be testing and training muscle strength in cerebral palsy? *Developmental Medicine and Child Neurology, 44,* 68–72.

Darrah, J., Fan, J.S., Chen, L.C., Nunwieler, J., & Watkins, B. (1997). Review of the effects of progressive resisted muscle strengthening in children with cerebral palsy: A clinical consensus exercise. *Pediatric Physical Therapy, 9,* 12–17.

Darrah, J., Watkins, B., Chen, L., & Bonin, C., for the AACPDM. (2004). Conductive education intervention for children with cerebral palsy: An AACPDM evidence report. *Developmental Medicine and Child Neurology, 46,* 187–203.

Dawson, G., & Osterling, J. (1997). Early intervention in autism. In M.J. Guralnick (Ed.), *The effectiveness of early intervention* (pp. 307–326). Baltimore: Paul H. Brookes Publishing Co.

DeLuca, S.C., Echols, K., Ramey, S.L., & Taub, E. (2003). Pediatric constraint-induced movement therapy for a young child with cerebral palsy: Two episodes of care. *Physical Therapy, 83,* 1003–1013.

Denhoff, E. (1981). Current status of infant stimulation or enrichment programs for children with developmental disabilities. *Pediatrics, 67,* 32–37.

Diggle, T., McConachie, H.R., & Randle, V.R. (2003). Parent-mediated early intervention for young children with autism spectrum disorder. *Cochrane Database of Systematic Reviews,* (1), CD003496.

Dihoff, R.E., Brosvic, G.M., Kafer, L.B., McEwan, M., Carpenter, L., Rizzuto, G.E., et al. (1994). Efficacy of part- and full-time early intervention. *Perceptual and Motor Skills, 79,* 907–911.

Dodd, K.J., Taylor, N.F., & Damiano, D.L. (2002). A systematic review of the effectiveness of strength-training programs for people with cerebral palsy. *Archives of Physical Medicine and Rehabilitation, 83,* 1157–1164.

Dodd, K.J., Taylor, N.F., & Graham, H.K. (2003). A randomized clinical trial of strength training in young people with cerebral palsy. *Developmental Medicine and Child Neurology, 45,* 652–657.

Drew, A., Baird, G., Baron-Cohen, S., Cox, A., Slonims, V., Wheelwright, S., et al. (2002). A pilot randomised control trial of a parent training intervention for pre-school children with autism: Preliminary findings and methodological challenges. *European Child and Adolescent Psychiatry, 11,* 266–272.

Dunst, C.J., & Rheingrover, R.M. (1981). An analysis of the efficacy of infant intervention programs with organically handicapped children. *Evaluation and Program Planning, 4,* 287–323.

Eagleton, M., Iams, A., McDowell, J., Morrison, R., & Evans, C.L. (2004). The effects of strength training on gait in adolescents with cerebral palsy. *Pediatric Physical Therapy, 16,* 22–30.

Education for All Handicapped Children Act of 1975, PL 94-142, 20 U.S.C. §§ 1400 *et seq.*

Education of the Handicapped Act Amendments of 1986, PL 99-457, 20 U.S.C. §§ 1400 *et seq.*

Eliasson, A.C., Bonnier, B., & Krumlinde-Sundholm, L. (2003). Clinical experience of constraint induced movement therapy in adolescents with hemiplegic cerebral palsy—a day camp model. *Developmental Medicine and Child Neurology, 45,* 357–359.

Eliasson, A.C., Krumlinde-Sundholm, L., Shaw, K., & Wang, C. (2005). Effects of constraint-induced movement therapy in young children with hemiplegic cerebral palsy: An adapted model. *Developmental Medicine and Child Neurology, 47,* 266–275.

Farran, D.C. (1990). Effects of intervention with disadvantaged and disabled children: A decade review. In S.J. Meisels & J.P. Shonkoff (Eds.), *Handbook of early childhood intervention* (pp. 501–539). New York: Cambridge University Press.

Farran, D.C. (2000). Another decade of intervention for disadvantaged and disabled children: What do we know now? In J.P. Shonkoff & S.J. Meisels (Eds.), *Handbook of early childhood intervention* (2nd ed., pp. 510–548). New York: Cambridge University Press.

Feldman, A.B., Haley, S.M., & Coryell, J. (1990). Concurrent and construct validity of the Pediatric Evaluation of Disability Inventory. *Physical Therapy, 70,* 602–610.

Fenske, E.C., Zalenski, S., Krantz, P.J., & McClannahan, L.E. (1985). Age at intervention and treatment outcome for autistic children in a comprehensive treatment program. *Analysis and Intervention in Developmental Disabilities, 5,* 49–58.

Foreman, P., & Crews, G. (1998). Using augmentative communication with infants and young children with Down syndrome. *Down Syndrome Research and Practice, 5,* 16–25.

Gibson, D., & Harris, A. (1988). Aggregated early intervention effects for Down's syndrome persons: Patterning and longevity of benefits. *Journal of Mental Deficiency Research, 32,* 1–17.

Gibson, J.J. (1979). *The ecological approach to visual perception.* Boston: Houghton-Mifflin.

Glass, G.V. (1976). Primary, secondary and meta-analysis of research. *Educational Researcher, 5,* 3–8.

Gordon, A.M., Charles, J., & Wolf, S.L. (2005). Methods of constraint-induced movement therapy for children with hemiplegic cerebral palsy: Development of a child-friendly intervention for improving upper-extremity function. *Archives of Physical Medicine and Rehabilitation, 86,* 837–844.

Gordon, A.M., Charles, J., & Wolf, S.L. (2006). Efficacy of constraint-induced movement therapy on involved upper-extremity use in children with hemiplegic cerebral palsy is not age-dependent. *Pediatrics, 117,* e363–e373.

Greenspan, S.I., & Wieder, S. (1997). Developmental patterns and outcomes in infants and children with disorders in relating and communicating: A chart review of 200 cases of children with autistic spectrum diagnoses. *Journal of Developmental and Learning Disorders, 1,* 87–141.

Guralnick, M.J. (1991). The next decade of research on the effectiveness of early intervention. *Exceptional Children, 58,* 174–183.

Guralnick, M.J. (1997). Second-generation research in the field of early intervention. In M.J. Guralnick

(Ed.), *The effectiveness of early intervention* (pp. 3–20). Baltimore: Paul H. Brookes Publishing Co.

Harris, S.L., Handleman, J.S., Gordon, R., Kristoff, B., & Fuentes, F. (1991). Changes in cognitive and language functioning of preschool children with autism. *Journal of Autism and Developmental Disorders, 21,* 281–290.

Harris, S.R. (1990). Therapeutic exercise for children with neurodevelopmental disabilities. In J.V. Basmajian & S.L. Wolf (Eds.), *Therapeutic exercise* (5th ed., pp. 163–176). Baltimore: Lippincott, Williams & Wilkins.

Harris, S.R. (1997). The effectiveness of early intervention for children with cerebral palsy and related motor disabilities. In M.J. Guralnick (Ed.), *The effectiveness of early intervention* (pp. 327–347). Baltimore: Paul H. Brookes Publishing Co.

Harris, S.R., Atwater, S.W., & Crowe, T.K. (1988). Accepted and controversial neuromotor therapies for infants at high risk for cerebral palsy. *Journal of Perinatology, 8,* 3–13.

Hines, S., & Bennett, F. (1996). Effectiveness of early intervention for children with Down syndrome. *Mental Retardation and Developmental Disabilities, 2,* 96–101.

Horak, F.B. (1991). Assumptions underlying motor control for neurologic rehabilitation. In M. Lister (Ed.), *Contemporary management of motor control problems: Proceedings of the II-STEP Conference* (pp. 11–27). Alexandria, VA: Foundation for Physical Therapy.

Howlin, P. (2003). Can early interventions alter the course of autism? *Novartis Foundation Symposium, 251,* 250–265, 281–297.

Hoyson, M., Jamieson, B., & Strain, P.S. (1984). Individualized group instruction of normally developing and autistic-like children: The LEAP curriculum model. *Journal of the Division for Early Childhood, 8,* 157–172.

Individuals with Disabilities Education Act Amendments of 1991, PL 102-119, 20 U.S.C. §§ 1400 *et seq.*

Individuals with Disabilities Education Act Amendments of 1997, PL 105-17, 20 U.S.C. §§ 1400 *et seq.*

Individuals with Disabilities Education Act (IDEA) of 1990, PL 101-476, 20 U.S.C. §§ 1400 *et seq.*

Individuals with Disabilities Education Improvement Act of 2004, PL 108-446, 20 U.S.C. §§ 1400 *et seq.*

Infant Health and Development Program. (1990). Enhancing the outcomes of low-birth-weight, premature infants: A multisite, randomized trial. *JAMA, 263,* 3035–3042.

Irwin, K.C. (1989). The school achievement of children with Down's syndrome. *New Zealand Medical Journal, 860,* 11–13.

Jacobs, S.E., Sokol, J., & Ohlsson, A. (2002). The Newborn Individualized Developmental Care and Assessment Program is not supported by meta-analyses of the data. *Journal of Pediatrics, 140,* 699–706.

Jocelyn, L.J., Casiro, O.G., Beattie, D., Bow, J., & Kneisz, J. (1998). Treatment of children with autism: A randomized controlled trial to evaluate a caregiver-based intervention program in community day-care centers. *Journal of Developmental and Behavioral Pediatrics, 19,* 326–334.

Kaiser, A.P., Yoder, P.J., & Keetz, A. (1992). Evaluating milieu teaching. In S.F. Warren & J. Reichle (Series & Vol. Eds.), *Communication and language intervention series: Vol. 1. Causes and effects in communication and language intervention* (pp. 9–48). Baltimore: Paul H. Brookes Publishing Co.

Kanda, T., Pidcock, F.S., Hayakawa, K., Yamori, Y., & Shikata, Y. (2004). Motor outcome differences between two groups of children with spastic diplegia who received different intensities of early onset physiotherapy followed for 5 years. *Brain and Development, 26,* 118–126.

Kasari, C. (2002). Assessing change in early intervention programs for children with autism. *Journal of Autism and Developmental Disorders, 32,* 447–461.

Kelso, J.A.S. (1995). *Dynamic patterns: The self-organization of brain and behavior.* Cambridge, MA: MIT Press.

Ketelaar, M., Vermeer, A., Hart, H., van Petegem-van Beek, E., & Helders, P.J. (2001). Effects of a functional therapy program on motor abilities of children with cerebral palsy. *Physical Therapy, 81,* 1534–1545.

Knox, V., & Evans, A.L. (2002). Evaluation of the functional effects of a course of Bobath therapy in children with cerebral palsy: A preliminary study. *Developmental Medicine and Child Neurology, 44,* 447–460.

Law, M., Cadman, D., Rosenbaum, P., Walter, S., Russell, D., & DeMatteo, C. (1991). Neurodevelopmental therapy and upper-extremity inhibitive casting for children with cerebral palsy. *Developmental Medicine and Child Neurology, 33,* 379–387.

Lord, C., Rutter, M., Goode, S., Heemsbergen, J., Jordan, H., Mawhood, L., et al. (1989). Autism Diagnostic Observation Schedule: A standardized observation of communicative and social behavior. *Journal of Autism and Developmental Disorders, 19*(2), 185–212.

Lovaas, O.I. (1987). Behavioral treatment and normal educational and intellectual functioning in young autistic children. *Journal of Consulting and Clinical Psychology, 55,* 3–9.

Mahoney, G., Robinson, C., & Fewell, R.R. (2001). The effects of early motor intervention on children with Down syndrome or cerebral palsy: A field-based study. *Journal of Developmental and Behavioral Pediatrics, 22,* 153–162.

Majnemer, A. (1998). Benefits of early intervention for children with developmental disabilities. *Seminars in Pediatric Neurology, 5,* 62–69.

Mayo, N.E. (1991). The effect of physical therapy for children with motor delay and cerebral palsy: A randomized clinical trial. *American Journal of Physical Medicine and Rehabilitation, 70,* 258–267.

McBurney, H., Taylor, N.F., Dodd, K.J., & Graham, H.K. (2003). A qualitative analysis of the benefits of strength training for young people with cerebral palsy. *Developmental Medicine and Child Neurology, 45,* 658–663.

McCarton, C.M., Brooks-Gunn, J., Wallace, I.F., Bauer, C.R., Bennett, F.C., Bernbaum, J.C., et al. (1997). Results at age 8 years of early intervention for low-birth-weight premature infants: The Infant Health and Development Program. *JAMA, 277,* 126–132.

McCormick, M.C., McCarton, C., Brooks-Gunn, J., Belt, P., & Gross, R.T. (1998). The Infant Health and Development Program: Interim summary. *Journal of Developmental and Behavioral Pediatrics, 19,* 359–370.

McCormick, M.C., McCarton, C., Tonascia, J., & Brooks-Gunn, J. (1993). Early educational intervention for very low birth weight infants: Results from the Infant Health and Development Program. *Journal of Pediatrics, 123,* 527–533.

McCubbin, J.A., & Shasby, G.B. (1985). Effects of isokinetic exercise on adolescents with cerebral palsy. *Adapted Physical Activity Quarterly, 2,* 56–64.

McEachin, J.J., Smith, T., & Lovaas, O.I. (1993). Long-term outcome for children with autism who received early intensive behavioral treatment. *American Journal on Mental Retardation, 97,* 359–372.

Morton, J.F., Brownlee, M., & McFadyen, A.K. (2005). The effects of progressive resistance training for children with cerebral palsy. *Clinical Rehabilitation, 19,* 283–289.

Naganuma, G.M. (1987). Early intervention for infants with Down syndrome: Efficacy research. *Physical & Occupational Therapy in Pediatrics, 7,* 81–92.

Naylor, C.E., & Bower, E. (2005). Modified constraint-induced movement therapy for young children with hemiplegic cerebral palsy: A pilot study. *Developmental Medicine and Child Neurology, 47,* 365–369.

Paine, R.S. (1962). On the treatment of cerebral palsy: The outcome of 177 patients, 74 totally untreated. *Pediatrics, 29,* 605–616.

Palisano, R., Rosenbaum, P., Walter, S., Russell, D., Wood, E., & Galuppi, B. (1997). Development and reliability of a system to classify gross motor function in children with cerebral palsy. *Developmental Medicine and Child Neurology, 39,* 214–223.

Palmer, F.B., Shapiro, B.K., Wachtel, R.C., Allen, M.C., Hiller, J.E., Harryman, S.E., et al. (1988). The effects of physical therapy on cerebral palsy: A controlled trial in infants with spastic diplegia. *New England Journal of Medicine, 318,* 803–808.

Parette, H.P. Jr., & Hourcade, J.J. (1984). A review of therapeutic intervention research on gross and fine motor progress in young children with cerebral palsy. *American Journal of Occupational Therapy, 38,* 462–468.

Piper, M.C. (1990). Efficacy of physical therapy: Rate of motor development in children with cerebral palsy. *Pediatric Physical Therapy, 2,* 126–130.

Piper, M.C., Gosselin, C., Gendron, M., & Mazer, B. (1986). Developmental profile of Down syndrome infants receiving early intervention. *Child: Care, Health and Development, 12,* 183–194.

Pretis, M. (2000). Early intervention in children with Down's syndrome: From evaluation to methodology. *Infants & Young Children, 12*(3), 23–31.

Provence, S. (1985). On the efficacy of early intervention programs. *Journal of Developmental and Behavioral Pediatrics, 6,* 363–366.

Ramey, C.T., Bryant, D.M., Wasik, B.H., Sparling, J.J., Fendt, K.H., & LaVange, L.M. (1992). Infant Health and Development Program for low birth weight, premature infants: Program elements, family participation, and child intelligence. *Pediatrics, 89,* 454–465.

Ramey, C.T., & Campbell, F.A. (1991). Poverty, early childhood education, and academic competence: The Abecedarian experiment. In A.C. Huston (Ed.), *Children in poverty* (pp. 190–221). Cambridge, England: Cambridge University Press.

Ramey, C.T., & Ramey, S.L. (1998). Prevention of intellectual disabilities: Early interventions to improve cognitive development. *Preventive Medicine, 27,* 224–232.

Reddihough, D.S., King, J., Coleman, G., & Catanese, T. (1998). Efficacy of programmes based on conductive education for young children with cerebral palsy. *Developmental Medicine and Child Neurology, 40,* 763–770.

Reynolds, A.J., Temple, J.A., Robertson, D.L., & Mann, E.A. (2001). Long-term effects of an early childhood intervention on educational achievement and juvenile arrest: A 15-year follow-up of low-income children in public schools. *JAMA, 285,* 2339–2346.

Richards, C.L., Malouin, F., Dumas, F., Marcoux, S., Lepage, C., & Menier, C. (1997). Early and intensive treadmill locomotor training for young children with cerebral palsy: A feasibility study. *Pediatric Physical Therapy, 9,* 158–165.

Rogers, S.J. (1998). Empirically supported comprehensive treatments for young children with autism. *Journal of Clinical Child Psychology, 27,* 168–179.

Rogers, S.J., & DiLalla, D. (1991). Comparative study of a developmentally based preschool curriculum on young children with autism and young children with other disorders of behavior and development. *Topics in Early Childhood Special Education, 11,* 29–48.

Ruskin, E.M., Kasari, C., Mundy, P., & Sigman, M. (1994). Attention to people and toys during social and object mastery in children with Down syndrome. *American Journal on Mental Retardation, 99,* 103–111.

Russell, D.J., Rosenbaum, P.L., Cadman, D.T., Gowland, C., Hardy, S., & Jarvis, S. (1989). The Gross Motor Function Measure: A means to evaluate the effects of physical therapy. *Developmental Medicine and Child Neurology, 31,* 341–352.

Sallows, G.O., & Graupner, T.D. (2005). Intensive behavioral treatment for children with autism: Four-year outcome and predictors. *American Journal of Mental Retardation, 110,* 417–438.

Sameroff, A.J., & Fiese, B.H. (1990). Transactional regulation and early intervention. In S.J. Meisels & J.P. Shonkoff (Eds.), *Handbook of early childhood intervention* (pp. 119–149). Cambridge, England: Cambridge University Press.

Scherzer, A.L., & Tscharnuter, I. (1990). *Early diagnosis and therapy in cerebral palsy: A primer on infant developmental problems* (2nd ed.). New York: Marcel Dekker.

Schindl, M.R., Forstner, C., Kern, H., & Hesse, S. (2000). Treadmill training with partial body weight support in nonambulatory patients with cerebral palsy. *Archives of Physical Medicine and Rehabilitation, 81,* 301–306.

Schweinhart, L., Berrueta-Clement, J., Barnett, S., Epstein, A., & Weikart, D. (1985). Effects of the Perry Preschool Program on youths through age 19: A summary. *Topics in Early Childhood Special Education, 5,* 26–35.

Sheinkopf, S.J., & Siegel, B. (1998). Home-based behavioral treatment of young children with autism. *Journal of Autism and Developmental Disorders, 23,* 15–23.

Shonkoff, J.P., & Hauser-Cram, P. (1987). Early intervention for disabled infants and their families: A quantitative analysis. *Pediatrics, 80,* 650–658.

Shonkoff, J.P., Hauser-Cram, P., Krauss, M.W., & Upshur, C.C. (1988). Early intervention efficacy research: What have we learned and where do we go from here? *Topics in Early Childhood Special Education, 8,* 81–93.

Shonkoff, J.P., Hauser-Cram, P., Krauss, M.W., & Upshur, C.C. (1992). Development of infants with disabilities and their families. *Monographs of the Society for Research in Child Development, 57*(6, Serial No. 230).

Simeonsson, R.J., Cooper, D.H., & Schemer, A.P. (1982). A review and analysis of the effectiveness of early intervention programs. *Pediatrics, 69,* 635–641.

Simeonsson, R.J., Leonardi, M., Lollar, D., Bjorck-Akesson, E., Hollenweger, J., & Martinuzzi, A. (2003). Applying the International Classification of Functioning, Disability and Health (ICF) to measure childhood disability. *Disability and Rehabilitation, 25,* 602–610.

Simeonsson, R.J., Olley, J.G., & Rosenthal, S.L. (1987). Early intervention for children with autism. In M.J. Guralnick & F.C. Bennett (Eds.), *The effectiveness of early intervention for at-risk and handicapped children* (pp. 275–296). San Diego: Academic Press.

Skeels, H., & Dye, H. (1939). A study of the effects of differential stimulation on mentally retarded children. *Proceedings of the American Association on Mental Deficiency, 44,* 114–136.

Smith, T., Groen, A.D., & Wynn, J.W. (2000). A randomized trial of intensive early intervention for children with pervasive developmental disorder. *American Journal on Mental Retardation, 5,* 269–285.

Spiker, D., & Hopmann, M.R. (1997). The effectiveness of early intervention for children with Down syndrome. In M.J. Guralnick (Ed.), *The effectiveness of early intervention* (pp. 271–305). Baltimore: Paul H. Brookes Publishing Co.

Steultjens, E.M., Dekker, J., Bouter, L.M., van de Nes, J.C., Lambregts, B.L., & van den Ende, C.H. (2004). Occupational therapy for children with cerebral palsy: A systematic review. *Clinical Rehabilitation, 18,* 1–14.

Strain, P.S., Hoyson, M.H., & Jamieson, B.J. (1985). Normally developing preschoolers as intervention agents for autistic-like children: Effects on class deportment and social interactions. *Journal of the Division for Early Childhood, 9,* 105–115.

Sung, I.Y., Ryu, J.S., Pyun, S.B., Yoo, S.D., Song, W.H., & Park, M.J. (2005). Efficacy of forced-use therapy in hemiplegic cerebral palsy. *Archives of Physical Medicine and Rehabilitation, 86*(11), 2195–2198.

Symington, A., & Pinelli, J. (2006). Developmental care for promoting development and preventing morbidity in preterm infants. *Cochrane Database of Systematic Reviews, 2,* CD001814.

Taub, E., Ramey, S.L., DeLuca, S., & Echols, K. (2004). Efficacy of constraint-induced movement therapy for children with cerebral palsy with asymmetric motor impairment. *Pediatrics, 113,* 305–312.

Thelen, E., & Smith, L.B. (1994). *A dynamic systems approach to the development of cognition and action.* Cambridge, MA: MIT Press.

Tirosh, E., & Rabino, S. (1989). Physiotherapy for children with cerebral palsy. *American Journal of Diseases of Children, 143,* 552–555.

Tonge, B., Brereton, A., Kiomall, M., Mackinnon, A., King, N., & Rinehart, N. (2006). Effects on parental mental health of an education and skills training program for parents of young children with autism: A randomized controlled trial. *Journal of the American Academy of Child and Adolescent Psychiatry, 45,* 561–569.

Tsorlakis, N., Evaggelinou, C., Grouios, G., & Tsorbatzoudis, C. (2004). Effect of intensive neurodevelopmental treatment in gross motor function of children with cerebral palsy. *Developmental Medicine and Child Neurology, 46,* 740–745.

Turnbull, J.D. (1993). Early intervention for children with or at risk of cerebral palsy. *American Journal of Diseases of Children, 147,* 54–59.

Ulrich, D.A., Ulrich, B.D., Angulo-Kinzler, R.M., & Yun, J. (2001). Treadmill training of infants with Down syndrome: Evidence-based developmental outcomes. *Pediatrics, 108,* E84.

Wieder, S., & Greenspan, S.I. (2003). Climbing the symbolic ladder in the DIR model through floor time/interactive play. *Autism, 7,* 425–435.

Willis, J.K., Morello, A., Davie, A., Rice, J.C., & Bennett, J.T. (2002). Forced use treatment of childhood hemiparesis. *Pediatrics, 110*(1 Pt. 1), 94–96.

Wishart, J.G. (1986). The effects of step-by-step training on cognitive performance in infants with Down's syndrome. *Journal of Mental Deficiency Research, 30*(Pt. 3), 233–250.

Wishart, J.G. (1993). The development of learning difficulties in children with Down's syndrome. *Journal of Intellectual Disability Research, 3,* 389–403.

Yoder, P., & Stone, W.L. (2006). Randomized comparison of two communication interventions for preschoolers with autism spectrum disorders. *Journal of Consulting and Clinical Psychology, 74*(3), 426–435.

27

Behavior Management

SUNGWOO KAHNG AND ISER G. DELEON

Individuals with developmental disabilities frequently engage in debilitating challenging behaviors such as self-injurious behavior (SIB), aggression, and property destruction. Numerous topographies or forms of behavior, which range in severity from mild to life threatening, have been reported. For example, the most common topographies of SIB tend to be head hitting, head banging, and self-biting (Griffin, Williams, Stark, Altmeyer, & Mason, 1986), but the specific response forms are often idiosyncratic and include relatively rare forms of SIB such as aerophagia, polydipsia, and stuffing objects into orifices (Rojahn & Esbensen, 2002). Topographies of aggression typically include hitting, biting, kicking, and scratching others, while common topographies of property destruction include throwing or tearing objects (Bruininks, Olson, Larson, & Lakin, 1994).

Approximately 10%–15% of individuals with developmental disabilities engage in some form of challenging behavior (Borthwick-Duffy, 1994; Emerson et al., 2001). Estimates of the prevalence of individuals with developmental disabilities who engage in challenging behaviors may vary significantly when considering specific factors such as residential settings, geographic location, functioning level, and gender. For example, Borthwick-Duffy (1994) examined data from the California Department of Developmental Disabilities (DDS). The data sample consisted of 91,164 individuals receiving services through DDS in 1987. Borthwick-Duffy indicated that approximately 14% of the sample was reported to engage in one or more challenging behavior and that individuals with severe (22%) and profound

(33%) disabilities as well as dual diagnoses (31%) tended to engage in challenging behavior. Furthermore, there was a higher prevalence of individuals residing in larger, institutional settings (48%) who engaged in challenging behavior than those individuals who lived independently (3%) or in a parental home (8%).

Individuals with developmental disabilities who engage in challenging behaviors may pose significant hazards to self, others, and property. Hyman, Fisher, Mercugliano, and Cataldo (1990) reviewed the medical records of 97 individuals admitted to an inpatient unit specializing in the assessment and treatment of SIB. Their results indicated that physical injury was documented in 76% of cases. The most frequently reported injuries were soft tissue lacerations and contusions, and the most severe injuries consisted of permanent damage to the eye (e.g., cataract formation, perforation, retinal detachment), which was reported in approximately 5% of these patients.

Challenging behaviors exhibited by individuals with developmental disabilities may also lead to indirect adverse effects. Oftentimes, individuals who engage in the most severe forms of challenging behavior are unable to participate in therapeutic activities such as educational, community, and/or vocational activities (Hill & Bruininks, 1984). Furthermore, challenging behaviors may limit an individual's opportunities for placement in community settings as well as contribute to failure in community placement and/or readmission to larger residential facilities (Anderson, Lakin, Hill, & Chen, 1992; Bruininks et al., 1994). Finally, physical and chemical restraints are sometimes used for protection, further limiting participation by these individuals in alternative activities as well as risking adverse side effects (Favell et al., 1982).

Given the relatively high frequency of individuals with developmental disabilities who engage in challenging behaviors as well as the adverse risks associated with these behaviors, there has been an abundance of research examining behaviorally based treatments (Foxx, 1996; Matson, Benavidez, Compton, Paclawskyj, & Baglio, 1996; Scotti, Ujcich, Weigle, Holland, & Kirk, 1996). These treatments are based on the principles of *behavior analysis* (sometimes referred to as *applied behavior analysis*) and consist of extensive behavior assessments and multiple behavioral treatment options.

BASIC BEHAVIORAL PRINCIPLES

Prior to discussing behavior assessments and treatments, we provide a brief introduction to the principles that serve as their foundation.

Reinforcement

Reinforcement is the presentation or removal of an event or stimulus following a behavior that results in strengthening of that behavior (Cooper, Heron, & Heward, 1987). In other words, a *reinforcer* is defined by its effect on behavior and always increases the future probability of the occurrence of that behavior. A distinction is made between *positive* and *negative* reinforcement.

Positive reinforcement is the *presentation* of a stimulus following a behavior that results in the strengthening of that behavior. Figure 27.1 shows the relationship between an antecedent event (the presentation of a math problem), the resulting behavior (completing the math problem), and the consequence

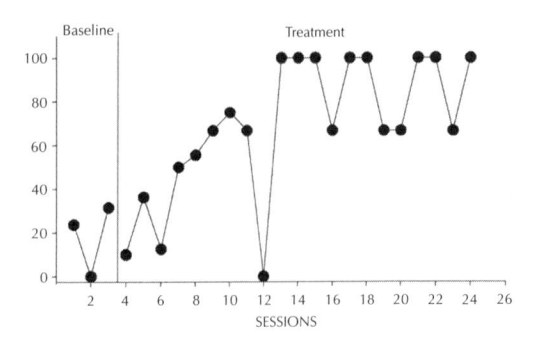

Figure 27.2. Increased compliance as a result of positive reinforcement.

(presentation/delivery of praise). Assuming that praise is an effective reinforcer, this sequence of actions will result in an increased probability of a child completing a math problem when presented with similar problems in the future.

Figure 27.2 is an example of the effects of positive reinforcement on compliance with a task. The individual was a 16-year-old girl diagnosed with mild intellectual disabilities and seizure disorder, and the target behavior was cleaning up the table after meals. During the no-intervention period (i.e., baseline), she seldom cleaned up after a meal. Treatment consisted of providing her with a preferred activity (playing with a ball) after she successfully cleaned up. Positive reinforcement resulted in a gradual increase in her compliance.

Negative reinforcement is the *removal* of a stimulus following some behavior that results in the strengthening of that behavior. Negative reinforcement is oftentimes erroneously confused with punishment. Much as positive reinforcement is positive to the extent that a stimulus is presented, negative reinforcement is negative only in the sense that a stimulus is removed contingent on a behavior. Figure 27.3

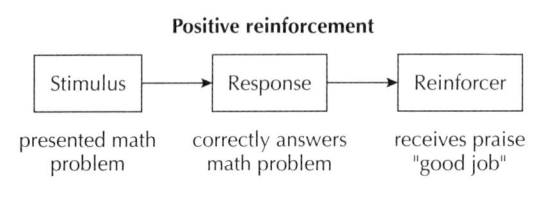

Figure 27.1. Sequence of events for positive reinforcement.

Negative reinforcement

| Stimulus | → | Response | → | Reinforcer |

presented math problem — correctly answers math problem — math problems removed (i.e., earns break)

Figure 27.3. Sequence of events for negative reinforcement.

shows the relationship between the same antecedent event as mentioned earlier (math problem), the resulting behavior (completing the math problem), and the consequence, in this case removal or break from schoolwork. In this figure, an event (schoolwork) is removed following the completion of the math problem, which will increase the future probability of completing math problems.

An example of the effects of negative reinforcement is presented in Figure 27.4. A behavioral treatment was developed for the previously described individual to increase her compliance during academic tasks such as coin identification, matching objects, and identifying days of the week, which she rarely completed during baseline. The treatment consisted of giving her a break from work (i.e., removing schoolwork) after she completed a certain number of tasks. Therefore, if she successfully completed the tasks, she was permitted to take a break for 30 seconds. These breaks from work resulted in an increase in compliance with the academic tasks.

Extinction

Extinction is the termination of reinforcement of a previously reinforced behavior that results in a decrease in that behavior. Extinction typically results in a gradual change in responding. When a behavior is reinforced by positive reinforcement, extinction would involve no longer providing a consequence for the behavior. For example, if the praise that was delivered following the completion of a math problem led to the increase of math problem completion,

no longer delivering praise would result in a decrease in completing math problems (i.e., the behavior is extinguished).

Extinction of a behavior reinforced by negative reinforcement is procedurally different from extinction of a behavior reinforced by positive reinforcement. Whereas extinction for a positively reinforced behavior involves not providing consequences, extinction for a negatively reinforced behavior involves not terminating the event (i.e., continuing with the task or activity). For example, if a break (i.e., escape) was delivered following the completion of a math problem and that break led to the increase of math problem completion, not providing a break (i.e., continuing to make the child work) may result in a decrease in completing math problems in the future (i.e., the behavior is extinguished).

The use of extinction is sometimes associated with side effects such as bursts in responding and indirect side effects (Lerman & Iwata, 1996; Lerman, Iwata, & Wallace, 1999). Extinction bursts are characterized by an initial increase in frequency, intensity, and/or duration of a behavior. This increase is temporary and in most instances brief. Indirect side effects of extinction include possible increases in aggressive responding (extinction-induced aggression), which may be elicited by the removal of the reinforcer, and increases in emotional behaviors such as crying or pouting, which may be a product of frustration at no longer receiving reinforcement.

Figure 27.5 is an example of extinction. The individual was an 11-year-old boy diagnosed with autism and moderate intellectual

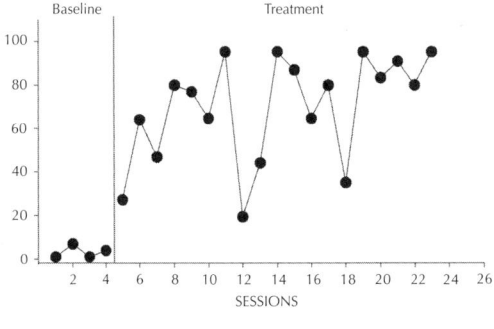

Figure 27.4. Increased compliance as a result of negative reinforcement.

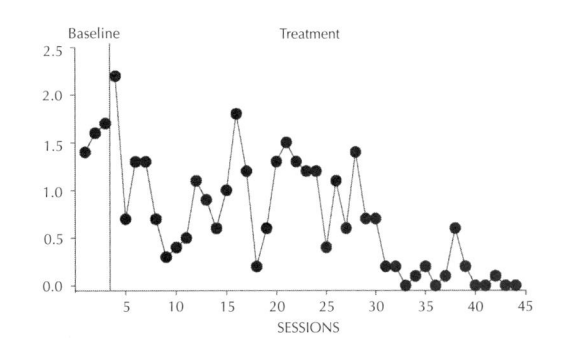

Figure 27.5. Decreased aggression as a result of extinction.

disabilities. His presenting problem behavior was aggression, which occurred at high levels during baseline. Extinction consisted of not providing any attention for his aggressive behavior (i.e., ignoring the aggression). His first exposure to extinction resulted in an increase in aggression (i.e., extinction burst). After that initial burst (i.e., extinction burst), aggression gradually decreased as this individual was exposed to extinction.

Punishment

Punishment is the presentation or removal of some stimulus following a behavior that results in a decrease in the future probability of that behavior. Punishment is defined by its effect on behavior and not by whether or not a stimulus is unpleasant, annoying, or painful. What one person finds unpleasant (e.g., verbal reprimand) may have little effect on another's behavior. Alternatively, what one person finds pleasurable (e.g., peanuts) may decrease the behavior of another (e.g., a person who has a peanut allergy).

Research suggests that punishment is an effective means of reducing unwanted behavior, particularly when that behavior has been resistant to other behavioral interventions. When utilizing punishment, clinicians should ensure that other, less intrusive procedures have been attempted (Carr & Lovaas, 1983; Favell et al., 1982). Furthermore, combining punishment of unwanted behavior with reinforcement of appropriate behavior oftentimes results in the most successful treatment outcome (Thompson, Iwata, Conners, & Roscoe, 1999).

Figure 27.6 provides an example of punishment. The individual was a 15-year-old girl with moderate intellectual disabilities who engaged in aggressive behavior. Following baseline during which aggression occurred at high levels, an initial treatment (Treatment 1) consisting of providing attention contingent on appropriate communication resulted in a modest reduction in aggression. The addition of a time-out procedure (Treatment 2) resulted in a reduction in aggression to clinically acceptable levels. When the time-out procedure was temporarily discontinued, aggressions increased,

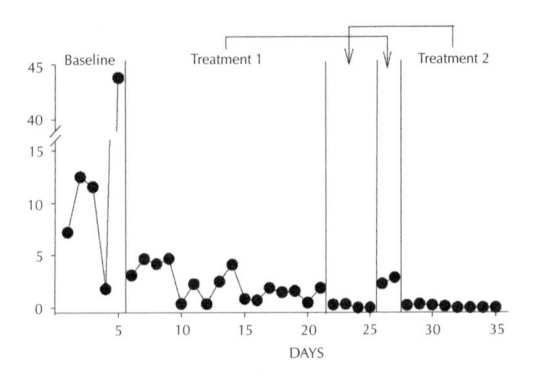

Figure 27.6.   Decreased aggression as a result of punishment.

indicating that the time-out procedure was necessary to reduce aggression. The reintroduction of the time-out procedure resulted in a clinically significant reduction in aggression.

Behavioral principles of reinforcement, extinction, and punishment serve as the foundation for behavior assessments and treatments for problem behaviors. An abundance of scientific evidence supports the application of these principles to address all forms of problems, particularly as they relate to individuals with developmental disabilities.

BEHAVIOR ASSESSMENT

The general strategy in the use of behavior management for treatment of behavior disorders has been one of decreasing aberrant behavior while increasing levels of adaptive responses. This strategy has not changed significantly since its inception; however, the approach has become far more sophisticated. Whereas many early studies relied on punishment and nonspecific reinforcers to reward appropriate alternative behaviors, changes in assessment technology set the stage for interventions based on empirically derived hypotheses regarding the specific consequences that serve to reinforce the challenging behaviors in the natural environment—the *functional reinforcers* (Carr, 1994; Mace, 1994). These assessment procedures have collectively been referred to as *functional assessment* (or *functional behavioral assessment*).

Functional assessment methods have permitted researchers and clinicians to identify highly specific antecedent stimuli and consequences involved in giving rise to and reinforcing challenging behaviors. Thus, behavioral management plans can be tailored to the observed functions. Functional assessment shows us that there is often a "purpose" to the behavior. Interventions can then disrupt the functional relations that maintain the challenging behaviors, train alternative means for achieving that "purpose," or both.

Common Behavioral Functions

Although there is evidence to suggest that some forms of challenging behaviors (e.g., SIB) may be induced through neurobiological mechanisms (e.g., Nyhan, 2002), decades of research suggest that these are often learned behaviors maintained through operant contingencies (Iwata, Pace, et al., 1994; National Institutes of Health, 1991) or interactions between the behaviors and environmental variables, particularly the functional outcomes of the behavior. The sorts of environmental variables often examined in functional assessments are derived from a landmark paper by Carr (1977). In that paper, Carr described three general classes of reinforcement contingencies that could maintain the SIB of individuals with developmental disabilities. These included positive, social reinforcement; negative reinforcement in the form of escape from or avoidance of aversive stimulation; and sensory stimulation, in which the behavior is purported to produce its own reinforcement independent of socially mediated outcomes—an effect now often referred to as automatic reinforcement (Vaughn & Michael, 1982; Vollmer, 1994).

Positive Reinforcement Events or stimuli that follow the occurrence of a behavior may function to strengthen that behavior. Often, these consequences are socially mediated (i.e., delivered by other individuals) and take the form of the delivery of attention or tangible items (e.g., toys, food). For example, a common response by parents when their child engages in less intensive forms of SIB (or stereotypic behavior) may be to provide a verbal reprimand (e.g., "don't do that") or physical comfort (e.g., soothing the child). Although these consequences may lead to a temporary

decrease in the challenging behavior, repeated pairing of either consequence with the challenging behavior may inadvertently result in future increase in both the frequency and intensity of this behavior. Alternatively, a parent or caregiver may provide a child with a preferred toy or other item in an effort to calm or redirect the child following an instance of challenging behavior. Over time the child may learn to exhibit the challenging behavior specifically because it results in the delivery of a desirable item.

Negative Reinforcement The removal of some unwanted or aversive event contingent on a behavior may result in strengthening of that behavior. In the most studied example, a teacher may present a student with a challenging academic task, and the child may refuse to comply or otherwise avoid completion of the task. If the teacher persists in his or her attempts to produce compliance, the child's behavior may escalate into a more severe form of behavior such as aggression. This aggressive behavior may eventually result in the teacher terminating the task and providing the student a break so that he or she will "calm down." In the short run, providing escape may lead to a temporary reduction of aggression; however, reinforcement of the aggressive response with a break from academic instruction may result in an increase in the future likelihood of aggression by the student. Thus, over many repetitions of this scenario, the child may learn that aggression will reliably result in escape from or avoidance of academic demands when confronted with similarly challenging tasks.

Automatic Reinforcement (Sensory Reinforcement) Some forms of challenging behavior, particularly SIB and other stereotypic movements, seem to occur independent of environmental or socially mediated consequences (Vollmer, 1994). These behaviors are often said to be self-stimulatory, and a variety of biological explanations have been suggested. These include biochemical deficiencies, insensitivity to pain, and the body's response to opiate-like substances (Cataldo & Harris, 1982). These contingencies have collectively become referred to as automatic reinforcement (Vaughan & Michael, 1982). The term *automatic reinforcement* refers to an arrangement in which behavior is reinforced through operations that are independent of the social environment. Thus, with respect to behavior problems, automatic reinforcement generally implies a situation in which the physical response products of the behavior itself suffice to perpetuate the behavior in the absence of any reaction from caregivers. The specific reinforcers are typically characterized as some form of sensory stimulation, leading some investigators to refer to this arrangement as sensory reinforcement. Hypotheses regarding the specific sort of stimulation that would maintain such aberrant behaviors have flourished (e.g., Cataldo & Harris, 1982; Guess & Carr, 1991).

Functional Assessment Methods

The goal of a functional assessment is to identify the antecedent variables and environmental consequences that give rise to and maintain challenging behaviors. Functional assessment, regardless of the method, focuses on both antecedents, or triggers, for the target behavior and sensory outcomes or caregiver reactions that serve to reinforce the challenging behavior. Researchers have developed several methods for determining which among these variables contributes most to the maintenance of the challenging behavior. These methods have come to be known as indirect assessment (e.g., checklists and rating scales), descriptive or naturalistic assessments (e.g., antecedent–behavior–consequence observation; Bijou, Peterson, & Ault, 1968; Touchette, MacDonald, & Langer, 1985), and experimental or functional analyses (Carr & Durand, 1985; Iwata, Dorsey, Slifer, Bauman, & Richman, 1982/1994). Each of these methods is discussed in greater detail in this section. For the sake of the following discussion, we should note that experimental analyses are considered to be the most rigorous method and the only method on which direct causal conclusions can be reached regarding the relations between challenging behavior and environmental variables. Thus, they are often used as a standard to assess the validity of the other methods.

Indirect (Informant-Based) Assessment

Indirect assessment instruments are the simplest method of gathering information regarding behavioral function. Assessment instruments typically ask caregivers to answer a series of questions regarding the targeted challenging behaviors and the circumstances under which the behaviors do and do not occur. Often, the instruments provide decision rules for deriving hypotheses about behavioral function based on the answers to the questions. This method has several purported advantages over other assessment methodologies, including ease of administration (Kennedy & Haring, 1992), and minimal time (Reid, 1992) and training (Sturmey, 1994) requirements relative to the other assessment methods.

A number of assessment instruments have been developed to assist in identifying the function of behavior problems. Early efforts include the Motivation Assessment Scale (MAS; Durand & Crimmins, 1988), the Contingency Analysis Questionnaire (Wieseler, Hanson, Chamberlain, & Thompson, 1985), the Stimulus Control Checklist (Van Houten & Rolider, 1991), and the Behavioral Diagnosis and Treatment Information Form (Bailey & Pyles, 1989). More recent years have seen the development of the Functional Assessment Screening Tool (Iwata & DeLeon, 1996), the Questions About Behavioral Function (QABF; Matson & Vollmer, 1995), and the Problem Behavior Questionnaire (Lewis, Scott, & Sugai, 1994).

Only two of these instruments, the MAS and QABF, have been researched in any extensive manner. The MAS consists of 16 questions designed to determine if the challenging behavior is maintained by one of four functions: escape from instructional demands, access to attention, access to tangible reinforcers, or sensory consequences. Informants are asked to rate the likelihood that behavior occurs in response to these functions as described by each of the 16 questions (4 questions per function). Informants respond by selecting a score on a 7-point Likert scale that ranges from never to always. Functional hypotheses are then developed by averaging the responses to each of the questions pertaining to each possible function, with the highest average suggesting the most likely function of the challenging behavior.

In their initial report on the MAS, Durand and Crimmins (1988) administered the instrument to teachers and assistant teachers regarding the behavioral challenges of 50 students with developmental disabilities. Separate assessments were completed by each of two raters (one teacher and one assistant teacher) for each child. The investigators found that correlation coefficients for the mean functional category scores ranged from .80 to .95 and rank-order correlation coefficients ranged from .66 to .81. Furthermore, test–retest reliability measures on individual items ranged from .89 to .98. Finally, for a subset of eight students, the order of functions as determined by the MAS (i.e., highest to lowest mean category score) corresponded well with the order of challenging behavior levels (highest to lowest across conditions) observed during additional behavioral assessments, producing an overall rank-order correlation coefficient of .99. According to these authors, then, the MAS produced highly reliable information with exceptional concurrent validity when compared with a more rigorous analysis.

The results of subsequent evaluations have yielded more variable results. In marked contrast to the initial reports, Zarcone, Rodgers, Iwata, Rourke, and Dorsey (1991) evaluated interrater reliability of the MAS for 55 subjects, a sample mixed with respect to setting (school and residential) and challenging behavior, and found that mean score correlation coefficients on categories ranged from $-.80$ to .99 ($M = .41$). Furthermore, these authors calculated exact agreement scores and adjacent agreement scores (where an agreement was counted if one rater's score fell within ± 1 of the other rater's score) and found agreement percentages with means of 20% and 48%, respectively.

Several other studies have assessed the reliability of the MAS (Conroy, Fox, Bucklin, & Good, 1996; Crawford, Brockel, Schauss, & Miltenberger, 1992; Kearney, 1994; Newton & Sturmey, 1991; Sigafoos, Kerr, & Roberts, 1994; Spreat & Connelly, 1996) with reliability estimates that often fell short of those reported by Durand and Crimmins (1988). From a clinical perspective, however, the most important measure of reliability may be agreement on

primary function. Intervention approaches ultimately will be based on this result. Of the studies mentioned, three reported agreement measures on primary function, again with varied results. Zarcone et al. (1991) found that raters agreed on the primary function of the behavior in only 16 of the 55 administrations (29.1%). Sigafoos et al. (1994) found agreement for 8 of 18 pairs (44.44%). Finally, Spreat and Connelly (1996) found agreement for 33 of 47 pairs (70.2%).

Another study of note was conducted by Arndorfer, Miltenberger, Woster, Rortvedt, and Gaffaney (1994), who measured test–retest reliability (after 1–2 weeks) of the MAS using correlation coefficients and the adjacent agreement method described by Zarcone et al. (1991). For a sample of seven MAS administrations on six subjects, they found a high degree of correlation (r ranged from .77 to .99) for test–retest reliability. Adjacent agreement scores ranged from 56% to 69%. This study was notable in two other respects. First, it included a small-scale replication of the concurrent validity of the MAS. These authors conducted descriptive functional assessments of challenging behavior and found that the MAS matched the primary function in only two of five cases. Because of the extremely small sample size and the questionable properties of naturalistic analyses (see later), the results must be viewed with caution. Nevertheless, the study suggested that the moderately high degree of item adjacent agreement and test–retest reliability did not translate into similarly high measures of concurrent validity.

Evaluations of the QABF have fared somewhat better, but the results have again been mixed. For example, analysis of test–retest reliability on the QABF revealed that percent agreement on each item was good, with 96% of the 25 items exceeding 80% agreement. Still, perhaps the most meaningful way of validating assessment methods is to determine whether they result in effective treatments. Matson, Bamburg, Cherry, and Paclawskyj (1999) compared treatments effects (the percentage reduction of SIB during treatment relative to baseline levels) when those treatments were 1) based on functional hypotheses derived from the QABF or 2) standard treatments involving interruption, blocking, and re-direction of challenging behavior, in the absence of any information about behavioral function. For each of three response class groups (SIB, aggression, and stereotypy; $n = 30$ for each treatment and control group), the treatments based on the QABF resulted in markedly greater reductions of the challenging behavior. This result suggested that the QABF was useful in developing better interventions relative to the standard intervention; however, the study lacked sufficient detail to thoroughly evaluate the interventions themselves. In addition, no other form of functional assessment was included, so no determination was made about whether a different form of assessment would have produced even better results. In relation to these results, Paclawskyj, Matson, Rush, Smalls, and Vollmer (2001) observed that the QABF and experimental analyses agreed in only 7 of 13 cases for individuals displaying self-injury, aggression, tantrums, or stereotypy.

Substantial research will be required to identify the conditions under which valid and reliable information can be consistently extracted from indirect assessment interviews. Often, suggestions as to these conditions have involved informant characteristics (Conroy et al., 1996; Sigafoos et al., 1994). For example, Lennox and Miltenberger (1989) pointed out that the information sought in indirect assessments is ultimately a product of informants' recollections of events and may therefore be influenced by forgetting, lack of exposure to relevant events, and idiosyncratic interpretation of those events. Sturmey (1994) added that informant characteristics, such as the sorts of interactions that the informant typically has with the individual with behavior disorder, may also affect the utility of the information provided.

In light of the questionable reliability and validity of assessment questionnaires, numerous authors, including some who developed the assessments, have advised using indirect assessments only as an initial part of the process of generating hypotheses about the functions of inappropriate behavior. As such, their primary utility might be in cases in which 1) because of temporal restrictions, it is advanta-geous to preselect one or two assessment conditions for more rigorous determination of function, or 2) no other form of assessment is feasible. As examples of the latter case, Sturmey (1994) suggested that behavior that occurs too infrequently to permit accurate analyses through other means or behavior that may be too severe to ethically expose to experimental analysis conditions may be more reasonably examined through indirect assessment. Under such conditions, it may be preferable to rely on questionable assessment techniques than on no assessment at all in designing treatments for behavioral challenges.

Descriptive Assessment or Naturalistic Observation

Descriptive analyses involve direct observation of the individual's behavior as well as its antecedent events and consequences under naturalistic conditions (e.g., Bijou et al., 1968; Lerman, & Iwata, 1993). Typically, these assessments seek to determine the degree of correspondence or correlation between a behavior and various environmental events. Hypotheses regarding the variables that give rise to and maintain challenging behavior are formulated on the basis of differentially high correlations between the behavior of interest and specific environmental events.

Descriptive assessments have been arranged in two ways. In one variation, a period of time is specified, and observers record all relevant events as they occur during the specified time interval. Alternatively, recording is sometimes based on the events themselves. That is, recording of data occurs only when the target behavior occurs. Often, these events are categorized as antecedents, behaviors, and consequence, thus lending the method one of the terms often used to refer to it: A-B-C assessments. Although the assessment formats are often open-ended, sometimes only specific events, predetermined by the clinician or researcher, are coded. The sorts of events that are recorded typically mirror antecedents and consequences that most commonly surround the challenging behavior (i.e., the same sorts of events that are inquired about in indirect assessments). Thus, for example, Lerman and Iwata (1993) used descriptive assessments in analyzing the challenging behavior of six adults diagnosed with profound intellectual disabilities. These investigators recorded the following sorts of antecedent events: instruction delivery; the presence of various materials or stimuli, including food, games, and training tasks; the presence of staff; and various forms of ambient stimuli. The sorts of consequences recorded in the same study included attention delivery, attention removal, instruction removal, reprimands contingent on the participant's behavior, and delivery of materials.

Hypotheses are typically drawn from descriptive assessments through the use of conditional probabilities. Four sorts of calculations are relevant: 1) the probability of challenging behavior given the relevant antecedent; 2) the probability of a given antecedent given that challenging behavior occurred; 3) the probability that each given instance of challenging behavior was followed by the relevant consequence; and 4) the probability that each time the given consequence was delivered, it was preceded by the challenging behavior. Relative conditional probabilities between the behavior and its antecedents and consequences can then be determined to identify a relationship between the challenging behavior and environmental events. For example, if the assessment reveals that challenging behavior is most likely to occur given periods of low attention as an antecedent, or that the probability of attention is greater following challenging behavior than are other sorts of consequences, or both, it would suggest that the behavior was maintained by attention. More recent variants of conditional probability analysis include lag sequential analysis (Emerson et al., 1996) and comparisons of conditional probabilities to background probabilities of events to ensure that the purported contingency is actually a positive one (Vollmer, Borrero, Wright, Van Camp, & Lalli, 2001).

Descriptive functional assessments are said to have a variety of advantages over other methods, including ecological validity (insofar as they are typically arranged in the environments in which behavioral challenges naturally occur) and permitting therapists to examine a fuller range of antecedents and consequences surrounding the behavior (i.e., certain variables may be overlooked in other

assessment methods). As with indirect assessments, however, results of descriptive analysis have not always been in agreement with more rigorous experimental analyses. For five of the six individuals assessed in the study by Lerman and Iwata (1993), the outcomes of the descriptive and experimental assessments were inconsistent. Similarly, Mace and Lalli (1991) conducted a descriptive analysis that suggested that the bizarre speech of a man with intellectual disabilities was sensitive to both escape and attention, but a subsequent experimental analysis confirmed only the attention function. More recently, Hall (2005) observed that agreement between descriptive and experimental functional assessment was reached in only one of four cases.

Erroneous descriptive assessment conclusions may be drawn for a variety of reasons, not the least of which is the possibility that, even though a specific event is highly correlated with challenging behavior, it does not necessarily follow that they are causally related. For example, severe self-injury maintained by automatic reinforcement is likely to receive attention even though that attention is not functionally related to the maintenance of the challenging behavior. Lerman and Iwata (1993) suggested that, in some cases, a relevant controlling variable might be masked by the more frequent occurrence of an irrelevant controlling variable.

As for indirect assessment, several authors have suggested that descriptive assessment be used as a method to augment more rigorous, experimental analysis (Anderson & Long, 2002; Mace & Lalli, 1991) primarily because together they may provide initial hypotheses that may not be otherwise considered. Indirect assessments typically inquire about a limited number of contexts, and experimental analyses typically test a limited number of contexts that may maintain behavior. By contrast, naturalistic observations may suggest detailed information about idiosyncratic kinds of antecedents and consequences (discussed in more detail later). In addition, certain circumstances surrounding the targeted behavior may make it difficult to accurately assess via experimental analyses, as in the case when the target behavior is very serious but occurs at a very low rate.

Experimental Analyses or Analogue Assessment   The most convincing demonstration of the effects of antecedents and consequences on challenging behaviors consists of the controlled manipulation of these events. The experimental or functional analysis of challenging behavior involves replication and direct manipulation of these controlling variables. Although various procedures for conducting a functional analysis have been described (e.g., Durand & Carr, 1992), the most commonly used are the procedures described by Iwata, Dorsey, et al. (1982/1994). This experiment described a set of conditions involving repeated observations of the target behavior under each condition, designed to identify controlling variables by manipulating both antecedent and consequent events for challenging behavior. Subsequently, similar procedures, often with slight modifications, have been used in numerous studies to experimentally identify the variables that maintain challenging behaviors.

A typical functional analysis might involve five conditions (alone, attention, demand, tangible, and play) conducted in accordance with a multi-element, single-case experimental design. In this design, experimental conditions, usually lasting between 10 and 15 minutes, are randomly assigned to successive sessions and are alternated in rapid fashion (e.g., Session 1 might be an alone condition, Session 2 a demand condition, Session 3 a play condition). During the *alone* condition, the participant is placed in the assessment setting alone without toys or materials to simulate an environment devoid of other potential sources of stimulation. This condition is designed to determine whether the challenging behavior occurs in the absence of social consequences (i.e., is maintained by automatic reinforcement).

In the *demand* condition, the therapist presents continuous academic tasks using sequential verbal, gestural, and physical prompts. Compliance with either the verbal or the gestural prompt results in brief praise (e.g., "nice working"), while the target behavior results in termination of the task for 30 seconds (escape). This condition is designed to determine whether challenging behavior is maintained by escape from demands.

During the *social attention* condition, the participant is given toys and asked to play quietly. The therapist engages in an independent activity (e.g., reading) but discontinues this activity and provides attention, usually in the form of a mild verbal reprimand (e.g., "Don't do that, you'll hurt me."), contingent on the target behavior. This condition determines whether social attention is the functional reinforcer. During the *tangible* condition, the participant is given free access to preferred objects for 2 minutes prior to the start of the session. When the session begins, the therapist withdraws the preferred objects and returns them for 30 seconds contingent on the target behavior. This condition is designed to determine whether challenging behavior is maintained by the delivery of preferred items.

Finally, in the *play* condition, a variety of toys are freely available, and the therapist interacts with the participant by providing praise once every 30 seconds at minimum. No demands are issued, and all target responses are ignored. The play condition is arranged as a control condition, theoretically devoid of the antecedents and consequences that give rise to and maintain challenging behaviors in the other conditions.

Functional analyses are interpreted by comparing rates of the target behavior during the test conditions with those observed during the control condition. The results of each session are plotted on the same line graph, with sessions on the horizontal axis and rates (response per minute) on the vertical axis. An example is depicted in Figure 27.7, a functional analysis of a 15-year-old girl with mild intellectual disabilities who engaged in SIB, aggres-

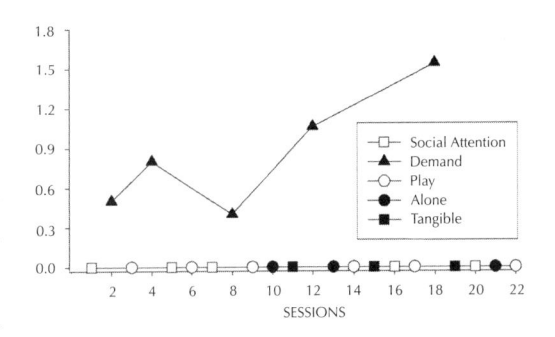

Figure 27.7.   Functional analysis of challenging behavior.

sion, and property destruction. Typically, data analysis is done via visual inspection in accordance with single-case experimental designs, although investigators have designed statistical analyses for interpreting functional analysis data (Hagopian et al., 1997). Elevated levels of the target behavior in any of the other conditions relative to the play condition are indicative of behavioral maintenance by the consequence tested in that condition. Thus, comparison of the levels of the challenging behavior across conditions in Figure 27.7 would suggest that challenging behaviors were sensitive to negative reinforcement in the form of escape from demands.

Of course, not all functional analyses produce results as clear as these data. For instance, functional analyses sometimes result in high levels of the target behavior across all conditions (undifferentiated results). Such results may occur for a variety of reasons (Vollmer, Marcus, & LeBlanc, 1994). In some cases, undifferentiated patterns are interpreted as being indicative of automatic reinforcement (Healey, Ahearn, Graff, & Libby, 2001; Lalli, Livezey, & Kates, 1996). That is, the behavior occurs independent of social variables such that the socially mediated contingencies arranged in the demand, attention, and control conditions have little influence on relative rates of the challenging behavior. Alternatively, the challenging behavior may be maintained by multiple functions (more than one set of controlling antecedent and consequent operations give rise to and maintain the behavior). It is also possible that the individuals do not respond differentially across conditions because the contingencies arranged in these conditions are alternating so rapidly that the patient has difficulty in making the sorts of discriminations that would facilitate differential responding.

Several investigators have suggested that experimental functional analyses may also have inherent limitations (Axelrod, 1987; Hall, 2005). One oft-cited potential problem is the risk that the analysis produces false positives by training behavior–consequence relationships that did not exist in the natural environment. For example, an individual may enter a functional analysis with no history of receiving tangible reinforcers contingent on challenging behavior; however, because this contingency is arranged during the analysis, over repeated sessions the individual may simply learn that the target behavior will consistently result in delivery of the items in question. Only a single instance of this sort of false-positive outcome has been reported (Shirley, Iwata, & Kahng, 1999), so it is difficult to determine whether it occurs with any regularity. Conceivably, this sort of learning could be detected by examining response patterns across sessions for learning curves characteristic of the acquisition of new response–reinforcer relationships (e.g., a steady increase in response rates).

Another possible limitation is that the challenging behavior is maintained by events that are simply not tested by the conditions arranged in a given functional analysis (Carr, 1994; Sturmey, 1995a) or that the analysis fails to identify the specific, often idiosyncratic, features of a situation that evoke the challenging behavior. As noted previously, this sort of limitation can sometimes be successfully addressed by combining descriptive and experimental functional assessment procedures. Moreover, as discussed later, researchers and clinicians have become increasingly adept at using functional analytic methods to identify highly specific critical features of the behavior–environment relationship.

Another reported limitation has been that the analysis as described by Iwata, Dorsey, et al. (1982/1994) may be too complex for many individuals in clinical settings to use or to replicate faithfully. For example, Spreat and Connelly (1996) suggested that the complexity of functional analysis impedes its use in typical treatment settings because staff members in these settings may lack the professional training needed to conduct such analyses. Studies, however, have suggested that it may be relatively easy to train individuals to implement a functional analysis of challenging behaviors in both clinical (Iwata, et al., 2000) and educational (Moore et al., 2002; Wallace, Doney, Mintz-Resudek, & Tarbox, 2004) settings. Thus, although some level of instruction is needed to produce proficiency in performing the analysis, these studies suggest that the training requirements may be minimal.

Impact of Functional Assessment Methods

The development of functional assessment tools has had a clear impact on the treatment of behavior disorders in individuals with developmental disabilities. The tools have become widely adopted, as indicated by a recent survey of members of the Psychology Division of the American Association on Intellectual and Developmental Disabilities ($n = 125$), who indicated that their treatment decisions were always (47%) or often (46%) based on a functional assessment (Desrochers, Hile, & Williams-Mosely, 1997). Furthermore, several studies have indicated that treatment is more effective following functional assessment (Iwata, Pace, et al., 1994; Sternberg, Taylor, & Babkie, 1994). Kahng, Iwata, and Lewin (2002), for example, examined 706 cases of SIB in people with developmental disabilities with specific regard to interventions that involved reinforcement alone, reinforcement plus extinction, or extinction alone. When conducted without a functional analysis, these interventions produced mean reductions in SIB of 61.6%, 47.5%, and 47.0%, respectively, relative to baseline levels. By contrast, the same interventions, when preceded by a functional analysis, all produced reductions exceeding 80%.

In addition, functional assessment may have altered general patterns of treatment selection. Prior to the advent of functional assessment, researchers and clinicians often attempted to decrease challenging behaviors without consideration of their causes. In most cases, this resulted in the arbitrary selection of treatment components. When these treatments failed, individuals resorted to default technologies, such as punishment (Iwata, 1988). More recently, a review of the behavioral treatment literature conducted by Pelios, Morren, Tesch, and Axelrod (1999) noted an increase in studies that relied on reinforcement-based procedures rather that punishment-based procedures since the early 1980s, roughly corresponding to the period in which functional analytic methods were being developed and reported. These authors suggested that the use of functional analyses increased the probability with which researchers chose less intrusive, perhaps less objectionable, reinforcement-based procedures.

This increased interest in functional assessments has been fueled in large part by its use as a treatment development tool. That is, this systematic use of functional assessment technology to identify the variables that maintain challenging behavior has the potential to aid in the development of effective behavioral interventions in several ways (Iwata, Vollmer, & Zarcone, 1990; Mace, Lalli, & Lalli, 1991). First, the antecedent conditions that influence challenging behavior can be identified and changed to reduce the likelihood of challenging behavior. Second, the source of reinforcement for the challenging behavior can be minimized or eliminated once identified. Third, the reinforcer that maintains the challenging behavior can be used in the behavioral intervention to reduce that behavior. Fourth, identification of behavioral function may permit one to eliminate unnecessary or irrelevant components of a treatment. Finally, when behavioral treatment fails to produce a positive outcome, functional assessment has provided information on factors responsible for the failure. For example, treatment failure may be a result of a mismatch between factors maintaining the challenging behavior and treatment (Durand & Kishi, 1987; Repp, Felce, & Barton, 1988) or a change in these factors over time (Lerman, Iwata, Smith, Zarcone, & Vollmer, 1994).

Trends in Functional Behavioral Assessment

Specificity of Behavioral Function   Thus far, we have reviewed methods largely in relation to those behavioral functions that are observed most commonly. As already noted, these few categories of behavioral function have accounted for the majority of cases. For example, in their analysis of 152 cases, Iwata, Pace, et al. (1994) found that 88% were accounted for by attention, escape from task demands, automatic reinforcement, or some combination of these functions. A literature review of 706 cases of self-injury conducted by Kahng et al.

(2002) revealed a similar percentage (85.2%) in which these functions were evident.

Still, some authors have commented that one of the drawbacks of experimental functional analyses is that they may fail to capture the full range of variables that maintain challenging behaviors in the natural environment (Sturmey, 1995a). Carr (1994) noted that, although attention seeking, escape, sensory reinforcement, and tangible events are key variables in any analysis of challenging behavior, they are not the only variables. Horner similarly remarked,

> To date, efforts to design functional assessment procedures have often focused on a four-part taxonomy of the variables that maintain challenging behavior (tangible, attention, escape, automatic). In the future, I believe we will need to be more specific about the stimuli that control challenging behaviors. (1994, p. 402)

Researchers have increasingly begun to explore complex, specific, and often idiosyncratic relations in an effort to better understand the motivations underlying challenging behavior and to provide more refined treatments for behavior disorders. To illustrate, several studies have employed functional analytic approaches to explore idiosyncratic behavior–environment relationships for challenging behavior that occurs during demand contexts but perhaps are not as straightforward as the general case of escape-maintained behavior. Differential effects are sometimes observed as a function of stimuli associated with the work. For example, Progar et al. (2001) observed that rates of challenging behavior were consistently higher in the presence of two specific staff members who had a history of presenting instructional tasks to the participants. Other investigators have found that certain features regarding the manner in which tasks are presented can alter the probability of escape-maintained behavior, presumably by modifying the extent to which the demands are deemed aversive (Smith, Iwata, Goh, & Shore, 1995).

Although escape from academic or other sorts of instructional demands has been by far the most commonly reported class of negative reinforcement contingency, a wide variety of stimuli or contexts have been shown to evoke escape-maintained behavior in individuals with developmental disabilities. For example, intrusive or painful stimulation arising from necessary medical procedures has set the occasion for escape-maintained behavior in some individuals (Iwata, Dorsey, et al., 1982/1994; Hagopian, Crockett, & Keeney, 2001). For others, certain simple forms of ambient environmental stimuli have evoked aberrant behavior (McCord, Iwata, Galensky, Ellingson, & Thomson, 2001). Transitions among activities have also been known to give rise to escape-related behavior (McCord, Thomson, & Iwata, 2001; Tustin, 1995). Still other individuals displayed challenging behavior that was occasioned by social interaction in general, a phenomenon that has come to be known as social avoidance or social escape (Hagopian, Wilson, & Wilder, 2001; Taylor & Carr, 1992).

Deviations of this sort, of course, have been identified in relation to each of the common behavior functions. Challenging behavior maintained by caregiver attention has been shown to be differentially sensitive to, among other factors, the content of attention (Piazza et al., 1999), the quality of attention (Richman & Hagopian, 1999), and divided or "diverted" attention, an interesting phenomenon in which attention-maintained challenging behavior is more likely to occur if the caregiver is already directing his or her attention elsewhere (e.g., Taylor, Sisson, McKelvey, & Trefelner, 1993; O'Reilly, Lancioni, King, Lally, & Dhomhnaill, 2000). The range of tangible stimuli that maintain challenging behavior has, of course, also been widely idiosyncratic. Specific stimuli have included food items (e.g., Goh, Iwata, & DeLeon, 2000; Kern, Carberry, & Haidara, 1997); various toy items (e.g., DeLeon, Fisher, Herman, & Crosland, 2000; Hagopian, Crockett, van Stone, DeLeon, & Bowman, 2000); various activities such as being pushed in a wheelchair (DeLeon, Kahng, Rodriguez-Catter, Sveinsdóttir, & Sadler, 2003); and, in some interesting cases, access to self-restraint or mechanical restraint (Smith, Lerman, & Iwata, 1996; Vollmer & Vorndran, 1998).

What binds most of these instances together is the powerful, single-case experimental methodology used to isolate the specific variables that give rise to and maintain challenging behavior. The term *functional analysis of challenging behavior* has, over the years, perhaps been assumed to mean a particular set of procedures, most specifically, those described by Iwata, Dorsey, et al. (1982/1994); however, it is clearly far more than this. More accurately, a functional analysis is being conducted anytime researchers or clinicians directly manipulate variables in a systematic and controlled fashion to isolate causal relations between behavior and its antecedents and consequences. As exemplified by the studies mentioned previously, this methodology has grown into a powerful tool for identifying highly specific controlling variables.

Functional Assessment and Pharmacological Intervention Behavior management based on learning theory has become part of the standard of care for the behavior disorders of individuals with developmental disabilities (DeLeon, Rodriguez-Catter, & Cataldo, 2002). Still, pharmacological interventions continue to be just as, if not more, common. Recent estimates suggest that between 12% and 43% of individuals with intellectual disabilities were receiving at least one psychoactive medication (Rinck, 1998). Unfortunately, numerous authors have suggested that pharmacological intervention for behavior disorders is, at best, imprecise (Baumeister, Todd, & Sevin, 1993; Matson, Bielecki, Mayville, & Matson, 2003). The basis for the use of such medications is often not as clear when it is evident that the challenging behavior is maintained by environmental contingencies. Schaal and Hackenberg noted that, although treatment with virtually every class of psychotropic drug has been attempted with individuals with developmental disabilities, these drugs are administered with little regard to the pharmacological basis for their effectiveness, leading the authors to conclude that "researchers and clinicians are still largely unable to specify with certainty what a drug should be given for, to whom it should be given, and why it should be expected to help" (1994, p. 124). They further commented that perhaps the most troubling aspect of pharmacological treatment research is that participants are selected for trials of one drug or another based on topographical (e.g., hand-to-head SIB, self-biting), rather than functional features of the problem behavior (e.g., SIB maintained by escape from demands).

To the extent that the drugs interact with environmental variables, it is possible that the interaction involves a modification of the individual's motivation to gain access to one form of reinforcement or another. For example, a variety of related hypotheses have implicated the endogenous opioid system in the maintenance of SIB, either through an addiction-like dependence on endogenous opiates (endorphins, enkephalins) or through abnormalities of the system that result in excessive basal levels of endogenous opiates (Cataldo & Harris, 1982; Sandman & Hetrick, 1995). Endogenous opiates, released subsequent to painful stimulation, can produce analgesic and euphoric effects similar to those produced by the opiate class of manufactured drugs (Snyder, 1977; Veith, Sandman, Walker, Coy, & Kastin, 1978). Based on these hypotheses, several studies have examined the effects of naloxone (Narcan) and naltrexone (ReVia), drugs that block opiate receptors, on SIB. The rationale behind this approach is that, if self-injury results in euphoric effects stemming from the continuous delivery of endogenous opiates, then opiate antagonists should result in the extinction of SIB (the response occurs, but the functional consequence does not). If the hypothesis is correct, it may suggest that opiate antagonists may have selective effects on SIB that is maintained by sensory reinforcement.

In other cases, a drug's effects may involve making aversive situations less aversive and, therefore, modifying the individual's motivation to escape from those situations. Alternatively, the drug effect may be a stimulus control phenomenon. For example, perhaps the drug's effects are to modify the saliency, from the individual's perspective, of stimuli associated with the availability and unavailability of reinforcement. By correlating behavior measures of these variables with drug effects on challenging behavior, it may be possible to discover the circumstances surrounding the specific behavioral effects of the drug and begin to make informed determinations regarding the functional characteristics of behaviors that are likely to respond to varying pharmacological interventions.

Several investigators have begun to explore the combination of functional assessment and pharmacological intervention with the goal of determining whether certain medications are differentially effective for certain forms or functions of behavior disorders. To date, most of these evaluations have involved specific drug actions. For example, DiCesare, McAdam, Toner, and Varrell (2005) examined the disruptive behavior of a man diagnosed with intellectual disabilities and attention-deficit/hyperactivity disorder by conducting a functional analysis with and without methylphenidate. They observed that challenging behavior was differentially sensitive to attention as a reinforcer when the man was not medicated, replicating similar finding in individuals without developmental disabilities (Northup et al., 1997). This finding suggests that drug effects involved an alteration of the value of attention, although other mechanisms are certainly possible (e.g., methylphenidate resulted in an increase in the probability of alternative, and competing, behavior).

Similar approaches have been taken with other drugs, including naltrexone (Garcia & Smith, 1999; Gibson, Hetrick, Taylor, Sandman, & Touchette, 1995); risperidone (Risperdal) (Crosland et al., 2003; Zarcone et al., 2004); and haloperidol (Haldol) (Fisher, Piazza, & Page, 1989). The results of these and related studies have provided only mild consistencies regarding interactions between the effects of the drug and behavioral function. For example, when Garcia and Smith (1999) combined functional analysis with a double-blind, placebo-controlled trial of naltrexone, the results for one participant appeared to show selective effects of the drug on response topography. One response form (head slapping) decreased during the functional analysis demand condition, whereas another (head banging) did not change significantly. In addition, levels of both behaviors remained unaffected in the functional analysis alone condition, casting doubt on the notion that naltrexone would selectively affect automatically reinforced behavior. Similarly, Crosland et al. (2003) observed that risperidone selectively decreased

challenging behavior during functional analysis demand conditions, whereas levels of the same behavior remained unaffected by the drug during the tangible condition for one of their participants. For a second participant, risperidone appeared to decrease SIB during the functional analysis attention condition, although levels of aggressive behavior remained relatively constant across drug and no-drug phases.

By contrast, when Zarcone et al. (2004) combined functional analysis with double-blind, placebo-controlled trials of risperidone, no differential effects with respect to function were found. Risperidone was either effective or not, independent of the variables hypothesized to maintain challenging behavior in children. Therefore, no differentially prescriptive knowledge was gained with respect to which children would benefit most from the drug as a function of the variables that maintained their challenging behavior. That study, however, included only 13 individuals, 10 of whom responded to the drug, and the vast majority of functional analyses determined that challenging behavior was maintained by automatic reinforcement.

Other investigators have taken a more comprehensive approach to the interaction of pharmacological agents and behavioral function. For example, researchers have begun to discuss and evaluate biobehavioral treatment decision models based jointly on the formal properties of SIB, its similarities to symptomology of other psychiatric diagnoses, and the possible role of environmental determinants of the behavior (e.g., Mace & Mauk, 1995; Sturmey, 1995b). In the model suggested by Mace and Mauk, pharmacological treatment becomes the focus when environmental determinants of SIB have been ruled out (i.e., for cases of automatic reinforcement). Automatic reinforcement may have emerged as a ''default'' category, indicating that no clear relationship between social variables and challenging behavior can be identified. It is perhaps in this functional category that the merger of biological and behavioral approaches to assessment and treatment can be most fruitfully exploited. In any event, although results of such analysis have thus far provided mixed results, the methodology nonetheless appears to have great potential along several lines. Functional analysis methods in combination with drug trials could

1. More clearly determine if sensory reinforcement results of a functional analysis serve as useful predictors of drug response

2. Possibly provide indications of when treatment with certain drugs is contraindicated (e.g., when behavior is clearly and exclusively maintained by social contingencies)

3. Provide insight into the interaction of drug treatment and learned functions (e.g., by systematically manipulating drug regimens in the course of functional analyses)

4. Possibly shed light on the accuracy of the hypotheses previously described

Anecdotally, it currently seems that researchers involved in environmental manipulation approaches to behavior disorder treatment rarely consider neurochemical mechanisms of challenging behavior maintenance or pharmacological treatment as a viable intervention. Alternatively, those who study pharmacological treatment interventions often ignore environmental determinants of challenging behavior. The use of functional analyses in evaluations of drug effects might be one way to promote a more comprehensive understanding of challenging behavior, a phenomenon of heterogeneous organic and environmental etiologies, and profitably combine environmental and neurochemical approaches to treatment.

BEHAVIORAL TREATMENT

More than 30 years of research on the treatment of challenging behavior exhibited by individuals with developmental disabilities indicates that treatments based on behavior analysis or applied behavior analysis are effective in reducing these challenging behaviors (Campbell, 2003, Didden, Duker, & Korzilius, 1997; Kahng et al., 2002; Lundervold & Bourland, 1988). Furthermore, research suggests that those behavioral treatments that are based on behavioral function (i.e., functional assess-

ment) are more effective than those that are not (Iwata, Pace, et al., 1994).

Treatments Based on Behavioral Function

Antecedent-Based Interventions Antecedent-based interventions alter variables that might affect the motivation to engage in challenging behavior. Thus, these types of behavioral interventions attempt to prevent challenging behavior from occurring. One common antecedent-based intervention is *noncontingent reinforcement* (NCR; Hagopian, Fisher, & Legacy, 1994; Vollmer, Iwata, Zarcone, Smith, & Mazaleski, 1993). NCR consists of the delivery of the reinforcer maintaining the challenging behavior independent of that challenging behavior. For example, if the challenging behavior is maintained by adult attention (as determined by a functional assessment), NCR would involve providing attention throughout the day regardless of what the individual is doing.

Vollmer et al. (1993) treated severe SIB exhibited by three individuals with developmental disabilities using NCR. Their functional analysis indicated that these individuals engaged in SIB maintained by adult attention. During their NCR treatment, Vollmer et al. provided continuous attention (e.g., positive comments not related to SIB) throughout the treatment period. This resulted in an immediate decrease in SIB for all individuals. Furthermore, they successfully decreased the need to deliver continuous attention by gradually reducing the periods of attention.

Differential Reinforcement Reinforcement-based interventions have been used to decrease challenging behavior. These interventions typically consist of differentially reinforcing more appropriate behaviors. For example, *differential reinforcement of alternative behavior* (DRA) consists of reinforcing an appropriate behavior that is an alternative to the challenging behavior. Although in some cases these alternative, appropriate behaviors are incompatible with challenging behavior (e.g., if a child is typing on a computer, he or she cannot engage in SIB), this is not a necessary requirement for DRA to be effective.

Pace, Iwata, Cowdery, Andree, and McIntyre (1993) conducted a treatment evaluation of SIB exhibited by three individuals with developmental disabilities. Their functional analysis indicated that these individuals' SIB was maintained by negative reinforcement in the form of escape from demands. Treatment consisted of DRA, which consisted of providing negative reinforcement (i.e., a brief break) only when the individuals accurately completed the task. Therefore, the experimenters provided reinforcement contingent on appropriate behavior (compliance). This resulted in a significant decrease in SIB and an increase in compliance with the tasks. The experimenters gradually increased the amount of work the individuals had to complete before receiving a break.

A specific type of DRA is *functional communication training* (FCT). FCT consists of teaching the individual a more appropriate means of communicating for the reinforcer that maintains challenging behavior. For example, if an individual engages in challenging behavior that is maintained by adult attention, the goal of FCT would be to teach the individual a more appropriate communicative response such as verbally asking for attention. Carr and Durand (1985) used FCT to reduce SIB, aggression, tantrums, and noncompliance exhibited by four children with developmental disabilities. The results of their functional assessment indicated that their participants' challenging behaviors were maintained by escape from demands, attention, or both. Treatment consisted of teaching the participants to either request help during demands or request attention, while no longer providing escape or attention for challenging behavior. This FCT treatment resulted in lower levels of challenging behavior and high levels of appropriate communication.

Another reinforcement-based intervention is *differential reinforcement of other behavior* (DRO). DRO consists of providing a reinforcer contingent on the absence of challenging behavior during a prespecified time period. For example, Mazaleski, Iwata, Vollmer, Zarcone, and Smith (1993) used DRO to treat SIB exhibited by three individuals with developmental

disabilities. Their functional assessment showed that SIB for all individuals was maintained by attention. The DRO intervention consisted of providing attention if the individuals did not engage in SIB for a specific time period. Initially, the time period during which they did not have to engage in challenging behavior was very short. This time interval was gradually increased as the participants progressed.

Extinction Research suggests that behavioral interventions are often unsuccessful unless the contingency between the challenging behavior and its functional consequences is disrupted (Fisher et al., 1993; Mazaleski et al., 1993; Shirley, Iwata, Kahng, Mazaleski, & Lerman, 1997). Therefore, in most cases, terminating the reinforcement that the individual receives for challenging behavior (i.e., extinction) is an important component of behavioral interventions. For example, Shirley et al. (1997) evaluated whether or not extinction was necessary when using FCT as a treatment for SIB. They compared two treatment conditions, one in which the participants received reinforcement for appropriate communication and for challenging behavior (i.e., challenging behaviors were not on extinction) and another in which the individuals only received reinforcement for appropriate communication (i.e., challenging behaviors were on extinction). The results of that study showed that FCT was only effective when challenging behaviors were on extinction. Those data highlight the importance of manipulating the consequences for challenging behavior to produce positive outcomes.

Other Behavioral Treatments

Although behavioral treatments that are based on the function of the challenging behavior have proved to be the most effective at reducing that behavior, it is sometimes necessary to use other behavioral treatments that are not based on the variables maintaining challenging behavior. In some cases, the presentation of *competing stimuli* can result in the reduction of challenging behavior. When using competing stimuli as a treatment of challenging behavior, preferred items that result in low levels of challenging behavior are identified. The individual is then provided continuous (or near-continuous) access to these preferred competing stimuli. It is generally thought that, if the child is actively engaged with some competing stimuli, he or she will not engage in challenging behavior.

Fisher, DeLeon, Rodriguez-Catter, and Keeney (2004) used competing stimuli to treat aggression and SIB exhibited by four individuals with developmental disabilities. They initially permitted the individuals to sample a variety of stimuli in order to identify items and activities with which the individuals had high levels of engagement and low levels of challenging behavior. They then provided continuous access to these stimuli. This treatment resulted in an immediate and near-complete suppression of challenging behavior.

In some instances, the severity, intensity, and the imminent risk of injury from behavior such as SIB may necessitate the use of *protective equipment* such as helmets or arm restraints. Protective equipment may be used programmatically rather than merely as a means to prevent injury. That is, protective equipment is oftentimes placed on an individual regardless of whether or not he or she is engaging in challenging behavior because of the need to prevent injury; however, it is possible to use protective equipment as a treatment for challenging behavior by placing it on the individual for a certain period of time only when he or she engages in the challenging behavior. Mazaleski, Iwata, Rodgers, Vollmer, and Zarcone (1994) used protective equipment to decrease self-injurious hand mouthing exhibited by two individuals with profound intellectual disabilities. They placed mitts on the individuals' hands for brief periods each time the individuals engaged in hand mouthing. This resulted in near-complete suppression of hand mouthing.

An alternative approach to using protective equipment programmatically for the treatment of challenging behavior is to gradually fade its use. This would allow for continued protection from injury, yet provide the individual with the least restrictive intervention possible. For example, Oliver, Hall, Hales, Murphy, and Watts (1998) used arm splints to prevent SIB exhibited by three adults with developmental disabilities. Although the arm splints prevented SIB and reduced the possibility of injury, they also restricted the individuals' ability to move their arms. Therefore, Oliver et al. examined whether or not they could gradually increase arm flexion while maintaining low levels of SIB. Their arm splints used hinge-like devices on the elbow to control flexion in the arm. They very gradually and systematically increased flexion, allowing their participants more movement of their arms while maintaining low levels of SIB. They were eventually able to increase flexion so that the individuals had full or near-full mobility in their arms. Furthermore, they were able to physically remove portions of the arm splints for one participant.

In some instances, less restrictive interventions may fail to reduce challenging behavior. In these cases, *punishment* might be necessary to reduce potentially harmful behavior. As previously mentioned, punishment is the presentation or removal of some stimulus that results in a decrease in the future probability of that behavior. Therefore, punishment is defined by its effects on behavior and not by whether or not it is unpleasant. Examples of punishment procedures used to decrease challenging behavior include overcorrection, which consists of either restoring the environment to its previous condition or having the individual repeatedly practice an appropriate behavior (Foxx & Azrin, 1972); time-out, which involves loss of access to positive reinforcers for a specified period of time (Wolf, Risley, & Mees, 1964); and response cost, which is the loss of a specific amount of reinforcement (Axelrod, 1973).

Dunlap et al. (1994) conducted a treatment evaluation of two boys diagnosed with developmental disabilities who were disruptive in a self-contained special education classroom. During treatment, the teachers provided the children with points that were exchangeable for preferred items. Challenging behavior resulted in a loss of points (i.e., response cost). Excessive disruptions resulted in the removal of the child from the classroom (i.e., time-out). These punishment procedures were used in combination with providing access to preferred items. This behavioral treatment resulted in lower levels of disruptive behavior.

Other Treatment Issues

Positive Behavioral Support   Positive behavioral support (PBS) is a service delivery model firmly rooted in applied behavior analysis (Horner, 2000; Sugai et al., 1999). PBS is characterized by person-centered planning, functional assessment, positive reinforcement strategies, multifaceted interventions, and a focus on environments, meaningful outcomes, ecological validity, and systems-level intervention (Anderson & Freeman, 2000; Carr et al., 2002)—factors that are all based on applied behavior analysis (Carr & Sidener, 2002). For example, Baer, Wolf, and Risley (1968) stressed the importance of examining the behavior of the individual (e.g., person-centered planning), working toward the goal of producing socially significant behavior change (e.g., meaningful outcome), and examining behavior across multiple situations (e.g., ecological validity). Furthermore, as previously mentioned, applied behavior analysis is guided by the philosophy of least restrictive yet effective treatment for individuals with developmental disabilities (e.g., positive intervention strategies; Van Houten et al., 1988). Finally, functional assessment of challenging behaviors exhibited by individuals with developmental disabilities is considered the standard of care (Pelios et al., 1999) and has been central to applied behavior analysis for more than two decades (Iwata, Dorsey, et al., 1982/1994).

Behavior Analyst Certification Board

Assessing and treating challenging behaviors (particularly those most severe forms) can be a daunting task for individuals without the necessary training. Equally challenging can be identifying a qualified professional to provide these services. The Behavior Analyst Certification Board (BACB; http://www.bacb.com) was developed, in part, to meet the needs of consumers of behavioral services (Moore & Shook, 2001). BACB issues credentials for Board Certified Behavior Analysts (BCBAs) and Board Certified Associate Behavior Analysts (BCABAs), professionals who are trained to assess

and treat challenging behaviors exhibited by individuals with developmental disabilities. The BCBA and BCABA credentials are based on uniform standards that allow for a high level of quality control.

CONCLUSION

Individuals with developmental disabilities are at significant risk for developing challenging behaviors. Fortunately, over three decades of research suggests that behavioral treatments are effective in reducing these unwanted behaviors. Currently, best practice dictates that treatment consists of the identification of the causes of these challenging behaviors through functional assessments. Once these causes are known, there are a number of behavioral interventions designed to reduce these challenging behaviors that can be developed by trained professionals.

REFERENCES

Anderson, C.M., & Freeman, K.A. (2000). Positive behavior support: Expanding the application of applied behavior analysis. *The Behavior Analyst, 23,* 85–94.

Anderson, C.M., & Long, E.S. (2002). Use of a structured descriptive assessment methodology to identify variables affecting problem behavior. *Journal of Applied Behavior Analysis, 35,* 137–154.

Anderson, D.J., Lakin, K.C., Hill, B.K., & Chen, T.H. (1992). Social integration of older persons with mental retardation in residential facilities. *American Journal on Mental Retardation, 96,* 488–501.

Arndorfer, R.E., Miltenberger, R.G., Woster, S.H., Rortvedt, A.K., & Gaffaney, T. (1994). Home-based descriptive and experimental analysis of problem behaviors in children. *Topics in Early Childhood Special Education, 14,* 64–87.

Axelrod, S. (1973). Comparison of individual and group contingencies in two special classes. *Behavior Therapy, 4,* 83–90.

Axelrod, S. (1987). Functional and structural analyses of behavior: Approaches leading to reduced use of punishment procedures? *Research in Developmental Disabilities, 8,* 165–178.

Baer, D.M., Wolf, M.M., & Risley, T.R. (1968). Some current dimensions of applied behavior analysis. *Journal of Applied Behavior Analysis, 1,* 91–97.

Bailey, J.S., & Pyles, D.A.M. (1989). Behavioral diagnostics. In E. Cipani (Ed.), *The treatment of severe behavior disorders: Behavior analysis approach* (pp. 85–107). Washington, DC: AAMR.

Baumeister, A.A., Todd, M.E., & Sevin, J.A. (1993). Efficacy and specificity of pharmacological therapies for behavioral disorders in persons with mental retardation. *Clinical Neuropharmacology, 16,* 271–294.

Bijou, S.W., Peterson, R.F., & Ault, M.H. (1968). A method to integrate descriptive and experimental field studies at the level of data and empirical concepts. *Journal of Applied Behavior Analysis, 1,* 175–191.

Borthwick-Duffy, S.A. (1994). Prevalence of destructive behaviors: A study of aggression, self-injury, and property destruction. In T. Thompson & D.B. Gray (Eds.), *Destructive behavior in developmental disabilities* (pp. 3–23). Thousand Oaks, CA: Sage Publications.

Bruininks, R.H., Olson, K.M., Larson, S.A., & Lakin, K.C. (1994). Challenging behaviors among persons with mental retardation in residential settings. In T. Thompson & D.B. Gray (Eds.), *Destructive behavior in developmental disabilities* (pp. 24–48). Thousand Oaks, CA: Sage Publications.

Campbell, J.M. (2003). Efficacy of behavioral interventions for reducing problem behavior in persons with autism: A quantitative synthesis of single-subject research. *Research in Developmental Disabilities, 24,* 120–138.

Carr, E.G. (1977). The motivation of self-injurious behavior: A review of some hypotheses. *Psychological Bulletin, 84,* 800–816.

Carr, E.G. (1994). Emerging themes in the functional analysis of problem behavior. *Journal of Applied Behavior Analysis, 27,* 393–399.

Carr, E.G., Dunlap, G., Horner, R.H., Koegel, R.L., Turnbull, A.P., Sailor, W., et al. (2002). Positive behavior support: Evolution of an applied science. *Journal of Positive Behavior Interventions, 4,* 4–20.

Carr, E.G., & Durand, V.M. (1985). Reducing behavior problems through functional communication training. *Journal of Applied Behavior Analysis, 18,* 111–126.

Carr, E.G., & Lovaas, O.I. (1983). Contingent electric shock as a treatment for severe behavior problems. In S. Axelrod & J. Apsche (Eds.), *The effects of punishment on human behavior* (pp. 221–245). San Diego: Academic Press.

Carr, J.E., & Sidener, T.M. (2002). On the relation between applied behavior analysis and positive behavioral support. *The Behavior Analyst, 25,* 245–253.

Cataldo, M.F., & Harris, J. (1982). The biological basis of self-injury in the mentally retarded. *Analysis and Intervention in Developmental Disabilities, 2,* 21–39.

Conroy, M.A., Fox, J.J., Bucklin, A., & Good, W. (1996). An analysis of the reliability and stability of the Motivation Assessment Scale in assessing the challenging behaviors of persons with developmental disabilities. *Education and Training in Mental Retardation and Developmental Disabilities, 31,* 243–259.

Cooper, J.O., Heron, T.E., & Heward, W.L. (1987). *Applied behavior analysis.* Columbus, OH: Charles E. Merrill.

Crawford, J., Brockel, B., Schauss, S., & Miltenberger, R.G. (1992). A comparison of methods for the functional assessment of stereotypic behavior. *Journal of The Association for Persons with Severe Handicaps, 17,* 77–86.

Crosland, K.A., Zarcone, J.R., Lindauer, S.E., Valdovinos, M.G., Zarcone, T., Hellings, J.A., et al. (2003). Use of functional analysis methodology in the evaluation of medication effects. *Journal of Autism and Developmental Disorders, 33,* 271–279.

DeLeon, I.G., Fisher, W.W., Herman, K.M., & Crosland, K.C. (2000). Assessment of a response bias for aggression over functionally equivalent appropriate behavior. *Journal of Applied Behavior Analysis, 33,* 73–77.

DeLeon, I.G., Kahng, S., Rodriguez-Catter, V., Sveinsdóttir, I., & Sadler, C. (2003). Assessment of aberrant behavior maintained by wheelchair movement in children with developmental disabilities. *Research in Developmental Disabilities, 24,* 381–390.

DeLeon, I.G., Rodriguez-Catter, V. & Cataldo, M.F. (2002). Treatment: Current standards of care and their research implications. In S. Schroeder, M.L. Oster-Granite, & T. Thompson (Eds.), *Self-injurious behavior: Gene-brain-behavior relationships* (pp. 81–91). Washington, DC: American Psychological Association.

Desrochers, M.N., Hile, M.G., & Williams-Mosely, T.L. (1997). Survey of functional assessment procedures used with individuals who display mental retardation and severe problem behaviors. *American Journal on Mental Retardation, 101,* 535–546.

Dicesare, A., McAdam, D.B., Toner, A., & Varrell, J. (2005). The effects of methylphenidate on a functional analysis of disruptive behavior: A replication and extension. *Journal of Applied Behavior Analysis, 38,* 125–128.

Didden, R., Duker, P.C., & Korzilius, H. (1997). Meta-analytic study on treatment effectiveness for problem behaviors with individuals who have mental retardation. *American Journal on Mental Retardation, 101,* 387–399.

Dunlap, G., dePerczel, M., Clarke, S., Wilson, D., Wright, S., White, R., et al. (1994). Choice making to promote adaptive behavior for students with emotional and behavioral challenges. *Journal of Applied Behavior Analysis, 27,* 505–518.

Durand, V.M., & Carr, E.G. (1992). An analysis of maintenance following functional communication training. *Journal of Applied Behavior Analysis, 25,* 777–794.

Durand, V.M., & Crimmins, D.B. (1988). Identifying the variables maintaining self-injurious behavior. *Journal of Autism and Developmental Disorders, 18,* 99–117.

Durand, V.M., & Kishi, G. (1987). Reducing severe behavior problems among persons with dual sensory impairments: An evaluation of a technical assistance model. *Journal of The Association for Persons with Severe Handicaps, 12,* 2–10.

Emerson, E., Kiernan, C., Alborz, A., Reeves, D., Mason, H., Swarbrick, R., et al. (2001). The prevalence of challenging behaviors: A total population study. *Research in Developmental Disabilities, 22,* 77–93.

Emerson, E., Reeves, D., Thompson, S., Henderson, D., Robertson, J., & Howard, D. (1996). Time-based lag sequential analysis and the functional assessment of challenging behaviour. *Journal of Intellectual Disability Research, 40,* 260–274.

Favell, J.E., Azrin, N.H., Baumeister, A.A., Carr, E.G., Dorsey, M.F., Forehand, R., et al. (1982). The treatment of self-injurious behavior. *Behavior Therapy, 13,* 529–554.

Fisher, W.W., DeLeon, I.G., Rodriguez-Catter, V., & Keeney, K.M. (2004). Enhancing the effects of extinction on attention-maintained behavior through noncontingent delivery of attention or stimuli identified via a competing stimulus assessment. *Journal of Applied Behavior Analysis, 37,* 171–184.

Fisher, W., Piazza, C., Cataldo, M., Harrell, R., Jefferson, G., & Conner, R. (1993). Functional communication training with and without extinction and punishment. *Journal of Applied Behavior Analysis, 26,* 23–36.

Fisher, W.W., Piazza, C.C., & Page, T.J. (1989). Assessing independent and interactive effects of behavioral and pharmacological interventions for a client with dual diagnosis. *Journal of Behavior Therapy and Experimental Psychiatry, 20,* 241–250.

Foxx, R.M. (1996). Twenty years of applied behavior analysis in treating the most severe problem behavior: Lessons learned. *The Behavior Analyst, 19,* 225–235.

Foxx, R.M., & Azrin, N.H. (1972). Restitution: A method of eliminating aggressive-disruptive behavior of retarded and brain damaged patients. *Behaviour Research and Therapy, 10,* 15–27.

Garcia, D., & Smith, R.G. (1999). Using analog baselines to assess the effects of naltrexone on self-injurious behavior. *Research in Developmental Disabilities, 20,* 1–21.

Gibson, A.K., Hetrick, W.P., Taylor, D.V., Sandman, C.A., & Touchette, P. (1995). Relating the efficacy of naltrexone in treating self-injurious behavior to the Motivation Assessment Scale. *Journal of Developmental and Physical Disabilities, 7,* 215–220.

Goh, H., Iwata, B.A., & DeLeon, I.G. (2000). Competition between noncontingent and contingent reinforcement schedules during response acquisition. *Journal of Applied Behavior Analysis, 33,* 195–205.

Griffin, J.C., Williams, D.E., Stark, M.T., Altmeyer, B.K., & Mason, M. (1986). Self-injurious behavior: A state-wide prevalence survey of the extent and circumstances. *Applied Research in Mental Retardation, 7,* 105–116.

Guess, D., & Carr, E. (1991). Emergence and maintenance of stereotypy and self-injury. *American Journal on Mental Retardation, 96,* 299–319.

Hagopian, L.P., Crockett, J.L., & Keeney, K.M. (2001). Multicomponent treatment for blood-injury-injection phobia in a young man with mental retardation. *Research in Developmental Disabilities, 21,* 141–149.

Hagopian, L.P., Crockett, J.L., van Stone, M., DeLeon, I.G., & Bowman, L.G. (2000). Effects of noncontingent reinforcement on problem behavior and stimulus engagement: The role of satiation, extinction, and alternative reinforcement. *Journal of Applied Behavior Analysis, 33,* 433–449.

Hagopian, L.P., Fisher, W.W., & Legacy, S.M. (1994). Schedule effects of noncontingent reinforcement on attention-maintained destructive behavior. *Journal of Applied Behavior Analysis, 27,* 317–325.

Hagopian, L.P., Fisher, W.W., Thompson, R.H., Owen-DeSchryver, J., Iwata, B.A., & Wacker, D.P. (1997). Toward the development of structured criteria for interpretation of functional analysis data. *Journal of Applied Behavior Analysis, 30,* 313–326.

Hagopian, L.P., Wilson, D.M., & Wilder D.A. (2001). Assessment and treatment of problem behavior maintained by negative reinforcement in the form of escape from interactive play. *Journal of Applied Behavior Analysis, 34,* 229–232.

Hall, S.S. (2005). Comparing descriptive, experimental, and informant-based assessments of problem behaviors. *Research in Developmental Disabilities, 26,* 514–526.

Healey, J.J., Ahearn, W.H., Graff, R.B., & Libby, M.E. (2001). Extended analysis and treatment of self-injurious behavior. *Behavioral Interventions, 16,* 185–195.

Hill, B.K., & Bruininks, R.H. (1984). Maladaptive behavior of mentally retarded individuals in residential facilities. *American Journal of Mental Deficiency, 88,* 380–387.

Horner, R.H. (1994). Functional assessment: Contributions and future directions. *Journal of Applied Behavior Analysis, 27,* 401–404.

Horner, R.H. (2000). Positive behavior supports. *Focus on Autism and Other Developmental Disabilities, 15,* 97–105.

Hyman, S.L., Fisher, W., Mercugliano, M., & Cataldo, M.F. (1990). Children with self-injurious behavior. *Pediatrics, 85,* 437–441.

Iwata, B.A. (1988). The development and adoption of controversial default technologies. *The Behavior Analyst, 11,* 149–157.

Iwata, B.A., & DeLeon, I.G. (1996). *The Functional Analysis Screening Tool (FAST).* Gainesville: University of Florida, Florida Center on Self-Injury.

Iwata, B.A., Dorsey, M.F., Slifer, K.J., Bauman, K.E., & Richman, G.S. (1994). Toward a functional analysis of self-injury. *Journal of Applied Behavior Analysis, 27,* 197–209. (Reprinted from Iwata, B.A., Dorsey, M.F., Slifer, K.J., Bauman, K.E., & Richman, G.S. [1982]. *Analysis and Intervention in Developmental Disabilities, 2,* 3–20.)

Iwata, B.A., Pace, G.M., Dorsey, M.F., Zarcone, J.R., Vollmer, T.R., Smith, R.G., et al. (1994). The functions of self-injurious behavior: An experimental-epidemiological analysis. *Journal of Applied Behavior Analysis, 27,* 215–240.

Iwata, B.A., Vollmer, T.R., & Zarcone, J.R. (1990). The experimental (functional) analysis of behavior disorders: Methodology, applications, and limitations. In A.C. Repp & N.N. Singh (Eds.), *Perspectives on the use of nonaversive and aversive interventions for persons with developmental disabilities* (pp. 301–330). Sycamore, IL: Sycamore Publishing Co.

Iwata, B.A., Wallace, M.D., Kahng, S., Lindberg, J.S., Roscoe, E.M., Conners, J., et al. (2000). Skill acquisition in the implementation of functional analysis methodology. *Journal of Applied Behavior Analysis, 33,* 181–194.

Kahng, S., Iwata, B.A., & Lewin, A.B. (2002). Behavioral treatment of self-injury, 1964–2000. *American Journal on Mental Retardation, 107,* 212–221.

Kearney, C.A. (1994). Interrater reliability of the Motivation Assessment Scale: Another, closer look. *Journal of The Association for Persons with Severe Handicaps, 24,* 293–304.

Kennedy, C.H., & Haring, T.G. (1992). Reducing the serious behavior problems of people with developmental disabilities living in the community. *Behavioral Residential Treatment, 7,* 81–98.

Kern, L., Carberry, N., & Haidara, C. (1997). Analysis and intervention with two topographies of challenging behavior exhibited by a young woman with autism. *Research in Developmental Disabilities, 18,* 275–287.

Lalli, J.S., Livezey, K., & Kates, K. (1996). Functional analysis and treatment of eye poking with response blocking. *Journal of Applied Behavior Analysis, 29,* 129–132.

Lennox, D.B., & Miltenberger, R.G. (1989). Conducting a functional assessment of problem behavior in applied settings. *Journal of The Association of Persons with Severe Handicaps, 14,* 304–311.

Lerman, D.C., & Iwata, B.A. (1993). Descriptive and experimental analysis of variables maintaining self-injurious behavior. *Journal of Applied Behavior Analysis, 26,* 293–319.

Lerman, D.C., & Iwata, B.A. (1996). Developing a technology for the use of operant extinction in clinical settings: An examination of basic and applied research. *Journal of Applied Behavior Analysis, 29,* 345–382.

Lerman, D.C., Iwata, B.A., Smith, R.G., Zarcone, J.R., & Vollmer, T.R. (1994). Transfer of behavioral function as a contributing factor in treatment relapse. *Journal of Applied Behavior Analysis, 27,* 357–370.

Lerman, D.C., Iwata, B.A., & Wallace, M.D. (1999). Side effects of extinction: Prevalence of bursting and aggression during the treatment of self-injurious behavior. *Journal of Applied Behavior Analysis, 32,* 1–8.

Lewis, T.J., Scott, T.M., & Sugai, G. (1994). The Problem Behavior Questionnaire: A teacher-based instrument to develop functional hypotheses of problem behavior in general education classrooms. *Diagnostique, 19,* 103–115.

Lundervold, D., & Bourland, G. (1988). Quantitative analysis of treatment of aggression, self-injury, and property destruction. *Behavior Modification, 12,* 590–617.

Mace, F.C. (1994). The significance and future of functional analysis methodologies. *Journal of Applied Behavior Analysis, 27,* 385–384.

Mace, F.C., & Lalli, J.S. (1991). Linking descriptive and experimental analysis in the treatment of bizarre speech. *Journal of Applied Behavior Analysis, 24,* 553–562.

Mace, F.C., Lalli, J.S., & Lalli, E.P. (1991). Functional analysis and treatment of aberrant behavior. *Research in Developmental Disabilities, 12,* 155–180.

Mace, F.C., & Mauk, J.E. (1995). Bio-behavioral diagnosis and treatment of self-injury. *Mental Retardation and Developmental Disabilities Research Reviews, 2,* 104–110.

Matson, J.L., Bamburg, J.W., Cherry, K.E., & Paclawskyj, T.R. (1999). A validity study on the Questions About Behavioral Function (QABF) scale: Predicting treatment success for self-injury, aggression, and stereotypies. *Research in Developmental Disabilities, 20,* 163–176.

Matson, J.L., Bielecki, J., Mayville, S.B., & Matson, M.L. (2003). Psychopharmacology research for individuals with mental retardation: Methodological issues and suggestions. *Research in Developmental Disabilities, 24,* 149–157.

Matson, J.L., Benavidez, D.A., Compton, L.S., Paclawskyj, T., & Baglio, C. (1996). Behavioral treatment of autistic persons: A review of research from 1980 to the present. *Research in Developmental Disabilities, 17,* 433–465.

Matson, J.L., & Vollmer, T.R. (1995). *User's guide: Questions About Behavioral Function (QABF).* Baton Rouge, LA: Scientific Publishers.

Mazaleski, J.L., Iwata, B.A., Rodgers, T.A., Vollmer, T.R., & Zarcone, J.R. (1994). Protective equipment as treatment for stereotypic hand mouthing: Sensory extinction or punishment effects? *Journal of Applied Behavior Analysis, 27,* 345–355.

Mazaleski, J.L., Iwata, B.A., Vollmer, T.R., Zarcone, J.R., & Smith, R.G. (1993). Analysis of the reinforcement and extinction components in DRO contingencies with self-injury. *Journal of Applied Behavior Analysis, 26,* 143–156.

McCord, B.E., Iwata, B.A., Galensky, T.L., Ellingson, S.A., & Thomson, R.J. (2001). Functional analysis and treatment of problem behavior evoked by noise. *Journal of Applied Behavior Analysis, 34,* 447–462.

McCord, B.E., Thomson, R.J., & Iwata, B.A. (2001). Functional analysis and treatment of self-injury associated with transitions. *Journal of Applied Behavior Analysis, 34,* 195–210.

Moore, J., & Shook, G.L. (2001). Certification, accreditation, and quality control in behavior analysis. *The Behavior Analyst, 24,* 45–55.

Moore, J.W., Edwards, R.P., Sterling-Turner, H.E., Riley, J., DuBard, M., & McGeorge, A. (2002). Teacher acquisition of functional analysis methodology. *Journal of Applied Behavior Analysis, 35,* 73–77.

National Institutes of Health. (1991). *Treatment of destructive behaviors in persons with developmental disabilities.* Washington, DC: U.S. Department of Health and Human Services.

Newton, J.T., & Sturmey, P. (1991). The Motivation Assessment Scale: Interrater reliability and internal consistency in a British sample. *Journal of Mental Deficiency Research, 35,* 472–474.

Northup, J., Jones, K., Broussard, C., DiGiovanni, G., Herring, M., Fusilier, I., et al. (1997). A preliminary analysis of interactive effects between common classroom contingencies and methylphenidate. *Journal of Applied Behavior Analysis, 30,* 121–125.

Nyhan, W.L. (2002). Lessons from Lesch-Nyhan syndrome. In S. Schroeder, M.L. Oster-Granite, & T. Thompson (Eds). *Self-injurious behavior: Gene-brain-behavior relationships* (pp. 251–267). Washington, DC: American Psychological Association.

Oliver, C., Hall, S., Hales, J., Murphy, G., & Watts, D. (1998). The treatment of severe self-injurious behavior by the systematic fading of restraints: Effects on self-injury, self-restraint, adaptive behavior, and behavioral correlates of affect. *Research in Developmental Disabilities, 19,* 143–165.

O'Reilly, M.F., Lancioni, G.E., King, L., Lally, G., & Dhomhnaill, O.N. (2000). Using brief assessments to evaluate aberrant behavior maintained by attention. *Journal of Applied Behavior Analysis, 33,* 109–112.

Pace, G.M., Iwata, B.A., Cowdery, G.E., Andree, P.J., & McIntyre, T. (1993). Stimulus (instructional) fading during extinction of self-injurious escape behavior. *Journal of Applied Behavior Analysis, 26,* 205–212.

Paclawskyj, T.R., Matson, J.L., Rush, K.S., Smalls, Y., & Vollmer, T.R. (2001). Assessment of the convergent validity of the Questions About Behavioral Function scale with analogue functional analysis and the Motivation Assessment Scale. *Journal of Intellectual Disability Research, 45,* 484–494.

Pelios, L., Morren, J., Tesch, D., & Axelrod, S. (1999). The impact of functional analysis methodology on treatment choice for self-injurious and aggressive behavior. *Journal of Applied Behavior Analysis, 32,* 185–195.

Piazza, C.C., Bowman, L.G., Contrucci, S.A., Delia, M.D., Adelinis, J.D., & Goh, H. (1999). An evaluation of the properties of attention as reinforcement for destructive and appropriate behavior. *Journal of Applied Behavior Analysis, 32,* 437–449.

Progar, P.R., North, S.T., Bruce, S.S., DiNovi, B.J., Nau, P.A., Eberman, E.M., et al. (2001). Putative behavioral history effects and aggression maintained by escape from therapists. *Journal of Applied Behavior Analysis, 34,* 69–72.

Reid, D.H. (1992). Recent developments in treating severe behavior disorders: Advances or impediments for residential services? *Behavioral Residential Treatment, 7,* 181–197.

Repp, A.C., Felce, D., & Barton, L.E. (1988). Basing the treatment of stereotypic and self-injurious behaviors on hypotheses of their causes. *Journal of Applied Behavior Analysis, 21,* 281–289.

Richman, D.M., & Hagopian, L.P. (1999). On the effects of "quality" of attention in the functional analysis of destructive behavior. *Research in Developmental Disabilities, 20,* 51–62.

Rinck C. 1998. Epidemiology and psychoactive medication. In S. Reiss & M. Aman (Eds.), *Psychotropic medication and developmental disabilities: The international consensus handbook* (pp. 31–44). Columbus: Ohio State University.

Rojahn, J., & Esbensen, A.J. (2002). Epidemiology of self-injurious behavior in mental retardation. In S. Schroeder, M.L. Oster-Granite, & T. Thompson (Eds.), *Self-injurious behavior: Gene-brain-behavior relationships* (pp. 41–77). Washington, DC: American Psychological Association.

Sandman, C.A., & Hetrick, W.P. (1995). Opiate mechanisms in self-injury. *Mental Retardation and Developmental Disabilities Research Reviews, 1,* 130–136.

Schaal, D.W., & Hackenberg, T. (1994). Toward a functional analysis of drug treatment for behavior problems of people with developmental disabilities. *American Journal on Mental Retardation, 99,* 123–140.

Scotti, J.R., Ujcich, K.J., Weigle, K.L., Holland, C.M., & Kirk, K.S. (1996). Interventions with challenging behavior of persons with developmental disabilities: A review of current research practices. *Journal of The Association for Persons with Severe Handicaps, 21,* 123–134.

Shirley, M.J., Iwata, B.A., & Kahng, S. (1999). False-positive maintenance of self-injurious behavior by access to tangible reinforcers. *Journal of Applied Behavior Analysis, 32,* 201–204.

Shirley, M.J., Iwata, B.A., Kahng, S., Mazaleski, J.L., & Lerman, D.C. (1997). Does functional communication training compete with ongoing contingencies of reinforcement? An analysis during response acquisition and maintenance. *Journal of Applied Behavior Analysis, 30,* 93–104.

Sigafoos, J., Kerr, M., & Roberts, D. (1994). Interrater reliability of the Motivation Assessment Scale: Failure to replicate with aggressive behavior. *Research in Developmental Disabilities, 15,* 333–342.

Smith, R.G., Iwata, B.A., Goh, H., & Shore, B.A. (1995). Analysis of establishing operations for self-injury maintained by escape. *Journal of Applied Behavior Analysis, 28,* 515–535.

Smith, R.G., Lerman, D.C., & Iwata, B.A. (1996). Self-restraint as positive reinforcement for self-injurious behavior. *Journal of Applied Behavior Analysis, 29,* 99–102.

Snyder, S.H. (1977). Opiate receptors in the brain. *New England Journal of Medicine, 296,* 266–271.

Spreat, S., & Connelly, L. (1996). Reliability analysis of the Motivation Assessment Scale. *American Journal of Mental Retardation, 100,* 528–532.

Sternberg, L., Taylor, R.L., & Babkie, A. (1994). Correlates of interventions with self-injurious behaviour. *Journal of Intellectual Disability Research, 38,* 475–485.

Sturmey, P. (1994). Assessing the functions of aberrant behaviors: A review of psychometric instruments. *Journal of Autism and Developmental Disorders, 24,* 293–304.

Sturmey, P. (1995a). Analog baselines: A critical review of the methodology. *Research in Developmental Disabilities, 16,* 269–284.

Sturmey, P. (1995b). Diagnostic-based pharmacological treatment of behavior disorders in persons with developmental disabilities: A review and decision-making typology. *Research in Developmental Disabilities, 16,* 235–252.

Sugai, G., Horner, R.H., Dunlap, G., Hieneman, M., Lewis, T.J., Nelson, C.M., et al. (1999). *Applying positive behavioral support and functional behavioral assessment in schools* (Technical Assistance Guide 1, Version 1.4.3). Eugene, OR: OSEP Technical Assistance Center on Positive Behavioral Interventions & Supports.

Taylor, J.C., & Carr, E.G. (1992). Severe behavior problems related to social interactions. I: Attention seeking and social avoidance. *Behavior Modification, 16,* 305–335.

Taylor, J.C., Sisson, L.A., McKelvey, J.L., & Trefelner, M.F. (1993). Situation specificity in attention-seeking problem behavior. *Behavior Modification, 17,* 474–497.

Thompson, R.H., Iwata, B.A., Conners, J., & Roscoe, E.M. (1999). Effects of reinforcement for alternative behavior during punishment of self-injury. *Journal of Applied Behavior Analysis, 32,* 317–328.

Touchette, P.E., MacDonald, R.F., & Langer, S.N. (1985). A scatter plot for identifying stimulus control of problem behavior. *Journal of Applied Behavior Analysis, 18,* 343–351.

Tustin, R.D. (1995). The effects of advance notice of activity transitions on stereotypic behavior. *Journal of Applied Behavior Analysis, 28,* 91–92.

Van Houten, R., Axelrod, S., Bailey, J.S., Favell, J.E., Foxx, R.M., Iwata, B.A., et al. (1988). The right to effective behavioral treatment. *Journal of Applied Behavior Analysis, 21,* 381–384.

Van Houten, R., & Rolider, A. (1991). Applied behavior analysis. In J.L. Matson & J.A. Mulick (Eds.), *Handbook of mental retardation* (2nd ed., pp. 569–585). New York: Pergamon Press.

Vaughn, M.E., & Michael, J.L (1982). Automatic reinforcement: An important but ignored concept. *Behaviorism, 10,* 217–228.

Veith, J.L. Sandman, C.A., Walker, J.M., Coy, D.H., & Kastin, A.J. (1978). Systemic administration of endorphins selectively alters open field behavior of rats. *Physiology and Behavior, 20,* 539–542.

Vollmer, T.R. (1994). The concept of automatic reinforcement: Implications for behavioral research in developmental disabilities. *Research in Developmental Disabilities, 15,* 187–207.

Vollmer, T.R., Borrero, J.C., Wright, C.S., Van Camp, C., & Lalli, J.S. (2001). Identifying possible contingencies during descriptive analyses of severe behavior disorders. *Journal of Applied Behavior Analysis, 34,* 269–287.

Vollmer, T.R., Iwata, B.A., Zarcone, J.R., Smith, R.G., & Mazaleski, J.L. (1993). The role of attention in the treatment of attention-maintained self-injurious behavior: Noncontingent reinforcement and differential reinforcement of other behavior. *Journal of Applied Behavior Analysis, 26,* 9–21.

Vollmer, T.R., Marcus, B.A., & LeBlanc, L. (1994). Treatment of self-injury and hand mouthing following inconclusive functional analyses. *Journal of Applied Behavior Analysis, 27,* 331–344.

Vollmer, T.R., & Vorndran, C.M. (1998). Assessment of self-injurious behavior maintained by access to self-restraint materials. *Journal of Applied Behavior Analysis, 31,* 647–650.

Wallace, M.D., Doney, J.K., Mintz-Resudek, C.M., & Tarbox, R.S.F. (2004). Training educators to implement functional analyses. *Journal of Applied Behavior Analysis, 37,* 89–92.

Wieseler, N.A., Hanson, R.H., Chamberlain, T.P., & Thompson, T. (1985). Functional taxonomy of stereotypic and self-injurious behavior. *Mental Retardation, 23,* 230–234.

Wolf, M.M., Risley, T., & Mees, H. (1964). Application of operant conditioning procedures to the behavior problems of an autistic child. *Behaviour Research and Therapy, 1,* 305–312.

Zarcone, J.R., Lindauer, S.E., Morse, P.S., Crosland, K.A., Valdovinos, M.G., McKerchar, T.L., et al. (2004). Effects of Risperidone on destructive behavior of persons with developmental disabilities: III. Functional analysis. *American Journal of Mental Retardation, 109,* 310–321.

Zarcone, J.R., Rodgers, T.A., Iwata, B.A., Rourke, D.A., & Dorsey, M.F. (1991). Reliability analysis of the Motivation Assessment Scale: A failure to replicate. *Research in Developmental Disabilities, 12,* 349–362.

28

Psychopharmacology

An Approach to Management in Autism and Intellectual Disabilities

SCOTT M. MYERS AND THOMAS D. CHALLMAN

Physicians who treat children with neurodevelopmental disabilities utilize a variety of tools and strategies, including pharmacological interventions. Psychopharmacology is the study and use of psychotropic medications to produce behavioral, emotional, or cognitive changes. This chapter focuses on the use of psychotropic medications in children with significant cognitive disabilities, including intellectual disabilities (ID) and autism spectrum disorders (ASD). Pharmacological interventions that are generally not considered to be within the realm of psychopharmacology but may produce significant changes in behavior, such as treatment of seizures or headaches, reduction of muscle tone, and management of associated problems such as constipation, gastroesophageal reflux, thyroid dysfunction, and menstrual problems, are beyond the scope of this chapter.

ASD and ID are common diagnoses among children cared for by specialists in neurodevelopmental disabilities. In recent large studies utilizing multiple administrative sources for ascertainment, the prevalence of ID has been found to be 12–14 per 1,000 (Leonard, Petterson, Bower, & Sanders, 2003; Murphy, Yeargin-Allsopp, Decoufle, & Drews, 1995). In an analysis of data from the National Health Interview survey, Fujiura (2003) estimated a prevalence of ID of 12.7 per 1,000. Recent studies suggest that the prevalence of ASD, as currently defined and operationally diagnosed, is approximately 3–6 per 1,000 (Chakrabarti &

Fombonne, 2005; Fombonne, 2003, 2005; Gurney et al., 2003; Lauritsen, Pedersen, & Mortensen, 2004; Yeargin-Allsopp et al., 2003). Using population estimates for the year 2000, it has been estimated that, in the United States, 220,000–483,000 people younger than age of 20 have a pervasive developmental disorder (Fombonne, 2005).

Estimates of the prevalence of ASD among individuals with ID vary widely (3%–50%), but a recent study found that 7.8%–19.8% of children and adolescents with ID also had ASD, depending on the criteria used for diagnosis (de Bildt, Sytema, Kraijer, & Minderaa, 2005). Using multiple sources of information and criteria in the *Diagnostic and Statistical Manual of Mental Disorders, Fourth Edition, Text Revision* (American Psychiatric Association, 2000), these investigators found that the prevalence of ASD in children with ID was 16.7%. Most individuals with autism have significantly subaverage general intellectual functioning and adaptive deficits that manifest before age 18 (and therefore meet criteria for ID), and the intelligence quotient (IQ) scores tend to be as stable as in other populations (Bryson, Clark, & Smith, 1988; Lord & Schopler, 1989). In a recent epidemiological study in Japan, Honda, Shimizu, Imai, and Nitto (2005) found that 75% of children with autism had IQ scores below 70, and 86% of this population had IQ scores below 85. Some authors, however, have suggested that, when the entire spectrum is considered, less than half of individuals with

ASD are expected to have ID (defined as IQ scores < 70 on standardized testing) (Bryson & Smith, 1998).

Approximately 10%–20% of individuals with ID exhibit very significant challenging behaviors such as aggression, self-injury, and destructive behaviors (Emerson et al., 2001; Jacobson, 1982; Kiernan & Kiernan, 1994; McClintock, Hall, & Oliver, 2003; Oliver, Murphy, & Corbett, 1987). Aggression is more common in males, and more severe intellectual impairment is associated with increased likelihood of self-injury and stereotypy. Among individuals with ID, those who also have a diagnosis of autism are more likely to exhibit aggression, self-injury, and disruptive behavior (McClintock et al., 2003). Bradley, Summers, Wood, and Bryson (2004) found that individuals with autism and IQ scores less than 40 had more clinically significant behavior disturbances than controls matched for age, gender, and IQ score. Specific vulnerability to anxiety, mood disturbance, sleep problems, and repetitive motor behaviors was described. When the issue of maladaptive behavior in children and adolescents with developmental disabilities is examined in terms of comorbid psychiatric diagnoses, higher estimates of prevalence (15%–52%) are reported (Baker & Cantwell, 1987; Chess & Hassibi, 1970; Cormack, Brown, & Hastings, 2000; Dekker, Koot, van der Ende, & Verhulst, 2002; Eaton & Menolascino, 1982; Hardan & Sahl, 1997; Ruedrich & Menolascino, 1984; Rutter, Tizard, Yule, Graham, & Whitmore, 1976; Tonge & Einfeld, 2000). Using the Developmental Behavior Checklist (Einfeld & Tonge, 1995) as the primary measure of psychiatric disturbance, Tonge and Einfeld (2000) found that 40% of children and adolescents with ID had psychiatric disorders that persisted for more than 4 years. Kerker, Owens, Zigler, and Horwitz (2004) reviewed the literature and found methodological limitations of previous research and inconsistent estimates of the prevalence of mental health disorders in individuals with ID, but it is generally agreed that people with ID are more likely to develop challenging behaviors and psychiatric illnesses than the general population.

The use of psychotropic medication is a common component of the approach to the management of maladaptive behaviors and psychiatric comorbidities in individuals with ASD, ID, or both. In the general population, there has been a trend toward increased use of psychotropic medications in children, including the preschool age group, and the use of atypical antipsychotics for a variety of indications has increased dramatically in recent years (Cooper, Hickson, Fuchs, Arbogast, & Ray, 2004; Curtis et al., 2005; Gadow, 1997; Zito et al., 2000). Caregiver surveys conducted in Ohio in 1999 (Aman, Lam, & Collier-Crespin, 2003) and in North Carolina in 2001 (Langworthy-Lam, Aman, & Van Bourgondien, 2002) revealed that 45% of individuals with ASD were taking psychotropic medication. In North Carolina, the prevalence of psychotropic use in this population increased from 30% in 1992–1993 to 45% in 2001 (Aman, Lam, & Van Bourgondien, 2005). Seltzer, Shattuck, Abbeduto, and Greenberg (2004) reported that 75% of a population of adults with autism were prescribed at least one psychotropic medication. Increased age, lower level of functioning, and living away from the parental home are associated with increased use of psychotropic medication (Aman et al., 2005; Seltzer et al., 2004). Studies of the prevalence of psychotropic medication use in people with ID tend to focus on the adult population. In a 1993 review, Baumeister, Todd, and Sevin reported that the mean prevalence of psychotropic use among individuals with ID ranged from 22% in school-based samples to 57% in institutions.

Many studies have found higher rates of psychotropic use, particularly among individuals residing in residential settings (Baumeister et al., 1993; Gadow, 1997; Rinck, 1998). Studies conducted between 1986 and 1995 revealed prevalence rates in the community (for adults and children analyzed together) of 19%–29% for psychotropics alone and 35%–45% when anticonvulsants were included (Singh, Ellis, & Wechsler, 1997). More recent studies continue to reveal high rates of psychotropic use in adults with ID. For example, Holden and Gitlesen (2004) found a prevalence rate of 37% in one Scandinavian country. Polypharmacy, defined as the concurrent use of two or more psychotropic medications, is common in people with ID and those with ASD (Lott et al., 2004; Martin, Scahill, Klin, & Volkmar, 1999; Stolker, Heerdink, Leufkens, Clerkx, & Nolen, 2001; Stolker, Koedoot, Heerdink, Leufkens, & Nolen, 2002).

EVIDENCE BASE

Literature regarding pediatric psychopharmacology began to appear in 1937, with observations of the effects of benzedrine on behavior and intellectual performance (Bradley, 1937; Molitch & Eccles, 1937); however, more scientifically rigorous clinical research in pediatric psychopharmacology did not appear until the early 1960s, and more widespread acceptance of the use of psychotropic medications in children in the United States did not emerge until the late 1980s (Riddle, 1995).

Evidence-based medicine refers to the use of treatments or interventions for which there is scientific evidence of effectiveness and safety for a given indication and population. Independently replicated randomized controlled clinical trials with adequate sample sizes and defined study populations are the "gold standard" of evidence-based pharmacotherapy. In the field of pediatric psychopharmacology, there has been a deficiency of well-designed, controlled studies with adequate sample size and statistical power. Problems with syndrome definition, clinical heterogeneity, comorbidity, determination of appropriate outcome targets and measures, ethical concerns, self-selection of participants, and issues of funding and sample size present practical barriers to the design and implementation of scientifically ideal clinical trials (Hollander et al., 2004).

Much of the pediatric psychopharmacology literature available to guide clinical practice has for many years consisted of controlled clinical trials in adults and small open-label studies and case reports in children and adolescents. One notable exception is the extensive literature documenting the effectiveness of stimulant medications in the treatment of attention-deficit/hyperactivity disorder (ADHD) (American Academy of Pediatrics, 2001; Greenhill, Halperin, & Abikoff, 1999; Greenhill, Pliszka, et al. 2002; McClellan & Werry,

2003). Since the 1990s, however, substantial numbers of well-designed controlled clinical trials for conditions other than ADHD have been published. In reviewing the literature from 1995 through June 2005, excluding ADHD studies unless they explicitly included patients with ID, ASD, or Tourette syndrome, we were able to find more than 90 published double-blind, controlled trials in pediatric psychopharmacology involving nearly 4,000 patients. In recent years, large, multisite, randomized controlled trials have helped to establish the efficacy of various stimulants for ADHD (Arnold et al., 2004; Biederman, Lopez, Boellner, & Chandler, 2002; Gillberg et al., 1997; Greenhill, Findling, Swanson, & the ADHD Study Group, 2002; MTA Cooperative Group, 1999; Wolraich et al., 2001); atomoxetine for ADHD (Biederman, Heiligenstein, et al., 2002; Kelsey et al., 2004; Michelson et al., 2001); selective serotonin reuptake inhibitors for anxiety and obsessive-compulsive disorder (OCD) (March et al., 1998; Riddle et al., 2001; RUPP Anxiety Study Group, 2001); and risperidone for disruptive behaviors in children with ASD (McCracken et al., 2002; Shea et al., 2004).

The history of psychopharmacological treatment of individuals with ID dates back to at least the 1800s (bromides and chloral hydrate), and barbiturates were introduced in the early 20th century (Schroeder et al., 1998). Reports of pharmacological manipulation of the neurochemistry of patients with autism first appeared in the literature approximately 50 years ago. The psychomimetic effects of the serotonergic hallucinogen lysergic acid diethylamide (LSD) stimulated speculation about the role of serotonin in a variety of disorders, including autism, and the discovery of elevated whole-blood serotonin in children with autism led to attempts at pharmacological reduction (Schain & Freedman, 1961). LSD was initially administered, both because of the potential to "break through autistic defenses" and because of theoretical interest in serotonin modulation (Bender, Faretra, & Cobrinik, 1963; Bender, Goldschmidt, & Sankar, 1962; Freedman, Ebin, & Wilson, 1962; Simmons, Leiken, Lovaas, Schaeffer, & Perloff, 1966). Subsequently, a wide variety of agents that act on serotonergic, dopaminergic, noradrenergic, opioid, and other neurotransmitter systems have been studied (Zimmerman, Bonfardin, & Myers, 2000).

The best evidence of efficacy of psychotropic medications in children and adolescents with ID or ASD comes from the relatively few randomized controlled clinical trials in these populations. Other sources of potentially useful information include open-label trials in children or adolescents, controlled clinical trials in adults, case series and individual reports, clinical experience, and emerging information about the neurobiology of the disorders. Although prevalence estimates of psychopathology are higher in children and adolescents with developmental disabilities than in the general population, most trials examining pharmacological treatment of depression, anxiety, OCD, bipolar disorder, schizophrenia, and ADHD exclude individuals with ID or ASD. This literature can also be a useful source of information, but it must be recognized that the generalizability of information provided by these studies to the ID/ASD population is often unestablished. Studies directly investigating the use of several classes of psychotropic agents in children with ASD or ID are summarized in this chapter. This review is limited to agents that are currently available and commonly utilized in clinical practice.

Central Nervous System Stimulants

Central nervous system stimulants—including methylphenidate, d-amphetamine, and mixed amphetamine salts—enhance dopaminergic and noradrenergic neurotransmission and are the treatment of choice for otherwise typically developing children with ADHD. Many of the early studies in individuals with ID, however, were negative but difficult to interpret because of issues such as the use of target outcomes unrelated to ADHD symptoms and other factors (Gadow, 1985). The research literature on stimulant use for patients with ID or ASD prior to 1997 has been comprehensively reviewed by Arnold, Gadow, Pearson, and Varley (1998). Stimulants have been shown to ameliorate inattention, impulsivity, and hyperactivity in a subset of this population, but effects

on IQ score and behavior unrelated to ADHD are not significant. Most studies documenting efficacy included patients with mild or moderate ID; the benefit of stimulants in individuals with severe or profound ID is not as well documented.

Aman, Buican, and Arnold (2003) published an aggregated analysis of three independent, placebo-controlled methylphenidate trials that included 90 children with low IQ scores and ADHD. They documented superiority of methylphenidate to placebo in reducing inattention, hyperactivity, and conduct problems in 67% of patients. There was an improvement of at least 30% in target symptoms in 44% of the patients. Although statistically and clinically significant, the effect sizes were smaller than those seen in typically developing children, and there was a more heterogeneous response in patients with IQ scores less than 50 (Aman, Buican, & Arnold, 2003). Other studies have not found a clear relationship between IQ score and response to stimulants (Handen, Janosky, McAuliffe, Breaux, & Feldman, 1994; Mayes, Crites, Bixler, Humphrey, & Mattison, 1994). Some studies have found high rates of side effects in children with ID, especially at higher doses (Arnold et al., 1998; Handen, Feldman, Gosling, Breaux, & McAuliffe, 1991; Handen, Feldman, Lurier, & Murray, 1999). However, in a double-blind, placebo-controlled crossover trial, Pearson and colleagues found that higher doses of methylphenidate (0.60 mg/kg/dose) were more effective than lower doses (0.15 mg/kg/dose and 0.30 mg/kg/dose), and the ratio of children with substantial behavioral improvement to those with substantial behavioral decline at the highest dose was 5:1 (Pearson et al., 2003; Pearson, Lane, et al., 2004; Pearson, Santos, et al., 2004).

Early trials of d-amphetamine and l-amphetamine in children with autism suggested that any decrease in hyperactivity noted was often outweighed by negative effects such as increased irritability and stereotypy (Campbell, Fish, David, et al., 1972; Campbell, Fish, Shapiro, & Floyd, 1972; Campbell et al., 1976). These early studies led many authors to conclude that stimulants are contraindicated in patients with ASD (Aman, 1982; Volkmar, Hoder, & Cohen, 1985), but subsequent studies have suggested that some children with autism respond favorably (Birmaher, Quintana, & Greenhill, 1988; Di Martino, Melis, Cianchetti, & Zuddas, 2004; Geller, Guttmacher, & Bleeg, 1981; Handen, Johnson, & Lubetsky, 2000; Quintana et al., 1995; RUPP Autism Network, 2005; Schmidt, 1982; Strayhorn, Rapp, Donina, & Strain, 1988; Vitriol & Farber, 1981). In a double-blind, placebo-controlled crossover study, Quintana et al. (1995) found modest but statistically significant improvement in hyperactivity in 10 children with autism treated with methylphenidate without associated worsening of behavior or stereotypic movements. In another small double-blind, controlled methylphenidate trial, Handen et al. (2000) demonstrated at least a 50% reduction of hyperactivity and inattention in 8 of 13 patients with ASD.

In the largest controlled trial of a stimulant medication in this population, which involved 72 children between the ages of 5 and 14, methylphenidate was superior to placebo for ADHD symptoms (RUPP Autism Network, 2005). The response rate was 49%, but there was an 18% discontinuation rate due to adverse effects. Reviewers have concluded that a subgroup of children with ASD and ADHD symptoms is likely to benefit from stimulants, but the response rate seems to be substantially lower than the 75%–90% response rate in children without autism who have ADHD and normal IQ scores (Aman, 2004; Aman & Langworthy, 2000). This conclusion is consistent with the clinical experience of the authors. However, Ishizaki and Sugama (2001) studied 141 patients with hyperactivity, including a subset with ASD, and found that methylphenidate was effective in 93% of individuals with IQ scores > 80 and in 70% with IQ scores < 80. There was no difference in response between those with ASD and those without ASD. Ninety-nine of the patients were followed for 1–5 years. Adverse effects were documented in 23%, but no serious events occurred. Di Martino et al. (2004) suggested that administering a single methylphenidate test dose may be useful in identifying children with ASD who may benefit from ongoing treatment with the medication.

Amantadine is an antiviral agent that also enhances dopaminergic neurotransmissionand blocks glutamate N-methyl-D-aspartate (NMDA) receptors (Farnebo, Fuxe, Goldstein, Hamberger, & Ungerstedt, 1971; Kornhuber, Weller, Schoppmeyer, & Riederer, 1994). Open-label studies have suggested benefits of amantadine for symptoms such as hyperactivity, impulsivity, agitation, irritability, and self-injury in patients with ADHD (Masters, 1997; Mattes, 1980), other developmental disabilities including ID and ASD (Chandler, Barnhill, & Gualtieri, 1991; King et al., 2001), and traumatic brain injury (Gualtieri, Chandler, Coons, & Brown, 1989). In a randomized, double-blind, placebo-controlled clinical trial in 39 children with ASD, amantadine (5 mg/kg/day) was not superior to placebo on parent-rated Aberrant Behavior Checklist (ABC; Aman, Singh, Stewart, & Field, 1985) Hyperactivity and Irritability subscales (King et al., 2001). However, masked investigator-rated ABC Hyperactivity scores from videotaped Autism Diagnostic Observation Schedule (Lord, Rutter, DiLavore, & Risi, 1999) sessions at baseline and after 4 weeks of treatment did reveal a significant difference favoring amantadine ($p < .05$). Adverse effects reported in the open and controlled amantadine studies included exacerbation of behavior problems, transient sedation, anorexia, weight loss, and insomnia.

Atypical Antipsychotics

Atypical, or second-generation, antipsychotic medications currently available in the United States include clozapine, risperidone, olanzapine, quetiapine, ziprasidone, and aripiprazole. Evidence suggests that this class of medication is efficacious in the treatment of children and adolescents with psychosis, bipolar disorder, and Tourette syndrome and potentially useful in conduct disorder and severe ADHD (Cheng-Shannon, McGough, Pataki, & McCracken, 2004). In the 1990s, controlled trials suggested benefits of risperidone on behavioral disturbances in adults with ID and ASD (McDougle et al., 1998; Vanden Borre et al., 1993). Subsequently, several small double-blind, placebo-controlled pilot studies demonstrated the short-term efficacy of risperidone for disruptive behaviors in children and adolescents with subaverage intellectual functioning (Buitelaar, van der Gaag, Cohen-Kettenis, & Melman, 2001; Van Bellinghen & De Troch, 2001; Zarcone et al., 2001). The literature regarding the use of risperidone in children with ASD was also positive, but prior to the Research Units on Pediatric Psychopharmacology (RUPP) Autism Network trial (McCracken et al., 2002), this was limited to open-label trials and case series (Barnard, Young, Pearson, Geddes, & O'Brien, 2002). The RUPP trial and other large multisite, randomized controlled trials have confirmed the short-term efficacy of risperidone for severe disruptive behaviors in children and adolescents with ID or ASD, and open-label studies have suggested long-term benefits and tolerance (Table 28.1).

The Nisonger Child Behavior Rating Form (NCBRF) (Aman, Tasse, Rojahn, & Hammer, 1996; Tasse, Aman, Hammer, & Rojahn, 1996), the ABC (Aman, Singh, Stewart, & Field, 1985; Brown, Aman, & Havercamp, 2002; Marshburn & Aman, 1992), and other tools with appropriate psychometric properties for use as outcome measures in medication trials in children and adolescents with disabilities have been used to demonstrate statistically and clinically significant improvement in severe behavioral symptoms such as aggression, self-injury, tantrums, irritability, destructive behavior, and hyperactivity in children with subaverage intelligence or ASD in randomized, double-blind, placebo-controlled risperidone trials (see Table 28.1). Severity ratings of parent-determined primary target symptoms, either by parent-completed visual analogue scales or by blinded clinician ratings based on semistructured interviews have also been shown to improve significantly with risperidone relative to placebo (Aman et al., 2002; Arnold et al., 2003; Shea et al., 2004; Snyder et al., 2002; Van Bellinghen & De Troch, 2001). The target symptoms most commonly chosen by parents at baseline, and monitored throughout the controlled trials and associated longer term open-label studies, were aggression, tantrums/negative mood, hyperactive/impulsive/agitated behavior, stereotypy, and self-injury (Findling,

Aman, et al., 2004; Turgay, Binder, Snyder, & Fisman, 2002). The benefits of treatment with risperidone seem to be independent of the presence or absence of sedation, particular disruptive behavior disorder diagnosis, psychostimulant use, and IQ score (Aman, Binder, & Turgay, 2004).

Although randomized, double-blind, placebo-controlled trials are the gold standard for establishing short-term efficacy, open-label extensions of these trials and other large, well-designed open-label studies have been important in beginning to demonstrate sustained effectiveness and tolerability of risperidone after 6–12 months of treatment (Croonenberghs et al., 2005; Findling, Aman, et al., 2004; McCracken et al., 2002; Turgay et al., 2002). In a study that may have the advantage of more closely resembling the conditions encountered in clinical practice, Croonenberghs et al. (2005) prospectively followed more than 500 children with disruptive behavior disorders and subaverage intelligence for 1 year and found that risperidone was generally safe and effective. Masi, Cosenza, Mucci, and Brovedani (2003) studied a group of 45 preschool children with ASD for up to 32 months (mean, 8 months), and 47% were considered to be responders at a mean dose of 0.55 mg/day.

Prosocial behaviors, as measured by the Compliant/Calm and Adaptive/Social subscales of the NCBRF, have also been noted to improve in patients with ID/subaverage IQ scores treated with risperidone, although it is possible that parents may have recognized overall improvement related primarily to reduction in severe maladaptive behaviors (Aman et al., 2002; Snyder et al., 2002). An important question in ASD research is whether medications can alter the core deficits, which include 1) qualitative impairment in reciprocal social interaction; 2) qualitative impairment in communication; and 3) restricted, repetitive, and stereotyped patterns of behavior, interests, and activities. In the RUPP trial, risperidone did improve the restricted, repetitive, and stereotyped patterns of behavior but did not significantly change deficits in reciprocal social interaction or communication (McDougle et al., 2005). The effect of risperi-

Table 28.1. Large, multicenter clinical trials demonstrating efficacy of risperidone for disruptive behaviors in children and adolescents with intellectual disabilities (ID) or autism spectrum disorders (ASD)

Reference	Population	Study design	Age (years)	Dose	N	Duration (wk)	Outcome measures
Aman et al. (2002)	ID or subaverage intelligence quotient (IQ) score (36–84)	DBPCRCT	5–12	0.02–0.06 mg/kg, mean 1.16 mg/day	118	6	NCBRF*, ABC, CGI, VAS/S
McCracken et al. (2002); and Arnold et al. (2003); and McDougle et al. (2005)	ASD	DBPCRCT	5–17	0.5–3.5 mg/day, mean 1.8 mg/day	101	8	ABC*, CGI*, CRPDTS, CYBOCS, MRFRLRS
Snyder et al. (2002)	ID or subaverage IQ score (36–84)	DBPCRCT	5–12	0.02–0.06 mg/kg/day, mean 0.98 mg/day	110	6	NCBRF*, ABC, BPI, CGI, VAS/S
Turgay, Binder, Snyder, and Fisman (2002)	Extension of Snyder et al. (2002) study; ID or subaverage IQ score (36–84)	OLCT	5–12	0.02–0.06 mg/kg/day, mean 1.38 mg/day	77	48	NCBRF*, CGI, VAS/S
Findling, Aman, et al. (2004)	Extension of Aman et al. (2002) study; ID or subaverage IQ score (36–84)	OLCT	5–12	0.02–0.06 mg/kg/day, mean 1.51 mg/day	107	48	NCBRF*, CGI, VAS/S
Shea et al. (2004)	ASD	DBPCRCT	5–12	Mean 0.04 mg/kg/day, or 1.17 mg/day	77	8	ABC*, NCBRF, CGI
Croonenberghs et al. (2005)	ID or subaverage IQ score (36–84)	OLCT	5–14	0.1–4.3 mg/day, mean 1.6 mg/day	504	52	NCBRF*, ABC, CGI, VAS/S

*Primary outcome measure.

Key: ABC, Aberrant Behavior Checklist (Aman, Singh, Stewart, & Field, 1985); BPI, Behavior Problems Inventory (Rojahn, Matson, Lott, Esbensen, & Smalls, 2001); CGI, Clinical Global Impression Scale (Guy, 1976c); CRPDTS, clinician ratings of parent-defined target symptoms on a 9-point scale (from semistructured interviews); CYBOCS, Children's Yale-Brown Obsessive-Compulsive Scale (Scahill et al., 1997); DBPCRCT, double-blind, placebo-controlled, randomized clinical trial; MRFRLRS, modified Ritvo-Freeman Real Life Rating Scale (Freeman, Ritvo, Yokota, & Ritvo, 1986); NCBRF, Nisonger Child Behavior Rating Form (Aman, Tasse, Rojahn, & Hammer, 1996); OLCT, open-label clinical trial; VAS/S, visual analogue scale rating of an individual target symptom for each patient.

done on the ABC Lethargy/Social Withdrawal subscale, which rates social isolation and interest in communicating with others, was significant in one controlled trial (Shea et al., 2004) but not in the other (McCracken et al., 2002). Even in the Canadian study, which did show benefit of risperidone on social withdrawal on the ABC, improvement on the NCBRF Self-isolated/Ritualistic subscale did not reach statistical significance. Although risperidone has not been proved to have significant beneficial effects on cognition or the core social and communication deficits of ASD, reduction of interfering maladaptive behaviors such as tantrums, aggression, and self-injury may allow an individual to be more available for social interaction.

In contrast to risperidone, evidence of efficacy of clozapine (Chen, Bedair, McKay, Bowers, & Mazure, 2001; Zuddas, Ledda, Fratta, Muglia, & Cianchetti, 1996), olanzapine (Horrigan, Barnhill, & Courvoisie, 1997; Kemner, Willemsen-Swinkels, de Jonge, Tuynman-Qua, & van Engeland, 2002; Malek-Ahmadi & Simonds, 1998; Malone, Cater, Sheikh, Choudhury, & Delaney, 2001; Potenza, Holmes, Kanes, & McDougle, 1999; Rubin, 1997; Stavrakaki, Antochi, & Emery, 2004), quetiapine (Corson, Barkenbus, Posey, Stigler, & McDougle, 2004; Findling, McNamara, et al., 2004; Hardan, Jou, & Handen, 2005; Martin, Koenig, Scahill, & Bregman, 1999), ziprasidone (McDougle, Kem, & Posey, 2002), and aripiprazole (Stigler, Posey, & McDougle, 2004) in children or adolescents with ID or ASD is limited to small open-label trials, retrospective chart reviews, and case reports.

First-generation antipsychotics, or neuroleptics, have also been reported to be helpful in reducing maladaptive behaviors in individuals with ID (Baumeister, Sevin, & King, 1998), and there is evidence of efficacy of haloperidol (Anderson et al., 1984, 1989; Campbell et al., 1978; Cohen et al., 1980; Perry, Campbell, Adams, & Lynch, 1989) and pimozide (Ernst, Magee, Gonzalez, & Locascio, 1992; Naruse et al., 1982) in children with ASD. Significant side effects, however, including dyskinesias or extrapyramidal symptoms, are common (Armenteros, Adams, Campbell, & Eisenberg, 1995;

Campbell et al., 1997). Atypical antipsychotics are characterized by their decreased propensity to cause these side effects, which may be due to their increased affinity for serotonin (5-hydroxytryptamine, 5HT) type 2A (5HT2A) receptors relative to dopamine type 2 (D2) receptors. In the controlled clinical trials outlined in Table 28.1, assessments of extrapyramidal symptoms using the Extrapyramidal Symptom Rating Scale (ESRS; Chouinard & Margolese, 2005) or the Abnormal Involuntary Movement Scale (Guy, 1976a) did not reveal any differences between the risperidone and placebo groups (Aman et al., 2002; McCracken et al., 2002; Shea et al., 2004; Snyder et al., 2002). Turgay et al. (2002) reported that 26% of patients in their 48-week open-label study experienced some type of extrapyramidal symptom, but none was severe and no patients withdrew for this reason. Extrapyramidal symptoms were less common in the 48-week open-label study by Findling, Aman, et al. (2004), and mean scores on the ESRS did not change significantly from baseline. Neither study reported any new onset of tardive dyskinesia. Croonenberghs et al. (2005) also found a low incidence of extrapyramidal symptoms in their large, 12-month open-label study. Two patients developed tardive dyskinesia, which resolved a few weeks after the risperidone was discontinued.

The most troublesome adverse effect in risperidone studies in children and adolescents has been excessive weight gain (Stigler, Potenza, Posey, & McDougle, 2004). In the controlled risperidone trials in patients with ID/subaverage IQ score or ASD, which lasted only 6 or 8 weeks, mean weight gain ranged from 2.0 to 2.7 kg in the risperidone groups (Aman et al., 2002; McCracken et al., 2002; Shea et al., 2004; Snyder et al., 2002). In the long-term open-label extension studies, weight gain was reported as an adverse event in 21% (mean weight increase, 5.5 kg; Findling, Aman, et al., 2004) to 36% (mean weight gain, 8.5 kg; Turgay et al., 2002) of participants. Almost half of the weight gain was attributable to normal growth, and the excessive weight gain is largely attributable to increased appetite. Weight gain tends to be most rapid in the first 3 months and then to level off as treatment progresses.

Among the atypical antipsychotics, clozapine and olanzapine are associated with high risk of excessive weight gain, risperidone and quetiapine with moderate risk, and ziprasidone and aripiprazole with low risk for this adverse effect. Somnolence or sedation is also commonly reported, but it tends to be mild and transient and not associated with cognitive decline.

The only notable laboratory abnormality reported in risperidone trials in the ID and ASD populations is an asymptomatic increase in prolactin levels (Aman et al., 2002; Croonenberghs et al., 2005; Findling, Aman, et al., 2004; Masi et al., 2003; Snyder et al., 2002; Turgay et al., 2002). In a pooled database of five studies including 700 children treated with risperidone for 11–12 months, mean prolactin levels were found to increase and peak in the first 1–2 months and then return to normal or near normal by 3–5 months, with no associated delay in growth or progression through Tanner stages (Dunbar, Kusumakar, Daneman, & Schulz, 2004; Findling, Kusumakar, et al., 2003). Increased triglycerides and insulin resistance are also of concern, particularly in patients who gain weight excessively on atypical antipsychotics (Cheng-Shannon et al., 2004). Treatment of children and adolescents with ASD or ID with risperidone has not been associated with significant electrocardiographic (ECG) changes in the larger trials (McCracken et al., 2002; Shea et al., 2004). Corrected Q-T interval (QTc) prolongation has been reported with risperidone, olanzapine, quetiapine, and ziprasidone, but a study in adults found no prolongation beyond the threshold generally accepted as being associated with risk of torsade de pointes (Harrigan et al., 2004). Among the atypical antipsychotics, ziprasidone is associated with the greatest degree of QTc prolongation, and preliminary findings in children suggest that ECG monitoring is warranted (Blair, Scahill, State, & Martin, 2005).

Antidepressants/Anxiolytics

Selective serotonin reuptake inhibitors (SSRIs) include fluoxetine, sertraline, fluvoxamine, paroxetine, citalopram, and escitalopram. The tricyclic antidepressant (TCA) clomipramine is also a potent, though nonselective, inhibitor of serotonin reuptake, and many other antidepressants and anxiolytics such as bupropion, trazodone, venlafaxine, mirtazapine, and buspirone modulate serotonin as well. The pharmacological treatment of depression in children and adolescents is controversial, and the effectiveness of cognitive behavior therapy (CBT) is more strongly supported by the scientific literature (Compton et al., 2004). Although TCAs are beneficial in adults, there is substantial evidence from controlled trials that they are no more effective than placebo for depressed children and adolescents (Hazell, O'Connell, Heathcote, & Henry, 2002; Hazell, O'Connell, Heathcote, Robertson, & Henry, 1995). Some studies, however, suggest that SSRIs may be effective and well tolerated (Emslie et al., 1997, 2002; Keller et al., 2001; Wagner et al., 2003, 2004). The issue remains controversial because unpublished data cast doubt on the effectiveness of all of the SSRIs except fluoxetine for depression in children and adolescents (Whittington et al., 2004). Controlled trials have demonstrated the efficacy of SSRIs in treating OCD and other anxiety disorders in children and adolescents (March et al., 1998; Riddle et al., 2001; RUPP Anxiety Study Group 2001). A meta-analysis of controlled trials in pediatric OCD showed that clomipramine, fluoxetine, fluvoxamine, sertraline, and paroxetine were significantly more effective than placebo (Geller et al., 2003). Although highly significant, the effect sizes for medication were modest. The recent Pediatric OCD Treatment Study (POTS) found that the combination of CBT and sertraline was superior to CBT alone and to sertraline alone (Pediatric OCD Treatment Study [POTS] Team, 2004).

The limited literature regarding the use of antidepressants, including SSRIs, to treat depression, OCD and other repetitive behaviors, aggression, and self-injury in children and adults with ID has been reviewed by Sovner et al. (1998) and Antochi, Stavrakaki, and Emery (2003). Two small double-blind, placebo-controlled clomipramine trials, including a total of 18 adults with ID, found significant improvement in self-injurious behavior or repetitive behavior (Lewis, Bodfish, Powell, & Golden, 1995; Lewis, Bodfish, Powell, Parker, & Golden, 1996). In an open-label trial, Cook, Rowlett, Jaselskis, and Leventhal (1992) found fluoxetine to be effective in reducing Clinical Global Impression Scale (CGI; Guy, 1976c) ratings of clinical severity in children and adults with ASD or ID and problematic perseverative behavior. In a retrospective chart review study, Branford, Bhaumik, and Naik (1998) found fluoxetine and paroxetine to be effective in 25% of adults with intellectual disability and autistic traits. Masi, Marcheschi, and Pfanner (1997) described significant improvement in self-injurious behavior and depressive symptoms in four of seven adolescents with mild ID treated with paroxetine. Additional small open-label trials have suggested some efficacy of paroxetine for aggression and citalopram for depression in adults with ID (Davanzo, Belin, Widawski, & King, 1998; Verhoeven, Veendrik-Meekes, Jacobs, van den Berg, & Tuinier, 2001). Response to buspirone for self-injury and other maladaptive behaviors in adults with developmental disabilities has been mixed. Small open-label studies have shown some positive results and some negative results, including worsening in a significant subgroup of adults with ID and ASD (King & Davanzo, 1996; Ratey, Sovner, Mikkelsen, & Chmielinski, 1989; Ricketts et al., 1994).

Many lines of evidence suggest that serotonin metabolism is dysregulated in patients with ASD (Anderson, 2005; Chugani, 2005), and pharmacological modulators of serotonergic neurotransmission studied in children with ASD have included LSD and methysergide in the 1960s; L-dopa in the 1970s; fenfluramine in the 1980s; and clomipramine, buspirone, and SSRIs in the 1990s (Zimmerman et al., 2000). SSRIs have continued to be a focus of investigation, and it is likely that the role of SSRIs in ASD will be clarified further in the present decade.

SSRIs are commonly prescribed for children with ASD (Aman et al., 2005; Martin et al., 1999); however, only three published double-blind, placebo-controlled trials have examined the efficacy of SSRIs in ASD, and one of these studies included only adults. In a well-designed trial, McDougle et al. (1996) studied fluvoxamine in adults with ASD and found that it was superior to placebo in decreasing maladaptive behaviors and improving social relatedness and communication with minimal side effects. Eight of 15 patients were positive responders to fluvoxamine, whereas none of the 15 patients randomized to placebo responded. The same group suggested that fluvoxamine may not be effective or well tolerated in children and adolescents (McDougle, Kresch, & Posey, 2000); however, Sugie et al. (2005) reported a double-blind crossover trial demonstrating improvements by CGI rating in 10 of 18 children with ASD treated with fluvoxamine. Fluoxetine at a mean dose of 10 mg/day has been shown to be superior to placebo in the treatment of repetitive behaviors in 45 children and adolescents with ASD in a double-blind, placebo-controlled crossover study (Hollander et al., 2005). A global improvement composite score of 2 (much improved) or better was achieved in 56% of patients during the fluoxetine phase.

In a large open-label, retrospective study of fluoxetine, DeLong, Ritch, and Burch (2002) found that 69% of 129 young children (ages 2–8) responded positively to fluoxetine at doses of 0.15–0.5 mg/kg/day. The most highly functioning children seemed to benefit most. Smaller open-label trials and retrospective chart review studies in children with ASD have provided some evidence of efficacy of sertraline (Steingard, Zimnitzky, DeMaso, Bauman, & Bucci, 1997), fluoxetine (Peral, Alcami, & Gilaberte, 1999), fluvoxamine (Martin, Koenig, Anderson, & Scahill, 2003), citalopram (Couturier & Nicolson, 2002; Namerow, Thomas, Bostic, Prince, & Monuteaux, 2003), and escitalopram (Owley et al., 2005). Evidence for paroxetine is limited to case reports. These and other case reports and open-label studies of the use of SSRIs in children and adults with ASD have been reviewed recently by Moore, Eichner, and Jones (2004). Open-label trials of SSRIs in children and adults with ASD reported response rates of 55%–73% but are highly susceptible to publication bias (Connor, Ozbayrak, Benjamin, Ma, & Fletcher, 1997; DeLong, Teague, & McSwain Kamran, 1998; DeLong et al., 2002; Hellings, Kelley, Gabrielli, Kilgore, & Shah, 1996; Namerow et al., 2003). Improvements have been reported in repetitive behaviors, irritability, depressive symptoms, tantrums, anxiety, aggression, difficulty with transitions, social interaction, and language; however, additional well-designed controlled trials are needed to establish effectiveness of SSRIs in children and adolescents with ASD.

Other antidepressants that inhibit serotonin reuptake or otherwise modulate serotonergic neurotransmission have been found to be beneficial in open-label trials in children and adolescents with ASD. These include venlafaxine (Hollander, Kaplan, Cartwright, & Reichman, 2000), mirtazapine (Posey, Guenin, Kohn, Swiezy, & McDougle, 2001), and buspirone (Buitelaar, van der Gaag, & van der Hoeven, 1998; Realmuto, August, & Garfinkel, 1989). Published experience with trazodone in this population is limited to case reports (Benjamin, Seek, Tresise, Price, & Gagnon, 1995; Gedye, 1991; Kem, Posey, & McDougle, 2002). Controlled trials with adequate sample size to evaluate these agents are lacking.

In a double-blind, placebo-controlled crossover trial, clomipramine was shown to be superior to placebo and desipramine on a variety of measures (Gordon, State, Nelson, Hamburger, & Rapoport, 1993). In a similar study, clomipramine was not superior to placebo or haloperidol in the intent-to-treat analysis but was superior to placebo and comparable to haloperidol in patients who completed the trial (Remington, Sloman, Konstantareas, Parker, & Gow, 2001). Only 37.5% of patients were able to complete a full therapeutic trial of clomipramine because of side effects and lack of efficacy. Significant side effects, including seizures, behavior deterioration, weight changes, constipation, sedation, and ECG changes, have also been common in open-label trials (Brasic, Barnett, Sheitman, & Tsaltas, 1997; Sanchez et al., 1996). Significant side effects are less common with SSRIs, but include behavior activation, agitation, appetite suppression, insomnia, headaches, mild sedation, gastrointestinal complaints, and lip dyskinesia (Moore et al., 2004; Namerow et al., 2003). In the placebo-controlled trial of fluoxetine in children with ASD, treatment-emergent side effects did not differ between the SSRI and placebo groups (Hollander et al., 2005).

Adrenergic Agents

Alpha-Adrenergic Agonists Clonidine and guanfacine are presynaptic $alpha_2$-adrenergic receptor agonists, which modulate norepinephrine neurotransmission. There is some evidence to support the use of $alpha_2$ agonists in children with ADHD (Connor, Fletcher, & Swanson, 1999; Hunt, Arnsten, & Asbell, 1995); tics or Tourette syndrome with or without ADHD (Gaffney et al., 2002; Leckman et al., 1991; Scahill et al., 2001; Singer et al., 1995; Steingard, Biederman, Spencer, Wilens, & Gonzalez, 1993; Tourette's Syndrome Study Group, 2002); aggression or conduct disorder (Connor, Barkley, & Davis, 2000; Kemph, DeVane, Levin, Jarecke, & Miller, 1993; Schvehla, Mandoki, & Sumner, 1994); and sleep disturbances in ADHD (Prince, Wilens, Biederman, Spencer, & Wozniak, 1996).

Data regarding the benefits of $alpha_2$ agonists in children or adolescents with ID or ASD are limited. In a small double-blind, placebo-controlled crossover trial involving 10 children with ID, Agarwal, Sitholey, Kumar, and Prasad (2001) found clonidine treatment to be associated with a dose-related reduction in hyperactivity, impulsivity, and inattention. Reviews of records from two large clinics suggested that clonidine and guanfacine can also be helpful for targeting hyperactivity and impulse control problems in patients with fragile X syndrome (Berry-Kravis & Potanos, 2004). Two small double-blind, placebo-controlled trials involving a total of only 17 patients have documented modest benefits of transdermal and oral clonidine in reducing hyperarousal symptoms, including hyperactivity, irritability and outbursts, impulsivity, and repetitive behaviors, in children with ASD (Fankhauser, Karumanchi, German, Yates, & Karumanchi, 1992; Jaselskis, Cook, Fletcher, & Leventhal, 1992). Mehta, Patel, and Castello (2004) found clonidine to be effective for sedation for electroencephalography in 27 children with ASD. Lofexidine, an $alpha_2$ agonist available in Europe but not in the United States, has also been found to reduce hyperactivity in children with ASD in a double-blind, placebo-controlled crossover study (Niederhofer, Staffen, & Mair, 2002b). A systematic retrospective review of the medical records of 80 children and adolescents with ASD treated with guanfacine in an open-label fashion showed that treatment was effective in 24%, with a trend for patients without comorbid ID to be more likely to respond (Posey, Puntney, Sasher, Kem, & McDougle, 2004). Improvement was noted in target symptoms including hyperactivity, inattention, insomnia, and tics.

Common side effects of alpha$_2$ agonists include sedation, decrease in blood pressure, dry mouth, and irritability (Connor et al., 1999; Fankhauser et al., 1992; Jaselskis et al., 1992). Drowsiness tends to improve over time (Agarwal et al., 2001), but tolerance to therapeutic effects also developed after 6–8 weeks of good response in four of six patients followed in an open-label extension of the Jaselskis et al. (1992) study. Guanfacine may have less sedating and hypotensive effects, and it was well tolerated by the patients studied by Posey, Puntney, et al. (2004), who reported no significant changes in blood pressure or heart rate. A systematic review of the ECGs of 42 patients treated with clonidine (with or without concurrent treatment with a stimulant) for ADHD or tic disorder found no systemic effects on PR or QTc intervals (Kofoed, Tadepalli, Oesterheld, Awadallah, & Shapiro, 1999), and it is not among the medications for which the American Heart Association recommended ECG monitoring in children (Gutgesell et al., 1999). Others have recommended baseline and treatment ECG monitoring, and the issue has been controversial (Blackman, Samson-Fang, & Gutgesell, 1996; Blair, Taggart, & Martin, 2004). Unintentional ingestions or overdoses can be dangerous, and proper caution and storage of the medication are important (Michael & Sztajnkrycer, 2004; Spiller et al., 2005).

Beta-Adrenergic Antagonists Beta-adrenergic antagonists (beta-blockers) have been shown to be beneficial for migraine prophylaxis and neurally mediated syncope in children and adolescents (Linde & Rossnagel, 2004; Riddle et al., 1999). Literature regarding their use for anxiety in children and adolescents is limited to case reports and small open-

label studies. There is also evidence to support the use of beta-blockers for agitation and aggression in adults with traumatic brain injury (Fleminger, Greenwood, & Oliver, 2003). Beta-blockers vary in their affinity for B$_1$ versus B$_2$ receptors and in their lipid solubility, which determines their ability to cross the blood–brain barrier. For example, propranolol readily enters the brain and therefore has central and peripheral effects, whereas nadolol and atenolol cross the blood–brain barrier only in small amounts and have effects primarily in the periphery (Steingard, Connor, & Trang, 2005).

Propranolol, nadolol, metoprolol, and pindolol have been reported to reduce aggression and self-injury in adults with ID or ASD in several trials reporting objective outcome measures (Kastner, Burlingham, & Friedman, 1990; Luchins & Dojka, 1989; Ratey & Lindem, 1991; Ratey et al., 1986, 1987). Decreased stereotypy and aggressive outbursts have been reported in a man with fragile X syndrome and ASD who was treated with long-acting propranolol and placebo in a double-blind, crossover design (Cohen, Tsiouris, & Pfadt, 1991). In a prospective open-label trial, Connor et al. (1997) found nadolol to be beneficial in 10 of 12 children, adolescents, and young adults with ID. Ratings of aggression and clinical improvement and severity improved, but no significant effects on inattention or hyperactivity were demonstrated. Sleep disturbance associated with Smith-Magenis syndrome is related to dysregulation of melatonin secretion, and acebutolol has been used to suppress diurnal melatonin secretion and improve sleep and disruptive behavior (de Leersnyder et al., 2001). Hypotension, bradycardia, bronchoconstriction, peripheral vasoconstriction, fatigue, depression, and sleep disturbance are potential side effects of beta-blockers (Fraser, Ruedrich, Kerr, & Levitas, 1998).

Mood Stabilizers

Use in Children and Adolescents with Bipolar Disorder
Mood-stabilizing medications are those that are effective in treating or preventing mania or depression associated with bipolar

disorder. Only lithium has been clearly demonstrated to treat and prevent both mania and depression in adults with bipolar disorder, but several anticonvulsants and atypical antipsychotics have been shown to be effective for either depression or mania (Bauer & Mitchner, 2004; Berk & Dodd, 2005; Macritchie et al., 2003; Rendell, Gijsman, Keck, Goodwin, & Geddes, 2005). The diagnosis of bipolar disorder in children and adolescents is challenging and controversial but increasingly common (Carlson, 2005; National Institute of Mental Health, 2001; Wagner, 2004; Wozniak, 2005). Some small controlled trials have suggested efficacy of lithium for mania symptoms and bipolar disorder in youth (DeLong & Nieman, 1983; Geller et al., 1998; McKnew et al., 1981), but most of the evidence comes from open-label trials (Findling, McNamara, et al., 2003; Kafantaris, Coletti, Dicker, Padula, & Kane, 2003; Kowatch et al., 2000; Pavuluri et al., 2004). A double-blind, placebo-controlled discontinuation study did not support a large effect for lithium continuation treatment of adolescents with acute mania (Kafantaris et al., 2004).

There are no controlled studies documenting the efficacy of anticonvulsant monotherapy for mood stabilization in children and adolescents with bipolar disorder. Some potential benefit of topiramate for mania was suggested in a double-blind, placebo-controlled trial, but the results were inconclusive because the study was terminated prematurely because of failure of adult topiramate trials to demonstrate efficacy (Delbello et al., 2005). Otherwise, evidence of efficacy of anticonvulsants for mood stabilization comes from open-label trials and chart reviews (Carandang, Maxwell, Robbins, & Oesterheld, 2003; Chang et al., 2003; Findling, McNamara, et al., 2003; Henry, Zamvil, Lam, Rosenquist, & Ghaemi, 2003; Kafantaris et al., 1992; Kowatch et al., 2000; Papatheodorou & Kutcher, 1993; Papatheodorou, Kutcher, Katic, & Szalai, 1995; Pavuluri, Henry, Carbray, Naylor, & Janicak, 2005; Scheffer & Niskala Apps, 2004; Wagner et al., 2002; West, Keck, & McElroy, 1995; West, Keck, McElroy, & Strakowski, 1994).

Combinations of two or more mood-stabilizing agents are frequently utilized, and there is some support for enhanced efficacy (Delbello, Kowatch, et al., 2002; Delbello, Schwiers, Rosenberg, & Strakowski, 2002; Kowatch, Sethuraman, Hume, Kromelis, & Weinberg, 2003; Pavuluri et al., 2004). Small controlled trials have documented superiority of lithium and valproate to placebo for aggression and explosive behavior associated with oppositional defiant disorder or conduct disorder (Campbell et al., 1984, 1995; Donovan et al., 2000; Malone, Delaney, Luebbert, Cater, & Campbell, 2000).

Use in Individuals with Developmental Disabilities

Several double-blind, placebo-controlled trials have demonstrated efficacy of lithium for aggression in adults with ID (Craft et al., 1987; Naylor, Donald, Le Poidevin, & Reid, 1974; Tyrer, Walsh, Edwards, Berney, & Stephens, 1984), and open-label studies suggest efficacy for aggression and self-injury in this population (Glue, 1989; Langee, 1990; Luchins & Dojka, 1989; Micev & Lynch, 1974; Pary, 1991; Poindexter et al., 1998; Smith & Perry, 1992). Campbell, Fish, Korein, et al. (1972) compared lithium to chlorpromazine in a controlled crossover study of 10 "severely disturbed" young children with hyperactivity. They found no significant differences between lithium and chlorpromazine and concluded that neither was particularly efficacious in this group of patients. They did, however, note a trend toward decreased explosiveness, aggressiveness, hyperactivity, and "psychotic speech" with lithium and suggested that it deserved further study. Several case reports describe children and adolescents with autism and atypical bipolar disorder or mania who responded well to open treatment with lithium (DeLong, 1994; Kerbeshian, Burd, & Fisher, 1987; Steingard & Biederman, 1987).

In addition to their role in seizure management, traditional anticonvulsants such as valproate and carbamazepine and newer agents such as lamotrigine, topiramate, and gabapentin have been reported to have positive behavioral effects in some patients with developmental disabilities (Antochi et al., 2003; Crawford, Brown, Kerr, & the Parke Davis Clinical Trials Group, 2001; Hardan, Jou, &

Handen, 2004; McKee et al., 2003; Sovner, 1991). In open-label trials in children and adults with ID, valproate has been found to be effective for aggression, self-injury, irritability, and behavioral cycling (Kastner, Finesmith, & Walsh, 1993; Kastner, Friedman, Plummer, Ruiz, & Henning, 1990; Ruedrich, Swales, Fossaceca, Toliver, & Rutkowski, 1999; Sovner, 1989).

Some open-label studies have suggested that treatment with valproate may be associated with significant improvement in both electroencephalographic recordings and subjective clinical status in patients with ASD (Chez, Memon, & Hung, 2004). In small open-label trials, valproate, levetiracetam, and topiramate were effective in reducing symptoms such as aggression, impulsivity, hyperactivity, conduct problems, and mood lability in children with ASD (Hardan et al., 2004; Hollander, Dolgoff-Kaspar, Cartwright, Rawitt, & Novotny, 2001; Rugino & Samsock, 2002). In an open-label valproate trial and several case reports, improvements in language and social skills were also described (Childs & Blair, 1997; Plioplys, 1994); however, Hellings and colleagues (2005) were not able to demonstrate a significant difference between valproate and placebo for treatment of aggression and irritability in a study of 30 young people with ASDs (ages 6–20 years). It was noted that 10 of 16 subjects (62%) who entered an open trial of valproate after the double-blind phase demonstrated a sustained response and attempted tapering in four subjects was associated with relapse in irritability and aggression, which improved when the medication was resumed. In another small ($n = 13$) double-blind, controlled trial, divalproex sodium was found to be superior to placebo in reducing repetitive behaviors (Hollander, Soorya, Wasserman et al., 2005). Uvebrant and Bauziene (1994) reported a decrease in "autistic symptoms" in 8 of 13 individuals with autism treated with lamotrigine for intractable epilepsy, regardless of efficacy in controlling the seizures; however, in a double-blind, placebo-controlled trial, Belsito, Law, Kirk, Landa, and Zimmerman (2001) did not find significant differences between lamotrigine and placebo in the treatment of children with ASD.

Adverse Effects Surveillance for potential side effects is important during therapy with anticonvulsants or lithium. Hepatotoxicity has been reported in association with the use of most of the major anticonvulsants. The risk is highest among children younger than age 2 treated with valproate, particularly in combination with other anticonvulsants (Bryant & Dreifuss, 1996). Acute pancreatitis is an additional rare but potentially serious side effect. Weight gain and sedation are the most common adverse effects of valproate, but hematologic side effects, including thrombocytopenia, are also relatively common. Baseline liver function tests and complete blood count should be obtained prior to the initiation of treatment with valproate and periodically thereafter (Stahl, 2005). Lithium use is also associated with weight gain and sedation, as well as thyroid dysfunction, tremor, and ataxia. Lithium has a narrow therapeutic index, increasing the risk of lithium toxicity and highlighting the need for close monitoring of lithium blood levels in addition to serum electrolytes, renal function tests, and thyroid function tests (Timmer & Sands, 1999).

Naltrexone

Naltrexone is an opiate receptor antagonist that is used in the treatment of opiate and alcohol dependence. Because opioidergic systems are thought to play a role in self-injurious behavior (Sandman, 1991), naltrexone has been studied and utilized clinically; however, reviewers of the same literature have come to contradictory conclusions ranging from ineffective or clinically insignificant effects to quite effective in a substantial percentage of patients. Symons, Thompson, and Rodriguez (2004) published a quantitative synthesis of the literature regarding the use of naltrexone for self-injury in individuals with ID or ASD. Overall, 80% of individuals in published reports from which data could be extracted and pooled for analysis experienced reductions in self-injurious behavior, with 47% experiencing at least a 50% reduction. Some reports suggest long-term benefits of naltrexone on self-injury (Casner, Weinheimer, & Gualtieri, 1996; Crews, Bonaventura, Rowe, & Bonsie, 1993;

Sandman et al., 2000). Limitations of the data were reviewed and recommendations were provided regarding the design of future studies to clarify the efficacy of naltrexone for self-injury among individuals with developmental disabilities (Symons et al., 2004).

A number of controlled trials have investigated the value of naltrexone in ASD (Bouvard et al., 1995; Campbell et al., 1990, 1993; Feldman, Kolmen, & Gonzaga, 1999; Kolmen, Feldman, Handen, & Janosky, 1995, 1997; Leboyer et al., 1992; Scifo, Batticane, Quattropani, & Spoto, 1991; Symons et al., 2001; Willemsen-Swinkels, Buitelaar, Nijhof, & van England, 1995; Willemsen-Swinkels, Buitelaar, & van Engeland, 1996; Willemsen-Swinkels, Buitelaar, Weijnen, & van Engeland, 1995). The most consistent finding is a modest reduction in hyperactivity, without clear benefit on learning or on the core social and communication deficits of autism. Naltrexone has a bitter taste and can be difficult to administer, but otherwise it is generally well tolerated. Increased liver enzymes have been noted in other populations at higher doses, but studies in patients with ID or ASD in which liver enzymes were monitored did not find any evidence of liver toxicity (Symons et al., 2004).

TREATMENT PRINCIPLES

ID and ASD are behaviorally defined neurobiological conditions that generally are not "curable." The primary goals of treatment are to maximize functional independence and quality of life and alleviate family distress by facilitating development and learning, promoting socialization, and reducing interfering maladaptive behaviors. Behavioral and educational interventions and associated habilitative therapies are the cornerstones of management of ID and ASD (Bodfish, 2004; Campbell, 2003; Goldstein, 2002; Horner, Carr, Strain, Todd, & Reed, 2002; Howlin, 1998; Jacobson & Mulick, 1996; Koegel, 2000; Koegel, Koegel, & McNerney, 2001; Matson, Benavidez, Compton, Paclawskyj, & Baglio, 1996; Mesibov, Shea, & Schopler, 2005; Rogers, 1998, 2000; Smith, Eikeseth, Klevstrand, & Lovaas, 1997). These interventions address communication, social skills, daily living skills, play/leisure skills, academic achievement, and aberrant behaviors. Individualization of the habilitation plan, treatment of the specific impairments rather than the diagnosis, provision of early and sustained intervention, and involvement of parents are guiding principles in the management of children with developmental disabilities.

Optimization of medical care is also likely to have a positive impact on habilitative progress and quality of life. Management of associated deficits such as seizures, motor impairment, and vision or hearing impairment may be particularly important. Medications have not been proved to correct the core deficits of ASD or ID; however, associated maladaptive behaviors or psychiatric comorbidities may interfere with educational and therapeutic progress, socialization, health or safety, and quality of life. These behaviors may be amenable to psychopharmacological intervention or, in some cases, to treatment of underlying medical conditions that are causing or exacerbating the behaviors. Effective medical management is likely to allow an individual to benefit more optimally from educational, behavioral, social, and other habilitative interventions.

General guidelines regarding the clinical "art" of pharmacological management of behavioral problems associated with ID and ASD are outlined in Table 28.2. Before initiating a trial of psychotropic medication, it is important to search for environmental and medical factors that may be causing or exacerbating the maladaptive behaviors. Maladaptive behaviors are often inadvertently reinforced by parents, teachers, therapists, or other caregivers, and in such cases the most appropriate and effective interventions are based on the principles of operant conditioning and applied behavior analysis. In some instances, a mismatch between educational or behavioral expectations and cognitive ability of the child is responsible for disruptive behavior, and adjustment of the expectations is the most appropriate intervention. This may occur, for example, when the diagnosis of ID has not been recognized.

Standard treatment of medical conditions may also eliminate the need for psychopharmacological agents in some cases. For example, in the case of an acute onset or exacerbation of aggressive or self-injurious behavior, an occult

Table 28.2. Principles for the use of psychotropic medication as an adjunct to behavioral and educational treatment in individuals with intellectual disabilities or autism spectrum disorder

Identify and assess target symptoms and evaluate for patterns of behavior that might guide choice of treatment.
• Interview
  Intensity
  Duration
  Exacerbating factors/triggers (e.g., time, setting/location, demand situations, denials, transitions)
  Ameliorating factors and response to behavioral interventions
  Time trends (increasing, decreasing, stable)
  Degree of interference with functioning
• Baseline behavior rating scales
• Baseline performance measures/direct observational data
 	
Assess existing and available supports.
• Behavioral services
• Educational services
• Respite care
• Family psychosocial supports
• Habilitative therapies
 	
Consider medication based on the presence of
• Evidence that the target symptoms are interfering substantially with learning/academic progress, socialization, health/safety (of the patient and/or others around him or her), or quality of life
• Suboptimal response to available behavioral interventions and environmental modifications
• Research evidence that the target behavioral symptoms or comorbid psychiatric diagnoses are amenable to pharmacological intervention
 	
Search for medical factors that may be causing or exacerbating target behavior(s).
• Consider occult sources of pain or discomfort (e.g., infectious, gastrointestinal, dental)
	• Consider other medical causes or contributors (e.g., sleep disorders, seizures, nutritional deficiencies)
	• Complete any medical tests that may have a bearing on treatment choice
	
	Choose a medication based on
	• Likely efficacy for the specific target symptoms
	• Potential adverse effects
	• Practical considerations such as formulations available, dosing schedule, cost, and requirement for laboratory or electrocardiographic monitoring
	• Informed consent from parent/guardian and, when possible, assent from the patient
	
	Establish a plan for monitoring of effects.
	• Identify outcome measures
	• Discuss time course of expected effects
	• Arrange follow-up telephone contact, completion of rating scales, reassessment of behavioral data, and visits accordingly
	• Outline a plan regarding what might be tried next if there is a negative or suboptimal response or to address additional target symptoms
	  Change to a different medication
	  Add another medication to augment a partial or suboptimal therapeutic response to the initial medication (same target symptoms)
	  Add a different medication to address additional target symptoms that remain problematic
	• Obtain baseline laboratory data, if necessary, for the drug being prescribed, and plan appropriate follow-up monitoring
	
	Explore the reasonable dose range for a single medication for an adequate length of time before changing to or adding a different medication.
	Monitor for side effects systematically.
	Consider careful withdrawal of the medication after 6–12 months of therapy to determine whether it is still needed.

source of pain or discomfort, such as otitis media, sinusitis, dental abscess, constipation, fracture, headache, esophagitis, gastritis, or allergic rhinitis, may be identified and treated. Obstructive sleep apnea may contribute to sleep disorders and related behavior deterioration, and extreme food selectivity can lead to malnutrition. Pica secondary to deficiency of iron or zinc may be responsive to treatment with supplements (Lofts, Schroeder, & Maier, 1990; Rose, Porcerelli, & Neale, 2000; Singhi, Ravishanker, Singhi, & Nath, 2003). In some cases, completion of laboratory tests or other studies may affect the choice of medication. For example, if staring spells and aggressive behav-

ior are both of concern, electroencephalography might lead to the choice of an appropriate anticonvulsant as first-line treatment for both a seizure disorder and behavioral outbursts.

Therapeutic Trials of Medication

After it has been determined that a maladaptive behavior or cluster of behaviors is causing significant impairment and that there is no treatable exacerbating medical factor or modifiable environmental cause, it is often appropriate to consider a therapeutic trial of medication. The parents and, whenever possible, the patient should be involved in this decision. The clinician must first provide information about the diagnoses and target behaviors and the various treatment options. Some level of discussion of the pertinent neurobiology and how the medications are thought to work in the central nervous system is often appropriate. The clinician draws on knowledge of the ID- and ASD-specific literature, inferences from literature pertaining to conditions with similar target symptoms (e.g., ADHD, OCD, mood disorders, anxiety disorders), and clinical experience to provide the basis for making treatment decisions. Theoretical considerations based on current knowledge and working hypotheses regarding the neurobiology of specific ID syndromes, ASD, and related behaviors may also help to determine which neurotransmitters to manipulate pharmacologically. The number of potential medications is narrowed down by formulating hypotheses regarding the origins of the behaviors and considering the specific issues associated with each medication, such as side effects, preparations available, dosing schedules, cost, and monitoring requirements. For some families, the need for ECG or laboratory monitoring with the use of certain medications is a major deterrent.

In order to obtain informed consent, the potential benefits and medical and behavioral side effects must be discussed. Provision of written materials is desirable. A substantial investment of time and effort is required to select an initial medication and dose, outline the timetable for titration of the dose and expected therapeutic response, collect baseline data regarding behaviors and somatic complaints, and broadly review potential strategies for dealing with treatment failure or partial response. This initial investment is important in establishing a lasting therapeutic alliance. It is important to have some quantifiable means of assessing the efficacy of the medication and to obtain input from a variety of sources, such as parents, teachers, therapists, and aides. Validated, treatment-sensitive rating scales, quantitative data collected systematically by caregivers (e.g., number of self-injurious acts per defined time period and situation), and individualized Likert scales for specific target behaviors can be utilized. The CGI is often utilized to quantify assessment of global functioning (Aman, No-

votny, et al., 2004). A wide variety of outcome measures have been utilized in research trials and in clinical practice (Aman, 1991a, 1991b). The instruments recommended by an expert review panel for use in measuring maladaptive behavioral treatment effects in clinical drug trials in ASD are listed in Table 28.3. Medication-specific side effects scales are also available, and their regular use is encouraged (Kutcher, 1997).

Whenever possible, only one change should be made at a time in order to be able to judge the treatment effect. For example, the first week of implementation of a new behavioral treatment plan would not be an ideal time to institute a trial of medication or make a change in medication because it would be diffi-

Table 28.3. Standardized rating instruments recommended for assessing target behavioral symptoms in autism spectrum disorder

Aberrant Behavior Checklist (Aman, Singh, Stewart, & Field, 1985)

Anxiety, Depression, and Mood Scale (Esbensen, Rojahn, Aman, & Ruedrich, 2003)

Behavior Problems Inventory (Rojahn, Matson, Lott, Esbensen, & Smalls, 2001)

Children's Yale-Brown Obsessive-Compulsive Scale (Scahill et al., 1997); Yale-Brown Obsessive-Compulsive Scale (Goodman et al., 1989)

Children's Psychiatric Rating Scale (adapted) (Guy, 1976b)

Developmental Behaviour Checklist (Einfeld & Tonge, 1995)

Diagnostic Assessment for the Severely Handicapped–Version II (Matson, 1995)

Early Childhood Inventory (Gadow & Sprafkin, 2000); Child Symptom Inventory (Gadow & Sprafkin, 2002); Adolescent Symptom Inventory (Gadow & Sprafkin, 1998)

Emotional Disorders Rating Scale (Feinstein, Kaminer, Barrett, & Tylenda, 1988)

Fear Survey Schedule for Children–Revised (Ollendick, 1983); Fear Survey for Children With and Without Mental Retardation (Ramirez & Kratochwill, 1990)

Nisonger Child Behavior Rating Form (Aman, Tasse, Rojahn, & Hammer, 1996)

Preschool Behavior Questionnaire (Behar, 1977)

Repetitive Behavior Scale–Revised (Lam, 2004)

Self Injurious Behavior Questionnaire (Schroeder, Rojahn, & Reese, 1997)

Stereotypic Behavior Scale (Bojahn, Matlock, & Tassé, 2000)

From Aman, M.G., Novotny, S., Samango-Sprouse, C., Lecavalier, L., Leonard, E., Gadow, K.D., et al. (2004). Outcome measures for clinical drug trials in autism. *CNS Spectrums, 9*(1), 36–47; adapted by permission.

cult to judge the source of effects, positive or negative. It is usually best to begin with a low dose of medication and titrate to the initial target dose or effect incrementally in order to minimize the risk of treatment-emergent adverse events. If a particular medication is found to be ineffective after appropriate titration or associated with intolerable side effects, the medication should be discontinued. Gradual tapering may be warranted, depending on the medication. This is particularly important with certain agents such as antipsychotics because of the risk of withdrawal dyskinesias.

One of the most difficult aspects of pharmacological management is allowing enough time after a target dose is reached to observe for therapeutic effects. In the case of partial or suboptimal response, the clinician and family must decide whether to substitute another agent or add a second medication. Although monotherapy is desirable, augmentation or combination strategies must sometimes be utilized in the management of ASD or ID, particularly in the setting of significant mood instability and severe aggression or self-injury. The clinician must be aware of potential interactions between drugs and monitor accordingly. Periodic setbacks or exacerbations are to be expected, and it is prudent to avoid quickly adding another medication to treat each behavior that arises. Careful withdrawal of a medication should be considered after 6–12 months of therapy so that it is possible to determine whether the medication is still needed.

Treatment Options for Common Target Symptoms

Discussion of potential pharmacological intervention often arises in the setting of problematic aggression, self-injurious behavior, repetitive behaviors (e.g., obsessions, compulsions, stereotypy, or perseveration), mood lability, irritability, anxiety, sleep disturbance, hyperactivity, inattention, destructive behavior, or other disruptive behaviors. Guidelines for medication choices based on target symptoms are provided in Table 28.4. These are based on the literature reviewed in this chapter and on clinical experience; however, it must be understood that the literature available at this time is not sufficient to establish a consensus, evi-

dence-based approach to pharmacological management of ID and ASD.

In some cases, the diagnosis of a comorbid disorder such as major depression, bipolar disorder, or an anxiety disorder can be reasonably made and the patient can be treated with the medications that are useful for treating these conditions in typically developing children and adolescents. Modifications to diagnostic criteria may be necessary to account for clinical presentations of psychiatric conditions in individuals with developmental disabilities (Perry, Marston, Hinder, Munden, & Roy, 2001; Szymanski et al., 1998). For example, behavioral cycling with rages and euphoria, decreased need for sleep, manic-like hyperactivity, irritability, aggression, self-injury, sexual behaviors, and strong family history of bipolar disorder may suggest a bipolar phenotype and potential response to mood-stabilizing anticonvulsants, atypical antipsychotics, or lithium. More often, specific behavioral symptoms are targeted in the absence of a clear psychiatric diagnosis. Aggressive or self-injurious outbursts in children with ASD or ID may respond to alpha$_2$ agonists, atypical antipsychotics, or mood stabilizers such as valproate or lithium; however, the contexts in which the behaviors occur must be considered. For example, if these behaviors occur primarily in response to interruption of compulsive rituals or rigid routines, an SSRI may be more appropriate and effective. Excessive fear or anxiety, behavioral rigidity, and resistance to change can interfere substantially with daily functioning and may respond to treatment with an SSRI, buspirone, or another anxiolytic medication.

For ADHD symptoms, stimulant medications are effective in some individuals without associated increases in stereotypy or irritability. There are several advantages to stimulants, including the long-term safety record, lack of requirement for laboratory monitoring, and potential for rapid titration and discontinuation (including on/off trials to clearly demonstrate efficacy). Alpha$_2$ agonists and atypical antipsychotics may also be beneficial, particularly for hyperactivity and impulsivity. Atomoxetine, a presynaptic norepinephrine reuptake inhibitor, has been shown to be effective for ADHD, and a retrospective study suggested that it may

Table 28.4. Potential psychopharmacological treatment options for common target symptoms

Target symptom cluster	Drug
Repetitive behavior, behavioral rigidity, obsessive-compulsive symptoms	SSRI Clomipramine Atypical antipsychotic
Hyperactivity, impulsivity, inattention	Stimulant Alpha$_2$ agonist Atomoxetine Atypical antipsychotic
Aggression, explosive outbursts, self-injury	Atypical antipsychotic Alpha$_2$ agonist Anticonvulsant mood stabilizer Lithium SSRI Beta-blocker
Sleep dysfunction	Melatonin Antihistamine Clonidine Trazodone Amitriptyline Zolpidem
Anxiety	SSRI Buspirone
Depressive phenotype (marked change from baseline, including symptoms, e.g., social withdrawal, irritability, sadness or crying spells, decreased energy, anorexia, weight loss, sleep dysfunction)	SSRI Venlafaxine Mirtazapine
Bipolar phenotype (behavioral cycling with rages and euphoria, decreased need for sleep, manic-like hyperactivity, irritability, aggression, self-injury, sexual behaviors)	Anticonvulsant mood stabilizer Lithium Atypical antipsychotic

Key: SSRI, selective serotonin reuptake inhibitor.

be effective for similar symptoms in ASD (Jou, Handen, & Hardan, 2005). Controlled trials in children with ASD and ID are warranted.

Relatively little information is available on the pharmacological management of sleep problems in children with or without developmental disabilities, but behavioral interventions are often effective (Meltzer & Mindell, 2004; Pelayo, Chen, Monzon, & Guilleminault, 2004). Sleep problems are common in children with ID, ASD, other developmental disabilities, and psychiatric conditions (Didde & Sigafoos, 2001; Ivanenko, Crabtree, & Gozal, 2004; Polimeni, Richdale, & Francis, 2005; Quine, 1991; Stores, 1999), and melatonin may be effective for improving sleep onset in children with and without disabilities (Jan & Freeman, 2004; Phillips & Appleton, 2004; Smits et al., 2003; Stores, 2003; Turk, 2003). Some children re-

spond to antihistamines such as diphenhydramine or hydroxyzine, whereas others have paradoxical responses with behavioral activation (Reed & Findling, 2002; Russo, Gururaj, & Allen, 1976; Tsai, 1999). Clonidine can also be helpful for inducing sleep in children with developmental disabilities (Ferber & Kryger, 1995; Ingrassia & Turk, 2005; Prince et al., 1996; Reed & Findling, 2002).

FUTURE CONSIDERATIONS

In recent years, tremendous progress has been made in understanding the neuroscience of brain development and its aberrations. The quantity and quality of psychopharmacological studies have increased but much important information needed to guide clinical practice is still lacking. Future studies are likely to address the need for 1) more rigorous evaluation of the safety and efficacy of psychotropic agents in children with ID or ASD, 2) the value of combining behavioral and medical interventions, 3) delineation of clinical and biological subgroups of patients that may be responsive to particular treatments, and 4) the role of psychopharmacology in treating core deficits such as cognition, language, and social interaction and the potential to alter the neural substrate during early critical periods to affect brain development and future function in a positive way.

Rigorous evaluation of psychotropic agents in large randomized, double-blind, placebo-controlled studies of adequate duration is essential. These studies should include appropriate case definitions and choices of control groups, randomization practices, choice of outcome measures, assessment of generality of treatment effects across settings, and measurement of treatment acceptability and cost (Bodfish, 2004). In addition to the use of rating scales with appropriate psychometric properties, performance-based measures should be utilized. Well-designed, long-term open-label studies have a role in establishing duration of effect, detecting adverse effects, and closing the gap between research and clinical practice by studying patients under more naturalistic circumstances. There is a need to study polypharmacy, which is common in clinical practice but rarely examined in research studies. In a group of higher-functioning children, adolescents, and adults with ASD, Martin, Scahill, et al. (1999) found that 29% were taking two or more medications simultaneously.

It will be important to examine further the interactions between behavioral and medical interventions. The RUPP Autism Network is currently investigating the combination of risperidone and behavior therapy compared with pharmacological treatment alone (Vitiello & Wagner, 2004). In the future, it would be helpful to determine whether short-term pharmacological treatment can allow behavioral interventions to be successful more rapidly, reduce overall cost of intensive behavioral interventions, or improve effectiveness by increasing parent or caregiver compliance because of more rapid and robust response. Re-search may lead the way to a more integrated approach to treatment. Also, behavioral techniques such as functional analysis methodology are likely to prove to be important tools for evaluating medication effects clinically and in research trials (Crosland et al., 2003; Valdovinos et al., 2002; Zarcone et al., 2004).

Delineation of clinical or biological subgroups of patients may allow differentiation of treatment effects and adverse effects by subgroup. For example, DeLong et al. (2002) have observed that children with autism who have a strong family history of affective disorders are more likely to respond positively to SSRIs, and it has been reported that the clinical response to fluvoxamine may depend on genetic polymorphism in the serotonin transporter promoter region (Sugie et al., 2005). New insights regarding the neurobiology of specific syndromes associated with ID or ASD may also lead to pharmacological intervention strategies. Already, in individuals with Smith-Magenis syndrome, it has been found that pineal secretion of melatonin is dysregulated, and de Leersnyder et al. (2001) showed that administration of a single morning dose of acebutolol lowered daytime plasma melatonin levels, decreased motor hyperactivity, controlled outbursts, reduced daytime naps, and improved nocturnal sleep. The addition of an evening dose of controlled-release melatonin increased nocturnal melatonin levels and further improved sleep (de Leersnyder et al., 2003). Much is now known about the functions of the fragile X mental retardation protein (FMRP; see Chapter 7, this volume), and it is possible that directed pharmacological interventions will be developed to address specific neurochemical and synaptic deficits caused by the absence of FMRP (Aschrafi, Cunningham, Edelman, & Vanderklish, 2005; Berry-Kravis & Potanos, 2004; Dolen & Bear, 2005). Knowledge of the role of histone acetylation in disorders such as fragile X syndrome and Rubinstein-Taybi syndrome is accumulating, and this may lead to pharmacological interventions targeting this process (Timmermann, Lehrmann, Polesskaya, & Harel-Bellan, 2001).

The question of whether core deficits such as impaired cognition, language, or social interaction can be addressed pharmacologically has not been answered. The effectiveness of treatment of children with Down syndrome with nootropic agents such as piracetam has generally not been supported by preclinical or clinical data (Lobaugh et al., 2001; Moran et al., 2002; Salman, 2002), but an open-label trial suggested that donepezil may improve expressive language (Heller et al., 2004). Donepezil and other cholinergic medications used to treat Alzheimer's disease, including galantamine and rivastigmine, have also been reported to improve language in children and adults with ASD (Chez, Aimonovitch, Buchanan, Mrazek, & Tremb, 2004; Chez, Memon, & Hung, 2004; Chez et al., 2003; Hardan & Handen, 2002; Hertzman, 2003). Galantamine has also been found to be associated with modest behavior improvements, particularly in irritability (Niederhofer, Staffen, & Mair, 2002a). A preliminary investigation suggested benefits of the glutamate NMDA antagonist memantine, including improvements in language and eye contact, in children and adolescents with ASD (Chez, Memon, & Hung, 2004). D-Cycloserine, a partial NMDA agonist, has been reported to improve social withdrawal in a small group of children and adults with ASD (Posey, Kem, et al., 2004). There has also been interest in studying modulators of glutamate AMPA receptors in patients with ID or ASD (des Portes, Hagerman, & Hendren, 2003). The issue of efficacy of pharmacological treatment of core cognitive, language, and social deficits remains to be settled by large, well-designed trials. A related issue is whether psychotropic agents can be used early in life to alter the neural substrate during critical periods and to enhance brain development and future function. For example, there is evidence of abnormality in the developmental regulation of serotonin in ASD (Anderson, 2005; Chugani, 2005), and it has been postulated that the early use of SSRIs might promote more normal neuronal growth and differentiation (Zimmerman et al., 2000).

CONCLUSION

Psychotropic medications are useful as adjuncts to behavioral and educational interventions for some children and adolescents with ID or ASD. Although many questions remain to be answered, there is a substantial and growing body of useful literature to guide clinicians in the use of these medications to target certain maladaptive behaviors that are causing significant impairment in order to allow the child to benefit more fully from other interventions and ultimately to improve functional independence and quality of life. It is possible that, in the future, the use of pharmacological agents will move beyond the role of improving associated maladaptive behaviors to modifying the neural substrate and treating the core deficits of ID and ASD.

REFERENCES

Agarwal, V., Sitholey, P., Kumar, S., & Prasad, M. (2001). Double-blind, placebo-controlled trial of clonidine in hyperactive children with mental retardation. *Mental Retardation, 39,* 259–267.

Aman, M.G. (1982). Stimulant drug effects in developmental disorders and hyperactivity—toward a resolution of disparate findings. *Journal of Autism and Developmental Disorders, 12,* 385–398.

Aman, M.G. (1991a). *Assessing psychopathology and behavior problems in persons with mental retardation: A review of available instruments* (DHHS Publication no. [ADM] 91-1712). Rockville, MD: U.S. Department of Health and Human Services.

Aman, M.G. (1991b). Review and evaluation of instruments for assessing emotional and behavioural disorders. *Australian and New Zealand Journal of Developmental Disabilities, 17,* 127–145.

Aman, M.G. (2004). Management of hyperactivity and other acting-out problems in patients with autism spectrum disorder. *Seminars in Pediatric Neurology, 11,* 225–228.

Aman, M.G., Binder, C., & Turgay, A. (2004). Risperidone effects in the presence/absence of psychostimulant medicine in children with ADHD, other disruptive behavior disorders, and subaverage IQ. *Journal of Child and Adolescent Psychopharmacology, 14,* 243–254.

Aman, M.G., Buican, B., & Arnold, L.E. (2003). Methylphenidate treatment in children with borderline IQ and mental retardation: Analysis of three aggregated studies. *Journal of Child and Adolescent Psychopharmacology, 13,* 29–40.

Aman, M.G., De Smedt, G., Derivan, A., Lyons, B., Findling, R.L., & the Risperidone Disruptive Behavior Study Group. (2002). Double-blind, placebo-controlled study of risperidone for the treatment of disruptive behaviors in children with subaverage intelligence. *American Journal of Psychiatry, 159,* 1337–1346.

Aman, M.G., Lam, K.S., & Collier-Crespin, A. (2003). Prevalence and patterns of use of psychoactive medicines among individuals with autism in the Autism Society of Ohio. *Journal of Autism and Developmental Disorders, 33,* 527–534.

Aman, M.G., Lam, K.S., & Van Bourgondien, M.E. (2005). Medication patterns in patients with autism: Temporal, regional, and demographic influences. *Journal of Child and Adolescent Psychopharmacology, 15,* 116–126.

Aman, M.G., & Langworthy, K.S. (2000). Pharmacotherapy for hyperactivity in children with autism and other pervasive developmental disorders. *Journal of Autism and Developmental Disorders, 30,* 451–459.

Aman, M.G., Novotny, S., Samango-Sprouse, C., Lecavalier, L., Leonard, E., Gadow, K.D., et al. (2004). Outcome measures for clinical drug trials in autism. *CNS Spectrums, 9*(1), 36–47.

Aman, M.G., Singh, N.N., Stewart, A.W., & Field, C.J. (1985). The Aberrant Behavior Checklist: A behavior rating scale for the assessment of treatment effects. *American Journal of Mental Deficiency, 89,* 485–491.

Aman, M.G., Tasse, M.J., Rojahn, J., & Hammer, D. (1996). The Nisonger CBRF: A child behavior rating form for children with developmental disabilities. *Research in Developmental Disabilities, 17,* 41–57.

American Academy of Pediatrics Subcommittee on Attention-Deficit/Hyperactivity Disorder and Committee on Quality Improvement. (2001). Clinical practice guideline: Treatment of the school-aged child with attention-deficit/hyperactivity disorder. *Pediatrics, 108,* 1033–1044.

American Psychiatric Association. (2000). *Diagnostic and statistical manual of mental disorders* (4th ed., Text rev.). Washington, DC: Author.

Anderson, G.M. (2005). Serotonin in autism. In M.L. Bauman & T.L. Kemper (Eds.), *The neurobiology of autism* (2nd ed., pp. 303–318). Baltimore: The Johns Hopkins University Press.

Anderson, L.T., Campbell, M., Adams, P., Small, A.M., Perry, R., & Shell, J. (1989). The effects of haloperidol on discrimination learning and behavioral symptoms in autistic children. *Journal of Autism and Developmental Disorders, 19,* 227–239.

Anderson, L.T., Campbell, M., Grega, D.M., Perry, R., Small, A.M., & Green, W.H. (1984). Haloperidol in the treatment of infantile autism: Effects on learning and behavioral symptoms. *American Journal of Psychiatry, 141,* 1195–1202.

Antochi, R., Stavrakaki, C., & Emery, P.C. (2003). Psychopharmacological treatments in persons with dual diagnosis of psychiatric disorders and developmental disabilities. *Postgraduate Medical Journal, 79,* 139–146.

Armenteros, J.L., Adams, P.B., Campbell, M., & Eisenberg, Z.W. (1995). Haloperidol-related dyskinesias

and pre- and perinatal complications in autistic children. *Psychopharmacology Bulletin, 31,* 363–369.

Arnold, L.E., Gadow, K.D., Pearson, D.A., & Varley, C.K. (1998). Stimulants. In S. Reiss & M.G. Aman (Eds.), *Psychotropic medications and developmental disabilities: The international consensus handbook* (pp. 229–257). Columbus: The Ohio State University, Nisonger Center.

Arnold, L.E., Lindsay, R.L., Conners, C.K., Wigal, S.B., Levine, A.J., Johnson, D.E., et al. (2004). A double-blind, placebo-controlled withdrawal trial of dexmethylphenidate hydrochloride in children with attention deficit hyperactivity disorder. *Journal of Child and Adolescent Psychopharmacology, 14,* 542–554.

Arnold, L.E., Vitiello, B., McDougle, C., Scahill, L., Shah, B., Gonzalez, N.M., et al. (2003). Parent-defined target symptoms respond to risperidone in RUPP autism study: Customer approach to clinical trials. *Journal of the American Academy of Child and Adolescent Psychiatry, 42,* 1443–1450.

Aschrafi, A., Cunningham, B.A., Edelman, G.M., & Vanderklish, P.W. (2005). The fragile X mental retardation protein and group I metabotropic glutamate receptors regulate levels of mRNA granules in brain. *Proceedings of the National Academy of Sciences of the United States of America, 102,* 2180–2185.

Baker, L., & Cantwell, D.P. (1987). Factors associated with the development of psychiatric illness in children with early speech/language problems. *Journal of Autism and Developmental Disorders, 17,* 499–510.

Barnard, L., Young, A.H., Pearson, J., Geddes, J., & O'Brien, G. (2002). A systematic review of the use of atypical antipsychotics in autism. *Journal of Psychopharmacology, 16,* 93–101.

Bauer, M.S., & Mitchner, L. (2004). What is a "mood stabilizer"? An evidence-based response. *American Journal of Psychiatry, 161,* 3–18.

Baumeister, A.A., Sevin, J.A., & King, B.H. (1998). Neuroleptic medications. In S. Reiss & M.G. Aman (Eds.), *Psychotropic medication and developmental disabilities: The international consensus handbook* (pp. 133–150). Columbus: The Ohio State University, Nisonger Center.

Baumeister, A.A., Todd, M.E., & Sevin, J.A. (1993). Efficacy and specificity of pharmacological therapies for behavioral disorders in persons with mental retardation. *Clinical Neuropharmacology, 16,* 271–294.

Behar, L.B. (1977). The Preschool Behaviour Questionaire. *Journal of Abnormal Psychology, 5,* 265–275.

Belsito, K.M., Law, P.A., Kirk, K.S., Landa, R.J., & Zimmerman, A.W. (2001). Lamotrigine therapy for autistic disorder: A randomized, double-blind, placebo-controlled trial. *Journal of Autism and Developmental Disorders, 31,* 175–181.

Bender, L., Faretra, G., & Cobrinik, L. (1963). LSD and UML treatment of hospitalized disturbed children. *Recent Advances in Biological Psychiatry, 5,* 84–92.

Bender, L., Goldschmidt, L., & Sankar, D.V.S. (1962). Treatment of autistic schizophrenic children with LSD-25 and UML-491. *Recent Advances in Biological Psychiatry, 4,* 170–177.

Benjamin, S., Seek, A., Tresise, L., Price, E., & Gagnon, M. (1995). Case study: Paradoxical response to naltrexone treatment of self-injurious behavior. *Journal of the American Academy of Child and Adolescent Psychiatry, 34,* 238–242.

Berk, M., & Dodd, S. (2005). Efficacy of atypical antipsychotics in bipolar disorder. *Drugs, 65,* 257–269.

Berry-Kravis, E., & Potanos, K. (2004). Psychopharmacology in fragile X syndrome—present and future. *Mental Retardation and Developmental Disabilities Research Reviews, 10,* 42–48.

Biederman, J., Heiligenstein, J.H., Faries, D.E., Galil, N., Dittmann, R., Emslie, G.J., et al. (2002). Efficacy of atomoxetine versus placebo in school-age girls with attention-deficit/hyperactivity disorder. *Pediatrics, 110,* e75.

Biederman, J., Lopez, F.A., Boellner, S.W., & Chandler, M.C. (2002). A randomized, double-blind, placebo-controlled, parallel-group study of SLI381 (Adderall XR) in children with attention-deficit/hyperactivity disorder. *Pediatrics, 110*(2 Pt. 1), 258–266.

Birmaher, B., Quintana, H., & Greenhill, L.L. (1988). Methylphenidate treatment of hyperactive autistic children. *Journal of the American Academy of Child and Adolescent Psychiatry, 27,* 248–251.

Blackman, J.A., Samson-Fang, L., & Gutgesell, H. (1996). Clonidine and electrocardiograms. *Pediatrics, 98*(6 Pt. 1), 1223–1224.

Blair, J., Scahill, L., State, M., & Martin, A. (2005). Electrocardiographic changes in children and adolescents treated with ziprasidone: A prospective study. *Journal of the American Academy of Child and Adolescent Psychiatry, 44,* 73–79.

Blair, J., Taggart, B., & Martin, A. (2004). Electrocardiographic safety profile and monitoring guidelines in pediatric psychopharmacology. *Journal of Neural Transmission, 111,* 791–815.

Bodfish, J.W. (2004). Treating the core features of autism: Are we there yet? *Mental Retardation and Developmental Disabilities Research Reviews, 10,* 318–326.

Bouvard, M.P., Leboyer, M., Launay, J.M., Recasens, C., Plumet, M.H., Waller-Perotte, D., et al. (1995). Low-dose naltrexone effects on plasma chemistries and clinical symptoms in autism: A double-blind, placebo-controlled study. *Psychiatry Research, 58,* 191–201.

Bradley, C. (1937). The behavior of children receiving benzedrine. *American Journal of Psychiatry, 94,* 577–585.

Bradley, E.A., Summers, J.A., Wood, H.L., & Bryson, S.E. (2004). Comparing rates of psychiatric and behavior disorders in adolescents and young adults with severe intellectual disability with and

without autism. *Journal of Autism and Developmental Disorders, 34,* 151–161.

Branford, D., Bhaumik, S., & Naik, B. (1998). Selective serotonin re-uptake inhibitors for the treatment of perseverative and maladaptive behaviours of people with intellectual disability. *Journal of Intellectual Disability Research, 42*(Pt. 4), 301–306.

Brasic, J.R., Barnett, J.Y., Sheitman, B.B., & Tsaltas, M.O. (1997). Adverse effects of clomipramine. *Journal of the American Academy of Child and Adolescent Psychiatry, 36,* 1165–1166.

Brown, E.C., Aman, M.G., & Havercamp, S.M. (2002). Factor analysis and norms for parent ratings on the Aberrant Behavior Checklist–Community for young people in special education. *Research in Developmental Disabilities, 23,* 45–60.

Bryant, A.E., III, & Dreifuss, F.E. (1996). Valproic acid hepatic fatalities: III. U.S. experience since 1986. *Neurology, 46,* 465–469.

Bryson, S.E., Clark, B.S., & Smith, I.M. (1988). First report of a Canadian epidemiological study of autistic syndromes. *Journal of Child Psychology and Psychiatry and Allied Disciplines, 29,* 433–445.

Bryson, S.E., & Smith, I.M. (1998). Epidemiology of autism: Prevalence, associated characteristics, and implications for research and service delivery. *Mental Retardation and Developmental Disabilities Research Reviews, 4,* 97–103.

Buitelaar, J.K., van der Gaag, R.J., Cohen-Kettenis, P., & Melman, C.T. (2001). A randomized controlled trial of risperidone in the treatment of aggression in hospitalized adolescents with subaverage cognitive abilities. *Journal of Clinical Psychiatry, 62,* 239–248.

Buitelaar, J.K., van der Gaag, R.J., & van der Hoeven, J. (1998). Buspirone in the management of anxiety and irritability in children with pervasive developmental disorders: Results of an open-label study. *Journal of Clinical Psychiatry, 59,* 56–59.

Campbell, J.M. (2003). Efficacy of behavioral interventions for reducing problem behavior in persons with autism: A quantitative synthesis of single-subject research. *Research in Developmental Disabilities, 24,* 120–138.

Campbell, M., Adams, P.B., Small, A.M., Kafantaris, V., Silva, R.R., Shell, J., et al. (1995). Lithium in hospitalized aggressive children with conduct disorder: A double-blind and placebo-controlled study. *Journal of the American Academy of Child and Adolescent Psychiatry, 34,* 445–453.

Campbell, M., Anderson, L.T., Meier, M., Cohen, I.L., Small, A.M., Samit, C., et al. (1978). A comparison of haloperidol and behavior therapy and their interaction in autistic children. *Journal of the American Academy of Child Psychiatry, 17,* 640–655.

Campbell, M., Anderson, L.T., Small, A.M., Adams, P., Gonzalez, N.M., & Ernst, M. (1993). Naltrexone in autistic children: Behavioral symptoms and attentional learning. *Journal of the American Academy of Child and Adolescent Psychiatry, 32,* 1283–1291.

Campbell, M., Anderson, L.T., Small, A.M., Locascio, J.J., Lynch, N.S., & Choroco, M.C. (1990). Naltrexone in autistic children: A double-blind and placebo-controlled study. *Psychopharmacology Bulletin, 26,* 130–135.

Campbell, M., Armenteros, J.L., Malone, R.P., Adams, P.B., Eisenberg, Z.W., & Overall, J.E. (1997). Neuroleptic-related dyskinesias in autistic children: A prospective, longitudinal study. *Journal of the American Academy of Child and Adolescent Psychiatry, 36,* 835–843.

Campbell, M., Fish, B., David, R., Shapiro, T., Collins, P., & Koh, C. (1972). Response to triiodothyronine and dextroamphetamine: A study of preschool schizophrenic children. *Journal of Autism and Childhood Schizophrenia, 2,* 343–358.

Campbell, M., Fish, B., Korein, J., Shapiro, T., Collins, P., & Koh, C. (1972). Lithium and chlorpromazine: A controlled crossover study of hyperactive severely disturbed young children. *Journal of Autism and Childhood Schizophrenia, 2,* 234–263.

Campbell, M., Fish, B., Shapiro, T., & Floyd, A., Jr. (1972). Acute responses of schizophrenic children to a sedative and a "stimulating" neuroleptic: A pharmacologic yardstick. *Current Therapeutic Research, Clinical and Experimental, 14,* 759–766.

Campbell, M., Small, A.M., Collins, P.J., Friedman, E., David, R., & Genieser, N. (1976). Levodopa and levoamphetamine: A crossover study in young schizophrenic children. *Current Therapeutic Research, Clinical and Experimental, 19,* 70–86.

Campbell, M., Small, A.M., Green, W.H., Jennings, S.J., Perry, R., Bennett, W.G., et al. (1984). Behavioral efficacy of haloperidol and lithium carbonate: A comparison in hospitalized aggressive children with conduct disorder. *Archives of General Psychiatry, 41,* 650–656.

Carandang, C.G., Maxwell, D.J., Robbins, D.R., & Oesterheld, J.R. (2003). Lamotrigine in adolescent mood disorders. *Journal of the American Academy of Child and Adolescent Psychiatry, 42,* 750–751.

Carlson, G.A. (2005). Early onset bipolar disorder: Clinical and research considerations. *Journal of Clinical Child and Adolescent Psychology, 34,* 333–343.

Casner, J.A., Weinheimer, B., & Gualtieri, C.T. (1996). Naltrexone and self-injurious behavior: A retrospective population study. *Journal of Clinical Psychopharmacology, 16,* 389–394.

Chakrabarti, S., & Fombonne, E. (2005). Pervasive developmental disorders in preschool children: Confirmation of high prevalence. *American Journal of Psychiatry, 162,* 1133–1141.

Chandler, M., Barnhill, L.J., & Gualtieri, C.T. (1991). Amantadine: Profile of use in the developmentally disabled. In J.J. Ratey (Ed.), *Mental retardation: Developing pharmacotherapies* (Progress in Psychiatry, no. 32, pp. 139–162). Washington, DC: American Psychiatric Association.

Chang, K.D., Dienes, K., Blasey, C., Adleman, N., Ketter, T., & Steiner, H. (2003). Divalproex mono-

therapy in the treatment of bipolar offspring with mood and behavioral disorders and at least mild affective symptoms. *Journal of Clinical Psychiatry, 64,* 936–942.

Chen, N.C., Bedair, H.S., McKay, B., Bowers, M.B.J., & Mazure, C. (2001). Clozapine in the treatment of aggression in an adolescent with autistic disorder. *Journal of Clinical Psychiatry, 62,* 479–480.

Cheng-Shannon, J., McGough, J.J., Pataki, C., & McCracken, J.T. (2004). Second-generation antipsychotic medications in children and adolescents. *Journal of Child and Adolescent Psychopharmacology, 14,* 372–394.

Chess, S., & Hassibi, M. (1970). Behavior deviations in mentally retarded children. *Journal of the American Academy of Child Psychiatry, 9,* 282–297.

Chez, M.G., Aimonovitch, M., Buchanan, T., Mrazek, S., & Tremb, R.J. (2004). Treating autistic spectrum disorders in children: Utility of the cholinesterase inhibitor rivastigmine tartrate. *Journal of Child Neurology, 19,* 165–169.

Chez, M.G., Buchanan, T.M., Becker, M., Kessler, J., Aimonovitch, M.C., & Mrazek, S.R. (2003). Donepezil hydrochloride: A double-blind study in autistic children. *Journal of Pediatric Neurology, 1,* 83–88.

Chez, M.G., Memon, S., & Hung, P.C. (2004). Neurologic treatment strategies in autism: An overview of medical intervention strategies. *Seminars in Pediatric Neurology, 11,* 229–235.

Childs, J.A., & Blair, J.L. (1997). Valproic acid treatment of epilepsy in autistic twins. *Journal of Neuroscience Nursing, 29,* 244–248.

Chouinard, G., & Margolese, H.C. (2005). Manual for the Extrapyramidal Symptom Rating Scale (ESRS). *Schizophrenia Research, 76*(2–3), 247–265.

Chugani, D.C. (2005). Positron emission tomography studies of autism. In M.L. Bauman & T.L. Kemper (Eds.), *The neurobiology of autism* (2nd ed., pp. 164–176). Baltimore: The Johns Hopkins University Press.

Cohen, I.L., Campbell, M., Posner, D., Small, A.M., Triebel, D., & Anderson, L.T. (1980). Behavioral effects of haloperidol in young autistic children: An objective analysis using a within-subjects reversal design. *Journal of the American Academy of Child Psychiatry, 19,* 665–677.

Cohen, I.L., Tsiouris, J.A., & Pfadt, A. (1991). Effects of long-acting propranolol on agonistic and stereotyped behaviors in a man with pervasive developmental disorder and fragile X syndrome: A double-blind, placebo-controlled study. *Journal of Clinical Psychopharmacology, 11,* 398–399.

Compton, S.N., March, J.S., Brent, D., Albano A.M., 5th, Weersing, R., & Curry, J. (2004). Cognitive-behavioral psychotherapy for anxiety and depressive disorders in children and adolescents: An evidence-based medicine review. *Journal of the American Academy of Child and Adolescent Psychiatry, 43,* 930–959.

Connor, D.F., Barkley, R.A., & Davis, H.T. (2000). A pilot study of methylphenidate, clonidine, or the combination in ADHD comorbid with aggressive oppositional defiant or conduct disorder. *Clinical Pediatrics, 39,* 15–25.

Connor, D.F., Fletcher, K.E., & Swanson, J.M. (1999). A meta-analysis of clonidine for symptoms of attention-deficit hyperactivity disorder. *Journal of the American Academy of Child and Adolescent Psychiatry, 38,* 1551–1559.

Connor, D.F., Ozbayrak, K.R., Benjamin, S., Ma, Y., & Fletcher, K.E. (1997). A pilot study of nadolol for overt aggression in developmentally delayed individuals. *Journal of the American Academy of Child and Adolescent Psychiatry, 36,* 826–834.

Cook, E.H., Jr., Rowlett, R., Jaselskis, C., & Leventhal, B.L. (1992). Fluoxetine treatment of children and adults with autistic disorder and mental retardation. *Journal of the American Academy of Child and Adolescent Psychiatry, 31,* 739–745.

Cooper, W.O., Hickson, G.B., Fuchs, C., Arbogast, P.G., & Ray, W.A. (2004). New users of antipsychotic medications among children enrolled in TennCare. *Archives of Pediatrics and Adolescent Medicine, 158,* 753–759.

Cormack, K.F., Brown, A.C., & Hastings, R.P. (2000). Behavioural and emotional difficulties in students attending schools for children and adolescents with severe intellectual disability. *Journal of Intellectual Disability Research, 44*(Pt. 2), 124–129.

Corson, A.H., Barkenbus, J.E., Posey, D.J., Stigler, K.A., & McDougle, C.J. (2004). A retrospective analysis of quetiapine in the treatment of pervasive developmental disorders. *Journal of Clinical Psychiatry, 65,* 1531–1536.

Couturier, J.L., & Nicolson, R. (2002). A retrospective assessment of citalopram in children and adolescents with pervasive developmental disorders. *Journal of Child and Adolescent Psychopharmacology, 12,* 243–248.

Craft, M., Ismail, I.A., Krishnamurti, D., Mathews, J., Regan, A., Seth, R.V., et al. (1987). Lithium in the treatment of aggression in mentally handicapped patients: A double-blind trial. *British Journal of Psychiatry, 150,* 685–689.

Crawford, P., Brown, S., Kerr, M., & the Parke Davis Clinical Trials Group. (2001). A randomized open-label study of gabapentin and lamotrigine in adults with learning disability and resistant epilepsy. *Seizure, 10,* 107–115.

Crews, W.D., Jr., Bonaventura, S., Rowe, F.B., & Bonsie, D. (1993). Cessation of long-term naltrexone therapy and self-injury: A case study. *Research in Developmental Disabilities, 14,* 331–340.

Croonenberghs, J., Fegert, J.M., Findling, R.L., De Smedt, G., Van Dongen, S., & the Risperidone Disruptive Behavior Study Group. (2005). Risperidone in children with disruptive behavior disorders and subaverage intelligence: A 1-year, open-label study of 504 patients. *Journal of the American Academy of Child and Adolescent Psychiatry, 44,* 64–72.

Crosland, K.A., Zarcone, J.R., Lindaucr, S.E., Valdovinos, M.G., Zarcone, T.J., Hellings, J.A., et al. (2003). Use of functional analysis methodology in the evaluation of medication effects. *Journal of Autism and Developmental Disorders, 33,* 271–279.

Curtis, L.H., Masselink, L.E., Ostbye, T., Hutchison, S., Dans, P.E., Wright, A., et al. (2005). Prevalence of atypical antipsychotic drug use among commercially insured youths in the United States. *Archives of Pediatrics and Adolescent Medicine, 159,* 362–366.

Davanzo, P.A., Belin, T.R., Widawski, M.H., & King, B.H. (1998). Paroxetine treatment of aggression and self-injury in persons with mental retardation. *American Journal on Mental Retardation, 102,* 427–437.

de Bildt, A., Sytema, S., Kraijer, D., & Minderaa, R. (2005). Prevalence of pervasive developmental disorders in children and adolescents with mental retardation. *Journal of Child Psychology and Psychiatry and Allied Disciplines, 46,* 275–286.

de Leersnyder, H., Bresson, J.L., de Blois, M.C., Souberbielle, J.C., Mogenet, A., Delhotal-Landes, B., et al. (2003). Beta₁-adrenergic antagonists and melatonin reset the clock and restore sleep in a circadian disorder, Smith-Magenis syndrome. *Journal of Medical Genetics, 40,* 74–78.

de Leersnyder, H., de Blois, M.C., Vekemans, M., Sidi, D., Villain, E., Kindermans, C., et al. (2001). Beta₁-adrenergic antagonists improve sleep and behavioural disturbances in a circadian disorder, Smith-Magenis syndrome. *Journal of Medical Genetics, 38,* 586–590.

Dekker, M.C., Koot, H.M., van der Ende, J., & Verhulst, F.C. (2002). Emotional and behavioral problems in children and adolescents with and without intellectual disability. *Journal of Child Psychology and Psychiatry and Allied Disciplines, 43,* 1087–1098.

Delbello, M.P., Findling, R.L., Kushner, S., Wang, D., Olson, W.H., Capece, J.A., et al. (2005). A pilot controlled trial of topiramate for mania in children and adolescents with bipolar disorder. *Journal of the American Academy of Child and Adolescent Psychiatry, 44,* 539–547.

Delbello, M.P., Kowatch, R.A., Warner, J., Schwiers, M.L., Rappaport, K.B., Daniels, J.P., et al. (2002). Adjunctive topiramate treatment for pediatric bipolar disorder: A retrospective chart review. *Journal of Child and Adolescent Psychopharmacology, 12,* 323–330.

Delbello, M.P., Schwiers, M.L., Rosenberg, H.L., & Strakowski, S.M. (2002). A double-blind, randomized, placebo-controlled study of quetiapine as adjunctive treatment for adolescent mania. *Journal of the American Academy of Child and Adolescent Psychiatry, 41,* 1216–1223.

DeLong, G.R., & Nieman, G.W. (1983). Lithium-induced behavior changes in children with symptoms suggesting manic-depressive illness. *Psychopharmacology Bulletin, 19,* 258–265.

DeLong, G.R., Ritch, C.R., & Burch, S. (2002). Fluoxetine response in children with autistic spectrum disorders: Correlation with familial major affective disorder and intellectual achievement. *Developmental Medicine and Child Neurology, 44,* 652–659.

DeLong, G.R., Teague, L.A., & McSwain Kamran, M. (1998). Effects of fluoxetine treatment in young children with idiopathic autism. *Developmental Medicine and Child Neurology, 40,* 551–562.

DeLong, R. (1994). Children with autistic spectrum disorder and a family history of affective disorder. *Developmental Medicine and Child Neurology, 36,* 674–687.

des Portes, V., Hagerman, R.J., & Hendren, R.L. (2003). Pharmacotherapy. In S. Ozonoff, S.J. Rogers, & R.L. Hendren (Eds.), *Autism spectrum disorders: A research review for practitioners* (pp. 161–186). Washington, DC: American Psychiatric Publishing.

Di Martino, A., Melis, G., Cianchetti, C., & Zuddas, A. (2004). Methylphenidate for pervasive developmental disorders: Safety and efficacy of acute single dose test and ongoing therapy. An open-pilot study. *Journal of Child and Adolescent Psychopharmacology, 14,* 207–218.

Didde, R., & Sigafoos, J. (2001). A review of the nature and treatment of sleep disorders in individuals with developmental disabilities. *Research in Developmental Disabilities, 22,* 255–272.

Dolen, G., & Bear, M.F. (2005). Courting a cure for fragile X. *Neuron, 45,* 642–644.

Donovan, S.J., Stewart, J.W., Nunes, E.V., Quitkin, F.M., Parides, M., Daniel, W., et al. (2000). Divalproex treatment for youth with explosive temper and mood lability: A double-blind, placebo-controlled crossover design. *American Journal of Psychiatry, 157,* 818–820.

Dunbar, F., Kusumakar, V., Daneman, D., & Schulz, M. (2004). Growth and sexual maturation during long-term treatment with risperidone. *American Journal of Psychiatry, 161,* 918–920.

Eaton, L.F., & Menolascino, F.J. (1982). Psychiatric disorders in the mentally retarded: Types, problems, and challenges. *American Journal of Psychiatry, 139,* 1297–1303.

Einfeld, S.L., & Tonge, B. J. (1995). The Developmental Behaviour Checklist: The development and validation of an instrument to assess behavioural and emotional disturbance in children and adolescents with mental retardation. *Journal of Autism and Developmental Disorders, 25*(2), 81–104.

Emerson, E., Kiernan, C., Alborz, A., Reeves, D., Mason, H., Swarbrick, R., et al. (2001). The prevalence of challenging behaviors: A total population study. *Research in Developmental Disabilities, 22,* 77–93.

Emslie, G.J., Heiligenstein, J.H., Wagner, K.D., Hoog, S.L., Ernest, D.E., Brown, E., et al. (2002). Fluoxetine for acute treatment of depression in children and adolescents: A placebo-controlled, randomized clinical trial. *Journal of the American Academy of Child and Adolescent Psychiatry, 41,* 1205–1215.

Emslie, G.J., Rush, A.J., Weinberg, W.A., Kowatch, R.A., Hughes, C.W., Carmody, T., et al. (1997). A double-blind, randomized, placebo-controlled trial of fluoxetine in children and adolescents with depression. *Archives of General Psychiatry, 54,* 1031–1037.

Ernst, M., Magee, H.J., Gonzalez, N.M., & Locascio, J.J. (1992). Pimozide in autistic children. *Psychopharmacology Bulletin, 28,* 187–191.

Esbensen, A.J., Rojahn, J., Aman, M.G., & Ruedrich, S. (2003). Reliability and validity of an instrument for anxiety, depression, and mood among individuals with mental retardation. *Journal of Autism and Developmental Disorders, 33*(6), 617–629.

Fankhauser, M.P., Karumanchi, V.C., German, M.L., Yates, A., & Karumanchi, S.D. (1992). A double-blind, placebo-controlled study of the efficacy of transdermal clonidine in autism. *Journal of Clinical Psychiatry, 53,* 77–82.

Farnebo, L.O., Fuxe, K., Goldstein, M., Hamberger, B., & Ungerstedt, U. (1971). Dopamine and noradrenaline releasing action of amantadine in the central and peripheral nervous system: A possible mode of action in Parkinson's disease. *European Journal of Pharmacology, 16,* 27–38.

Feinstein, C., Kaminer, Y., Barrett, R.P., & Tylenda, B. (1988). The assessment of mood and affect in developmentally disabled children and adolescents: The Emotional Disorders Rating Scale. *Research in Developmental Disabilities, 9*(2), 109–121.

Feldman, H.M., Kolmen, B.K., & Gonzaga, A.M. (1999). Naltrexone and communication skills in young children with autism. *Journal of the American Academy of Child and Adolescent Psychiatry, 38,* 587–593.

Ferber, R., & Kryger, M. (1995). *Principles and practice of sleep medicine in the child.* Philadelphia: W.B. Saunders.

Findling, R.L., Aman, M.G., Eerdekens, M., Derivan, A., Lyons, B., & the Risperidone Disruptive Behavior Study Group. (2004). Long-term, open-label study of risperidone in children with severe disruptive behaviors and below-average IQ. *American Journal of Psychiatry, 161,* 677–684.

Findling, R.L., Kusumakar, V., Daneman, D., Moshang, T., De Smedt, G., & Binder, C. (2003). Prolactin levels during long-term risperidone treatment in children and adolescents. *Journal of Clinical Psychiatry, 64,* 1362–1369.

Findling, R.L., McNamara, N.K., Gracious, B.L., O'Riordan, M.A., Reed, M.D., Demeter, C., et al. (2004). Quetiapine in nine youths with autistic disorder. *Journal of Child and Adolescent Psychopharmacology, 14,* 287–294.

Findling, R.L., McNamara, N.K., Gracious, B.L., Youngstrom, E.A., Stansbrey, R.J., Reed, M.D., et al. (2003). Combination lithium and divalproex sodium in pediatric bipolarity. *Journal of the Ameri-*

can *Academy of Child and Adolescent Psychiatry, 42,* 895–901.

Fleminger, S., Greenwood, R.J., & Oliver, D.L. (2003). Pharmacological management for agitation and aggression in people with acquired brain injury. *Cochrane Database of Systematic Reviews,* (1), CD003299.

Fombonne, E. (2003). Epidemiological surveys of autism and other pervasive developmental disorders: An update. *Journal of Autism and Developmental Disorders, 33,* 365–382.

Fombonne, E. (2005). The epidemiology of pervasive developmental disorders. In M.L. Bauman & T.L. Kemper (Eds.), *The neurobiology of autism* (2nd ed., pp. 3–22). Baltimore: The Johns Hopkins University Press.

Fraser, W.I., Ruedrich, S., Kerr, M., & Levitas, A. (1998). Beta-adrenergic blockers. In S. Reiss & M.G. Aman (Eds.), *Psychotropic medication and developmental disabilities: The international consensus handbook* (pp. 271–290). Columbus: The Ohio State University Nisonger Center.

Freedman, A.M., Ebin, E.V., & Wilson, E.A. (1962). Autistic schizophrenic children: An experiment in the use of d-lysergic acid diethylamide (LSD-25). *Archives of General Psychiatry, 6,* 203–213.

Freeman, B.J., Ritvo, E.R., Yokota, A., & Ritvo, A. (1986). A scale for rating symptoms of patients with symptoms of autism in real life settings. *Journal of the American Academy of Child and Adolescent Psychiatry, 25*(1), 130–136.

Fujiura, G.T. (2003). Continuum of intellectual disability: Demographic evidence for the "forgotten generation." *Mental Retardation, 41,* 420–429.

Gadow, K.D. (1985). Prevalence and efficacy of stimulant drug use with mentally retarded children and youth. *Psychopharmacology Bulletin, 21,* 291–303.

Gadow, K.D. (1997). An overview of three decades of research in pediatric psychopharmacoepidemiology. *Journal of Child and Adolescent Psychopharmacology, 7,* 219–236.

Gadow, K.D., & Sprafkin, J. (1998). *Adolescent Symptom Inventory-4: Norms manual.* Stony Brook, NY: Checkmate Plus.

Gadow, K.D., & Sprafkin, J. (2000). *Early Childhood Inventory–4: Screening manual.* Stony Brook, NY: Checkmate Plus.

Gadow, K.D., & Sprafkin, J. (2002). *Child Symptom Inventory–4: Screening and norms manual.* Stony Brook, NY: Checkmate Plus.

Gaffney, G.R., Perry, P.J., Lund, B.C., Bever-Stille, K.A., Arndt, S., & Kuperman, S. (2002). Risperidone versus clonidine in the treatment of children and adolescents with Tourette's syndrome. *Journal of the American Academy of Child and Adolescent Psychiatry, 41,* 330–336.

Gedye, A. (1991). Trazodone reduced aggressive and self-injurious movements in a mentally handicapped male patient with autism. *Journal of Clinical Psychopharmacology, 11,* 275–276.

Geller, B., Cooper, T.B., Sun, K., Zimerman, B., Frazier, J., Williams, M., et al. (1998). Double-blind and placebo-controlled study of lithium for adolescent bipolar disorders with secondary substance dependency. *Journal of the American Academy of Child and Adolescent Psychiatry, 37,* 171–178.

Geller, B., Guttmacher, L.B., & Bleeg, M. (1981). Coexistence of childhood onset pervasive developmental disorder and attention deficit disorder with hyperactivity. *American Journal of Psychiatry, 138,* 388–389.

Geller, D.A., Biederman, J., Stewart, S.E., Mullin, B., Martin, A., Spencer, T., et al. (2003). Which SSRI? A meta-analysis of pharmacotherapy trials in pediatric obsessive-compulsive disorder. *American Journal of Psychiatry, 160,* 1919–1928.

Gillberg, C., Melander, H., von Knorring, A.L., Janols, L.O., Thernlund, G., Hagglof, B., et al. (1997). Long-term stimulant treatment of children with attention-deficit hyperactivity disorder symptoms: A randomized, double-blind, placebo-controlled trial. *Archives of General Psychiatry, 54,* 857–864.

Glue, P. (1989). Rapid cycling affective disorders in the mentally retarded. *Biological Psychiatry, 26,* 250–256.

Goldstein, H. (2002). Communication intervention for children with autism: A review of treatment efficacy. *Journal of Autism and Developmental Disorders, 32,* 373–396.

Goodman, W.K., Price, L.H., Rasmussen, S.A., Mazure, C., Fleischmann, R.L., Hill, C.L., et al. (1989). The Yale-Brown Obsessive Compulsive Scale, I: Development, use, and reliability. *Archives of General Psychiatry, 46,* 1006–1011.

Gordon, C.T., State, R.C., Nelson, J.E., Hamburger, S.D., & Rapoport, J.L. (1993). A double-blind comparison of clomipramine, desipramine, and placebo in the treatment of autistic disorder. *Archives of General Psychiatry, 50,* 441–447.

Greenhill, L.L., Findling, R.L., Swanson, J.M., & the ADHD Study Group. (2002). A double-blind, placebo-controlled study of modified-release methylphenidate in children with attention-deficit/hyperactivity disorder. *Pediatrics, 109,* e39.

Greenhill, L.L., Halperin, J.M., & Abikoff, H. (1999). Stimulant medications. *Journal of the American Academy of Child and Adolescent Psychiatry, 38,* 503–512.

Greenhill, L.L., Pliszka, S., Dulcan, M.K., Bernet, W., Arnold, V., Beitchman, J., et al. (2002). Practice parameter for the use of stimulant medications in the treatment of children, adolescents, and adults. *Journal of the American Academy of Child and Adolescent Psychiatry, 41*(2 Suppl.), 26S–49S.

Gualtieri, T., Chandler, M., Coons, T.B., & Brown, L.T. (1989). Amantadine: A new clinical profile for traumatic brain injury. *Clinical Neuropharmacology, 12,* 258–270.

Gurney, J.G., Fritz, M.S., Ness, K.K., Sievers, P., Newschaffer, C.J., & Shapiro, E.G. (2003). Analysis of prevalence trends of autism spectrum disorder in Minnesota. *Archives of Pediatrics and Adolescent Medicine, 157,* 622–627.

Gutgesell, H., Atkins, D., Barst, R., Buck, M., Franklin, W., Humes, R., et al. (1999). AHA scientific statement: Cardiovascular monitoring of children and adolescents receiving psychotropic drugs. *Journal of the American Academy of Child and Adolescent Psychiatry, 38,* 1047–1050.

Guy, W. (1976a). Abnormal Involuntary Movement Scale. In *ECDEU assessment manual for psychopharmacology.* Rockville, MD: National Institute for Mental Health.

Guy W. (1976b). Children's Psychiatric Rating Scale. In *ECDEU assessment manual for psychopharmacology.* Rockville, MD: National Institute for Mental Health.

Guy, W. (1976c). Clinical Global Impressions. In *ECDEU assessment manual for psychopharmacology* (pp. 218–222). Rockville, MD: National Institute for Mental Health.

Handen, B.L., Feldman, H., Gosling, A., Breaux, A.M., & McAuliffe, S. (1991). Adverse side effects of methylphenidate among mentally retarded children with ADHD. *Journal of the American Academy of Child and Adolescent Psychiatry, 30,* 241–245.

Handen, B.L., Feldman, H.M., Lurier, A., & Murray, P.J. (1999). Efficacy of methylphenidate among preschool children with developmental disabilities and ADHD. *Journal of the American Academy of Child and Adolescent Psychiatry, 38,* 805–812.

Handen, B.L., Janosky, J., McAuliffe, S., Breaux, A.M., & Feldman, H. (1994). Prediction of response to methylphenidate among children with ADHD and mental retardation. *Journal of the American Academy of Child and Adolescent Psychiatry, 33,* 1185–1193.

Handen, B.L., Johnson, C.R., & Lubetsky, M. (2000). Efficacy of methylphenidate among children with autism and symptoms of attention-deficit hyperactivity disorder. *Journal of Autism and Developmental Disorders, 30,* 245–255.

Hardan, A.Y., & Handen, B.L. (2002). A retrospective open trial of adjunctive donepezil in children and adolescents with autistic disorder. *Journal of Child and Adolescent Psychopharmacology, 12,* 237–241.

Hardan, A.Y., Jou, R.J., & Handen, B.L. (2004). A retrospective assessment of topiramate in children and adolescents with pervasive developmental disorders. *Journal of Child and Adolescent Psychopharmacology, 14,* 426–432.

Hardan, A.Y., Jou, R.J., & Handen, B.L. (2005). Retrospective study of quetiapine in children and adolescents with pervasive developmental disorders. *Journal of Autism and Developmental Disorders, 35,* 387–391.

Hardan, A.Y., & Sahl, R. (1997). Psychopathology in children and adolescents with developmental disorders. *Research in Developmental Disabilities, 18,* 369–382.

Harrigan, E.P., Miceli, J.J., Anziano, R., Watsky, E., Reeves, K.R., Cutler, N.R., et al. (2004). A randomized evaluation of the effects of six antipsychotic agents on QTc, in the absence and presence of metabolic inhibition. *Journal of Clinical Psychopharmacology, 24,* 62–69.

Hazell, P., O'Connell, D., Heathcote, D., & Henry, D. (2002). Tricyclic drugs for depression in children and adolescents. *Cochrane Database of Systematic Reviews, 2,* CD002317.

Hazell, P., O'Connell, D., Heathcote, D., Robertson, J., & Henry, D. (1995). Efficacy of tricyclic drugs in treating child and adolescent depression: A meta-analysis. *BMJ, 310,* 897–901.

Heller, J.H., Spiridigliozzi, G.A., Doraiswamy, P.M., Sullivan, J.A., Crissman, B.G., & Kishnani, P.S. (2004). Donepezil effects on language in children with Down syndrome: Results of the first 22-week pilot clinical trial. *American Journal of Medical Genetics. Part A, 130,* 325–326.

Hellings, J.A., Weckbaugh, M., Nickel, E.J., Cain, S.E., Zarcone, J.R., Reese, R.M., et al. (2005). A double-blind, placebo-controlled study of valproate for aggression in youth with pervasive developmental disorders. *Journal of Child and Adolescent Psychopharmacology, 15,* 682–692.

Hellings, J.A., Kelley, L.A., Gabrielli, W.F., Kilgore, E., & Shah, P. (1996). Sertraline response in adults with mental retardation and autistic disorder. *Journal of Clinical Psychiatry, 57,* 333–336.

Henry, C.A., Zamvil, L.S., Lam, C., Rosenquist, K.J., & Ghaemi, S.N. (2003). Long-term outcome with divalproex in children and adolescents with bipolar disorder. *Journal of Child and Adolescent Psychopharmacology, 13,* 523–529.

Hertzman, M. (2003). Galantamine in the treatment of adult autism: A report of three clinical cases. *International Journal of Psychiatry in Medicine, 33,* 395–398.

Holden, B., & Gitlesen, J.P. (2004). Psychotropic medication in adults with mental retardation: Prevalence, and prescription practices. *Research in Developmental Disabilities, 25,* 509–521.

Hollander, E., Dolgoff-Kaspar, R., Cartwright, C., Rawitt, R., & Novotny, S. (2001). An open trial of divalproex sodium in autism spectrum disorders. *Journal of Clinical Psychiatry, 62,* 530–534.

Hollander, E., Kaplan, A., Cartwright, C., & Reichman, D. (2000). Venlafaxine in children, adolescents, and young adults with autism spectrum disorders: An open retrospective clinical report. *Journal of Child Neurology, 15,* 132–135.

Hollander, E., Phillips, A., Chaplin, W., Zagursky, K., Novotny, S., Wasserman, S., et al. (2005). A placebo controlled crossover trial of liquid fluoxetine on repetitive behaviors in childhood and adolescent autism. *Neuropsychopharmacology, 30,* 582–589.

Hollander, E., Phillips, A., King, B.H., Guthrie, D., Aman, M.G., Law, P., et al. (2004). Impact of recent findings on study design of future autism clinical trials. *CNS Spectrums, 9*(1), 49–56.

Hollander, E., Soorya, L., Wasserman, S., Esposito, K., Chaplin, W., & Anagnostou, E. (2005). Divalproex sodium vs. placebo in the treatment of repetitive behaviours in autism spectrum disorder. *International Journal of Neuropsychopharmacology, 9*(2), 209–213.

Honda, H., Shimizu, Y., Imai, M., & Nitto, Y. (2005). Cumulative incidence of childhood autism: A total population study of better accuracy and precision. *Developmental Medicine and Child Neurology, 47,* 10–18.

Horner, R.H., Carr, E.G., Strain, P.S., Todd, A.W., & Reed, H.K. (2002). Problem behavior interventions for young children with autism: A research synthesis. *Journal of Autism and Developmental Disorders, 32,* 423–446.

Horrigan, J.P., Barnhill, L.J., & Courvoisie, H.E. (1997). Olanzapine in PDD. *Journal of the American Academy of Child and Adolescent Psychiatry, 36,* 1166–1167.

Howlin, P. (1998). Practitioner review: Psychological and educational treatments for autism. *Journal of Child Psychology and Psychiatry and Allied Disciplines, 39,* 307–322.

Hunt, R.D., Arnsten, A.F., & Asbell, M.D. (1995). An open trial of guanfacine in the treatment of attention-deficit hyperactivity disorder. *Journal of the American Academy of Child and Adolescent Psychiatry, 34,* 50–54.

Ingrassia, A., & Turk, J. (2005). The use of clonidine for severe and intractable sleep problems in children with neurodevelopmental disorders—a case series. *European Child and Adolescent Psychiatry, 14,* 34–40.

Ishizaki, A., & Sugama, M. (2001). Methylphenidate therapy in 141 patients with hyperkinetic disorder or with pervasive developmental disorder and hyperkinesia. *No to Hattatsu [Brain and Development], 33,* 323–328.

Ivanenko, A., Crabtree, V.M., & Gozal, D. (2004). Sleep in children with psychiatric disorders. *Pediatric Clinics of North America, 51,* 51–68.

Jacobson, J.W. (1982). Problem behavior and psychiatric impairment within a developmentally disabled population: I. Behavior frequency. *Applied Research in Mental Retardation, 3,* 121–139.

Jacobson, J.W., & Mulick, J.A. (1996). *Manual of diagnosis and professional practice in mental retardation.* Washington, DC: American Psychological Association.

Jan, J.E., & Freeman, R.D. (2004). Melatonin therapy for circadian rhythm sleep disorders in children with multiple disabilities: What have we learned in the last decade? *Developmental Medicine and Child Neurology, 46,* 776–782.

Jaselskis, C.A., Cook, E.H., Jr., Fletcher, K.E., & Leventhal, B.L. (1992). Clonidine treatment of hyperactive and impulsive children with autistic disorder. *Journal of Clinical Psychopharmacology, 12,* 322–327.

Jou, R.J., Handen, B.L., & Hardan, A.Y. (2005). Retrospective assessment of atomoxetine in children and adolescents with pervasive developmental disorders. *Journal of Child and Adolescent Psychopharmacology, 15,* 325–330.

Kafantaris, V., Campbell, M., Padron-Gayol, M.V., Small, A.M., Locascio, J.J., & Rosenberg, C.R. (1992). Carbamazepine in hospitalized aggressive conduct disorder children: An open pilot study. *Psychopharmacology Bulletin, 28,* 193–199.

Kafantaris, V., Coletti, D.J., Dicker, R., Padula, G., & Kane, J.M. (2003). Lithium treatment of acute mania in adolescents: A large open trial. *Journal of the American Academy of Child and Adolescent Psychiatry, 42,* 1038–1045.

Kafantaris, V., Coletti, D.J., Dicker, R., Padula, G., Pleak, R.R., & Alvir, J.M. (2004). Lithium treatment of acute mania in adolescents: A placebo-controlled discontinuation study. *Journal of the American Academy of Child and Adolescent Psychiatry, 43,* 984–993.

Kastner, T., Burlingham, K., & Friedman, D.L. (1990). Metoprolol for aggressive behavior in persons with mental retardation. *American Family Physician, 42,* 1585–1588.

Kastner, T., Finesmith, R., & Walsh, K. (1993). Long-term administration of valproic acid in the treatment of affective symptoms in people with mental retardation. *Journal of Clinical Psychopharmacology, 13,* 448–451.

Kastner, T., Friedman, D.L., Plummer, A.T., Ruiz, M.Q., & Henning, D. (1990). Valproic acid for the treatment of children with mental retardation and mood symptomatology. *Pediatrics, 86,* 467–472.

Keller, M.B., Ryan, N.D., Strober, M., Klein, R.G., Kutcher, S.P., Birmaher, B., et al. (2001). Efficacy of paroxetine in the treatment of adolescent major depression: A randomized, controlled trial. *Journal of the American Academy of Child and Adolescent Psychiatry, 40,* 762–772.

Kelsey, D.K., Sumner, C.R., Casat, C.D., Coury, D.L., Quintana, H., Saylor, K.E., et al. (2004). Once-daily atomoxetine treatment for children with attention-deficit/hyperactivity disorder, including an assessment of evening and morning behavior: A double-blind, placebo-controlled trial. *Pediatrics, 114,* e1–e8.

Kem, D.L., Posey, D.J., & McDougle, C.J. (2002). Priapism associated with trazodone in an adolescent with autism. *Journal of the American Academy of Child and Adolescent Psychiatry, 41,* 758.

Kemner, C., Willemsen-Swinkels, S.H., de Jonge, M., Tuynman-Qua, H., & van Engeland, H. (2002). Open-label study of olanzapine in children with pervasive developmental disorder. *Journal of Clinical Psychopharmacology, 22,* 455–460.

Kemph, J.P., DeVane, C.L., Levin, G.M., Jarecke, R., & Miller, R.L. (1993). Treatment of aggressive children with clonidine: Results of an open pilot study. *Journal of the American Academy of Child and Adolescent Psychiatry, 32,* 577–581.

Kerbeshian, J., Burd, L., & Fisher, W. (1987). Lithium carbonate in the treatment of two patients with infantile autism and atypical bipolar symptomatology. *Journal of Clinical Psychopharmacology,* 7, 401–405.

Kerker, B.D., Owens, P.L., Zigler, E., & Horwitz, S.M. (2004). Mental health disorders among individuals with mental retardation: Challenges to accurate prevalence estimates. *Public Health Reports,* 119, 409–417.

Kiernan, C., & Kiernan, D. (1994). Challenging behaviour in schools for pupils with severe learning difficulties. *Mental Handicap Research,* 7, 177–201.

King, B.H., & Davanzo, P. (1996). Buspirone treatment of aggression and self-injury in autistic and nonautistic persons with severe mental retardation. *Developmental Brain Dysfunction,* 90, 22–31.

King, B.H., Wright, D.M., Handen, B.L., Sikich, L., Zimmerman, A.W., McMahon, W., et al. (2001). Double-blind, placebo-controlled study of amantadine hydrochloride in the treatment of children with autistic disorder. *Journal of the American Academy of Child and Adolescent Psychiatry,* 40, 658–665.

Koegel, L.K. (2000). Interventions to facilitate communication in autism. *Journal of Autism and Developmental Disorders,* 30, 383–391.

Koegel, R.L., Koegel, L.K., & McNerney, E.K. (2001). Pivotal areas in intervention for autism. *Journal of Clinical Child Psychology,* 30, 19–32.

Kofoed, L., Tadepalli, G., Oesterheld, J.R., Awadallah, S., & Shapiro, R. (1999). Case series: Clonidine has no systematic effects on PR or QTc intervals in children. *Journal of the American Academy of Child and Adolescent Psychiatry,* 38, 1193–1196.

Kolmen, B.K., Feldman, H.M., Handen, B.L., & Janosky, J.E. (1995). Naltrexone in young autistic children: A double-blind, placebo-controlled crossover study. *Journal of the American Academy of Child and Adolescent Psychiatry,* 34, 223–231.

Kolmen, B.K., Feldman, H.M., Handen, B.L., & Janosky, J.E. (1997). Naltrexone in young autistic children: Replication study and learning measures. *Journal of the American Academy of Child and Adolescent Psychiatry,* 36, 1570–1578.

Kornhuber, J., Weller, M., Schoppmeyer, K., & Riederer, P. (1994). Amantadine and memantine are NMDA receptor antagonists with neuroprotective properties. *Journal of Neural Transmission, Supplementum,* 43, 91–104.

Kowatch, R.A., Sethuraman, G., Hume, J.H., Kromelis, M., & Weinberg, W.A. (2003). Combination pharmacotherapy in children and adolescents with bipolar disorder. *Biological Psychiatry,* 53, 978–984.

Kowatch, R.A., Suppes, T., Carmody, T.J., Bucci, J.P., Hume, J.H., Kromelis, M., et al. (2000). Effect size of lithium, divalproex sodium, and carbamazepine in children and adolescents with bipolar disorder. *Journal of the American Academy of Child and Adolescent Psychiatry,* 39, 713–720.

Kutcher, S.P. (1997). *Child and adolescent psychopharmacology.* Philadelphia: W.B. Saunders.

Lam, K.S., (2004). *The repetitive behavior scale–revised: Independent validation and the effects of subject variables.* Unpublished doctoral dissertation, The Ohio State Univerty.

Langee, H.R. (1990). Retrospective study of lithium use for institutionalized mentally retarded individuals with behavior disorders. *American Journal of Mental Retardation,* 94, 448–452.

Langworthy-Lam, K.S., Aman, M.G., & Van Bourgondien, M.E. (2002). Prevalence and patterns of use of psychoactive medicines in individuals with autism in the Autism Society of North Carolina. *Journal of Child and Adolescent Psychopharmacology,* 12, 311–321.

Lauritsen, M.B., Pedersen, C.B., & Mortensen, P.B. (2004). The incidence and prevalence of pervasive developmental disorders: A Danish population-based study. *Psychological Medicine,* 34, 1339–1346.

Leboyer, M., Bouvard, M.P., Launay, J.M., Tabuteau, F., Waller, D., Dugas, M., et al. (1992). Brief report: A double-blind study of naltrexone in infantile autism. *Journal of Autism and Developmental Disorders,* 22, 309–319.

Leckman, J.F., Hardin, M.T., Riddle, M.A., Stevenson, J., Ort, S.I., & Cohen, D.J. (1991). Clonidine treatment of Gilles de la Tourette's syndrome. *Archives of General Psychiatry,* 48, 324–328.

Leonard, H., Petterson, B., Bower, C., & Sanders, R. (2003). Prevalence of intellectual disability in Western Australia. *Paediatric and Perinatal Epidemiology,* 17, 58–67.

Lewis, M.H., Bodfish, J.W., Powell, S.B., & Golden, R.N. (1995). Clomipramine treatment for stereotype and related repetitive movement disorders associated with mental retardation. *American Journal on Mental Retardation,* 100, 299–312.

Lewis, M.H., Bodfish, J.W., Powell, S.B., Parker, D.E., & Golden, R.N. (1996). Clomipramine treatment for self-injurious behavior of individuals with mental retardation: A double-blind comparison with placebo. *American Journal of Mental Retardation,* 100, 654–665.

Linde, K., & Rossnagel, K. (2004). Propranolol for migraine prophylaxis. *Cochrane Database of Systematic Reviews,* 2, CD003225.

Lobaugh, N.J., Karaskov, V., Rombough, V., Rovet, J., Bryson, S., Greenbaum, R., et al. (2001). Piracetam therapy does not enhance cognitive functioning in children with Down syndrome. *Archives of Pediatrics and Adolescent Medicine,* 155, 442–448.

Lofts, R.H., Schroeder, S.R., & Maier, R.H. (1990). Effects of serum zinc supplementation on pica behavior of persons with mental retardation. *American Journal on Mental Retardation,* 95, 103–109.

Lord, C., Rutter, M., DiLavore, P.C., & Risi, S. (1999). *Autism Diagnostic Observation Schedule.* Los Angeles: Western Psychological Services.

Lord, C., & Schopler, E. (1989). Stability of assessment results of autistic and non-autistic language-impaired children from preschool years to early school age. *Journal of Child Psychology and Psychiatry and Allied Disciplines,* 30, 575–590.

Lott, I.T., McGregor, M., Engelman, L., Touchette, P., Tournay, A., Sandman, C., et al. (2004). Longitudinal prescribing patterns for psychoactive medications in community-based individuals with developmental disabilities: Utilization of pharmacy records. *Journal of Intellectual Disability Research, 48*(Pt. 6), 563–571.

Luchins, D.J., & Dojka, D. (1989). Lithium and propranolol in aggression and self-injurious behavior in the mentally retarded. *Psychopharmacology Bulletin, 25,* 372–375.

Macritchie, K., Geddes, J.R., Scott, J., Haslam, D., de Lima, M., & Goodwin, G. (2003). Valproate for acute mood episodes in bipolar disorder. *Cochrane Database of Systematic Reviews, 1,* CD004052.

Malek-Ahmadi, P., & Simonds, J.F. (1998). Olanzapine for autistic disorder with hyperactivity. *Journal of the American Academy of Child and Adolescent Psychiatry, 37,* 902.

Malone, R.P., Cater, J., Sheikh, R.M., Choudhury, M.S., & Delaney, M.A. (2001). Olanzapine versus haloperidol in children with autistic disorder: An open pilot study. *Journal of the American Academy of Child and Adolescent Psychiatry, 40,* 887–894.

Malone, R.P., Delaney, M.A., Luebbert, J.F., Cater, J., & Campbell, M. (2000). A double-blind placebo-controlled study of lithium in hospitalized aggressive children and adolescents with conduct disorder. *Archives of General Psychiatry, 57,* 649–654.

March, J.S., Biederman, J., Wolkow, R., Safferman, A., Mardekian, J., Cook, E.H., et al. (1998). Sertraline in children and adolescents with obsessive-compulsive disorder: A multicenter randomized controlled trial. *JAMA, 280,* 1752–1756.

Marshburn, E.C., & Aman, M.G. (1992). Factor validity and norms for the Aberrant Behavior Checklist in a community sample of children with mental retardation. *Journal of Autism and Developmental Disorders, 22,* 357–373.

Marson, J.L. (1995). *Manual for the Diagnostic Assessment for the Severely Handicapped-II.* Baton Rouge: Louisianna State University Press.

Martin, A., Koenig, K., Anderson, G.M., & Scahill, L. (2003). Low-dose fluvoxamine treatment of children and adolescents with pervasive developmental disorders: A prospective, open-label study. *Journal of Autism and Developmental Disorders, 33,* 77–85.

Martin, A., Koenig, K., Scahill, L., & Bregman, J. (1999). Open-label quetiapine in the treatment of children and adolescents with autistic disorder. *Journal of Child and Adolescent Psychopharmacology, 9,* 99–107.

Martin, A., Scahill, L., Klin, A., & Volkmar, F.R. (1999). Higher-functioning pervasive developmental disorders: Rates and patterns of psychotropic drug use. *Journal of the American Academy of Child and Adolescent Psychiatry, 38,* 923–931.

Masi, G., Cosenza, A., Mucci, M., & Brovedani, P. (2003). A 3-year naturalistic study of 53 preschool children with pervasive developmental disorders treated with risperidone. *Journal of Clinical Psychiatry, 64,* 1039–1047.

Masi, G., Marcheschi, M., & Pfanner, P. (1997). Paroxetine in depressed adolescents with intellectual disability: An open label study. *Journal of Intellectual Disability Research, 41*(Pt. 3), 268–272.

Masters, K.J. (1997). Alternative medications for ADHD. *Journal of the American Academy of Child and Adolescent Psychiatry, 36,* 301–302.

Matson, J.L., Benavidez, D.A., Compton, L.S., Paclawskyj, T., & Baglio, C. (1996). Behavioral treatment of autistic persons: A review of research from 1980 to the present. *Research in Developmental Disabilities, 17,* 433–465.

Mattes, J. (1980). A pilot trial of amantadine in hyperactive children. *Psychopharmacology Bulletin, 16,* 67–69.

Mayes, S.D., Crites, D.L., Bixler, E.O., Humphrey, F.J., 2nd, & Mattison, R.E. (1994). Methylphenidate and ADHD: Influence of age, IQ and neurodevelopmental status. *Developmental Medicine and Child Neurology, 36,* 1099–1107.

McClellan, J.M., & Werry, J.S. (2003). Evidence-based treatments in child and adolescent psychiatry: An inventory. *Journal of the American Academy of Child and Adolescent Psychiatry, 42,* 1388–1400.

McClintock, K., Hall, S., & Oliver, C. (2003). Risk markers associated with challenging behaviours in people with intellectual disabilities: A meta-analytic study. *Journal of Intellectual Disability Research, 47*(Pt. 6), 405–416.

McCracken, J.T., McGough, J., Shah, B., Cronin, P., Hong, D., Aman, M.G., et al. (2002). Risperidone in children with autism and serious behavioral problems. *New England Journal of Medicine, 347,* 314–321.

McDougle, C.J., Holmes, J.P., Carlson, D.C., Pelton, G.H., Cohen, D.J., & Price, L.H. (1998). A double-blind, placebo-controlled study of risperidone in adults with autistic disorder and other pervasive developmental disorders. *Archives of General Psychiatry, 55,* 633–641.

McDougle, C.J., Kem, D.L., & Posey, D.J. (2002). Case series: Use of ziprasidone for maladaptive symptoms in youths with autism. *Journal of the American Academy of Child and Adolescent Psychiatry, 41,* 921–927.

McDougle, C.J., Kresch, L.E., & Posey, D.J. (2000). Repetitive thoughts and behavior in pervasive developmental disorders: Treatment with serotonin reuptake inhibitors. *Journal of Autism and Developmental Disorders, 30,* 427–435.

McDougle, C.J., Naylor, S.T., Cohen, D.J., Volkmar, F.R., Heninger, G.R., & Price, L.H. (1996). A double-blind, placebo-controlled study of fluvoxamine in adults with autistic disorder. *Archives of General Psychiatry, 53,* 1001–1008.

McDougle, C.J., Scahill, L., Aman, M.G., McCracken, J.T., Tierney, E., Davies, M., et al. (2005). Risperidone for the core symptom domains of autism: Results from the study by the Autism Network of the Research Units on Pediatric Psychopharmacology. *American Journal of Psychiatry, 162,* 1142–1148.

McKee, J.R., Sunder, T.R., FineSmith, R., Vuong, A., Varner, J.A., Hammer, A.E., et al. (2003). Lamotrigine as adjunctive therapy in patients with refractory epilepsy and mental retardation. *Epilepsy and Behavior, 4,* 386–394.

McKnew, D.H., Cytryn, L., Buchsbaum, M.S., Hamovit, J., Lamour, M., Rapoport, J.L., et al. (1981). Lithium in children of lithium-responding parents. *Psychiatry Research, 4,* 171–180.

Mehta, U.C., Patel, I., & Castello, F.V. (2004). EEG sedation for children with autism. *Journal of Developmental and Behavioral Pediatrics, 25,* 102–104.

Meltzer, L.J., & Mindell, J.A. (2004). Nonpharmacologic treatments for pediatric sleeplessness. *Pediatric Clinics of North America, 51,* 135–151.

Mesibov, G.B., Shea, V., & Schopler, E. (2005). *The TEACCH approach to autism spectrum disorders.* New York: Kluwer/Plenum.

Micev, V., & Lynch, D.M. (1974). Effect of lithium on disturbed severely mentally retarded patients [letter]. *British Journal of Psychiatry, 125,* 110.

Michael, J.B., & Sztajnkrycer, M.D. (2004). Deadly pediatric poisons: Nine common agents that kill at low doses. *Emergency Medicine Clinics of North America, 22,* 1019–1050.

Michelson, D., Faries, D., Wernicke, J., Kelsey, D., Kendrick, K., Sallee, F.R., et al. (2001). Atomoxetine in the treatment of children and adolescents with attention-deficit/hyperactivity disorder: A randomized, placebo-controlled, dose-response study. *Pediatrics, 108,* e83.

Molitch, M., & Eccles, A.K. (1937). The effect of benzedrine sulfate on the intelligence scores of children. *American Journal of Psychiatry, 94,* 587–590.

Moore, M.L., Eichner, S.F., & Jones, J.R. (2004). Treating functional impairment of autism with selective serotonin-reuptake inhibitors. *Annals of Pharmacotherapy, 38,* 1515–1519.

Moran, T.H., Capone, G.T., Knipp, S., Davisson, M.T., Reeves, R.H., & Gearhart, J.D. (2002). The effects of piracetam on cognitive performance in a mouse model of Down's syndrome. *Physiology and Behavior, 77,* 403–409.

MTA Cooperative Group. (1999). 14-month randomized clinical trial of treatment strategies for attention-deficit/hyperactivity disorder. *Archives of General Psychiatry, 56,* 1073–1086.

Murphy, C.C., Yeargin-Allsopp, M., Decoufle, P., & Drews, C.D. (1995). The administrative prevalence of mental retardation in 10-year-old children in metropolitan Atlanta, 1985 through 1987. *American Journal of Public Health, 85,* 319–323.

Namerow, L.B., Thomas, P., Bostic, J.Q., Prince, J., & Monuteaux, M.C. (2003). Use of citalopram in pervasive developmental disorders. *Journal of Developmental and Behavioral Pediatrics, 24,* 104–108.

Naruse, H., Nagahata, M., Nakane, Y., Shirahashi, K., Takesada, M., & Yamazaki, K. (1982). A multicenter double-blind trial of pimozide (Orap), halo-peridol and placebo in children with behavioral disorders, using crossover design. *Acta Paedopsychiatrica, 48,* 173–184.

National Institute of Mental Health. (2001). National Institute of Mental Health research roundtable on prepubertal bipolar disorder. *Journal of the American Academy of Child and Adolescent Psychiatry, 40,* 871–878.

Naylor, G.J., Donald, J.M., Le Poidevin, D., & Reid, A.H. (1974). A double-blind trial of long-term lithium therapy in mental defectives. *British Journal of Psychiatry, 124,* 52–57.

Niederhofer, H., Staffen, W., & Mair, A. (2002a). Galantamine may be effective in treating autistic disorder. *BMJ, 325,* 1422.

Niederhofer, H., Staffen, W., & Mair, A. (2002b). Lofexidine in hyperactive and impulsive children with autistic disorder. *Journal of the American Academy of Child and Adolescent Psychiatry, 41,* 1396–1397.

Oliver, C., Murphy, G.H., & Corbett, J.A. (1987). Self-injurious behaviour in people with mental handicap: A total population study. *Journal of Mental Deficiency Research, 31*(Pt. 2), 147–162.

Ollendick, T.H. (1983). Reliability and validity of the Revised Fear Survey Schedule for Children (FSSC-R). *Behaviour Research and Therapy, 21*(6), 685–692

Owley, T., Walton, L., Salt, J., Guter, S.J., Jr., Winnega, M., Leventhal, B.L., et al. (2005). An open-label trial of escitalopram in pervasive developmental disorders. *Journal of the American Academy of Child and Adolescent Psychiatry, 44,* 343–348.

Papatheodorou, G., & Kutcher, S.P. (1993). Divalproex sodium treatment in late adolescent and young adult acute mania. *Psychopharmacology Bulletin, 29,* 213–219.

Papatheodorou, G., Kutcher, S.P., Katic, M., & Szalai, J.P. (1995). The efficacy and safety of divalproex sodium in the treatment of acute mania in adolescents and young adults: An open clinical trial. *Journal of Clinical Psychopharmacology, 15,* 110–116.

Pary, R.J. (1991). Towards defining adequate lithium trials for individuals with mental retardation and mental illness. *American Journal on Mental Retardation, 95,* 681–691.

Pavuluri, M.N., Henry, D.B., Carbray, J.A., Naylor, M.W., & Janicak, P.G. (2005). Divalproex sodium for pediatric mixed mania: A 6-month prospective trial. *Bipolar Disorders, 7,* 266–273.

Pavuluri, M.N., Henry, D.B., Carbray, J.A., Sampson, G., Naylor, M.W., & Janicak, P.G. (2004). Open-label prospective trial of risperidone in combination with lithium or divalproex sodium in pediatric mania. *Journal of Affective Disorders, 82*(Suppl. 1), S103–S111.

Pearson, D.A., Lane, D.M., Santos, C.W., Casat, C.D., Jerger, S.W., Loveland, K.A., et al. (2004). Effects of methylphenidate treatment in children with mental retardation and ADHD: Individual variation in medication response. *Journal of the Ameri-*

can Academy of Child and Adolescent Psychiatry, 43, 686–698.

Pearson, D.A., Santos, C.W., Casat, C.D., Lane, D.M., Jerger, S.W., Roache, J.D., et al. (2004). Treatment effects of methylphenidate on cognitive functioning in children with mental retardation and ADHD. Journal of the American Academy of Child and Adolescent Psychiatry, 43, 677–685.

Pearson, D.A., Santos, C.W., Roache, J.D., Casat, C.D., Loveland, K.A., Lachar, D., et al. (2003). Treatment effects of methylphenidate on behavioral adjustment in children with mental retardation and ADHD. Journal of the American Academy of Child and Adolescent Psychiatry, 42, 209–216.

Pediatric OCD Treatment Study (POTS) Team. (2004). Cognitive-behavior therapy, sertraline, and their combination for children and adolescents with obsessive-compulsive disorder: The Pediatric OCD Treatment Study (POTS) randomized controlled trial. JAMA, 292, 1969–1976.

Pelayo, R., Chen, W., Monzon, S., & Guilleminault, C. (2004). Pediatric sleep pharmacology: You want to give my kid sleeping pills? Pediatric Clinics of North America, 51, 117–134.

Peral, M., Alcami, M., & Gilaberte, I. (1999). Fluoxetine in children with autism. Journal of the American Academy of Child and Adolescent Psychiatry, 38, 1472–1473.

Perry, D.W., Marston, G.M., Hinder, S.A., Munden, A.C., & Roy, A. (2001). The phenomenology of depressive illness in people with a learning disability and autism. Autism, 5, 265–275.

Perry, R., Campbell, M., Adams, P., & Lynch, N. (1989). Long-term efficacy of haloperidol in autistic children: Continuous versus discontinuous drug administration. Journal of the American Academy of Child and Adolescent Psychiatry, 28, 87–92.

Phillips, L., & Appleton, R.E. (2004). Systematic review of melatonin treatment in children with neurodevelopmental disabilities and sleep impairment. Developmental Medicine and Child Neurology, 46, 771–775.

Plioplys, A.V. (1994). Autism: Electroencephalogram abnormalities and clinical improvement with valproic acid. Archives of Pediatrics and Adolescent Medicine, 148, 220–222.

Poindexter, A.R., Cain, N., Clarke, D.J., Cook, E.H., Corbett, J.A., & Levitas, A. (1998). Mood stabilizers. In S. Reiss & M.G. Aman (Eds.), Psychotropic medications and developmental disabilities: The international consensus handbook (pp. 215–227). Columbus: Ohio State University, Nisonger Center.

Polimeni, M.A., Richdale, A.L., & Francis, A.J. (2005). A survey of sleep problems in autism, Asperger's disorder and typically developing children. Journal of Intellectual Disability Research, 49(Pt. 4), 260–268.

Posey, D.J., Guenin, K.D., Kohn, A.E., Swiezy, N.B., & McDougle, C.J. (2001). A naturalistic open-label study of mirtazapine in autistic and other pervasive developmental disorders. Journal

of Child and Adolescent Psychopharmacology, 11, 267–277.

Posey, D.J., Kem, D.L., Swiezy, N.B., Sweeten, T.L., Wiegand, R.E., & McDougle, C.J. (2004). A pilot study of D-cycloserine in subjects with autistic disorder. American Journal of Psychiatry, 161, 2115–2117.

Posey, D.J., Puntney, J.I., Sasher, T.M., Kem, D.L., & McDougle, C.J. (2004). Guanfacine treatment of hyperactivity and inattention in pervasive developmental disorders: A retrospective analysis of 80 cases. Journal of Child and Adolescent Psychopharmacology, 14, 233–241.

Potenza, M.N., Holmes, J.P., Kanes, S.J., & McDougle, C.J. (1999). Olanzapine treatment of children, adolescents, and adults with pervasive developmental disorders: An open-label pilot study. Journal of Clinical Psychopharmacology, 19, 37–44.

Prince, J.B., Wilens, T.E., Biederman, J., Spencer, T.J., & Wozniak, J.R. (1996). Clonidine for sleep disturbances associated with attention-deficit hyperactivity disorder: A systematic chart review of 62 cases. Journal of the American Academy of Child and Adolescent Psychiatry, 35, 599–605.

Quine, L. (1991). Sleep problems in children with mental handicap. Journal of Mental Deficiency Research, 35(Pt. 4), 269–290.

Quintana, H., Birmaher, B., Stedge, D., Lennon, S., Freed, J., Bridge, J., et al. (1995). Use of methylphenidate in the treatment of children with autistic disorder. Journal of Autism and Developmental Disorders, 25, 283–294.

Ramirez, S.Z., & Kratochwill, T.R. (1990). Development of the Fear Survey for Children With and Without Mental Retardation. Behavioral Assessment, 12, 457–470.

Ratey, J.J., & Lindem, K.J. (1991). Beta-blockers as primary treatment for aggression and self-injury in the developmentally disabled. In J.J. Ratey (Ed.), Mental retardation: Developing pharmacotherapies (pp. 51–81). Washington, DC: American Psychiatric Press.

Ratey, J.J., Mikkelsen, E.J., Smith, G.B., Upadhyaya, A., Zuckerman, H.S., Martell, D., et al. (1986). Beta-blockers in the severely and profoundly mentally retarded. Journal of Clinical Psychopharmacology, 6, 103–107.

Ratey, J.J., Mikkelsen, E., Sorgi, P., Zuckerman, H.S., Polakoff, S., Bemporad, J., et al. (1987). Autism: The treatment of aggressive behaviors. Journal of Clinical Psychopharmacology, 7, 35–41.

Ratey, J.J., Sovner, R., Mikkelsen, E., & Chmielinski, H.E. (1989). Buspirone therapy for maladaptive behavior and anxiety in developmentally disabled persons. Journal of Clinical Psychiatry, 50, 382–384.

Realmuto, G.M., August, G.J., & Garfinkel, B.D. (1989). Clinical effect of buspirone in autistic children. Journal of Clinical Psychopharmacology, 9, 122–125.

Reed, M.D., & Findling, R.L. (2002). Overview of current management of sleep disturbances in children: I—pharmacotherapy. *Current Therapeutic Research, 63*(Suppl. B), B18–B37.

Remington, G., Sloman, L., Konstantareas, M., Parker, K., & Gow, R. (2001). Clomipramine versus haloperidol in the treatment of autistic disorder: A double-blind, placebo-controlled, crossover study. *Journal of Clinical Psychopharmacology, 21*, 440–444.

Rendell, J.M., Gijsman, H.J., Keck, P., Goodwin, G.M., & Geddes, J.R. (2005). Olanzapine alone or in combination for acute mania. *Cochrane Database of Systematic Reviews, 3*, CD004040.

Ricketts, R.W., Goza, A.B., Ellis, C.R., Singh, Y.N., Chambers, S., Singh, N.N., et al. (1994). Clinical effects of buspirone on intractable self-injury in adults with mental retardation. *Journal of the American Academy of Child and Adolescent Psychiatry, 33*, 270–276.

Riddle, M.A. (1995). Pediatric psychopharmacology: I. Preface. *Child and Adolescent Psychiatric Clinics of North America, 4*, xii–xv.

Riddle, M.A., Bernstein, G.A., Cook, E.H., Leonard, H.L., March, J.S., & Swanson, J.M. (1999). Anxiolytics, adrenergic agents, and naltrexone. *Journal of the American Academy of Child and Adolescent Psychiatry, 38*, 546–556.

Riddle, M.A., Reeve, E.A., Yaryura-Tobias, J.A., Yang, H.M., Claghorn, J.L., Gaffney, G., et al. (2001). Fluvoxamine for children and adolescents with obsessive-compulsive disorder: A randomized, controlled, multicenter trial. *Journal of the American Academy of Child and Adolescent Psychiatry, 40*, 222–229.

Rinck, C. (1998). Epidemiology and psychoactive medication. In S. Reiss & M.G. Aman (Eds.), *Psychotropic medication and developmental disabilities: The international consensus handbook* (pp. 3–18). Columbus: The Ohio State University, Nisonger Center.

Rogers, S.J. (1998). Empirically supported comprehensive treatments for young children with autism. *Journal of Clinical Child Psychology, 27*, 168–179.

Rogers, S.J. (2000). Interventions that facilitate socialization in children with autism. *Journal of Autism and Developmental Disorders, 30*, 399–409.

Rojahn, J., Matlock, S.T., & Tassé, M.J. (2000). The Stereotyped Behavior Scale: Psychometric properties and norms. *Research in Developmental Disabilities, 21*(6), 437–454.

Rojahn, J., Matson, J.L., Lott, D., Esbensen, A.J., & Smalls, Y. (2001). The Behavior Problems Inventory: An instrument for the assessment of self-injury, stereotyped behavior, and aggression/destruction of individuals with developmental disorders. *Journal of Autism and Developmental Disorders, 31*(6), 577–588.

Rose, E.A., Porcerelli, J.H., & Neale, A.V. (2000). Pica: Common but commonly missed. *Journal of the American Board of Family Practice, 13*, 353–358.

Rubin, M. (1997). Use of atypical antipsychotics in children with mental retardation, autism, and other developmental disabilities. *Psychiatric Annals, 27*, 219–221.

Ruedrich, S., & Menolascino, F.J. (1984). Dual diagnosis of mental retardation and mental illness: An overview. In F.J. Menolascino & J.A. Starks (Eds.), *Handbook of mental illness in the mentally retarded* (pp. 45–81). New York: Plenum.

Ruedrich, S., Swales, T.P., Fossaceca, C., Toliver, J., & Rutkowski, A. (1999). Effect of divalproex sodium on aggression and self-injurious behaviour in adults with intellectual disability: A retrospective review. *Journal of Intellectual Disability Research, 43*(Pt. 2), 105–111.

Rugino, T.A., & Samsock, T.C. (2002). Levetiracetam in autistic children: An open-label study. *Journal of Developmental and Behavioral Pediatrics, 23*, 225–230.

Research Units on Pediatric Psychopharmacology (RUPP) Autism Network (2002). Randomized, controlled, crossover trial of methylphenidate in pervasive developmental disorders with hyperactivity. *Archives of General Psychiatry, 62*, 1266–1274.

RUPP Anxiety Study Group. (2001). Fluvoxamine for the treatment of anxiety disorders in children and adolescents. *New England Journal of Medicine, 344*, 1279–1285.

Russo, R.M., Gururaj, V.J., & Allen, J.E. (1976). The effectiveness of diphenhydramine HCl in pediatric sleep disorders. *Journal of Clinical Pharmacology, 16*, 284–288.

Rutter, M., Tizard, J., Yule, W., Graham, P., & Whitmore, K. (1976). Research report: Isle of Wight studies, 1964–1974. *Psychological Medicine, 6*, 313–332.

Salman, M. (2002). Systematic review of the effect of therapeutic dietary supplements and drugs on cognitive function in subjects with Down syndrome. *European Journal of Paediatric Neurology, 6*, 213–219.

Sanchez, L.E., Campbell, M., Small, A.M., Cueva, J.E., Armenteros, J.L., & Adams, P.B. (1996). A pilot study of clomipramine in young autistic children. *Journal of the American Academy of Child and Adolescent Psychiatry, 35*, 537–544.

Sandman, C.A. (1991). The opiate hypothesis in autism and self-injury. *Journal of Child and Adolescent Psychopharmacology, 1*, 237–248.

Sandman, C.A., Hetrick, W., Taylor, D.V., Marion, S.D., Touchette, P., Barron, J.L., et al. (2000). Long-term effects of naltrexone on self-injurious behavior. *American Journal on Mental Retardation, 105*, 103–117.

Scahill, L., Chappell, P.B., Kim, Y.S., Schultz, R.T., Katsovich, L., Shepherd, E., et al. (2001). A placebo-controlled study of guanfacine in the treatment of children with tic disorders and attention deficit hyperactivity disorder. *American Journal of Psychiatry, 158*, 1067–1074.

Scahill, L., Riddle, M.A., McSwiggin-Hardin, M., Ort, S.I., King, R.A., Goodman, W.K., et al. (1997). Children's Yale-Brown Obsessive-Compulsive Scale: Reliability and validity. *Journal of the Ameri-*

can Academy of Child and Adolescent Psychiatry, 36(6), 844–852.

Schain, R.J., & Freedman, D.X. (1961). Studies on 5-hydroxyindole metabolism in autistic and other mentally retarded children. Journal of Pediatrics, 58, 315–320.

Scheffer, R.E., & Niskala Apps, J.A. (2004). The diagnosis of preschool bipolar disorder presenting with mania: Open pharmacological treatment. Journal of Affective Disorders, 82(Suppl. 1), S25–S34.

Schmidt, K. (1982). The effect of stimulant medication in childhood-onset pervasive developmental disorder—a case report. Journal of Developmental and Behavioral Pediatrics, 3, 244–246.

Schroeder, S.R., Bouras, N., Ellis, C.R., Reid, A.H., Sandman, C., Werry, J.S., et al. (1998). Past research on psychopharmacology of people with mental retardation and developmental disabilities. In S. Reiss & M.G. Aman (Eds.), Psychotropic medication and developmental disabilities: The international consensus handbook (pp. 19–30). Columbus: The Ohio State University, Nisonger Center.

Schroeder, S.R., Rojahn, J., & Reese, R.M. (1997). Reliability and validity of instruments for assessing psychotropic medication effects on self-injurious behavior in mental retardation. Journal of Autism and Developmental Disorders, 27(1), 89–102.

Schvehla, T.J., Mandoki, M.W., & Sumner, G.S. (1994). Clonidine therapy for comorbid attention deficit hyperactivity disorder and conduct disorder: Preliminary findings in a children's inpatient unit. Southern Medical Journal, 87, 692–695.

Scifo, R., Batticane, N., Quattropani, M.C., & Spoto, G. (1991). A double-blind trial with naltrexone in autism. Brain Dysfunction, 4, 301–307.

Seltzer, M.M., Shattuck, P., Abbeduto, L., & Greenberg, J.S. (2004). Trajectory of development in adolescents and adults with autism. Mental Retardation and Developmental Disabilities Research Reviews, 10, 234–247.

Shea, S., Turgay, A., Carroll, A., Schulz, M., Orlik, H., Smith, I., et al. (2004). Risperidone in the treatment of disruptive behavioral symptoms in children with autistic and other pervasive developmental disorders. Pediatrics, 114, e634–e641.

Simmons, J.Q., 3rd, Leiken, S.J., Lovaas, O.I., Schaeffer, B., & Perloff, B. (1966). Modification of autistic behavior with LSD-25. American Journal of Psychiatry, 122, 1201–1211.

Singer, H.S., Brown, J., Quaskey, S., Rosenberg, L.A., Mellits, E.D., & Denckla, M.B. (1995). The treatment of attention-deficit hyperactivity disorder in Tourette's syndrome: A double-blind placebo-controlled study with clonidine and desipramine. Pediatrics, 95, 74–81.

Singh, N.N., Ellis, C.R., & Wechsler, H. (1997). Psychopharmacoepidemiology of mental retardation: 1966 to 1995. Journal of Child and Adolescent Psychopharmacology, 7, 255–266.

Singhi, S., Ravishanker, R., Singhi, P., & Nath, R. (2003). Low plasma zinc and iron in pica. Indian Journal of Pediatrics, 70, 139–143.

Smith, D.A., & Perry, P.J. (1992). Nonneuroleptic treatment of disruptive behavior in organic mental syndromes. Annals of Pharmacotherapy, 26, 1400–1408.

Smith, T., Eikeseth, S., Klevstrand, M., & Lovaas, O.I. (1997). Intensive behavioral treatment for preschoolers with severe mental retardation and pervasive developmental disorder. American Journal on Mental Retardation, 102, 238–249.

Smits, M.G., van Stel, H.F., van der Heijden, K., Meijer, A.M., Coenen, A.M., & Kerkhof, G.A. (2003). Melatonin improves health status and sleep in children with idiopathic chronic sleep-onset insomnia: A randomized placebo-controlled trial. Journal of the American Academy of Child and Adolescent Psychiatry, 42, 1286–1293.

Snyder, R., Turgay, A., Aman, M., Binder, C., Fisman, S., Carroll, A., et al. (2002). Effects of risperidone on conduct and disruptive behavior disorders in children with subaverage IQs. Journal of the American Academy of Child and Adolescent Psychiatry, 41, 1026–1036.

Sovner, R. (1989). The use of valproate in the treatment of mentally retarded persons with typical and atypical bipolar disorders. Journal of Clinical Psychiatry, 50(Suppl.), 40–43.

Sovner, R. (1991). Use of anticonvulsant agents for treatment of neuropsychiatric disorders in the developmentally disabled. In J.J. Ratey (Ed.), Mental retardation: Developing pharmacotherapies (pp. 83–106). Washington, DC: American Psychiatric Association.

Sovner, R., Pary, R.J., Dosen, A., Gedye, A., Barrera, F.J., Cantwell, D.P., et al. (1998). Antidepressant drugs. In S. Reiss & M.G. Aman (Eds.), Psychotropic medications and developmental disabilities: The international consensus handbook (pp. 179–200). Columbus: The Ohio State University, Nisonger Center.

Spiller, H.A., Klein-Schwartz, W., Colvin, J.M., Villalobos, D., Johnson, P.B., & Anderson, D.L. (2005). Toxic clonidine ingestion in children. Journal of Pediatrics, 146, 263–266.

Stahl, S.M. (2005). Essential psychopharmacology: The prescriber's guide. Cambridge, UK: Cambridge University Press.

Stavrakaki, C., Antochi, R., & Emery, P.C. (2004). Olanzapine in the treatment of pervasive developmental disorders: A case series analysis. Journal of Psychiatry and Neuroscience, 29, 57–60.

Steingard, R., & Biederman, J. (1987). Lithium responsive manic-like symptoms in two individuals with autism and mental retardation. Journal of the American Academy of Child and Adolescent Psychiatry, 26, 932–935.

Steingard, R., Biederman, J., Spencer, T., Wilens, T., & Gonzalez, A. (1993). Comparison of clonidine response in the treatment of attention-deficit hyperactivity disorder with and without comorbid tic disorders. Journal of the American Academy of Child and Adolescent Psychiatry, 32, 350–353.

Steingard, R.J., Connor, D.F., & Trang, A. (2005). Approaches to psychopharmacology. In M.L. Bauman & T.L. Kemper (Eds.), *The neurobiology of autism* (2nd ed., pp. 79–102). Baltimore: The Johns Hopkins University Press.

Steingard, R.J., Zimnitzky, B., DeMaso, D.R., Bauman, M.L., & Bucci, J.P. (1997). Sertraline treatment of transition-associated anxiety and agitation in children with autistic disorder. *Journal of Child and Adolescent Psychopharmacology, 7,* 9–15.

Stigler, K.A., Posey, D.J., & McDougle, C.J. (2004). Aripiprazole for maladaptive behavior in pervasive developmental disorders. *Journal of Child and Adolescent Psychopharmacology, 14,* 455–463.

Stigler, K.A., Potenza, M.N., Posey, D.J., & McDougle, C.J. (2004). Weight gain associated with atypical antipsychotic use in children and adolescents: Prevalence, clinical relevance, and management. *Paediatric Drugs, 6*(1), 33–44.

Stolker, J.J., Heerdink, E.R., Leufkens, H.G., Clerkx, M.G., & Nolen, W.A. (2001). Determinants of multiple psychotropic drug use in patients with mild intellectual disabilities or borderline intellectual functioning and psychiatric or behavioral disorders. *General Hospital Psychiatry, 23,* 345–349.

Stolker, J.J., Koedoot, P.J., Heerdink, E.R., Leufkens, H.G., & Nolen, W.A. (2002). Psychotropic drug use in intellectually disabled group-home residents with behavioural problems. *Pharmacopsychiatry, 35*(1), 19–23.

Stores, G. (1999). Children's sleep disorders: Modern approaches, developmental effects, and children at special risk. *Developmental Medicine and Child Neurology, 41,* 568–573.

Stores, G. (2003). Medication for sleep-wake disorders. *Archives of Disease in Childhood, 88,* 899–903.

Strayhorn, J.M., Jr., Rapp, N., Donina, W., & Strain, P.S. (1988). Randomized trial of methylphenidate for an autistic child. *Journal of the American Academy of Child and Adolescent Psychiatry, 27,* 244–247.

Sugie, Y., Sugie, H., Fukuda, T., Ito, M., Sasada, Y., Nakabayashi, M., et al. (2005). Clinical efficacy of fluvoxamine and functional polymorphism in a serotonin transporter gene on childhood autism. *Journal of Autism and Developmental Disorders, 35,* 377–385.

Symons, F.J., Tapp, J., Wulfsberg, A., Sutton, K.A., Heeth, W.L., & Bodfish, J.W. (2001). Sequential analysis of the effects of naltrexone on the environmental mediation of self-injurious behavior. *Experimental and Clinical Psychopharmacology, 9,* 269–276.

Symons, F.J., Thompson, A., & Rodriguez, M.C. (2004). Self-injurious behavior and the efficacy of naltrexone treatment: A quantitative synthesis. *Mental Retardation and Developmental Disabilities Research Reviews, 10,* 193–200.

Syzmanski, L.S., King, B., Goldberg, B., Reid, A.H., Tonge, B.J., & Cain, N. (1998). Diagnosis of mental disorders in people with mental retardation. In S. Reiss & M.G. Aman (Eds.), *Psychotropic medications and developmental disabilities: The international consensus handbook* (pp. 3–17). Columbus: The Ohio State University, Nisonger Center.

Tasse, M.J., Aman, M.G., Hammer, D., & Rojahn, J. (1996). The Nisonger Child Behavior Rating Form: Age and gender effects and norms. *Research in Developmental Disabilities, 17,* 59–75.

Timmer, R.T., & Sands, J.M. (1999). Lithium intoxication. *Journal of the American Society of Nephrology, 10,* 666–674.

Timmermann, S., Lehrmann, H., Polesskaya, A., & Harel-Bellan, A. (2001). Histone acetylation and disease. *Cellular and Molecular Life Sciences, 58,* 728–736.

Tonge, B., & Einfeld, S. (2000). The trajectory of psychiatric disorders in young people with intellectual disabilities. *Australian and New Zealand Journal of Psychiatry, 34,* 80–84.

Tourette's Syndrome Study Group. (2002). Treatment of ADHD in children with tics: A randomized controlled trial. *Neurology, 58,* 527–536.

Tsai, L.Y. (1999). Psychopharmacology in autism. *Psychosomatic Medicine, 61,* 651–665.

Turgay, A., Binder, C., Snyder, R., & Fisman, S. (2002). Long-term safety and efficacy of risperidone for the treatment of disruptive behavior disorders in children with subaverage IQs. *Pediatrics, 110,* e34.

Turk, J. (2003). Melatonin supplementation for severe and intractable sleep disturbance in young people with genetically determined developmental disabilities: Short review and commentary. *Journal of Medical Genetics, 40,* 793–796.

Tyrer, S.P., Walsh, A., Edwards, D.E., Berney, T.P., & Stephens, D.A. (1984). Factors associated with a good response to lithium in aggressive mentally handicapped subjects. *Progress in Neuro-Psychopharmacology and Biological Psychiatry, 8,* 751–755.

Uvebrant, P., & Bauziene, R. (1994). Intractable epilepsy in children: The efficacy of lamotrigine treatment, including non-seizure-related benefits. *Neuropediatrics, 25,* 284–289.

Valdovinos, M.G., Napolitano, D.A., Zarcone, J.R., Hellings, J.A., Williams, D.C., & Schroeder, S.R. (2002). Multimodal evaluation of risperidone for destructive behavior: Functional analysis, direct observations, rating scales, and psychiatric impressions. *Experimental and Clinical Psychopharmacology, 10,* 268–275.

Van Bellinghen, M., & De Troch, C. (2001). Risperidone in the treatment of behavioral disturbances in children and adolescents with borderline intellectual functioning: A double-blind, placebo-controlled pilot trial. *Journal of Child and Adolescent Psychopharmacology, 11,* 5–13.

Vanden Borre, R., Vermote, R., Buttiens, M., Thiry, P., Dierick, G., Geutjens, J., et al. (1993). Risperidone as add-on therapy in behavioural disturbances in mental retardation: A double-blind placebo-controlled cross-over study. *Acta Psychiatrica Scandinavica, 87,* 167–171.

Verhoeven, W.M., Veendrik-Meekes, M.J., Jacobs, G.A., van den Berg, Y.W., & Tuinier, S. (2001). Citalopram in mentally retarded patients with depression: A long-term clinical investigation. *European Psychiatry: The Journal of the Association of European Psychiatrists, 16,* 104–108.

Vitiello, B., & Wagner, A. (2004). Government initiatives in autism clinical trials. *CNS Spectrums, 9*(1), 66–70.

Vitriol, C., & Farber, B. (1981). Stimulant medication in certain childhood disorders. *American Journal of Psychiatry, 138,* 1517–1518.

Volkmar, F.R., Hoder, E.L., & Cohen, D.J. (1985). Inappropriate uses of stimulant medications. *Clinical Pediatrics, 24,* 127–130.

Wagner, K.D. (2004). Diagnosis and treatment of bipolar disorder in children and adolescents. *Journal of Clinical Psychiatry, 65*(Suppl. 15), 30–34.

Wagner, K.D., Ambrosini, P., Rynn, M., Wohlberg, C., Yang, R., Greenbaum, M.S., et al. (2003). Efficacy of sertraline in the treatment of children and adolescents with major depressive disorder: Two randomized controlled trials. *JAMA, 290,* 1033–1041.

Wagner, K.D., Robb, A.S., Findling, R.L., Jin, J., Gutierrez, M.M., & Heydorn, W.E. (2004). A randomized, placebo-controlled trial of citalopram for the treatment of major depression in children and adolescents. *American Journal of Psychiatry, 161,* 1079–1083.

Wagner, K.D., Weller, E.B., Carlson, G.A., Sachs, G., Biederman, J., Frazier, J.A., et al. (2002). An open-label trial of divalproex in children and adolescents with bipolar disorder. *Journal of the American Academy of Child and Adolescent Psychiatry, 41,* 1224–1230.

West, S.A., Keck, P.E., & McElroy, S.L. (1995). Oral loading doses in the valproate treatment of adolescents with mixed bipolar disorder. *Journal of Child and Adolescent Psychopharmacology, 5,* 225–231.

West, S.A., Keck, P.E., McElroy, S.L., & Strakowski, S.M. (1994). Open trial of valproate in the treatment of adolescent mania. *Journal of Child and Adolescent Psychopharmacology, 4,* 263–267.

Whittington, C.J., Kendall, T., Fonagy, P., Cottrell, D., Cotgrove, A., & Boddington, E. (2004). Selective serotonin reuptake inhibitors in childhood depression: Systematic review of published versus unpublished data. *Lancet, 363,* 1341–1345.

Willemsen-Swinkels, S.H., Buitelaar, J.K., Nijhof, G.J., & van England, H. (1995). Failure of naltrexone hydrochloride to reduce self-injurious and autistic behavior in mentally retarded adults: Double-blind placebo-controlled studies. *Archives of General Psychiatry, 52,* 766–773.

Willemsen-Swinkels, S.H., Buitelaar, J.K., & van Engeland, H. (1996). The effects of chronic naltrexone treatment in young autistic children: A double-blind placebo-controlled crossover study. *Biological Psychiatry, 39,* 1023–1031.

Willemsen-Swinkels, S.H., Buitelaar, J.K., Weijnen, F.G., & van Engeland, H. (1995). Placebo-controlled acute dosage naltrexone study in young autistic children. *Psychiatry Research, 58,* 203–215.

Wolraich, M.L., Greenhill, L.L., Pelham, W., Swanson, J., Wilens, T., Palumbo, D., et al. (2001). Randomized, controlled trial of OROS methylphenidate once a day in children with attention-deficit/hyperactivity disorder. *Pediatrics, 108,* 883–892.

Wozniak, J. (2005). Recognizing and managing bipolar disorder in children. *Journal of Clinical Psychiatry, 66*(Suppl. 1), 18–23.

Yeargin-Allsopp, M., Rice, C., Karapurkar, T., Doernberg, N., Boyle, C., & Murphy, C. (2003). Prevalence of autism in a US metropolitan area. *JAMA, 289,* 49–55.

Zarcone, J.R., Hellings, J.A., Crandall, K., Reese, R.M., Marquis, J., Fleming, K., et al. (2001). Effects of risperidone on aberrant behavior of persons with developmental disabilities: I. A double-blind crossover study using multiple measures. *American Journal on Mental Retardation, 106,* 525–538.

Zarcone, J.R., Lindauer, S.E., Morse, P.S., Crosland, K.A., Valdovinos, M.G., McKerchar, T.L., et al. (2004). Effects of risperidone on destructive behavior of persons with developmental disabilities: III. Functional analysis. *American Journal on Mental Retardation, 109,* 310–321.

Zimmerman, A.W., Bonfardin, B., & Myers, S.M. (2000). Neuropharmacological therapy in autism. In P.J. Accardo, C. Magnusen, & A.J. Capute (Eds.), *Autism: Clinical and research issues* (pp. 241–302). Baltimore: York Press.

Zito, J.M., Safer, D.J., dosReis, S., Gardner, J.F., Boles, M., & Lynch, F. (2000). Trends in the prescribing of psychotropic medications to preschoolers. *JAMA, 283,* 1025–1030.

Zuddas, A., Ledda, M.G., Fratta, A., Muglia, P., & Cianchetti, C. (1996). Clinical effects of clozapine on autistic disorder. *American Journal of Psychiatry, 153,* 738.

29

Traumatic Brain Injury

JAMES CHRISTENSEN,
MELISSA K. TROVATO, CYNTHIA SALORIO, EWA BRANDYS,
OLGA MOROZOVA, CRISTINA SADOWSKY, AND FRANK S. PIDCOCK

Acquired brain injuries (ABIs) in children and adolescents are caused by a wide variety of etiologies, including trauma, central nervous system (CNS) infections, noninfectious disorders (epilepsy, hypoxia-ischemia, genetic/metabolic disorders), CNS tumors, and vascular disorders (Tojo & Nitta, 2003). Of course, there are major differences between pediatric and adult ABIs. Many of these disorders are unique to the pediatric population (e.g., certain genetic/metabolic disorders) or have different differential diagnoses as compared with those for adults (e.g., pediatric stroke). Also, the acquisition of an ABI during development and growth results in different outcomes and in the need for different rehabilitation approaches.

Although there are many causes of ABI in children, traumatic brain injury (TBI) is by far the most common. The incidence of acute stroke in children has been reported as between 1.29 (Earley et al., 1998) and 13.02 per 100,000 per year (Giroud et al., 1995), and the incidence of new CNS tumors is 2.94 per 100,000 children (birth to 14 years of age) (Ries et al., 2004). When these causes are compared with the incidence of TBI, which varies from 100 to 400 per 100,000 (depending on age and sex), the importance of TBI is obvious. Also, TBI comprises a majority of those cases admitted for acute inpatient rehabilitation after ABI, resulting in a large percentage of health care resources dedicated to this problem. Because of these issues, and the overlap that some of the other disorders have with other chapters in this text, we focus on TBI in this chapter.

Acquired spinal cord injuries are discussed in Chapter 30 of this volume.

BRAIN INJURY RESULTING FROM TRAUMA

Trauma is the leading cause of pediatric morbidity and mortality, and brain injury is the most common cause of mortality and the most important determinant of the severity of injury and outcome. When compared with other possible etiologies of acquired nervous system injuries, the relative importance of trauma is overwhelmingly evident.

Neurological function and development can be subtly or dramatically disrupted after TBI. In the literature, the extent of recovery of children and adolescents after TBI has sometimes been overestimated, which can result in residual disabilities being overlooked or minimized. The range of possible neurological deficits secondary to TBI is very wide, but specific disability profiles unique to this group distinguish it from the groups with congenital or other acquired disabilities. These differences are related to the type and distribution of the injury, as well as the stage of neurodevelopment at the time of acquisition. It is important that professionals working with children who have sustained TBIs recognize and appreciate these deficit patterns so that recommendations and management are appropriate.

DEFINITIONS

Head injury classification is usually divided into closed and open head injuries. *Closed head injury,* the most common type, refers to blunt traumatic injuries that result in the acute transfer of mechanical energy to the head but do not penetrate the brain or dura mater. *Open head injury* refers to blunt or penetrating blows that penetrate the dura mater and possibly the brain. This chapter primarily focuses on TBI associated with closed head injury because it is the most common type of injury in children and adolescents. Head injury, by definition, includes injuries other than those to the brain, such as facial, scalp, and skull injuries. Consequently, literature that uses this definition will report significantly higher incidences than literature that reports brain injury only.

Traumatic brain injury refers to any head injury with evidence of brain involvement, as demonstrated by altered level of consciousness (i.e., drowsiness, lethargy, confusion, coma) or focal neurological signs. The depth and duration of objective brain dysfunction correlate strongly with outcome after TBI. Consequently, the periods of coma and posttraumatic amnesia (PTA) are often quantified for prognostic purposes.

Disorders of consciousness (DOC), including coma, have been defined differently in different settings. During recovery, the emergence of consciousness is very important, serving as a marker for prognosis and for determining rehabilitation management. This milestone is determined by evidence of meaningful interaction with the environment, often defined operationally as "following simple commands." Be-

cause of the importance of this milestone, it has been previously used in the rehabilitation setting as the definition of the end of coma and is currently referred to as the "time to follow commands" (TFC). This previous definition was in variance with the strict neurosurgical definition of coma, and failed to distinguish between the period of unwakeful unconsciousness coma and wakeful unconsciousness vegetative state. Consequently, attempts to standardize the terminology of DOC have led to the following lexicon. *Coma* is defined as a state of complete unconsciousness, without eye opening, without sleep–wake cycles, and with no evidence of purposeful behavior or communication (Plum & Posner, 1982). The *vegetative state* is evidenced by spontaneous or stimulus-induced arousal, sleep–wake cycles, and intermittent eye opening but no behavioral signs of environmental or self-awareness and no ability to interact with others (Jennett & Plum, 1972; The Multi-Society Task Force Report on PVS, 1994). To distinguish between the beginning stages of consciousness and full consciousness, the *minimally conscious state* has been defined as the "condition of severely altered consciousness in which minimal but definite behavioral evidence of self or environmental awareness is demonstrated" (Giacino & Trott, 2004, p. 255). Early signs of the transition from vegetative state to minimally conscious state are visual fixation and sustained visual pursuit. Table 29.1 compares the behavioral features of DOC.

Table 29.1. Comparison of behavioral features of disorders of consciousness

Behavior	MCS[a]	VS[b]	Coma
Eye opening	Spontaneous	Spontaneous	None
Spontaneous movement	Automatic behavior Object manipulation	Reflexive/patterned	None
Response to pain	Localization	Posturing/withdrawal	Posturing/none
Visual response	Object recognition Visual pursuit	Startle Visual pursuit (rare)	None
Affective response	Contingent	Random	None
Command following	Inconsistent	None	None
Verbalization	Intelligible words	Random vocalization	None
Communication	Unreliable	None	None

From Giacino, J.T., & Trott, C.T. (2004). Rehabilitative management of patients with disorders of consciousness: Grand rounds. *Journal of Head Trauma Rehabilitation, 19*(3), 254–265; reprinted by permission.
[a]Minimally conscious state.
[b]Vegetative state.

Memory disorders are very common after TBI. *Posttraumatic amnesia* is that period of time after injury during which the patient has no continuous memory (also referred to as anterograde amnesia); however, it is not, as the definition might suggest, simply a period of impaired memory. It is also a time of confusion and often agitation, comparable to an organic delirium. Some authors will time the period of PTA from the initial trauma, and others from the end of the coma. Its end often correlates historically with the point at which the family states that the patient "woke up" or "came to him- or herself." PTA does not end abruptly, but rather gradually resolves. Objective measures have therefore been developed to document the period of PTA. The most commonly used measures are the Galveston Orientation and Amnesia Test (GOAT; Levin, O'Donnell, & Grossman, 1979) for adults and the Children's Orientation and Amnesia Test (COAT; Ewing-Cobbs, Levin, Fletcher, Miner, & Eisenberg, 1990). The COAT is normed on typically developing children 3–15 years of age, and the termination of PTA is considered to have occurred when the patient scores within 2 standard deviations of the mean for age on 2 consecutive days. There may also be a period of retrograde amnesia for events before and up to the time of the injury. This period of amnesia usually gradually shrinks with time and is not prognostically useful.

Severity of injury is defined by the depth, duration, or both of objective nervous system dysfunction. The Glasgow Coma Scale (GCS) score is used for depth of dysfunction. Severe TBI is defined as a GCS score of 3–8, moderate TBI as a GCS score of 9–12, and mild TBI as a GCS score of 13–15. Length of coma, PTA, or both are used to define the duration of dysfunction. There are discrepancies in the criteria used, both in the literature and in reference manuals; however, severe TBI is usually defined as coma of 6 hours or more or PTA of 24 hours or more (Jennett & Teasdale, 1981).

EPIDEMIOLOGY

In the general population, approximately 1.5 million Americans sustain a TBI each year, and approximately one-quarter million are hospitalized and survive (National Center for Injury Prevention and Control, 1999). It is an important public health issue, as illustrated by the estimated lifetime costs of TBI in the United States, which are staggering, totaling approximately $56.3 billion in 1995 (Thurman, 2001).

In the pediatric population, trauma is the major cause of morbidity and mortality, and head trauma is the single most important determinant of the severity of injury and outcome. A sobering statistic is that the estimated cumulative risk of brain injury for American children through age 15 years is 4% in boys and 2.3% in girls (Rivara & Mueller, 1986).

Because of lack of previous long-term surveillance systems, we often need to use different data sets for looking at the changing epidemiology of TBI. This is possible because data on mortality, hospitalization, and incidence mirror each other. Of course, because most TBI is mild, the hospitalization rate will always be less than the incidence.

In 1984, Kraus et al. reported that the incidence of TBI was highest in males ages 10–29 years, with the peak incidence between 15 and 19 years. Incidence for boys increased steadily from about 150–200 per 100,000 for those younger than 5 years old to greater than 400 per 100,000 for those age 15 years. Incidence for girls reached a peak of approximately 200 per 100,000 (Kraus et al., 1984).

Fortunately, mortality and hospitalizations have been declining, related to improved injury prevention measures and changes in hospitalization admission practices. According to National Hospital Discharge Survey data, the annual incidence rate of TBI hospitalizations has been declining since 1975, when it peaked at 234 per 100,0000 (approximately 230,000 cases; Thurman, Alverson, Dunn, Guerrero, & Sniezek, 1999). TBI surveillance data for 1997 show an age-adjusted TBI-related hospital discharge rate of 69.7 per 100,000 (Table 29.2). The highest incidence is in 15- to 19-year-olds and those 65 years of age or older. Within those populations, the highest incidence (139.9 per 100,000) is in 15- to 19-year-old males (Langlois et al., 2003). These studies report an approximately 2:1 male-to-female ratio, compatible with the literature.

Table 29.2. Traumatic brain injury–related hospital discharge rates (per 100,000 population) by selected causes

	Total	All traffic	Motor-cycle	MV[a] Occupant	Pedal cyclist	Pedes-trian	Falls	Struck by/ against	Assault	Self-inflicted
All ages	69.3	28.0	1.7	19.8	1.3	4.2	22.1	2.6	7.4	0.3
0–4	64.0	12.8	—	7.8	0.3	4.5	36.3	3.3	5.1	—
5–14	48.1	19.1	0.6	8.1	3.5	6.5	13.1	4.1	1.2	—
15–19	103.5	62.7	2.5	49.9	2.3	5.4	9.6	5.3	12.1	0.5

Adapted from tables in Langlois, J.A., Kegler, S.R., Butler, J.A., Gotsch, K.E., Johnson, R.L., Reichard, A.A., et al. (2003). Traumatic brain injury-related hospital discharges: Results from a 14-state surveillance system, 1997. *Morbidity and Mortality Weekly Report: CDC Surveillance Summaries, 52*(4), 1–20.

[a]Motor vehicle.

Injury does not occur randomly in the population. Race and ethnicity are markers for risk factors for injuries (e.g., socioeconomic status) (Centers for Disease Control and Prevention, 1993). Overall, age-adjusted rates are highest for American Indians/Alaska Natives and African Americans, but substantial variation by age and sex occurs (Langlois et al., 2003). Inner-city African Americans have a higher incidence of head injuries than those in the suburbs (Whitman, Coonley-Hoganson, & Desai, 1984). As noted by Rivara,

For all races, injury death rates are inversely related to income level, and much, if not all, of the difference seen in death rates between racial groups may be the result of differences in income. . . . The reasons for the increased risk of poor children probably include both decreased supervision, lower levels of information about and use of prevention strategies (such as bicycle helmets), and exposure to more hazardous environments such as high-rise tenements (leading to falls from windows) and higher volume, faster moving traffic (resulting in pedestrian injuries). (1994, p. 14)

Children with premorbid learning difficulties and attention and behavior problems are also more prone to injuries. Although many early studies failed to show that children with head injuries have significantly more premorbid emotional and behavior problems than other children in the community (Pelco, Sawyer, Duffield, Prior, & Kinsella, 1992), other studies have shown a higher than expected number of head-injured patients with premorbid behavior and learning problems (Mahoney et al., 1983). In one study, premorbid prevalence of attention-deficit/hyperactivity disorder (ADHD) was 0.20, significantly higher than

in a reference population (Gerring et al., 1998). Substance abuse also clearly is associated with many severe injuries, especially in the adolescent and adult populations.

MECHANISM OF INJURY

The mechanism of TBI varies with age at time of injury and with severity of injury. The major causes of pediatric brain injury are falls, motor vehicle crashes, recreational accidents, and assaults. Falls constitute a much larger percentage of mild than severe injuries, and the opposite is true for motor vehicle–related injuries. Based on hospital discharges, motor vehicle crashes, falls, and assaults are also the leading causes of TBI for the general population. From a pediatric perspective, hospital discharge data show the following: 15- to 19-year-olds have the highest rate related to motor vehicle crashes; birth to 4-year-olds have a high rate of falls (surpassed only by those $\geq$ 65 years of age); 15- to 19-year-olds have the second highest rate of assaults (surpassed only by 20- to 24-year-olds); birth to 4-year-olds have a higher rate of assaults than 5- to 14-year-olds, related to inflicted trauma; and motor vehicle–related crashes as a cyclist or pedestrian are more common in the pediatric age range, especially in 5- to 14-year-olds (Langlois et al., 2003).

Sports and recreational activities are also an important cause of TBI. The age-related incidence mirrors that of other causes, with a similar peak in the adolescent and young adult ages. Of those head injuries (most of which are mild) that result from competitive sports and were evaluated in an emergency department, the majority are associated with basketball, baseball, and football. This relates to both the frequency of participation in these sports and the inherent risks in each. Among noncompetitive recreational activities resulting in an emergency department visit, playground activities were the most common cause (Thurman, Branche, & Sniezek, 1998).

TYPE OF INJURY

Injuries sustained as a result of mechanical forces that are imparted to the brain can be divided into two groups: primary (immediate) and secondary (delayed). Primary injuries are divided into contusions and diffuse axonal injury (DAI). Second insults are those factors such as hypoxia and hypotension. Secondary injuries are the brain's response to the events following the primary injury and second insults and are mediated through factors such as excitotoxicity, inflammation, apoptosis or delayed cell death, lipid peroxidation, and protein synthesis. Second insults and secondary injuries are now known to be major contributors to worsened morbidity and mortality (Kochanek, Clark, Benn, Whalen, & Adelson, 1998; Levin et al., 1992). These injuries and their distribution are unique to TBI and result in disability profiles that are also unique, distinguishing them from disability profiles of other groups of children with organic brain injury.

Contusions are areas of bruising or local tissue injury. A *coup injury* is a focal contusion, occurring at the point of contact when a moving object strikes the head (e.g., in a fight) or the moving head strikes an object (e.g., with a fall), resulting in low-velocity, short-duration forces. The *contrecoup lesion* occurs 180 degrees opposite to the coup injury (although the concept of contrecoup has been questioned); however, the distribution of contusions in severe TBI, related to long-duration, high-velocity forces, does not follow the coup-contrecoup distribution. Instead, contusions occur where the brain decelerates on bony prominences, classically in the orbitofrontal and anterotemporal regions, as well as the brain stem (Auerbach, 1986) (Figure 29.1). A Contusion Index exists for quantification of injury (Adams et al., 1985).

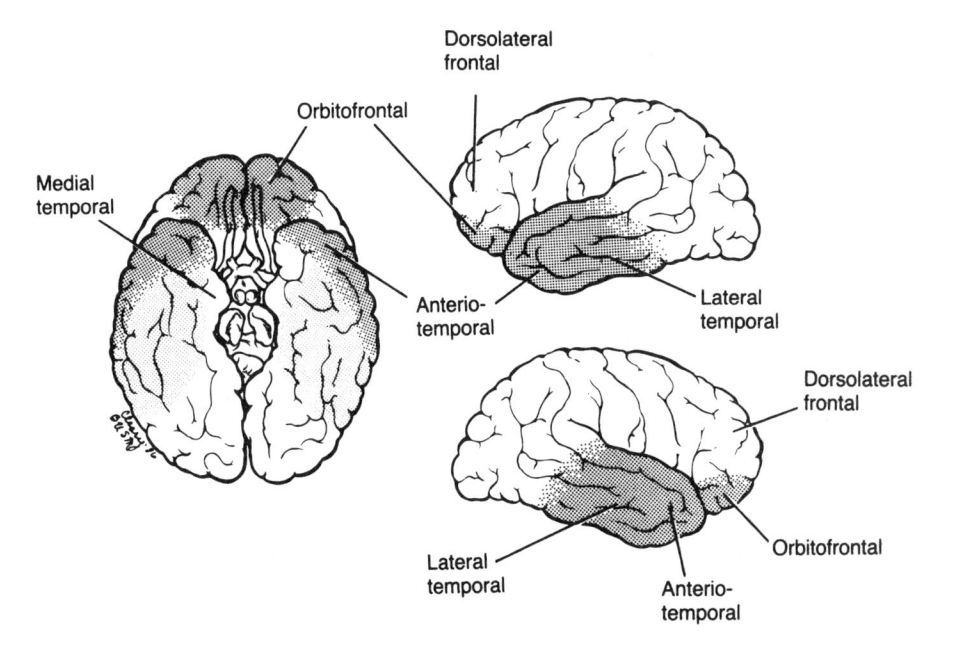

Figure 29.1.   Areas predominantly affected by cortical contusions. Darker shading represents more frequently involved areas. Anterotemporal and orbitofrontal regions are particularly involved. Note relative sparing of dorsolateral frontal lobe and medial temporal lobe. (From Auerbach, S.H. [1986]. Neuroanatomical correlates of attention and memory disorders in traumatic brain injury: An application of neurobehavioral subtypes. *Journal of Head Trauma Rehabilitation, 1*[3], 1–12; reprinted by permission.)

DAI, or shearing injury, may result in a physical interruption of axons. It occurs with long-duration trauma associated with acceleration-deceleration and rotational forces. Its most common distribution is in the corpus callosum, subcortical white matter, midbrain, and cerebellar peduncles (Auerbach, 1986) (Figure 29.2). Histologically, three grades of DAI have been identified:

> In grade 1 there is histological evidence of axonal injury in the white matter of the cerebral hemispheres, the corpus callosum, the brain stem and, less commonly, the cerebellum; in grade 2 there is also a focal lesion in the corpus callosum; and in grade 3 there is in addition a focal lesion in the dorsolateral quadrant or quadrants of the rostral brain stem. The focal lesions can often only be identified microscopically. (Adams et al., 1989, p. 49)

Originally, the physical discontinuity of the axons and resultant neuronal death was thought to result from the physical forces at the time of the injury. It is now recognized that some, if not most, of the axonal damage noted on light microscopy is a consequence of complicated pathological processes that begin with the initial trauma and then proceed to ultrastructural changes and interruption of axonal transport. This may later culminate in axonal transection and formation of neuroaxonal spheroids. The initial insults appear to cause transient alteration of the integrity of the axonal membrane, associated with changes in ionic (calcium, sodium, potassium) concentrations, axonal transport disruption, excitotoxic transmitter effect, free radical formation, and lipid peroxidation. Mitochondrial dysfunction also develops (McArthur, Chute, & Villablanca, 2004).

In addition to neuronal death, glial cell death related to contusions and DAI also contributes to the overall pathology of TBI, and the dying neural cells can exhibit either an apoptotic or necrotic morphology. Although processes such as increases in excitatory amino acids and intracellular calcium and free radicals can cause necrotic cell death, they can also cause cells to undergo apoptosis. In addition, there may be many other pathways that lead to apoptotic cell death after TBI, in light of the effect of TBI on cellular expression of survival promoting–proteins and death-inducing proteins (Raghupathi, 2004).

Other immediate injuries relate to disruption of blood vessels and secondary bleeding, resulting in subarachnoid, intraventricular, or intracerebral hemorrhage. Delayed injuries or effects of TBI include delayed bleeding, resulting in epidural or subdural hematomas; edema with secondary focal or diffuse increased pressure or both, resulting in hypoperfusion injuries or herniation syndromes associated with focal infarcts (posterior cerebral artery, mesial

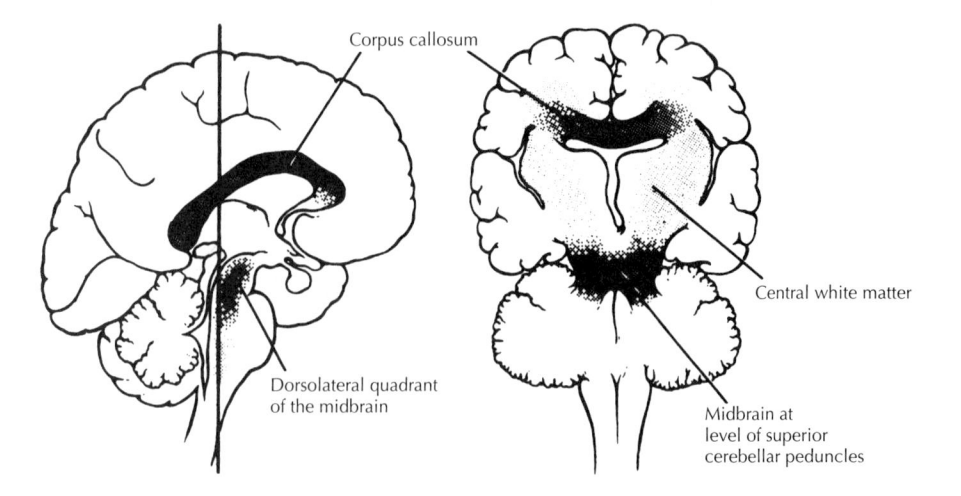

Figure 29.2. Brain regions particularly involved by diffuse axonal injury, including corpus callosum and parasagittal white matter, as well as dorsolateral quadrants of the midbrain. (From Auerbach, S.H. [1986]. Neuroanatomical correlates of attention and memory disorders in traumatic brain injury: An application of neurobehavioral subtypes. *Journal of Head Trauma Rehabilitation, 1*[3], 1–12; reprinted by permission.)

temporal lobe, brain stem); and hydrocephalus. Of course, additional related injuries can also be sustained. Cardiopulmonary arrest or shock may result in a hypoxic-ischemic encephalopathy superimposed on the traumatic injury, which will change the injury and the prognosis for the worse.

PROGNOSIS

Multiple factors predict outcome, including individual and family characteristics and markers of injury severity and trajectory of recovery.

Injury Severity Factors and Trajectory of Recovery

The previously described classification of severity is based on clinical markers that have been shown to exhibit a "dose-response" relationship between severity of injury, trajectory of recovery, and outcome. These factors—GCS score, TFC, and duration of PTA—are the best predictors of long-term outcome.

In general, children and adolescents with mild uncomplicated TBI (GCS scores of 13–15) have good long-term outcomes. Most studies examining cohorts of children and adolescents with mild TBI have failed to show differences from control groups on a variety of long-term outcome measures, including cognition, language, achievement, intellect, adaptive problem solving, memory, motor skills, independent living, and social skills (Bijur, Haslum, & Golding, 1990; Fay et al., 1993; Jordan, Cannon, & Murdoch, 1992). A review of the literature confirmed this and concluded that there was consistent and methodologically sound evidence that the prognosis in children after mild TBI is good, with quick resolution of symptoms and little evidence of residual cognitive, behavioral, or academic deficits (Carroll et al., 2004); however, mild TBI may have at least temporary effects, and these need to be addressed appropriately. One study demonstrated that, after 4–6 weeks, 23 of 98 patients still exhibited posttraumatic complaints of headache, fatigue, sleep disturbances, anxiety, and affect instability (Korinthenberg, Schreck, Weser, & Lehmkuhl, 2004). Slowed response time and balance deficits have been shown to

persist until 12 weeks postinjury, which can have educational and recreational implications (Gagnon, Swaine, Friedman, & Forget, 2004a, 2004b). Also, there may be some long-lasting effects. In a recent population study, children with a negative psychiatric history for the year preceding their mild TBI were at significantly increased risk for psychiatric illness for the 3 subsequent years, particularly hyperactivity in the first year after injury (Massagli et al., 2004). Clinical pathways to improve the quality and consistency of care provided to children after mild TBI are available and stress the need for standardized discharge instructions, identification of high-risk children, and appropriate patient/family education (Kamerling, Lutz, Posner, & Vanore, 2003).

One group at high risk for persisting problems and who should be identified early and followed more closely is those with previous head injury; preexisting learning difficulties; or neurological, psychiatric, or family problems (Ponsford et al., 1999). Concerning interventions, family/patient education has been demonstrated to lower the incidence of ongoing problems after mild TBI. In one study, families of children with mild TBI who were given an information booklet outlining symptoms associated with mild TBI and suggested coping strategies reported fewer symptoms overall and were less stressed 3 months after injury (Ponsford et al., 2001).

Exceptions to the rule of good outcome after mild TBI certainly exist. Some of these exceptions are explained by "complicated" mild TBIs (e.g., with depressed skull fracture, intracranial lesion, focal neurological signs), which for prognostic purposes should be clustered with moderate TBI (Williams, Levin, & Eisenberg, 1990). Other exceptions are explained by inaccurate classification, usually because of reliance on GCS score and length of coma, and failure to reclassify based on prolonged PTA. Also, whether those with a GCS score of 13 should be considered to have mild or moderate TBI has recently been questioned, based on a study reporting that 33.8% of patients with a GCS score of 13 had an intracranial lesion and 10.8% required emergency surgery (Stein, 2001).

After both moderate and severe TBI, children have persisting and comprehensive neurobehavioral deficits that have an impact on real-life functioning as evidenced by school achievement tests and grades (Fay et al., 1994). Also, there is a strong correlation between severity and neurobehavioral outcome (Jaffe, Polissar, Fay, & Liao, 1995).

Outcome in severe TBI has a very wide range, in part because of the wide variation of severity within the category designated as "severe." It is intuitively obvious that the severity of injury is different between someone with a coma duration of 6 hours as compared with 3 months, yet both will be described as having severe TBI. Consequently, it is important to examine the two ends of the spectrum and to have different outcome expectations.

At the severe end of the severe TBI category, one can be optimistic that recovery will occur but that there will be significant long-term impairments. In one cohort with a median duration of coma (TFC) between 5 and 6 weeks, 73% regained independence in ambulation and self-care, 10% remained partially dependent in self-care and achieved only limited ambulation, 9% regained consciousness but were totally dependent, and 8% remained comatose. When the length of coma (TFC) was less than 6 weeks, 94% of the patients had the better outcome. On neurological examination, 10% were said to be "normal," but in this group intellectual deficits and severe emotional problems were common; only 28% of this "normal" group scored within 1 standard deviation of the mean on intelligence testing within 1 year of injury (Brink, Imbus, & Woo-Sam, 1980).

The length of PTA correlates strongly with long-term outcome (McDonald et al., 1994) and is often a better indicator of outcome than is coma, especially for the milder end of the severe TBI category. This is in part because of the difficulty in determining the length of coma accurately in patients who are pharmacologically sedated or paralyzed as part of their acute medical treatment and in part because the duration of PTA can vary widely in patients with short or even absent coma. Rutter, Chadwick, Brown, and their colleagues (Brown, Chadwick, Shaffer, Rutter, & Traub, 1981; Chad-

wick, Rutter, Brown, Shaffer, & Traub, 1981; Rutter, Chadwick, Shaffer, & Brown, 1980) described the milder end of the severe TBI spectrum. In their study, cognitive evaluations showed evidence of transient intellectual impairment in a minority of subjects with PTA of less than 2 weeks and in a majority of subjects with PTA of 2–3 weeks. Although the general measures of intelligence for the severe TBI group were within the "normal" range at long-term follow-up, persistent intellectual impairment was observed in a majority with PTA of 3 weeks or more. Of these individuals, 77.8% had persistent schoolwork difficulties ($2\frac{1}{2}$-year follow-up). In addition, more than half of those with PTA of 1 week or more developed new and persistent psychiatric sequelae. These psychiatric disorders attributable to head injuries were different when compared with those of controls in that there was increased social disinhibition and a slight tendency for the disorders to show greater persistence over time. From these studies of severe TBI, it can be appreciated that cognitive and behavioral problems are the rule and that physical problems are common in the more severely injured patients.

In addition to the length of coma or PTA as a predictor, the depth of coma within the severe category is also useful. Massagli et al. (1996) reported greater impairment in those patients with initial GCS score of 3–5, and Kraus, Fife, and Conroy (1987) found that 100% of those patients with an initial GCS score of 3 or 4 had at least moderate disability, whereas only 65% of those with a GCS score of 5–8 had this outcome.

Neuroimaging and Outcome

A variety of imaging techniques and parameters have been shown to correlate with severity of injury, prognosis, and specific outcomes. The depth of lesion correlates with severity (GCS score) and functional outcome (Disability Rating Scale) (Grados et al., 2001). The number and volume of lesions on magnetic resonance imaging (MRI) relate to severity of injury parameters (Tong et al., 2004). On MRI volumetric studies, greater preservation of volume of frontotemporal tissue is related to better functional recovery (Wilde et al., 2005). On magnetic resonance spectroscopy, N-acetylaspartate/choline concentration was lower in TBI patients than in control subjects; cognition was lower in the TBI group than the control group and correlated with N-acetylaspartate levels (Hunter et al., 2005).

Lesion–deficit correlation studies have described the relationship between lesion size/location and cognitive and behavioral/psychiatric outcomes. Cognitive outcome studies have shown the following: the size of frontal lobe lesion enhanced the relationship between cognitive performance and the severity of injury (Levin et al., 1993); greater extrafrontal lesion volume and total number of lesions were predictive of worse performance on letter fluency (Slomine et al., 2002); and the area of the corpus callosum that sustained injury correlated strongly with measures involving processing speed and visuospatial function (Verger et al., 2001).

Behavioral and psychiatric studies have shown the following: greater damage to the orbitofrontal cortex is associated with decreased risk for anxiety (Vasa et al., 2004); lesions in the right limbic system may inhibit subsequent manifestation of the reexperiencing symptoms of posttraumatic stress disorder (Herskovits, Gerring, Davatzikos, & Bryan, 2002); there is an association between secondary ADHD (S-ADHD) and injury in either the thalamus or the basal ganglia or both (Gerring et al., 2000); and the presence and volume of unilateral frontal lesions adversely affect psychosocial outcome (Levin et al., 2004).

Individual and Family Factors Affecting Prognosis

Although age has been cited as an important predictor of outcome, its importance should not be exaggerated. It is clear that pediatric mortality related to trauma is less than that for adults (Tepas, DiScala, Ramenofsky, & Barlow, 1990), but the degree of residual disability in children seems no less than that in adults with trauma of similar severity (Costeff, Groswasser, & Goldstein, 1990). Within the pediatric age range, some studies have shown no difference in morbidity with age (Chadwick et al.,

1981), but many have shown that older children do better than younger children (Brink, Garrett, Hale, Woo-Sam, & Nickel, 1970; Levin, Eisenberg, Wigg, & Kobayashi, 1982; Slomine et al., 2002; Verger et al., 2000).

The fact that prognosis after TBI is better in older than younger children does not follow the general rule in pediatric brain injury—that outcome is better with earlier insults. There are many possible explanations for this difference. Plasticity, which is so important in recovery from focal brain injuries (i.e., infantile strokes), may be at a disadvantage because of the diffuse nature of the injuries. The younger brain may be more susceptible to the effects of trauma because of its different physical (i.e., less myelinated) and neurochemical (i.e., increased excitatory amino acids) properties. Mechanism of injury is different depending on age, which may result in differences in the primary injury. Another explanation is related to the negative effects of TBI on neuropsychological processes required for new learning, the effects of which are more devastating to the younger child who still has much to learn, as contrasted with an adolescent who has already learned and retained large stores of knowledge and overlearned skills.

The role of gender is being investigated because of the apparent protective effect of the sex hormones estrogen and progesterone. In a review of data from the National Pediatric Trauma Registry on nonpenetrating traumatic brain injury, there were no statistically significant differences between boys and girls in total hospital length of stay, functional outcome, and discharge location; however, for every outcome there was a trend toward girls having worse outcomes, which was the opposite of the hypothesized effect of gender (Morrison, Arbelaez, Fackler, De Maio, & Paidas, 2004).

Factors that reflect family and individual functioning are also important in determining outcome. As a general rule, recovery is better for children who have better preinjury individual functioning (cognitive and behavioral) and whose families have more resources and less stress and can provide more structure. In a study by Yeates et al. (1997), measures of the preinjury family environment accounted for approximately 25% of the variance in behavioral outcomes 6 and 12 months after moderate and severe TBI. Interestingly, the effect of pre-injury functioning may be variable, depending on the outcome assessed. In a study by Rivara et al. (1994), most of the variation in behavioral outcomes was explained by preinjury child or family factors, whereas poor academic and cognitive outcomes were primarily associated with injury severity and, to a lesser degree, poor preinjury family and child functioning.

OUTCOME

Cognition

During the first year after moderate and severe TBI, measures of intellectual abilities usually improve to within the normal range but not to pretraumatic levels and then subsequently plateau (Jaffe, Polissar, Fay, & Liao, 1995). Because general measures of intelligence usually return to within the normal range, they cannot be used as the sole measure when evaluating someone with posttraumatic academic, cognitive, and behavioral problems. Instead, evaluations need to assess specific neuropsychological processes known to be affected by TBI. Although any process can be affected, those most affected by trauma are memory, attention, speed, and executive function. Impairments in any of these areas can create havoc in vocational and avocational pursuits, in spite of well-preserved skills and fund of knowledge.

Memory impairment has been reported to be the most common cognitive deficit following pediatric TBI, seen in almost half of patients (Levin & Eisenberg, 1979). It is seen after both moderate and severe TBI and is often a disabling problem. It results in impairments in learning and remembering new information, abilities that are essential for good academic performance (Levin, 1989; Miller & Donders, 2003; Van Zomeren & Van Den Berg, 1985; Yeates, 2000). Although memory significantly improves during the first year following TBI in children, persisting deficits in memory can be found 6 months (Catroppa & Anderson, 2002), 1 year, 3 years (Jaffe et al., 1992, 1993, 1995), and 4–5 years (Yeates et al., 2002) postinjury.

Disorders of attention are also common after TBI. In one study, 19% of the study population developed S-ADHD postinjury, and this percentage excluded the 20% with preinjury ADHD. Children who developed S-ADHD had significantly greater premorbid psychosocial adversity, posttraumatic affective lability and aggression, posttraumatic psychiatric comorbidity, and overall disability than children who did not develop S-ADHD (Gerring et al., 1998). In another study in which 52% of the study population was cases with mild TBI, the development of ADHD symptoms in the first 2 years after injury was significantly related to injury severity and to the degree of family dysfunction (Max, Arndt, et al., 1998). Attentional sequelae after TBI, including sustained, selective, and shifting attention and slower speed of processing, show worse performance with increasing severity of injury. Also, the deficits are most evident on more complex and timed tasks, which is important to remember when one is evaluating the patient in a controlled, one-on-one clinic setting (Catroppa & Anderson, 2005).

Speed of response is a significant problem for people after TBI and may pervade all functions/responses. Speed of information processing often underlies the poor performance on cognitive and linguistic tasks. This is illustrated by its negative effect on new learning on a memory task (the California Verbal Learning Test–Children's Version [CVLT-C; Dolis, Kramer, Kaplan, & Ober, 1994]) after pediatric TBI (Donders & Minnema, 2004). Slow motor response time has been noted with all degrees of severity of TBI, as previously discussed. The importance of speed of response should not be underestimated. It is one of the factors that correlates highly with real-life outcomes such as social autonomy, ability to work, and vocational outcome (Mazaux et al., 1997; Nybo & Koskiniemi, 1999).

Executive function is defined as the capacity for self-direction and self-control/regulation. It is described as those mental processes necessary for the formulation of goals, the planning of how to achieve them, and then carrying out the plans effectively (Lezak, 1982, 1995). Executive function can also be thought of as those processes that allow mental flexibility—the ability to initiate and sustain thoughts and plans appropriately, inhibit unwanted thoughts and actions, and yet mentally "shift gears" when appropriate. The frontal lobes are linked to executive function (Auerbach, 1986), and, because of the unique distribution of injury sustained with TBI, executive function is particularly vulnerable and often impaired. Like other neuropsychological processes, executive function changes and becomes more complex with development (Levin et al., 1996; Welsh, Pennington, & Groisser, 1991). After TBI, a failure or arrest in the expected development of executive function is not unusual in children, given the frontal lobe injuries. Clinically, this can appear as if "new" deficits and problems are emerging. These "new" problems often manifest themselves during times of increased expectations for self-direction and self-control/regulation. This often occurs during transition from one school level to another, such as from a highly structured elementary classroom to a less structured middle school. Anticipatory guidance is critical during these transitions.

Those individuals who do not return to within normal limits of general intelligence are the exceptions after TBI and are usually those with extremely severe injuries and those who are young. In a retrospective study of patients with severe brain injury (ages 2–18 years, with average duration of coma of 7 weeks), there was a direct relationship between general measures of intelligence (intelligence quotient [IQ] score) and severity of injury in severe brain injury, with IQ score being depressed for the more severe end of the severe brain injury spectrum. Also, children younger than 10 years of age (most of whom were younger than 6 years of age) had more severe reduction in intelligence than did children older than 10, given the same length of coma (Brink et al., 1970). Others have also confirmed a "dose–response curve" between measures of intellectual functioning and severity of injury (Chadwick et al., 1981; Jaffe et al., 1992, 1993).

Communication Effects

Verbal communication may be impaired secondary to speech or language dysfunction or both. Motor speech disorders are common after TBI and tend to show improvement with time. They include mutism (Dayer, Roulet, Maeder, & Deonna, 1998; Levin et al., 1983), aprosodia (Wymer, Lindman, & Booksh, 2002), oral-motor apraxia, dysarthria, and difficulties with breath control resulting in short length of utterance, whispering, or a monotone voice (Massagli & Jaffe, 1994). Recent studies utilizing quantitative analyses of speech and articulation have revealed different underlying articulatory kinematic profiles that have important implications for the treatment of speech rate disturbances in children with dysarthria following TBI (Murdoch & Goozee, 2003). These quantitative techniques have also shown that, even in those patients who did not have dysarthria after TBI, there were significant impairments in many areas of oral-motor function (Cahill, Murdoch, & Theodoros, 2002).

Language function may be impaired secondary to cognitive dysfunction or to specific language deficits. TBI has direct adverse effects on language development (Morse et al., 1999), including lexical development, discourse processes (Chapman et al., 2004; Ewing-Cobbs, Brookshire, Scott, & Fletcher, 1998), and reading. Young children who sustain severe TBI are particularly vulnerable to linguistic deficits at both the lexical and discourse levels, whereas TBI in older children and adolescents preferentially disrupts higher order discourse functions (Ewing-Cobbs & Barnes, 2002). Although the classic aphasias associated with strokes are not seen in uncomplicated TBI, aphasic symptoms are seen, including inability to name objects or remember names, word retrieval problems, and auditory and reading comprehension deficits (Carney & Schoenbrodt, 1994).

Impaired cognition plays an important role in the language problems after TBI. "Attention, memory, conceptual organization, speed of processing, and analysis and synthesis of such things as environmental cues and conversation are all related to language formulation. These executive functions support language processing, and when they are disrupted, language is impaired" (Carney & Schoenbrodt, 1994, p. 49).

Academic Effects

Academic function is affected by the cognitive, language, behavior, and motor impairments related to TBI. Injury severity and neuropsychological performance (both early and late) are related to need for special education after TBI (Kinsella et al., 1997) and to academic performance (Fay et al., 1994). Miller and Donders (2003) reported that children who obtained a low score on the CVLT-C during initial postinjury neuropsychological assessment were 8–13 times more likely to be placed in special education 12–24 months later compared with children who obtained higher scores. In another study, 76% of children with TBI who had significant behavioral problems had difficulties with schoolwork and scored lower on IQ tests (Hawley, 2004).

More specifically, tests of academic achievement show that both reading and mathematics can be affected. One study measured reading ability in a group of 88 children who sustained depressed skull fractures. At least 2 years postinjury, 55% were reading 1 or more years below their age peers; 33% performed more than 3 years behind their chronological ages. Reading disability was also more common in those injured before 9 years of age (Shaffer, Bijur, Chadwick, & Rutter, 1980). The educational management of these issues, including the issue of discrepant performance related to overlearned rote skills versus novel tasks, in discussed in Chapter 31 of this volume.

Psychiatric/Behavioral Effects

The posttraumatic psychiatric sequelae of TBI, both behavioral and emotional, vary with the severity and location of injury, the phase of recovery, the premorbid personality of the patient, and the psychosocial environment. Persistent psychiatric problems are very common after severe head injury, and their presence contributes significantly to a poor late outcome. Brown et al. (1981) reported that slightly more than half of their group of children and adolescents with severe head injury with 1 or more weeks of PTA developed persistent psychiatric problems (through $2\frac{1}{2}$ years of follow-up). They found that the types of behavior profiles were not dissimilar to those of other children with behavior problems, with the exception of symptoms of increased disin-

hibition. This high percentage of psychiatric problems continues to be reported. Max, Koele, et al. (1998) noted that, of those children who sustained a severe TBI and did not have a premorbid psychiatric history, 63% had psychiatric disorders at 2-year follow-up. They also reported that approximately 40% of their severe TBI subjects had ongoing persistent personality changes (on follow-up at an average of 2 years postinjury) (Max et al., 2000; Max, Robertson, & Lansing, 2001). The personality changes described were the labile subtype of personality change (49%), aggressive and disinhibited subtypes (38% each), apathy (14%), and paranoia (5%) (Max et al., 2000). As noted previously in the section on attention, S-ADHD is a common problem after TBI. Also, a variety of postinjury anxiety disorders, including posttraumatic stress disorder, overanxious disorder, separation anxiety disorder, obsessive-compulsive disorder, and simple phobia, develop after childhood TBI (Vasa et al., 2002).

Motor Effects

The degree and type of motor impairment are related to the severity and location of injury. Much of the severe, permanent motor impairment is related to injury of the subcortical gray and white matter, including the brain stem and cerebellar peduncles. Although motor outcome in the mild end of the severe TBI group is generally good, abilities rarely return to normal. Even if the classic motor examination appears normal, there will usually be deficits related to speed of performance (Chaplin, Deitz, & Jaffe, 1993). In the best of recoveries, this is usually enough to take away any competitive edge in fine motor performance (athletics, instrumental music). Significant improvements in motor abilities are expected after moderate to severe TBI, yet on follow-up, differences in measures such as gait velocity, stride length, and hand function of children with brain injuries versus controls are still present at 8 months postinjury, and hand motor skills improved less than gait (Kuhtz-Buschbeck et al., 2003).

In those children with more severe injuries, there is usually significant long-term motor impairment. In Brink et al.'s (1980) group (average coma 5–6 weeks), neurological assessment revealed that most children had spasticity (38%), ataxia (8%), or a combination of both (39%). The combination of ataxia and spasticity is often related to a brain stem/cerebellar outflow tract injury, secondary to the susceptibility of this region to DAI and contusions. If this injury is asymmetrical, as it often is, it will result in contralateral spasticity and ipsilateral ataxia.

Balance problems are very common after TBI, as previously noted, even in children with mild TBI for a period of time (Gagnon et al., 2004a). Posttraumatic tremor is not uncommon with severe brain injury. In a survey of 289 children with severe head injury, prevalence of tremor was at least 45%, presenting up to 18 months postinjury and subsiding spontaneously in at least 50% of cases (Johnson & Hall, 1992). Intention tremor (associated with other symptoms of ataxia) is the most common type of significant tremor seen. Postural or action tremors, resting tremors, and other associated movements (myoclonus, *mouvemente oppositionniste*) can also be seen, usually in combination with other signs of ataxia, and are related to the brain stem injury involving the cerebellar outflow tracts, including the red nucleus, dentate nucleus, and thalamus (Harmon, Long, & Shirtz, 1991; Saitoh, Ueki, Yamada, Mori, & Iwasa, 1991). The list of potential medications to use is long, and these tremors are difficult to treat pharmacologically. Neurosurgical procedures have been used in selected cases (Krauss, Mohadjer, Nobbe, & Mundinger, 1994).

Dystonia may occur secondary to TBI. Although it may be present during the acute period, it may also present in a delayed fashion. Lee, Rinne, Ceballos-Baumann, Thompson, and Marsden (1994) reported 18 cases with severe head injury whose onset of dystonia was at 18 months on average (range, 1 month to 9 years), and 11 cases with mild head injury with onset at 14 days on average (range, 3 days to 5 years). In these delayed cases, the dystonia usually started as a focal dystonia but usually progressed and spread over several months or years, developing into segmental, hemifocal, multifocal, or generalized dystonia. On brain imaging studies (computed tomography or MRI), the most frequent lesion site was in the contralateral basal ganglia or thalamus (Lee et al., 1994). Peripheral nerve injuries were reported in 7% of a group prospectively studied, and included those acquired both at the time of the injury and during the acute postinjury course (Philip & Philip, 1992).

Although motor recovery in children with TBI is generally good, the effects of motor impairment should not be minimized. The residual impairments interfere not only with mobility and athletics but also with acceptance by peers, compounding these children's difficulty with socialization.

Medical Effects

Trauma can result in isolated brain injury or in multiple system injuries. Even without multiple system injuries, almost every system within the body will be affected as a result of a neurological injury. Many of the effects will be isolated to the acute period, but others will persist.

The *musculoskeletal system* will be affected in many ways following neurological injury. Acutely there may be orthopedic fractures related to the incident. These can include long bone fractures that require open reduction and internal fixation, as well as rib fractures and skull fractures. Secondary orthopedic issues may include abnormal bone growth as a result of growth plate injury, leading to limb length discrepancies, scoliosis, joint subluxation/dislocation, and contractures. Disuse osteoporosis can be significant in this population, leading to iatrogenic fractures. Bed rest has been shown to produce significant decreases in bone mineral density in the lumbar spine, femoral neck, tibia, and calcaneous (LeBlanc, Schneider, Evans, Engelbretson, & Krebs, 1990.) Muscle will also be affected as a result of the prolonged bed rest and inactivity that follow a more severe brain injury. Changes in muscle mass begin to develop within 4–6 weeks of bed rest; this can be associated with a decrease of up to 40% in muscle strength (Bloomfield, 1997). Bed rest and inactivity also lead to deconditioning of the cardiovascular system, with decrease in stoke volume, cardiac output, oxygen uptake, and orthostatic tolerance (Convertino, Bloomfield, & Greenleaf, 1997).

Heterotopic ossification (HO), the formation of new bone in soft tissue, is a potential problem. It typically presents as warm swelling of a joint or leg, pain, or restricted mobility. Clinically significant HO occurs in 10%–20% of cases (Kwai-Tung, 2005). It is usually seen in children older than 11 years of age. Major risk factors include immobility, limb spasticity, and prolonged coma. The hip and knee are the most common sites of HO, followed by the elbow and nonjoint sites. Although pain secondary to HO may limit progress in acute rehabilitation, the long-term functional limitations are a result of limitation of range of motion, and this depends on the extent and location of the new bone. In a study of children and adolescents, HO was diagnosed in 32 of 643 patients after TBI, near drowning, strangulation, cerebral hemorrhage, hydrocephalus, or spinal cord injury. Mean age was 14.8 years, and average time of onset was 4 months. Only six of these patients underwent surgery for removal of HO because of severely restricted joint mobility (Kluger, Kochs, & Holthausen, 2000).

Deep venous thrombosis (DVT) is not common in childhood but has the potential for serious complications such as pulmonary embolism. The incidence of DVT in childhood is 1 in 100,000 children (van Ommen & Peters, 2003). Risk factors are acquired or congenital. Acquired risk factors include presence of a central venous catheter, infection, malignancy, immobilization, trauma, and surgery. Clinical presentation may include swelling, pain, and discoloration of the extremity. Children who have gone through puberty should be considered for anticoagulant prophylaxis. Pediatric patients with uncomplicated DVTs are usually treated for 3 months (van Ommen & Peters 2003).

The *immune system* is affected acutely. Cell-mediated immunity is severely depressed, including T-cell function and cytokine production. This may be responsible for the high incidence of infection following severe head injury. No significant decrease in immunoglobulin levels is noted (Miller, Quattrocchi, Frank, Issel, & Wagner, 1991; Pepe & Barba, 1999).

With severe TBI, early *feeding* intolerance can be a problem. This is in part related to changes in gastric motility. During the first week, there is a delay in gastric emptying. By the second week, there is an abnormal biphasic response to gastric emptying, with gastric emptying faster than normal during the early stage but prolonged later. By the third week, this biphasic response is still present but improving (Ott et al., 1991). A study by Thor et al. (2003) also noted what they described as "gastric dysrrhythmias." Gastric myoelectric activity was recorded as a marker of gastric motility. Following TBI, there was an increased percentage of time with bradygastria and tachygastria and the duration of normogastria was decreased. The dysrrhythmias were correlated with GCS score. A lower GCS score was associated with a higher percentage of dysrrhythmias, and a higher GCS score was associated with normal frequency (Thor et al., 2003). Gastroesophageal reflux is common following brain injury, even in patients without nasogastric tubes (Vane, Shiffler, & Grosfeld, 1982).

Nutritional needs change after a severe brain injury. There is an initial 1- to 2-week hypermetabolic period, with daily calorie and protein needs possibly reaching 2 times the normal predicted amount. A hypercatabolic period is also present, with resultant increase in protein turnover and increase in glucose utilization by glucose-dependent organs. Following TBI, a patient can lose up to 1,000 g of muscle tissue per day, which will affect muscle mass and contribute to generalized weakness (Pepe & Barba, 1999).

Dysphagia is a common problem in children after severe brain injury. The incidence of swallowing problems increases with severity of brain injury. A retrospective chart review noted that 68% of severely brain-injured children had dysphagia in the acute care setting (Morgan, Ward, Murdoch, Kennedy, & Murison 2003). The modified barium swallow is a clinically useful tool for identify swallowing abnormalities as well as aspiration. In a review of 608 swallowing studies, only 10.4% were normal, and 32.4% revealed aspiration. An additional 57.2% of studies revealed a swallowing abnormality without aspiration (Martin-Harris, Logemann, McMahon, Schleicher, &

Sandidge, 2000). Other factors that contribute to dysphagia include impairment of cognition, behavioral and oral sensitivity issues, and postural deficits (Morgan, Ward, & Murdoch, 2004). The outcome for pediatric swallowing disorders is not well documented in the literature; however, the outcome is probably comparable to that in adults, if developmental differences are taken into account. Findings in adults include oral feeding and pharyngeal swallowing problems that typically occur in combination—reduced lingual control and bolus manipulation in the mouth, delayed triggering of the pharyngeal swallow, and inefficient transport of food through the mouth and pharynx (Ylvisaker & Weinstein, 1989).

Neurological Effects

Neurological complications, in addition to those mentioned previously, include posttraumatic seizures, hydrocephalus, sensory impairments, and endocrine and autonomic dysfunction.

Posttraumatic seizures are divided into early (first 7 days) and late (after the first 7 days) seizures. Early seizures, especially those that occur on impact, are not uncommon with all degrees of severity of head injury in children, and, therefore, do not have significant prognostic utility. The risk of posttraumatic epilepsy (recurrent late posttraumatic seizures) is increased with increasing severity of head injury. In a population-based study, the cumulative 5-year probability of seizures was 0.5% for mild injuries, 1.2% for moderate injuries, and 10% for severe injuries (Annegers, Hauser, Coan, & Rocca, 1998). Late posttraumatic seizures are more likely in patients with biparietal contusions, dural penetration with bone and metal fragments, multiple intracranial operations, multiple subcortical contusions, subdural hematoma with evacuation, midline shift greater than 5 mm, or multiple or bilateral cortical contusions (Englander et al., 2003). Englander et al. (2003) also noted that, of the individuals they studied who developed late posttraumatic seizures, 79% had generalized seizures and 21% had focal seizures. Anticonvulsant prophylaxis with phenytoin (Dilantin) has been shown to be efficacious only for the first week postinjury (Temkin et al., 1990). Ongoing treatment should be reserved for those patients with diagnosed late posttraumatic seizures.

Hydrocephalus is a complication of TBI. The incidence varies in the literature but ranges from 0.7% to 29% (Guyot & Michael, 2000). It can occur acutely with ventricular system obstruction related to intraventricular hemorrhage or external compression. Communicating hydrocephalus may occur later, secondary to a decreased resorption of cerebrospinal fluid related to subarachnoid hemorrhages or infections. The most common cause for progressive ventricular enlargement is cortical atrophy, but progressive hydrocephalus must be ruled out. Symptomatic hydrocephalus is likely to improve with shunting. The risk of hydrocephalus increases with longer duration of coma, increased age, and decompressive craniotomy (Mazzini et al., 2003). For patients manifesting new neurological deficits, worsening spasticity, or cessation of neurological improvement, reimaging of the brain is indicated to rule out treatable problems that are impeding recovery, such as hydrocephalus (Licata, Cristofori, Gambin, Vivenza, & Turazzi, 2001).

Autonomic instability is often noted with very severe brain injuries, manifesting with hypertension, tachycardia, hyperthermia, tachypnea, and hypertonia and decerebrate posturing. The pathophysiology is linked to dysfunction of the thalamus or hypothalamus and the connections to the cortical, subcortical, and brain stem areas that mediate autonomic functions. The drugs most commonly used for treatment include morphine sulfate, bromocriptine, propranolol, clonidine, lorazepam, and dantrolene (Blackman, Patrick, Buck, & Rust, 2004).

Endocrine abnormalities may be transient or permanent and are linked to the severity of head trauma. Dysregulation of antidiuretic hormone can present either with syndrome of inappropriate antidiuretic hormone secretion (seen during the acute posttraumatic period) or diabetes insipidus (which may rarely persist after the acute period). Hypogonadism, cortisol hyporesponsiveness, and hypothyroidism are common in the acute period (Dimopoulou et al., 2004).

Sensory deficits are not uncommon after TBI and can have obvious deleterious effects on function. A national household survey of adults with TBI estimated a prevalence rate of 19.6 for hearing disability per 100,000 adults (Lubinski, Moscato, & Willer, 1997). A retrospective chart review of 62 children ages 2–18 years (3 with mild and 59 with moderate or severe TBI), found that 25 (40%) had hearing deficits, of which 15 were persistent. Sixteen percent of the entire sample had conductive hearing loss, 13% sensorineural hearing loss, and 16% central auditory processing problems (Cockrell & Gregory, 1992).

Visual deficits are also common after severe TBI and include strabismus, convergence deficit, accommodation dysfunction, absence of stereopsis, reduction of visual acuity, visual field defects, and fundus alterations. In a study evaluating 56 children younger than the age of 12 with TBI (Poggi et al., 2000), 75% of the patients had at least one ophthalmological lesion, with visual acuity changes being the most frequent. The fundus was normal in 78.6%. Fifty percent had convergence issues (correlated with a longer duration of coma and brain stem lesions); 42.9% had strabismus, and 21.4% had nystagmus. Thirty nine percent had saccades and pursuit disorders, and 41% had fixation disorders (both correlated with longer duration of coma and brain stem lesions). Forty-one percent had visual field deficits (Poggi et al., 2000). Retinal hemorrhages occur in infants and toddlers, usually as a result of inflicted trauma. Transient cortical blindness can also occur after mild to severe head injury and can confuse the patient's management during the early period if not recognized (Woodward, 1990). Permanent cortical blindness is uncommon and usually occurs as a result of secondary complications.

Urinary incontinence is common after moderate and severe neurological injuries. This may result from cognitive/behavioral issues, brain injury, associated injury to the spinal cord, or direct bladder injury. Oostra, Everaert, and Van Laere (1996) examined urinary incontinence following brain injury. Fifty percent of patients were found to be incontinent at admission to a rehab facility. Correlation was noted with length of coma and frontal lobe in-

jury. Frontal lobe injury results in loss of inhibition of the brain stem detrusor nucleus. Improvements are typically seen in the first 6 months following injury.

The *bowel* is also frequently affected with neurological injuries. Commonly, constipation is noted, requiring a consistent program of laxatives, suppositories, or both. Incontinence has also been noted and may be associated with loose stools or constipation. In the brain injury literature, a retrospective study examined the incidence, risk factors, and outcome of fecal incontinence following acute brain injury (Foxx-Orenstein et al., 2003). The incidence of fecal incontinence was noted to be 68% at admission to acute rehabilitation, 12.4% at discharge, and 5.2% at 1 year follow-up. Fecal incontinence was associated with severity of brain injury, length of coma and PTA, length of stay, incidence of urinary tract infection, and frontal contusion.

ACUTE MEDICAL MANAGEMENT

The acute medical management of TBI is directed toward minimizing or preventing second insults related to factors such as decreased cerebral perfusion pressure, increased intracranial pressure, shock, hypoxia, expanding intracranial mass lesions, temperature elevations, and infection. Adelson et al. (2003) have published their "Guidelines for the Acute Medical Management of Severe Traumatic Brain Injury in Infants, Children, and Adolescents," highlighting the state of evidenced-based medicine in this area. There has been considerable improvement in the care of children after TBI, related to imaging techniques and neurosurgical and intensive care interventions, and this has resulted in decreased mortality. At least in those patients with very severe injury (GCS score of 3 or 4), however, current improvements in mortality may be at the expense of unchanged morbidity (Kumar, West, Quirke, Hall, & Taylor, 1991).

Currently, there is a great deal of interest and investigation into ways to minimize secondary injury. This includes interventions such as neuroprotective medications and hypothermia (Adelson et al., 2005; Faden & Salzman, 1992). If successful, these strategies will hopefully lead to the improvement of morbidity as well as mortality.

REHABILITATION

The rehabilitation needs of patients who have sustained TBIs vary according to the severity of injury and secondary deficits, and range from reassurance and anticipatory guidance to extensive intervention. Because mild, uncomplicated TBI is not expected to result in long-term deficits, reassurance and family/patient education on postconcussional symptoms and suggested coping strategies are indicated, as long as this is coupled with appropriate medical follow-up to detect any unanticipated secondary problems. Although children with moderate and complicated mild TBI are expected to do relatively well, as a group they have cognitive and behavioral changes relative to their preinjury status and consequently must be followed closely and be assisted in their return to school. With severe TBI, because of the resultant cognitive and physical impairment, there is often need for inpatient rehabilitation followed by outpatient rehabilitation and planned school reintegration and for long-term follow-up. Types of rehabilitation intervention are discussed in Chapter 31 of this volume.

Rehabilitation should begin during the acute hospitalization, not when a patient is discharged to the rehabilitation unit. Early management of the patient with physical impairment is directed toward prevention of complications related to abnormal muscle tone and prolonged bed rest/immobility, such as contractures and decubitus ulcers. When tolerated, range-of-motion exercises and appropriate positioning (bed positioning, adaptive seating systems, splinting, and serial casting) should be begun as needed. When the patient is able to participate actively in the rehabilitation, active retraining is beneficial for motor disorders (Massagli & Jaffe, 1994). The motor impairment that continues in the patient with very severe injury is sometimes trivialized by referring to the cognitive and behavioral impairments as the major determinants of outcome. The motor impairment and related disabilities should not be minimized because they may have far-reaching effects on socialization, self-esteem, and independence. When the acute rehabilitation process has ended, the patient should be assisted in finding appropriate avenues for physical activity, such as adaptive physical education/training and encouragement of individual (rather than team) sports.

PREVENTION

Although the improvement of care and treatment of the patient with TBI is advancing, prevention is the most effective "treatment." The main principles of brain injury prevention include the following:

1. Anything that can decrease the amount and rate of energy transfer will decrease the severity of injury to the brain, if not prevent it entirely.

2. Methods that rely as much as possible on "passive" or automatic strategies are likely to be more effective than those based solely on behavior changes, especially because behavior changes are hardest to achieve in the population at most risk (e.g., adolescents, the poor, the intoxicated).

3. Strategies and recommendations should be focused and specific (e.g., telling parents and children to use a car seat, to buy and use a bike helmet, and to throw out the baby walker).

Because of the limitations of education and other strategies in isolation, prevention must be approached from multiple simultaneous angles—passive strategies, education, financial incentives (e.g., bicycle helmet coupons/subsidies), and "mandatory use" legislation (Rivara, 1994). Prevention should be given highest priority by any professional working with children.

CONCLUSION

Since traumatic brain injury is so common, it should always be considered in the differential diagnosis of children being evaluated for learning and behavior problems. The unique nature of the deficits, related to the type and distribution of injury, must be stressed, and evaluations, recommendations, and treatment must be adapted to meet each patient's needs.

REFERENCES

Adams, J.H., Doyle, D., Ford, I., Gennarelli, T.A., Graham, D.I., & McLellan, D.R. (1989). Diffuse axonal injury in head injury: Definition, diagnosis and grading. *Histopathology, 15,* 49–59.

Adams, J.H., Doyle, D., Graham, D.I., Lawrence, A.E., McLellan, D.R., Gennarelli, T.A., et al. (1985). The Contusion Index: A reappraisal in human and experimental non-missile head injury. *Neuropathology and Applied Neurobiology, 11,* 299–308.

Adelson, P.D., Bratton, S.L., Carney, N.A., Chesnut, R.M., du Coudray, H.E., Goldstein, B., et al. (2003). Guidelines for the acute medical management of severe traumatic brain injury in infants, children, and adolescents. *Pediatric Critical Care Medicine, 4*(3 Suppl.), S2–S75.

Adelson, P.D., Ragheb, J., Kanev, P., Brockmeyer, D., Beers, S.R., Brown, S.D., et al. (2005). Phase II clinical trial of moderate hypothermia after severe traumatic brain injury in children. *Neurosurgery, 56,* 740–754.

Annegers, J.F., Hauser, W.A., Coan, S.P., & Rocca, W.A. (1998). A population-based study of seizures after traumatic brain injuries. *New England Journal of Medicine, 338,* 20–42.

Auerbach, S.H. (1986). Neuroanatomical correlates of attention and memory disorders in traumatic brain injury: An application of neurobehavioral subtypes. *Journal of Head Trauma Rehabilitation, 1*(3), 1–12.

Bijur, P.E., Haslum, M., & Golding, J. (1990). Cognitive and behavioral sequelae of mild head injury in children. *Pediatrics, 86,* 337–344.

Blackman, J.A., Patrick, P.D., Buck, M.L., & Rust, R.S. (2004). Paroxysmal autonomic instability with dystonia after brain injury. *Archives of Neurology, 61,* 321–328.

Bloomfield, S.A. (1997). Changes in musculoskeletal structure and function with prolonged bed rest. *Medicine and Science in Sports and Exercise, 29,* 197–206.

Brink, J.D., Garrett, A.L., Hale, W.R., Woo-Sam, J., & Nickel, V.L. (1970). Recovery of motor and intellectual function in children sustaining severe head injuries. *Developmental Medicine and Child Neurology, 12,* 565–571.

Brink, J.D., Imbus, C., & Woo-Sam, J. (1980). Physical recovery after severe closed head trauma in children and adolescents. *Journal of Pediatrics, 97,* 721–727.

Brown, G., Chadwick, O., Shaffer, D., Rutter, M., & Traub, M. (1981). A prospective study of children with head injuries: III. Psychiatric sequelae. *Psychological Medicine, 11,* 63–78.

Cahill, L.M., Murdoch, B.E., & Theodoros, D.G. (2002). Perceptual analysis of speech following traumatic brain injury in childhood. *Brain Injury, 16,* 415–446.

Carney, J., & Schoenbrodt, L. (1994). Educational implications of traumatic brain injury. *Pediatric Annals, 23,* 47–52.

Carroll, L.J., Cassidy, J.D., Peloso, P.M., Borg, J., von Holst, H., Holm, L., et al. & the WHO Collaborating Centre Task Force on Mild Traumatic Brain Injury. (2004). Prognosis for mild traumatic brain injury: Results of the WHO Collaborating Centre Task Force on Mild Traumatic Brain Injury. *Journal of Rehabilitation Medicine, 43*(Suppl.), 84–105.

Catroppa, C., & Anderson, V. (2002). Recovery in memory function in the first year following TBI in children. *Brain Injury, 16,* 369–384.

Catroppa, C., & Anderson, V. (2005). A prospective study of the recovery of attention from acute to 2 years following pediatric traumatic brain injury. *Journal of the International Neuropsychological Society, 11,* 84–98.

Centers for Disease Control and Prevention. (1993). Use of race and ethnicity in public health surveillance: Summary of the CDC/ATSDR workshop. *MMWR: Recommendations and Reports, 42*(No. RR-10).

Chadwick, O., Rutter, M., Brown, G., Shaffer, D., & Traub, M. (1981). A prospective study of children with head injuries: II. Cognitive sequelae. *Psychological Medicine, 11,* 49–61.

Chaplin, D., Deitz, J., & Jaffe, K.M. (1993). Motor performance in children after traumatic brain injury. *Archives of Physical Medicine and Rehabilitation, 74,* 161–164.

Chapman, S.B., Sparks, G., Levin, H.S., Dennis, M., Roncadin, C., Zhang, L., et al. (2004). Discourse macrolevel processing after severe pediatric traumatic brain injury. *Developmental Neuropsychology, 25,* 37–60.

Cockrell, J.L., & Gregory, S.A. (1992). Audiological deficits in brain-injured children and adolescents. *Brain Injury, 6,* 261–266.

Convertino, V.A., Bloomfield, S.A., & Greenleaf, J.E. (1997). An overview of the issues: Physiological effects of bed rest and restricted physical activity. *Medicine and Science in Sports and Exercise, 29,* 187–190.

Costeff, H., Groswasser, Z., & Goldstein, R. (1990). Long-term follow-up review of 31 children with severe closed head trauma. *Journal of Neurosurgery, 73,* 684–687.

Dayer, A., Roulet, E., Maeder, P., & Deonna, T. (1998). Post-traumatic mutism in children: Clinical characteristics, pattern of recovery and clinico-pathological correlations. *European Journal of Paediatric Neurology, 2,* 109–116.

Dimopoulou, I., Tsagarakis, S., Theodorakopoulou, M., Douka, E., Zervou, M., Kouyialis, A.T., et al. (2004). Endocrine abnormalities in critical care patients with moderate to severe head trauma: Incidence, pattern and predisposing factors. *Intensive Care Medicine, 30,* 1051–1057.

Dolis, D.C., Kramer, J.H., Kaplan, E., & Ober, B.A. (1994). *California Verbal Learning Test–Children's Version.* San Antonio, TX: Harcourt Assessment.

Donders, J., & Minnema, M.T. (2004). Performance discrepancies on the California Verbal Learning Test–Children's Version (CVLT-C) in children with traumatic brain injury. *Journal of the International Neuropsychological Society, 10,* 482–488.

Earley, C.J., Kittner, S.J., Feeser, B.R., Gardner, J., Epstein, A., Wozniak, M.A., et al. (1998). Stroke in children and sickle-cell disease: Baltimore-Washington Cooperative Young Stroke Study. *Neurology, 51,* 169–176.

Englander, J., Bushnik, T., Duong, T.T., Cifu, D.X., Zafonte, R., Wright, J., et al. (2003). Analyzing risk factors for late posttraumatic seizures: A prospective, multicenter investigation. *Archives of Physical Medicine and Rehabilitation, 84,* 365–373.

Ewing-Cobbs, L., & Barnes, M. (2002). Linguistic outcomes following traumatic brain injury in children. *Seminars in Pediatric Neurology, 9,* 209–217.

Ewing-Cobbs, L., Brookshire, B., Scott, M.A., & Fletcher, J.M. (1998). Children's narratives following traumatic brain injury: Linguistic structure, cohesion, and thematic recall. *Brain and Language, 61,* 395–419.

Ewing-Cobbs, L., Levin, H.S., Fletcher, J.M., Miner, M.E., & Eisenberg, H.M. (1990). The Children's Orientation and Amnesia Test: Relationship to severity of acute head injury and to recovery of memory. *Neurosurgery, 27,* 683–691.

Faden, A.I., & Salzman, S. (1992). Pharmacological strategies in CNS trauma. *Trends in Pharmacological Sciences, 13,* 29–35.

Fay, G.C., Jaffe, K.M., Polissar, N.L., Liao, S., Martin, K.M., Shurtleff, H.A., et al. (1993). Mild pediatric traumatic brain injury: A cohort study. *Archives of Physical Medicine and Rehabilitation, 74,* 895–901.

Fay, G.C., Jaffe, K.M., Polissar, N.L., Liao, S., Rivara, J.B., & Martin, K.M. (1994). Outcome of pediatric traumatic brain injury at three years: A cohort study. *Archives of Physical Medicine and Rehabilitation, 75,* 733–741.

Foxx-Orenstein, A., Kolakowsky-Hayner, S., Marwitz, J., Cifu, D.X., Dunbar, A., Englander, J., et al. (2003). Incidence, risk factors, and outcomes of fecal incontinence after acute brain injury: Findings from the Traumatic Brain Injury Model Systems national database. *Archives of Physical Medicine and Rehabilitation, 84,* 231–237.

Gagnon, I., Swaine, B., Friedman, D., & Forget, R. (2004a). Children show decreased dynamic balance after mild traumatic brain injury. *Archives of Physical Medicine and Rehabilitation, 85,* 444–452.

Gagnon, I., Swaine, B., Friedman, D., & Forget, R. (2004b). Visuomotor response time in children with a mild traumatic brain injury. *Journal of Head Trauma Rehabilitation, 19*(5), 391–404.

Gerring, J., Brady, K., Chen, A., Quinn, C., Herskovits, E., Bandeen-Roche, K., et al. (2000). Neuroimaging variables related to development of secondary attention deficit hyperactivity disorder after closed head injury in children and adolescents. *Brain Injury, 14,* 205–218.

Gerring, J.P., Brady, K.D., Chen, A., Vasa, R., Grados, M., Bandeen-Roche, K.J., et al. (1998). Premorbid prevalence of ADHD and development of secondary ADHD after closed head injury. *Journal of the American Academy of Child and Adolescent Psychiatry, 37,* 647–654.

Giacino, J.T., & Trott, C.T. (2004). Rehabilitative management of patients with disorders of consciousness: Grand rounds. *Journal of Head Trauma Rehabilitation, 19*(3), 254–265.

Giroud, M., Lemesle, M., Gouyon, J.B., Nivelon, J.L., Milan, C., & Dumas, R. (1995). Cerebrovascular disease in children under 16 years of age in the city of Dijon, France: A study of incidence and clinical features from 1985 to 1993. *Journal of Clinical Epidemiology, 48,* 1343–1348.

Grados, M.A., Slomine, B.S., Gerring, J.P., Vasa, R., Bryan, N., & Denckla, M.B. (2001). Depth of lesion model in children and adolescents with moderate to severe traumatic brain injury: Use of SPGR MRI to predict severity and outcome. *Journal of Neurology, Neurosurgery, and Psychiatry, 70,* 350–358.

Guyot, L.L., & Michael, D.B. (2000). Post-traumatic hydrocephalus. *Neurological Research, 22,* 25–28.

Harmon, R.L., Long, D.F., & Shirtz, J. (1991). Treatment of posttraumatic midbrain resting-kinetic tremor with combined levodopa/carbidopa and carbamazepine. *Brain Injury, 5,* 213–218.

Hawley, C.A. (2004). Behaviour and school performance after brain injury. *Brain Injury, 18,* 645–659.

Herskovits, E.H., Gerring, J.P., Davatzikos, C., & Bryan, R.N. (2002). Is the spatial distribution of brain lesions associated with closed-head injury in children predictive of subsequent development of posttraumatic stress disorder? *Radiology, 224,* 345–351.

Hunter, J.V., Thornton, R.J., Wang, Z.J., Levin, H.S., Roberson, G., Brooks, W.M., et al. (2005). Late proton MR spectroscopy in children after traumatic brain injury: Correlation with cognitive outcomes. *AJNR: American Journal of Neuroradiology, 26,* 482–488.

Jaffe, K.M., Fay, G.C., Polissar, N.L., Martin, K.M., Shurtleff, H., Rivara, J.B., et al. (1992). Severity of pediatric traumatic brain injury and early neurobehavioral outcome: A cohort study. *Archives of Physical Medicine and Rehabilitation, 73,* 540–547.

Jaffe, K.M., Fay, G.C., Polissar, N.L., Martin, K.M., Shurtleff, H.A., Rivara, J.B., et al. (1993). Severity of pediatric traumatic brain injury and neurobehavioral recovery at 1 year—a cohort study. *Archives of Physical Medicine and Rehabilitation, 74,* 587–595.

Jaffe, K.M., Polissar, N.L., Fay, G.C., & Liao, S. (1995). Recovery trends over three years following pediatric traumatic brain injury. *Archives of Physical Medicine and Rehabilitation, 76,* 17–26.

Jennett, B., & Plum, F. (1972). Persistent vegetative state after brain damage: A syndrome in search of a name. *Lancet, 1,* 734–737.

Jennett, B., & Teasdale, G. (1981). *Management of head injuries* (6th ed., pp. 89–90, 318–319). Philadelphia: F. A. Davis.

Johnson, S.L., & Hall, D.M. (1992). Post-traumatic tremor in head injured children. *Archives of Diseases in Childhood, 67,* 227–228.

Jordan, F.M., Cannon, A., & Murdoch, B.E. (1992). Language abilities of mildly closed head injured (CHI) children 10 years post-injury. *Brain Injury, 6,* 39–44.

Kamerling, S.N., Lutz, N., Posner, J.C., & Vanore, M. (2003). Mild traumatic brain injury in children: Practice guidelines for emergency department and hospitalized patients. The Trauma Program, The Children's Hospital of Philadelphia, University of Pennsylvania School of Medicine. *Pediatric Emergency Care, 19,* 431–440.

Kinsella, G.J., Prior, M., Sawyer, M., Ong, B., Murtagh, D., Eisenmajer, R., et al. (1997). Predictors and indicators of academic outcome in children 2 years following traumatic brain injury. *Journal of the International Neuropsychological Society, 3,* 608–616.

Kluger, G., Kochs, A., & Holthausen, H. (2000). Heterotopic ossification in childhood and adolescence. *Journal of Child Neurology, 15,* 406–413.

Kochanek, P.M., Clark, R.S.B., Benn, M.J., Whalen, M.J., & Adelson, P.D. (1998). Severe traumatic injury in children: Epidemiology, pathophysiology, monitoring, and management. In O.F. Mohan & D.M. Steinhorn (Eds.), *Current concepts in pediatric critical care* (pp. 1–14). Anaheim, CA: Society of Critical Care Medicine.

Korinthenberg, R., Schreck, J., Weser, J., & Lehmkuhl, G. (2004). Post-traumatic syndrome after minor head injury cannot be predicted by neurological investigations. *Brain and Development, 26,* 113–117.

Kraus, J.F., Black, M.A., Hessol, N., Ley, P., Rokaw, W., Sullivan, C., et al. (1984). The incidence of acute brain injury and serious impairment in a defined population. *American Journal of Epidemiology, 119,* 186–201.

Kraus, J.F., Fife, D., & Conroy, C. (1987). Pediatric brain injuries: The nature, clinical course and early outcomes in a defined United States population. *Pediatrics, 79,* 501–507.

Krauss, J.K., Mohadjer, M., Nobbe, F., & Mundinger, F. (1994). The treatment of posttraumatic tremor by stereotactic surgery: Symptomatic and functional outcome in a series of 35 patients. *Journal of Neurosurgery, 80,* 810–819.

Kuhtz-Buschbeck, J.P., Hoppe, B., Golge, M., Dreesmann, M., Damm-Stunitz, U., & Ritz, A. (2003). Degree of impairment increased with trauma severity. Sensorimotor recovery in children after traumatic brain injury: Analyses of gait, gross motor, and fine motor skills. *Developmental Medicine and Child Neurology, 45,* 821–828.

Kumar, R., West, C.G., Quirke, C., Hall, L., & Taylor, R. (1991). Do children with severe head injury benefit from intensive care? *Child's Nervous System, 7,* 299–304.

Kwai-Tung, C. (2005). Heterotopic ossification in traumatic brain injury. *American Journal of Physical Medicine and Rehabilitation, 84,* 145–146.

Langlois, J.A., Kegler, S.R., Butler, J.A., Gotsch, K.E., Johnson, R.L., Reichard, A.A., et al. (2003). Traumatic brain injury-related hospital discharges: Results from a 14-state surveillance system, 1997. *Morbidity and Mortality Weekly Report: CDC Surveillance Summaries, 52*(4), 1–20.

LeBlanc, A., Schneider, V., Evans, H., Engelbretson, D., & Krebs, J. (1990). Bone mineral loss and recovery after 17 weeks of bed rest. *Journal of Bone Mineral Research, 5,* 843–850.

Lee, M.S., Rinne, J.O., Ceballos-Baumann, A., Thompson, P.D., & Marsden, C.D. (1994). Dystonia after head trauma. *Neurology, 44,* 1374–1378.

Levin, H.S. (1989). Memory deficit after closed head injury. *Journal of Clinical and Experimental Neuropsychology, 12,* 129–153.

Levin, H.S., Aldrich, E.F., Saydjari, C., Eisenberg, H.M., Foulkes, M.A., Bellefleur, M., et al. (1992). Severe head injury in children: Experience of the Traumatic Coma Data Bank. *Neurosurgery, 31,* 435–444.

Levin, H.S., Culhane, K.A., Mendelsohn, D., Lilly, M.A., Bruce, D., Fletcher, J.M, et al. (1993). Cognition in relation to magnetic resonance imaging in head-injured children and adolescents. *Archives of Neurology, 50,* 897–905.

Levin, H.S., & Eisenberg, H.M. (1979). Neuropsychological impairment after closed head injury in children and adolescents. *Journal of Pediatric Psychology, 4,* 389–402.

Levin, H.S., Eisenberg, H.M., Wigg, N.R., & Kobayashi, K. (1982). Memory and intellectual ability after head injury in children and adolescents. *Neurosurgery, 11,* 668–673.

Levin, H.S., Fletcher, J.M., Kufera, J.A., Harward, H., Lilly, M.A, Mendelsohn, D., et al. (1996). Dimensions of cognition measured by the Tower of London and other cognitive tasks in head-injured children and adolescents. *Developmental Neuropsychology, 12,* 17–34.

Levin, H.S., Madison, C.F., Bailey, C.B., Meyers, C.A., Eisenberg, H.M., & Guinto, F.C. (1983). Mutism after closed head injury. *Archives of Neurology, 40,* 601–606.

Levin, H.S., O'Donnell, V.M., & Grossman, R.G. (1979). The Galveston Orientation and Amnesia Test: A practical scale to assess cognition after head injury. *Journal of Nervous and Mental Disease, 167*(11), 675–684.

Levin, H.S., Zhang, L., Dennis, M., Ewing-Cobbs, L., Schachar, R., Max, J., et al. (2004). Psychosocial outcome of TBI in children with unilateral frontal lesions. *Journal of the International Neuropsychological Society, 10*, 305–316.

Lezak, M.D. (1982). The problem of assessing executive functions. *International Journal of Psychology, 17*, 281–297.

Lezak, M. (1995). *Neuropsychological assessment* (3rd ed.). New York: Oxford University Press.

Licata, C., Cristofori, L., Gambin, R., Vivenza, C., & Turazzi, S. (2001). Post-traumatic hydrocephalus. *Journal of Neurosurgical Sciences, 45*, 141–149.

Lubinski, R., Moscato, B.S., & Willer, B.S. (1997). Prevalence of speaking and hearing disabilities among adults with traumatic brain injury from a national household survey. *Brain Injury, 11*, 103–114.

Mahoney, W.J., D'Souza, B.J., Haller, J.A., Rogers, M.C., Epstein, M.H., & Freeman, J.M. (1983). Long-term outcome of children with severe head trauma and prolonged coma. *Pediatrics, 71*, 756–761.

Martin-Harris, B., Logemann, J.A., McMahon, S., Schleicher, M., & Sandidge, J. (2000). Clinical utility of the modified barium swallow. *Dysphagia, 15*, 136–141.

Massagli, T.L., Fann, J.R., Burington, B.E., Jaffe, K.M., Katon, W.J., & Thompson, R.S. (2004). Psychiatric illness after mild traumatic brain injury in children. *Archives of Physical Medicine and Rehabilitation, 85*, 1428–1434.

Massagli, T.L., & Jaffe, K.M. (1994). Pediatric traumatic brain injury: Prognosis and rehabilitation. *Pediatric Annals, 23*, 29–36.

Massagli, T.L., Jaffe, K.M., Fay, G.C., Polissar, N.L., Liao, S., & Rivara, J.B. (1996). Neurobehavioral sequelae of severe pediatric traumatic brain injury: A cohort study. *Archives of Physical Medicine and Rehabilitation, 77*, 223–231.

Max, J.E., Arndt, S., Castillo, C.S., Bokura, H., Robin, D.A., Lindgren, S.D., et al. (1998). Attention-deficit hyperactivity symptomatology after traumatic brain injury: A prospective study. *Journal of the American Academy of Child and Adolescent Psychiatry, 37*, 841–847.

Max, J.E., Koele, S.L., Castillo, C.C., Lindgren, S.D., Arndt, S., Bokura, H., et al. (2000). Personality change disorder in children and adolescents following traumatic brain injury. *Journal of the International Neuropsychological Society, 6*, 279–289.

Max, J.E., Koele, S.L., Smith, W.L., Jr., Sato, Y., Lindgren, S.D., Robin, D.A., et al. (1998). Psychiatric disorders in children and adolescents after severe traumatic brain injury: A controlled study. *Journal of the American Academy of Child and Adolescent Psychiatry, 37*, 832–840.

Max, J.E., Robertson, B.A., & Lansing, A.E. (2001). The phenomenology of personality change (PC) due to traumatic brain injury in children and adolescents. *Journal of Neuropsychiatry and Clinical Neurosciences, 13*, 161–170.

Mazaux, J.M., Masson, F., Levin, H.S., Alaoui, P., Maurette, P., & Barat, M. (1997). Long-term neuropsychological outcome and loss of social autonomy after traumatic brain injury. *Archives of Physical Medicine and Rehabilitation, 78*, 1316–1320.

Mazzini, L., Campini, R., Angelino, E., Rognone, F., Pastore, I., & Oliveri, G. (2003). Post-traumatic hydrocephalus: A clinical, neuroradiologic and neuropsychologic assessment of long term outcome. *Archives of Physical Medicine and Rehabilitation, 84*, 1637–1641.

McArthur, D.L., Chute, D.J., & Villablanca, J.P. (2004). Moderate and severe traumatic brain injury: Epidemiologic, imaging and neuropathologic perspectives. *Brain Pathology, 14*, 185–194.

McDonald, C.M., Jaffe, K.M., Fay, G.C., Polissar, N.L., Martin, K.M., Liao, S., et al. (1994). Comparison of indices of traumatic brain injury severity as predictors of neurobehavioral outcome in children. *Archives of Physical Medicine and Rehabilitation, 75*, 328–337.

Miller, C.H., Quattrocchi, K.B., Frank, E.H., Issel, B.W., & Wagner, F.C., Jr. (1991). Humoral and cellular immunity following severe head injury: Review and current investigations. *Neurological Research, 13*, 117–124.

Miller, L.J., & Donders, J. (2003). Prediction of educational outcome after pediatric traumatic brain injury. *Rehabilitation Psychology, 48*, 237–241.

Morgan, A., Ward, E., & Murdoch, B. (2004). Clinical characteristics of acute dysphagia in pediatric patients following traumatic brain injury. *Journal of Head Trauma Rehabilitation, 19*(3), 226–240.

Morgan, A., Ward, E., Murdoch, B., Kennedy, B., & Murison, R. (2003). Incidence, characteristics, and predictive factors for dysphagia after pediatric traumatic brain injury. *Journal of Head Trauma Rehabilitation, 18*(3), 239–251.

Morrison, W.E., Arbelaez, J.J., Fackler, J.C., De Maio, A., & Paidas, C.N. (2004). Gender and age effects on outcome after pediatric traumatic brain injury. *Pediatric Critical Care Medicine, 5*, 145–151.

Morse, S., Haritou, F., Ong, K., Anderson, V., Catroppa, C., & Rosenfeld, J. (1999). Early effects of traumatic brain injury on young children's language performance: A preliminary linguistic analysis. *Pediatric Rehabilitation, 3*, 139–148.

Multi-Society Task Force Report on PVS, The. (1994). Medical aspects of the persistent vegetative state. *New England Journal of Medicine, 330*, 1499–1508, 1572–1579.

Murdoch, B.E., & Goozee, J.V. (2003). EMA analysis of tongue function in children with dysarthria following traumatic brain injury. *Brain Injury, 17*, 79–93.

National Center for Injury Prevention and Control. (1999). *Traumatic brain injury in the United States: A report to Congress.* Atlanta: Centers for Disease Control and Prevention.

Nybo, T., & Koskiniemi, M. (1999). Cognitive indicators of vocational outcome after severe traumatic brain injury (TBI) in childhood. *Brain Injury, 13,* 759–766.

Oostra, K., Everaert, K., & Van Laere, M. (1996). Urinary incontinence in brain injury. *Brain Injury, 10,* 459–464.

Ott, L., Young, B., Phillips, R., McClain, C., Adams, L., Dempsey, R., et al. (1991). Altered gastric emptying in the head-injured patient: Relationship to feeding intolerance. *Journal of Neurosurgery, 74,* 738–742.

Pelco, L., Sawyer, M., Duffield, G., Prior, M., & Kinsella, G. (1992). Premorbid emotional and behavioral adjustment in children with mild head injuries. *Brain Injury, 6,* 29–37.

Pepe, J.L., & Barba, C.A. (1999). The metabolic response to acute traumatic brain injury and implications for nutritional support. *Journal of Head Trauma Rehabilitation, 14*(5), 462–474.

Philip, P.A., & Philip, M. (1992). Peripheral nerve injuries in children with traumatic brain injury. *Brain Injury, 6,* 53–58.

Plum, F., & Posner, J. (1982). *The diagnosis of stupor and coma* (3rd ed.). Philadelphia: F. A. Davis.

Poggi, G., Calori, G., Mancarella, G., Colombo, E., Profice, P., Martinell, F., et al. (2000). Visual disorders after traumatic brain injury in developmental age. *Brain Injury, 14,* 833–845.

Ponsford, J., Willmott, C., Rothwell, A., Cameron, P., Ayton, G., Nelms, R., et al. (1999). Cognitive and behavioral outcome following mild traumatic head injury in children. *Journal of Head Trauma Rehabilitation, 14*(4), 360–372.

Ponsford, J., Willmott, C., Rothwell, A., Cameron, P., Ayton, G., Nelms, R., et al. (2001). Impact of early intervention on outcome after mild traumatic brain injury in children. *Pediatrics, 108,* 1297–1303.

Raghupathi, R. (2004). Cell death mechanisms following traumatic brain injury. *Brain Pathology, 14,* 215–222.

Ries, L.A.G., Eisner, M.P., Kosary, C.L., Hankey, B.F., Miller, B.A., Clegg, L., et al. (Eds.). (2004). *SEER cancer statistics review, 1975–2001.* Bethesda, MD: National Cancer Institute.

Rivara, F.P. (1994). Epidemiology and prevention of pediatric traumatic brain injury. *Pediatric Annals, 23,* 12–17.

Rivara, F.P., & Mueller, B.A. (1986). The epidemiology and prevention of pediatric head injury. *Journal of Head Trauma Rehabilitation, 1*(4), 7–15.

Rivara, J.B., Jaffe, K.M., Polissar, N.L., Fay, G.C., Martin, K.M., Shurtleff, H.A., et al. (1994). Family functioning and children's academic performance and behavior problems in the year following traumatic brain injury. *Archives of Physical Medicine and Rehabilitation, 75,* 369–379.

Rutter, M., Chadwick, O., Shaffer, D., & Brown, G. (1980). A prospective study of children with head injuries: I. Design and methods. *Psychological Medicine, 10,* 633–645.

Saitoh, T., Ueki, A., Yamada, N., Mori, S., & Iwasa, H. (1991). Hyperkinesie volitionnelle following head injury. *Rinsho-Shinkeigaku [Clinical Neurology], 31,* 738–741.

Shaffer, D., Bijur, P., Chadwick, O.F.D., & Rutter, M.L. (1980). Head injury and later reading disability. *American Journal of Child Psychiatry, 19,* 592–610.

Slomine, B.S., Gerring, J.P., Grados, M.A., Vasa, R., Brady, K.D., Christensen, J.R., et al. (2002). Performance on measures of executive function following pediatric traumatic brain injury. *Brain Injury, 16,* 759–772.

Stein, S.C. (2001). Minor head injury: 13 is an unlucky number. *Journal of Trauma, Injury, Infection and Critical Care, 50,* 759–760.

Temkin, N.R., Dikmen, S.S., Wilensky, A.J., Keihm, J., Chabal, S., & Winn, H.R. (1990). A randomized, double-blind study of phenytoin for the prevention of post-traumatic seizures. *New England Journal of Medicine, 323,* 497–502.

Tepas, J.J., III, DiScala, C., Ramenofsky, M.L., & Barlow, B. (1990). Mortality and head injury: The pediatric perspective. *Journal of Pediatric Surgery, 25,* 92–95.

Thor, P.J., Goscinski, I., Kolasinska-Kloch, W., Madroszkiewicz, D., Madroszkiewicz, E., & Furgala, A. (2003). Gastric myoelectric activity inpatients with closed head brain injury. *Medical Science Moniter, 9*(9), CR392–CR395.

Thurman, D.J. (2001). The epidemiology and economics of head trauma. In L.P. Miller & R.L. Hayes (Eds.), *Head trauma therapeutics: Basic, preclinical and clinical aspects* (pp. 327–347). New York: John Wiley & Sons.

Thurman, D.J., Alverson, C., Dunn, K.A., Guerrero, J., & Sniezek, J.E. (1999). Traumatic brain injury in the United States: A public health perspective. *Journal of Head Trauma Rehabilitation, 14*(6), 602–615.

Thurman, D.J., Branche, C.M., & Sniezek, J.E. (1998). The epidemiology of sports-related traumatic brain injuries in the United States: Recent developments. *Journal of Head Trauma Rehabilitation, 13*(2), 1–8.

Tojo, M., & Nitta, H. (2003). Clinico-etiological study of 116 children with acquired damage to the central nervous system during the last decade in Niigata Prefecture. *No To Hattatsu [Brain and Development], 35,* 292–296.

Tong, K.A., Ashwal, S., Holshouser, B.A., Nickerson, J.P., Wall, C.J., Shutter, L.A., et al. (2004). Diffuse axonal injury in children: Clinical correlation with hemorrhagic lesions. *Annals of Neurology, 56,* 36–50.

Van Ommen, C.H., & Peters, M. (2003). Venous thromboembolic disease in childhood. *Seminars in Thrombosis and Hemostasis, 29,* 391–403.

Van Zomeren, A.H., & Van Den Berg, W. (1985). Residual complaints of patients two years after severe head injury. *Journal of Neurology, Neurosurgery and Psychiatry, 48,* 21–28.

Vane, D., Shiffler, M., & Grossfeld, J. (1982). Reduced lower esophageal sphincter pressure after acute and chronic brain injury. *Journal of Pediatric Surgery, 17,* 960–964.

Vasa, R., Gerring, J.P., Grados, M., Slomine, B., Christensen, J.R., Rising, W., et al. (2002). Anxiety after severe pediatric closed head injury. *Journal of the American Academy of Child and Adolescent Psychiatry, 41,* 148–156.

Vasa, R.A., Grados, M., Slomine, B., Herskovits, E.H., Thompson, R.E., Salorio, C., et al. (2004). Neuroimaging correlates of anxiety after pediatric traumatic brain injury. *Biological Psychiatry, 55,* 208–216.

Verger, K., Junque, C., Jurado, M.A., Tresserras, P., Bartumeus, F., Nogues, P., et al. (2000). Age effects on long-term neuropsychological outcome in paediatric traumatic brain injury. *Brain Injury, 14,* 495–503.

Verger, K., Junque, C., Levin, H.S., Jurado, M.A., Perez-Gomez, M., Bartres-Faz, D., et al. (2001). Correlation of atrophy measures on MRI with neuropsychological sequelae in children and adolescents with traumatic brain injury. *Brain Injury, 15,* 211–221.

Welsh, M.C., Pennington, B.F., & Groisser, D.B. (1991). A normative-developmental study of executive functioning: A window on prefrontal functioning in children. *Developmental Neuropsychology, 7,* 131–149.

Whitman, S., Coonley-Hoganson, R., & Desai, B.T. (1984). Comparative head injury experiences in two socioeconomically different Chicago-area communities: A population study. *American Journal of Epidemiology, 119,* 570–580.

Wilde, E.A., Hunter, J.V., Newsome, M.R., Scheibel, R.S., Bigler, E.D., Johnson, J.L., et al. (2005). Frontal and temporal morphometric findings on MRI in children after moderate to severe traumatic brain injury. *Journal of Neurotrauma, 22,* 333–344.

Williams, D.H., Levin, H.S., & Eisenberg, H.M. (1990). Mild head injury classification. *Neurosurgery, 27,* 422–428.

Woodward, G.A. (1990). Posttraumatic cortical-blindness: Are we missing the diagnosis in children? *Pediatric Emergency Care, 6,* 289–292.

Wymer, J.H., Lindman, L.S., & Booksh, R.L. (2002). A neuropsychological perspective of aprosody: Features, function, assessment, and treatment. *Applied Neuropsychology, 9,* 37–47.

Yeates, K.O. (2000). Closed-head injury. In K.O. Yeates, M.D. Ris, & H.G. Taylor (Eds.), *Pediatric neuropsychology: Research, theory and practice* (pp. 92–116). New York: Guilford Press.

Yeates, K.O., Taylor, H.G., Drotar, D., Wade, S.L., Klein, S., Stancin, T., et al. (1997). Preinjury family environment as a determinant of recovery from traumatic brain injuries in school-age children. *Journal of the International Neuropsychological Society, 3,* 617–630.

Yeates, K.O., Taylor, H.G., Wade, S.L., Drotar, D., Stancin, T., & Minich, N. (2002). A prospective study of short- and long-term neuropsychological outcomes after traumatic brain injury in children. *Neuropsychology, 16,* 514–523.

Ylvisaker, M., & Weinstein, M. (1989). Recovery of oral feeding after pediatric head injury. *Journal of Head Trauma Rehabilitation, 4*(4), 51–63.

30

Acquired Spinal Cord Dysfunction

CRISTINA SADOWSKY,
FRANK S. PIDCOCK, EWA BRANDYS,
OLGA MOROZOVA, MELISSA K. TROVATO,
CYNTHIA SALORIO, AND JAMES CHRISTENSEN

Spinal cord injuries (SCIs) are regarded as irreversible, catastrophic events that carry a significant physiological, functional, and social burden. Until recently, individuals with SCIs were given extremely conservative outcome predictions, and the rehabilitative treatment consisted mostly of adapting to the neurological function present in the acute/subacute stage. Little was done to promote long-term rehabilitative habits because neurological recovery was considered a spontaneous, preordained process not significantly influenced by active interventions. Today, clinicians recognize that they can substantially modify function restoration by implementing modalities that parallel physiological neurological development.

ETIOLOGY AND EPIDEMIOLOGY

Traumatic Injuries

The most common cause of traumatic SCI is motor vehicle accidents. Violence can be equally responsible in urban populations (Haffner, Hoffer, & Wiedbusch, 1993). Falls and sports injuries are also common causes, with diving accounting for about two thirds of the sports-related injuries and football for only 2%–3% (Go, DeVivo, & Richards, 1995). Some etiologies are specific for the pediatric population: lap-belt injuries for children between 40 and 60 lb, because the lap belt riding above the pelvic brim becomes an anterior fulcrum for flexion/distraction forces that act on the mid-lumbar spine; birth injuries, which affect the upper cervical spine as a result of torsional forces applied during delivery or the lower cervical or upper thoracic spine as a result of breech delivery; and child abuse–induced injuries, the true incidence of which is not known.

In children younger than 10 years of age, SCI may occur without signs of damage on radiographs or computed tomography scans. This entity was termed *spinal cord injury without radiographic abnormality* (SCIWORA) by Pang and Wilberger (1982). They estimated that up to 67% of children with SCI will present with SCIWORA, and these injuries will be more severe (Pang & Pollack, 1989). Today, with the frequent use of magnetic resonance imaging (MRI) in the assessment of the traumatized spine, MRI abnormalities (anterior or posterior longitudinal ligament rupture, end plate fractures, intradisk abnormalities, spinal cord hemorrhage or edema) are commonly seen in individuals with SCIWORA (Grabb & Pang, 1994; Shimada & Tokioka, 1995). Unlike in the adult population with SCI, in children, MRI abnormalities correlate with the severity of the neurological deficit and the prognosis for recovery.

The neurological level and degree of completeness vary with age, with younger children more likely to have paraplegia and a complete lesion (Vogel & DeVivo, 1997). Upper cervical injuries are more common in infants and young children because of their proportionately larger heads, less developed neck musculature, a horizontal orientation of the facet joints, presence of a cartilaginous uncinate process that only ossifies at the age of 7, and relative ligamentous laxity. The fulcrum of spinal flexion is located at C2–3 in infancy, shifting to C3–4 for 3- to 8-year-olds, C4–5 for 9- to 11-year-olds, and C5–6 in children older than 11 years of age and adults.

The male–female ratio varies according to age: from birth to 3 years old it is 1:1; from 4 to 8 years old, 60:40; from 9 to 15 years old, 70:30; and from 16 to 20 years old, 85:15. The last value is similar to that in the adult SCI population (Masagli, 2000). Twenty percent to 50% of children with vertebral column injuries will have a neurological deficit; one third to one half of them will have a complete SCI (Hadley, Zabramski, Browner, Rekate, & Sonntag, 1988; Hamilton & Myles, 1992).

Nontraumatic Injuries

Nontraumatic causes of spinal cord dysfunction include Down syndrome (atlantoaxial instability), skeletal dysplasias such as achondroplasia and Morquio syndrome (associated with myelopathy secondary to stenosis or instability), juvenile rheumatoid arthritis (C1–2 instability secondary to facet synovitis and fusion of cervical vertebra), C1–2 rotary subluxation caused by tonsilopharyngitis (Grisel's syndrome) (Wilberger, 1986), and transverse myelitis (Knebusch, Strassburg, & Reiners, 1998).

PATHOPHYSIOLOGY

Trauma to the spine in children creates significantly different patterns of injury compared with those in the adult spine because of the anatomic differences between the young and the adult spine. Before 8–10 years of age, spinal ligaments are more elastic, facet joints have a more shallow and horizontal orientation, vertebral bodies have anterior wedging, ossification centers are not fused, and uncinate processes are poorly developed.

Applying Denis's (1983) three-column theory allows injuries to be divided into four major types: 1) compression fractures (failure of the anterior column with an intact middle column); 2) burst fractures (failure of the anterior and middle columns under compression);

3) seat belt fractures (anterior column compression injury with distraction of the middle and posterior columns); and 4) fracture-dislocations (failure of all three columns). Fractures can also be classified according to the mechanism of injury, attributed to predominant force vectors acting on the spine (Harris, Edeiken-Monroe, & Kopaniky, 1986):

1. Flexion force, resulting in anterior subluxation, bilateral facet dislocation, simple wedge compression fracture, and flexion teardrop fracture

2. Flexion rotation force, resulting in unilateral facet dislocation

3. Extension rotation force, resulting in pillar fractures

4. Vertical compression force, resulting in burst fractures

5. Hyperextension force, resulting in hyperextension/dislocation, avulsion fracture of the anterior arch of the atlas, extension teardrop fracture of the atlas, fracture of the posterior arch of the atlas, laminar fracture, traumatic spondylolisthesis, and hyperextension fracture-dislocation

6. Lateral flexion force, resulting in uncinate process fractures (in children older than 10 years old)

OUTCOME MEASURES

Neurological Measures

The most common scale employed in defining traumatic SCIs is the International Standards for Neurological and Functional Classification of Spinal Cord Injury, developed by the American Spinal Injury Association (ASIA) in 1982, and subsequently revised multiple times (last revision in 2002). The ASIA Impairment Scale is the result of systematic examination of dermatomes and myotomes in the body in order to determine the cord segments affected by the SCI. Several measures of neurological damage can be generated: Neurological Level, Sensory Level, and Motor Level (on right and left sides); Sensory Scores (Pin Prick and Light Touch); Motor Score; and Zone of Partial Preservation.

The ASIA Impairment Scale grades the degree of impairment in five different subgroups:

- *A*—Complete: no sensory or motor function is preserved in sacral segments S4–5.

- *B*—Incomplete: sensory but not motor function is preserved below the neurological level and includes sacral segments S4–5.

- *C*—Incomplete: motor function is preserved below the neurological level, and more than half of key muscles below the neurological level have a muscle grade less than 3 (grades 0–2).

- *D*—Incomplete: motor function is preserved below the neurological level and at least half of key muscles below the neurological level have a muscle grade greater than or equal to 3.

- *E*—Normal: sensory and motor functions are normal.

Functional Measures

The Functional Independence Measure for Children (WeeFIM; Msall et al., 1994) was adapted from the adult Functional Independence Measure (FIM; Keith, Granger, Hamilton, & Sherwin, 1987) in 1987 to provide uniform assessment of rehabilitation outcomes, the severity of disability, and the burden of care in children older than 6 months of age. The FIM focuses on six areas of functioning (self-care, sphincter control, mobility, locomotion, communication, social cognition), with each of the items evaluated on level of assistance (in terms of dependence on others and assistive devices) using a 7-point scale, where 7 denotes independence and 1 complete dependence (Kidd et al., 1995).

The Pediatric Evaluation of Disability Inventory (PEDI; Haley, Coster, Ludlow, Haltiwanger, & Andrellos, 1992) is a discipline-free, judgment-based assessment of functional capabilities and performance in the domains of self-care, mobility, and social function that consists of 210 test items that can be administered by observation or parent interview. It assesses children between 6 months and 7.5 years of age who have physical limitations or

a combination of physical and cognitive limitations.

ACUTE INJURIES

Treatment

Immobilization requires the use of a backboard and other devices immobilizing the cervical spine (cervical collar or sandbags and taping). Because young children have larger heads in comparison with the rest of their bodies, use of a mattress to raise the torso in relationship to the head is recommended (Herzenberg, Hensinger, Dedrick, & Phillips, 1989).

Airway management is imperative. The technique of intubation is controversial. Comparison of oral versus nasal intubation in adults with cervical spine fractures showed no neurological deterioration attributed to the intubation technique. In-line traction and fiberoptic-guided intubation tend to minimize spinal motion.

Pharmacological treatment includes high-dose methylprednisolone and vasopressors for spinal shock–induced hypotension. The use of high-dose methylprednisolone in adults suffering SCIs is controversial (Bracken et al., 1990, 1997; Nesathurai, 1998). Managing the spinal shock mainly with fluids runs the risk of neurogenic pulmonary edema development.

Stabilization can be accomplished through external or internal (surgical) means. External stabilization devices include hard collars and halos for cervical injuries. Halo use in the pediatric population has a higher rate of pin loosening and infection and requires the use of multiple pins to minimize torque to the thin skull (Baum, Hanley, & Pullekines, 1989). For thoracolumbar fractures, bracing is advocated. Surgical stabilization can be done early or late. Indications for early surgery include nonreducible fracture-dislocations, progression of neurological deficit, and compound wounds. Early fusion of the developing spine creates loss of longitudinal trunk growth, postoperative curve progression and vertebral rotation, and progressive lordosis resulting from anterior vertebral growth after posterior fusion ("crankshaft phenomenon") (Dubousset, Herring, & Shufflebarger, 1989; Lancourt, Dickson, & Carter, 1981).

Complications

Respiratory Complications The primary structures involved in breathing are the diaphragm, with C3–5 innervation by the phrenic nerve, and the intercostal muscles, innervated by T1–11 segmental spinal nerves. Accessory breathing muscles are the trapezium, innervated by cranial nerve XI and the C3–4 spinal nerves; the sternocleidomastoid muscle, innervated by cranial nerve XI and the C1–2 spinal nerves; the scalene muscles, innervated by spinal nerves C1–4; the pectoralis muscles, innervated by C5–8 roots; and the abdominal muscles, with T6–L1 innervation. Respiratory centers are located in the medulla, regulating respiratory depth and rhythmicity, and in the cortex, regulating volitional breathing and breathing during speech.

The primary respiratory dysfunction in children with SCI is restrictive respiratory insufficiency induced by muscle paralysis. There is a smaller obstructive component in children with high cervical injuries in which there is vagal nerve predominance, predisposing to airway hyperreactivity. Pneumococcal vaccine should be given to children with respiratory dysfunction older than 2 years of age, and influenza vaccination should be given yearly for children older than 6 months. Children who require lifelong ventilatory support and have a neurological lesion at C3 or above may be candidates for diaphragmatic pacing, which should be performed bilaterally to avoid mediastinal shifts (Weese-Mayer, Hunt, Brouillette, & Silvestri, 1992).

Cardiovascular Complications Deep venous thrombosis (DVT) occurs in 2.5%–17.5% of children and adolescents with SCIs (Radecki & Gaebler-Spira, 1994), and pulmonary embolism occurs in up to 2.3% (Warning & Karunas, 1991). Children who have gone through puberty should be considered for anticoagulant prophylaxis. Prophylaxis and treatment for DVT in children and adolescents with SCI is similar to that for adults (Consortium for Spinal Cord Medicine, 1999) (Table 30.1).

Autonomic dysreflexia (AD) manifests with sweating, facial flushing, headaches, hypertension, and piloerection. Whereas school-age children are able to report headache or discomfort, younger children are not, so a high index of suspicion needs to be maintained. Blood pressure varies with body size and age, so appropriate values need to be determined, and appropriate-size cuffs need to be used. Baseline blood pressure needs to be established, because children with cervical injuries will exhibit

Table 30.1. Deep venous thrombosis prophylaxis clinical practice guidelines

	Level of risk		
	Motor incomplete	Motor complete	Motor complete with other risk[a]
Intensity of prophylaxis			
Low	Compression hose	Compression hose	Compression hose
	Compression boots *and*	Compression boots *and*	Compression boots *and*
Intermediate	Unfractionated heparin 5000 units every 12 hours	Unfractionated heparin (dose adjusted to high-normal APTT)	Unfractionated heparin (dose adjusted to high-normal APTT)
	or LMWH	*or* LMWH	*or* LMWH *and*
High	—	—	Inferior vena cava filter in certain situations
Duration of prophylaxis			
Compression boots	2 weeks	2 weeks	2 weeks
Anticoagulants	ASIA D: while in hospital ASIA C: up to 8 weeks	At least 8 weeks	12 weeks or until discharge from rehabilitation

From Consortium for Spinal Cord Medicine. (1999). *Clinical practice guidelines: Prevention of thromboembolism in spinal cord injury* (2nd ed.). Washington, DC: Paralyzed Veterans of America; adapted by permission.

[a]Other risk factors: lower extremity fractures, previous thrombosis, cancer, heart failure, obesity.

Key: APTT, activated partial thromboplastin time; ASIA, American Spinal Injury Association; LMWH, low-molecular-weight heparin.

lower values than those without SCI. The mechanism of AD involves unopposed sympathetic outflow below the injury level and parasympathetic outflow above the injury level. There is accumulation of substance P and inhibitory neurotransmitter deficit (e.g., γ-aminobutyric acid, norepinephrine, 5-hydroxytryptamine) below the injury, with resultant supersensitivity of spinal alpha and peripheral adrenoreceptors. There is also carotid sinus and aortic arch baroreceptor insensitivity for very high or very low blood pressure values ($<$ 60 or $>$ 160 mm Hg).

The treatment of AD is symptomatic, including sitting the individual upright and identifying the precipitating factor; lower urinary tract irritants account for 75%–85% of AD episodes and anorectal stimulation for 13%–19%. Other causes, including gastrointestinal (GI) factors, cutaneous stimuli, trauma, fracture, DVT, and drugs, should also be considered. For those individuals not responding to conservative measures, hypertension treatment using short-acting drugs with rapid onset (e.g., sublingual nifedipine; sublingual, paste, or intravenous nitroglycerin; intravenous hydralazine) should be considered. Individuals with recurrent AD may be treated with adrenergic antagonist agents such as clonidine (5–7 mcg/kg/24 hours divided every 6–12 hours to a maximum dose of 0.9 mg/24 hours); prazosin (25–150 mcg/kg/24 hours divided every 6 hours); or terazosin (1–5 mg/24 hours). Most important in the treatment and prevention of AD is patient and family education.

Fever Fever is common in the acute and subacute phases of SCI. Differential diagnosis include infections (e.g., urinary tract infections, surgical site infections, epididymitis, sinusitis, otitis media), DVT/phlebitis, pressure ulcers, pulmonary disorders, heterotopic ossification, and pathological fractures. In 8%–11% of cases, no etiology is found and the fever is presumed to be secondary to thermoregulatory abnormalities (Beraldo et al., 1993).

Gastrointestinal Complications Gastrointestinal dysfunction mechanisms are multifactorial in individuals with SCI. Direct GI trauma, neuroendocrine response to stress, and changes in neurological control are all potential contributors. Gastrointestinal trauma accompanies 6.8% of SCIs in adults. Signs and symptoms are late (decreased hematocrit) or absent, so a high index of suspicion must be maintained for anorexia, nausea, vomiting, fever, and abdominal distension. Neuroendocrine response to stress induces ulcers in 22% of individuals during the first month. Significant bleeding occurs most frequently in the first 4–10 days after the injury in 5% of cases, with higher incidence in complete, high lesions. The mortality rate can be very high (up to 80%) secondary to loss of sympathetic compensatory response. Prophylaxis and treatment with histamine$_2$ receptor blockers is advocated. The GI system has parasympathetic innervation originating in the brain stem and spinal nerves S2–4 (vagus nerve and pelvic nerves, respectively), sympathetic innervation from T5 to L2 through the superior and inferior mesenteric and hypogastric nerves, and somatic innervation from spinal nerves S2–4 through the pudendal nerve. Each segment of the tract exhibits specific dysfunctions: gastroesophageal reflux disease and hiatal hernia in high injuries (esophagus), dissociation of antral and duodenal motility, and decreased gastric emptying secondary to lack of pacesetting action from the antrum in high injuries (stomach), increased incidence of cholelithiasis in injuries above T10 (gallbladder), and paralytic ileus (bowel).

Genitourinary Complications Genitourinary system manifestations in the acute phase consist mainly of urinary retention secondary to nervous system dysfunction and urinary tract infections related to bladder instrumentation. The peripheral pathways to the genitourinary system are parasympathetic (vagus nerve for the kidneys, S2–4 for the bladder), sympathetic (hypogastric nerve [T12–L2] to the bladder), and somatic (pudendal nerve [S3–4] to the pelvic diaphragm). There is also a central component involving the cortex, midbrain-pons, and sacral nuclei.

Dermatological Complications Skin/pressure ulcerations can occur after only 1–2 hours of immobilization on a backboard in a neurocompromised individual. As many as 32% of adults with SCI develop pressure ulcerations during acute care and rehabilitation (Stover, DeLisa, & Whiteneck, 1995). The incidence in pediatric SCI is not known.

Nutritional and Metabolic Complications Nutritional and metabolic abnormalities in the acute phase include changes in energy requirements (decreased to 54% of normal), loss of body proteins, decreased lean body mass and increased fat percentage, loss of intracellular water with increased extracellular-intracellular ratio, increased response to diuretics, nocturnal natriuresis with negative sodium balance and propensity to hyponatremia, hyperphosphaturia, hypermagnesuria, and hyperuricosuria. Immobilization hypercalcemia is almost unique to children and occurs in 10%–23% of young individuals with SCI (Tori & Hill, 1978). The decreased motility following SCI triggers an increase in bone resorption, with subsequent dumping of calcium into the blood. The ensuing hypercalcemia depresses renal function and further increases the blood calcium level. The elevation in calcium can occur as early as 2 weeks following the SCI but is most common at the 4- to 8-week mark (Maynard & Imai, 1977). There is an associated depressed parathyroid hormone level. The management of immobilization hypercalcemia includes hydration, furosemide (0.5–2 mg/kg/24 hours every 6–12 hours), and bisphosphonates (e.g., pamidronate, 1 mg/kg in a single dose, up to a maximum of 60 mg over 4 hours or 90 mg over 24 hours) (Bilezikian, 1992; Lteif & Zimmermand, 1998). Complications of hypercalcemia include urolithiasis, nephrocalcinosis, and renal failure.

In the chronic phase, lipid and glucose metabolism are most notably affected. There is a decrease in the high-density lipoprotein level with development of accelerated or premature coronary artery disease (Bauman & Spungen, 1994; Bauman et al., 1992, 1999; Breanes, Dearwater, Shapera, LaPorte, & Collins, 1986). Seventy percent of individuals with SCI have an abnormal response to an oral glucose load and hyperinsulinemia after glucose administration, indicating tissue resistance to endogenous insulin.

CHRONIC INJURIES

Treatment and Rehabilitation

The treatment of chronic SCI has a medicosurgical component that addresses prevention or correction of complications related to the neurological deficit (see Complications later) and a rehabilitative component. The principles of rehabilitation of a neurological injury have been presented elsewhere in this volume (see Chapter 31). Typical interventions are multidisciplinary and include mobility and activities of daily living (ADLs) training; initiation of bowel, bladder, and skin regimens/prevention programs; patient and family education; community reintegration; education, leisure, and recreation interventions; vocational and psychological counseling; social work involvement; and resource identification. The key is to achieve maximal function at any given time in the individual's life. This can only be accomplished by providing ongoing examination of function and impairments and adjusting therapeutic interventions, goals, and target outcomes according to age and ever-changing neurological and functional status. The concept of ongoing rehabilitative care has its roots in neurodevelopment. Maintaining neural activity below the injury level has theoretically multiple positive consequences.

Establishment and Maintenance of Neuronal Connections (Synapses) The dependence of nervous system development on electrical activity has been demonstrated in many situations, perhaps most prominently in vision (Shatz, 1990; Wisel & Hubel, 1965; Wong, Herrmann & Shatz, 1991). Some of the strongest evidence is for synapse formation, or the establishment and maintenance of connections between neurons during development. For example, neuronal activity is necessary for the full development and maintenance of inhibitory circuitry (Baker & Ruijter, 1991; Corner & Ramakers, 1992; Furshpan, 1991; Ramakers, Corner, & Habets, 1990; Ruijter, Baker, De Jong, & Romijn, 1991; Rutherford, DeWan, Lauer, & Turrigiano, 1997; Seil & Drake-Baumann, 1994; Seil, Drake-Baumann, Leiman, Herndon, & Tiekotter, 1994). Chemical inhibition of neural activity in cell cultures and in animals results in reduced numbers of inhibitory synapse connections and can result in nervous system overactivity (e.g., spasticity) once the blockade is partially removed. New synapse formation and stabilization of excitatory synapses may also require coincident neural input to maintain connections and refine connection selectivity.

Myelination: Formation and Maintenance of Myelin

If myelin is damaged, it impairs information transmission between neurons; such demyelination occurs after nervous system injury and contributes to the functional deficits (Blight, 1983, 1985; Bunge, Bunge, & Ris, 1961; Bunge, Puckett, Becerra, Marcillo, & Quencer, 1993; Gledhill, Harrison, & McDonald, 1973a, 1973b; Griffiths & McCulloch, 1983). Remyelination of axons that have been demyelinated secondary to injury is dependent on optimal electrical activity in the nerve being myelinated (Demerens et al., 1996). The strongest evidence is in the peripheral nervous system, but strong data also exist for the central nervous system (Barres & Raff, 1993).

Birth of New Neural Cells from Stem Cells

Stem cells exist in the ventricle lining of the brain and spinal cord of adults. These stem cells are capable of birthing new neurons, oligodendrocytes, and astrocytes (Gage, 1998; Kempermann & Gage, 1999). Although these are early days in research and we do not yet have a good handle on how to stimulate the dormant stem cells to birth new cells, recent work from several laboratories, including that of Rusty Gage, Ph.D., has shown that patterned neural activity created by enhancing walking activity in rodents can lead to overall greater production and survival of newly born cells (Kempermann & Gage, 1999). The survival of injured or newly developed neurons and glia has been shown to be partly dependent on optimal levels of neural activity (Barres & Raff, 1993).

Promotion of Functional Recovery

Activity is known to promote functional recovery after nervous system insults such as trauma or stroke (Chollet et al., 1991; Elbert et al., 1994; Jenkins & Merzenich, 1987). New interest has developed in incorporating patterned neural (motor or sensory) activation of the lower limbs in the rehabilitative program of individuals with neurological injuries. Partial weight-supported walking has the best documented scientific background (Barbeau & Funga, 2001; Barbeau, Ladoucer, Norman, Pepin, & Leroux, 1999), but other modalities can be employed to achieve patterned activity: functional electrical stimulation (FES) bicycling (utilizing commercially available FES-assisted lower extremity ergometers, e.g., ERGYS and the RT 300) or walking (utilizing surface-stimulated systems, e.g., Parastep), assisted movements such as motorized bicycling, or utilization of continuous passive movement devices.

Activity below the injury level can also be produced in a nonpatterned manner. Recruitment and strengthening of the muscle fibers can be done with traditional isotonic, isometric, and isokinetic strengthening; electrically stimulated recruitment and strengthening; recruitment in a gravity-eliminated environment (i.e., aquatic therapy); and muscle recruitment and motor reeducation using biofeedback. Patterned sensory activation of neural circuitry seated below the injury level can be done with massage therapy or sustained vibratory stimulation of a targeted structure (i.e., the upper extremity in individuals with tetraplegia).

A typical rehabilitative prescription should involve all components coordinated into a supervised program: stretching; strengthening through traditional, electrically stimulated, gravity-eliminated, or biofeedback methods; balance training; mobility and ADL training; gait training utilizing the over-the-ground method, but also body weight–supported or FES-assisted techniques and aquatic therapy–facilitated gait training; and endurance building employing methods such as FES-assisted bicycling, aquatic therapy, and wheelchair sports. Such a program applied in the acute/subacute SCI rehabilitative phase accomplishes functional training and limits the onset of secondary complications related to the neurological deficit (muscle atrophy, contractures, spasticity, bone loss, glucose- and lipid-related metabolic changes) (Hjeltnes et al., 1997; Mohr et al., 1997; Skold et al., 2002; Sloan, Bremner, Byrne, Day, & Scull, 1994). If the program is applied in the chronic phase, it partially restores muscle mass, reverses or minimizes bone and metabolic changes, and even improves neurological function (McDonald et al., 2002).

Complications

The child with an SCI above T6 is essentially poikilothermic because of autonomic nervous system dysfunction. The hypothalamus is "disconnected" from the periphery, and the sensory input from the skin is diminished. Exposure to cold and use of medication that increases blood flow to the skin (cholinergics, alpha blockers) may predispose to hypothermia, and exposure to high temperatures induces fever.

Latex allergy is more prevalent in children with SCIs, myelomeningocele, and congenital genitourinary abnormalities (Konz et al., 1995). Spasticity is less prevalent in children with SCIs compared with adults. The principles of diagnosis and treatment are nevertheless the same (Vogel, 1996). Physical modalities (range of motion, mobilization) remain the least invasive method of management, with pharmacological and surgical interventions carrying a higher risk of complications and side effects.

The incidence of *heterotopic ossification* in children with SCI is reported at 3%, in contrast to 20% reported in adults with SCI (Betz, 1997; Garland, 1991). It has a later onset (14 months compared with 1–4 months) (Garland, Shimoyama, Lugo, Barras, & Gilgoff, 1989), and the hip is most commonly involved. Treatment with etidronate or postoperative use of radiation therapy is contraindicated in children prior to puberty.

Osteopenia and *osteoporosis* are consequences of immobility, lack of weight bearing, and muscle torque on the bone. Following onset of paralysis, there is an initial increase in osteoclastic activity, followed by a decrease in the osteoblastic rate. This, coupled with the massive negative calcium balance present in the first 12–18 months after the injury, leads to an average 40% loss of bone density in children with SCI compared with normal age- and sex-matched controls. A combination of standing, stepping, and FES may increase the bone

mineral density by 25% (Betz et al., 1991). Pathological fractures are reported to have a 14% incidence in children (Betz, 1997) compared with 7% in adults.

Hip instability and deformities are common in children who are injured prior to puberty. Children with spasticity develop posterior subluxation, whereas those with flaccid lower extremities have a shallow acetabulum. Surgical correction is advocated if FES-assisted ambulation is entertained (Betz, Mulcahey, Smith, Triolo, & McMarthy, 2001).

Spine deformities, specifically neurogenic scoliosis, develop in 98% of children injured prior to skeletal maturity; 67% of them require surgery (Dearolf et al., 1990). Bracing with a thoracolumbo-sacral orthosis is recommended for skeletally immature children with curves between 20 and 45 degrees (Lubicky & Betz, 1996). Children older than 10 years old with curves greater than 40 degrees should undergo fusion (Betz & Mulcahey, 1994). Children younger than 10 years of age can tolerate up to 80 degrees of curvature if the curve is flexible and can be decreased while braced.

Syringomyelia can occur in up to 51% of pediatric SCI cases (Backe, Betz, Mesgarzadeh, Beck, & Clancy, 1991). Clinically it may present as a decrease in neurological function, rapid progression of the scoliotic curve, increased spasticity, an ascending sensory level, and increase in or new onset of pain. Surgical shunting can be combined with curve repair, if the latter is indicated.

CONCLUSION

Children with SCI are not just small adults. The time of injury onset and the changing nature of the child's anatomy and physiology create specific circumstances that make pediatric SCI unique. Although some features and interventions can be adapted from the practice of SCI medicine in adults, there are numerous differences that require customization of the process to children in general and to each child and each time frame in that child's development in particular. The focus of rehabilitative interventions changes with age, and the process is extended beyond the family and health care world to the school and community. Although an SCI is devastating no matter the age, the still-developing nervous system in children allows for a greater degree of neurological restoration if clinicians follow neurodevelopmental principles in their therapeutic approach.

Neurorehabilitation has grown and changed immensely over the last several decades. Much of the need for its development has been the result of modern medical/trauma systems that allow individuals with significant neurological injuries to survive, but often with disabilities. Although our understanding of these injuries and their medical and rehabilitation management has been rapidly progressing, large gaps remain in our knowledge of the efficiency and efficacy of rehabilitation interventions. With the explosion of new interventions and outcome measures (ranging from clinical scales of neurological function to noninvasive methods of documenting central nervous system reorganization), however, the ability to answer these important questions is now possible.

REFERENCES

Backe, H.A., Betz, R.R., Mesgarzadeh, M., Beck, T., & Clancy, M. (1991). Post traumatic spinal cord cysts evaluated by magnetic resonance imaging. *Paraplegia, 29,* 607–612.

Baker, R.E., & Ruijter, J.M. (1991). Chronic blockade of bioelectric activity in neonatal rat neocortex in vitro: Physiological effects. *International Journal of Developmental Neuroscience, 9,* 321–329.

Barbeau, H., & Funga, J. (2001). The role of rehabilitation in the recovery of walking in the neurological populations. *Current Opinions in Neurology, 14,* 735–740.

Barbeau, H., Ladoucer, M., Norman, K.E., Pepin, A., & Leroux, A. (1999). Walking after spinal cord injury: Evaluation, treatment and functional recovery. *Archives of Physical Medicine and Rehabilitation, 80,* 225–235.

Barres, B.A., & Raff, M.C. (1993). Proliferation of oligodendrocyte precursor cells depends on electrical activity in axons. *Nature, 361,* 258–260.

Baum, I.A., Hanley, E.N., & Pullekines, I. (1989). Comparison of halo complications in adults and children. *Spine, 14,* 251–252.

Bauman, W.A., Adkins, R.H., Spungen, A.M., Herbert, R., Schechter, C., Smith, D., et al. (1999). Is immobilization associated with an abnormal lipoprotein profile? Observations from a diverse cohort. *Spinal Cord, 37,* 485–490.

Bauman, W.A., & Spungen, A.M. (1994). Disorders of carbohydrate and lipid metabolism in veterans with paraplegia or quadriplegia: A model of premature aging. *Metabolism, 43,* 749–756.

Bauman, W.A., Spungen, A.M., Zhong, Y.G., Rothstein, J.L., Petry, C., & Gordon, S.K. (1992). Depressed serum HDL cholesterol levels in veterans with spinal cord injury. *Paraplegia, 30,* 697–703.

Beraldo, P.S., Neves, E.G., Alves, C.M., Khan, P., Cirilo, A.C., & Alencar, M.R. (1993). Pyrexia in hospitalized spinal cord injury patients. *Paraplegia, 31,* 186–191.

Betz, R.R. (1997). Orthopedic problems in the child with spinal cord injury. *Topics in Spinal Cord Injury Rehabilitation, 3,* 9–19.

Betz, R.R., & Mulcahey, M.J. (1994). Spinal cord injury rehabilitation. In S.L. Weinstein (Ed.), *The pediatric spine: Principles and practice* (pp. 781–810). New York: Raven Press.

Betz, R.R., Mulcahey, M.J., Smith, B.T., Triolo, R.J., & McMarthy, J.J. (2001). Implications of hip subluxation for FES-assisted mobility in patients with spinal cord injury. *Orthopedics, 24,* 181–184.

Betz, R.R., Triolo, R.J., Hermida, V.M., Moynahan, M., Gardner, A., Cook, S.D., et al. (1991). The effects of functional neuromuscular stimulation on the bone mineral content in the lower limbs of spinal cord injured children. *Journal of the American Paraplegia Society, 14,* 65–66.

Bilezikian, J.P. (1992). Management of acute hypercalcemia. *New England Journal of Medicine, 326,* 1196–1203.

Blight, A.R. (1983). Cellular morphology of chronic spinal cord injury in the cat: Analysis of myelinated axons by line sampling. *Neuroscience, 10,* 521–543.

Blight, A.R. (1985). Delayed demyelination and macrophage invasion: A candidate for secondary cell damage in spinal cord injury. *Central Nervous System Trauma, 2,* 299–315.

Bracken, M.B., Shepard, M.J., Collins, W.F., Holford, T.R., Young, W., Baskin, D.S., et al. (1990). A randomized controlled trial of methylprednisolone or naloxone in the treatment of acute spinal cord injury. *New England Journal of Medicine, 322,* 1405–1411.

Bracken, M.B., Shepard, M.J., Holford, T.R., Leo-Summers, L., Aldrich, E.F., Fazl, M., et al. (1997). Administration of methylprednisolone for 24 or 48 hours or tirilizad mesylate for 48 hours in the treatment of acute spinal cord injury. *JAMA, 277,* 1597–1604.

Breanes, G., Dearwater, S., Shapera, R., LaPorte, R.E., & Collins, E. (1986). HDL cholesterol concentrations in physically active and sedentary spinal cord injured patients. *Archives of Physical Medicine and Rehabilitation, 67,* 445–450.

Bunge, M.B., Bunge, R.P., & Ris, H. (1961). Ultrastructural study of remyelination in an experimental lesion in adult cat spinal cord. *Journal of Biophysical and Biochemical Cytology, 10,* 67–94.

Bunge, R.P., Puckett, W.R., Becerra, J.L., Marcillo, A., & Quencer, R.M. (1993). Observations on the pathology of human spinal cord injury: A review and classification of 22 new cases with details from a case of chronic cord compression with extensive focal demyelination. *Advances in Neurology, 59,* 75–89.

Chollet, F., DiPiero, V., Wise, R.J., Brooks, D.J., Dolan, R.J., & Frackowiak, R.S. (1991). The functional anatomy of motor recovery after stroke in humans: A study with positron emission tomography. *Annuals of Neurology, 29,* 63–71.

Consortium for Spinal Cord Medicine. (1999). *Clinical practice guidelines: Prevention of thromboembolism in spinal cord injury* (2nd ed.). Washington, DC: Paralyzed Veterans of America.

Corner, M.A., & Ramakers, G.J. (1992). Spontaneous firing as an epigenetic factor in brain development—physiological consequences of chronic tetrodotoxin and picrotoxin exposure on cultured rat neocortex neurons. *Brain Research: Developmental Brain Research, 65,* 57–64.

Dearolf, W.W., III, Betz, R.R., Vogel, L.C., Levin, J., Clancy, M., & Steel, H.H. (1990). Scoliosis in pediatric spinal cord injured patients. *Journal of Pediatric Orthopedics, 10,* 214–218.

Demerens, C., Stankoff, B., Logak, M., Anglade, P., Allinquant, B., Couraud, F., et al. (1996). Induction of myelination in the central nervous system by electrical activity. *Proceedings of the National Academy of Sciences of the United States of America, 93,* 9887–9892.

Denis, F. (1983). The three-column spine and its significance in the classification of acute thoracolumbar spinal injuries. *Spine, 8,* 817–831.

Dubousset, J., Herring, J.A., & Shufflebarger, H. (1989). The crankshaft phenomenon. *Journal of Pediatric Orthopedics, 9,* 541–550.

Elbert, T., Flor, H., Birbaumer, N., Knecht, S., Hampson, S., Larbig, W., et al. (1994). Extensive reorganization of the somatosensory cortex in adult humans after nervous system injury. *NeuroReport, 5,* 2593–2597.

Furshpan, E.J. (1991). Seizure-like activity in cell culture. *Epilepsy Research, 10,* 24–32.

Gage, F.H. (1998). Stem cells of the central nervous system. *Current Opinion in Neurobiology, 8,* 671–676.

Garland, D.A. (1991). A clinical perspective on common forms of acquired heterotopic ossification. *Clinical Orthopedics and Related Research, 263,* 13–29.

Garland, D.E., Shimoyama, S.T., Lugo, C., Barras, D., & Gilgoff, I. (1989). Spinal cord insults and heterotopic ossification in the pediatric population. *Clinical Orthopedics and Related Research, 245,* 303–310.

Gledhill, R.F., Harrison, B.M., & McDonald, W.I. (1973a). Demyelination and remyelination after acute spinal cord compression. *Experimental Neurology, 38,* 472–487.

Gledhill, R.F., Harrison, B.M., & McDonald, W.I. (1973b). Pattern of remyelination in the CNS. *Nature, 244,* 443–444.

Go, B.K., DeVivo, M.J., & Richards, J.S. (1995). The epidemiology of spinal cord injury. In S.L. Stover, J.A. DeLisa, & G.G. Whiteneck (Eds.), *Spinal cord injury: Clinical outcomes from the model systems* (pp. 21–25). Gaithersburg, MD: Aspen Publications.

Grabb, P.A., & Pang, D. (1994). Magnetic resonance imaging in the evaluation of spinal cord injury without radiographic abnormality in children. *Neurosurgery, 35,* 406–413.

Griffiths, I.R., & McCulloch, M.C. (1983). Nerve fibres in spinal cord impact injuries. Part 1: Changes in the myelin sheath during the initial 5 weeks. *Journal of Neurological Sciences, 58,* 335–349.

Hadley, N.M., Zabramski, I.M., Browner, C.M., Rekate, H., & Sonntag, V.K. (1988). Pediatric spinal trauma: Review of 122 cases of spinal cord and vertebral column injuries. *Journal of Neurosurgery, 68,* 18–24.

Haffner, D.L., Hoffer, M.M., & Wiedbusch, R.W. (1993). Etiology of children's spinal injuries at Ranchos Los Amigos. *Spine, 18,* 679–684.

Haley, S.M., Coster, W.J., Ludlow, L.H., Haltiwanger, J.T., & Andrellos, P.J. (1992). *Pediatric Evaluation of Disability Inventory (PEDI): Development, standardization and administration manual.* Boston: New England Medical Center Hospital PEDI Research Group.

Hamilton, M.G., & Myles, S.T. (1992). Pediatric spinal injury: Review of 174 hospital admissions. *Journal of Neurosurgery, 77,* 700–704.

Harris, J.H., Edeiken-Monroe, B., & Kopaniky, D.R. (1986). A practical classification of acute cervical spine injuries. *Orthopedic Clinics of North America, 17,* 15–30.

Hawley, C.A. (2004). Behaviour and school performance after brain injury. *Brain Injury, 18,* 645–659.

Herzenberg, J.E., Hensinger, R.N., Dedrick, D.K., & Phillips, W.A. (1989). Emergency transport and positioning of young children who have an injury of the cervical spine: The standard backboard may be hazardous. *Journal of Bone and Joint Surgery: American Volume, 71,* 15–22.

Hjeltnes, N., Aksnes, A.K., Birkeland, K.I., Johansen, J., Lannem, A., & Wallberg-Henriksson, H. (1997). Improved body composition after 8 weeks of electrically stimulated leg cycling in tetraplegic patients. *American Journal of Physiology, 273*(3 Pt. 2), R1072–R1079.

Jenkins, W.M., & Merzenich, M.M. (1987). Reorganization of neocortical representations after brain injury: A neurophysiological model of the bases of recovery from stroke. *Progress in Brain Research, 71,* 249–266.

Keith, R.A., Granger, C.V., Hamilton, B.B., & Sherwin, F.S. (1987). The Functional Independence Measure: A new tool for rehabilitation. *Advances in Clinical Rehabilitation, 1*, 6–18.

Kempermann, G., & Gage, F.H. (1999). New nerve cells for the adult brain. *Scientific American, 280*, 48–53.

Kidd, D., Stewart, G., Baldry, J., Johnson, J., Rossiter, D., Petruckevitch, A., et al. (1995). The Functional Independence Measure: A comparative validity and reliability study. *Disability and Rehabilitation, 17*, 10–14.

Knebusch, M., Strassburg, H.M., & Reiners, K. (1998). Acute transverse myelitis in childhood: Nine cases and review of the literature. *Developmental Medicine and Child Neurology, 40*, 631–639.

Konz, K.R., Chia, J.K., Kurup, V.P., Resnick, A., Kelly, K.J., & Fink, J.N. (1995). Comparison of latex hypersensitivity among patients with neurologic defects. *Journal of Allergy and Clinical Immunology, 95*(5 Pt. 1), 950–954.

Lancourt, J.E., Dickson, J.H., & Carter, R.E. (1981). Paralytic spinal deformity following traumatic spinal cord injury in children and adolescents. *Journal of Bone and Joint Surgery, 63*(A), 47–53.

Lteif, A.N., & Zimmermand, D. (1998). Biphosphonates for treatment of childhood hypercalcemia. *Pediatrics, 102*, 990–993.

Lubicky, J.P., & Betz, R.R. (1996). Spinal deformities in children and adolescents after spinal cord injury. In R.R. Betz, & M.J. Mulcahey (Eds.), *The child with a spinal cord injury* (pp. 363–370). Rosemont, IL: American Academy of Orthopedic Surgeons.

Massagli, T.L. (2000). Medical and rehabilitation issues in the care of children with spinal cord injuries. *Physical Medicine and Rehabilitation Clinics of North America, 11*, 169–182.

Maynard, F.M., & Imai, K. (1977). Immobilization hypercalcemia in spinal cord injury. *Archives of Physical Medicine and Rehabilitation, 58*, 16–24.

McDonald, J.W., Becker, D., Sadowsky, C., Jane, J.A., Conturo, T.E., & Schultz, L.M. (2002). Late recovery following spinal cord injury: Case report and review of the literature. *Journal of Neurosurgery: Spine, 97*, 252–265.

Mohr, T., Andersen, J., Biering-Sorensen, F., Galbo, H., Bangsbo, J., Wagner, A., et al. (1997). Longterm adaptation to electrically induced cycle training in severe spinal cord injured individuals. *Spinal Cord, 35*, 1–16.

Msall, M.E., DiGaudio, K., Rogers, B.T., LaForest, S., Catanzaro, N.L., Campbell, J., et al. (1994). The Functional Independence Measure for Children (WeeFIM): Conceptual basis and pilot use in children with developmental disabilities. *Clinical Pediatrics, 33*, 431–438.

Nesathurai, S. (1998). Steroids and spinal cord injury: Revisiting the NASCIC 2 and NASCIS 3 trials. *Journal of Trauma, 45*, 1088–1093.

Pang, D., & Pollack, I.F. (1989). Spinal cord injury without radiographic abnormality in children—the SCIWORA syndrome. *Journal of Trauma, 29*, 654–664.

Pang, D., & Wilberger, J.E (1982). Spinal cord injury without radiographic abnormalities in children. *Journal of Neurosurgery, 57*, 114–129.

Radecki, R.T., & Gaebler-Spira, D. (1994). Deep vein thrombosis in the disabled pediatric population. *Archives of Physical Medicine and Rehabilitation, 75*, 248–250.

Ramakers, G.J., Corner, M.A., & Habets, A.M. (1990). Development in the absence of spontaneous bioelectric activity results in increased stereotyped burst firing in cultures of dissociated cerebral cortex. *Experimental Brain Research, 79*, 157–166.

Ruijter, J.M., Baker, R.E., De Jong, B.M., & Romijn, H.J. (1991). Chronic blockade of bioelectric activity in neonatal rat cortex grown in vitro: Morphological effects. *International Journal of Developmental Neuroscience, 9*, 331–338.

Rutherford, L.C., DeWan, A., Lauer, H.M., & Turrigiano, G.G. (1997). Brain-derived neurotrophic factor mediates the activity-dependent regulation of inhibition in neocortical cultures. *Journal of Neuroscience, 17*, 4527–4535.

Seil, F.J., & Drake-Baumann, R. (1994). Reduced cortical inhibitory synaptogenesis in organotypic cerebellar cultures developing in the absence of neuronal activity. *Journal of Comparative Neurology, 342*, 366–377.

Seil, F.J., Drake-Baumann, R., Leiman, A.L., Herndon, R.M., & Tiekotter, K.L (1994). Morphological correlates of altered neuronal activity in organotypic cerebellar cultures chronically exposed to anti-GABA agents. *Developmental Brain Research, 77*, 123–132.

Shatz, C.J. (1990). Impulse activity and the patterning of connections during CNS development. *Neuron, 5*, 745–756.

Shimada, K., & Tokioka, T. (1995). Sequential MRI studies in patients with cervical cord injury but without bony injury. *Paraplegia, 33*, 573–578.

Skold, C., Lonn, L., Harms-Ringdahl, K., Hultling, C., Levi, R., Nash, M., et al. (2002). Effects of functional electrical stimulation training for six months on body composition and spasticity in motor complete tetraplegic spinal cord-injured individuals. *Journal of Rehabilitation Medicine, 34*, 25–32.

Sloan, K.E., Bremner, L.A., Byrne, J., Day, R.E., & Scull, E.R. (1994). Musculoskeletal effects of an electrical stimulation induced cycling programme in the spinal injured. *Paraplegia, 32*, 407–415.

Stover, S.L., DeLisa, J.A., & Whiteneck, G.G. (1995). *Spinal cord injury: Clinical outcomes from the model systems.* Gaithersburg, MD: Aspen Publications.

Tori, J.A., & Hill, L.L. (1978). Hypercalcemia in children with spinal cord injury. *Archives of Physical Medicine and Rehabilitation, 59,* 443–447.

Vogel, L.C. (1996). Spasticity: Diagnostic workup and medical management. In R.R. Betz, & M.J. Mulcahey (Eds.), *The child with spinal cord injury* (pp. 261–268). Rosemont, IL: American Academy of Orthopedic Surgeons.

Vogel, L.C., & DeVivo, M.J. (1997). Pediatric spinal cord injury issues: Etiology, demographics, and pathophysiology. *Topics in Spinal Cord Injury Rehabilitation, 31,* 1–8.

Warning, W.P., & Karunas, R.S. (1991). Acute spinal cord injuries and the incidence of clinically occurring thromboembolic disease. *Paraplegia, 29,* 8–16.

Weese-Mayer, D.E., Hunt, C.E., Brouillette, R.T., & Silvestri, J.M. (1992). Diaphragm pacing in infants and children. *Journal of Pediatrics, 120,* 1–8.

Wilberger, J.E., Jr. (1986). Clinical aspects of specific spinal injuries. In J.E. Wilberger, Jr. (Ed.), *Spinal cord injuries in children* (pp. 69–95). Mount Kisco, NY: Futura.

Wisel, T.N., & Hubel, D.H. (1965). Comparison of the effects of unilateral and bilateral eye closure on cortical unit responses in kittens. *Journal of Neurophysiology, 28,* 1029–1040.

Wong, R.O., Herrmann, K., & Shatz, C.J. (1991). Remodeling of retinal ganglion cell dendrites in the absence of action potential activity. *Journal of Neurobiology, 22,* 685–697.

31

Neurorehabilitation

CYNTHIA SALORIO,
EWA BRANDYS, OLGA MOROZOVA,
FRANK S. PIDCOCK, MELISSA K. TROVATO,
CRISTINA SADOWSKY, AND JAMES CHRISTENSEN

The process of rehabilitation for a child who has an acquired neurological injury ideally begins in the intensive care unit. Potentially disabling complications such as plantar flexion ankle contractures can begin at this stage and have a devastating effect on the success of rehabilitation efforts later in the recovery phase. Although the first priority is ensuring medical stability and optimizing recovery of neurological function, preventative measures can be started during the first week of treatment following injury. The early initiation of bedside therapies can be a key component to the overall success of treatment.

A pediatric rehabilitation medicine (PRM) physician may be consulted at this stage. A PRM physician has completed residency training in the specialty of physical medicine and rehabilitation; many have also completed pediatric training as well. The PRM field focuses on restoring function and aiding patients and their families in understanding and utilizing the resources and therapeutic specialties that will be encountered during the recovery phase after an acute neurological injury.

A major priority of a rehabilitation consultation at the early stage of treatment for a neurological injury is to provide recommendations that aid in preventing medical complications that may adversely affect subsequent efforts to optimize functional recovery. This includes advice about skin protection, a bowel program to avoid constipation, prevention of urinary tract infections, gastric protection, bracing, and spasticity management.

An important role of the PRM physician during the early stage of treatment for a serious neurological injury is to meet with the family and discuss the potential issues to be faced during the rehabilitation phase of recovery. An explanation of the expected sequence of returning skills with an approximation of timing as best as can be determined should be shared with families. The perspective of the rehabilitation physician can help the family understand better what challenges are coming up after the patient leaves the intensive care setting. The roles of therapists and other team members should be explained to families because this is likely their first experience with a rehabilitation model of care, which is more team oriented and interactive than the typical medical model of care.

The PRM physician also assists in the determination of the appropriate level of care required for rehabilitation after medical stability has been achieved. This is often intensive inpatient rehabilitation either in a freestanding facility or in a unit of an acute care hospital. The PRM physician will often be the attending physician on this service and will provide direction to the therapy team.

When a patient who is recovering from an injury to the neurological system is admitted to a neurorehabilitation unit, a whole new team of people is introduced to the patient and family (Table 31.1). This is a very complex and stressful time for the family. Well-organized scheduling of initial evaluations and feedback to the family by the entire team is an important

Table 31.1. Members of the neurorehabilitation team

Child life specialists
Dietitians
Educators
Nurses
Occupational therapists
Physicians
Physical therapists
Psychologists
Social workers
Speech-language therapists
Therapeutic recreation specialists
Vocational services workers

step in ensuring a smooth transition. A crucial issue to address soon after admission is the discharge plan because often it will require time and effort to secure the correct resources, equipment, family training, and finances. There are often issues that families have not thought about because the previous focus has been on medical recovery. A sensitive and clear approach to family discussions from the beginning of an admission to the rehabilitation unit will facilitate a smooth transition for the family as they adjust to a new set of priorities.

A comprehensive neurorehabilitation program consists of at least eight essential components (Cope, 1995):

1. Medical and nursing expertise in directing and providing rehabilitation care that takes into account the consequences of neuropathology as it has an impact on the domain of human function.

2. Prevention of secondary deterioration through an organized approach that is not reliably found in a nonrehabilitation setting (Rusk, Block, & Lowman, 1969; Rusk, Lowman, & Block, 1966).

3. Optimization of the natural course of recovery through the prevention of injudicious interventions such as premature oral feeding resulting in aspiration and pneumonia.

4. Providing appropriately graded therapeutic goals that challenge patients to achieve relevant functional gains without overwhelming them. Specific techniques and goal setting should be applied by experts in mobility, self-care, communication, and feeding.

5. An optimal environment for fostering neurological recovery. This may include controlling excessive sensory stimulation during early recovery, protecting the patient from harm during the agitated stages of recovery, and addressing function in "real-world" settings as the patient progresses toward volitional activities.

6. Teaching of compensatory techniques, including cognitive, behavioral, and motor strategies for areas in which recovery is incomplete.

7. Providing the appropriate equipment for assisting in skills and reentry to the community. Examples include wheelchairs, outdoor ramps, braces, shower chairs, and adaptive utensils, to name a few.

8. Home, school, and community assessments and interventions to maximize the successful return to social and personal life. A rehabilitation discharge manager or medical social worker will often work with families to order equipment, schedule follow-up appointments, deal with the insurance companies, and implement other aspects of the discharge plan as needed.

THERAPEUTIC REHABILITATION APPROACHES

The age of a child and the type and severity of injury to the central nervous system (CNS) are key factors in selecting appropriate intervention methods, selecting a treatment strategy, and setting rehabilitation goals. Patients with traumatic brain injury or spinal cord injury sustained during infancy or early childhood may respond favorably to therapies that were originally developed for children with prenatal insult to the CNS (e.g., cerebral palsy, spina bifida). Development of scientific evidence supporting rehabilitative practices is in its early stage, and more clinical research is needed to suggest specific protocols for specific diagnoses or neurological impairments. "Gold standards" for rehabilitative treatment in specific dysfunctions are not well established, and further research will be required to draw conclusions regarding the most effective rehabilitation method for a particular diagnosis or dysfunction.

In the following sections, rehabilitation approaches to neurological dysfunction are reviewed. Although the approaches may be appropriate to both congenital and acquired disorders, this chapter has an emphasis on acquired disorders. Acquired brain (primarily traumatic brain injury) and spinal cord dysfunction are discussed in depth elsewhere in this volume (see Chapters 29 and 30).

COGNITION

Individuals with neurological injuries frequently experience changes in neurocognitive abilities after injury. The nature and extent of these cognitive changes depend on a number of factors, including preinjury characteristics such as overall intelligence and family functioning; age at onset; and aspects of the injury itself, including etiology, type of lesion, extent of injury, and location of injury in the brain. Because of the heterogeneity of individual cognitive strengths and weaknesses during the rehabilitation phase and beyond, careful assessment of these neuropsychological strengths and weaknesses is crucial (Trexler & Thomas, 1983).

Pediatric rehabilitation strives not only to help a child regain functional skill and return to "baseline" status but also to promote continued successful growth and development in the future. In children with neurological injuries during development, psychoeducational assessments that provide general developmental quotients or an overall intelligence quotient (IQ) score may not be the most useful in describing a child's abilities and impairments because confounding factors such as a child's language or motor deficits may differentially affect his or her overall score (Lezak, 1995). With the exception of the most severe neurological injuries, measures of general intelligence frequently return to pretrauma levels. In spite of this, there are usually significant specific neuropsychological deficits that interfere with optimal functioning. Therefore, careful and comprehensive assessment of the child's neuropsychological strengths and weaknesses, academic status, adaptive skills, motor skills, and psychological status may be crucial in educational and treatment planning for children with neurological conditions (Baron, 2003; Yeates, Ris, & Taylor, 1999). The goal of identifying these deficits is then to develop strategies for minimizing their impact. It is obvious how critical these functions are to new learning as well as daily performance (be it school, work, or socialization) and how impairment of these abilities can lead to significant disability in spite of "normal" general intelligence.

Postinjury cognitive deficits may be seen in a number of domains, including attention, visuospatial perception, language, memory, and executive function (including reasoning, mental flexibility, initiation, inhibitory control, goal-directed behavior, problem solving, planning ahead, organization, and behavioral regulation). Depending on the areas of cognitive dysfunction after injury, an individualized approach to cognitive rehabilitation can be designed. Most approaches to cognitive rehabilitation can be classified as using either remediation strategies or compensatory strategies. Regarding cognitive rehabilitation, Ylvisaker et al. (2005) noted that there has been a shift over the past two decades from "restorative" approaches to more "contextual" or "functional" approaches. Traditional restorative approaches make use of cognitive exercises and repetitive rehearsal, with the idea of remediating the neurological injury or cognitive process. A more contextual approach focuses on functional participation, that is, changing the child's environment and engaging family and teachers with the goal of finding ways to best allow the child to engage in valued activities.

Research focused on direct retraining of specific neuropsychological functions such as memory or attention is mixed. Although some studies have shown efficacy in specific areas (e.g., attention after seizures; Engelberts et al., 2002), the literature generally does not support the use of retraining strategies for cognitive impairments as the most successful approach. Rather, cognitive therapy should be directed toward performance of specific functional tasks, and using compensatory strategies (e.g., Park & Ingles, 2001).

For difficulties with memory, compensatory strategies may include repetition and rehearsal of information, providing information in context, use of a memory journal, written "recipes" and checklists for task completion, use of electronic pagers or alarms, and increased structure and routine. A specific issue related to memory—the definition and management of posttraumatic amnesia—is discussed elsewhere in this volume (see Chapter 29).

Modification of the environment at home and at school can be helpful for attention deficits. In addition, providing more frequent breaks during tasks, the use of timers for task persistence, and getting a child's attention prior to giving instructions are methods that can help maximize attentional capacity.

Difficulties with executive function can be supported by providing assistance with breaking tasks into smaller component parts, cues for where to begin and how to approach tasks, warnings prior to transitions or changes in schedule, breaks in between topics or lessons, and the use of organizational devices, interim deadlines for task completion, and increased structure.

Other examples of compensatory strategies include allowance for untimed test taking, assistance of a "note-taking buddy" or copies of teacher lecture plans in the classroom, the use of graph paper and lined paper, and the use of assistive devices as indicated (e.g., computer, dictation software, calculator, augmentative communication device).

The development of strategies and accommodations that work best for any given child is likely to be an ongoing, potentially lifelong process. It is obvious that the success of any rehabilitation program is measured by its ability to generalize to the child's daily life. Consequently, the training of the family in the needs of their child and ways to help meet those needs is essential. It is also important that reevaluations of neuropsychological strengths and weaknesses be done periodically, for various reasons. Initially, more frequent evaluations are needed to appreciate and adjust to the ongoing recovery that occurs. Later, periodic evaluations may be needed to detect deficits that become apparent as anticipated higher-level developmental skills fail to develop, or to detect failure of new learning as a result of specific neuropsychological deficits (Carney & Schoenbrodt, 1994).

COMMUNICATION

Verbal communication may be impaired secondary to speech or language dysfunction or both. Treatment for the motor or speech dysfunction is focused on oral motor strengthening, exercises designed to practice speech and vocalization activities, and recovery over time. Children with neurological injuries typically do not demonstrate global aphasias, and the distinction between *fluent* and *nonfluent* aphasia does not fit the pediatric population well (Bates et al., 2001). Still, children may demonstrate difficulties in expressive and/or receptive language after neurological injury, and these difficulties may be persistent (Nass & Trauner, 2004).

If a child has expressive language difficulties after an injury, therapists will initially focus on developing a consistent mode of communication for the child. This may include a picture board, thumbs-up/thumbs-down responding, use of switches, or use of eye gaze to allow the child to communicate basic needs. As recovery progresses, therapy may turn to facilitating fluency, elaboration of information to be communicated, initiation of communication, pragmatics, and organizational skills. Notably, although there is a reasonable body of literature supporting the efficacy of treatment for expressive and phonological language difficulties, there is mixed or minimal evidence showing efficacy for treatment of receptive difficulties (Law, Garrett, & Nye, 2004).

The use of compensatory strategies is helpful for ongoing language difficulties, such as the use of circumlocution (describing the word) for word-finding deficits, repetition of instructions, breaking instructions into smaller steps, providing multiple choice response formats and sound cues, and asking simple yes/no (as opposed to open-ended) questions.

EDUCATION

One of the primary tasks for children and adolescents is attending school. Rehabilitation professionals frequently assist with the integration or reintegration of a child into a school setting. Careful evaluation of the medical, mobility, behavioral, psychological, and cognitive factors that may affect the success of the transition back to school and future academic function is important. It is the rehabilitation team's responsibility to ascertain that appropriate referrals are made, that information from evaluations and ongoing treatment is communicated, that the individualized education program is appropriate, and that the educators within the school understand the student's deficits and the peculiarities of cognitive and behavioral dysfunction after neurological injury.

Law and policy in the United States is ever changing. The Education for All Handicapped Children Act (PL 94-142), passed in 1976 and reauthorized in 1990 (PL 101-476, as the Individuals with Disabilities Education Act), mandated that a *free appropriate public education* be provided in the *least restrictive environment* for children with disabilities. This law requires the development of an individualized education program for children between 3 and 21 years of age to address needs and modifications required to ensure that the student will succeed in the educational environment. In 1986, the Education of the Handicapped Act Amendments (PL 99-457) Part H expanded these rights to include early intervention services for infants and toddlers. In addition, Section 504 of the Rehabilitation Act of 1973 (PL 93-112) states that it is illegal to discriminate against a person with a disability solely because of the disability and that individuals with disabilities must have equal access to programs and services. These and other federal laws provide mechanisms by which children can be provided with school services and accommodations, including educationally relevant physical, occupational, and speech therapy.

After a neurological injury, children often show a discrepancy between performance related to overlearned rote skills and performance on novel tasks requiring new learning. Impaired new learning, as measured by the California Verbal Learning Test–Children's Version (Delis, Kramer, Kaplan, & Ober, 1994), has been shown to be predictive of the need for special education services after traumatic brain injury in children (Miller & Donders, 2003). It has been noted clinically that reading recognition returns to pretraumatic levels quickly, presumably because it is so overlearned. Reading comprehension, however, continues to be problematic, most likely because of disruption of executive function or working memory (i.e., the ability to "hold" information "on-line" during a task). Similarly, basic mathematical calculation skills are usually less affected or improve more quickly than the application of mathematical reasoning (Carney & Schoenbrodt, 1994).

This performance discrepancy leads to wide variations in apparent abilities that, if not understood, can be interpreted as lack of motivation or resistance, resulting in inappropriate management. In addition, behavior changes after injury, including increased impulsivity and decreased initiation, are often misinterpreted by caregivers and educators as a child being a troublemaker or unmotivated.

EMOTION AND BEHAVIOR

Children in need of rehabilitation have a greater risk for adjustment problems (Wallander & Thompson, 1995), and children with disabilities have been shown to have more social and behavior problems than children without disabilities (Cadman, Boyle, Szatmari, & Offord, 1987; Werner & Smith, 1992). Psychological adjustment in the child is often closely tied with family factors such as cohesiveness, resilience, family support, maternal stress and coping, and parental reactions to injury or illness (Harper, 1984; Wallander, Varni, Babani, Banis, & Wilcox, 1989; Wells & Schwebel, 1987; Werner & Smith, 1992). The posttraumatic psychiatric sequelae of neurological injury, both behavioral and emotional, vary with the severity, type, and location of injury; the phase of recovery; the premorbid personality of the patient; and the psychosocial environment (Felton & Revenson, 1984).

Premorbid psychiatric symptoms can potentially be made worse by neurological events. Frontal lobe dysfunction, which is common in neurological injuries, particularly traumatic brain injury, may lead to symptoms such as aggression, disinhibition, demandingness, childishness, euphoria, overtalkativeness, disregard for social convention, carelessness in personal hygiene and dress, and impulsivity. Apathy, slowness of movement, and decreased speech production may also be attributed to focal frontal lobe damage (Anderson, Damasio, Tranel, & Damasio, 2000).

Postinjury emotional, behavior, and psychiatric impairments are seen in many individuals with neurological injury. The problems may begin in the acute rehabilitation setting but often occur later, after discharge. It is essential to anticipate and try to prevent the occurrence of undesirable behaviors. Mood disturbances, such as depression and anxiety, are frequent after neurological injury and are thought to arise from both the neurobiological changes related to the injury and the psychological adjustment to changes in abilities (Anderson, Catroppa, Haritou, Morse, & Rosenfeld, 2005; Felton & Revenson, 1984). With appropriate expectations and modifications at home and at school, many problems secondary to frustration (of the patient, parent, and educator) may be avoided. Neurobehavioral treatment programs include behavior modification techniques, patient and family counseling, social skills training, therapeutic recreation to facilitate the productive use of leisure, treatment of substance abuse, and the prescribing of medication as needed (for problems, e.g., severe anxiety, depression, psychosis, disruptive behavior). The primary goals are to replace maladaptive behaviors with positive behaviors that generalize to everyday life and to eliminate pathological emotional states (Gerring & Carney, 1992).

Behavior modification does not require that the person whose behavior is being targeted is aware of the behavior or the intervention; thus, these principles can be used in young children and in individuals with cognitive impairments. The use of these principles in conjunction with the individual's efforts to modify his or her own behaviors or cognitive responses to stimuli is the basis for cognitive-behavioral therapy techniques and cognitive rehabilitation (see Cognition, earlier; see also Chapter 29). Behavior modification assumes that all behavior is maintained, changed, or shaped by the consequences of that behavior. *Reinforcers* are consequences that strengthen behavior. *Punishments* are consequences that weaken behavior (Premack, 1959).

Techniques used clinically to increase desired behaviors include positive reinforcement (presenting something positive in response to the behavior), negative reinforcement (removing something negative in response to the behavior), and a token economy (presenting points or small tokens in response to the behavior that can be exchanged for rewards). Techniques used clinically to develop a new desired behavior include shaping (waiting for the appropriate target behavior or something close to that behavior to occur before reinforcing the behavior), and modeling (demonstration of the target behavior via a model). This model can be a parent, a therapist, another patient, or a peer.

Techniques used clinically to decrease undesired behaviors include punishment (presenting something negative in response to the behavior), extinction (removing the reinforcement of or ignoring the behavior), time-out (removing all positive environmental stimuli in response to the undesired behavior), response cost (requiring the individual to give up something positive when the undesired behavior occurs), and differential reinforcement of other or incompatible behaviors (providing positive reinforcement of other behaviors and ignoring the undesired behavior, or reinforcing behaviors that are incompatible with the undesired behavior). Applied behavior analysis is a set of techniques used to eliminate very problematic or dangerous behaviors (e.g., head banging). This method focuses more on the antecedents than the consequences of the behaviors in order to predict when the behavior will occur and eliminate it quickly (Cooper, Heron, & Heward, 1987).

During the acute period after a severe traumatic brain injury, a patient typically goes through a predictable progression of recovery. The Rancho Los Amigos Scale of Cognitive Recovery (RLAS) was designed as a standardized way to measure and track a patient's cognitive and behavioral progress through this early recovery period and is based on behavioral observations of a patient's response to his or her environment. The progression of recovery includes an emergence from coma, a gradual increase in awareness of the environment, and increasing purposeful activity. There is often a period of posttraumatic amnesia, which includes disorientation and confusion, and psychiatrically is described as delirium. During this stage of recovery (Rancho level IV, confused/agitated), behavior varies widely, ranging from calmness to fearfulness, disruptiveness, or agitation and aggression. Symptoms and signs usually include impairment of the sleep-wake cycle, inattention, illusions and hallucinations, agitation, and disinhibition. The problems of this period usually abate but may be replaced at any time, even months or years later, by new behavior or emotional problems. The best treatment for this stage of recovery is time and an increased environmental structure with a focus on safety (Hagan, Malkmus, & Durham, 1979; Ylvisaker et al., 2005).

MOTOR FUNCTION

Motor Consequences of the Upper Motor Neuron Lesion

Upper motor neuron (UMN) lesions result in a constellation of clinical symptoms, including altered muscle tone, hyperactive reflexes, weakness, poor coordination, and sensory discrimination deficits. In individuals with spinal cord pathology, additional involvement of lower motor neurons, with hypotonia and muscle atrophy, contributes to the complexity of the clinical presentation. The loss of suprasegmental inhibitory inputs, resulting in increased excitability of gamma and alpha motor neurons and hyperactive segmental spinal reflex arcs, is believed to be responsible for the clinical signs of muscle spasticity, hyperreflexia, and clonus (Mayer, 1997). Children with CNS dysfunction encounter multiple challenges in performing gross and fine motor tasks, such as lack of anticipatory motor control, poor agonist and antagonist muscle interaction, and poor postural control, as well as difficulties with motor skill learning. During the past two decades, advances in treatment of muscle tone (spasticity and dystonia) and better understanding of the principles underlying motor learning have contributed to progress in neurorehabilitation therapies. Management of spasticity has also become an important part of the interdisciplinary approach in management of children with brain or spinal cord injury. Effective management of muscle hypertonia can improve a child's tolerance of therapeutic exercises, facilitate progress in rehabilitative therapies, and result in more satisfactory outcomes.

Spasticity

According to the definition introduced by Lance (1981), *spasticity* is a motor disorder characterized by velocity-dependent increase in tonic stretch reflex (muscle tone) with exaggerated deep tendon jerks resulting from hyperexcitability of the stretch reflexes, as one component of the UMN syndrome. Spasticity has neurophysiological and muscular components. Chronic spasticity leads to secondary changes in the muscle filaments (actin and myosin) and connective tissue elements and, in consequence, to muscle fibrosis and atrophy (Tilton, 2003). Abnormal muscle tone not only impairs function but also interferes with a child's growth and development. Muscle tone imbalance across joints may result in shortening of myotendinous units, joint contractures, subluxation or dislocation, and ultimately bony deformities if left untreated.

Along with the advances in treatment methods to reduce spasticity, it has become clear that increased muscle tone (positive symptom of the UMN syndrome) frequently is masking underlying weakness, poor endurance, and impaired selective muscle control and speed (negative symptoms). The decision to treat spasticity, therefore, should be preceded by a thorough evaluation of its severity and effects on the child's function and should be driven by clearly stated goals. The family's role in this process cannot be overstated. In children with severe spasticity, the reduction of spasticity may help improve hygiene and daily care, as well as the child's comfort. Spasticity management goals may include better control of pain and spasms; increased range of motion;

ease in use of orthoses; decreased progression of contractures; decreased need for orthopedic surgeries; facilitation of rehabilitative therapies; and improved positioning, mobility, and performance of activities of daily living (ADLs). Other goals such as improved appearance (e.g., improved hand and wrist posture) and comfort (e.g., improved sleep after spasms reduction) may also be of sufficient importance to justify treatment. Dystonia can coexist with spasticity and may be resistant to physical medicine approaches. This should be considered while setting therapeutic strategies and functional goals. Pharmacological treatment of dystonia along with therapy for spasticity may be necessary to maximize results. Thorough assessment of various components of muscle tone is vital for developing a realistic and efficient treatment strategy.

When aggressive reduction in hypertonia is considered, one needs to make sure that increased muscle tone is not assisting the patient's performance. The antigravity effects of spasticity in the lower limbs and trunk may in fact support some functional abilities. The child who is primarily using hypertonia to maintain sitting, support transfers, or walk may lose these functions after the tone is effectively reduced. It is therefore helpful when selecting therapeutic interventions to differentiate between the positive and negative elements of the UMN syndrome in order to optimize desirable results. In a child with significant weakness and lack of selective muscle control, reduction in muscle tone without other interventions will not improve functional performance (Tilton, 2003). When improved functional activity is the primary goal, the reduction in spasticity is usually only the first step in the therapeutic strategy and should be followed by aggressive rehabilitative therapies.

A variety of methods can be used to reduce spasticity. Any intervention, however, should begin with elimination of potentially aggravating factors such as pain, anxiety, discomfort, skin breakdown, and infection. The choices of treatment depend on the severity and the distribution of spasticity. For mild and moderate spasticity, therapeutic exercises supplemented by the use of orthoses and adaptive equipment should be considered prior to more invasive methods. For local spasticity that is difficult to manage with exercises and orthotic devices alone, nerve blocks and motor point (point where the nerve enters the muscle, intramuscular nerve) blocks may be effective. In diffuse spasticity, the child may benefit from oral pharmacotherapy, intrathecal baclofen pump placement, or selective dorsal rhizotomy. In selected patients, orthopedic surgery may be the most effective approach. Usually a combination of several methods is necessary to achieve desired goals.

Physical Medicine's Role in Spasticity Management The peripheral consequences of spasticity (e.g., shortening of the muscles and tendons) can be addressed by rehabilitative interventions including passive stretching of the tight muscles, coupled with strengthening (if possible) of their antagonists. Early introduction of orthotic devices (e.g., ankle–foot orthosis [AFO]) should be considered to secure functional position of the affected muscles and joints and to prolong the effects of stretching exercises. The length of time required for effective stretch may vary. The severity of the contracture and the level of hypertonia, as well as the child's age and functional goals, may be taken under consideration when the intensity and frequency of a stretching program are prescribed. It has been shown that prolonged stretch (6 hours/day) is beneficial in preventing contractures (Tardieu, Lespargot, Tabary, & Bret, 1988). Early mobilization and performing functional activities can also positively affect and normalize muscle tone. Orthoses (e.g., hinged AFO) can assist in balancing muscle forces across joints during therapy and daily activities. Topical cold or other physical modalities applied prior to stretching exercises can diminish muscle tone and facilitate stretching (Braddom, 2000). Use of electrical stimulation has been shown to provide decrease in spasticity that can persist for several hours after a treatment session (Braddom, 2000).

Pharmacological Treatment of Spasticity If rehabilitative modalities are insufficient in controlling muscle tone, pharmacological and surgical treatment should be considered. Monitoring the treatment results and balancing possible side effects to ensure optimal results requires close cooperation of the family and all team members involved in the child's care (Goldstein, 2001).

Oral Agents Oral pharmacological therapy is usually recommended if general reduction of muscle tone is desired. Benzodiazepines, baclofen (Lioresal), alpha$_2$ agonists, and dantrolene (Dantrium) are the common choices. Baclofen, benzodiazepines (diazepam [Valium], clonazepam [Klonopin]), and alpha$_2$ agonists (tizanidine [Zanaflex], clonidine) decrease excitability of the reflexes by targeting the CNS. Their nonselective action affects all muscle groups as well as the CNS, with frequent cognitive side effects. Common side effects include sedation, generalized weakness, and fatigue, which all affect function of the child. Titration of the dose to achieve desired tone reduction without an unacceptable adverse reaction is an important and challenging task. Dantrolene acts at the skeletal muscle level by inhibition of calcium release from the muscle sarcoplasmic reticulum and weakens contraction. General weakness and potential hepatic toxicity are the possible disadvantages of dantrolene (Goldstein, 2001).

Intrathecal Baclofen Intrathecal baclofen (ITB) was introduced in the 1980s for spinal-origin spasticity and was followed by use in cerebral palsy and traumatic brain injury. It is recommended for patients who have multisegmental or more extensive spasticity and for whom oral medications are not effective or not appropriate. Baclofen acts at the spinal cord level, primarily by inhibiting the release of excitatory neurotransmitters. ITB decreases spasticity through a direct effect on the CNS without the systemic side effects observed in the oral therapy. A continuous supply of medication is delivered by an infusion system that uses a catheter in the intrathecal space, a pump implanted in the abdominal wall, and telemetry programming. Required doses are approximately one thirtieth of the effective doses used in oral therapy.

ITB therapy was originally reported effective in patients with severe involvement who did not ambulate, but current indications have included patients who are ambulatory whose spasticity interferes with ambulation and function. Selection of appropriate candidates for ITB pump placement requires setting of realistic goals, a thorough analysis of the potential for patient compliance with refills and dose adjustments, and planning for management of complications. Financial and geographic factors may also play a role when considering ITB pump placement. The dosage of ITB is titrated according to its efficacy on positive and negative symptoms of UMN syndrome.

Reduction in spasticity without excessive muscle weakness is the desired outcome. Potential complications include those related to the surgical procedure (e.g., infection), device-related problems (e.g., battery, catheter problems), and drug overdose or withdrawal. An evidence-based analysis of 14 studies of ITB therapy concluded that the treatment reduces lower extremity spasticity, appears to improve function and ease of care, and has common but manageable complications (Butler & Campbell, 2000).

Phenol Phenol alcohol at a concentration of 3%–7% denatures protein and causes tissue necrosis. It has been used to reduce spasticity since the 1960s. The use of phenol has been significantly limited since the introduction of botulinum toxin, but in selected cases and in experienced hands it is still a valuable option to consider. Transcutaneous injection may target either motor nerves (obturator, musculocutaneous nerves) or motor points of the spastic muscles. Both techniques require precise localization with the use of a nerve stimulator. Because it is a tedious procedure, patient cooperation or sedation is required. In the "era" of botulinum neurotoxin use, phenol is sometimes used as an adjunct combined with botulinum neurotoxin when injection of multiple muscles during one session is the goal. Common adverse reactions include pain during injection and local tenderness at injection site believed to be secondary to local tissue necrosis and inflammation. Less commonly reported complications include postinjection neuralgia, interstitial fibrosis, sensory loss, deep venous thrombosis, and muscle necrosis (Mooney, Koman, & Smith, 2003). The advantages of phenol use include early onset of action (immediately after injection); longer duration, anecdotally reported as up to 18 months (Wood, 1978); low cost; and absence of antigenicity.

Botulinum Neurotoxin   Since the 1980s, botulinum neurotoxin has become a treatment of choice for local chemodenervation in children. Botulinum A toxin, the most popular serotype used in the United States, interacts at the presynaptic cholinergic terminals in the neuromuscular junction. It prevents presynaptic vesicles containing acetylcholine from fusing with the synaptic membrane and in consequence functionally produces chemical denervation.

The neuromuscular blockade is achieved by a direct injection into the target muscle. Localization may be aided by using anatomic landmarks and palpation, electromyography, electrical stimulation, ultrasonography, and combinations of these methods. The toxin diffuses approximately 2–3 cm from the injection point (Koman, Smith, & Balkrishnan, 2003). Selectivity of botulinum neurotoxin to the neuromuscular junction, and the fact that it does not affect axons or peripheral nerves, enhances its safety and minimizes side effects.

The injection can be performed using reassurance and restraint, topical cold spray or lidocaine cream, conscious sedation, or general anesthesia. When making the decision as to whether or not sedation or anesthesia is necessary, the number of injections, their sites, and the comfort level of the patient and the practitioner should be considered. Conscious sedation or anesthesia may be appropriate for complex injections, such as to the iliopsoas muscle, or in multilevel procedures (Koman et al., 2003).

In clinical trials, botulinum toxin has been shown effective in reducing muscle tone and painful spasms and improving limb function. Current indications for use of botulinum neurotoxin are treating equinus foot deformity and crouched gait, enhancing range of motion, improving upper extremity deformity, eliminating pain associated with spasticity, and serving as an alternative or adjunct to serial casting (Mooney et al., 2003). Side effects are rare but may include pain during injection, infection, allergic reaction, antibody formation, flulike symptoms, weakness, and fatigue (Goldstein, 2001).

The therapeutic effect after injection is usually observed within 48 hours, with maximum results seen in 2–3 weeks. Spasticity reduction is usually present for 6–12 weeks, with a positive response (improved muscle balance across the joints) maintained for 3–6 months. Intensive rehabilitative therapy consisting of stretching, strengthening, functional training, use of orthoses, and electrical stimulation can enhance results.

Selective Dorsal Rhizotomy   Before the introduction of ITB therapy, selective dorsal rhizotomy (SDR) was frequently recommended to decrease diffuse spasticity in children with cerebral palsy. In SDR, 25%–60% of dorsal rootlets are usually cut. Postoperatively, the child requires intensive physical therapy 4–5 times per week and occupational therapy once or twice per week for strengthening and functional training. Randomized clinical trials have reported reduction in spasticity, and some also reported significant improvement in function. Long-term effects of SDR are yet to be established. Because SDR is irreversible, appropriate patient selection is critical. Most commonly, the ideal candidate is described as a child with spastic diplegia who walks, has pure spasticity and good selective motor control and muscle strength, is between the ages of 4 and 8 years, is cognitively intact, and has a strong social structure (Gormley, 2001).

Therapeutic Approaches: Neurophysiological Bases and Evolution

Many popular therapies for children with CNS injury evolved empirically from clinical experience. Along with the progress in medicine and neurosciences, new therapies have emerged complementing the traditional rehabilitative approaches.

Better understanding of how motor control in humans develops and reaches the level of precise and purposeful movements is vital to designing effective rehabilitative interventions. Classic neurophysiological theories popular during the 20th century served as scientific justification for many traditional therapeutic methods, some of which are still in use in rehabilitation practice today. At the beginning of the 20th century, Sherrington hypothesized that coordination of single excitatory and inhibitory reflexes (reflex chaining) leads to a development of purposeful movements. Based on his experiments on deafferented monkeys, he also concluded that sensation is essential for movement and that sensory input and feedback influence motor control and motor learning (Lundy-Ekman, 1998).

During the second half of the 20th century, motor and developmental disabilities in children with CNS lesions were frequently attributed to spasticity, abnormal movement synergies, and persistent primitive reflexes. These beliefs resulted in the development of numerous therapies that attempted to balance these abnormalities, hoping that motor control would be normal if the spasticity and primitive reflexes were successfully reduced. Therapeutic interventions such as Rood's method, Brunnstrom's therapy, Kabat's Proprioceptive Neuromuscular Facilitation (PNF), and the Bobaths' Reflex Inhibition Method (a prototype of neurodevelopmental treatment [NDT]) represent only several examples. As a group, these rehabilitative approaches are sometimes classified as *neurodevelopmental therapies.* They focus on muscle tone normalization using exercise and positioning protocols, and on training of physiological movements and postural patterns that are believed to underlie functional skills (Helsel, McGee, & Graveline, 2001). Some of these therapies have changed their objectives over time as new scientific evidence became available.

Neurodevelopmental Treatment A good example of such an "evolving" therapy is NDT. Since its creation by the Bobaths in the 1950s, the treatment strategy has changed several times. The original emphasis of NDT was on normalization of muscle tone and postural reactions and promoting physiological movement patterns following the developmental sequence; the child was a relatively passive recipient of the therapy. Over time, the Bobaths concluded that there was no carryover into

function. The importance of the child's active participation and taking control over the voluntary movement was recognized, and the NDT approach was broadened to include systematic preparation for specific functional tasks. It is by far the most common approach used in the United States by therapists working with young children, particularly with infants and toddlers. To date, however, there is no convincing evidence that NDT improves function or is more effective than other neurodevelopmental approaches (Butler & Darrah, 2001).

Alternative Therapies Other therapies for children with cerebral palsy and CNS dysfunction that evolved empirically from clinical experience and are still in popular use include Conductive Education (CE), Patterning or the Doman-Delacato method, and the Vojta method. Some elements of the Brunnstrom, Rood, and PNF methods may also be seen incorporated in the more complex rehabilitative interventions practiced by therapists familiar with these techniques. In search of alternatives to improve function in children with CNS diseases, new therapeutic systems constantly are developed. Among many, the myofascial release technique, Awareness Through Movement (Feldenkrais), craniosacral therapy, and the Adeli suit (Euromed Rehabilitation Institute, Poland) serve as examples of such attempts. There is no convincing published evidence, however, to support or refute any of these approaches.

Conductive Education CE, also known as the Petö method, was developed in the 1940s in Hungary. This therapy integrates educational and rehabilitation goals into one program. The Conductor assigned to each child provides all educational and therapeutic needs. This is a problem-solving approach emphasizing development of functional independence. The group format utilizes highly structured activities and goal-oriented tasks representing intentional activity rather than an isolated exercise program.

Rhythm, music, rhyme, and songs are used as means of facilitating motor action and learning. Orthotic devices and adaptive equipment such as wheelchairs were not recommended in the original method; instead, a system of specially design furniture was used to assist children with their movements. The current CE approach represents a variety of interventions in different countries; however, the group format with structured and goal-oriented training and the use of rhythm and CE-specific equipment are common features of this program in various countries. An evidence-based report published by the American Academy for Cerebral Palsy and Developmental Medicine (AACPDM) concluded that there is no convincing evidence to support or refute the effectiveness of CE (Darrah, Watkins, Chen, & Binin, 2004).

Doman-Delacato (Patterning) Method
The Doman-Delacato (Patterning) Method has originated from Fay's Evolutionary Pattern Movements method. Fay's therapy was designed as an adjunct to the Phelps therapeutic protocols. The method involves utilization of certain primitive nervous system patterns that the cerebral injury has not destroyed. The patterning refers to passively guiding the child's body through certain movement patterns. The method recommends periods of carbon dioxide rebreathing (masking) and fluid restriction that raise concern about its safety.

Vojta Method
The Vojta method is a diagnostic and therapeutic protocol popularized in Germany. The therapy is preceded by diagnostic screening of several specific postural reflexive responses in the child. Treatment consists of stimulative manipulations to provoke reflexive movement patterns that are believed to activate reflex locomotion, isolate and strengthen muscle groups, and contribute to development of postural ontogenesis and mobility (Molnar & Alexander, 1999).

Motor Control: Neurophysiological Bases of Neurorehabilitation

Advances in neuroscience and neuroimaging techniques as well as the results of animal studies have begun revealing the complexity and diversity of the neural processes underlying

motor performance. It has been shown that "movement is orchestrated by the coordinated action of the peripheral, spinal, brain stem, cerebellar, and cerebral regions, shaped by a specific context, and directed by the intentions of the performer" (Lundy-Ekman, 1998, p. 150).

Learning new motor skills as well as modification of already mastered skills involves integrated activity of many regions of the CNS. Each motor action starts with a decision made by the individual (anterior frontal lobe). This leads to activation of the motor planning system and control circuits (cerebellum, basal ganglia). Motor planning systems and control circuits regulate the action of the descending motor pathways, which transmit signals to the spinal interneurons and alpha motor neurons. As a result, appropriate muscle groups contract and relax in a precise and coordinated fashion.

Sensory information influences and navigates CNS function in each step involved in motor performance. The activity of motor planning areas, control circuits, and descending pathways is integrated with sensory information to provide instructions to the lower motor neurons (Lundy-Ekman, 1998). Proprioceptive feedback works as an integral component in gross motor control, such as posture and locomotion, as well as in fine movements in humans. The basal ganglia are active in comparing proprioceptive information and movement commands, sequencing movements, and regulating muscle tone and muscle force (Hallet, 1993). If proprioception is impaired, visual information can partially substitute for the deficit and may play an important role in rehabilitative training (Pearson, 2000).

The physical properties of the limbs and body (e.g., musculoskeletal mechanics) are represented in the CNS by internal models, and learning plays an essential role in the formation and maintenance of these models. Improvement in reaching movements in infants has been attributed to the change of the internal model of the arm as a result of learning (Konczak, Borutta, & Dichgans, 1997). The cerebellum is considered to be a critical structure in motor learning and to be one of the locations of the internal models. Individuals with cerebellar dysfunction clinically present with decomposition of multijoint limb movements. The primary motor cortex plays an important role in controlling voluntary arm movements, muscle force, and joint torque, and in sensorimotor transformations as well as cognitive aspects of movement control (Pearson, 2000). The parietal cortex, by providing an interface between cognitive processes (e.g., attention and inattention) and the motor system, participates in guiding movements and has a critical role in reaching and in fine motor skills.

The dynamics and plasticity of the CNS are active throughout the entire human life span, allowing constant learning and reorganization. Cortical representations are constantly adjusting to environmental and body changes. Studies on limb deafferentation in nonhuman primates and in humans have demonstrated expansion of the adjacent cortical representations into the cortical territory of the deafferented body parts. Cortical representations constantly change their size depending on their use. Learning a new motor skill, such as finger opposition, increases cortical representations of the involved fingers. Inactivity has the converse effect. Immobilization of the ankle joint without peripheral nerve dysfunction results in diminished cortical representation of the inactive tibialis anterior muscle (Hallett, 2001).

One of the most significant changes in neurorehabilitation practice since the 1980s resulted from current concepts of motor learning that favor a task-specific approach. In order to learn a specific motor skill, it is necessary to practice this given task. For example, to learn how to walk, it is necessary to practice walking. Neurorehabilitation in all preparatory stages to ambulation, such as balance training while sitting or standing (a classic focus of NDT), were shown to improve balance but not gait (Winstein, Gardner, McNeal, Barto, & Nicholson, 1989). Task-specific and goal-oriented functional training is now considered the most effective rehabilitative approach to improve performance in children and adults with CNS lesion.

An exciting and promising discovery related to motor system function is that of central pattern generators found in animals and humans (e.g., respiratory rhythm, spinal locomotor rhythm). These rhythmic motor systems have been shown to be able to generate patterned activity in the absence of afferent feedback. Research on cats with spinal lesions has contributed to the development of new therapies for humans with spinal cord injury. Additional studies on the physiological paradigms of new skills acquisition in the context of the underlying neural mechanism are promising and will support further development of more effective neurorehabilitative therapies.

Current Standard Approaches in Motor Dysfunction

Rehabilitation of children with motor impairment should be developmentally oriented. Early intervention therapies can incorporate handling, positioning, and play intended to challenge postural and movement responses that are fundamental for gross and fine motor development. Therapy should begin as early as possible after the injury, and intensity of the treatment should be adjusted according to the child's needs and abilities. As children learn to follow instructions and are able to cooperate, therapy becomes more structured (Molnar, 1991).

Current standard of care in neurological motor impairments may include muscle tone modification, exercises to improve muscle strength and maintain range of motion, muscle and cardiovascular endurance training, goal-oriented functional training (bed mobility, transfers, static and dynamic balance, ambulation, self-care skills, vocational skills), and training in use of orthotic devices and mobility or ADL aids. In younger children, appropriate games, play therapy, and stimulative toys may be used to facilitate program objectives. The main goal of rehabilitative therapies is to improve the quality of life of the children and their families. As was already emphasized in this chapter, many disciplines are involved in rehabilitation of a child to optimize functional abilities and ensure the best possible quality of life.

Occupational and Physical Therapy
The occupational therapy approach concentrates on development of skills necessary to perform ADLs. ADLs in children are age spe-

cific and may include play, self-care (dressing, grooming, feeding), and fine motor tasks such as drawing or writing. Optimal performance, specific for the child's age and severity of impairment is usually achieved by training in sensorimotor and fine motor functions. Comprehensive occupational therapy assessment also focuses on cognitive and perceptual skills (e.g., visual, visual-motor function) and their role in specific ADLs. The occupational therapist will incorporate in the therapeutic intervention proper exercises; training in use of assistive devices; and necessary rehabilitation equipment, including an optimal seating arrangement to promote upper limb function (Steultjens et al., 2004).

The physical therapy approach focuses on enhancement of gross motor skills and functional mobility (e.g., transfers, walking, wheelchair use). Physical therapists assess the neuromuscular and musculoskeletal systems in respect to existing impairments and abilities and analyze how they affect function. Based on the assessment, short- and long-term goals for therapy are developed. Physical therapists use various physical exercise strategies with the assistance of rehabilitative equipment if indicated (e.g., walking aids, wheelchairs, orthoses) to maximize functional independence and prevent secondary impairments (e.g., joint deformities). Some of the goals of physical therapy are to improve range of motion, strength, neuromuscular control, coordination, balance, mobility, muscle tone, and cardiopulmonary endurance.

There are many common goals and strategies in the therapeutic approaches of both disciplines; therefore, a combination of occupational and physical therapy is often prescribed to maximize functional outcome. Complementary to applied exercises and functional activity training, physical and occupational therapy management commonly includes use of adjunctive physical modalities (e.g., therapeutic cold, electrical stimulation), orthotic devices, mobility equipment, and ADL aids to assist with function and therapeutic goals. Parental and family advising is also an important part of the occupational and physical therapy treatment strategy.

Therapeutic Exercises Therapeutic exercises are widely used in pediatric rehabilitation to preserve or improve range of motion, improve coordination, increase strength, and enhance muscle and cardiopulmonary endurance. Many factors should be taken under consideration when developing an exercise program for a child. The child's age, type and extent of injury and impairments, anticipated functional goals, cognitive capacity, home and school environment, and family and community support will all contribute to the selection of a suitable rehabilitative intervention.

Range of Motion Range of motion of the joints is extremely important in optimizing a child's mobility and function, facilitating ease of care, and improving comfort and self-esteem. Muscle and joint contractures can lead to permanent deformities and limit the functional potential of a child. Restrictions in flexibility of the limbs or spine can result in difficulty in positioning, and may cause skin problems and premature joint degeneration, all of which can contribute to decreased quality of life and suffering. A daily stretching program is a crucial factor in contracture prevention. Many techniques, as solitary approaches or in combination, can be implemented to achieve this goal. A strategy aiming to preserve joint flexibility can consist of active and passive range-of-motion exercises, manual stretching, and application of orthoses (e.g., AFOs, serial casting). Clinical practice and scientific evidence indicate that slow, gentle, and prolonged stretching is more effective than vigorous intermittent stretching (Molnar & Alexander, 1999; Tardieu et al., 1988).

Muscle Strength A very important component of effective motor control, muscle strength is usually diminished in individuals with disabilities. If not aggressively treated, weakness and impairment of voluntary movements present in the acute stage of the CNS injury will inevitably progress to secondary muscle dysfunction caused by disuse and decreased physical activity. Historically, in the 1950s, Phelps emphasized strengthening as a vital element of therapy for children with cerebral palsy. Clinicians, however, have had a tendency to fear that any improvement in power of the spastic muscle may exacerbate its tightness and tone, worsening functional outcomes.

Current review of clinical studies conducted in children and young adults with cerebral palsy between 1966 and 2000 suggests that strength training may in fact provide benefits for this population, including improved motor activity and functional abilities. Empirical evidence presented in these studies does not support common clinical beliefs that strength training may increase spasticity and muscle tightness (Dodd, Taylor, & Damiano, 2002). Individually tailored strengthening programs may result in improved functional outcomes.

In children with spastic cerebral palsy, strength training targeting lower limb muscles resulted in significant improvements in gross motor skills such as standing, walking, running, and jumping (Damiano & Abel, 1998; MacPhail & Kramer, 1995); however, velocity and efficiency of walking remained unchanged in the studied population (MacPhail & Kramer, 1995). Strengthening of the upper limb and trunk muscles can improve general endurance, sitting posture, and biomechanical and energy efficiency in wheelchair or mobility aids use. A variety of exercise paradigms (e.g., isometric, isotonic, progressive resistive) as well as play activities may serve as rehabilitative techniques to improve muscle strength in children. In patients with profound weakness, use of electrical stimulation with or without assistive therapeutic equipment (e.g., orthoses) may facilitate functional activation and strengthening of selected muscle groups.

Orthoses   An orthosis is defined as any externally applied device used to modify structural and functional characteristics of the neuromuscular skeletal system (Braddom, 2000). In general, orthotic devices can be used to protect, correct, and assist with function. An appropriate orthosis can contribute to prevention of contracture and deformity (e.g., resting hand splints, AFO, spinal braces), protect body parts and prevent injury or facilitate healing, and correct body dynamics by providing accurate guidance of motion (e.g., hinged AFO), all of which can improve function. An orthotic device may also compensate for muscle weak-

ness, influence muscle length, and help modify abnormal muscle tone. Upper and lower limb as well as spine and trunk position and function may be assisted by application of appropriate orthoses.

In order to meet this broad spectrum of goals, orthotic devices use a variety of designs, materials, and mechanical characteristics. Full description of the complexity and variety of orthoses prescribed for children is not within the scope of this chapter; however, in simplistic terms, one may divide orthoses into two groups: rigid restrictive braces (e.g., solid AFO) and more complex mechanical devices allowing for certain motion of the embraced body parts (e.g., hinged AFO). In contrast to passive restriction of motion, *dynamic orthoses* apply elastic force, allowing some movement in order to increase motion or improve function (e.g., posterior leaf-spring AFO, elbow Dynasplint, reciprocating gait orthosis).

When prescribing a device, careful consideration should be given to the differences in the design of the orthosis and the potential effects on short- and long-term outcome. Buckon et al. (2001) studied the effectiveness of three types of AFOs in maintaining ankle range of motion and gait dynamics and in general functional performance in children with spastic hemiplegia. The three types of AFOs compared were hinged (HAFO), posterior leaf-spring (PLS), and solid (SAFO). The majority of children gained the greatest benefit from the HAFO or PLS. The HAFO offered better control of knee hyperextension in the stance phase of gait, whereas the PLS was superior in promoting knee extension in children with a tendency to more than 10 degrees of knee flexion in the stance phase. The majority of children demonstrated more natural ankle motion during walking, improved dorsiflexion, improved energy efficiency, and better functional mobility while using the HAFO or PLS configurations (Buckon et al., 2001).

When prescribing an orthosis, the child's age, functional capacity and motor control, type of deformity, and commitment to use, as well as the patient's and family's goals, should be taken into consideration. Any device should be simple, lightweight, durable, and easy to use and should optimize functional independence.

The aesthetic aspect also plays an important role, particularly in older children and teens.

Serial Casting Serial casting can be used as an adjunct to management of children with neuromuscular disorders in order to prevent loss of or restore joint range of motion, to improve muscle extensibility in the presence of increased tone, or both (Singer, Singer, & Allison, 2001). While a gentle manual force is stretching the joint, a cast is applied to secure this position in its terminal but easily achievable range. The force should be sufficient but not excessive because muscle, nerve, vascular, and skin injury may occur and adversely affect outcome. Usually the cast is removed and the process is repeated at weekly intervals until gradually the desired joint position is achieved. Two to three sequential weeks of casting (serial casting) are usually sufficient to improve joint flexibility. In addition to constant gentle tension applied to the shortened soft tissue elements, a slight elevation in tissue temperature under the cast may facilitate collagen fiber extensibility. Research on animal models indicates that tissue growth and remodeling are induced by prolonged low-load mechanical strain (Fess, Gentle, Philips, & Janson, 2005). Reduction of sensory input during serial casting treatment may also contribute to reduction of hyperactivity of the spastic muscles and improve flexibility.

Adaptive and Mobility Equipment A wide variety of assistive devices are available to ensure proper positioning, maximize functional mobility, improve independence, and facilitate daily care provided by families and caregivers.

Transfer Aids Overhead trapeze bars can facilitate transfers and position changes (rolling, sitting up) in bed. Transfer boards may be used for bed, chair, car, or commode transfers by providing a bridge between two surfaces. Different types of commercially available lifts facilitate safe and effortless transfers in older children and children who are more affected.

Standing Frames and Other Standing Devices Standing frames and other standing devices provide therapeutic benefits to children who cannot achieve or maintain a standing position on their own. Experience of gravity forces and body weight bearing while in the upright position has stimulative effects on posture development and may improve head and trunk control. Sustained muscle stretch assists in maintenance of trunk and lower limb passive range of motion.

A classic example is the parapodium, with or without swivel modification, used in young children with paraplegia and good head and trunk control. These devices allow the child to stand or walk. Walking in a parapodium with swivel does not require gait aids and allows free use of the upper limbs for other activities.

A supine stander gives posterior support to the child and is appropriate for a child with significant extensor tone with posturing and poor head control. It can be positioned from a horizontal plane to approximately 90 degrees upright. Prone standers give anterior support to the child and have a tray that can be placed in front of the child. This design promotes antigravity head control, upper limb weight bearing, and functional use of the hand (Molnar & Alexander, 1999). Numerous models of commercially available standers with dynamic features offer independence in mobility as well as assisted transition from sitting to standing in addition to the therapeutic benefits of standing. This enables children who do not ambulate to explore their environment while being at eye level with their peers.

Gait Aids Canes, crutches, and walkers can facilitate functional independence, improve balance and posture, decrease energy expenditure, and alleviate pain. Good upper limb strength is needed in order to use most of the gait aids. A reciprocal gait pattern is easily achieved with the use of a straight cane when muscle strength and control are sufficient. A quad cane can provide a better base of support and assist balance.

Two types of crutches, axillary and forearm (Lofstrand), are being used with children. The risk and symptoms of compressive radial neuropathy with improper use of axillary crutches should be explained to the child and family. Forearm crutches provide less trunk support than axillary crutches; however, they offer increased functional independence and allow the child to reach with his or her hands.

Several types of walkers are appropriate for children. Forward walkers promote trunk flexion; they come with or without wheels and with handles or platforms. Reverse or posterior walkers (posture-control walkers) endorse an erect posture and are widely used for children. Gait trainers represent a third category of walkers and offer independent mobility to children with poor pelvic and trunk control who cannot use other walking aids. Gait trainers may serve as transition devices in ambulation training or as a valuable means of independent mobility for children with more severe mobility challenges (Molnar & Alexander, 1999).

Mobility Devices   Scooters, adapted tricycles, and wheelchairs allow children who do not ambulate to be more independent in daily activities and in exploring the environment, enhancing their social skills and self-esteem. A variety of manual and powered wheelchairs are available to meet the individual needs of a child. Children with adequate cognitive, visual, and spatial discrimination abilities can learn how to operate a motorized device at 3 years of age (Molnar, 1991). Many factors should be taken into consideration when choosing a wheelchair for a child. The type and extent of disability, the potential for growth and development, the specific child's needs, and the motor as well as functional and cognitive capacity of the child should be carefully considered prior to prescribing a certain type of mobility device.

Adjunctive Therapeutic Interventions

Interventions such as electrical nerve and muscle stimulation, hippotherapy, aquatic therapy, and music therapy can be used in conjunction with traditional physical and occupational therapies in pediatric rehabilitation practice.

Threshold Electrical Stimulation   Threshold electrical stimulation (TES) is a low-level electrical stimulus of subcontraction intensity, at the sensory threshold. TES is applied during sleep and has been proposed to treat muscle

atrophy. Initially TES was reported to improve strength and function; however, further research reported no statistically significant effects (Kerr, McDowell, & McDonough, 2004).

Neuromuscular Electrical Stimulation
Neuromuscular electrical stimulation (NMES) consists of application of electric current to elicit muscle contraction. The goals are strengthening and spasticity reduction, and NMES is often used with other therapies. When applied to support specific functional activity, the treatment is referred to as functional electric stimulation (FES). FES of the peroneal nerve in patients with hemiplegia who are ambulatory can assist ankle dorsiflexion and suppress plantar flexor tone via reciprocal inhibition (Braddom, 2000). FES of the peripheral nerves may be used in patients with paraplegia to enhance exercise and functional training. Review of 12 studies revealed two randomized, controlled trials demonstrating statistically significant improvement in strength and range of motion (Kerr et al., 2004).

There is more evidence to support the use of NMES than TES; however, the studies had insufficient statistical power to provide conclusive evidence for or against these modalities. Variations in stimulation parameters and incomplete information make the comparison difficult.

Hippotherapy   Horseback-riding therapy, or hippotherapy, is an enjoyable activity that results in significant improvements in gross motor skills. In a heterogeneous group of children with mild to severe cerebral palsy, this type of intervention demonstrated clinical improvement in walking, running, and jumping (Sterba, Rogers, France, & Vokes, 2002). The emotional, sensory, and motor benefits that hippotherapy may provide should be considered in the management of children with neurological disorders or developmental disabilities.

Aquatic Therapy   Water creates an amusing environment for children. Elimination of the effect of gravity in the water reduces efforts to create certain movements (e.g., walking) but may also provide mild resistance (e.g., respiratory muscles). The therapy can improve muscle strength, increase range of motion, alter abnormal muscle tone, and increase muscle endurance and cardiopulmonary fitness, simultaneously providing multiple sensory stimuli. Pool therapy can be a valuable option for increasing physical activity of a child and may serve as an adjunct to conventional therapies. Scientific evidence of efficacy, however, is limited in the pediatric population (Dumas & Francesconi, 2001).

Music Therapy Music can facilitate rhythmic physical activity as well as influence and fulfill emotional, social, psychological, and spiritual needs of people of all ages (Kennelly, 2000). In the pediatric setting, music creates a fun, enjoyable, and attractive atmosphere, helping children to accept therapy as part of play activity. This type of therapy can be used in conjunction with other therapies to promote gross and fine motor skills, motor sensory skills, speech and language, communication, and social development.

New Therapies

Promising rehabilitative techniques are emerging following advances in understanding motor learning principles and the importance of behavioral and cognitive components affecting new skill acquisition.

Locomotor Therapy Treadmill training with partial body weight support represents a task-specific therapy that enables individuals with profound weakness to practice complex gait cycles repetitively (Schindl, Forstner, Kern, & Hesse, 2000). Several studies have shown its potential in patients after stroke, spinal cord injury, cerebral palsy, and Parkinson disease. Treadmill therapy with partial body weight support was compared to physical therapy using early therapy-assisted ambulation with support of orthoses and assistive devices in patients after stroke. Intensity, frequency, and overall length of treatment in both groups were matched (45 minutes daily, 5 days per week, until the patient could walk over the ground unassisted). The overall outcome did not differ, except for patients with major hemi-

spheric stroke who were difficult to mobilize using physiotherapy alone (Kosak & Reding, 2000).

Constraint-Induced Movement Therapy Constraint-induced movement therapy (CIMT) was developed by Taub et al. (1966, 1973, 1975) using a primate model. Deafferentation of the upper limb in monkeys by posterior rhizotomy resulted in complete cessation of motor use of that limb. The animals began to use the deafferented extremity only when the unaffected limb was restricted. Taub et al. concluded that loss of sensation causing difficulty in effective use of the limb contributed to development of a learned nonuse phenomenon. This approach was then transferred to human subject experiments and disproved the common belief that hand function has only a narrow time window for improvement after stroke. Since the first published trials in the 1990s on adults who experienced chronic stroke, CIMT has been applied in adults with acute stroke, in children and adults with traumatic brain injury, and in children with cerebral palsy, including infants. A randomized, controlled trial on 18 children with cerebral palsy demonstrated significant improvement in skills of the treated upper extremity (Taub, Ramey, DeLuca, & Echols, 2004). The therapy in the CIMT group consisted of immobilization of the unaffected (or less affected) upper limb for a period of 3 weeks using a bivalved cast. The treatment group received intensive therapy, 6 hours daily for 21 consecutive days (mass practice), with training procedures using frequent positive reinforcement (shaping). The control group was assigned to conventional occupational therapy for a mean of 2.2 hours/week. At the completion of the 3 weeks of therapy and at 6 months follow-up, the CIMT group showed significant improvement in the use of the trained extremity (Taub et al., 2004).

The CIMT approach has been reported as a promising treatment for the upper extremity affected by stroke, traumatic brain injury, and cerebral palsy. Although the results of CIMT have been reproduced in several centers with a limited sample size, it is too early to justify standard use of this approach. Several elements of CIMT may have contributed to its success, one of which is the intensity of the therapy. Randomized, controlled studies with control groups undergoing therapy of comparable intensity would add to a better understanding of the mechanisms of CIMT efficacy. From a pragmatic point of view, CIMT in its current paradigm (3 weeks of intense therapy given daily for 6 hours) may be difficult to fit into the existing health care system. Also, long-term results of the CIMT approach have not been reported.

Virtual Reality Virtual reality is a computer technology that allows creation of detailed three-dimensional visual situations, which can be examined and manipulated and within which one can move (Rose, Johnson, & Attree, 1997). This approach can be used in the pediatric population to optimize skills necessary for daily activities in controlled and danger-free virtual settings, such as the home, city, supermarket, or public transportation. The technology may be utilized to enhance motor control and to improve social participation and the quality of life. Using virtual reality technology, an individual exercise program can be designed to address motor and sensory impairments of the particular patient (Sveistrup et al., 2003).

Summary

The treatment plan for a child with motor dysfunction secondary to CNS injury should be customized with succinct, definable, and realistic therapeutic objectives. All parties should agree on the goals. Depending on the child's potential, the goals may include improvement in ambulation and daily living skills, facilitation of hygiene, contracture prevention, improved sleep and comfort, and improved appearance, all of which should contribute to a better quality of patients' and their families' lives.

COMMUNITY REINTEGRATION

The rehabilitation needs of patients who have sustained neurological injury vary according to the severity of injury and secondary deficits and range from reassurance and anticipatory guidance to extensive intervention. Children with more severe injuries must be followed more closely and may require neuropsychological and educational evaluations to assist in successful return to school. Because of the resultant cognitive and physical impairment with severe neurological injury, there is often a need for inpatient rehabilitation followed by outpatient rehabilitation and planned school reintegration. The type and intensity of rehabilitation will in part be dictated by the rate of recovery, which will be most rapid initially (first 3 months after coma resolution) but will continue at a slower rate for at least 1 year and probably longer (2–5 years). Based on the time course of recovery and the nature of the long-term disabilities, the need for services (both evaluations and treatments) will continue over an extended period of time. Some of this rehabilitation will be accomplished through the medical system, but, in the pediatric population, the educational system should assist in the rehabilitation of those impairments that are education related. Rehabilitation, as well as education, should be done within the least restrictive environment.

CONCLUSION

Advances in health sciences and the trend to practice evidenced-based medicine have challenged the traditional neurorehabilitative approaches and have called for thorough reevaluation of the methods used in children and adults with CNS diseases. As a result, rehabilitation therapies are transforming from isolated exercises and pure neurodevelopmental approaches to comprehensive, goal-oriented treatment paradigms involving the patient's motor, cognitive, emotional, perceptual, and behavioral dimensions.

REFERENCES

Anderson, S.W., Damasio, H., Tranel, D., & Damasio, A.R. (2000). Long-term sequelae of prefrontal cortex damage acquired in early childhood. *Developmental Neuropsychology, 18,* 281–296.

Anderson, V.A., Catroppa, C., Haritou, F., Morse, S., & Rosenfeld, J.V. (2005). Identifying factors contributing to child and family outcome 30 months after traumatic brain injury in children.

Journal of Neurology, Neurosurgery and Psychiatry, 76, 401–408.

Baron, I.S. (2003). *Neuropsychological evaluation of the child.* New York: Oxford University Press.

Bates, E., Reilly, J., Wulfeck, B., Dronkers, N., Opie, M., Fenson, J., et al. (2001). Differential effects of unilateral lesions on language production in children and adults. *Brain and Language, 79,* 223–265.

Braddom, R.L. (2000). *Physical medicine and rehabilitation* (2nd ed.). Philadelphia: W.B. Saunders.

Buckon, C.E., Thomas, S.S., Jakobson-Huston, S., Moor, M., Sussman, M., & Aiona, M. (2001). Comparison of three ankle-foot orthosis configurations for children with spastic diplegia. *Developmental Medicine and Child Neurology, 43,* 371–378.

Butler, C., & Campbell, S. (2000). Evidence of the effects of intrathecal baclofen for spastic and dystonic cerebral palsy. AACPDM Treatment Outcome Committee Review Panel. *Developmental Medicine and Child Neurology, 42,* 634–645.

Butler, C., & Darrah, J. (2001). Effects of neurodevelopmental treatment (NDT) for cerebral palsy: An AACPDM evidence report. *Developmental Medicine and Child Neurology, 43,* 778–790.

Cadman, D., Boyle, B., Szatmari, P., & Offord, D.R. (1987). Chronic illness, disability and mental and social well-being: Findings of the Ontario Child Heath Study. *Pediatrics, 79,* 805–813.

Carney, J., & Schoenbrodt, L. (1994). Educational implications of traumatic brain injury. *Pediatric Annals, 23,* 47–52.

Cooper, J.O., Heron, T.E., & Heward, W.L. (1987). *Applied behavior analysis.* Upper Saddle River, NJ: Prentice-Hall.

Cope, D.N. (1995). The effectiveness of traumatic brain injury rehabilitation: A review. *Brain Injury, 9,* 649–670.

Damiano, D.L., & Abel, M.F. (1998). Functional outcomes of strength training in spastic cerebral palsy. *Archives of Physical Medicine and Rehabilitation, 79,* 119–125.

Darrah, J., Watkins, B., Chen, L., & Binin, C. (2004). Conductive education intervention for children with cerebral palsy: An AACPDM evidence report. *Developmental Medicine and Child Neurology, 46,* 187–203.

Delis, D.C., Kramer, J.H., Kaplan, E., & Ober, B.A. (1994). *California Verbal Learning Test–Children's Version.* San Antonio, TX: Psychological Corporation.

Dodd, K.J., Taylor, N.F., & Damiano, D.L. (2002). A systematic review of the effectiveness of strength-training programs for people with cerebral palsy. *Archives of Physical Medicine and Rehabilitation, 83,* 1157–1164.

Dumas, H., & Francesconi, S. (2001). Aquatic therapy in pediatrics: Annotated bibliography. *Physical & Occupational Therapy in Pediatrics, 20*(4), 63–78.

Education for All Handicapped Children Act of 1975, PL 94-142, 20 U.S.C. §§ 1400 *et seq.*

Education of the Handicapped Act Amendments of 1986, PL 99-457, 20 U.S.C. §§ 1400 *et seq.*

Engelberts, N.H.J., Klein, M., Ader, H.J., Heimans, J.J., Trenite, D.G.A.K., & van der Ploeg, H.M. (2002). The effectiveness of cognitive rehabilitation for attention deficits in focal seizures: A randomized controlled study. *Epilepsia, 43,* 587–595.

Fehlings, D., Rang, M., Glazier, J., & Steele, C. (2001). Botulinum toxin type A injections in the spastic upper extremity of children with hemiplegia: Child characteristics that predict a positive outcome. *European Journal of Neurology, 8*(Suppl. 5), 145–149.

Felton, B.J., & Revenson, T.A. (1984). Coping with chronic illness: A study of controllability and the influence of coping strategies on psychological adjustment. *Journal of Consulting and Clinical Psychology, 53,* 343–353.

Fess, E.E., Gentle, K.S., Philips, C.A., & Janson, J.R. (2005). Soft tissue remodeling. In E.E. Fess, K.S. Gentle, C.A. Philips, & J.R. Janson (Eds.), *Hand and upper extremity splinting principles and methods* (pp. 112–116). St. Louis: Elsevier Mosby.

Gerring, J.P., & Carney, J.M. (1992). *Head trauma: Strategies for educational reintegration.* San Diego: Singular Publishing Group.

Goldstein, E.M. (2001). Spasticity management: An overview. *Journal of Child Neurology, 16,* 16–23.

Gormley, M.E., Jr. (2001). Treatment of neuromuscular and musculoskeletal problems in cerebral palsy. *Pediatric Rehabilitation, 4,* 5–16.

Hagan, C., Malkmus, D., & Durham, P. (1979). *Levels of cognitive function. Rehabilitation of the head injured adult: Comprehensive physical management.* Downey, CA: Professional Staff Association of Rancho Los Amigos Hospital.

Hallett, M. (1993). Physiology of basal ganglia disorders: An overview. *Canadian Journal of Neurological Sciences, 20,* 177–183.

Hallett, M. (2001). Plasticity of the human motor cortex and recovery from stroke. *Brain Research Reviews, 36,* 169–174.

Harper, D.C. (1984). Child behavior toward the parent: A factor analysis of mothers' reports of disabled children. *Journal of Autism and Developmental Disorders, 14,* 165–182.

Helsel, P., McGee, J., & Graveline, C. (2001). Physical management of spasticity. *Journal of Child Neurology, 16,* 24–30.

Individuals with Disabilities Education Act of 1990, PL 101-476, 20 U.S.C. §§ 1400 *et seq.*

Kennelly, J. (2000). The specialist role of the music therapist in developmental programs for hospitalized children. *Journal of Pediatric Health Care, 14,* 56–59.

Kerr, C., McDowell, B., & McDonough, S. (2004). Electrical stimulation in cerebral palsy: A review of effects on strength and motor function. *Developmental Medicine and Child Neurology, 46,* 205–213.

Koman, A.L., Mooney, J.F., III, Smith, B.P., Walker, F., & Leon, J.M. (2000). Botulinum toxin type A neuromuscular blockade in the treatment of lower extremity spasticity in cerebral palsy: A randomized, double-blind, placebo-controlled trial. *Journal of Pediatric Orthopedics, 20,* 108–115.

Koman, A.L., Smith, B.P., & Balkrishnan, R. (2003). Spasticity associated with cerebral palsy in children: Guidelines for use of botulinum A toxin. *Pediatric Drugs, 5*(1), 11–23.

Konczak, J., Borutta, M., & Dichgans, J. (1997). The development of goal-directed reaching in infants: II. Learning to produce task-adequate patterns of joint torque. *Experimental Brain Research, 113,* 465–474.

Kosak, M.C., & Reding, M.J. (2000). Comparison of partial body weight-supported treadmill gait training versus aggressive bracing assisted walking post stroke. *Neurorehabilitation and Neural Repair, 14,* 13–19.

Lance, J.W. (1981). Disordered muscle tone and movement. *Clinical and Experimental Neurology, 18,* 27–35.

Law, J., Garrett, Z., & Nye, C. (2004). The efficacy of treatment for children with developmental speech and language delay/disorder: A meta-analysis. *Journal of Speech, Language, and Hearing Research, 47,* 924–943.

Lezak, M. (1995). *Neuropsychological assessment* (3rd ed.). New York: Oxford University Press.

Lundy-Ekman, L. (1998). *Neuroscience fundamentals for rehabilitation.* Philadelphia: W.B. Saunders.

MacPhail, H.E., & Kramer, J.F. (1995). Effect of isokinetic strength-training on functional ability and walking efficiency in adolescents with cerebral palsy. *Developmental Medicine and Child Neurology, 37,* 763–775.

Mayer, N.H. (1997). Clinicophysiologic concepts of spasticity and motor dysfunction in adults with an upper motoneuron lesion. *Muscle and Nerve, 6,* S1–S13.

Miller, L.J., & Donders, J. (2003). Prediction of educational outcome after pediatric traumatic brain injury. *Rehabilitation Psychology, 48,* 237–241.

Molnar, G.E. (1991). Rehabilitation in cerebral palsy. *Western Journal of Medicine, 154,* 569–572.

Molnar, G.E., & Alexander, M.A. (1999). *Pediatric rehabilitation* (3rd ed.). Philadelphia: Hanley & Belfus.

Mooney, J.F., III, Koman, L.A., & Smith, B.P. (2003). Pharmacologic management of spasticity in cerebral palsy. *Journal of Pediatric Orthopedics, 23,* 679–686.

Nass, R.D., & Trauner, D. (2004). Social and affective impairments are important in recovery after acquired stroke in childhood. *CNS Spectrums, 9,* 420–434.

Park, N.W., & Ingles, J.L. (2001). Effectiveness of attention rehabilitation after an acquired brain injury. *Neuropsychology, 15,* 199–210.

Pearson, K. (2000). Motor systems. *Current Opinion in Neurobiology, 10,* 649–654.

Premack, D. (1959). Toward empirical behavioral laws: I. Positive reinforcement. *Psychological Review, 66,* 219–233.

Rehabilitation Act of 1973, PL 93-112, 29 U.S.C. §§ 701 *et seq.*

Rose, F.D., Johnson, D.A., & Attree, E.A. (1997). Rehabilitation of the head-injured child: Basic research and new technology. *Pediatric Rehabilitation, 1,* 3–7.

Rusk, H.A., Block, J.M., & Lowman, E.W. (1969). Rehabilitation following traumatic brain damage. *Medical Clinics of North America, 53,* 677–684.

Rusk, H.A., Lowman, E.W., & Block, J.M. (1966). Rehabilitation for the patient with head injuries. *Clinical Neurology, 12,* 312–323.

Schindl, M.R., Forstner, C., Kern, H., & Hesse, S. (2000). Treadmill training with partial body weight support in nonambulatory patients with cerebral palsy. *Archives of Physical Medicine and Rehabilitation, 81,* 301–306.

Singer, B., Singer, K.P., & Allison, G. (2001). Serial plaster casting to correct equino-varus deformity of the ankle following acquired brain injury in adults. *Disability and Rehabilitation, 23,* 829–836.

Sterba, J.A., Rogers, B.T., France, A.P., & Vokes, D.A. (2002). Horseback riding in children with cerebral palsy: Effect on gross motor function. *Developmental Medicine and Child Neurology, 44,* 301–308.

Steultjens, E.M.J., Dekker, J., Bouter, L.M., van de Nes, J.C.M., Lambregts, B.L.M., & van den Ende, C.H.M. (2004). Occupational therapy for children with cerebral palsy: A systematic review. *Clinical Rehabilitation, 18,* 1–14.

Sveistrup, H., McComas, J., Thornton, M., Marshall, S., Finestone, H., McCormick, A., et al. (2003). Experimental studies of virtual reality-delivered compared to conventional exercise programs for rehabilitation. *CyberPsychology & Behavior, 6,* 245–249.

Tardieu, C., Lespargot, A., Tabary, C., & Bret, M.D. (1988). For how long must the soleus muscle be stretched each day to prevent contracture? *Developmental Medicine and Child Neurology, 30,* 3–10.

Taub, E., Ellman, S.J., & Berman, A.J. (1966). Deafferentation in monkeys: Effect on conditioned grasp response. *Science, 151,* 593–594.

Taub, E., Goldberg, I.A., & Taub, P.B. (1975). Deafferentation in monkeys: Pointing at a target without visual feedback. *Experimental Neurology, 46,* 178–186.

Taub, E., Perrella, P.N., & Barro, G. (1973). Behavioral development following forelimb deafferentiation on day of birth in monkeys with and without blinding. *Science, 181,* 959–960.

Taub, E., Ramey, S.L., DeLuca, S., & Echols, K. (2004). Efficacy of constraint-induced movement therapy for children with cerebral palsy with asymmetric motor impairment. *Pediatrics, 113,* 305–312.

Tilton, A.H. (2003). Approach to the rehabilitation of spasticity and neuromuscular disorders in children. *Neurologic Clinics, 21,* 853–881.

Trexler, L.E., & Thomas, J.D. (1983). Behavioral and cognitive deficits in cerebrovascular accident and closed head injury: Implications for cognitive rehabilitation. In L.E. Trexler (Ed.), *Cognitive rehabilitation: Conceptualization and intervention* (pp. 27–62). New York: Plenum.

Wallander, J.L., & Thompson, R.J. (1995). Psychosocial adjustment of children with chronic physical conditions. In M.C. Roberts (Ed.), *Handbook of pediatric psychology* (2nd ed., pp. 124–141). New York: Guilford Press.

Wallander, J.L., Varni, J.W., Babani, L., Banis, H.T., & Wilcox, K.T. (1989). Family resources as resistance factors for psychological maladjustment in chronically ill and handicapped children. *Journal of Pediatric Psychiatry, 14,* 157–173.

Wells, R.D., & Schwebel, A. (1987). Chronically ill children and their mothers: Predictors of resilience and vulnerability to hospitalization and surgical stress. *Journal of Developmental and Behavioral Pediatrics, 8,* 83–89.

Werner, E., & Smith, R. (1992). *Overcoming the odds: High-risk children from birth to adulthood.* New York: Cornell University Press.

Winstein, C.J., Gardner, E.R., McNeal, D.R., Barto, P.S., & Nicholson, D.E. (1989). Standing balance training: Effect on balance and locomotion in hemiparetic adults. *Archives of Physical Medicine and Rehabilitation, 70,* 755–762.

Wood, K.M. (1978). The use of phenol as neurolytic agent: A review. *Pain, 5,* 205–229.

Yeates, K.O., Ris, M.D. & Taylor, H.G. (Eds.). (1999). *Pediatric neuropsychology: Research, theory and practice.* New York: Guilford Press.

Yvilsaker, M., Adelson, D., Braga, L.W., Burnett, S.M., Glang, A., Feeney, T., et al. (2005). Rehabilitation and ongoing support after pediatric TBI. *Journal of Head Trauma Rehabilitation, 20,* 95–109.

32

Sensory Integration

SHELLY J. LANE

The theory of sensory integration was first articulated by Dr. A. Jean Ayres in the late 1960s and early 1970s. Combining clinical expertise with children experiencing academic or motor difficulties or both and advanced training in neuroscience and educational psychology, Ayres developed the theory of sensory integration to explain the links between how the brain processes input and how the child expresses this processing in output (Ayres, 1972b). In her original work, Ayres sought to bring to the forefront an awareness of the issues related to learning disorders and to inspire others to find the most effective means of assessing and intervening with these children. The theory was put forward as provisional, knowing that, as a deeper understanding of both brain and behavior evolved, sensory integration theory would evolve as well (Ayres, 1972a, 1972b, 1972c).

The theory of sensory integration has always linked mind and body; it ties observable behavior with the input and processing of sensation from the environment (see Ayres, 1972b). This is the area where hard science (neuroscience) meets "soft" science (behavioral science). Sensory integration theory draws from neuroscience and behavior backgrounds, indicating that sensory information is processed within and between sensory systems (integrated) in regions in the brain and used by central nervous system (CNS) subsystems responsible for attention, emotion, learning, memory, and motor performance. This highly processed sensory information forms the foundation for output for interaction with the environment, from either a motor or a behavioral perspective. Understanding the processing re-quires an understanding of neuroscience. Understanding the behavior requires that we understand the neuroscience and its *potential* impacts on behavior. Ayres' oft-quoted definition of sensory integration is "the organization of sensory information for use" (1972b, p. 1). *Use* here is use by the person for interaction with the environment. There are leaps to be made between neuroscience and its application to behavior, but they are informed leaps.

The theory then links CNS processing of sensory input with the behavior of the person: a theory of brain–behavior relationships (Ayres, 1972b; Bundy & Murray, 2002). It postulates that environmental interaction depends on an individual's ability to take in and process sensation from the environment (both internal and external) and use the processed sensory information to plan and organize behavior. Thus, sensory input, processing, and integration lead to organized behavioral output. Furthermore, the theory postulates that, in individuals with deficits in the processing and integration of sensation, one may also see deficits in their ability to produce behavior that is planned and organized and to interact effectively with the environment. Ayres also proposed that, by providing intervention that emphasized enhanced sensory input, *as a part of meaningful activity requiring adaptive responses on the part of the child,* the ability to process sensory information could be improved and would result in improved planning and organization of behavior. Therefore, the theory relies on an understanding of CNS function and dysfunction in order to understand behavioral dysfunction and plan intervention.

UNDERSTANDING FUNCTION AND DYSFUNCTION

An understanding of function begins with an understanding of sensory systems. Sensory integration theory has emphasized the role that vestibular, tactile, and proprioceptive input plays in the development of early environmental interactions (e.g., Ayres, 1972b, 1979; Bundy & Murray, 2002). Input from the vestibular system coupled with that from proprioceptors in the muscles and joints is what guides a person in understanding movement through and position in space (Bear, Conners, & Paradiso, 2001). These systems together contribute to the development of body scheme. Postural responses, which form the foundation of many of our interactions with the environment, are the result of integrating information from the vestibular system and proprioceptors, along with input from the visual system. Proprioceptive input has been linked to the planning and execution of coordinated movement, or coordinated motor interaction with the environment (Gazzaniga, 1995). Proprioception is also seen as having a modulating influence over other senses (Blanche & Schaaf, 2001). Tactile input is one of our first sources of environmental information. It has been linked with the development of psychosocial skills and interpersonal relationships, emotional regulation, motor reflexes, and fine motor skills (Caulfield, 2001; Field, 2001, 2002a, 2002b; Stack, 2001; Weiss, Wilson, & Morrison, 2004; Weiss, Wilson, St. John Seed, & Paul, 2001). Proprioception is linked with both the vestibular system and the tactile system. Inputs that are proprioceptive in nature have already been mentioned in their relationship to postural responses, the development of body scheme, and movement through space. In addition, proprioception is often linked to tactile input during environmental interactions.

Although the visual and auditory systems have always been recognized as major means of interacting with the environment, they were not seen as the drivers of the integrative process in sensory integration theory. They are, however, closely linked functionally and structurally to the other sensory systems and, therefore, are considered part of the whole picture of the child.

Sensory Modulation and Dyspraxia

Current sensory integration theory holds that there are two broad manifestations of inadequate sensory integration—poor sensory modulation and inadequate planning and execution of movement—both of which are played out in behavioral interactions with the environment.

Deficits in Sensory Modulation Poor sensory modulation is a conceptualization that has only recently been clearly articulated (Lane, 2002; Miller, Anzalone, Osten, Lane, & Cermak, 2007). Ordinarily responses to sensation can be expected to fluctuate throughout the day in typically developing individuals. Responses to environmental input are influenced by context and are generally thought to be subject to the accumulation of sensory input across the day (Royeen & Lane, 1991). Thus, a stressful work or school day can diminish our ability to cope with loud music, crowded stores, and chaos at home. Modulation deficits are apparent when fluctuations within one person are extreme, or when someone tends to typically either overrespond to environmental inputs or underrespond. Although practitioners have recognized increased or decreased sensitivity to inputs such as touch and movement for years, historically we have not had the tools to identify these deficits by means other than observation. Clinically poor sensory modulation can be defined as "the [in]ability of an individual to regulate and organize responses to sensations in a graded and adaptive manner, congruent with the situational demand" (Miller, Reisman, McIntosh, & Simon, 2001, p. 57). Generally a sensory modulation disorder is identified when children have difficulty regulating and organizing the degree, intensity, and nature of their responses to sensory input in a way that allows them to interact with the environment in a graded and adaptive manner. What we see is that the child's response to sensory input does not fit the demands or expectations of the environment (Lane, 2002). As a result, the child cannot perform optimally and cannot adapt to the challenges of everyday life (Prudhomme, White, Mulligan, Merrill, & Wright, 2007).

Although we are making strides in our understanding of sensory modulation deficits, we remain limited in our ability to describe the full extent of difficulties in this realm. Work by Davies and Gavin (2007) has documented that children with sensory modulation deficits demonstrated limited auditory gating compared with typically developing children. These investigators suggested that children with sensory modulation deficits could be distinguished from typically developing children by comparing predicted with actual sensory gating. Thus, there is a growing understanding of central nervous system function related to sensory modulation deficits. Further, it has become clearer with recently developed clinical tools is that there are children who tend to overrespond to sensory input in one or more sensory channels. Their reactions are more intense, are more rapid in onset, and/or last longer than would be expected in the situation. There are also children who tend to underrespond to sensory input, who seem to be unaware of, or evidence limited responses to, input of typical intensity, frequency, or both. Clinicians also identify a third group of children, those showing labile responsiveness to sensory input, sometimes overresponding and other times underresponding (Miller, Cermak, Lane, Anzalone, & Osten, 2005; Miller, Anzalone, Osten, Lane, & Cermak, 2007; Miller & Lane, 2000; Miller et al., 2001).

Overresponsivity Children who overrespond to sensation may react to a light touch as though it were painful, be terrified to play on playground equipment, or cover their ears in the cafeteria because the sound of such chaos hurts their ears. Their responses to typical inputs, inputs that elicit little or no reaction from most of us, are negative and extreme. Responses such as those described may be most pronounced or apparent when the sensory input is unexpected. Furthermore, for these children, sensory input may be cumulative. That is, children with overresponsiveness may put forth effort to control and organize their behavior and reactions to sensory input they find disturbing until something that seems quite trivial sets off a sudden behavioral eruption (Lane, 2002; Miller et al., 2007). Sensory

overresponsiveness has been documented as a "stand-alone" condition by Reynolds and Lane (in press). These investigators presented preliminary evidence of children with sensory overresponsiveness, in the absence of comorbidities such as attention deficit, anxiety disorders, or mood swings.

Over time, clinicians have identified aspects of sensory overresponsiveness that reflect sensitivities in specific sensory systems, or in multiple sensory systems. Tactile defensiveness was the first form of overresponsiveness to be labeled (Ayres, 1965, 1966a). It is characterized by an overresponsiveness to touch sensations, particularly light or unexpected touch. Children with tactile defensiveness have an increased tendency to dislike certain textures of clothing, tags in the neck and waistband of clothes, seams on the top of socks, the feel of grass or sand on skin, light or unexpected touch, messy activities (e.g., fingerpainting), having their hair or teeth brushed, and the like. They respond with "anxiety, distractibility, restlessness, anger, throwing a tantrum, aggression, fear, and emotional distress" (Parham & Mailloux, 2001, p. 351).

Overresponsiveness to vestibular input has been characterized by two very different responses. *Gravitational insecurity* is one reflection of poor vestibular modulation, and the hallmark of this deficit in processing is fear of movement. Identification of gravitational insecurity is primarily observational; however, the Gravitational Insecurity Assessment Tool is under development and has been reported to be reliable and accurate in identifying children with gravitational insecurity (May-Benson & Koomar, 2007). Children with gravitational insecurity are described as being insecure in their relationship to gravity to the extent that they are overwhelmed by changes in head position relative to gravity (Ayres, 1972b; Parham & Mailloux, 2001). The expression of gravitational insecurity is fear of movement (particularly backward movement), fear of being out of upright position, and fear of heights (even when the height seems minimal). Children with gravitational insecurity will avoid activities that move them out of their comfort zone and will express anxiety or even panic if faced with a need to engage in such activities. There will be a tendency to move slowly and carefully, especially when they are moving through an unfamiliar environment or over uneven or unfamiliar terrain. Although such children may swing, they will keep their feet on the ground; they are unlikely to willingly engage in other playground activities or even other typical childhood activities such as bike riding and skateboarding.

A second type of clinically identifiable overresponsiveness is termed *aversiveness to movement* (Koomar & Bundy, 2002). Children with aversiveness to movement find movement sensation unpleasant because it causes them to feel ill or get a headache. Motion sickness when riding in a car, boat, or plane is an example of this overresponsiveness. Children with aversiveness to movement are not afraid to move; instead, movement makes them feel ill. They too may sometimes avoid certain activities, but their reasoning is very different. For instance, they may avoid the merry-go-round on the playground or an amusement park because the circular movement makes them ill.

A more general sensitivity to sensory input has been termed *sensory defensiveness* (Lane, 2002; Royeen & Lane, 1991). This could include overresponsivity to touch and movement, as described previously, but also to sound, visual input, taste, or smells. Children with sensory defensiveness may cover their ears in the cafeteria because the sound bouncing off the tile floors and nonacoustic ceilings is overwhelming; they may complain of light hurting their eyes. Sensory defensiveness may occur in response to sensory input in all sensory channels or only in a few. As with other forms of overresponsivity to sensation, sensory defensiveness is characterized by negative and emotional reactions that are out of proportion to the intensity of the sensory input.

When children experience overresponsivity to sensory stimuli, they may respond in one of two ways. One behavioral response seen is negativity and defiance, in an attempt to avoid becoming overloaded by their sensory environment. Children with this set of behaviors may be seen as aggressive or impulsive when faced with unexpected sensory input and may demonstrate tantrums and be difficult to con-

sole. The second behavioral reaction is to withdraw from the sensory environment. These children work to avoid interaction with potentially overwhelming input by avoiding engagement. They may become controlling and perfectionist in an attempt to control their environment and make it as comfortable as possible (Miller et al., 2007).

Underresponsivity Children identified as *underresponsive* to sensory input have behaviors that indicate they have not recognized the sensory input available to them and, as such, have not responded (Lane, 2002). This was termed a problem in *sensory registration* early in Ayres' work (1979), suggesting that children with underresponsiveness have not engaged in the initial step needed to process sensory input, that of recognizing that it is there. Thus, the child with poor registration "frequently fails to attend to or register relevant environmental stimuli" (Parham & Mailloux, 2001). Because *underresponsiveness* better captures what can be seen clinically than does *poor sensory registration*, the former term is used here.

Children who underrespond to sensation may be unaware of sound in their environment, not responding when their name is called; they may not be aware that their pants have been twisted on being pulled up, that their shirt is not buttoned properly, or that their shoes are on the wrong feet. They may also become very focused on irrelevant environmental stimuli, seeming to be deeply engaged in a visual or auditory pattern in the environment. Such a child may look to be withdrawn or difficult to engage, or potentially apathetic and lethargic. In a classroom or similar environment, this child may be overlooked because he or she does not cause trouble but instead will sit quietly, seeming to "behave" (Miller et al., in press).

There is some thought that children with modulation deficits may actually move from overresponsiveness to underresponsiveness, or their reactions to some sensory inputs may seem overresponsive while their reaction to other inputs may seem underresponsive (Miller et al., in press). Clinicians observing this seemingly paradoxical behavior have indicated that the underresponsiveness may be a mechanism by which some children cope with potential sensory overload. The labile nature of responsiveness was noted previously in the discussion of overresponsiveness as well.

Sensory Seekers An alternative modulation issue, perhaps related to underresponsiveness, is seen when children become seekers of sensory input. This sensory seeking exceeds what would be considered typical. Children described as sensory seekers tend to seek out more intense or greater frequency of sensory input, seemingly driven to engage the environment (Lane, 2002). According to Dunn,

> These children add sensory input to every experience in daily life. They make noises while working, fidget, rub or explore objects with their skin, chew on things, and wrap body parts around furniture or people as ways to increase input during tasks. (1999, p. 36)

Other behaviors that may be noted include constantly rocking in their chair in the classroom, spinning on the playground equipment for an entire recess period, or burying themselves in the sand pit each and every recess period. Children described as sensory seekers tend to be on the move, often crashing into things, climbing, and jumping. They may prefer loud sounds (television, music), seek strong visual input, and stare fixedly at stimulating objects or events. Behaviors that accompany such sensory seeking tend to be disruptive or inappropriate for a given environment. Thus, in contrast to the "very good" behavior of the child who is underresponsive but not sensory seeking, the sensory-seeking child may present problems in many environments because of his or her rowdy and often unsafe behavior (Miller et al., in press).

Empirical Support for Deficits in Sensory Modulation Evidence is mounting to support the existence of deficits in sensory modulation. In the development of an assessment tool designed to identify sensory modulation deficits. Two "families" of tools are currently available to identify sensory modulation and sensory processing disorders: the Sensory Processing Measure (Miller-Kuhanek, Henry, & Glennon, 2007; Miller-Kuhanek, Henry, Glennon, &

Mu, 2007; Parham & Ecker, 2007) and the Sensory Profile (Dunn, 1999). The Sensory Processing Measure is the newest of these tools and is designed to examine sensory processing across crucial child environments: the home and multiple environments related to the school. The Sensory Processing Measure was nationally standardized on a sample of more than 1,000 children, has adequate reliability and validity, and is effective in differentiating between typically developing children and those with sensory processing disorders. The Sensory Profile was the first tool available to identify sensory processing disorder. The Sensory Profile is now available as an infant/toddler version (Dunn, 2002), an adolescent/adult version (Brown & Dunn, 2002), and a school companion (Dunn, 2006).

Dunn and Westman (1997) compiled a list of 125 items to describe unusual responses to sensory inputs in the everyday life of children. The Sensory Profile was designed as a caregiver questionnaire that addresses sensory processing (auditory, visual, vestibular, touch, multisensory, and oral), modulation (related to aspects of daily life), and behavior and emotional responses believed to be reflective of sensory processing abilities. A sample of more than 1,000 children without disabilities was compiled, along with smaller samples of children with disabilities (attention-deficit/hyperactivity disorder [ADHD], pervasive developmental disorder [PDD], fragile X syndrome, and "other"). Cutoff scores were established from the group of children without disabilities, enabling the identification of children whose sensory responsivity shows "probable difference" from typically developing children and "definite difference" from typically developing children. Factor analysis of the sample groups resulted in nine identifiable factors, including sensory seeking, poor registration, and sensitivity (Dunn & Brown, 1997). Thus, within a population without disabilities there exists a small group of children responding with a definite difference to sensory stimuli in the environment than do their peers. These findings were substantiated by Reynolds and Lane (in press). Subsequent discriminate analysis of Dunn's work indicated that children with PDD and ADHD could be discriminated from children without disabilities and that the Sensory Profile provided different profiles for children with PDD and ADHD (Ermer & Dunn, 1998). The authors suggested that frequency or intensity of responsiveness to sensory stimuli was likely at the root of these differences. Tomchek and Dunn (2007) also found that children with autism spectrum disorder demonstrated sensory modulation deficits more often than did typically developing children. Their findings suggested that children on the autism spectrum showed sensory seeking behavior, along with auditory and tactile overresponsivity.

From the Sensory Profile, a short version was constructed to serve as a screening tool. The Short Sensory Profile (SSP; McIntosh, Miller, Shyu, & Dunn, 1999) consists of items taken from the Sensory Profile that have been subjected to further analysis. Factor analysis of the SSP defined a seven-factor structure that in this version separates sensory systems. Factors include tactile sensitivity, movement sensitivity, taste/smell sensitivity, auditory filtering, visual/auditory sensitivity, underresponsiveness/seeks sensation, and low energy/weak. Furthermore, children with and without sensory modulation deficits can be distinguished using this tool. Additional investigation of this tool has been undertaken to link deficits in sensory processing with differences in physiological responses to sensory challenges. Early findings indicated that children identified as having a deficit in sensory modulation showed a concomitant alteration in electrodermal responsiveness when given a sensory challenge (McIntosh, Miller, Shyu, & Dunn, 1999; McIntosh, Miller, Shyu, & Hagerman, 1999). These results have been repeated in children with ADHD (Mangeot et al., 2001) and fragile X syndrome (Miller et al., 1999).

An investigation of the potential prevalence of sensory modulation disorders was conducted by Ahn, Miller, Milberger, and McIntosh (2004). Parents of kindergarten students from a single suburban school district were asked to complete the SSP for their child. Thirty-nine percent of the SSPs were returned (703 of 1,796), and, of these, 96 children (13.7%) were identified as having a modulation disorder. The authors suggested using a much more conservative estimate, assuming

that the additional unreturned SSPs represented children without sensory modulation deficits. They therefore concluded that, in this population, approximately 5.3% of children demonstrated evidence of sensory modulation disorders.

Praxis and Dyspraxia

Originally called *developmental apraxia,* the term *dyspraxia* applies to a disorder in the ability to plan and execute unfamiliar or novel acts; it includes not knowing what to do and not knowing how to go about doing it (Ayres, 1979, 1985; Cermak, 1991). A broad look at mild motor disabilities is presented in Chapter 11 of Volume II; here we are addressing only dyspraxia that has a sensory integrative basis of dysfunction. This means that the dyspraxia must have, at its core, a deficit in the processing of vestibular, proprioceptive, and/or tactile sensation. The aspect of processing that is involved in dyspraxia is not sensory modulation, as was discussed previously, but rather sensory discrimination.

Sensory Discrimination Sensory discrimination is the process of interpreting the sensory qualities of a stimulus. Tactile discrimination includes such skills as localizing touch on the skin, identifying objects placed in the hand, and recognizing the direction of touch movement across the skin. Discrimination within the vestibular system includes such things as knowledge of position in space and movement through space, and the development of postural responses to environmental perturbations (seen in such things as equilibrium and balance). Proprioception contributes to these vestibular skills by providing feedback from muscles and joints that inform the CNS about muscle length and tension and joint position and movement. Visual perception underlies the child's ability to carry out skills such as distinguishing between *b, p, d,* and *q* and detecting objects within a busy visual background. Auditory discrimination forms the foundation for distinguishing among the nuances of phonemes, making language understandable (Miller et al., in press).

Dypraxia From a sensory integrative frame of reference, praxis is seen to depend on sensory discrimination abilities (Ayres, 1985; Dahl Reeves & Cermak, 2002; Miller, et al., in press). Dahl Reeves and Cermak suggested that there are two levels of dyspraxia, the least severe of which involves poor processing within the vestibular and proprioceptive systems, with the more significant involving deficits in the processing of tactile and proprioceptive sensations, as well as potential deficits in the processing of vestibular inputs.

When vestibular input and proprioception are compromised, postural deficits result, and the ability to move in a coordinated manner through the environment is challenged. Historically, vestibular and proprioceptive processing have been associated with the development of aspects of body scheme (Lackner & DiZio, 1988; Sirigu, Cohen, Duhamel, & Pillon, 1995). Thus, when a child has inadequate processing of vestibular and proprioceptive input and consequent poor body scheme, placement and movement of his or her body in space, through the environment, may appear uncoordinated (see Dahl Reeves & Cermak, 2002). It has also been suggested that inadequate processing of these sensations results in inefficiency in feed-forward mechanisms of the CNS, which are dependent on proprioception (Fisher, 1991). Feed-forward is linked to the ability to anticipate action, to set up the body for coordinated movement. Children with dyspraxia entailing inefficient feed-forward mechanisms may show relatively subtle difficulties in such things as bilateral skills and those activities that require anticipation of movement and setup of the body for action. In addition, because of compromised vestibular integration, children often demonstrate poor equilibrium and balance, poor postural stability, and muscle tone that is lower than normal, although not falling into the realm of true muscle hypotonicity as might be seen in a child with a specific neuromuscular deficit.

When proprioceptive, tactile, and (potentially) vestibular processing are all faulty, the child can be said to have a more severe form of dyspraxia, one that affects not only postural mechanisms and feed-forward but also feedback mechanisms. These children will appear qualitatively different from their counterparts with adequate somatosensory and vestibular processing. Children with a somatosensory-based dyspraxia can benefit neither from feedforward in the production of a motor act, nor from feedback once the act has been completed (Dahl Reeves & Cermak, 2002). In early factor analyses, Ayres (1965, 1966b, 1969, 1972b, 1972c, 1977) identified a link between tactile discrimination, kinesthesia, and praxis, leading to a description of dyspraxia as a problem in sensory integration that links impaired tactile and proprioceptive processing with difficulties in praxis. Ayres used the term *somatodyspraxia* to describe this combination of deficits (Ayres, 1989; Ayres, Mailloux, & Wendler, 1987). In a child with somatosensory-based dyspraxia, movements appear clumsy, transitioning from one position to another can be problematic, and accurate sequencing and timing of movement present challenges.

Because praxis is linked to inadequate integration of tactile and proprioceptive sensation, these children do not have a well-developed sense of themselves, or body scheme. They seem to not know where they are in space and are not able to move cleanly through space. When faced with a novel environment, these children may fail to come up with ideas for environmental interaction. Thus, taken to a playground with unfamiliar equipment, they may migrate toward the familiar—a swing, for instance—because they are unable to conceptualize how to manage the climbing structure made from rope or how to work the springy seesaw.

Shumway-Cook and Woollacott (2001) suggested not only that motor control relies on programs that drive muscle contraction and reflex action but also that coordinated movement is also dependent on feedback from muscles and joints as well as other perceptual systems. Ayres hypothesized that children with somatodyspraxia did not benefit from feedback from their bodies as they moved in space (Ayres, 1989; Ayres et al., 1987). Following a review of the motor learning and control literature, Guifridda (2001) came to much the same conclusion.

More recent factor analyses have indicated that, whereas children with dyspraxia often have a concomitant somatosensory processing problem, they will likely also have difficulty with vestibular and proprioceptive processing (Mulligan, 1998). Thus, the differentiation made previously may not exist, or it may represent different degrees of interference with motor planning ability (Lai, Fisher, Magalhaes, & Bundy, 1996; Mulligan, 1998). Until there is more clear evidence, it is probably best to consider dyspraxia to be a single arena of dysfunction, with probable different degrees of severity.

Empirical Support for Dyspraxia Dyspraxia as viewed here is considered a developmental motor coordination deficit, with a foundation in inadequate sensory processing. Children without problems in tactile, proprioceptive, and/or vestibular processing may also have praxis difficulties but would not be considered to have sensory integrative deficits in ideation, planning, and execution of movement. A wealth of literature is available on a broader concept, developmental coordination disorder (see, e.g., Cermak & Larkin, 2002). Current conceptualization holds that developmental coordination disorder includes deficits beyond those involved in sensory integration–based dyspraxia, deficits that encompass motor dysfunction that may not necessarily include a deficit in sensory processing.

Evidence supporting the existence of dyspraxia comes from a series of factor and cluster analytical studies conducted by Ayres using data from the original tests of sensory integrative function, the Southern California Sensory Integration Tests and the more current Sensory Integration and Praxis Tests (SIPT; Ayres, 1965, 1966a, 1966b, 1969, 1972a, 1972c, 1977, 1978, 1989). Some of these have been referenced previously. Throughout this array of work in which Ayres attempted to define sensory integrative deficits, a factor related to praxis consistently emerged. In the last of these studies (Ayres, 1989), the factor structure supported differentiating between vestibular-based praxis deficits and somatosensory-based praxis deficits.

Mulligan (1998) conducted a confirmatory factor analysis using Ayres' data from 1989 along with substantial additional data. In

this analysis, which included more than 10,000 subjects, Mulligan supported a five-factor solution that included the categories of praxis described here but concluded by indicating that a more generalized praxis dysfunction, or general sensory integrative dysfunction, better reflects the overall performance of children on the SIPT. She indicated that the specific patterns identified in this section could be viewed as components of the general sensory integrative dysfunction. A subsequent cluster analysis on a subset of the data supported differentiating among five clusters, with dyspraxia identified as a component in three of the five (Mulligan, 2000).

SCREENING/SUSPICION

Problems in sensory integration have the potential to interfere with the childhood occupations of play, learning, and activities of daily living. Screening should be multifaceted and include interviews, questionnaires, or both, designed to be done with the parents; observation of the child in play, school, or other learning environments and in activities of daily living; and the use of formal screening tools with the child. In all aspects of screening, and more formal assessment, it is critical to look at the *quality* of the child's interaction with the human and nonhuman environment. As with any screening or assessment of a child, age appropriateness of expectation must always be at the forefront. In addition, and also consistent with any type of screening or assessment, there must be a *meaningful cluster* of behaviors of concern (Bundy & Fisher, 2002).

Parental Report and Child Observation

Table 32.1 lists observations that can be made during the performance of activities. Such observations may be made by the parents and reported in an interview or on a questionnaire, or directly observed as the child engages in daily occupations. This table is meant to give a general idea of how observations would differ among the aspects of sensory integrative deficits presented earlier, and what a parent, teacher, or physician could look for or ask about when there is a question of inadequate sensory integration.

Table 32.1. Observation of sensory integrative deficits

	Sensory overresponsivity	Sensory underresponsivity	Sensory seeking	Dyspraxia
General description	Avoids, or expresses extreme dislike or fear of, typical sensory input in one or multiple sensory channels; may seem irritable, emotional	Needs intense and repeated input in one or more sensory channels in order to respond; may appear disengaged or unusually quiet	Actively seeks increased intensity and frequency of input and things, poor balance, and often a danger to self or others because of the intensity of input sought; may seem impulsive in seeking behavior and get in trouble for engaging in dangerous or "bad" behavior; may break toys or other materials because of difficulty modulating force	Overall clumsy in movement, frequent falls, bumps into things, poor balance, and preference for sedentary play; difficulty with fine motor skills, problems with timed and/or sequenced activities, and general disorganization
Examples of observations during play				
Playground swings	Avoids; sits on but moves only in rockinglike motion, keeping feet on the ground; may be very sensitive to movement backward	Comfortable swinging, but shows little or no joy with the activity; may not react to falls or scrapes	Swings high and fast; tries to spin repeatedly; likes to ride seated, on stomach, or laying way back	Trouble getting on and off; delayed development of ability to pump; grip on chains or ropes may seem ineffective and/or awkward
Playground merry-go-round	Avoids; shows fear with movement of the merry-go-round if strongly encouraged by adult to try; becomes ill with rotary movement while at the playground or develops a stomachache or headache later	Comfortable, although may not hold on tightly enough, but shows little or no joy with the activity; if movement is sufficiently intense or of sufficient duration, may show enjoyment	Cannot seem to get enough; wants faster and faster ride, well beyond the level that other children enjoy; wants to continue well beyond the length of time others are interested	Difficulty getting on and holding on; trouble maintaining balance when it begins to move or stops moving
Sandbox, garden play, beach	Avoids getting hands into sand or dirt, may play with objects in sand or dirt but uses only fingertips and is anxious to clean hands repeatedly during play and/or immediately at the end of the activity; dislikes walking barefoot on textured surfaces such as sand and grass	May become covered with sand or mud and seem unaware of it	Rolls in sand or dirt, buries self in sand, and may put it in his or her mouth; may destroy structures such as sand castles in order to meet internal need/drive for input	Trouble thinking of things to do; likes to crash things down instead of build things up; difficulty with use of trowel or other tools in digging and building

(continued)

Table 32.1. *(continued)*

	Sensory overresponsivity	Sensory underresponsivity	Sensory seeking	Dyspraxia
Examples of observations during playgroup or school				
Playgroup	Often plays alone and/or withdraws from group play, especially when it becomes "rowdy"; overreacts to inadvertent touch from a peer; avoids movement activities out of fear of or discomfort with movement	Physically present but appears disengaged; may need to be called to attend to an activity more than once before attention is gained; may invade the personal space of others due to a lack of awareness of his or her own position in space as well as that of others	Difficulty understanding concepts such as "inside voice"; overzealous in interactions; difficulty with social interactions; difficulty doing activities that are timed or that require alternating movements (e.g., clapping games); difficulty with anticipatory activities such as catching or kicking a ball	Whiny, manipulative, and easily frustrated with planned activities; difficulty with social interactions; difficulty doing activities that are timed or that require alternating movements (e.g., clapping games); difficulty with anticipatory activities such as catching or kicking a ball
School	Dislikes messy activities; overreacts to bumps from other children when lining up; covers ears when in cafeteria; avoids some movement activities during recess and/or physical education; may exhibit disruptive behavior when personal space is "invaded"	Seems overly quiet in the classroom; may seem to daydream	Difficulty understanding concepts such as "inside voice"; overzealous in interactions with others; may seek to be too close	Difficulty sitting still; always touching things; gets into materials, both his or hers and those belonging to others; louder than is appropriate in this environment in spite of reminders; rough and possibly dangerous play on the playground or in physical education
				Unusually clumsy in the classroom and may trip over feet or objects in the aisle; desk and/or locker are poorly organized; frequently cannot find all materials needed for a class or specific activity; non-age-appropriate difficulty with shoe tying, buttoning, and zipping; difficulty managing scissors and writing and drawing tools; play in physical education or on playground is unusually clumsy
Examples of observations during activities of daily living				
Activities of daily living	Strong dislike for such things as washing hair and face, brushing hair, cutting and cleaning nails, and brushing teeth; may have limited clothing preferences (soft, no tags, strictly long or short sleeved, no turtlenecks, socks with no seams); may express distress over sounds in the bathroom	Unaware of the need to wash when dirty, unaware of food or dirt on hands or face; may not realize that shoes are on wrong feet, clothes are on backward, or glasses are twisted or crooked on face	Uses very hot or very cold water to wash or shower; prefers washcloths or scrubbies that are very rough; brushes teeth with such vigor that gums may bleed	May show delays in development of independence in washing, toileting, tooth brushing, fastenings, and pouring liquids

Tools are available to guide clinical observation of sensory modulation and praxis. One such tool is the OTA Watertown Clinical Assessment Worksheet (Windsor, Roley, & Szklut, 2001). This tool offers clinicians a guide for observing the child during a session in a clinic outfitted with opportunities for sensory integrative activities. The child controls the session, and the clinician observes the child's interaction with people and things in the environment, drawing inferences about the child's ability to organize sensation, make adaptive responses, challenge him- or herself posturally, and respond to environmental demands. This information can be combined with less formal observation, as well as more formal assessment, to provide a complete picture.

Formal Screening and Assessment

The "gold standard" for assessment of sensory integration is the SIPT. As the name implies, this battery of 17 subtests examines many aspects of sensory integration and praxis, giving the examiner a great deal of insight into both sensory discrimination and praxis. It is a lengthy test to both give and score but provides valuable information that is not feasible to obtain using other assessment tools. Using the SIPT, one can obtain standardized information about visual perception and visual-motor skills, planning and execution of postural and oral motor skills, tactile discrimination, bilateral skills, and vestibular functions such as balance and equilibrium. It was standardized on children across the United States and Canada and has adequate reliability and validity (Ayres, 1989). The SIPT can be used with children ages 4 years, 10 months to 8 years, 11 months. There is a floor effect for some of the subtests and a ceiling effect for others, making use at the extremes of age range somewhat less reliable. The SIPT are designed to be used by occupational or physical therapists, and the user must be certified to administer and interpret the results of this tool.

One of the challenges inherent in identifying dyspraxia may be that the function of praxis is complex, involving ideation, planning, and execution. May-Benson and Cermak (2007) have begun development of a tool de-

signed to look specifically at one aspect of praxis—ideation. Initial analysis suggests that the tool, the Test of Ideational Praxis, is a valid and objective measure. Although further research is needed, such a tool may help better define aspects of dyspraxia in children with sensory processing disorders.

For children younger than 4 years, 10 months, the Miller Assessment for Preschoolers (MAP; Miller, 1982) and the FirstSTEP tool (Miller, 1993) may be used as screening tools for sensory discrimination and perception, and praxis. FirstSTEP is a short screening tool meant to indicate whether or not it would be prudent to follow-up with the longer MAP. Although the MAP was designed as a screening tool, it is longer than most and offers more detailed information than is generally obtainable in the screening process. Both of these screening tools have demonstrated reliability and validity.

Both FirstSTEP and the MAP focus on the presence or absence of developmental delays in the cognitive, communication, motor, social-emotional, and adaptive functioning domains. FirstSTEP is designed to be administered in 15 minutes or less as a "first step" in the assessment process. This tool includes an optional social-emotional scale and a parent–teacher scale. Although neither tool requires the degree of training and certification needed to administer and interpret the SIPT, both require that the user be familiar with test administration procedures and child development.

Conspicuously absent from the SIPT, the MAP, and FirstSTEP is the ability to formally assess sensory modulation. This has been a major shortcoming until recent years, when the Sensory Profile became available. Described earlier, the first Sensory Profile was designed to be applied to children ages 6–18 years. Both a short form and a long form of this tool were developed. Subsequently the Infant/Toddler Sensory Profile (Dunn, 2000) and the Adolescent/Adult Sensory Profile (Brown & Dunn, 2002) have become available. These tools guide clinicians in determining if a child's, adolescent's, or adult's responses to sensory input are like those of peers, probably different from peers, or definitely different from peers. Although the three age versions have somewhat different scoring, all can yield information about the sensory systems individually and, to a limited extent, about how sensory modulation influences other aspects of function and occupational performance. Unlike the SIPT, these tools are available to all professionals wishing to take the time to learn administration, scoring, and interpretation. It is helpful to have a background that includes knowledge of child development, sensory systems, and assessment, but no formal training or certification is required.

INTERVENTION

If assessment indicates that difficulties in sensory integration underlie difficulties in play, learning, or activities of daily living, intervention is indicated. If the assessment process did not identify deficits that interfere with performance of the child's occupational roles or activities within those roles, then intervention should not be pursued. Thus, the identification of tactile defensiveness alone is insufficient rationale for the recommendation of intervention. If the tactile defensiveness is interfering with the child's ability to play with peers on the playground or to manage self-care to the satisfaction of the child or his or her parents, then it should be addressed in a treatment program.

Armed with a synthesis of information obtained through formal and informal assessment, the therapist will meet with the child, parents, and potentially the teacher to establish goals designed to minimize difficulties identified. From global goals, objectives can be designed to more specifically address expected and desired changes: "we seek to learn, specifically, how the clients would *behave* differently or what they would like to be able to *do* after intervention that they cannot currently do" (Bundy & Fisher, 2002, p. 212). The overall design of the intervention plan will be based on the established goals and objectives.

Treatment can be carried out in a variety of environments and take different forms. Choice of environment should reflect the occupational roles and activities that are problematic and linked to the identified sensory integrative problem. Environment will be further influenced by the system in which therapist and child find themselves. Environmental options include the classroom or a separate clinic space within a school, a private clinic, a hospital inpatient or outpatient clinic, the home, or another community environment. *Direct intervention*, provided by a trained therapist, can take place in a private clinic, in the school, in the classroom, in the home, or in another environment. *Consultation* with parents, teacher, or both is a second form of intervention. It is often focused on environmental modifications and may include home programs.

Regardless of the intervention approach, the following principles for intervention are important (Parham & Mailloux, 2001):

1. Controlled sensory input can be used to elicit an adaptive response.

2. Registration of meaningful sensory input is necessary before an adaptive response can be made.

3. An adaptive response contributes to the development of sensory integration.

4. Better organization of adaptive responses enhances the child's general behavioral organization.

5. More mature and complex patterns of behavior are composed of consolidations of more primitive behaviors.

6. The more inner-directed a child's activities are, the greater the potential of the intervention activities for improving neural organization.

Direct Intervention

Direct intervention is typically carried out with a one-to-one therapist-to-child ratio, with the intent being to capitalize on the innate plasticity of the nervous system and influence the way sensory input is processed in the production of an adaptive response, or an adaptive environmental interaction. The one-to-one ratio allows the therapist to focus on the needs and strengths of a single child and match these to the demands of the environment.

A therapist skilled in sensory integration intervention will create an environment that addresses the established goals and objectives while also challenging the child to perform at a higher level than is currently comfortable. This environment will allow the child to sense that he or she is "in control," will tap into his or her inner drive toward mastery, and will promote a sense of playfulness. It is critical that the child be an active participant in the intervention process. To an uninformed observer, the process should appear to be interesting "play." A more informed observation would indicate that the therapist has designed activity options to improve postural stability through linear vestibular activities, or to improve bilateral skills in tasks that require the use of both sides of the body, or to improve praxis by offering opportunities for the child to problem-solve and plan for successful accomplishment of specific tasks. If it appears that the child is doing sensorimotor exercises rather than play, or if the therapist rather than the child is in control of when an activity starts, how it unfolds, and when it ends, then the session may be very good sensorimotor intervention, but it is not sensory integrative in nature.

Parham and colleagues (2007) have begun the process of developing a fidelity to treatment tool. This tool is designed to guide direct intervention sessions and ensure that intervention using a sensory integrative approach addresses what are considered the core elements of sensory integration theory. Once completed, this tool will provide a firm foundation for future carefully controlled studies of intervention effectiveness.

Consultation

Consultation with parents, the teacher, or both is a second form of intervention. Using a consultative model, a therapist might begin with an explanation of the child's behavior, strengths, and needs from a sensory integrative point of view. This reframing offers the parents or teacher a new and different way to conceptualize the child's behavior and needs. Whereas before a sensory integrative assessment the child's refusal to wear some clothes, eat certain foods, or walk barefoot in the grass and sand might have been construed as simple antagonism or acting-out behavior, from a sen-

sory integrative perspective it can be framed as tactile defensiveness. When viewed from this perspective, the problem is no longer a behavioral issue but is instead a sensory processing issue that requires different intervention. Offering the parents or teacher an alternative way to frame their behavioral observations can be powerful for the child as well as for the adults in the child's environment.

Beyond reframing, consultation can be used to focus on environmental modifications. Thus, for the child with tactile defensiveness, the teacher may move his or her desk out of the main thoroughfare in the classroom to a location that gets less child traffic. Less traffic means there is a decreased likelihood of unexpected touch and a lesser likelihood of an emotional outburst. At home, the parents can support the child's preferences for soft clothes, removal of tags from sweatshirts and T-shirts, and seamless socks.

Home programs are sometimes recommended as well, with either the child or the parents taking primary responsibility. The extent of the home program will be determined by the goals and objectives, as well as by the individual family's ability to carry out such a program. In some family contexts, a home program is exactly what the parents and child need; in other families, a busy work schedule, intense academic schedule, or other factors preclude an in-depth home program.

Sensory Diet

If a child has a sensory modulation disorder, a sensory "diet" may be recommended to augment direct intervention or consultation (Wilbarger & Wilbarger, 2002). A sensory diet is part of a treatment plan that includes providing the child with specific sensory activities throughout the day, in the context of daily occupations. First proposed by Ayres (1979) and later expanded by Wilbarger (1995), the sensory diet is geared primarily toward reducing defensive responses to sensation, although it could also be designed to address sensory underresponsivity. Activities are designed to be used throughout the day to meet the sensory needs of the child and are provided at regular intervals toward this end. Adaptations to the environment to reduce or enhance the sensation available are another component. Goals of the sensory diet are to be consistent with those developed for other aspects of intervention but designed to aid the child in maintaining a more consistent response to environment demand throughout the day.

Clinical Evidence

Research on the effectiveness of sensory integration intervention has demonstrated some important improvements in language, sensory processing, behavioral regulation, and gross motor performance (Ayres, 1972a, 1976; Cermak & Henderson, 1989; Magrun, McCue, Ottenbacher, & Keefe, 1981; Miller & Kinnealey, 1993; Ottenbacher, 1982, 1991; Ottenbacher & Short, 1985; Varga & Camilli, 1999). Of no surprise, it has been shown to be most effective when the child receiving therapy has been identified specifically as having sensory integrative deficits. Furthermore, the greatest effectiveness can be seen when this intervention is applied to younger children (Mulligan, 2002).

One randomized control trial is now published examining the effectiveness of occupational therapy intervention using a sensory integrative approach (Miller, Coll, & Schoen, 2007). Twenty-four children were randomized to one of three intervention groups: sensory integration, activities, and no treatment. Pre- and post-treatment assessments were conducted using the Leiter International Performance Scale–Revised (Roid & Miller, 1997). Outcomes indicated that children receiving sensory integration intervention made significantly more gains on the attention subscale and within the cognitive/social domain. Other outcomes were in a direction that favored sensory integration intervention, but the small sample size precluded statistical significance. This study provides the first randomized control trial using a fidelity tool as a guide to treatment. It lays the foundation for stronger methodology in future studies.

As is often pointed out, the research findings are not consistent and the effect sizes are not large. Part of the difficulty in demonstrating solid effectiveness comes from the variabil-

ity in populations under study and differing application of sensory integrative principles. Sensory integrative intervention, in its most true form, utilizes individualized and purposeful activities; capitalizes on enhanced vestibular, tactile, and proprioceptive sensation; is administered by an informed and skilled therapist; and leads to an adaptive (successful) environmental interaction (Mulligan, 2002). The overarching goal of intervention is "to facilitate appropriate physical and emotional adaptive responses by improving CNS processing rather than to teach specific skills" (Mulligan, 2002, p. 404). Studies of the effectiveness of sensory integrative intervention have not always held true to these concepts, instead examining the effects of such things as passively applied sensory stimulation, group interventions utilizing perceptual-motor rather than sensory integrative concepts, or combination therapies. Furthermore, participants in such studies may have undetermined sensory integrative deficits, making appropriate planning and implementation of treatment difficult.

It is beyond the intent of this chapter to delineate and critique the variety of studies that have been carried out; as noted previously, findings are generally mixed. Although outcomes heralding success are contested (Cummins, 1991) or at best viewed as neutral (Humphries, Wright, Snider, & McDougall, 1992; Wilson, Kaplan, Fellowes, Grunchy, & Faris, 1992), the most recent meta-analysis (Varga & Camilli, 1999) suggested that, overall, sensory integration intervention was shown to be as effective as alternative treatment approaches with similar populations. There is much to be done to provide a strong evidence base for this intervention.

REFERENCES

Ahn, R.R., Miller, L.J., Milberger, S., & McIntosh, D.N. (2004). Prevalence of parents' perceptions of sensory processing disorders among kindergarten children. *American Journal of Occupational Therapy, 58,* 287–293.

Ayres, A.J. (1965). Patterns of perceptual-motor dysfunction in children: A factor analytic study. *Perceptual and Motor Skills, 20,* 335–368.

Ayres, A.J. (1966a). Interrelations among perceptual-motor abilities in a group of normal children.

American Journal of Occupational Therapy, 20, 288–292.

Ayres, A.J. (1966b). Interrelationships among perceptual-motor functions in children. *American Journal of Occupational Therapy, 20,* 68–71.

Ayres, A.J. (1969). Deficits in sensory integration in educationally handicapped children. *Journal of Learning Disabilities 2,* 160–168.

Ayres, A.J. (1972a). Improving academic scores through sensory integration. *Journal of Learning Disabilities, 5,* 338–343.

Ayres, A.J. (1972b). *Sensory integration and learning disorders.* Los Angeles: Western Psychological Services.

Ayres, A.J. (1972c). Types of sensory integrative dysfunction among disabled learners. *American Journal of Occupational Therapy, 26,* 13–18.

Ayres, A.J. (1976). *The effect of sensory integrative therapy on learning disabled children: The final report of a research project.* Los Angeles: University of Southern California.

Ayres, A.J. (1977). Cluster analyses of measures of sensory integration. *American Journal of Occupational Therapy, 31,* 362–366.

Ayres, A.J. (1978). Learning disabilities and the vestibular system. *Journal of Learning Disabilities, 11,* 18–29.

Ayres, A.J. (1979). *Sensory integration and the child.* Los Angeles: Western Psychological Services.

Ayres, A.J. (1985). *Developmental dyspraxia and adult-onset apraxia.* Torrance, CA: Sensory Integration International.

Ayres, A.J. (1989). *Sensory Integration and Praxis Tests.* Los Angeles: Western Psychological Services.

Ayres, A.J., Mailloux, Z.K., & Wendler, C.L.W. (1987). Developmental dyspraxia: Is it a unitary function? *Occupational Therapy Journal of Research, 7,* 93–110.

Ayres, A.J., & Tickle, L. (1980). Hyper-responsivity to touch and vestibular stimulation as a predictor of responsivity to sensory integrative procedures in autistic children. *American Journal of Occupational Therapy, 34,* 375–381.

Bear, M.F., Connors, B.W., & Paradiso, M.A. (2001). *Neuroscience: Exploring the brain* (2nd ed.). Baltimore: Lippincott, Williams, & Wilkins.

Blanche, E.I., & Schaaf, R.C. (2001). *Proprioception: A cornerstone of sensory integration intervention.* In S.S. Roley, E.I. Blanche, & R.C. Schaaf (Eds.), *Understanding the nature of sensory integration with diverse populations.* San Antonio, TX: Therapy Skill Builders.

Brown, C.E., & Dunn, W. (2002). *Adolescent/Adult Sensory Profile.* San Antonio, TX: Psychological Corporation.

Bundy, A.C., & Fisher, A.G. (2002). Interpreting test scores and observations: A case example. In A.C. Bundy, S.J. Lane, & E.A. Murray (Eds.), *Sensory integration: Theory and practice* (pp. 199–209). Philadelphia: F.A. Davis.

Bundy, A.C., & Murray, E.A. (2002). Sensory integration: A. Jean Ayres' theory revisited. In A.C. Bundy, S.J. Lane, & E.A. Murray (Eds.), *Sensory integration: Theory and practice* (pp. 3–33). Philadelphia, PA: F.A. Davis.

Caulfield, R. (2001). Beneficial effects of tactile stimulation on early development. *Early Childhood Education Journal, 27,* 255–257.

Cermak, S.A. (1991). Somatodyspraxia. In A. Fisher, E. Murray, & A. Bundy (Eds.), *Sensory integration: Theory and practice* (pp. 137–165). Philadelphia: F.A. Davis.

Cermak, S.A., & Henderson, A. (1989). *The efficacy of sensory integration procedures. Sensory Integration Quarterly, XVII(3).* Torrance, CA: Sensory Integration International.

Cermak, S.A., & Larkin, D. (2002). *Developmental coordination disorder.* Albany, NY: Delmar.

Cummins, R. (1991). Sensory integration and learning disabilities: Ayres' factor analyses reappraised. *Journal of Learning Disabilities, 24,* 160–168.

Dahl Reeves, G., & Cermak, S.A. (2002). Disorders of praxis. In A. Fisher, E. Murray, & A. Bundy (Eds.), *Sensory integration: Theory and practice* (pp. 71–100). Philadelphia: F.A. Davis.

Davies, P.L., & Gavin, W.J. (2007). Validating the diagnosis of sensory processing disorders using EEG technology. *American Journal of Occupational Therapy, 6(2),* 176–189.

Dunn, W. (1999). *Sensory Profile.* San Antonio, TX: Psychological Corporation.

Dunn, W. (2000). *Infant/Toddler Sensory Profile.* San Antonio, TX: Psychological Corporation.

Dunn, W. (2006). *Sensory Profile School Companion.* San Antonio, TX: Psychological Corporation.

Dunn, W., & Brown, C. (1997). Factor analysis on the Sensory Profile from a national sample of children without disabilities. *American Journal of Occupational Therapy, 51,* 490–495.

Dunn, W., & Westman, K. (1997). The Sensory Profile: The performance of a national sample of children without disabilities. *American Journal of Occupational Therapy, 51,* 25–34.

Ermer, J., & Dunn, W. (1998). The Sensory Profile: A discriminate analysis of children with and without disabilities. *American Journal of Occupational Therapy, 52,* 283–290.

Field, T. (2001). *Touch.* Cambridge, MA: MIT Press.

Field, T. (2002a). Infants' need for touch. *Human Development, 45,* 100–103.

Field, T. (2002b). Violence and touch deprivation in adolescents. *Adolescence, 37,* 735–749.

Fisher, A.G. (1991). Vestibular-proprioceptive processing and bilateral integration and sequencing deficits. In C. Bundy, S.J. Lane, & E.A. Murray (Eds.), *Sensory integration: Theory and practice* (pp. 71–106). Philadelphia: F.A. Davis.

Gazzaniga, M.S. (1995). Principles of human brain organization derived from split-brain studies. *Neuron, 14(2),* 217–228.

Guiffrida, C. (2001). Praxis, motor planning, and motor learning. In S.S. Roley, E.I. Blanche, & R.C. Schaaf (Eds.), *Sensory integration with diverse populations* (pp. 133–162). San Antonio, TX: Therapy Skill Builders.

Humphries, T., Wright, M., Snider, L., & McDougall, B. (1992). A comparison of the effectiveness of sensory integration therapy and perceptual-motor training in treating children with learning disabilities. *Journal of Developmental and Behavioral Pediatrics, 13,* 31–40.

Kaplan, B., Polatajko, H., Wilson, B., & Faris, P. (1993). Reexamination of sensory integration treatment: A combination of two efficacy studies. *Journal of Learning Disabilities, 26,* 342–347.

Koomar, J.A., & Bundy, A.C. (2002). Creating direct intervention from theory. In A.C. Bundy, S.J. Lane, & E.A. Murray (Eds.), *Sensory integration: Theory and practice* (pp. 261–308). Philadelphia: F.A. Davis.

Lackner, J.R., & DiZio, P. (1988). Gravitational effects on nystagmus and perception of orientation. *Annals of the New York Academy of Sciences, 545,* 93–104.

Lai, J., Fisher, A., Magalhaes, L., & Bundy, A. (1996). Construct validity of the Sensory Integration and Praxis Tests. *Occupational Therapy Journal of Research, 16,* 75–97.

Lane, S.J. (2002). Sensory modulation. In C. Bundy, S.J. Lane, & E.A. Murray (Eds.), *Sensory integration: Theory and practice* (pp. 101–122). Philadelphia: F.A. Davis.

Magrun, W.M., McCue, S., Ottenbacher, K., & Keefe, R. (1981). Effects of vestibular stimulation on the spontaneous use of verbal language in developmentally delayed children. *American Journal of Occupational Therapy, 35,* 101–104.

Mangeot, S.D., Miller, L.J., McIntosh, D.N., McGrath-Clarke, J., Simon, J., Hagerman, R.J., et al. (2001). Sensory modulation dysfunction in children with attention-deficit-hyperactivity disorder. *Developmental Medicine and Child Neurology, 43,* 399–406.

May-Benson, T.A., & Cermak, S.A. (2007). Development of an assessment for ideational praxis. *American Journal of Occupational Therapy, 61*(2), 148–153.

May-Benson, T.A., & Koomar, J.A. (2007). Identifying gravitational insecurity in children: A pilot study. *American Journal of Occupational Therapy, 61*(2), 142–147.

McIntosh, D.N., Miller, L.J., Shyu, V., & Dunn, W. (1999). Overview of the Short Sensory Profile (SSP). In W. Dunn (Ed.), *Sensory profile: User's manual* (pp. 59–73). San Antonio, TX: Psychological Corporation.

McIntosh, D.N., Miller, L.J., Shyu, V., & Hagerman, R. (1999). Sensory modulation disruption, electrodermal responses, and functional behaviors. *Developmental Medicine and Child Neurology, 41,* 608–615.

Miller, L.J. (1982). *Miller Assessment for Preschoolers.* Littleton, CO: Foundation for Knowledge and Development.

Miller, L.J. (1993). *FirstSTEP: Screening test for evaluating preschoolers.* San Antonio, TX: Psychological Corporation.

Miller, L.J., Anzalone, M.E., Osten, E., Lane, S.J., & Cermak, S. (2007). Concept evolution in sensory integration: A proposed taxonomy. *American Journal of Occupational Therapy, 61*(2), 135–140.

Miller, L.J., Coll, J.R., & Schoen, S.A. (2007). A randomized controlled pilot study of the effectiveness of occupational therapy for children with sensory modulation disorder. *American Journal of Occupational Therapy, 61*(2), 228–238.

Miller, L.J., & Kinnealey, M. (1993). Researching the effectiveness of sensory integration. *Sensory Integration Quarterly, XXI*(2).

Miller, L.J., & Lane, S.J. (2000). Toward a consensus in terminology in sensory integration theory and practice. Part 1: Taxonomy of neurophysiologic processes. *Sensory Integration Special Interest Section Newsletter, 23*(1), 1–4.

Miller, L.J., Lane, S.J., Cermak, S., Anzalone, M., & Osten, E. (2005). Regulatory-sensory processing disorders. In S. Greenspan & S. Weider (Eds.), *ICDL diagnostic manual for infancy and early childhood.* Baltimore: ICDL.

Miller, L.J., McIntosh, D.N., McGrath, J., Shyu, V., Lampe, M., Taylor, A.K., et al. (1999). Electrodermal responses to sensory stimuli in individuals with fragile X syndrome: A preliminary report. *American Journal of Medical Genetics, 83,* 268–279.

Miller, L.J., Reisman, J.E., McIntosh, D.N., & Simon, J (2001). An ecological model of sensory modulation: Performance of children with fragile X syndrome, autistic disorder, attention-deficit/hyperactivity disorder, and sensory modulation dysfunction. In S.S. Roley, E.I. Blanche, & R.C. Schaaf (Eds.), *Sensory integration with diverse populations* (pp. 57–88). San Antonio, TX: Therapy Skill Builders.

Miller-Kuhanek, H., Henry, D.A., Glennon, T.J., & Mu, K. (2007). Development of the Sensory Processing Measure–School: Initial studies of reliability and validity. *American Journal of Occupational Therapy, 61*(2), 170–175.

Miller-Kuhanek, H., Henry, D.A., & Glennon, T.J. (2007). *Sensory Processing Measure: Main Classroom and Environmental Form.* Los Angeles: Western Psychological Services.

Mulligan, S. (1998). Patterns of sensory integration dysfunction: A confirmatory factor analysis. *American Journal of Occupational Therapy, 52,* 819–828.

Mulligan, S. (2000). Cluster analysis of scores of children on the Sensory Integration and Praxis Tests. *Occupational Therapy Journal of Research, 20*(4), 256–270.

Mulligan, S. (2002). Advances in sensory integration research. In A. Fisher, E. Murray, & A. Bundy

(Eds.), *Sensory integration: Theory and practice* (pp. 397–411). Philadelphia: F.A. Davis.

Ottenbacher, K. (1982). Sensory integration therapy: Affect or effect? *American Journal of Occupational Therapy, 36,* 571–578.

Ottenbacher, K. (1991). Research in sensory integration: Empirical perceptions and progress. In A. Fisher, E. Murray, & A. Bundy (Eds.), *Sensory integration: Theory and practice* (pp. 387–399). Philadelphia: F.A. Davis.

Ottenbacher, K., & Short, M.A. (1985). Sensory integration dysfunction in children: A review of theory and treatment. *Advances in Developmental and Behavioral Pediatrics, 6,* 287–329.

Ottenbacher, K., Short, M.A., & Watson, P.J. (1981). The effects of a clinically applied program of vestibular stimulation on the neuromotor performance of children with severe developmental delay. *Physical and Occupational Therapy in Pediatrics, 1*(3), 1–11.

Parham, L.D., & Ecker, C. (2007). *Sensory Processing Measure: Home Form.* Los Angeles: Western Psychological Services.

Parham, L.D., & Mailloux, Z. (2001). Sensory integration. In J. Case-Smith, A. Allen, & P. Pratt (Eds.), *Occupational therapy for children* (3rd ed.). St. Louis: Mosby.

Parham, L.D., Cohn, E.S., Spitzer, S.,Koomar, J.A., Miller, L.J., Burke, J.P., et al. (2007). Fidelity in sensory integration intervention research. *American Journal of Occupational Therapy, 61*(2), 216–227.

Prudhomme White, B., Mulligan, S., Merrill, K., & Wright, J. (2007). An examination of the relationships between motor and process skills and scores on the Sensory Profile. *American Journal of Occupational Therapy, 61*(2), 154–161.

Reynolds, S., & Lane, S.J. (in press). Diagnostic validity of sensory over-responsivity. *Journal of Autism and Developmental Disability.*

Roid, G.H., & Miller, L.J. (1997). *Leiter International Performance Scale–Revised.* Wood Dale, IL: Stoeling.

Royeen, C.B., & Lane, S.J. (1991). Tactile processing and sensory defensiveness. In C. Bundy, S.J. Lane, & E.A. Murray (Eds.), *Sensory integration: Theory and practice* (pp. 108–136). Philadelphia: F.A. Davis.

Shumway-Cook, A., & Woollacott, M.H. (2001). *Motor control—theory and practical applications.* Baltimore: Lippincott, Williams, & Wilkins.

Sirigu, A., Cohen, L., Duhamel, J., & Pillon, B. (1995). A selective impairment of hand posture for object utilization in praxis. *Cortex, 31,* 41–55.

Stack, D. (2001). The salience of touch and physical contact during infancy: Unraveling some of the mysteries of the somesthetic sense. In G. Bremner & A. Fogel (Eds.), *Blackwell handbooks of developmental psychology: Blackwell handbook of infant development* (pp. 351–378). Oxford, UK: Blackwell.

Tomchek, S.D., Dunn, W. (2007). Sensory processing in children with and without autism: a comparative study using the Short Sensory Profile. *American Journal of Occupational Therapy, 61*(2), 190–200.

Varga, S., & Camilli, G. (1999). A meta-analysis of research on sensory integration treatment. *American Journal of Occupational Therapy, 53,* 189–198.

Weiss, S.J., Wilson, P., & Morrison, D. (2004). Maternal tactile stimulation and the neurodevelopment of low birth weight infants. *Infancy, 5,* 85–107.

Weiss, S.J., Wilson, P., St. John Seed, M., & Paul, S.M. (2001). Early tactile experience of low birth weight children: Links to later mental health and social adaptation. *Infant and Child Development, 10,* 93–115.

Wilbarger, J., & Wilbarger, P. (2002). Clinical application of the sensory diet. In A.C. Bundy, S.J. Lane, & E.A. Murray (Eds.), *Sensory integration: Theory and practice* (pp. 339–341). Philadelphia: F.A. Davis.

Wilbarger, P. (1995). The sensory diet: Activity programs based on sensory processing theory. *Sensory Integration Special Interest Section Newsletter, 18*(2), 1–4.

Wilson, B., Kaplan, B., Fellowes, S., Grunchy, C., & Faris, P. (1992). The efficacy of sensory integration intervention compared to tutoring. *Physical and Occupational Therapy in Pediatrics, 12,* 1–37.

Windsor, M.M., Roley, S.S., & Szklut, S. (2001). Assessment of sensory integration and praxis. In S.S. Roley, E.I. Blanche, & R.C. Schaaf (Eds.), *Sensory integration with diverse populations* (pp. 215–246). San Antonio, TX: Therapy Skill Builders.

33

The Spectrum of Assistive and Augmentative Technology for Individuals with Developmental Disabilities

LARRY W. DESCH

In many places throughout these two volumes, the term *spectrum* is used, for example, *autism spectrum disorders.* In most of these instances, the term refers to the variability in severity of a particular disease or disorder. In this chapter, *spectrum* refers to the wide variation in the complexity of treatment modalities that can be used with people who have developmental disorders and disabilities. The purpose of this chapter is not to provide extensive information about the tens of thousands of available assistive devices, but rather to provide information about the categories of currently available technology and, more important, the process of evaluating their use and effectiveness. At the start, however, it should be emphasized that this chapter does not deal with complementary/alternative therapies, for example, devices using unproved or disproved methodologies, such as colored lenses for treatment of dyslexia (Committee on Children with Disabilities, 1998). The devices that are discussed in this chapter will have at least some empirical evidence that documents their effectiveness. Evaluation of the use of these devices is discussed later in this chapter; Chapter 34 of this volume discusses alternative and complementary treatments (the majority of which are not assistive devices).

Based on the 2003 American Community Survey from the U.S. Census Bureau (2005), approximately 15% of children (about 3.7 million) and about 25% of adults (about 73 million) in the United States today have some type of disabling condition. These problems range in extent from severe physical disabilities to mild learning disabilities. Many children with disabilities have been helped to be more functional in their day-to-day living abilities by the use of adaptive, augmentative, or assistive devices. Although definitions for these have varied somewhat by author, and these definitions overlap, there seems to be some consensus emerging.

Assistive devices are those that help alleviate the impact of a disability, lessening the functional limitations. An example would be use of tape-recorded lessons for students with reading disabilities. *Adaptive technology* is that which substitutes or makes up for the loss of functioning from a disability, for example, a sophisticated robotic feeding device for children with severe quadriplegia. Finally, *augmentative devices* are those that "augment" an area of functioning that is deficient, sometimes severely, but for which there is some residual ability. An example would be the use of a microchip-powered voice-output device for a child with dysarthria. In this situation, the child's speech might be readily understood by family members but the device would be needed when the child wanted to communicate with others. The most common context for the use of the term *augmentative* is in the field of speech and language (e.g., augmentative and alternative communication [AAC] devices). In this chapter, the general term *assistive technology* is used primarily because it has more of an overall meaning in all types of therapeutic areas and treatments.

OVERVIEW OF ASSISTIVE AND AUGMENTATIVE TECHNOLOGY

For many years, assistive technology has been thought of by many as referring only to microcomputers and microchip-enabled devices. Although such complicated devices may be the only answer for a particular problem, they represent only the higher end of the spectrum of assistive technology. Since at least 1986, assistive and augmentative technology has been thought of as low technology (*low tech*), middle technology (*mid-tech*), and high technology (*high tech*) and everything in between (Desch, 1986). Many people, even professionals working in the field, sometimes do not realize that they are using assistive technology on a daily basis with their clients or patients, or even themselves. For example, using a foam or rubber cushion over a pencil or pen to help you with your grip is making use of a type of low-technology assistive device. Table 33.1 gives

examples of the spectrum of assistive technology.

Low-tech devices are those that use low-cost materials and do not require batteries or other electrical sources to operate. Examples of low-tech devices include wheelchair ramps, ankle–foot orthoses, and printed picture communication boards. Mid-tech devices are generally more sophisticated devices that do require battery power or are more complex in their use, such as telecommunication devices (e.g., teletypewriter [TTY]) for individuals who are deaf or sophisticated manual wheelchairs for those with mobility limitations. Finally, high-tech devices are those that are quite complicated and, thus, often quite expensive to own and operate. Examples of these would be microchip-enabled voice-output devices and cochlear implants.

Despite the innovativeness of these low- and mid-tech devices, a child with a disability might have certain problems that can only be dealt with by an electronic or computerized assistive device. For example, many children with moderate or severe physical disabilities will have oral and written communication

Table 33.1.   Examples of available devices

Area of disability	Spectrum of technology		
	Low tech	Mid-tech	High tech
Physical	Swivel-spoon (and other feeding aids)	Reciprocating-gait orthosis	Electronically controlled/ adapted wheelchairs
	Wheelchair ramps	Lightweight wheelchairs	Environmental control units
	Adapted playgrounds	Adapted toys	Robotic devices
	Most orthotics		Functional electrical stimulation
	Grips for pencils		Voice-input and eye gaze–input devices
Communication	Simple picture/word boards	On/off light for yes/no responses	Adapted laptops
	Eye gaze picture boards	Digital voice recorder	Commercially available computerized devices (e.g., TouchTalker)
	Visual schedule/planner	Scanning light board	
Sensory	Magnifying lenses	Alerting systems (to movement/sound)	Digital hearing aids
	Large-print books	Braille typewriters	Cochlear implants
	Books on tape	Frequency modulation (FM) transmitting devices	Kurzweil 1000 reading software
			Voice-output computer
Learning	Color-coded notebooks	Talking calculators	Kurzweil 3000 reading software
	Self-stick note tags	Electronic speller/ dictionary	Hypertext learning programs
	Flashcards	Tape recorders	Software for cognitive/ attention rehabilitation
	Visual schedule/planner	Books on tape	

problems that can, at least partially, be remedied by use of an electronic assistive device. Devices such as computerized speech synthesizers or adapted computers are becoming more readily available to help these children with their communication needs.

Assistive devices, across the spectrum, are acquired in one of three different ways. They can be obtained by 1) direct purchase from commercial suppliers, who often also manufacture such devices; 2) development of an individualized, custom-made device (these can be simple, hand-made devices or complex, one-of-a-kind devices made by an engineer or technician for use by one person); or 3) modifying an existing device such as a computer, a telephone, or a typewriter (these modifications may also be commercially available items from a manufacturer). Some modified devices are constructed at rehabilitation centers at a high cost; however, in the past decade the availability of this technology overall has improved so that the purchase of commercial or commercially modified devices is becoming the most common way to acquire assistive devices.

These three approaches have their own advantages and disadvantages. Commercially available aids have the advantage of being specially designed and optimized to meet the needs of a large group of individuals or a specific type of disability. In addition, maintenance of the equipment is usually provided by the company. There are two disadvantages, however: 1) the aids may not meet individual needs because they must be designed for large groups of people, and 2) only aids needed by a large number of individuals can be produced economically.

The second group of devices, custom-built aids, have the advantage of being constructed to meet the needs of one individual; however, the cost of such aids can be extremely high, especially with respect to high-tech devices, because they are usually one-of-a-kind designs. Maintenance and repair are difficult because funding is often tenuous for universities, hospitals, or other agencies that make these complex devices. Even without these funding problems, there is often some turnover of personnel with subsequent changes in expertise.

The third approach, modifying or adapting common devices, has some of the advantages and disadvantages of the first two approaches. Using a microcomputer as an aid for a person with a disability (e.g., adapting an Apple or PC-type laptop microcomputer) falls into this category. Devices such as microcomputers are often easily adaptable for a particular person with a disability. This entails connecting various commercially produced keyboards, switches, microphones, or other electronic components that, generally, are readily available from several specialized companies. As soon as a more difficult modification or customization is needed, however, these modified systems quickly begin to resemble custom-built aids and also begin to take on the disadvantages of custom-built aids in terms of cost and maintenance. The next several sections address these three approaches to assistive devices in regard to different types of disabilities.

Assistive Devices for Physical Disabilities

In the usual therapeutic interventions for children with disabilities, the focus is mainly to normalize their abilities. Years may be spent in helping a child, for example, develop enough hand and arm control to feed him- or herself independently or to develop enough speech to be able to indicate even simple wants. The use of many assistive devices by children who have physical disabilities often entails a different style of intervention. These two differing approaches were described decades ago in a classic reference by Goldenberg (1979), in which he called the first approach the *exercise* model and the latter approach the *substitution* model. The exercise model concentrates on habilitation or rehabilitation that attempts to normalize functioning. The substitution model involves the development of alternative means of communication or control of objects, such as using electronic-controlled assistive devices.

Assistive devices at the lower end of the spectrum dominate what is used now and probably will be used in future. Such low-tech devices as ankle–foot orthoses, hand splints, spine braces, and adapted feeding equipment will always have an important role to improve functioning and lessen disability. Mid-tech devices such as electrical stimulators for functional electrical stimulation, treadmills with support frames to increase strength even in children who do not ambulate, and dynamic braces (e.g., for treatment of a hemiplegic arm) have been becoming increasingly available and likely will continue to have a major impact for years to come.

With all devices available in the three possible areas of acquisition—commercial, custom-made, and modified—the main issue is how a child with physical disabilities can use the device; how is the "input" achieved? Input consists of two components: the actual hardware used (e.g., keyboard, wheelchair controls and switches) and how the hardware can be used via a particular selection technique. Vanderheiden and Grilley (1976) described three categories of selection techniques: direct selection, scanning, and encoding.

To use direct selection, either a part of the child's body (e.g., finger, toe, elbow) or a special device (e.g., head stick, light pointer, mouth stick) is used to point to or push on or somehow select a specific single electronic or physical switch. The simplest method involves making direct contact with a group of switches (e.g., on an electric wheelchair), a specially built keyboard, or some other device.

Direct selection aids include mid-tech devices such as specialized joysticks, sip-and-puff (pneumatic) switches, or switches in slots for use with electric wheelchairs so that an "unusual" movement type can be used to control off/on and directional functions. For more high-tech devices, direct selection aids would include enlarged keyboards, touch screens, membrane switches, magnetic or optically activated keys, and voice selection of keys by using an electronic voice recognition system. Special magnetic field–sensitive switches can be used in a keyboard to respond to a magnet that is moved around. Membrane switches that respond to minimal pressure have been used quite successfully and are generally lower in cost than other methods. A keyboard consisting of electronic switches that respond to a focused light beam have also been used to replace standard input devices such as manual keyboards. Commercially available electronic communication aids that use the latter type of switches, include the LightWRITER sold by DynaVox Technologies. (See the appendix at the end of the chapter for a list of vendors.)

The most promising approach to direct selection is the use of voice input or speech recognition. Speech recognition is the ability of a computer to collect, process, interpret, and execute audible instructions. The commercial systems that are available at the present time, although highly useful and relatively low-cost because they are mass marketed, are unfortunately still somewhat inflexible and require some time to train the person in their use. One commercial device is the Dragon Naturally Speaking software for microcomputers from the Nuance Corporation (see the appendix). Mainly used by people without physical disabilities, some use of this technology has also been reported with children with learning disabilities (Wetzel, 1996). It is anticipated that, when further improved, speech recognition systems will be in wide use because they would be in much demand with all types of users.

Scanning, the second selection technique, is most commonly used in high-tech devices for children with severe physical impairments. In most cases, input is made by controlling a single switch; therefore, this is usually the slowest selection technique. The switch is either custom made or purchased from companies that produce this type of equipment for children with disabilities. Changes are made in the switch or the way it is mounted so that the user can easily activate it by a voluntarily controlled part of the body.

Scanning communication devices, often controlled by a single switch, exemplify the principles of the scanning method. On these mid-tech or high-tech devices, a light blinks in each square while moving across squares on boards that contain pictures, symbols, or letters of the alphabet; these sequential blinks stop when a switch is activated. The information or symbol on that particular square—for example, the letter *a*—then causes a signal representing the letter *a* to be sent to a computer or a printer. The types of switches that can be used to control such a device can often be activated by such slight movements as blowing or sucking on a tube (pneumatic switch), or by minimal contraction of a single muscle (myoelectric switch). These boards can also be used as a remote control input device to a computer. Several manufacturers, such as ZYGO Industries and the Prentke Romich Company, make this type of equipment (see the appendix).

Encoding, the third selection technique, used primarily with microprocessor-based assistive devices, is frequently used in communication aids for nonspeaking children. The main purpose of encoding is to speed up the selection or input process (Olson & Olson, 2003). Encoding is used with several commercially available devices, such as the LightWRITER AAC device mentioned previously or the Link spelling/voice-output devices from Assistive Technology (see the appendix). These devices use a voice synthesizer to create an artificial voice. The voice synthesizer produces words or phonemes—individual sound units of speech. In order to produce words that are not already stored in the device's memory, the user of this device can type on the machine's keyboard a series of codes for various phonemes. After all the codes are entered, the artificial voice then ''speaks'' the words or sentences.

Microcomputers, with the appropriate adaptations, can be very useful high-tech tools for children with physical disabilities. An important advancement in the adaptation of microcomputers for these individuals is the development of ''transparent modifications.'' Modifications to the microcomputer can be made by using added-on equipment and/or specialized software programs so that most commercial software programs, such as computer games, word-processing programs, and computerized instructional programs, can be used. With a transparent modification, neither the computer nor the standard software program being used is modified or interfered with. The best example of a transparent modification is the *keyboard emulator,* a device used to replace the keyboard on a microcomputer with another device such as a joystick (Platts & Fraser, 1993).

Keyboard emulators are electronic circuits that function by taking the output from a special keyboard or input device, altering this output appropriately, and then transmitting a standard signal format by wires to the appropriate connectors on the microcomputer. The emulator translates the original signal into a different format that the computer interprets as coming from its own keyboard. By having a keyboard emulator, a special keyboard or input device can be constructed or purchased to meet the individual needs of someone with a specific type of disability.

Besides multiple-use devices such as microcomputers, there are also many single-application devices designed or adapted for children with physical disabilities. Examples of these range from relatively simple mid-tech electronic feeding devices to elaborate environmental control units that can turn on and off lights and appliances and dial a telephone (Platts & Fraser, 1993). Environmental control units have recently begun to be marketed by such companies as ZYGO and Technical Aids and Systems for the Handicapped (see the appendix).

Children who have moderate to severe physical impairments involving the extremities always have some type of communication disability. These communication problems may mainly involve text production (written or typed), but many of these children also have some vocal communication problems. The next section discusses these and related concerns.

Communication Disabilities and Autism: The World of ACC

The simplest may be the most cumbersome.

Many types of communication devices can be used by a child who is unable to use speech as an effective means of communication (see Table 33.1). Symbols rather than words are often used in the development of communication techniques used by children who do not speak, such as those with autism. The use of symbols is especially helpful if the individual does not know how to read prior to using a communication board. Children with significant intellectual disabilities or autism, for example, may continue to use pictures or symbols as their only method of communication as they grow older.

Low-tech answers to communication disorders might include various lists of words or pictures that a child could point to in order to get the message across. Sometimes these low-tech measures are all that is needed with certain individuals. Low-tech communication boards are constructed by printing words or symbols on a flat surface, and they are used in face-to-face communication by pointing to the words.

A battery-operated scanning communication device (as described in the previous section) is an example of a mid-tech device. These have been successfully used by children with speech and language disorders as well as autism (Mirenda, 2001). Other mid-tech devices that can be used by these groups include portable voice-output storage devices, which require direct selection and hold only a few minutes of prerecorded sentences or phrases; however, all low-tech and mid-tech devices have two faults: 1) they represent a very slow or very limited method of communication, and 2) they cannot be used for "long-distance" communication.

Many high-tech electronic communication aids, often incorporating the use of symbols that may substitute for groups of words, are becoming more commercially available to children with disabilities. For individuals with severe physical and communicative disabilities, these high-tech aids commonly use the methods of scanning or encoding. Systems that allow direct selection are used with those children who have better control of movements.

Single-function voice-output communication devices have been found to be quite helpful, but their use has been curtailed by their cost and somewhat by their limited flexibility. Similar to what has been accomplished for children with physical disabilities, various companies have recently used less expensive laptop microcomputers as the core part of a communication system (see the appendix). The use of a laptop as the central part of the device has increased the versatility of these communication aids. Rather than being used only for person-to-person communications, these adapted laptops can be used for all types of communication—letter writing, telecommunications and electronic mail—and other personal uses such as for environmental control, as safety and security systems, or for just

playing computer games, even virtual-reality games (Weiss, Bialik, & Kizony, 2003).

The newfound flexibility in these "new-generation" communication devices is not necessarily a result of the sometimes extensive adaptations that are made to the laptop microcomputer. It is primarily the result of the fact that the typical microcomputer (desktop and laptop) was not designed for one particular use but for use by many people with many different purposes. One example is the tablet type of laptop computer (which has no keyboard), on which input is accomplished by touch screen or is pen-based (see the appendix). These commercial devices can easily be modified into an AAC device by adding the appropriate software, input hardware, and voice-output or other hardware. In other words, transparent modifications can easily be added. Most of these devices have utilized a certain degree of transparent modification in order to successfully adapt the microcomputer.

The main advantage of using a microcomputer-based aid over most dedicated communication aids is the greater flexibility of a microcomputer. In particular, for children whose communication skills will continue to improve, it is usually easier to change the amount and quality of the available vocabulary in a microcomputer-based aid than in most dedicated communication aids. A major barrier to using microcomputers as communication aids, if the intended user has significantly physical disabilities, is the custom interfacing needed to achieve optimum speed. Because using custom hardware with standard computers can eliminate many of the advantages of microcomputers, care must be taken in deciding between adapting a microcomputer or purchasing a specially designed but commercially available communication aid.

The development of electronic high-tech communications aids is a tremendous achievement, but there are still practical problems, especially in regard to speed in comparison to typical communication. Something even closely approximating normal speech production has yet to be achieved, and unfortunately this point has not always been emphasized. Neither commercially available, dedicated communication aids nor adapted microcomputers can attain rates of communication that even come close to the rates of person-to-person communication. Even when direct selection techniques are employed by experienced users who do not speak but have no other impairments, the rate of conversation is very slow—usually less than 10–15 words per minute.

A relatively recent attempt to solve this problem of communication rate is the development of new systems in which symbols represent not just words or small phrases but rather entire concepts. With these systems, of course, some sort of extensive translation must occur for effective communication with others to take place. An example of this approach is Min-Speak (minimum effort speech). MinSpeak is essentially a new language designed for people with disabilities who cannot express themselves through speech or hand signs. It is a *semantic interface* that utilizes microprocessor-based technology and speech synthesis in a system that reduces the time and effort required for communications (Baker, 1982; Dattilo & Camarata, 1991; van der Merwe & Alant, 2004). A child using a MinSpeak board with fewer than 50 keys can produce thousands of sentences with usually fewer than seven keystrokes for each sentence. Children using Min-Speak do not even have to know how to spell; they can produce complete sentences without selecting letters, phonemes, or words. The symbols on the MinSpeak board represent neither letters nor words, but generalized concepts. The Prentke Romich Company, for example, has for many years developed special electronic communication aids that implement the MinSpeak concept (see the appendix).

An alternative way to accelerate the rate of communication, besides using a new "language" such as MinSpeak, is to improve the way in which a specific language, such as English, can be used. English and other languages have certain grammatical rules, common phrases, and other syntactic constructs that are somewhat predictable. Methods have been developed that consider the statistical nature of the English language so that previously typed characters or words can be used to predict what should follow (e.g., the LightWRITER).

Spoken communication among individuals without disabilities is performed at such a high rate of speed that few have the patience necessary to communicate with an individual with disabilities using a slow manual communication aid such as a low-tech symbol, letter, or word board. Even though these methods are extremely slow, such boards should not be abandoned. As often as not, they are just as effective as high-tech devices in face-to-face communication, if not more so. Electronic devices are often limited by their need for some power source—batteries wear down and often a wall socket is not nearby—thus limiting the usefulness of the device in many situations. Therefore, a lower tech solution such as a word or picture board should always be available to use as a backup should the electronic device fail.

Many difficulties still need to be worked out to improve the clarity and usefulness of the spoken output devices. The number of words or phrases that these devices can store is finite, and the generation of new words by using phonemes is very time consuming. Improvements in acceleration and prediction software (as described previously), coupled with artificial intelligence computer programs, are probably the areas of greatest promise for the future.

Assistive Devices for Sensory Disabilities

Children with sensory disabilities have also been helped in many different and exciting ways with various assistive devices across the spectrum of sensory disability. For children with visual impairments, there are low-tech magnification devices and mid-tech aids such as alerting systems, laser canes, and books on tape or digitally recorded systems (Flax, Golembiewski, & McCaulley, 1993). Children with visual impairments are able to use microcomputers by the simple addition of extra-large type on video screens. Various devices using electronic technology have also been developed for blind people. Some devices, such as the Kurzweil-1000 Reading Machine, translate the written word to voice-synthesized output. Other devices make it possible for Braille readers who are deaf-blind to use a computer and produce Braille output, and there are refreshable Braille displays (e.g., ALVA Satellite) that substitute for a computer monitor with text (see the appendix).

An exciting technology, possibly available in the not-too-distant future, is the development of neural implants that take in visual information through some type of camera or similar imaging device and then send signals to the brain that can be interpreted as actual objects or perspectives in a person's environment. A review article by Eberhart Zrenner, a researcher from Germany, has outlined the research that is currently being done on microchip retinal implants as well as the many challenges to the successful clinical use of such technology (Zrenner, 2002).

The past two decades have seen an explosion in the complexity and efficacy of hearing aids for children who could benefit from amplified sounds. Digital programmable hearing aids have become more available, allowing for much improved "customization" for an individual's specific degree and range of hearing loss. Many mid-tech solutions for these children are also available, such as assistive listening devices using infrared or frequency modulation (FM) transmitters in movie theaters or assembly halls in schools, or palm-sized telecommunication devices for use with telephones.

For the child with severe hearing impairment, as well as for their families and others, there have been advances in better methods to learn lipreading or sign language by use of computer modeling programs. Also available are improved versions of the electronic cochlear implant, which for individuals with some types of hearing loss can restore a type of "hearing," or at least a better awareness of sounds. A number of studies have been done in young children documenting that the use of cochlear implants, coupled with intense therapies, can lead to near-normal language development (e.g., Zwolan et al., 2004). Although the majority of children being born in the United States with total deafness or profound bilateral hearing loss possibly will receive cochlear implants, this procedure is not universal and is not without controversy. For example, cochlear implants are more common in deaf children who have parents with normal hearing than in deaf children who have parents who are deaf themselves and are part of a community of deaf people (Eleweke & Rodda, 2000). Disparities have also been found related to ethnicity and socioeconomic status (Stern, Yueh, Lewis, Norton, & Sie, 2005). Although risks with a cochlear implant are uncommon, much caution and planning should be exercised with the use of this device with children, especially younger children, because the operation to insert the device destroys whatever residual hearing there might have been prior to the placement of the device, and there are neurological risks from cerebrospinal fluid or other infections (Cohen, Roland, & Marrinan, 2004).

Assistive Devices for Learning and Cognitive Disabilities

Large numbers of children who have special needs do not have physical or sensory disabilities, but have difficulties in learning—for example, with reading, writing, or mathematical skills. Although the needs of these children are usually covered for the most part by special education services, medical input into possible diagnosis or treatment of problems is often sought. This medical input may also require that an opinion be given about the appropriateness of certain services or assistive technologies.

Children who have learning disabilities have been helped by various low-tech through high-tech methods and devices (Day & Edwards, 1996; Raskind & Higgins, 1998). The assistive devices mainly utilized with this group of children employ software programs and microcomputers. Microcomputers can be extremely patient teachers and will not add more frustration for children with learning problems, who have had more than their fair share of frustration. Many software programs have been developed in the past two decades that use microcomputers to assist in special education instruction in reading, mathematics, and other subject areas. These programs range very widely in price and utility. The caveat for their use is that, even now, only a limited amount of research has been done to determine their effectiveness and generalizability, especially over the long term.

Microcomputer-based instruction has several unique advantages for teaching children with special needs, perhaps the most significant of which is the ease of individualization. Wide variation in the type and degree of learning problems is seen with these children. By using microcomputers, it is possible to build on the children's strengths and talents and develop alternative ways of learning. Individualization of the level of instruction in a microcomputer software program is possible through flexible branching in the program. Flexible branching allows students to start an instructional program at a point that is appropriate to the prior knowledge they have on the subject. Properly designed microcomputer material is also self-paced. The learner can cover the material as rapidly or as slowly as needed and can review it as well. Very few children with learning disabilities have their own personal teacher on a full-time basis. The use of a microcomputer allows these children to begin to develop independent learning skills.

A second advantage that microcomputer educational programs have is that they are an interactive medium. This interactivity provides students with immediate feedback regarding performance. This prevents the learner from practicing wrong responses until the teacher can provide remedial instruction. Microcomputers thus serve as important motivators for learning—an important factor in teaching some children who may need additional motivation because of frequent and repeated failures.

Most children who have learning disabilities do not have any significant motor disability, but changes often must be made to the microcomputer hardware, especially in the way information is entered. Children with severe dyslexia, for example, might need to use some form of input device to a microcomputer other than a conventional keyboard. These children would likely have problems recognizing the correct letters and might quickly lose interest in their work, leading to frustration and errors. Many devices can be creatively used in such situations to replace keyboard entry: joysticks,

touch screens, and graphic tablets are but three examples.

Often the output side of the computerized instructional environment also needs to be adapted. Presenting words on the computer screen is inappropriate for certain ages or with different types of learning problems. Graphic representations or pictures, especially for younger children, can provide motivation as well as instruction. DVD and CD-ROM players have been connected to computers to help teach various skills to very young children or for use by those with intellectual disabilities. Voice-synthesized output, a more expensive option, also has been frequently used.

Limited research has been done to try to determine if these microcomputer programs are truly a better way to teach children who have certain learning problems (Higgins, Boone, & Lovitt, 1996; Wilson, Majsterek, & Simmons, 1996). Unfortunately, conclusive results have not yet been published that give a final answer to the issue of effectiveness and generalizability. More research using larger numbers of students with longer follow-up is needed to further study these issues. The results of research published so far look very promising. Nonetheless, special education teachers and other educators are becoming much better trained and more aware of how microcomputers can be used in classroom situations with children who have learning disabilities.

These software programs are not a panacea for learning disabilities and should not be used without appropriate planning and consultation with educational specialists. Some features that are often incorporated into educational software, such as sound effects, can also create problems when used with certain children with learning disabilities (e.g., those who are easily distracted). Some software instructional programs, therefore, may be harmful or inappropriate. In the past, many microcomputer-based instructional programs were deficient and improperly designed. This occurred because some of the software that had been produced was designed not by educators but by computer programmers. This situation has changed, especially since the 1990s, as educators became more involved in the development of software programs.

To summarize this section, it is crucial that the educational strengths and needs of a student with disabilities be evaluated fully first; then, the assistive technology can be applied where it can best alleviate the appropriate problems. In all cases, however, low-tech and mid-tech solutions should be considered *first*. A high-tech solution is often *not* the best answer for a specific problem that a child is having in school.

ASSESSMENT ISSUES

It is of utmost importance that the assessment process and prescribing of any assistive device be done by knowledgeable individuals. Every child with a disability is different in his or her abilities and needs, and the process of selecting an assistive device nearly always requires extensive planning by an experienced team of professionals. This team approach is needed to properly evaluate both the child and the device in order to ensure that the device can be used effectively and will not interfere with other parts of the child's overall treatment, educational, or vocational plan. Depending on the type of assistive device to be prescribed, this team might include such individuals as speech-language therapists; physical therapists; occupational therapists; rehabilitation engineers; neurodevelopmental pediatricians; neurologists; physiatrists or other physicians; special educators; computer specialists; and others who, by their training or experience, are appropriate. If at all possible, this should be an *inter*disciplinary team, in which there are ongoing discussions among the team members and decisions are made jointly. Such a team is also usually needed to provide training in and monitor the use of the device.

The overall assessment process is shown in Figure 33.1. An important aspect of assessment is to always consider the entire spectrum of assistive technology that may be needed or could be useful. The best approach is always to begin with the low-tech devices and then, if needed, to assess mid-tech devices and, finally, high-tech devices. If a low-tech solution solves a particular problem, then it is never appropri-

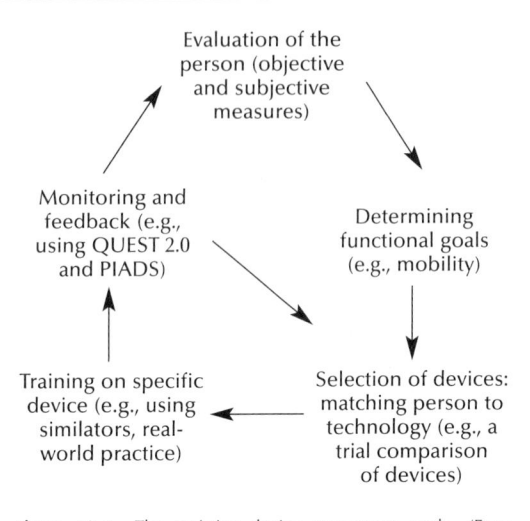

Figure 33.1. The assistive device assessment cycle. (From Desch, L.W. [2007]. Technological assistance. In M.L. Batshaw, L. Pellegrino, & N.J. Roizon [Eds.], *Children with disabilities* [6th ed., p. 563]. Baltimore: Paul H. Brookes Publishing Co; reprinted by permission.) (*Key:* QUEST 2.0, Quebec User Evaluation of Staisfaction with Assistive Technology, Version 2.0 [Demers, Weiss-Lambrou. & Ska, 2000]; PIADS, Psychosocial Impact of Assistive Devices Scale [Day, Jutai, & Campbell, 2002; Routhier, Vincent, Morrissette, & Desaulniers, 2001].)

ate to go any further in the process. For example, a child with a severe physical disability may actually get more benefit from ramps and wider doors and may actually have problems using an electric wheelchair to get around in the house.

Part of the assessment process is often done by having the child try out various possible devices; however, educated guesses based on prior assessments or experiences with other children are usually helpful. As complete an evaluation as possible should be done prior to actually ordering equipment so that devices that are unusable or inappropriate are not inadvertently purchased.

Functional Evaluation of the Individual

The ultimate goal for using an assistive device is to achieve the highest possible functioning. The first step, therefore, is to determine the child's current functional abilities, environmental situations, and personal preferences. One example of a way to determine the most complete picture of a child's health and abilities is to use the system devised by the World Health Organization (2001) known as the International Classification of Functioning, Disability and Health (ICFDH). Using this system, for example, one can classify and determine the extent of problems and strengths that a child has related to a disability that affects the Activities and Participation ICFDH domain. Within this domain there are subcategories such as Communication and Mobility, and using this ICFDH system may help lead to better planning for how a specific device might have an impact on these subcategories.

Since the 1970s, a number of other standardized instruments have been developed that can objectively evaluate the current functioning of children with various types of disabilities. These systems are less complex than the ICFDH system and have been found to be useful in longitudinal assessments to measure change. Two examples of such measurement instruments are the children's version of the Functional Independence Measure (WeeFIM; Ottenbacher et al., 1997) and the Pediatric Evaluation of Disability Inventory (PEDI; Haley, Coster, Ludlow, Haltiwanger, & Andrellos, 1992) (Bunch & Dvonch, 1994; Dodds, Martin, Stolov, & Deyo, 1993). These types of assessment measures should be used to establish baseline functioning because it is crucial to document over time the functional changes that occur after assistive technology is introduced.

Much more should be done to ensure success in using an assistive device. A number of studies have demonstrated that about a third of assistive devices are abandoned shortly after they are obtained; in some studies the proportion is as high as 75% (Galvin & Scherer, 1996; Phillips & Zhao, 1993). Since the 1980s, however, methods to improve matching assistive devices to children who have various types and degrees of impairments have been developed. Some of these techniques have been developed specifically to predict the successful use of assistive devices.

One person who has done considerable work in the prediction of successful use of assistive technology is Marcia Scherer, who developed the Matching Person and Technology (MPT) model (Scherer, 1998b). Table 33.2 summarizes the important factors associated with device abandonment as determined by this model. Essentially this model stresses the importance of three areas that must be addressed whenever assistive technology is being considered: environmental, personal, and technology. The environmental area includes issues such as family support and the school setting. The personal area consists primarily of the functional limitations but also includes motivation and coping skills and personality traits such as optimism. The technology area includes device characteristics such as reliability and ease of use, adaptability, and whether there is discomfort or stress with use. Scherer and colleagues have developed an assessment tool, the Assistive Technology Device Predisposition Assessment, that uses the MPT model in a systematic way to facilitate the "match" between device and child and to ensure the best long-term results (Scherer, 1998a, 1998b).

Two groups of researchers in Canada have also been doing considerable work in the past

Table 33.2. Factors associated with abandonment of an assistive device

Factor	Example
Improper or ineffective training on the use of a device	Single-session training without follow-up and feedback
Problems or obstacles in the environment preventing use of a device	Second-floor rooms inaccessible to an electric wheelchair user
Faults or failures in performance of the device	AAC device that is too sensitive to movement
Device size, weight, or appearance	AAC device decorated with pink roses for a boy to use
Motivational factors in the user/family members	Depression occurring after traumatic injuries
Perceived lack of or minimal need for the device	Decision made not to leave the house rather than using wheelchair
Functional abilities that worsen or improve	Progressive disorder or recovery

From Scherer, M.J. (1998). *Matching person and technology model and accompanying assessment forms* (3rd ed.). Webster, NY: Institute for Matching Person and Technology; adapted by permission.
Key: AAC, augmentative and alternative communication.

decade developing and evaluating assessment tools that specifically address the long-term use and acceptance of assistive technology by individuals using such devices. These types of assessment are very important during the training and the monitoring/feedback periods of the assessment cycle, as depicted in Figures 33.1 and 33.2. These two assessment tools are the Quebec User Evaluation of Satisfaction with Assistive Technology (QUEST), now the QUEST-2 (Demers, Weiss-Lambrou, & Ska, 1996, 2000), and the Psychosocial Impact of Assistive Devices Scale (PIADS; Day, Jutai, & Campbell, 2002). Although these measures have been standardized on adults with various disabilities, the QUEST was used successfully in at least one study in older children to evaluate their success with upper limb myoelectric prostheses (Routhier, Vincent, Morissette, & Desaulniers, 2001). Work is currently being done to adapt the PIADS for use with older children and teenagers (Day et al., 2002).

Both the QUEST-2 and the PIADS use a questionnaire format to evaluate new users of an assistive device on such issues as the device's physical aspects (weight and size) and services (repairs and training), but the PIADS additionally asks questions about "competency" and "self-esteem." In many ways these measures are complementary in how they assess the factors that seem to lead to successful use of assistive devices. In one research study evaluating a population of adults with multiple sclerosis, a positive correlation was found between the PIADS and QUEST-2 results. The highest association found was between the Competence subscale on the PIADS and the Device Characteristics subscale on the QUEST-2 (Demers, Monette, Lapierre, Arnold, & Wolfson, 2002).

Evaluation of Children with Physical and Communicative Disabilities

Children with moderate to severe physical and communicative limitations are the group who can possibly benefit most from the combined knowledge and experience of an interdisciplinary team of professionals. During the evaluation of these individuals, such a team's main task is to determine which movements can be consistently made and how these movements can be used

to control some type of device. Especially in regard to communication devices, decisions also have to be made about which output method would be the most acceptable and useful to both the child with disabilities and the receiver of the output information. For example, output information could be displayed on a monitor screen, typed out by a printer, or presented as synthesized speech. Most of the time, multiple output types are preferred.

There has been a recent emphasis in many areas of services and in various locations around the world on addressing what has been called *universal access* (Akoumianakis & Stephanidis, 2003). Within this viewpoint, systems are developed that can be easily used or easily adapted for use both by people without disabilities and by those who have a disability of whatever type or severity. In other words, in the initial plans to produce a device, often a high-tech device, steps are taken to ensure that the device can be used by the largest number of people possible, with or without disabilities. Even such a simple device as an alarm clock could be made so that a socket is present on the clock into which a cord to a vibrating pillow could be plugged. With this simple adaptation, that same alarm clock could be used by people with hearing impairments. Although universal access is increasing for many devices, it will take many years to make a significant impact, and evaluating how a person with a disability can use assistive technology often remains a time-consuming process.

Perhaps the most important part of the evaluation for a child with a significant physical disability is deciding on the input method, or the type of control switches that will be used with the assistive device or communication system. Many types of control switches are available for various situations so that the selection can easily be based on what is most appropriate to the child's needs and abilities. These interface devices may fall anywhere along the spectrum from low tech to high tech (Angelo, 1998). Several switching methods and types of switches have already been mentioned. Large switches are easier for some children to use, and some of these switches have been constructed to withstand rough treatment. This is especially helpful for children

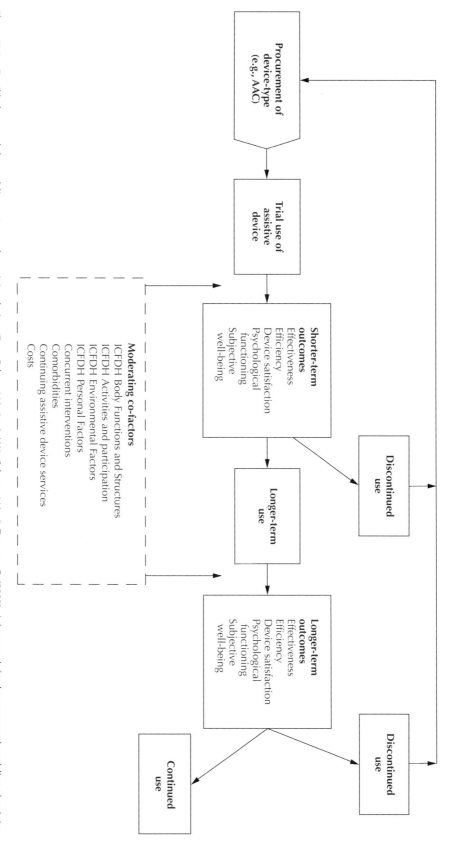

Figure 33.2. Possible framework for modeling outcomes for assistive devices (From Fuhrer, M.J., Jutai, J.W., Scherer, M.J., & Deruyter, F. [2003]. A framework for the conceptual modeling of assistive device outcomes. *Disability and Rehabilitation, 25,* 1243–1251; adapted by permission.) (*Key:* AAC, augmentative and alternative communication; ICFDH, International Classification of Functioning, Disability and Health [World Health Organization, 2001].)

with athetosis or other movement disorders. The ubiquitous joystick can also be used quite effectively as a type of multiple-switch input device. Joysticks are often employed when scanning input techniques are used to help increase the speed of input. Commercial switches have become more readily available from companies such as ZYGO Industries, the Prentke Romich Company, the J. A. Preston Corporation, and AbleNet, Inc. (see the appendix).

Selecting the best switch to use is often a difficult task, especially when working with individuals with severe disabilities who have very limited movement control. Fortunately, the vast majority of children with disabilities have at least one movement that is consistent and can be voluntarily controlled, even if it is only an eye movement or blink. Time must be spent to identify these useful voluntary movements, measure the strength and stamina of the movement (especially after continued use), and determine how the child reacts to the output of the device (e.g., loud noise may cause a startle reflex). The movement must be both consistent and unmistakable before it can be used to point, push a switch, or increase pressure. Sometimes a very unusual movement can be the most "normal" one for the child with a disability to make (Latash & Anson, 1996). Systematic assessment methods have been devised that, if time proves them successful, will facilitate the portion of the evaluation process concerned with selecting appropriate control switches (Akoumianakis & Stephanidis, 1999; Casali, 1995; Rahman & Springle, 1997; Shein, Lee, & Milner, 1983).

The difficulties that some children have in moving their hands or arms are sometimes caused by interference from uncontrolled primitive reflexes. Such a child may be able to send a weak neurosignal (myoelectric signal) that will not evoke reflex reactions but will still be recognized by an electronic sensor. Myoelectric switches, therefore, may ultimately offer the best way to achieve control for some individuals, especially for those with particular problems such as severe spasticity (Barreto, Scargle, & Adjouadi, 2000). There would be disadvantages in that only a few such switches could be used, and the switches would have to be directly connected to the child's body. This would cause some inconvenience for the user and would also require that an assistant be available to attach and remove the myoelectric sensors.

Because using switches to control a device requires an overt movement by some part of the body, assessment must take into account the possibility that this movement may cause serious positional problems. How a child is positioned relative to the device is an important factor that should always be addressed. When evaluating children with severe physical impairments, extra care must be taken in determining the proper body positioning and in trying to find the most controllable and appropriate motor movement. There are two reasons for this. First, the child should not become frustrated because the movement is too difficult or too inefficient. Second, the extended use of abnormal reflex patterns or movements may actually lead to or worsen significant physical deformities, such as contractures or scoliosis.

Training and Monitoring

The physicians or therapists who prescribe or recommend electronic assistive devices, or assistive devices in general, must also accept responsibility for seeing that the child receives proper training and monitoring (see Figure 33.2 and Table 33.2). Training is probably the most crucial factor in ensuring that a child with disabilities becomes comfortable with and properly uses any assistive device. Generally, the most appropriate approach to training and monitoring is to utilize the combined expertise of an interdisciplinary team of therapists and specialists.

A few tools and standardized measures are available to assist in the process of evaluating the efficacy and performance of assistive devices (Angelo, Buning, Schmeler, & Doster, 1997; Routhier, Vincent, Desrosiers, & Nadeau, 2003; Smith, 1996). One promising method was recently reported by a group that has developed a "10–step framework" that includes input from parents to help therapists and providers obtain assistive technology for young children (Long, Huang, Woodbridge, Woolverton, & Minkel, 2003). These tools are still in their early developmental phase, but researchers continue to further improve on the specific methods and criteria. The near future is very promising because only through scientific evaluation and monitoring of the users of these devices can it be determined whether a piece of equipment is improving function or other outcomes.

Simulators have been developed for some devices (e.g., simulated electric wheelchair controls), and others may be developed in the near future, that can help with training before the actual devices are ordered (Harrison, Derwent, Enticknap, Rose, & Attree, 2002). Simulation software has been developed to assist with selection of appropriate AAC devices (e.g., from Assistive Technology, Inc. and the Doug Dodgen Co.; see Appendix A). Simulators are especially helpful in evaluating reaction time, speed, and accuracy for the child trying out an expensive electronic-based AAC aid or even an electric wheelchair. Simulators may also reduce the costs to an evaluation center, because it would be unnecessary to have many different types of devices available for training and testing.

Case for Monitoring Using Single-Subject Designs

Notwithstanding the minimal data from controlled studies that have addressed the indications for and effectiveness of assistive devices for children with disabilities, there are methods clinicians can use that will, at the very least, lead to more evidence-based and, hopefully, more appropriate use of assistive devices. The best available method to determine the usefulness of such interventions is the careful implementation of what has been called a *single-subject research design* (Patrick, Mozzoni, & Patrick, 2000; Wolery & Harris, 1982; Zhan & Ottenbacher, 2001). This type of study, also called an "*N* of 1 trial" or "single-patient trial," essentially involves the determination of baseline abilities by an evaluation test or technique, followed by one or more interventions; the effectiveness of each intervention is also determined by the same evaluation test or technique (Larson, 1990). In the best of such studies, the evaluations are done by blinded evaluators; however, this is not critical. What has been very useful are what has been called *multiple baselines*, wherein the interventions are

spaced out by periods of "no intervention." Although multiple-baseline studies may be difficult to implement in a practical sense with children in a vocational, rehabilitation, or school environment, two or more types of interventions could easily be studied across time to determine which treatment or device (e.g., which AAC device) seems to be the most effective. Figure 33.1 includes a "bypass" between the "monitoring and feedback on the use of the device" step and the "selection of device(s)" step to allow for multiple baselines or even to go back and try out a new device if, during the monitoring step, the first device is found to be ineffective or is causing problems.

An essential part of the single-subject research design is the analysis of the results. This usually involves a comparison of the changes in the child's abilities following (or as a result of) the intervention compared with those of the baseline period. If appropriate and feasible, standardized functional assessments such as the WeeFIM should be used (see previous discussions). In the case of a multiple-intervention study, or for a comparison of different devices to determine which is most effective, analyses need to be done to evaluate the changes in the assessment results occurring as a result of the different interventions. An example of this would be a trial of two or three different assistive devices to determine which is the most effective solution to one specific problem. In this sense, with the use of single-subject research designs, the individual serves as his or her own control.

Although some statistical techniques can be used to determine whether a *true* change has occurred using a single-subject research design, all of these techniques are complex and much more complicated to use and interpret than the commonly used *t*-test or correlation coefficient determinations. In addition, depending on what type of functioning is being studied, sometimes standardized measures (e.g., the WeeFIM) are not available or not applicable.

A careful, unbiased, *visual analysis* of the data collected during a single-subject evaluation process, however, can be a very effective way of analyzing the results. In fact, it has been suggested that visual analysis of the data from a study actually can lead to "better interpretation of the clinical significance of the results" (Wolery & Harris, 1982, p. 446). In other words, if the evaluation test results *appear* to be much better after the intervention (e.g., more interactions with peers after acquiring an AAC), then it is very likely that the intervention was truly *clinically* useful (see Figures 33.1 and 33.2). If it can be appropriately constructed, a multiple-baseline study may also be more easily interpreted using visual analysis because such a study would help to control for effects that are only a result of the passage of time, rather than the result of the specific intervention occurring or the device being used. This is especially true for evaluations of children, wherein developmental and maturational changes might make it initially appear that the last device tried during the series was the most successful. In this scenario, one should expect some improvements just because time has passed.

FUNDING ISSUES

The situation regarding funding for assistive devices has been gradually improving, especially recently. Much of this change is due to federal and state legislation in response to intense lobbying from grass roots civil rights and disability advocacy groups. There are still frequent roadblocks to funding, however, and it is unfortunate that often it is easier to obtain funding for a wheelchair than it is for a communication device, even though the latter does more to improve functioning and quality of life for some children with disabilities.

Beginning in the mid-to-late 1970s, an important series of laws were implemented in the United States that directly affected the funding of assistive devices for people with disabilities. The first was Section 504 of the Rehabilitation Act of 1973 (PL 93–112), which prohibited discrimination against people with disabilities and mandated equal opportunities for children with disabilities. The second important law was the Education for All Handicapped Children Act of 1975 (EAHCA, PL 94–142), which requires public education systems to provide a *free appropriate public education* and related services to meet the unique needs of every child

with a disability. This educational service is to be provided in the *least restrictive environment* possible, an environment in which a child with a disability can have access to and interaction with typically developing peers. Section 602 of the law provides for the "use of instructional materials, including telecommunications, sensory and other technical aids and devices," which are intended to help the child with disabilities function more easily in the school environment. The third important law passed during that decade, the Rehabilitation Act Amendments of 1978, guaranteed access (primarily to adults) to any vocational or similar program that received federal funds, even if the person with disabilities would not be expected to eventually be employed.

Another extremely important law was passed in 1988 that, although written to affect mainly adults, also has proved to be quite beneficial to children. The Technology-Related Assistance for Individuals with Disabilities Act of 1988 (the "Tech Act"; PL 100–407) defined assistive technology but, more importantly, provided financial assistance to states to develop projects to improve each state's delivery of assistive technology devices and services. After several revisions to the law (e.g., major amendments in 1998) and with increased funding, by 1998 there were a total of 56 State Assistive Technology Projects Resource Centers (i.e., centers in all states and territories) (Bryant & Seay, 1998).

Although numerous other legal opinions were handed down and some minor changes to several disability laws were made during the 1980s, the more major changes came beginning in the 1990s with the passage of the Americans with Disabilities Act of 1990 (PL 101–336). This significant piece of civil rights legislation set in motion a major paradigm shift in how children and adults in the United States who happen to have disabilities should be seen by every facet of the educational and vocational systems and in nearly every other aspect of living as a person in the United States. Of course, with any law this encompassing, court cases continue to fine-tune what this law actually means and how its provisions should be enforced. Minimal funding is available from this law to support the changes that are sometimes mandated (e.g., changes to a building to allow for accessibility).

Also during the 1990s came the changing of the EAHCA to what it is now known as the Individuals with Disabilities Education Act (IDEA) of 1990 (PL 101–476). Over the years, IDEA and its amendments have led to increased services so that all children who have disabilities, from birth to 21 years, can receive some assistance, including (by specific inclusion in the law) appropriate assistive technology. This important law was last reauthorized in 2004, and although some controversial changes in IDEA were made, the sections related to assistive technology were essentially left intact.

Finally, perhaps the most important piece of legislation in the new millennium related to special education funding is the No Child Left Behind Act (NCLB) of 2001 (PL 107–110). Although written primarily with general education students in mind, this law undoubtedly affects special education students and their use of assistive technology because no group of students is exempted from the requirement within the law for "adequate yearly progress." The NCLB does provide some funding as well as emphasize evidence-based strategies, including strategies that incorporate assistive technology (Browder & Cooper-Duffy, 2003). Much more time and effort will be needed to determine whether the NCLB will turn out to be more of an opportunity than a hindrance to schools, especially regarding special education services and assistive technology.

School Funding

Locating funding for assistive devices and computer software, as well as for even nonadapted microcomputers and software, will continue to be frustrating for many school districts unless funding inequities between schools are somehow resolved. Fortunately, as noted before, there is a provision within EAHCA/IDEA as well as subsequent laws (e.g., the Tech Act) and legal opinions that specifically indicate that funding should be made available for "technological" devices, including software, to help children who have special education needs. Although these statements are part of public law,

which can create tremendous expectations on the part of knowledgeable parents for devices to be provided immediately, difficulties in actually finding funds to provide them will inevitably continue. Cooperative efforts between philanthropic agencies, school systems, and parents in some localities may be the best solution to finding appropriate funding. Parent groups concerned with children with special education needs may be able to effectively lobby for other sources of funding as well as to convince schools of the need for appropriate assistive devices. The last resort, but a laborious and slow one, is to work with lawyers and the court systems. It is quite unfortunate that, even today, in many school districts microcomputers continue to be provided mainly for gifted and talented students, while those with learning difficulties or other disabilities have minimal time to spend with microcomputers or cannot use them because of their disabilities.

Funding by schools for assistive devices is often more of a concern when dealing with devices for children with physical, communicative, or sensory disabilities, rather than with devices for children who have learning disabilities. At the present time, schools are usually willing to purchase microcomputers and software to be used by their students, some of whom have learning disabilities. On occasion, schools have purchased electronic communication aids for children with physical and/or communicative disabilities. Unfortunately, on too many occasions these devices are then kept at the school and are not allowed to be used at home. Specific provisions within the Tech Act and more recent authorizations of IDEA, as well as some subsequent legal opinions, have fortunately reduced this occurrence.

Despite this occasional funding by school systems, there continues to be debate as to whether assistive devices are *medically* or *educationally* necessary. If they could be shown to be medically necessary, it might then be possible to obtain money to pay for these devices from medical insurance companies. If they are truly educationally necessary, then perhaps the school systems should be required to purchase the needed devices. The Tech Act has tried to solve this problem in part by legally allowing Medicaid funding to be used by the schools to purchase assistive devices. The Tech Act further requires that schools allow such devices to be taken home by the children for "educationally related" purposes.

Third-Party Funding

Some devices, especially AAC devices, are gradually being seen as medically necessary in much the same way that a wheelchair can be determined to be a medical necessity. Most private and governmental medical coverage agencies have been willing for years to pay for the purchase of wheelchairs and gradually are beginning to fund assistive devices.

One source of reticence on the part of funding sources is the fact that the benefits from many assistive devices may not be immediate, even though tremendous benefits may occur after months or years of use. Although these benefits may result from actual improvements in physical health, they are more likely to be due to improved mental health, self-esteem, and independence.

As professionals gradually learned more about using these assistive devices, the evaluation and delivery system for such devices have improved greatly, especially over the last decade. These changes have helped funding agencies see that this equipment is *necessary* and that the child has been properly evaluated. What has happened in the past, especially in the absence of proper assessment, training, and monitoring, is that some adapted microcomputer or other assistive device has been purchased with financial assistance from an insurance company or government agency, and afterward the child is unable to use the device or it is found to be totally inappropriate. When this occurs, funding agencies have sometimes become more reluctant to pay for such devices again.

Physicians are often called on to send "medical necessity" letters and prescriptions to funding sources in order to help obtain funding. In most cases, this correspondence should be written only after conferring with several different therapists who have evaluated the child to obtain as much information as possible about his or her current abilities. Complete information, in this sense, does not mean a report of the physical examination findings or treatment, but rather a presentation of the findings that would be of most interest to the funding agency. As one is formulating the correspondence, it might be best to imagine oneself as the reviewer of the funding program and include only information that the reviewer would be specifically looking for, such as the child's current abilities and expected outcome from using the devices. Government agencies, private insurance companies, and charitable organizations all have limited funds, and those requests that clearly outline the specific needs of children whom they have never met are the types of requests best able to assist these agencies in more appropriately allocating the few dollars that they do have.

Patience and perseverance are frequently necessary in order for funding to be secured. Denials of payment are almost automatic by some funding sources. Sometimes a request for an assistive device is denied because the funding agency has never had any experience with such a device; however, denials of funding by most agencies are subject to appeal. The appeal process in these situations should not be taken lightly. The best results occur with a "good case" in which one is able to show that the child can benefit significantly from using the particular device. A failure of an appeal can sometimes make funding for a particular device (or even any device) unlikely, if not impossible, for other children with similar disabilities. Therefore, a successful appeal can be used as an important precedent for future requests. Many assistive devices and their related professional services are relatively new and specialized, and they usually are not included on lists of approved products eligible for funding. Many funding agencies need to be properly, but gently, instructed about the potential of these devices to improve functioning and independence for children with disabilities.

Funding for the purchase and training in the use of these devices is not easy to obtain in these days of frequent budget cuts or lack of expansion. To borrow a phrase from the real estate agencies, *creative financing* is what is needed at present. It is likely that physicians and therapists will need to become increasingly sophisticated to obtain funding for even the simplest low-tech devices. The issues surrounding responsibility for funding are complex and unclear, but several inroads have been made. Literature is becoming available that focuses on the specifics of funding for devices and their long-term cost-effectiveness (Creasey et al., 2000; DePape & Krause, 1980; O'Day & Corcoran, 1994). Unfortunately there is no final answer to the question of who should pay, and funding often requires a good deal of patience and creativity. In some cases, the best and quickest source of funding may be local philanthropic organizations (e.g., United Cerebral Palsy, Easter Seals, various social organizations).

RESEARCH INSIGHTS

Partially because of the relative newness and ever-changing nature of the technology, only limited research has been done on the benefits or detriments of assistive devices used with children with disabilities. This is especially true concerning the long-term use of this equipment by children who have physical disabilities. Until recently, most government, foundation, and corporate funding has generally gone toward the development of the devices, and very little has been used to determine their usefulness or to demonstrate how they have changed the lives of the children using them. Fortunately, in the last decade, such agencies as the National Institute for Disability and Rehabilitation Research have increased funding to support outcomes research (Fuhrer, 2001; Fuhrer, Jutai, Scherer, & Deruyter, 2003). Much of this change no doubt is the result of the recent emphasis on "evidence-based medicine" and similar changes in perspective (Evidenced-Based Medicine Working Group, 1992).

The opportunities for good research to be done, however, seem to be almost limitless. Assistive technology differs greatly from the usual forms of therapy for children with disabilities in that it compensates for or builds on those individual skills that each child already has. As mentioned previously, in the classic *exercise* type of therapy programs for children with disabilities, too much emphasis is often placed on developing skills that the child lost or never had. Changing the focus in treatment, some-

times very slightly, so that the child can *substitute* existing skills, as is often done with assistive devices, may lead to increased motivation, lead to more feelings of success and self-worth, and, hopefully, also improve function in some way (Goldenberg, 1979).

Basic psychological research being done on the ways that people learn, especially as infants and children, may also be affected by increased use of high-tech aids (Figure 33.3). Theorists such as Piaget and those who have followed his beliefs have hypothesized that most, if not all, of early learning is accomplished as the infant and child manipulates objects in his or her environment (Piaget, 1962). Notable among the theories related to this hypothesis are cause and effect, object permanence, and learning through use of objects as tools. More recently, researchers have provided some evidence that problems with intellectual development may occur when children

Physical disability leading to abnormal and atypical sensory and motor learning

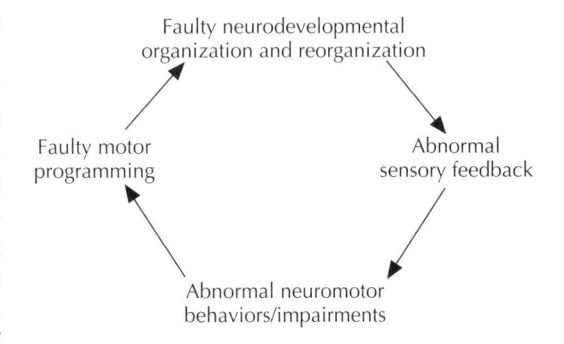

Substitutive manipulation leading to improved learning

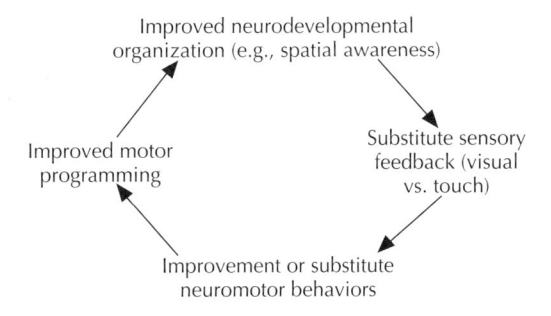

Figure 33.3. Impairments and their relationship to learning and possible improvements using assistive technology.

have limited mobility (Lane & Mistrett, 1996; Missiuna & Pollock, 1991; Perrin & Gerrity, 1984). If severe physical disabilities cause some children to be lacking in how or what they are learning, it should be possible to study what might be achieved by using an electronically controlled "manipulator" such as a robotic arm rather than their own arms and hands. They may also be able to learn through nonphysical representations on a monitor screen controlled by a computer interface (see Figure 33.3). Researchers and clinicians throughout the world are also beginning to evaluate how best to adapt toys for children who have disabilities. Several research projects have determined the positive effects of using adapted toys on intellectual development (Besio, 2002; Brodin, 1999).

Researchers may also be able to study how children with physical disabilities are able to progress through what have been called the emotional/maturational stages for typically developing children. For example, a study could be made of how children with disabilities demonstrate rebelliousness or acting-out behaviors. New technological devices may be found to help these children engage in more constructive outlets or behaviors. Children with severe disabilities, for example, have limited opportunity to fight with their peers or siblings, and the aggressive behaviors that they are capable of performing are somewhat counterproductive (e.g., biting, screaming, refusing to eat). Wheelchairs, especially electric wheelchairs, not only have offered some of these children mobility, but also have been used quite effectively in expressing aggression or anger.

Much uncertainty remains about the earliest age at which a child can successfully use an electronic assistive device, especially communication aids. Some pilot studies, however, have reported successful use of such aids by children younger than 5 years of age. For example, studies of electric wheelchair use demonstrated that children as young as 2 years can be quite successful in their use and reap considerable social benefits as well (Bottos, Bolcati, Sciuto, Ruggeri, & Feliciangeli, 2001; Butler, 1986, 1991). There are also some suggestions, based on limited research, that using wheel-

chairs beginning at a young age can help improve the cognitive abilities of some children who have meningomyelocele (Rendeli et al., 2002), but such an improvement in intelligence quotient (IQ) score was not found with children who have tetraplegia (Bottos et al., 2001). A possible cause for the difference between the results of these two studies may be that the children with tetraplegia, as a group, had a lower preintervention IQ scores compared with children with meningomyelocele.

The use of electronic or computer-based AAC devices may help researchers interested in studying language acquisition and cognitive development, especially in those children who use these devices. There has been at least some minimal evidence from one study that an AAC device will actually help to increase natural speech production in children who have that capacity (Blischak, 1999). In addition, the use of communication aids offers many opportunities for research into the interaction between children with disabilities who do not speak and those who are able to speak. An interesting, but limited, study by Buekelman and Mirenda (1992), for example, documents why the process of selecting and using communication devices for children needs to be studied much further. The results of their research suggested that, if AAC devices were *not* being successfully used by the first grade, the children using AAC devices would not be active participants in the classroom setting. If children were skilled and comfortable with their AAC device, communication between them and typically developing children occurred much more frequently.

Researchers have also begun studying the possible use of microcomputer-based artificial intelligence systems as aids for children who have head injuries or mild or moderate intellectual disabilities to help them with remembering and performing certain tasks. This idea offers seemingly endless opportunities for clinical research in these areas. A practical microcomputer-based cognitive prosthesis is not that far beyond the range of possibilities, and various prototypes are being studied at present (Bergman, 2002; Gorman, Dayle, Hood, & Rumrell, 2003).

ADVOCACY INFORMATION

It is impossible for a general pediatrician, physiatrist, or neurologist, or even a subspecialist in any of these three fields, to be completely knowledgeable about assistive devices. The best approach for these professionals is to serve as informed *advocates*. Families and other caregivers of children with disabilities sometimes may look toward this new high technology as a possible way to work miracles. They will try to find answers to their questions with or without support from health care professionals. Physicians who care for children with disabilities may often have a critical role in this process because caregivers, patients, or allied health professionals may initially come to them requesting their opinion or asking for prescriptions for some of these devices. These physicians should have a unique view of the situation because they are more apt to see the "whole child" in terms of the child's functional and personal skills and needs as well as the family and social environment. In order to provide realistic and appropriate answers, these physicians must keep generally informed about what is being developed and marketed and, more important, what local resources are available that can help provide more information and, hopefully, a proper assessment.

Even for those individuals who will not be actively involved in the selection of assistive technology, it must be noted that there are reasons to expand on the basic advocacy role. Taking active steps to inform children, parents, or others of places where they can find additional assistance, being open-minded about the usefulness of assistive devices, staying informed as much as possible and relaying this new information, and communicating actively with other professionals who are involved with children with disabilities are steps that can be easily taken but will do much to increase the number of children being properly evaluated for use of assistive devices. Keeping an appropriate perspective is important, however. It would be as incorrect to say that all children with severe disabilities should be using high-tech electronic assistive devices as it would to say that no child with severe disabilities should use them. As noted previously, each child's unique capabilities, situations, and interests must be carefully examined, and often low-tech or mid-tech solutions are the ones found to be the most appropriate.

Professionals who deal with children with disabilities are beginning to realize that using a multifaceted approach is probably the best therapeutic methodology available at the present time. Assistive technology is only one facet of treatment, and it may actually be the least important to make long-lasting gains in functional abilities. The ultimate aim of interventions with children with disabilities is to make them more functional and independent during childhood and later as adults. This is not the sole realm of health or education or any other single area; rather, it is a combined role. Any given physician, educator, or therapist cannot be expected to have the necessary skills or to be always up-to-date on what is currently available or the latest research findings.

Fortunately, more readily accessible sources of information have developed that can provide the latest in information about assistive technology. Sources such as regional Technological Assistance Services centers (Tech Act sites) are now available, and information from them is becoming more widely accessible. ABLEDATA, funded by the National Institute for Disability and Rehabilitation Research, is probably the best example of a large database that holds continuously updated information pertinent to many different disabilities. Various organizations and entities dealing with children with disabilities, such as the Council for Exceptional Children and *Exceptional Parent* magazine, have also developed services that can be used to obtain references and abstracts about many facets of disability, especially in regard to school-related services. Increasing numbers of web sites offer resources for people interested in assistive technology, although many of these are thinly disguised advertisements from companies or sites that propose *alternative therapies*; therefore, all web sites should be evaluated critically. The appendix contains a list of selected sources for information retrieval.

CONCLUSION

Although technical barriers to the development of improved assistive devices will always exist, they are continually being broken down by the rapid advances in technology. More important, though, are the financial and societal barriers that prevent the successful distribution and application of this technology. Jobs already exist that depend more on the manipulation of information than on physical manipulation. Many jobs, because they involve using computers, can be performed by people with even the most severe physical disabilities. Such jobs as editing, writing, computer programming, storing or analyzing information on a computer, or being a reference librarian do not depend on speed of output as much as on good judgment and reasoning abilities. Perhaps children who have severe physical disabilities but good cognitive skills can now look forward to a degree of independence in adult life with some possibility for an occupation that both is personally rewarding and allows financial security.

The expanding evolution of high-tech electronics, while it has increased the production of software programs and devices that are available to children with disabilities, has the paradoxical potential of widening the gap between these children and those without disabilities. Opportunities for high-tech professions are increasing, but unless proper provisions are made, children with disabilities will have increasingly *less* chance to compete for these jobs as adults when compared with the population without disabilities.

Perhaps the best way to ensure that vocational opportunities will be there in the future for children with disabilities is for these children to have access to appropriate assistive devices at an early age so that they will be proficient in the use of these devices by the time they are adults. Improved access to these devices has social implications as well. As children with disabilities become better able to use their assistive or communication devices, they likely will be less isolated and will have more contact with the community. It is up to the members of society who do not have disabilities to see that the expenditures and efforts that have been made regarding access will continue. Hopefully, these will also be expanded to include more children, and adults, with disabilities. In the not-too-distant future, with society's assistance, many more people with disabilities will themselves become productive, rather than dependent, members of society.

Undoubtedly, the future will bring many new and useful devices that can assist a child with a disability to be much more functional. In the future, new assistive devices should be used because they have been proved to be useful and not simply because they are high-tech and new. Appropriate use of the entire spectrum of assistive technology devices for children with disabilities is needed and is justifiable.

REFERENCES

Akoumianakis, D., & Stephanidis, C. (1999). Propagating experience-based accessibility guidelines to user interface development. *Ergonomics, 42,* 1283–1311.

Akoumianakis, D., & Stephanidis, C. (2003). Multiple metaphor environments: Designing for diversity. *Ergonomics, 46*(1–3), 88–113.

Americans with Disabilities Act of 1990, PL 101–336, 42 U.S.C. §§ 12101 *et seq.*

Angelo, J. (1998). Low technology interface devices. In S.J. Lane (Ed.), *Assistive technology for the rehabilitation specialist* (pp. 69–98). Philadelphia: F.A. Davis.

Angelo, J., Buning, M.E., Schmeler, M., & Doster, S. (1997). Identifying best practice in the occupational therapy assistive technology evaluation: An analysis of three focus groups. *American Journal of Occupational Therapy, 51,* 916–920.

Baker, B. (1982). MinSpeak. *Byte, 7*(9), 186–202.

Barreto, A.B., Scargle, S.D., & Adjouadi, M. (2000). A practical EMG-based human-computer interface for users with motor disabilities. *Journal of Rehabilitation Research and Development, 37,* 53–63.

Bergman, M.H. (2002). The benefits of a cognitive orthotic in brain injury rehabilitation. *Journal of Head Trauma Rehabilitation, 17,* 431–445.

Besio, S. (2002). An Italian research project to study the play of children with motor disabilities: The first year of activity. *Disability and Rehabilitation, 24,* 72–79.

Blischak, D.M. (1999). Increases in natural speech production following experience with synthetic speech. *Journal of Special Education Technology, 14,* 44–53.

Bottos, M., Bolcati, C., Scuito, L., Ruggeri, C., & Feliciangeli, A. (2001). Powered wheelchairs and independence in young children with tetraplegia. *Developmental Medicine and Child Neurology, 43,* 769–777.

Brodin, J. (1999). Play in children with severe multiple disabilities: Play with toys—a review. *Interna-*

tional Journal of Disability, Development and Education, 46, 25–34.

Browder, D.M., & Cooper-Duffy, K. (2003). Evidence-based practices for students with severe disabilities and the requirement for accountability in "No Child Left Behind". *Journal of Special Education, 37*, 157–163.

Bryant, B.R., & Seay, P.C. (1998). The Technology-Related Assistance to Individuals with Disabilities Act: Relevance to individuals with learning disabilities and their advocates. *Journal of Learning Disabilities, 31*, 4–15.

Buekelman, D.R., & Mirenda, P. (1992). *Augmentative and alternative communication: Management of severe communication disorders in children and adults.* Baltimore: Paul H. Brookes Publishing Co.

Bunch, W.H., & Dvonch V.M. (1994). The "value" of functional independence measure scores. *American Journal of Physical Medicine and Rehabilitation, 73*, 40–43.

Butler, C. (1986). Effects of powered mobility on self-initiated behaviors of very young children with locomotor disability. *Developmental Medicine and Child Neurology, 28*, 325–332.

Butler, C. (1991). Augmentative mobility: Why do it? *Physical Medicine and Rehabilitation Clinics of North America, 25*, 801–815.

Casali, S.P. (1995). A physical skills-based strategy for choosing an appropriate interface method. In A.D.N. Edwards (Ed.), *Extraordinary human computer interaction: Interfaces for people with disabilities* (pp. 315–342). Cambridge, UK: Cambridge University Press.

Cohen, N.L., Roland, J.T. Jr., & Marrinan, N. (2004). Meningitis in cochlear implant recipients: The North American experience. *Otology and Neurotology, 25*, 275–281.

Committee on Children with Disabilities. (1998). Learning disabilities, dyslexia and vision: A subject review. *Pediatrics, 102*, 1217–1219.

Creasey, G.H., Kilgore, K.L., Brown-Triolo, D.L., Dahlberg, J.E., Peckham, P.H., & Keith, M.W. (2000). Reduction of costs of disability using neuroprotheses. *Assistive Technology, 12*, 67–75.

Dattilo, J., & Camarata, S. (1991). Facilitating conversation through self-initiated augmentative communication treatment. *Journal of Applied Behavioral Analysis, 24*(2), 369–378.

Day, H., Jutai, J., & Campbell, K.A. (2002). Development of a scale to measure the psychosocial impact of assistive devices: Lessons learned and the road ahead. *Disability and Rehabilitation, 24*, 31–37.

Day, S.L., & Edwards, B.J. (1996). Assistive technology for postsecondary students with learning disabilities. *Journal of Learning Disabilities, 29*, 486–492.

Demers, L., Monette, M., Lapierre, Y., Arnold, D.L., & Wolfson, C. (2002). Reliability, validity and applicability of the Quebec User Evaluation of Satisfaction with Assistive Technology (QUEST 2.0) for adults with multiple sclerosis. *Disability and Rehabilitation, 24*, 21–30.

Demers, L., Weiss-Lambrou, R., & Ska, B. (1996). Development of the Quebec User Evaluation of Satisfaction with Assistive Technology (QUEST). *Assistive Technology, 8*, 3–13.

Demers, L., Weiss-Lambrou, R., & Ska, B. (2000). *Quebec User Evaluation of Satisfaction with Assistive Technology (QUEST Version 2.0): An outcome measure for assistive technology devices.* Webster, NY: Institute for Matching Person and Technology.

DePape, D.J., & Krause, L.A. (1980). *Guidelines for seeking funding for communication aids.* Madison, WI: Trace Research and Developmental Center.

Desch, L.W. (1986). High technology for handicapped children. *Pediatrics, 77*, 71–85.

Desch, L.W. (2007). Technological assistance. In M.L. Batshaw, L. Pellegrino, & N.J. Roizen (Eds.), *Children with disabilities* (6th ed., pp. 557–569). Baltimore: Paul H. Brookes Publishing Co.

Dodds, T.A., Martin, D.P., Stolov, W.C., & Deyo, R.A. (1993). A validation of the Functional Independence Measure and its performance among rehabilitation inpatients. *American Journal of Physical Medicine and Rehabilitation, 74*, 531–536.

Education for All Handicapped Children Act of 1975, PL 94–142, 20 U.S.C. §§ 1400 *et seq.*

Eleweke, C.J., & Rodda, M. (2000). Factors contributing to parent's selection of a communication mode to use with deaf children. *American Annals of the Deaf, 145*, 375–383.

Evidenced-Based Medicine Working Group. (1992). Evidenced-based medicine: A new approach to teaching the practice of medicine. *JAMA, 268*, 2420–2425.

Flax, M.E., Golembiewski, D.E., & McCaulley, B.L. (1993). *Coping with low vision.* San Diego: Singular Publishing Group.

Fuhrer, M.J. (2001). Assistive technology outcomes research: Challenges met and yet unmet. *American Journal of Physical Medicine and Rehabilitation, 80*, 528–535.

Fuhrer, M.J., Jutai, J.W., Scherer, M.J., & Deruyter, F. (2003). A framework for the conceptual modeling of assistive device outcomes. *Disability and Rehabilitation, 25*, 1243–1251.

Galvin, J.C., & Scherer, M.J. (Eds.). (1996). *Evaluating, selecting and using appropriate assistive technology.* Gaithersburg, MD: Aspen Publishers.

Goldenberg, E.P. (1979). *Special technology for special children* (pp. 30–32). Baltimore: University Park Press.

Gorman, P., Dayle, R., Hood, C.A., & Rumrell, L. (2003). Effectiveness of the ISAAC cognitive prosthetic system for improving rehabilitation outcomes with neurofunctional impairment. *NeuroRehabilitation, 18*, 57–67.

Haley, S.M., Coster, W.J., Ludlow, L.H., Haltiwanger, J.T. & Andrellos, P.J. (1992). *Pediatric Evaluation of Disability Inventory.* Boston: Trustees of Boston University

Harrison, A., Derwent, G., Enticknap, A., Rose, F.D., & Attree, E.A. (2002). The role of virtual reality technology in the assessment and training of inexperienced powered wheelchair users. *Disability and Rehabilitation, 24,* 599–607.

Higgins, K., Boone, R., & Lovitt, T.C. (1996). Hypertext support for remedial students and students with learning disabilities. *Journal of Learning Disabilities, 29,* 402–412.

Individuals with Disabilities Education Act of 1990, PL 101–476, 20 U.S.C. §§ 1400 *et seq.*

Korpela, R., Siirtola, T.O., & Koivikko, M.J. (1992). The cost of assistive devices for children with mobility limitation. *Pediatrics, 90,* 597–602.

Lane, S.J., & Mistrett, S.G. (1996). Play and assistive technology issues for infants and young children with disabilities: A preliminary evaluation. *Focus on Autism and Developmental Disabilities, 11,* 96–105.

Larson, E.B. (1990). *N* of 1 clinical trials: A technique for improving medical therapeutics. *Western Journal of Medicine, 152,* 52–58.

Latash, M.L., & Anson, G. (1996). What are "normal movements" in atypical populations? *Behavioral and Brain Sciences, 19,* 55–106.

Long, T., Huang, L., Woodbridge, M.M., Woolverton, M., & Minkel, J. (2003). Integrating assistive technology into an outcome-driven model of service delivery. *Infants & Young Children: An Interdisciplinary Journal of Special Care Practices, 16,* 272–284.

Mirenda, P. (2001). Autism, augmentative communication, and assistive technology: What do we really know? *Focus on Autism and Other Developmental Disabilities, 16,* 141–151.

Missiuna, C., & Pollock, N. (1991). Play deprivation in children with physical disabilities: The role of the occupational therapist in preventing secondary disability. *American Journal of Occupational Therapy, 45,* 882–888.

No Child Left Behind Act of 2001, PL 107–110, 20 U.S.C. §§ 6301 *et seq.*

O'Day, B.L., & Corcoran, P.J. (1994). Assistive technology: Problems and policy alternatives. *Archives of Physical Medicine and Rehabilitation, 75,* 1165–1169.

Olson, G.M., & Olson, J.S. (2003). Human-computer interaction: psychological aspects of the human use of computing. *Annual Reviews of Psychology, 54,* 491–516

Ottenbacher, K.J., Msall, M.E., Lyon, N.R., Duffy, L.C., Granger, C.V., & Braun, S. (1997). Interrater agreement and stability of the Functional Independence Measure for Children (WeeFim): Use in children with developmental disabilities. *Archives of Physical Medicine and Rehabilitation, 78*(12), 1309–1315.

Patrick, P.D., Mozzoni, M., & Patrick, S.T. (2000). Evidence-based care and the single-subject design. *Infants & Young Children: An Interdisciplinary Journal of Special Care Practices, 13,* 60–74.

Perrin, E.C., & Gerrity, P.S. (1984). Development of children with a chronic illness. *Pediatric Clinics of North America, 31,* 19–31

Phillips, B., & Zhao, H. (1993). Predictors of assistive technology abandonment. *Assistive Technology, 5,* 36–45.

Piaget, J. (1962). *Play, dreams and imitation in childhood.* New York: W.W. Norton.

Platts, R.G., & Fraser, M.H. (1993). Assistive technology in the rehabilitation of patients with high spinal cord lesions. *Paraplegia, 31*(5), 280–287.

Rahman, M.M., & Springle, S. (1997). Physical accessibility guidelines of consumer product controls. *Assistive Technology Journal, 9,* 3–14.

Raskind, M.H., & Higgins, E.L. (1998). Assistive technology for postsecondary students with learning disabilities: An overview. *Journal of Learning Disabilities, 31,* 27–40.

Rehabilitation Act Amendments of 1978, PL 95–602, 29 U.S.C. §§ 701 *et seq.*

Rehabilitation Act of 1973, PL 93–112, 29 U.S.C. §§ 701 *et seq.*

Rendeli, C., Salvaggio, E., Sciascia-Cannizzano, G., Bianchi, E., Caldarelli, M., & Gussetta, F. (2002). Does locomotion improve the cognitive profile of children with meningomyelocele? *Child's Nervous System, 18,* 231–234.

Routhier, F., Vincent, C., Desrosiers, J., & Nadeau, S. (2003). Mobility of wheelchair users: A proposed performance assessment framework. *Disability and Rehabilitation, 25,* 19–35.

Routhier, F., Vincent, C., Morrissette, M.J., & Desaulniers, L. (2001). Clinical results of an investigation of paediatric upper limb myoelectric prosthesis fitting at the Quebec Rehabilitation Institute. *Prosthetics and Orthotics International, 25,* 119–131.

Scherer, M.J. (1998a). The impact of assistive technology on the lives of people with disabilities. In D.B. Gray, L.A. Quatrano, & M.L. Lieberman (Eds.), *Designing and using assistive technology: The human perspective* (pp. 99–115). Baltimore: Paul H. Brookes Publishing Co.

Scherer, M.J. (1998b). *Matching person and technology model and accompanying assessment forms* (3rd ed.). Webster, NY: Institute for Matching Person and Technology.

Shein, F., Lee, K., & Milner, M. (1983). Systematic assessment of key factors to prescribe single-input interface controls. In *Proceedings of the Sixth Annual Conference on Rehabilitation Engineering* (p. 221). San Diego: IEEE Publishing.

Smith, R.O. (1996). Measuring the outcomes of assistive technology: Challenge and innovation. *Assistive Technology, 8,* 71–81.

Stern, R.E., Yueh, B., Lewis, C., Norton, S., & Sie, K.C. (2005). Recent epidemiology of pediatric cochlear implantation in the United States: Disparity among children of different ethnicity and socioeconomic status. *Laryngoscope, 115,* 125–131.

Technology-Related Assistance for Individuals with Disabilities Act of 1988, PL 100–407, 29 U.S.C. §§ 2201 *et seq.*

Udwin, O., & Yule, W. (1991). Augmentative communication systems taught to cerebral-palsied children—a longitudinal study. *British Journal of Disorders of Communication, 26*, 149–162.

U.S. Census Bureau. (2005). *Disability web site.* Retrieved January 15, 2005, from http://www.census.gov/hhes/www/disability/disability.html

Van der Merwe, E., & Alant, E. (2004). Associations with Minspeak icons. *Journal of Communication Disorders, 37(3)*, 255–274.

Vanderheiden, G.C., & Grilley, K. (Eds.). (1976). *Non-verbal communication techniques and aids for the severely physically handicapped.* Baltimore: University Park Press.

Weiss, P.L., Bialik, P., & Kizony, R. (2003). Virtual reality provides leisure time opportunities for young adults with physical and intellectual disabilities. *Cyberpsychology and Behavior, 6(3)*, 335–342.

Wetzel, K. (1996). Speech-recognizing computers: A written-communication tool for students with learning disabilities? *Journal of Learning Disabilities, 29*, 371–380.

Wilson, R., Majsterek, D., & Simmons, D. (1996). The effects of computer-assisted versus teacher-directed instruction on the multiplication performance of elementary students with learning disabilities. *Journal of Learning Disabilities, 29*, 382–390.

Wolery, M., & Harris, S.R. (1982). Interpreting results of single-subject research designs. *Physical Therapy, 62*, 445–452.

World Health Organization. (2001). *International classification of functioning, disability and health.* Geneva: Author.

Zhan, S., & Ottenbacher, K.J. (2001). Single subject research designs for disability research. *Disability and Rehabilitation, 23*, 1–9.

Zrenner, E. (2002). Will retinal implants restore vision? *Science, 295*, 1022–1025.

Zwolan, T.A., Ashbaugh, C.M., Alarfaj, A., Kileny, P.R., Arts, H.A., El-Kashlan, H.K., et al. (2004). Pediatric cochlear implant patient performance as a function of age at implantation. *Otology and Neurotology, 25*, 112–120.

Appendix

SELECTED RESOURCES FOR DEVICES AND SOFTWARE

AbleNet, Inc.
(Switch technology; low-tech and mid-tech AAC devices)
2808 Fairview Avenue
Roseville, MN 55113
800-322-0956
http://www.ablenetinc.com/

Advanced Multimedia Devices, Inc.
(Tech/Talk, Tech/Speak, and Tech/Touch AAC devices)
200 Frank Road
Hicksville, NY 11801
888-353-2634
http://www.amdi.net/

Apple Computers Accessibility
1 Infinite Loop
Cupertino, CA 95014
408-996-1010
http://www.apple.com/accessibility/

Assistive Technology, Inc.
(EvaluWare simulation for AAC; Link software; mini AAC that uses Apple ibook)
333 Elm Street
Dedham, MA 02026
800-793-9227
http://www.assistivetech.com/

Attainment Company, Inc.
(GoTalk mid-tech layered AAC device)
Post Office Box 930160
Verona, WI 53593
800-327-4269
http://www.attainmentcompany.com/

Augmentative Communication, Inc.
(Videos, books, and journals on AAC)
One Surf Way, #237
Monterey, CA 93940
831-649-3050
http://www.augcominc.com

Compex Technologies Inc.
(Functional electrical stimulation equipment)
1811 Old Highway 8
New Brighton, MN 55112
800-676-6489
http://www.compextechnologies.com/

Crestwood Communication Aids, Inc.
(Low- and mid-tech AAC aids; switch technology)
6625 N. Sidney Place
Milwaukee, WI 53209-3259
414-352-5678
http://www.communicationaids.com/

Don Johnston Developmental Equipment, Inc.
(Switch technology; adaptive keyboards; products for learning disabilities)
26799 West Commerce Drive
Volo, IL 60073
800-999-4660
http://www.donjohnston.com/

Doug Dodgen & Associates
(AAC Feature Match software; ActiveVoices simulator for AAC)
Post Office Box 173302
Arlington, TX 76003
817-572-6023
http://www.dougdodgen.com/

DynaVox Technologies (previously Sentient Systems Technologies)
(DynaVox and Dynamo dynamic display AAC devices)
2100 Wharton Street, Suite 400
Pittsburgh, PA 15203
800-396-2869
http://www.dynavoxtech.com/

Edmark software, *see* Riverdeep

EKEG Electronics Co. Ltd.
(Activity board, expanded keyboards)

26277 62nd Avenue
Aldergrove, BC V4W 1L8
Canada
604-857-0828
http://www.ekegelectronics.com/

EMPI
(Functional electrical stimulation; dynamic splinting)
599 Cardigan Road
St. Paul, MN 55126
800-328-2536
http://www.empi.com/

EnableMart
(All types of assistive technology)
4210 E. 4th Plain Boulevard
Vancouver, WA 98661
888-640-1999
http://www.enablemart.com/

Enabling Devices
(Seven-level Communication Builder AAC device with inputs for switches; adapted toys; independent living aids)
385 Warburton Avenue
Hastings-on-Hudson, NY 10706
800-832-8697
http://enablingdevices.com/

Frame Technologies, Inc.
(MicroVoice AAC with automatic leveling)
W677 Pearl Street
Oneida, WI 54155
920-869-2979
http://www.frame-tech.com/

George Adams Consulting
(Needs First selection software; yearly updates on AAC devices)
49 Overlook Road
Poughkeepsie, NY 12603
845-452-1850

IBM Human Ability and Accessibility Center
11400 Burnet Road

Austin, TX 78758
http://www-306.ibm.com/able/

IntelliTools
(IntelliKeys hardware, software for learning problems)
1720 Corporate Circle
Petaluma, CA 94954
800-899-6687
http://www.intellitools.com/

Mayer-Johnson LLC
(Board Maker software)
Post Office Box 1579
Solana Beach, CA 92075-1579
800-588-4548
http://www.mayer-johnson.com/

Microsoft Accessibility—Technology for Everyone
(Free newsletter and downloads)
http://www.microsoft.com/enable/

National Lekotek Center (sites throughout United States)
(Adapted toys and computers for children—some can be borrowed)
3204 W. Armitage Avenue
Chicago, IL 60647
773-276-5164
http://www.lekotek.org/

Nuance Corporation
(Dragon Naturally Speaking and related products)
1 Wayside Road
Burlington, MA 01803
781-565-5000
http://www.nuance.com

Optelec, Tieman Group
(Alva Satellite refreshable Braille devices)

3030 Enterprise Court, Suite C
Vista, CA 92081
800-826-4200
http://www.optelec.com/

Prentke Romich Company
(Pathfinder with dynamic display and MinSpeak AAC devices; switch technology)
1022 Heyl Road
Wooster, OH 44691
800-262-1984
http://www.prentrom.com/

J.A. Preston Corporation
(Adaptive furniture, walkers, positioning aids, and balls for infants and toddlers with motor dysfunctions)
60 Page Road
Clifton, NJ 07012
800-631-7277

Rehabilicare, see Compex Technologies

Riverdeep, Inc. (also in Ireland and England)
(TouchWindow hardware, Edmark House Series software for learning problems)
100 Pine Street, Suite 1900
San Francisco, CA 94111
415-659-2000
http://www.riverdeep.net/

Saltillo Corp.
(ChatBox AAC device with auditory scanning and MinSpeak; Chat PC-II adapted pocket PC with Mayer-Johnson PCS symbols)
2143 Township Road #112
Millersburg, OH 44654

800-382-8622
http://www.saltillo.com

Technical Aids and Systems for the Handicapped (TASH), Inc.
(Switch technology; environmental controls))
3512 Maryland Court
Richmond, VA 23233
800-463-5685
http://www.tashinc.com/

Toby Churchill Ltd.
(LightWRITER AAC device)
20 Panton Street
Cambridge CB2 1HP UK
44 (0) 1223 576117

Toys for Special Children, see Enabling Devices

Trace Research & Development Center
University of Wisconsin–Madison
2107 Engineering Centers Bldg.
1550 Engineering Drive
Madison, WI 53706
608-263-6966
http://trace.wisc.edu/

UltraFlex Systems, Inc.
(Dynamic bracing and orthoses)
237 South Street, Suite 200
Pottstown, PA 19464
800-220-6670
http://www.ultraflexsystems.com/

ZYGO Industries, Inc.
(Dialect dynamic display and other AAC devices; switch technology; environmental controls)
Post Office Box 1008
Portland, OR 97207
800-234-6006
http://www.zygo-usa.com/

ORGANIZATIONS AND RESOURCES WITH INFORMATION ABOUT ASSISTIVE TECHNOLOGY

Selected General Disability Organizations and Resources

ABLEDATA
(Large computerized databases of assistive technology and links to state Assistive Technology Projects Centers "Tech Act centers")
National Rehabilitation Information Center
8630 Fenton Street, Suite 930
Silver Spring, MD 20910
800-227-0216
http://www.abledata.com/

ACRES—American Council on Rural Special Education
2323 Anderson Avenue, Suite 226
Manhattan, KS 66502
785-532-2737
http://www.ksu.edu/acres/

Administration on Developmental Disabilities
HHH 405-D
370 L'Enfant Promenade, S.W.
Washington, DC 20447
202-690-6590
http://www.acf.dhhs.gov/programs/add/

American Association for People with Disabilities
1819 H Street, N.W., Suite 330
Washington, DC 20006
800-840-8844
http://www.aapd-dc.org/

Association of University Centers on Disabilities
1010 Wayne Avenue, Suite 920
Silver Spring, MD 20910

301-588-8252
http://www.aucd.org/

Clearinghouse on Disability Information
Office of Special Education and Rehabilitation Services
Room 3132, Switzer Building
330 C Street, N.W.
Washington, DC 20202
202-205-8241
http://www.ed.gov/offices/OSERS/

Closing the Gap
(Publications, database, conferences)
526 Main Street
Post Office Box 68
Henderson, MN 56044
507-248-3294
http://www.closingthegap.com/

Consortium for Children and Youth with Disabilities
(A National Rehabilitation Research and Training center)
3307 M Street, N.W., Suite 401
Washington, DC 20007
202-687-8617
http://www.consortiumnrrtc.org/

Council for Exceptional Children
(Publications, conferences, information services)
1110 N. Glebe Road, Suite 300
Arlington, VA 22201
800-328-0272
http://www.cec.sped.org/

Exceptional Parent Magazine
(Publication and annual resource guide)
EP Global Communications
551 Main Street
Johnstown, PA 15901
877-372-7368
http://www.eparent.com/

Family Center on Technology and Disability
Academy for Educational Development (AED)
1825 Connecticut Avenue, N.W.
7th Floor

Washington, DC 20009
202-884-8064
http://www.fctd.info/

National Center for Technology Innovation
(Yellow Pages search and printed materials)
http://www.nationaltechcenter.org/

National Center to Improve Practice (Special Education)
Education Development Center, Inc.
(Message board, printed materials and newsletter)
55 Chapel Drive
Newton, MA 02158
http://www2.edu.org/NCIP/

National Organization on Disability
910 Sixteenth Street, N.W., Suite 600
Washington, DC 20006
202-293-5960
http://www.nod.org/

National Rehabilitation Information Center
(REHABDATA database, publications)
1010 Wayne Avenue, Suite 800

Silver Spring, MD 20910
800-346-2742
http://www.naric.com/

Trace Research & Development Center
(Research and publications)
University of Wisconsin–Madison
2107 Engineering Centers Building
1550 Engineering Drive
Madison, WI 53706
608-263-6966
http://trace.wisc.edu/

Technical Resource Centre
(Information about adapted toys, microcomputer aids)
1349 County Home Road
Waterville, Nova Scotia B0P 1V0
Canada
902-538-3103
http://www.ncset.org/trc/

ERIC—Education Research Information Center
(Large federal computer database dealing with special education)
c/o Computer Science Corp.
4483-A Forbes Boulevard
Lanham, MD 20706
800-538-3742
http://www.eric.ed.gov/

Selected Organizations for Physical Disabilities

Functional Electrical Stimulation Information Center
http://feswww.fes.cwru.edu/

International Functional Electrical Stimulation Society, Inc.
25129 Rye Canyon Loop
Valencia, CA 91355
http://www.ifess.org/

United Cerebral Palsy Organizations
(One-Stop resource guide for all states, publications)
1600 L Street, N.W., Suite 700
Washington, DC 20036

800-872-5872
http://www.ucpa.org/

National Easter Seal Society
(Publication)
230 W. Monroe Street, Suite 1800
Chicago, IL 60606
800-221-6827
http://www.easter-seals.org/

National Lekotek Center (sites throughout United States)
(Adapted toys and computers for children—some can be borrowed)
3204 W. Armitage Avenue
Chicago, IL 60647

773-276-5164
http://www.lekotek.org/

American Spinal Injury Association
345 East Superior Street
Room 1436
Chicago, IL 60611
http://www.asia-spinalinjury.org/

Spina Bifida Association of America
4590 MacArthur Boulevard,
Suite 250
Washington, DC 20007
800-621-3141
http://www.sbaa.org/

Selected Organizations for Hearing and/or Visual Impairments

American Council of the Blind
1155 15th Street, N.W., Suite 1004
Washington, DC 20005
800-424-8666
http://acb.org/

American Foundation for the Blind
11 Penn Plaza, Suite 300
New York, NY 10001
800-232-5463
http://www.afb.org/

Bookshare
(Subscription service to ebooks in digital Braille, etc.)

480 California Avenue, Suite 201
Palo Alto, CA 94306
http://www.bookshare.org/

Canadian National Institute for the Blind
1929 Bayview Avenue
Toronto, ON M4G 4C8
Canada
416-480-2500
http://www.cnib.ca/

Helen Keller National Center for Deaf-Blind Youths and Adults
141 Middle Neck Road

Sands Point, NY 11050
516-944-8900
http://www.helenkeller.org/

Lighthouse International
(International vision services and advocacy)
111 East 5th Street
New York, NY 10022
http://www.lighthouse.org/

National Deaf Education Center
Gallaudet University
800 Florida Avenue, N.E.
Washington, DC 20002

202-651-5855
http://clerccenter.gallaudet.edu/

National Institute on Deafness and Other Communication Disorders
1 Communication Avenue

Bethesda, MD 20892
800-241-1044
http://www.nih.gov/nidcd/

Royal National Institute for the Blind

224 Great Portland Street
London, W1N 6AA
United Kingdom
(0171) 388-1266
http://www.rnib.org.uk/

Selected Organizations for Learning and Cognitive Disabilities

ACRES—American Council on Rural Special Education
2323 Anderson Avenue, Suite 226
Manhattan, KS 66502
785-532-2737
http://www.ksu.edu/acres/

American Association on Mental Retardation
44 N. Capitol Street, N.W., Suite 846
Washington, DC 20011
800-242-3680
http://www.aamr.org/

CHADD—Children and Adults with ADHD
8181 Professional Place, Suite 201
Landover, MD 20785
301-306-7070
http://www.chadd.org/

International Dyslexia Society
(Formally the Orton Dyslexia Society)
Chester Building, Suite 382
8600 LaSalle Road
Baltimore, MD 21286-2044
800-ABC-D123
http://www.interdys.org/

Learning Disabilities Association of America (LDA)
4156 Library Road
Pittsburgh, PA 15234
412-341-1515
http://www.ldanatl.org/

Learning Disabilities Association of Canada
323 Chapel Street
Ottawa, ON K1N 7Z2

Canada
613-238-5721
http://www.ldac-taac.ca/

National Center for Learning Disabilities, Inc.
381 Park Avenue South
Suite 1401
New York, NY 10016
888-575-7373
http://www.ncld.org/

National Resource Center for Traumatic Brain Injury
Post Office Box 980542
Richmond, VA 23908
804-828-9055
http://neuro.pmr.vcu.edu/

Selected Organizations and Resources for Communication Disabilities and Autism

American Speech, Language and Hearing Association (ASHA)
10801 Rockville Pike
Rockville, MD 20852
800-638-8255
http://www.asha.org/

Augmentative and Alternative Communication Centers
University of Nebraska–Lincoln
Departmet of Special Education and Communication Disorders
318R Barkley Memorial Center
Post Office Box 830738

Lincoln, NE 68583
402-472-9867
http://aac.unl.edu/

Autism Society of America
7910 Woodmont Avenue, Suite 650
Bethesda, MD 20814
800-3-AUTISM
http://www.autism-society.org/

National Institute on Deafness and Other Communication Disorders
31 Center Drive
MSC 2320

Bethesda, MD 20892
800-241-1044
http://www.nih.gov/nidcd/

Rehabilitation Engineering Research Center on Communication Enhancement
Division of Speech Pathology and Audiology
Duke University
DUMC 3888
Durham, NC 27770
919-681-9983
http://www.aac-rerc.com/

Selected Resources for Funding Information

Association for Blind Citizens Technology Fund
http://www.assocofblindcitizens.org/assistive.html

Disabled Children's Relief Fund
Post Office Box 7420
Freeport, NY 111520
http://www.dcrf.com/

Electronic Data Systems, Inc.
Technology Grants
http://www.eds.com/about/community/grants/

Equal Access to Software and Information

(Provider of information and training for "over 3 dozen countries" on accessible information technology including the e-journal Information Technology and Disabilities)
http://www.easi.cc/cd.htm

Hear Now
(Funding for hearing aids and cochlear implants)
9745 E. Hampden Avenue,
Suite 300
Denver, CO 80231
800-648-HEAR

TechGrants program
http://www.techfoundation.org/

Technology Grants for Schools
(Subscription service for grants newsletter)
http://www.technologygrantnews.com/

U.S. Department of Education
(E-grants searchable database)
http://e-grants.ed.gov/egWelcome.asp/
http://www.edu.gov/fund/landing.jhtml/

34

Nonstandard Therapies in Developmental Disabilities

THOMAS D. CHALLMAN,
ROBERT G. VOIGT, AND SCOTT M. MYERS

There is no alternative physics.
—Gunnar Stickler, M.D.

Neurodevelopmental disorders are chronic, often serious conditions for which curative treatments are not available. In many areas of health care in which treatment approaches are not dramatically effective, the use of therapies that fall outside the boundary of conventional medicine is common. Issues surrounding nonstandard therapies have affected the field of neurodevelopmental disabilities in a significant way.

Parents and caregivers of children with developmental disabilities will understandably pursue therapeutic interventions that they feel may present some hope of helping their children. Unfortunately, families are often exposed to unsubstantiated, pseudoscientific theories and practices that are at best ineffective and at worst can lead to physical, emotional, or financial harm. Time and effort wasted on ineffective therapies create an additional burden on already overwhelmed families. Parents may have considerable difficulty distinguishing between pseudoscientific interventions and validated treatment approaches. These problems have been compounded by the explosion in information technology and the propensity of questionable theories and practices to disseminate rapidly. It has become increasingly important for health care practitioners to recognize that their patients often use nonstandard therapies and that it is essential to have a framework through which these therapies can be critically analyzed.

The boundary between therapies considered conventional and those viewed as nonstandard can be poorly delineated. The possibility exists that a therapy initially deemed complementary or alternative may develop a sufficient evidence base that supports its use in the treatment of a particular disorder. In order for medical progress to continue, however, all hypotheses must be subject to the same level of scrutiny, and all proposed therapies for a disorder must be held to high standards of evidence prior to being accepted as worthwhile. Recent history has shown that in some cases rational medical investigation has been turned on its head, with scarce resources being expended out of necessity to prove the ineffectiveness of an intervention whose use has already become widespread. The main goals of this chapter are to review the most common categories of nonstandard therapies, to examine data on the use of these interventions in children with developmental disabilities, and to outline important issues practitioners must consider in analyzing nonstandard therapies in order to provide advice of high scientific quality to families.

DEFINITIONS

An unambiguous definition of what constitutes a "nonstandard" therapy is difficult to formulate; in this chapter, the terms *nonstandard therapy* and *complementary and alternative medicine* (CAM) are used interchangeably. There is no agreed-on set of methods or therapies that are considered "complementary" or "alternative." A variety of definitions of CAM have been used in the medical literature, including "interventions not taught widely in medical schools or generally available at U.S. hospitals" (Eisenberg et al., 1993, p. 246); "diagnosis, treatment and/or prevention which complements mainstream medicine by contributing to a common whole, by satisfying a demand not met by orthodoxy or by diversifying conceptual frameworks of medicine" (Ernst et al., 1995, p. 506); and "practices that are not accepted as correct, proper, or appropriate or are not in conformity with the beliefs and standards of the dominant group of medical practitioners in a society" (Gevitz, 1988, p. 1). The definition of CAM adopted by the Cochrane Collaboration is

> A broad domain of healing resources that encompasses all health systems, modalities, and practices and their accompanying theories and beliefs, other than those intrinsic to the politically dominant health systems of a particular society or culture in a given historical period. (Zollman & Vickers, 1999, p. 693).

One widely used definition categorizes CAM as practices that are "not presently considered an integral part of conventional medicine" (National Center for Complementary and Alternative Medicine [NCCAM], 2000, p. 10).

Not surprisingly, most definitions of CAM are inherently vague and require some interpretation as to which specific practices should be considered "nonstandard." There is an assumption that, when unproven practices acquire enough evidence of effectiveness, they will migrate into the realm of conventional medicine. The situation is further confounded by the fact that some practices presented as CAM are more appropriately viewed in the context of faith, spirituality, or cultural beliefs and may not be suited to categorization under the rubric of science or medicine (Figure 34.1). NCCAM has proposed a classification scheme for CAM therapies in an effort to provide some organization to the field, dividing CAM practices into four domains: mind–body medicine, manipulative and body-based practices, energy medicine, and biologically based practices. A fifth domain comprises alternative medical sys-

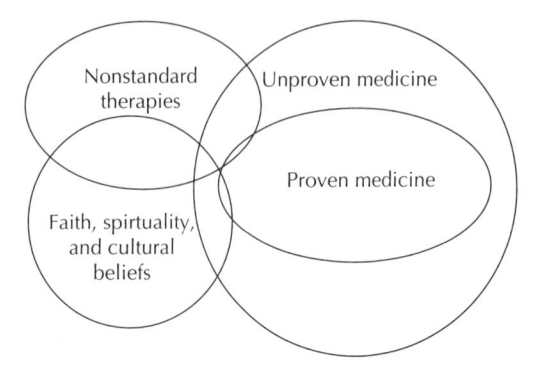

Figure 34.1. One view of the relationship between nonstandard therapies, medicine, and spirituality.

tems that may utilize therapies derived from any of the other four domains (Table 34.1). Regardless of whether one believes that there is any value in these interventions, this classification can be used as a framework through which nonstandard therapies can be examined.

Table 34.1. National Center for Complementary and Alternative Medicine classification of complementary and alternative practices, with examples

Alternative medical systems
Homeopathy
Naturopathy
Traditional Chinese medicine
Ayurvedic medicine

Mind–body medicine
Meditation
Biofeedback
Prayer
Hypnosis
Yoga

Manipulative and body-based practices
Chiropractic
Massage
Reflexology

Energy medicine
Therapeutic touch
Qi gong
Reiki
Magnet therapy
Acupuncture

Biologically based practices
Herbs
Diets
Vitamins and other supplements

Source: http://nccam.nih.gov/health/whatiscam/

PREVALENCE AND COST OF NONSTANDARD THERAPIES

Studies investigating the frequency of use of nonstandard therapies have been limited by ascertainment bias and significant variations in the definition of what constitutes CAM. The first national survey to determine patterns of use of unconventional medical therapies showed that the use of these practices among adults in the United States is common (Eisenberg et al., 1993). Approximately one third of the respondents reported using at least one unconventional therapy during the previous year; 10% saw a practitioner who provided nonstandard therapies. These therapies were used for a variety of chronic conditions, including back problems, anxiety, headaches, chronic pain, and cancer. A majority of patients did not inform their regular medical doctors about their use of these interventions.

The 1999 National Health Interview Survey (NHIS) estimated that 28.9% of U.S. adults used at least one CAM therapy in the previous year, with the most commonly used therapies consisting of spiritual healing or prayer, herbal medicine, and chiropractic (Ni, Simile, & Hardy, 2002). When prayer is included in the definition of CAM therapies, estimates of the use of these therapies is usually quite high—62% of respondents in the 2002 NHIS reported that they had used some form of CAM therapy in the previous 12 months (Barnes, Powell-Griner, McFann, & Nahin, 2004). Other studies have demonstrated both short-term and long-term temporal increases in the use of a variety of nonstandard therapies in the United States (Eisenberg et al., 1998; Kessler et al., 2001; Tindle, Davis, Phillips, & Eisenberg, 2005). The use of nonstandard therapies is particularly widespread in Europe (Schneider, Hanisch, & Weiser, 2004; Thomas, Nicholl, & Coleman, 2001).

Among pediatric populations, considerable variation in estimates of nonstandard therapy use has been reported, likely as a result of the same ascertainment bias, variations in definitions, and geographic or cultural factors also observed in adult studies (Ernst, 1999). In selected general pediatric outpatient and inpa-tient populations, estimates of prior or current CAM use have ranged from 11% to 53% (Fong & Fong, 2002; Madsen et al., 2003; Ottolini et al., 2001; Sawni-Sikand, Schubiner, & Thomas, 2002; Sibinga, Ottolini, Duggan, & Wilson, 2004; Simpson & Roman, 2001; Spigelblatt, Laine-Ammara, Pless, & Guyver, 1994; Wilson & Klein, 2002). More recent analysis of population-based data (from the 1996 Medical Expenditure Panel Survey) showed significantly lower use of CAM (1.8%–2.0%) among U.S. children and young adults (Davis & Darden, 2003; Yussman, Ryan, Auinger, & Weitzman, 2004). In children with various chronic medical conditions, however, the use of nonstandard therapies appears to be common (Feldman et al., 2004; Friedman et al., 1997; Johnston, Bilbao, & Graham-Brown, 2003; Junker, Oberwittler, Jackson, & Berger, 2004; Kelly, 2004; Markowitz et al., 2004; Orhan et al., 2003).

Among children with neurodevelopmental disabilities, similar high rates of nonstandard therapy use have been observed. In recently diagnosed children with autism, the prevalence of CAM use has been estimated to be 30% (Levy, Mandell, Merhar, Ittenbach, & Pinto-Martin, 2003). A substantial minority of these children were using therapies that could be harmful. Children with attention-deficit/hyperactivity disorder (ADHD) also appear to utilize nonstandard therapies, including nutritional supplements, special diets, herbal remedies, and biofeedback, at increased rates (Bussing, Zima, Gary, & Garvan, 2002; Gross-Tsur, Lahad, & Shalev, 2003; Miller, Brehaut, Raina, McGrail, & Armstrong, 2004; Sinha & Efron, 2005). Down syndrome, cerebral palsy, and spina bifida are additional conditions for which CAM use may be increased (Hurvitz, Leonard, Ayyangar, & Nelson, 2003; Prussing, Sobo, Walker, Dennis, & Kurtin, 2004; Sanders et al., 2003).

A variety of factors are associated with an increased likelihood of nonstandard therapy use in adults and children. Adults who utilize CAM are not necessarily dissatisfied with conventional medicine; rather, they may view these therapies as being more congruent with their specific values and underlying life philosophies (Astin, 1998; Eisenberg et al., 2001). Among pediatric users of nonstandard therapies, higher levels of parental education and increased parental rates of CAM use have been consistently observed (Bellas, Lafferty, Lind, & Tyree, 2005; Davis, Meaney, & Duncan, 2004; Fong & Fong, 2002; Ottolini et al., 2001; Sawni-Sikand et al., 2002; Spigelblatt et al., 1994; Yussman et al., 2004).

Annual out-of-pocket expenditures for CAM services in the U.S. population were conservatively estimated to be greater than $10 billion in 1990 (Eisenberg et al., 1993); by 1997, this had increased to $27 billion (Eisenberg et al., 1998). Although CAM services are often not covered by insurance, an overall increase in insurance coverage for these therapies has been observed, driven primarily by market and political forces (Lundgren & Ugalde, 2004). This should not be taken as evidence of scientific value; rather, the embracing of CAM by health plans should be properly recognized as a marketing tool designed to increase subscriber enrollment. Also as a result of strong political pressures, in October 1991 the U.S. Congress passed legislation creating the Office of Alternative Medicine (OAM)—whose primary mission was to evaluate alternative medicine practices—within the National Institutes of Health. OAM was elevated to the status of a National Institutes of Health Center in 1999 with the formation of the NCCAM. Funding for these entities has increased dramatically since the creation of OAM, from an initial OAM budget of $2 million to the 2005 fiscal year NCCAM appropriation of more than $120 million.

The stated mission of NCCAM encompasses research, training, and public education priorities, with particular emphasis on utilizing rigorous research methodologies to evaluate specific CAM practices. The rise in federal funding to study nonstandard therapies has been accompanied by a significant increase in the number of academic medical centers with research programs in CAM (NCCAM, 2004). Although some may view these academic affiliations as lending a certain amount of superficial credibility to nonstandard practices, strong consideration must also be given to the notion that the increased availability of federal funding, and not scientific merit, has created the interest in CAM among academic institutions. In the first 5 years of the existence of NCCAM, some progress has been made toward creating an infrastructure for higher-quality research into CAM practices, although clinically relevant results (proving or disproving the value of specific interventions) have thus far been quite limited (Atwood, 2003). Despite the fact that nonstandard therapies are commonly used in children, NCCAM has funded few studies assessing safety or efficacy of these interventions in children, and even fewer studies specific to children with disabilities (NCCAM, 2005).

NONSTANDARD THERAPY USE IN CHILDREN WITH DEVELOPMENTAL DISABILITIES

Evidence of effectiveness is extremely sparse for most of the therapies that fall under the NCAAM definition of *complementary and alternative medicine*. Certain herbal preparations do appear to confer some benefit in the treatment of specific conditions. Acupuncture may be effective in modulating certain pain syndromes, although there is evidence to suggest that this is a nonspecific effect of needling and not related to the proposed hypothetical framework of meridians and energy flow (Linde et al., 2005). Most clinical trials evaluating the effectiveness nonstandard therapies have been of very poor quality. Conclusions derived from the Cochrane Database of Systematic Reviews for various therapies (used in any medical condition) are summarized in Table 34.2.

In the field of developmental disabilities, evidence of effectiveness for any of these methods is even weaker or nonexistent. Table 34.3 presents the numbers of controlled clinical trials of various nonstandard therapies in developmental disabilities from the Cochrane Central Register of Controlled Clinical Trials. Although this is not a comprehensive listing, it does reveal the significant knowledge gaps that are present. Currently, there is no widely accepted role for virtually any of the therapies

Table 34.2. Reviews of selected nonstandard therapies (for any medical condition) in the Cochrane Database of Systematic Reviews

Therapy	Number of reviews	Review conclusions		
		Beneficial	Possibly beneficial	Ineffective or indeterminate
Alternative medical systems				
Acupuncture	14	2	2	10
Homeopathy	4	0	0	4
Mind–body medicine				
Biofeedback	6	1	1	4
Hypnosis	1	0	0	1
Meditation	1	0	0	1
Intercessory prayer	1	0	0	1
Manipulative and body-based practices				
Chiropractic	3	0	0	3
Massage	4	0	1	3
Energy medicine				
Therapeutic touch	1	0	0	1
Biologically based practices				
Herbal remedies	14	1	3	10
Vitamins for cognitive disorders	5	0	0	5

Note: Based on searches of the database (http://www.cochrane.org/).

considered nonstandard or complementary and alternative in the treatment of any developmental disorder.

Alternative Medical Systems

Alternative medical systems are defined as entire systems of theory and practice that developed separately from conventional medicine. Examples of alternative medical systems include traditional Chinese medicine, Ayurvedic medicine, homeopathy, and naturopathy. These systems generally incorporate a variety of the unconventional methods discussed further later in this section (e.g., manipulative practices, herbal remedies).

Traditional Chinese medicine relies heavily on the use of *energy*-based practices such as acupuncture or Qi gong, with the belief that the uninterrupted flow of energy through 20 meridians is necessary for health to be maintained (a view of health and disease that lacks empirical supporting evidence, despite the fact that these therapies have been used for centuries). As with most nonstandard therapies, the quality of clinical trials per-

formed to evaluate traditional Chinese medicine has been extremely poor (Tang, Zhan, & Ernst, 1999). There have been some studies of traditional Chinese medicine in the treatment of various developmental disabilities, including cerebral palsy, intellectual disabilities, and ADHD (Lai, Feng, Jin, & Zhang, 1999; Liu, Song, & Du, 1994; Lu, 1994; Sun, Ko, Wong, & Sun, 2004; Sun et al., 1994; Tian, Yuan, Ba, Chen, & Zhou, 1995; Zhang & Huang, 1990; Zhou & Zheng, 2005). Significant methodological shortcomings and biases in these studies prevent any interpretation of whether such methods are truly beneficial in these conditions.

Ayurvedic medicine, which originated on the Indian subcontinent, is based on Hindu philosophy utilizing dietary or herbal remedies and various mind–body therapies. There are no controlled trials indicating any benefit of any Ayurvedic practice in the treatment of any developmental disability. Likewise, although attempts have been made to study homeopathic interventions in ADHD and traumatic brain injury, there is no replicated experimental evidence showing these methods to be effective in treating any medical condition

Table 34.3. Trials of selected nonstandard therapies in developmental disabilities from the Cochrane Central Register of Controlled Trials

Therapy	Number of trials	Summary clinical recommendation for use of the therapy[a]
Alternative medical systems		
Homeopathy	1	No
Mind–body medicine		
Biofeedback, EEG/EMG biofeedback	21	Indeterminate
Meditation, relaxation techniques (excluding massage)	14	Indeterminate
Hypnosis	1	No
Music therapy	4	Indeterminate
Art therapy	0	No
Spiritual therapies	0	No
Manipulative and body-based practices		
Chiropractic	0	No
Massage	4	Indeterminate
Sensory integration therapy	6	Indeterminate
Auditory integration therapy	4	No
Vestibular stimulation	5	No
Vision therapy, visual perceptual training	1	No
Reflexology, neuroflexology	0	No
Craniosacral therapy	0	No
Patterning, Doman-Delacato method	3	No
Energy medicine		
Acupuncture	11	No
Therapeutic touch	0	No
Magnet therapy	0	No
Reiki, Qi gong	0	No
Biologically based practices		
Melatonin	4	Yes[b]
Pharmacological doses of vitamins and other supplements	32	No[c]
Oligoantigenic diets in ADHD	6	Indeterminate
Gluten-free, casein-free diet in autism	2	No
Herbal remedies	9	No
Chelation therapy	0	No
Secretin in autism	17	No
Hyperbaric oxygen	3	No
Antifungal agents	0	No

Note: Based on searches of the database (http://www.cochrane.org/). Search terms used were as follows: *developmental disabilities, autistic disorder, autism, pervasive developmental disorder, attention deficit disorder with hyperactivity, ADHD, learning disorders, mental retardation,* and *cerebral palsy.*

[a]Conclusion (yes, no, indeterminate) based on all available evidence: number and quality of clinical trials, replication, effect size, and potential adverse effects.

[b]Treatment of prolonged sleep latency.

[c]Excluding treatment of known metabolic disorders.

Key: ADHD, attention-deficit/hyperactivity disorder; EEG, electroencephalographic; EMG, electromyographic.

(Chapman, Weintraub, Milburn, Pirozzi, & Woo, 1999; Frei & Thurneysen, 2001). *Homeopathy* (which is based on the dubious theory that "like cures like" and that disease can be treated by the administration of extremely dilute solutions of various compounds) and *naturopathy* (whose practitioners use numerous highly questionable diagnostic and therapeutic methods that also lack biological plausibility and experimental validation; Atwood, 2004) should be actively avoided by caregivers of children with developmental disorders.

Mind–Body Medicine

This category of nonstandard therapy comprises practices that use mind-based activities, such as meditation, biofeedback, hypnosis, or prayer, in attempts to treat disease or improve physical or mental functioning. None of these methods currently has an accepted role in the treatment of children with developmental disabilities.

Studies of relaxation training or other meditation techniques in children with ADHD, cerebral palsy, or intellectual disabilities have been equivocal or limited by significant methodological issues (Jensen & Kenny, 2004; Mauersberger, Artz, Duncan, & Gurgevich, 2000; Uma, Nagendra, Nagarathna, Vaidehi, & Seethalakshmi, 1989), although short-term improvements in certain behavioral measures have been observed in some studies (Goldbeck & Schmid, 2003; McPhail & Chamove, 1989; Wachelka & Katz, 1999). Hypnosis has been proposed as a treatment modality for certain behavioral or learning disorders, but has not been validated as an effective therapeutic approach (Barabasz & Barabasz, 2000; Johnson, Johnson, Olson, & Newman, 1981). Although there has been an increase in the use of behavioral research designs in the investigation of music therapy interventions, and some benefits of music therapy have been reported in various populations, the exact role of these methods in the treatment of children with developmental disabilities remains unclear (Gregory, 2002; Kaplan & Steele, 2005; Overy, 2003; Overy, Nicolson, Fawcett, & Clarke, 2003; Rickson & Watkins, 2003; Whipple, 2004).

The modality within the category of mind–body interventions that has received the most public and research interest has been biofeedback, particularly electroencephalographic (EEG) biofeedback. In this technique, children try to learn to use brain electrical activity to control a video game–like interface, with the hope that this will improve attention in other settings. Electroencephalographic biofeedback has been promoted predominantly for the treatment of children with ADHD. Although early studies showed apparent effectiveness of this technique, criticisms have been raised regarding methodological deficiencies (Kline, Brann, & Loney, 2002; Ramirez, Desantis, & Opler, 2001). Failure to control for behavioral trends unrelated to the intervention and lack of "intent to treat" analysis may be contributing factors to the appearance of efficacy in some studies (Heywood & Beale, 2003). Although EEG biofeedback remains under investigation, it is not currently a recommended treatment approach for children with ADHD (American Academy of Pediatrics [AAP], 2001c; Monastra, 2005; Thornton & Carmody, 2005).

Manipulative and Body-Based Practices

Body-based methods rely on physical manipulation or the application of other forces (e.g., sound) to try to achieve a specific therapeutic goal. Examples of these methods include chiropractic manipulation, massage, sensory integration therapy, and sound-based interventions such as auditory integration training (AIT). Most of these methods are based on unproved and untenable hypotheses and are not validated approaches in the treatment of children with developmental disabilities.

Massage, not surprisingly, may confer short-term relaxation (and associated behavior) benefits in children with various developmental disorders (Dossetor, Couryer, & Nicol, 1991; Escalona, Field, Singer-Strunck, Cullen, & Hartshorn, 2001; Field, Quintino, Hernandez-Reif, & Koslovsky, 1998; Khilnani, Field, Hernandez-Reif, & Schanberg, 2003). There is no convincing evidence, however, that there are any developmental benefits of massage in preterm or low birth weight infants (Vickers, Ohlsson, Lacy, & Horsley, 2004). The concept of sensory integration dysfunction was proposed in the 1970s and postulates that abnormal or inefficient functioning in various central nervous system sensory pathways lies at the root of many developmental and behavioral disorders (Ayres, 1972). Although various *sensory integration* methods are widely used in the treatment of children with developmental disorders, particularly autism spectrum disorders, there remains a significant lack of empirical evidence indicating clinical benefit for any of these specific techniques (Case-Smith & Miller, 1999; Hoehn & Baumeister, 1994; Vargas & Camilli, 1999). AIT, which was developed by French physician Guy Berard in the 1960s, is based on a theory that abnormal auditory perception is a cause of various behavioral features in children with autism. As is the case with many of the nonstandard therapies reviewed in this chapter, widespread use of this therapy occurred in the absence of a sufficient body of evidence supporting its effectiveness. There is no convincing evidence that AIT is effective in the treatment of children with autism spectrum disorders (Sinha, Silove, Wheeler, & Williams, 2004), and its use in the treatment of children with these or other developmental disabilities is not recommended (AAP, 1998). Chiropractic manipulation, which also has no role in the treatment of any developmental disorder, may be particularly risky in children with certain conditions, such as Down syndrome (La Francis, 1990).

Energy Medicine

Energy therapies are among the most implausible of all the nonstandard therapies. These interventions are based on the theory that energy fields (*biofields*) exist around all living organisms and that a disruption in these fields is a primary cause of disease. Manipulation of these fields using various techniques restores *balance* and health. Many traditional Chinese practices (acupuncture, Qi gong) as well as practices of more recent vintage (e.g., therapeutic touch) are based on these beliefs.

There is limited evidence that acupuncture is effective in the treatment of certain pain syndromes, although equivalent benefit was seen from sham acupuncture in one study, indicating that the needling itself, and not the adjustment of "energy flow" along meridians, may be responsible for the observed pain relief (Furlan et al., 2005; Linde et al., 2005; Melchart et al., 2005). Reports of the use of acupuncture in children with developmental disabilities have typically been uncontrolled or have had ill-defined or unreliable outcome measures (Lai et al., 1999; Liu et al., 1994; Sanner & Sundequist, 1981; Sun et al., 2004; Svedberg, Nordahl, & Lundeberg, 2003; Tian et al., 1995; Zhou & Zheng, 2005). One study relied on parental perceptions of the therapeutic benefit of acupuncture in children with cerebral palsy—an outcome laden with potential bias (Duncan, Barton, Edmonds, & Blashill, 2004).

Therapeutic touch involves a practitioner performing smoothing movements above the body (without actually touching), thereby *massaging* the biofield around the human body. Believers in this therapy think that this balances the nonphysical *life energy* and restores the body to a state of good health. Practitioners believe that the intent of the healer to heal is a necessary element of the encounter. The existence of biofields that can be manually detected and manipulated has never been proved and would violate known laws of physics (Rosa, Rosa, Sarner, & Barrett, 1998); however, this is usually of no concern to believers in this technique. Therapeutic touch is ineffective as a method for accelerating wound healing (O'Mathuna & Ashford, 2003). There are no published controlled studies of therapeutic touch (which bears the characteristic hallmarks of a pseudoscientific intervention, as discussed later) in the treatment of developmental disabilities.

Biologically Based Therapies

Many different "biological" interventions (which include herbs, foods and vitamins) have been used over the years in an effort to treat various developmental disorders, accounting for the largest group of nonstandard therapies that have been utilized for this reason. Although not as overtly biologically implausible as many of the methods discussed previously (and there is a long history of effective medical therapies being derived from botanical agents), these interventions suffer from a similar lack of experimental evidence of effectiveness. Some of these therapies, such as chelation therapy in autism, manifest the highly unfavorable juxtaposition of absence of proven benefits and presence of potentially serious risks.

Orthomolecular treatments of ADHD that utilized vitamin or mineral supplementation were popularized in the 1970s, largely through the efforts of Linus Pauling (1968). Although anecdotal reports and uncontrolled studies have often been favorable to this approach, placebo-controlled trials have not replicated these positive results (Arnold, Christopher, Huestis, & Smeltzer, 1978; Haslam, Dalby, & Rademaker, 1984). Many other substances, such as docosahexaenoic acid, have been investigated in ADHD, without clear and convincing evidence of benefit (Hirayama, Hamazaki, & Terasawa, 2004; Voigt et al., 2001). Although there are continued investigations of various supplements in children with hyperactivity, there is currently no role for vitamin or other supplement treatment in children with ADHD (Torrioli et al., 1999; Van Oudheusden & Scholte, 2002). The use of various supplements and biological agents is also common in children with autism (Green et al., 2005). Vitamins and minerals (including vitamin B_6 and magnesium), probiotics, dimethylglycine, antifungals, and various immunological agents have all been used widely. The best available data do not support any benefit of vitamin B_6 and magnesium treatment (Findling et al., 1997; Tolbert, Haigler, Waits, & Dennis, 1993). There are currently no supplements that are accepted as safe and effective in the treatment of autism spectrum disorders (AAP, 2001b). Likewise, available evidence does not support a beneficial effect of supplements on cognitive functioning in children with Down syndrome (Centre for Reviews and Dissemination, 2005).

Dietary interventions also have a long history in the field of developmental disabilities. The Feingold diet (Feingold, 1975), based on the hypothesis that various food additives are the cause of hyperactive behavior, gained popularity in the 1970s in the absence of a convincing foundation of supporting evidence. Controlled trials of the Feingold diet have not shown any consistent benefit, although the possibility that certain food additives may exert some negative behavioral effect in subgroups of young children cannot be completely discounted (Bateman et al., 2004; Rowe, 1988; Rowe & Rowe, 1994; Wender, 1986). Oligoantigenic diets, which arose from a theory that ADHD is caused by a food allergy–mediated mechanism, have also been promoted as a therapeutic option. The Cochrane Central Register of Controlled Trials lists six clinical trials of oligoantigenic diets in ADHD between 1985 and 1997 (Boris & Mandel, 1994; Egger,

Carter, Graham, Gumley, & Soothill, 1985; Egger, Stolla, & McEwen, 1992; Schmidt et al., 1997; Schulte-Korne et al., 1996; Uhlig, Merkenschlager, Brandmaier, & Egger, 1997). These data have been reviewed both positively (Arnold, 2001) and negatively (Accardo, 2000); any observed positive effect does not appear to be robust and may only occur in a subset of children.

In children with autism, the main dietary intervention that has gained a large following has been the gluten- and casein-free diet (GF-CF). This diet arose from the (unproved and unlikely) hypothesis that peptides from gluten and casein exert a central nervous system effect that leads to the symptomatology seen in autism. The controlled trials of this diet that have been performed have had methodological limitations, including the fact that parents were not blinded to group assignment (Knivsberg, Reichelt, Hoien, & Nodland, 2002; Sponheim, 1991). The GF-CF diet is not currently a validated therapy in autism.

Hyperbaric oxygen therapy for children with cerebral palsy and other disorders developed a great deal of popularity in the 1990s. Promoters of this intervention have argued that oxygen delivered at high concentration and pressure can revive dormant brain tissue adjacent to areas of previous injury. Controlled trials of hyperbaric oxygen therapy in children with cerebral palsy have not shown any benefit compared with room air (although these studies were confounded by the fact that the control groups received room air at slightly increased atmospheric pressure) (Collet et al., 2001; Hardy et al., 2002). The Agency for Healthcare Research and Quality has concluded there is insufficient evidence to determine whether hyperbaric oxygen treatment improves functional outcome in children with cerebral palsy (McDonagh et al., 2003).

Example of Secretin

Although convincing evidence of efficacy and safety from controlled research trials should precede widespread clinical use of any therapy, in the case of CAM, the reverse is often true. There are numerous examples in which widespread publicity and adoption of a treatment has occurred prior to the performance of controlled research to appropriately evaluate efficacy. The use of secretin as a treatment for autism is one illustrative case.

In 1998, a published case series described improvement in communication and social behavior in three children with autism following intravenous administration of porcine secretin to assess pancreatic exocrine function during diagnostic gastrointestinal (GI) endoscopy (Horvath et al., 1998). In October of 1998, NBC's *Dateline* television news program featured a story about the dramatic improvement observed in one of these three patients. Almost immediately, there was widespread endorsement of the use of secretin on the Internet and in the lay press, and parents began to request secretin infusions for their children with autism. It is estimated that thousands of children with autism received this treatment outside of research trials, and the demand created a shortage of secretin for use in diagnostic GI procedures (Somogyi, Cintron, & Toskes, 2000).

Because of the public interest in and popularity of the treatment despite the lack of adequate evidence of efficacy, double-blind, randomized, controlled clinical trials were quickly designed and implemented. The results of the first trials, published in 1999, failed to detect any evidence that secretin was an effective treatment for autism (Owley et al., 1999; Sandler et al., 1999). Subsequently, more than a dozen separate double-blind, randomized, controlled trials involving more than 600 individuals with autism have been published, and the treatment has been shown to be no more effective than placebo (Esch & Carr, 2004; Sturmey, 2005). These studies have examined various types of secretin, single and multiple dosing regimens, and differential effects on subgroups of children with autism and GI problems. No consistent beneficial effects have been demonstrated, although one study suggested more improvement in some outcome measures in a subgroup of children with autism and GI problems when they received secretin as compared with placebo (Kern, Van Miller, Evans, & Trivedi, 2002; Sturmey, 2005). Repligen, the company that was developing secretin as a treatment for autism, halted development

in autism after a Phase III trial including 132 young children with autism failed to demonstrate benefit (Pollack, 2004).

The dramatic explosion of public interest in secretin resulted in exposure of thousands of children to a treatment that is not effective and necessitated the pursuit of a line of research at a cost of millions of dollars (Esch & Carr, 2004). This example illustrates the importance of adhering to the scientific paradigm of establishing efficacy and safety before instituting clinical use of a therapy and the powerful role that the media and the Internet can play in promoting the widespread use of a treatment with unproved benefit.

POTENTIAL RISKS IN THE USE OF NONSTANDARD THERAPIES

All therapeutic interventions, whether considered conventional or nonstandard, carry potential risks. Both direct and indirect risks are recognized for interventions in all of the categories of nonstandard therapy outlined previously (AAP, 2001a). Direct risks can include toxic effects of biological or manipulative techniques (Bakerink, Gospe, Dimand, & Eldridge, 1996; Bose, Vashistha, & O'Loughlin, 1983; Montoya-Cabrera, Rubio-Rodriguez, Velazquez-Gonzalez, & Avila Montoya, 1991; Saper et al., 2004; Shafrir & Kaufman, 1992; Yu & Yeung, 1987), interference with adequate nutrition, and interruption or postponement of conventional therapies known to be helpful (Coppes, Anderson, Egeler, & Wolff, 1998; Wilson et al., 2005). Financial burdens on the family, time demands that interfere with quality of life, and the risk of guilt related to imperfect treatment compliance are additional hazards. Alternative medicine practitioners may develop attitudes against conventional medical practices, such as vaccination, that are known to be effective (Busse, Kulkarni, Campbell, & Injeyan, 2002). Misleading or inaccurate information available on the Internet regarding nonstandard therapies has the potential for leading to direct physical harm (Walji et al., 2004). Health care providers should recognize that the endorsement of nonstandard therapies known to be potentially harmful, or the development of supervisory relationships with CAM providers, might have liability implications (Cohen & Kemper, 2005; Studdert et al., 1998).

PLACEBO RESPONSE AND NONSTANDARD THERAPIES

With the popularity of unproved and sometimes nonsensical therapies seemingly on the rise, it is instructive to examine some of the factors that may contribute to the illusion of effectiveness of various nonstandard therapies.

Placebos (a term derived from the Latin for "I shall please") have been used in the practice of medicine since the time of Hippocrates, although this term did not appear in medical parlance until the late 18th century. Hooper's Medical Dictionary of 1811 defined a placebo as "any medicine adapted more to please than benefit the patient" (Edwards, 2005). In addition to medications, placebo treatments have included dietary interventions, medical devices, surgeries, and other therapeutic procedures. In the 19th century, as some physicians became skeptical about the value of much of their existing medical armamentarium, the deliberate prescription of pharmacologically ineffective preparations became commonplace. Although current medical practice aspires to be driven by an evidence base, the use of placebos in clinical practice remains common (Nitzan & Lichtenberg, 2004), and physicians do not exclusively rely on empirically proved pharmacological and surgical interventions (Hardern, Leong, Page, Shepherd, & Teoh, 2003).

Across centuries of medical practice, patients have been successfully treated with agents that were inherently ineffective. The placebo effect has been defined as "a genuine psychological or physiological effect, which is attributable to receiving a substance or undergoing a procedure, but which is not due to the inherent powers of that substance or procedure" (Stewart-Williams & Podd, 2004). It is likely that in the past, when truly effective treatments were limited, the placebo effect was a main reason why people continued to seek medical care; however, physicians using placebos as treatment would be incorrect in assuming that the placebo itself was responsible for their patients' improvement—a common error

of human reasoning referred to as *post hoc, ergo propter hoc* ("after this, therefore because of this"). The term *placebo effect* implies an action of the placebo itself, but what actually is occurring is a post-therapeutic response that is then erroneously attributed to the placebo (Feinstein, 2002).

Toward the end of the 19th century and in the early 20th century, the use of placebos in clinical medical practice became increasingly viewed as paternalistic, dishonest, and fraudulent (Edwards, 2005). Recognition of the placebo effect, however, led to the acceptance in the 1950s of randomized controlled trials as a mainstay of therapeutic investigations. A randomized controlled trial that compares a new therapy to a placebo rather than to no treatment implicitly assumes that treatment with placebo exerts a true effect. This underlines a fundamental change in the understanding of the placebo, from an inactive therapy issued simply to placate a patient to a pharmacologically inert but psychologically and physiologically active preparation. Although recent meta-analyses have questioned the conventional wisdom that placebo effects are powerful and widespread across all medical conditions, there is less doubt that placebo effects exist for more subjective clinical outcomes, particularly in trials evaluating treatments in psychiatry, developmental disabilities, and other chronic conditions with fluctuating courses and highly subjective symptoms (Hrobjartsson & Gotzsche, 2004a, 2004b). In trials evaluating treatments for depression, the response rate to placebo has been reported to be as high as 50% (Carls, 2004). Trials of therapeutic interventions in autism also show a uniformly high rate of placebo response (Hollander et al., 2004).

There are no specific features (personality, cognitive style, or educational level) that make a patient more likely to respond to placebo, and therefore anyone may be susceptible to placebo effects with any treatment (Thompson, 2000). The placebo effect appears to be mediated by four primary factors: 1) natural biological healing; 2) the patient's psychic state, which can affect individual beliefs about cause and/or therapy; 3) patient and provider expectations; and 4) iatrotherapy produced by the provider's professional behavior (Feinstein, 2002).

Natural biological healing refers to the fact that most illnesses are self-limited and improve over time regardless of treatment, and even chronic conditions that have no cure typically exhibit significantly fluctuating symptoms. When symptoms of a chronic illness lessen following any type of treatment, that therapy may be credited with causing the improvement, although such improvement may have occurred anyway in the natural course of events. Patients with chronic conditions with unclear pathophysiology, fluctuating courses, highly subjective symptoms, and few effective evidenced-based treatments are most vulnerable to the placebo effect (Kaptchuk & Eisenberg, 1998). This is the case in children with developmental disabilities, which represent chronic, neurologically based conditions without any evidence-based cures. Children with even severe disabilities tend to make some developmental progress over time. These temporal developmental gains may be misinterpreted as being secondary to any treatment strategy that is employed coincident with this developmental progress. Children with disabilities often exhibit associated behavioral problems, which also tend to wax and wane. Any treatment strategy employed during a period of improving behavior may be given undeserved credit for producing the behavior change. Parents also tend to seek interventions during periods when behavior is at a nadir; the subsequent behavioral "regression to the mean" may create the impression of treatment efficacy.

Parental beliefs about the cause of their child's illness or about its treatment can be powerful factors in interpreting the effects of any treatment strategy. Even when no objective improvement occurs during the use of a particular therapy (whether conventional or nonstandard), parents with a strong psychological investment in the treatment strategy can convince themselves that it has been beneficial (Barrett, 2001). According to cognitive dissonance theory, when experiences contradict existing attitudes, feelings, knowledge, or core beliefs, mental distress is produced. If no improvement occurs after the commitment of significant time, money, and personal effort to a specific treatment strategy that parents

strongly believe in, they may still report some subjective benefit that is not supported by any objective data, rather than recognize that the treatment strategy was ineffective. The fields of psychoneuroimmunology and psychoneuroendocrinology are proposing mechanisms to explain how belief in benefit might affect treatment outcome, as a form of stress reduction with physiological consequences (Spiegel, 2004). Quantitative EEG and positron emission tomography scan studies have shown distinct physiological changes in patients who respond to placebo compared with those who do not respond (Leuchter, Cook, Witte, Morgan, & Abrams, 2002; Mayberg et al., 2002).

Expectations on the part of both caregivers and health care providers clearly contribute to the placebo effect. Benefits derived from the placebo effect are greater when patients or families have high expectations for improvement (Kirsch, 1985). In cases of children with developmental disabilities, caregivers with high expectations for improvement are more likely to misinterpret the usual variability in their children's behavior as evidence of effectiveness (Sandler & Bodfish, 2000).

The Hawthorne effect (named after the Hawthorne factory of Western Electric in Chicago) was first described following a series of experiments in which worker productivity progressively increased with a series of changes in working conditions, including a return to original conditions (Mayo, 1933). One explanation for these observations was that the act of observing the workers contributed directly to the improved performance. A similar phenomenon may occur in clinical trials and therapeutic interventions in developmental disabilities, wherein improvement in some aspect of functioning occurs as a direct consequence of the interest being focused on the child and family during the course of the intervention. The Hawthorne "effect" is more accurately viewed as a conglomeration of unmeasured social and psychological variables that have an impact on the outcome of a trial or therapeutic intervention (Wickstrom & Bendix, 2000).

A health care provider's professional behavior may be the most critical factor in producing a placebo effect, particularly in regard to unorthodox treatments. Providers who present themselves as willing to do everything in their power to heal their patients, regardless of how great that therapeutic power really is, will maximize positive expectations in patients (and their parents)—a phenomenon akin to the Hawthorne effect (Mackenback, 2005). These positive expectations may then produce placebo effects through anxiety reduction, more effective coping styles, or behavior change (Peck & Coleman, 1991; Turner, Deyo, Loeser, Von Korff, & Fordyce, 1994). Altruistic-appearing providers can more easily obtain families' confidence, promote disclosure of their emotions and fears, and provide them with emotional support—contextual factors that have been shown to contribute to the placebo effect. Physicians who adopt a warm, friendly, and reassuring manner are more effective than those who keep consultations formal and do not offer reassurance (Di Blasi, Harkness, Ernst, Georgiou, & Kleijnen, 2001). In today's high technology medical climate, physicians may neglect the role of good therapeutic style in the care of patients, whereas an "alternative" style of practice may be perceived as a kinder and gentler style that harnesses rather than eschews the placebo effect and engages caregivers as active participants in the treatment of their children (Coulehan, 1999; Spiegel, 2004).

Given the power and pervasiveness of these expectancy effects, particularly in regard to chronic disorders with subjective and fluctuating symptomatology such as developmental disabilities, no therapeutic intervention should be considered effective until it is proved to provide statistically significant benefits relative to placebo in randomized, double-blind, placebo-controlled clinical trials. Trials of nonstandard therapies should have strict inclusion criteria to make certain that the individuals studied truly have the disorder that the therapeutic intervention being studied is designed to treat. Randomization increases objectivity and prevents the potential bias of investigators preferentially assigning subjects to the treatment group whom they feel would more likely show a positive effect of the treatment. Double-blinding, when feasible, also eliminates the potential confounding effect of caregiver expectations of therapeutic benefit—a particu-larly important issue in outcomes that rely on parental report. Although complementary and alternative practices present unique challenges in the creation of well-designed clinical trials, rigorous research methodology is sorely needed (Margolin, Avants, & Kleber, 1998; Mason, Tovey, & Long, 2002).

PSEUDOSCIENCE AND NONSTANDARD THERAPIES

Although not all therapies currently considered complementary or alternative should be automatically rejected simply because they are unorthodox, providers must maintain a high level of skepticism and learn to recognize characteristic features that indicate a therapy is pseudoscientific. Proponents of nonstandard interventions often relate their practices to "the art of medicine"; however, art should begin where science ends, not substitute for science. The following characteristics of pseudoscience are common in many different nonstandard practices and should serve as warning signs that a particular CAM practice is questionable (Lilienfeld, Lynn, & Lohr, 2003):

1. *Overuse of ad hoc hypotheses designed to immunize claims from falsification:* When reduced hair mercury levels were reported in children with autism, the contention that mercury exposure causes autism was modified to include the hypothesis that children with autism might have impaired mercury excretion, without adequate consideration of other potential explanations for the data (Holmes, Blaxill, & Haley, 2003).

2. *Absence of self-correction:* Consumers of CAM may erroneously believe that ancient therapies must be effective simply because they have been used for centuries; however, this lack of substantive change over time may be evidence of a failure to weed out ineffective practices.

3. *Evasion of peer review:* This practice is illustrated by the paucity of controlled trials of many CAM methods in the medical literature.

4. *Emphasis on confirmation rather than refutation:* Such emphasis is often a hallmark of

investigations of practices linked to spiritual and cultural beliefs.

5. *Reversed burden of proof:* This characteristic often obligates the scientific community to disprove questionable therapies that have become widely used, as in the case of secretin therapy for autism.

6. *Absence of connectivity:* This feature is commonly seen in methods such as therapeutic touch that propose the existence of forces not verified by other scientific disciplines.

7. *Overreliance on testimonial and anecdotal evidence:* This is frequently observed in the Internet-driven spread of various biological interventions in autism.

8. *Use of obscurantist language:* Complicated and often meaningless scientific jargon is commonly used to describe a nonstandard therapy or theory.

9. *Absence of boundary conditions:* Claims may be made that a particular treatment, such as anti-yeast therapy (Crook, 1983), is useful in an exceptionally wide range of biologically diverse conditions.

10. *The mantra of "holism":* Pronouncements are made that a particular therapy cannot or should not be viewed in isolation, but only as part of a larger package of interventions and practices (Institute of Medicine, 2004).

COUNSELING FAMILIES REGARDING NONSTANDARD THERAPY USE

Children with developmental disabilities, and their families, deserve the very best that medicine has to offer. Choices that parents make regarding the interventions that they pursue for their children need to be respected; however, health care providers have a responsibility to provide families with accurate, evidenced-based guidance to help shape their decisions. When counseling families of children with disabilities regarding complementary and alternative therapies, providers need to be informed about various nonstandard

practices, critically analyze the merits of specific therapies, identify potential risks of different treatments, and provide education about different therapeutic options and the importance of studying nonstandard practices using rigorous scientific methodology (AAP, 2001a). Although it may be counterproductive and potentially offensive for providers to summarily dismiss families' questions regarding CAM practices, it is justifiable to use reasoned argument to actively dissuade families from pursuing any intervention with potential health risks or that may impart added time, financial, or emotional burdens on the family and child. Health care providers should place a high priority on taking the time to educate families about what is truly known regarding the etiology and treatment of a developmental disability—any void created by the absence of good information will likely be filled with faulty information.

CONCLUSION

A main hazard of the culture of *holism* is that it endorses an overly inclusive view of what should be considered medicine. Attempts to apply the tools of science to evaluate the value of these specific activities frequently lead to consternation on the side of both believers and skeptics. Supporters of a holistic approach to medical care embrace a worldview in which there is virtually no distinction between the scientific and the spiritual (Kaptchuk & Eisenberg, 1998). This invariably leads to conflict between those who believe in the value of a particular "therapy" and those who wish to critically analyze the effectiveness of that therapy. The abandonment of interventions that cannot be proved to have efficacy should be as much a part of evidence-based medicine as the adoption of practices that actually work. This is a central feature of the machinery of scientific investigation—the compelling necessity to disprove oneself (Sagan, 1995). If a practice will not be rejected by its proponents or consumers in the face of strong evidence of nonefficacy, then it is questionable whether that particular activity can even be considered part of science or medicine. It is highly unlikely, for instance, that people will abandon the use of prayer as a consequence of any clinical trial (even if perfectly designed and executed) that fails to show any benefits of prayer for a particular medical condition. The fervor with which some practitioners believe in the value of other CAM methods, such as therapeutic touch, also borders on the religious. It may ultimately be fruitless to expend time or resources (using scientific methods) to evaluate those interventions that have weak prima facie plausibility and a low likelihood, despite any amount of contrary evidence, of ever being rejected by believers; however, when extraordinary therapeutic claims are made (or when therapies are based on theories that violate proven scientific principles), extraordinary evidence should be demanded.

"Keeping an open mind is a virtue—but . . .not so open that your brains fall out" (Sagan, 1995, p. 187). We must always remember that there is no alternative physics, pseudoscience complements nothing, and magical thinking is not the foundation on which any therapeutic intervention should be based.

REFERENCES

Accardo, P.J. (2000). Other therapies. In P.J. Accardo, T.A. Blondis, B.Y. Whitman, & M.A. Stein (Eds.), *Attention deficits and hyperactivity in children and adults* (2nd ed., pp. 633–651). New York: Marcel Dekker.

American Academy of Pediatrics, Committee on Children with Disabilities. (1998). Auditory integration training and facilitated communication for autism. *Pediatrics, 102*(2 Pt. 1), 431–433.

American Academy of Pediatrics, Committee on Children with Disabilities. (2001a). Counseling families who choose complementary and alternative medicine for their child with chronic illness or disability. *Pediatrics, 107*(3), 598–601. [Published erratum appears in *Pediatrics, 108*, 507, 2001.]

American Academy of Pediatrics, Committee on Children with Disabilities. (2001b). The pediatrician's role in the diagnosis and management of autistic spectrum disorder in children. *Pediatrics, 107*, 1221–1226.

American Academy of Pediatrics, Subcommittee on Attention-Deficit/Hyperactivity Disorder and Committee on Quality Improvement. (2001c). Clinical practice guideline: Treatment of the school-aged child with attention-deficit/hyperactivity disorder. *Pediatrics, 108*, 1033–1044.

Arnold, L.E. (2001). Alternative/complementary treatments for attention deficit hyperactivity disorder. In B.T. Rogers, T.R. Montgomery, T.M. Lock, & P.J. Accardo (Eds.), *Attention deficit hyperactivity disorder: The clinical spectrum* (pp. 197–207). Baltimore: York Press.

Arnold, L.E., Christopher, J., Huestis, R.D., & Smeltzer, D.J. (1978). Megavitamins for minimal brain dysfunction: A placebo-controlled study. *JAMA, 240*, 2642–2643.

Astin, J.A. (1998). Why patients use alternative medicine: Results of a national study. *JAMA, 279*, 1548–1553.

Atwood, K.C., IV. (2003). The ongoing problem with the National Center for *Complementary and Alternative Medicine. Skeptical Inquirer, 27*(5).

Atwood, K.C., IV. (2004). Naturopathy: A monograph, part II. *Scientific Review of Alternative Medicine, 8*(2), 56–73.

Ayres, A.J. (1972). *Sensory integration and learning disorders.* Los Angeles: Western Psychological Services.

Bakerink, J.A., Gospe, S.M., Jr., Dimand, R.J., & Eldridge, M.W. (1996). Multiple organ failure after ingestion of pennyroyal oil from herbal tea in two infants. *Pediatrics, 98*, 944–947.

Barabasz, A., & Barabasz, M. (2000). Treating AD/HD with hypnosis and neurotherapy. *Child Study Journal, 30*(1), 25–42.

Barnes, P.M., Powell-Griner, E., McFann, K., & Nahin, R.L. (2004). Complementary and alternative medicine use among adults: United States, 2002. *Advance Data, 343*, 1–19.

Barrett, S. (2001). *Spontaneous remission and the placebo effect.* Retrieved June 30, 2005, from http://www.quackwatch.org/04ConsumerEducation/placebo.html

Bateman, B., Warner, J.O., Hutchinson, E., Dean, T., Rowlandson, P., Gant, C., et al. (2004). The effects of a double blind, placebo controlled, artificial food colourings and benzoate preservative challenge on hyperactivity in a general population sample of preschool children. *Archives of Disease in Childhood, 89*, 506–511.

Bellas, A., Lafferty, W.E., Lind, B., & Tyree, P.T. (2005). Frequency, predictors, and expenditures for pediatric insurance claims for complementary and alternative medical professionals in Washington State. *Archives of Pediatrics and Adolescent Medicine, 159*, 367–372.

Boris, M., & Mandel, F.S. (1994). Foods and additives are common causes of the attention deficit hyperactive disorder in children [Review]. *Annals of Allergy, 72*, 462–468.

Bose, A., Vashistha, K., & O'Loughlin, B.J. (1983). Azarcon por empacho—another cause of lead toxicity. *Pediatrics, 72*, 106–108.

Busse, J.W., Kulkarni, A.V., Campbell, J.B., & Injeyan, H.S. (2002). Attitudes toward vaccination: A survey of Canadian chiropractic students. *CMAJ, 166*, 1531–1534.

Bussing, R., Zima, B.T., Gary, F.A., & Garvan, C.W. (2002). Use of complementary and alternative medicine for symptoms of attention-deficit hyperactivity disorder. *Psychiatric Services, 53,* 1096–1102.

Carls, K.A. (2004). Role of the placebo effect in evaluating antidepressant efficacy. *American Journal of Health-System Pharmacy, 61,* 1059–1063.

Case-Smith, J., & Miller, H. (1999). Occupational therapy with children with pervasive developmental disorders. *American Journal of Occupational Therapy, 53,* 506–513.

Centre for Reviews and Dissemination. (2005). Systematic review of the effect of therapeutic dietary supplements and drugs on cognitive function in subjects with Down syndrome (structured abstract). *Database of Abstracts of Reviews of Effectiveness, 2.*

Chapman, E., Weintraub, R., Milburn, M., Pirozzi, T., & Woo, E. (1999). Homeopathic treatment of mild traumatic brain injury: A randomized, double-blind, placebo-controlled clinical trial. *Journal of Head Trauma Rehabilitation, 14,* 521–542.

Cohen, M.H., & Kemper, K.J. (2005). Complementary therapies in pediatrics: A legal perspective. *Pediatrics, 115,* 774–780.

Collet, J.P., Vanasse, M., Marois, P., Amar, M., Goldberg, J., Lambert, J., et al. (2001). Hyperbaric oxygen for children with cerebral palsy: A randomised multicentre trial. *Lancet, 357,* 582–586.

Coppes, M.J., Anderson, R.A., Egeler, R.M., & Wolff, J.E. (1998). Alternative therapies for the treatment of childhood cancer. *New England Journal of Medicine, 339,* 846–847.

Coulehan, J. (1999). An alternative view: Listening to patients. *Lancet, 354,* 1467–1468.

Crook, W.G. (1983). *The yeast connection: A medical breakthrough.* Jackson, TN: Professional Books.

Davis, M.F., Meaney, F.J., & Duncan, B. (2004). Factors influencing the use of complementary and alternative medicine in children. *Journal of Alternative and Complementary Medicine, 10,* 740–742.

Davis, M.P., & Darden, P.M. (2003). Use of complementary and alternative medicine by children in the United States. *Archives of Pediatrics and Adolescent Medicine, 157,* 393–396.

Di Blasi, Z., Harkness, E., Ernst, E., Georgiou, A., & Kleijnen, J. (2001). Influence of context effects on health outcomes: A systematic review. *Lancet, 357,* 757–762.

Dossetor, D.R., Couryer, S., & Nicol, A.R. (1991). Massage for very severe self-injurious behaviour in a girl with Cornelia de Lange syndrome. *Developmental Medicine and Child Neurology, 33,* 636–640.

Duncan, B., Barton, L., Edmonds, D., & Blashill, B.M. (2004). Parental perceptions of the therapeutic effect from osteopathic manipulation or acupuncture in children with spastic cerebral palsy. *Clinical Pediatrics, 43,* 349–353.

Edwards, M. (2005). Placebo. *Lancet, 365,* 1023.

Egger, J., Carter, C.M., Graham, P.J., Gumley, D., & Soothill, J.F. (1985). Controlled trial of oligoantigenic treatment in the hyperkinetic syndrome. *Lancet, 1,* 540–545.

Egger, J., Stolla, A., & McEwen, L.M. (1992). Controlled trial of hyposensitisation in children with food-induced hyperkinetic syndrome. *Lancet, 339,* 1150–1153.

Eisenberg, D.M., Davis, R.B., Ettner, S.L., Appel, S., Wilkey, S., Van Rompay, M., et al. (1998). Trends in alternative medicine use in the United States, 1990–1997: Results of a follow-up national survey. *JAMA, 280,* 1569–1575.

Eisenberg, D.M., Kessler, R.C., Foster, C., Norlock, F.E., Calkins, D.R., & Delbanco, T.L. (1993). Unconventional medicine in the United States: Prevalence, costs, and patterns of use. *New England Journal of Medicine, 328,* 246–252.

Eisenberg, D.M., Kessler, R.C., Van Rompay, M.I., Kaptchuk, T.J., Wilkey, S.A., Appel, S., et al. (2001). Perceptions about complementary therapies relative to conventional therapies among adults who use both: Results from a national survey. *Annals of Internal Medicine, 135,* 344–351.

Ernst, E. (1999). Prevalence of complementary/alternative medicine for children: A systematic review [Review]. *European Journal of Pediatrics, 158,* 7–11.

Ernst, E., Resch, K.L., Mills, S., Hill, R., Mitchell, A., Willoughby, M., et al. (1995). Complementary medicine—a definition. *British Journal of General Practice, 45,* 506.

Escalona, A., Field, T., Singer-Strunck, R., Cullen, C., & Hartshorn, K. (2001). Brief report: Improvements in the behavior of children with autism following massage therapy. *Journal of Autism and Developmental Disorders, 31,* 513–516.

Esch, B.E., & Carr, J.E. (2004). Secretin as a treatment for autism: A review of the evidence. *Journal of Autism and Developmental Disorders, 34,* 543–556.

Feingold, B.F. (1975). *Why your child is hyperactive.* New York: Random House.

Feinstein, A.R. (2002). Post-therapeutic response and therapeutic "style": Re-formulating the "placebo effect." *Journal of Clinical Epidemiology, 55,* 427–429.

Feldman, D.E., Duffy, C., De Civita, M., Malleson, P., Philibert, L., Gibbon, M., et al. (2004). Factors associated with the use of complementary and alternative medicine in juvenile idiopathic arthritis. *Arthritis and Rheumatism, 51,* 527–532.

Field, T.M., Quintino, O., Hernandez-Reif, M., & Koslovsky, G. (1998). Adolescents with attention deficit hyperactivity disorder benefit from massage therapy. *Adolescence, 33,* 103–108.

Findling, R.L., Maxwell, K., Scotese-Wojtila, L., Huang, J., Yamashita, T., & Wiznitzer, M. (1997). High-dose pyridoxine and magnesium administration in children with autistic disorder: An absence of salutary effects in a double-blind, placebo-controlled study. *Journal of Autism and Developmental Disorders, 27,* 467–478.

Fong, D.P., & Fong, L.K. (2002). Usage of complementary medicine among children. *Australian Family Physician, 31,* 388–391.

Frei, H., & Thurneysen, A. (2001). Treatment for hyperactive children: Homeopathy and methylphenidate compared in a family setting. *British Homoeopathic Journal, 90*(4), 183–188.

Friedman, T., Slayton, W.B., Allen, L.S., Pollock, B.H., Dumont-Driscoll, M., Mehta, P., et al. (1997). Use of alternative therapies for children with cancer. *Pediatrics, 100*, e1.

Furlan, A.D., van Tulder, M.W., Cherkin, D.C., Tsukayama, H., Lao, L., Koes, B.W., et al. (2005). Acupuncture and dry-needling for low back pain [Review]. *Cochrane Database of Systematic Reviews, 1*, CD001351.

Gevitz, N. (1988). *Other healers: Unorthodox medicine in America.* Baltimore: The Johns Hopkins University Press.

Goldbeck, L., & Schmid, K. (2003). Effectiveness of autogenic relaxation training on children and adolescents with behavioral and emotional problems. *Journal of the American Academy of Child and Adolescent Psychiatry, 42*, 1046–1054.

Green, V.A., Pituch, K.A., Itchon, J., Choi, A., O'Reilly, M., & Sigafoos, J. (2005). Internet survey of treatments used by parents of children with autism. *Research in Developmental Disabilities, 27*, 70–84.

Gregory, D. (2002). Four decades of music therapy behavioral research designs: A content analysis of Journal of Music Therapy articles [Review]. *Journal of Music Therapy, 39*, 56–71.

Gross-Tsur, V., Lahad, A., & Shalev, R.S. (2003). Use of complementary medicine in children with attention deficit hyperactivity disorder and epilepsy. *Pediatric Neurology, 29*, 53–55.

Hardern, R.D., Leong, F.T., Page, A.V., Shepherd, M., & Teoh, R.C. (2003). How evidence based are therapeutic decisions taken on a medical admissions unit? *Emergency Medicine Journal, 20*, 447–448.

Hardy, P., Collet, J.P., Goldberg, J., Ducruet, T., Vanasse, M., Lambert, J., et al. (2002). Neuropsychological effects of hyperbaric oxygen therapy in cerebral palsy. *Developmental Medicine and Child Neurology, 44*, 436–446.

Haslam, R.H., Dalby, J.T., & Rademaker, A.W. (1984). Effects of megavitamin therapy on children with attention deficit disorders. *Pediatrics, 74*, 103–111.

Heywood, C., & Beale, I. (2003). EEG biofeedback vs. placebo treatment for attention-deficit/hyperactivity disorder: A pilot study. *Journal of Attention Disorders, 7*, 43–55.

Hirayama, S., Hamazaki, T., & Terasawa, K. (2004). Effect of docosahexaenoic acid-containing food administration on symptoms of attention-deficit/hyperactivity disorder—a placebo-controlled double-blind study. *European Journal of Clinical Nutrition, 58*, 467–473.

Hoehn, T.P., & Baumeister, A.A. (1994). A critique of the application of sensory integration therapy to children with learning disabilities. *Journal of Learning Disabilities, 27*, 338–350.

Hollander, E., Phillips, A., King, B.H., Guthrie, D., Aman, M.G., Law, P., et al. (2004). Impact of recent findings on study design of future autism clinical trials [Review]. *CNS Spectrums, 9*(1), 49–56.

Holmes, A.S., Blaxill, M.F., & Haley, B.E. (2003). Reduced levels of mercury in first baby haircuts of autistic children. *International Journal of Toxicology, 22*, 277–285.

Horvath, K., Stefanatos, G., Sokolski, K.N., Wachtel, R., Nabors, L., & Tildon, J.T. (1998). Improved social and language skills after secretin administration in patients with autistic spectrum disorders. *Journal of the Association for Academic Minority Physicians, 9*(1), 9–15.

Hrobjartsson, A., & Gotzsche, P.C. (2004a). Is the placebo powerless? Update of a systematic review with 52 new randomized trials comparing placebo with no treatment [Review]. *Journal of Internal Medicine, 256*, 91–100.

Hrobjartsson, A., & Gotzsche, P.C. (2004b). Placebo interventions for all clinical conditions [Review]. *Cochrane Database of Systematic Reviews, 3*, 003974.

Hurvitz, E.A., Leonard, C., Ayyangar, R., & Nelson, V.S. (2003). Complementary and alternative medicine use in families of children with cerebral palsy. *Developmental Medicine and Child Neurology, 45*, 364–370.

Institute of Medicine. (2004). *Complementary and alternative medicine in the United States.* Washington, DC: National Academies Press.

Jensen, P.S., & Kenny, D.T. (2004). The effects of yoga on the attention and behavior of boys with attention-deficit/ hyperactivity disorder (ADHD). *Journal of Attention Disorders, 7*, 205–216.

Johnson, L.S., Johnson, D.L., Olson, M.R., & Newman, J.P. (1981). The uses of hypnotherapy with learning disabled children. *Journal of Clinical Psychology, 37*, 291–299.

Johnston, G.A., Bilbao, R.M., & Graham-Brown, R.A. (2003). The use of complementary medicine in children with atopic dermatitis in secondary care in Leicester. *British Journal of Dermatology, 149*, 566–571.

Junker, J., Oberwittler, C., Jackson, D., & Berger, K. (2004). Utilization and perceived effectiveness of complementary and alternative medicine in patients with dystonia. *Movement Disorders, 19*, 158–161.

Kaplan, R.S., & Steele, A.L. (2005). An analysis of music therapy program goals and outcomes for clients with diagnoses on the autism spectrum. *Journal of Music Therapy, 42*, 2–19.

Kaptchuk, T.J., & Eisenberg, D.M. (1998). The persuasive appeal of alternative medicine [Review]. *Annals of Internal Medicine, 129*, 1061–1065.

Kelly, K.M. (2004). Complementary and alternative medical therapies for children with cancer [Review]. *European Journal of Cancer, 40*, 2041–2046.

Kern, J.K., Van Miller, S., Evans, P.A., & Trivedi, M.H. (2002). Efficacy of porcine secretin in children with autism and pervasive developmental disorder. *Journal of Autism and Developmental Disorders, 32,* 153–160.

Kessler, R.C., Davis, R.B., Foster, D.F., Van Rompay, M.I., Walters, E.E., Wilkey, S.A., et al. (2001). Long-term trends in the use of complementary and alternative medical therapies in the United States. *Annals of Internal Medicine, 135,* 262–268.

Khilnani, S., Field, T., Hernandez-Reif, M., & Schanberg, S. (2003). Massage therapy improves mood and behavior of students with attention-deficit/hyperactivity disorder. *Adolescence, 38,* 623–638.

Kirsch, I. (1985). Response expectancy as a determinant of experience and behavior. *American Psychologist, 40,* 1189–1202.

Kline, J.P., Brann, C.N., & Loney, B.R. (2002). A cacophony in the brainwaves: A critical appraisal of neurotherapy for attention-deficit disorders. *Scientific Review of Mental Health Practice, 1*(1), 44–54.

Knivsberg, A.M., Reichelt, K.L., Hoien, T., & Nodland, M. (2002). A randomised, controlled study of dietary intervention in autistic syndromes. *Nutritional Neuroscience, 5,* 251–261.

La Francis, M.E. (1990). A chiropractic perspective on atlantoaxial instability in Down's syndrome [Review]. *Journal of Manipulative and Physiological Therapeutics, 13*(3), 157–160.

Lai, X., Feng, S., Jin, R., & Zhang, J. (1999). The effect of electroacupuncture on auditory P300 potential in mongolism cases. *Journal of Traditional Chinese Medicine, 19*(4), 259–263.

Leuchter, A.F., Cook, I.A., Witte, E.A., Morgan, M., & Abrams, M. (2002). Changes in brain function of depressed subjects during treatment with placebo. *American Journal of Psychiatry, 159,* 122–129.

Levy, S.E., Mandell, D.S., Merhar, S., Ittenbach, R.F., & Pinto-Martin, J.A. (2003). Use of complementary and alternative medicine among children recently diagnosed with autistic spectrum disorder. *Journal of Developmental and Behavioral Pediatrics, 24,* 418–423.

Lilienfeld, S.O., Lynn, S.J., & Lohr, J.M. (Eds.). (2003). *Science and pseudoscience in clinical psychology.* New York: The Guilford Press.

Linde, K., Streng, A., Jurgens, S., Hoppe, A., Brinkhaus, B., Witt, C., et al. (2005). Acupuncture for patients with migraine: A randomized controlled trial. *JAMA, 293,* 2118–2125.

Liu, Z.H., Song, Z.H., & Du, N.Q. (1994). [Study of treatment on acquired infantile mental retardation with traditional Chinese and Western medicine]. *Zhongguo Zhong Xi Yi Jie He Za [Chinese Journal of Integrated Traditional and Western Medicine], 14,* 730–732.

Lu, W. (1994). Prompt pressure applied to peculiar points in the treatment of spasmodic infantile cerebral palsy—a report of 318 cases. *Journal of Traditional Chinese Medicine, 14*(3), 180–184.

Lundgren, J., & Ugalde, V. (2004). The demographics and economics of complementary alternative medicine [Review]. *Physical Medicine and Rehabilitation Clinics of North America, 15,* 955–961.

Mackenback, J.P. (2005). On the survival of the altruistic trait in medicine: Is there a link with the placebo effect? *Journal of Clinical Epidemiology, 58,* 433–435.

Madsen, H., Andersen, S., Nielsen, R.G., Dolmer, B.S., Host, A., & Damkier, A. (2003). Use of complementary/alternative medicine among paediatric patients. *European Journal of Pediatrics, 162,* 334–341.

Margolin, A., Avants, S.K., & Kleber, H.D. (1998). Investigating alternative medicine therapies in randomized controlled trials. *JAMA, 280,* 1626–1628.

Markowitz, J.E., Mamula, P., delRosario, J.F., Baldassano, R.N., Lewis, J.D., Jawad, A.F., et al. (2004). Patterns of complementary and alternative medicine use in a population of pediatric patients with inflammatory bowel disease. *Inflammatory Bowel Diseases, 10,* 599–605.

Mason, S., Tovey, P., & Long, A.F. (2002). Evaluating complementary medicine: Methodological challenges of randomised controlled trials [Review]. *BMJ, 325,* 832–834.

Mauersberger, K., Artz, K., Duncan, B., & Gurgevich, S. (2000). Can children with spastic cerebral palsy use self-hypnosis to reduce muscle tone? A preliminary study. *Integrative Medicine, 2*(2), 93–96.

Mayberg, H.S., Silva, J.A., Brannan, S.K., Tekell, J.L., Mahurin, R.K., McGinnis, S., et al. (2002). The functional neuroanatomy of the placebo effect. *American Journal of Psychiatry, 159,* 728–737.

Mayo, E. (1933). *The human problems of an industrial civilization.* New York: Macmillan.

McDonagh, M., Carson, S., Ash, J., Russman, B.S., Stavri, P.Z., Krages, K.P., et al. (2003). *Hyperbaric oxygen therapy for brain injury, cerebral palsy, and stroke. Evidence Report/Technology Assessment No. 85* (AHRQ Publication No. 04-E003). Rockville, MD: Agency for Healthcare Research and Quality.

McPhail, C.H., & Chamove, A.S. (1989). Relaxation reduces disruption in mentally handicapped adults. *Journal of Mental Deficiency Research, 33*(Pt. 5), 399–406.

Melchart, D., Linde, K., Berman, B., White, A., Vickers, A., Allais, G., et al. (2005). Acupuncture for idiopathic headache. *Cochrane Database of Systematic Reviews, 1,* CD001218.

Miller, A.R., Brehaut, J.C., Raina, P., McGrail, K.M., & Armstrong, R.W. (2004). Use of medical services by methylphenidate-treated children in the general population. *Ambulatory Pediatrics, 4,* 174–180.

Monastra, V.J. (2005). Electroencephalographic biofeedback (neurotherapy) as a treatment for attention deficit hyperactivity disorder: Rationale and empirical foundation [Review]. *Child and Adolescent Psychiatric Clinics of North America, 14,* 55–82.

Montoya-Cabrera, M.A., Rubio-Rodriguez, S., Velazquez-Gonzalez, E., & Avila Montoya, S. (1991). Mercury poisoning caused by a homeopathic drug. *Gaceta Medica De Mexico, 127,* 267–270.

National Center for Complementary and Alternative Medicine. (2000). *Expanding horizons of healthcare: Five year strategic plan 2001–2005.* Washington, DC: U.S. Department of Health and Human Services.

National Center for Complementary and Alternative Medicine. (2004). *NCCAM's research centers program.* Retrieved May 30, 2005, from http://nccam.nih.gov/training/centers/index.htm

National Center for Complementary and Alternative Medicine. (2005). *NCCAM-funded research for FY 2004.* Retrieved May 30, 2005, from http://nccam.nih.gov/research/extramural/awards/2004/index.htm

Ni, H., Simile, C., & Hardy, A.M. (2002). Utilization of complementary and alternative medicine by United States adults: Results from the 1999 National Health Interview Survey. *Medical Care, 40,* 353–358.

Nitzan, U., & Lichtenberg, P. (2004). Questionnaire survey on use of placebo. *BMJ, 329,* 944–946.

O'Mathuna, D.P., & Ashford, R.L. (2003). Therapeutic touch for healing acute wounds [Review]. *Cochrane Database of Systematic Reviews, 4,* CD002766.

Orhan, F., Sekerel, B.E., Kocabas, C.N., Sackesen, C., Adalioglu, G., & Tuncer, A. (2003). Complementary and alternative medicine in children with asthma. *Annals of Allergy, Asthma, and Immunology, 90,* 611–615.

Ottolini, M.C., Hamburger, E.K., Loprieato, J.O., Coleman, R.H., Sachs, H.C., Madden, R., et al. (2001). Complementary and alternative medicine use among children in the Washington, DC area. *Ambulatory Pediatrics, 1,* 122–125.

Overy, K. (2003). Dyslexia and music: From timing deficits to musical intervention [Review]. *Annals of the New York Academy of Sciences, 999,* 497–505.

Overy, K., Nicolson, R.I., Fawcett, A.J., & Clarke, E.F. (2003). Dyslexia and music: Measuring musical timing skills. *Dyslexia, 9,* 18–36.

Owley, T., Steele, E., Corsello, C., Risi, S., McKaig, K., Lord, C., et al. (1999). *A double-blind, placebo-controlled trial of secretin for the treatment of autistic disorder. MedGenMed, October 6, 1999.* Retrieved from http://www.medscape.com/viewarticle/408013

Pauling, L. (1968). Orthomolecular psychiatry: Varying the concentrations of substances normally present in the human body may control mental disease. *Science, 160,* 265–271.

Peck, C., & Coleman, G. (1991). Implications of placebo theory for clinical research and practice in pain management [Review]. *Theoretical Medicine, 12,* 247–270.

Pollack, A. (2004, January 6). Trials end parents' hope for autism drug. *The New York Times,* p. 14.

Prussing, E., Sobo, E.J., Walker, E., Dennis, K., & Kurtin, P.S. (2004). Communicating with pediatricians about complementary/alternative medicine: Perspectives from parents of children with Down syndrome. *Ambulatory Pediatrics, 4,* 488–494.

Ramirez, P.M., Desantis, D., & Opler, L.A. (2001). EEG biofeedback treatment of ADD: A viable alternative to traditional medical intervention? [Review]. *Annals of the New York Academy of Sciences, 931,* 342–358.

Rickson, D.J., & Watkins, W.G. (2003). Music therapy to promote prosocial behaviors in aggressive adolescent boys—a pilot study. *Journal of Music Therapy, 40,* 283–301.

Rosa, L., Rosa, E., Sarner, L., & Barrett, S. (1998). A close look at therapeutic touch. *JAMA, 279,* 1005–1010.

Rowe, K.S. (1988). Synthetic food colourings and ''hyperactivity'': A double-blind crossover study. *Australian Paediatric Journal, 24,* 143–147.

Rowe, K.S., & Rowe, K.J. (1994). Synthetic food coloring and behavior: A dose response effect in a double-blind, placebo-controlled, repeated-measures study. *Journal of Pediatrics, 125*(5 Pt. 1), 691–698.

Sagan, C. (1995). *The demon-haunted world: Science as a candle in the dark.* New York: Random House.

Sanders, H., Davis, M.F., Duncan, B., Meaney, F.J., Haynes, J., & Barton, L.L. (2003). Use of complementary and alternative medical therapies among children with special health care needs in Southern Arizona. *Pediatrics, 111,* 584–587.

Sandler, A.D., & Bodfish, J.W. (2000). Placebo effects in autism: Lessons from secretin. *Journal of Developmental and Behavioral Pediatrics, 21,* 347–350.

Sandler, A.D., Sutton, K.A., DeWeese, J., Girardi, M.A., Sheppard, V., & Bodfish, J.W. (1999). Lack of benefit of a single dose of synthetic human secretin in the treatment of autism and pervasive developmental disorder. *New England Journal of Medicine, 341,* 1801–1806.

Sanner, C., & Sundequist, U. (1981). Acupuncture for the relief of painful muscle spasms in dystonic cerebral palsy. *Developmental Medicine and Child Neurology, 23,* 544–545.

Saper, R.B., Kales, S.N., Paquin, J., Burns, M.J., Eisenberg, D.M., Davis, R.B., et al. (2004). Heavy metal content of ayurvedic herbal medicine products. *JAMA, 292,* 2868–2873.

Sawni-Sikand, A., Schubiner, H., & Thomas, R.L. (2002). Use of complementary/alternative therapies among children in primary care pediatrics. *Ambulatory Pediatrics, 2,* 99–103.

Schmidt, M.H., Mocks, P., Lay, B., Eisert, H.G., Fojkar, R., FritzSigmund, D., et al. (1997). Does oligoantigenic diet influence hyperactive/conduct-disordered children—a controlled trial. *European Child and Adolescent Psychiatry, 6,* 88–95.

Schneider, B., Hanisch, J., & Weiser, M. (2004). Complementary medicine prescription patterns in Germany. *Annals of Pharmacotherapy, 38,* 502–507.

Schulte-Korne, G., Deimel, W., Gutenbrunner, C., Hennighausen, K., Blank, R., Rieger, C., et al. (1996). [Effect of an oligo-antigen diet on the behavior of hyperkinetic children]. *Zeitschrift fur Kinder- und Jugendpsychiatrie und Psychotherapie, 24,* 176–183.

Shafrir, Y., & Kaufman, B.A. (1992). Quadriplegia after chiropractic manipulation in an infant with congenital torticollis caused by a spinal cord astrocytoma. *Journal of Pediatrics, 120*(2 Pt. 1), 266–269.

Sibinga, E.M., Ottolini, M.C., Duggan, A.K., & Wilson, M.H. (2004). Parent-pediatrician communication about complementary and alternative medicine use for children. *Clinical Pediatrics, 43,* 367–373.

Simpson, N., & Roman, K. (2001). Complementary medicine use in children: Extent and reasons. A population-based study. *British Journal of General Practice, 51,* 914–916.

Sinha, D., & Efron, D. (2005). Complementary and alternative medicine use in children with attention deficit hyperactivity disorder. *Journal of Paediatrics and Child Health, 41,* 23–26.

Sinha, Y., Silove, N., Wheeler, D., & Williams, K. (2004). Auditory integration training and other sound therapies for autism spectrum disorders [Review]. *Cochrane Database of Systematic Reviews, 1,* CD003681.

Somogyi, L., Cintron, M., & Toskes, P.P. (2000). Synthetic porcine secretin is highly accurate in pancreatic function testing in individuals with chronic pancreatitis. *Pancreas, 21,* 262–265.

Spiegel, D. (2004). Placebos in practice. *BMJ, 329,* 927–928.

Spigelblatt, L., Laine-Ammara, G., Pless, I.B., & Guyver, A. (1994). The use of alternative medicine by children. *Pediatrics, 94*(6 Pt. 1), 811–814.

Sponheim, E. (1991). [Gluten-free diet in infantile autism: A therapeutic trial]. *Tidsskrift for Den Norske Laegeforening, 111,* 704–707.

Stewart-Williams, S., & Podd, J. (2004). The placebo effect: Dissolving the expectancy versus conditioning debate [Review]. *Psychological Bulletin, 130,* 324–340.

Studdert, D.M., Eisenberg, D.M., Miller, F.H., Curto, D.A., Kaptchuk, T.J., & Brennan, T.A. (1998). Medical malpractice implications of alternative medicine. *JAMA, 280,* 1610–1615.

Sturmey, P. (2005). Secretin is an ineffective treatment for pervasive developmental disabilities: A review of 15 double-blind randomized controlled trials [Review]. *Research in Developmental Disabilities, 26,* 87–97.

Sun, J.G., Ko, C.H., Wong, V., & Sun, X.R. (2004). Randomised control trial of tongue acupuncture versus sham acupuncture in improving functional outcome in cerebral palsy. *Journal of Neurology, Neurosurgery and Psychiatry, 75,* 1054–1057.

Sun, Y., Wang, Y., Qu, X., Wang, J., Fang, J., & Zhang, L. (1994). Clinical observation and treatment of hyperkinesia in children by traditional Chinese medicine. *Journal of Traditional Chinese Medicine, 14,* 105–109.

Svedberg, L., Nordahl, G., & Lundeberg, T. (2003). Electro-acupuncture in a child with mild spastic hemiplegic cerebral palsy. *Developmental Medicine and Child Neurology, 45,* 503–504.

Tang, J.L., Zhan, S.Y., & Ernst, E. (1999). Review of randomised controlled trials of traditional Chinese medicine. *BMJ, 319,* 160–161.

Thomas, K.J., Nicholl, J.P., & Coleman, P. (2001). Use and expenditure on complementary medicine in England: A population based survey. *Complementary Therapies in Medicine, 9*(1), 2–11.

Thompson, W.G. (2000). Placebos: A review of the placebo response [Review]. *American Journal of Gastroenterology, 95,* 1637–1643.

Thornton, K.E., & Carmody, D.P. (2005). Electroencephalogram biofeedback for reading disability and traumatic brain injury [Review]. *Child and Adolescent Psychiatric Clinics of North America, 14,* 137–162.

Tian, L., Yuan, S., Ba, E., Chen, H., & Zhou, Z. (1995). Composite acupuncture treatment of mental retardation in children. *Journal of Traditional Chinese Medicine, 15,* 34–37.

Tindle, H.A., Davis, R.B., Phillips, R.S., & Eisenberg, D.M. (2005). Trends in use of complementary and alternative medicine by US adults: 1997–2002. *Alternative Therapies in Health & Medicine, 11*(1), 42–49.

Tolbert, L., Haigler, T., Waits, M.M., & Dennis, T. (1993). Brief report: Lack of response in an autistic population to a low dose clinical trial of pyridoxine plus magnesium. *Journal of Autism and Developmental Disorders, 23,* 193–199.

Torrioli, M.G., Vernacotola, S., Mariotti, P., Bianchi, E., Calvani, M., De Gaetano, A., et al. (1999). Double-blind, placebo-controlled study of L-acetylcarnitine for the treatment of hyperactive behavior in fragile X syndrome. *American Journal of Medical Genetics, 87,* 366–368.

Turner, J.A., Deyo, R.A., Loeser, J.D., Von Korff, M., & Fordyce, W.E. (1994). The importance of placebo effects in pain treatment and research [Review]. *JAMA, 271,* 1609–1614.

Uhlig, T., Merkenschlager, A., Brandmaier, R., & Egger, J. (1997). Topographic mapping of brain electrical activity in children with food-induced attention deficit hyperkinetic disorder. *European Journal of Pediatrics, 156,* 557–561.

Uma, K., Nagendra, H.R., Nagarathna, R., Vaidehi, S., & Seethalakshmi, R. (1989). The integrated approach of yoga: A therapeutic tool for mentally retarded children. A one-year controlled study. *Journal of Mental Deficiency Research, 33*(Pt. 5), 415–421.

Van Oudheusden, L.J., & Scholte, H.R. (2002). Efficacy of carnitine in the treatment of children with attention-deficit hyperactivity disorder. *Prostaglandins, Leukotrienes and Essential Fatty Acids, 67,* 33–38.

Vargas, S., & Camilli, G. (1999). A meta-analysis of research on sensory integration treatment. *American Journal of Occupational Therapy, 53,* 189–198.

Vickers, A., Ohlsson, A., Lacy, J.B., & Horsley, A. (2004). Massage for promoting growth and development of preterm and/or low birth-weight infants [Review]. *Cochrane Database of Systematic Reviews, 2,* CD000390.

Voigt, R.G., Llorente, A.M., Jensen, C.L., Fraley, J.K., Berretta, M.C., & Heird, W.C. (2001). A randomized, double-blind, placebo-controlled trial of docosahexaenoic acid supplementation in children with attention-deficit/hyperactivity disorder. *Journal of Pediatrics, 139,* 189–196.

Wachelka, D., & Katz, R.C. (1999). Reducing test anxiety and improving academic self-esteem in high school and college students with learning disabilities. *Journal of Behavior Therapy and Experimental Psychiatry, 30,* 191–198.

Walji, M., Sagaram, S., Sagaram, D., Meric-Bernstam, F., Johnson, C., Mirza, N.Q., et al. (2004). Efficacy of quality criteria to identify potentially harmful information: A cross-sectional survey of complementary and alternative medicine web sites. *Journal of Medical Internet Research, 6*(2), e21.

Wender, E.H. (1986). The food additive-free diet in the treatment of behavior disorders: A review. *Journal of Developmental and Behavioral Pediatrics, 7,* 35–42.

Whipple, J. (2004). Music in intervention for children and adolescents with autism: A meta-analysis. *Journal of Music Therapy, 41,* 90–106.

Wickstrom, G., & Bendix, T. (2000). The "Hawthorne effect"—what did the original Hawthorne studies actually show? *Scandinavian Journal of Work, Environment and Health, 26,* 363–367.

Wilson, K., Busse, J.W., Gilchrist, A., Vohra, S., Boon, H., & Mills, E. (2005). Characteristics of pediatric and adolescent patients attending a naturopathic college clinic in Canada. *Pediatrics, 115,* e338–e343.

Wilson, K.M., & Klein, J.D. (2002). Adolescents' use of complementary and alternative medicine. *Ambulatory Pediatrics, 2,* 104–110.

Yu, E.C., & Yeung, C.Y. (1987). Lead encephalopathy due to herbal medicine. *Chinese Medical Journal, 100,* 915–917.

Yussman, S.M., Ryan, S.A., Auinger, P., & Weitzman, M. (2004). Visits to complementary and alternative medicine providers by children and adolescents in the United States. *Ambulatory Pediatrics, 4,* 429–435.

Zhang, H., & Huang, J. (1990). [Preliminary study of traditional Chinese medicine treatment of minimal brain dysfunction: Analysis of 100 cases]. *Zhong Xi Yi Jie He Za Zhi [Chinese Journal of Modern Developments in Traditional Medicine], 10*(5), 278–279.

Zhou, X.J., & Zheng, K. (2005). Treatment of 140 cerebral palsied children with a combined method based on traditional Chinese medicine (TCM) and Western medicine. *Journal of Zhejiang University. Science. B, 6*(1), 57–60.

Zollman, C., & Vickers, A. (1999). What is complementary medicine? [Review]. *BMJ, 319,* 693–696.

35

Ethical Issues in Disabilities

PETER J. SMITH

The goals of this chapter are 1) to review the history of medical ethics, including outlines of the major paradigms used in the analysis of ethical dilemmas; 2) to present a new theoretical paradigm within bioethics that is based on the perspective of individuals with disabilities; and 3) to examine one current moral dilemma (genetic counseling during pregnancy). It must be stated at the onset that this chapter has been written from an early 21st-century, North American perspective. This does not imply that this perspective is in any way superior to other systems; rather, it reflects the limits of both the author of the chapter and the space restrictions inherent in this type of enterprise.

BRIEF HISTORY OF MEDICAL ETHICS

Natural Law

Within the Western tradition, medicine often is traced back to the Greek physician Hippocrates and the community gathered around him. It is not clear from current evidence who precisely created the code of conduct that is represented by the oath that bears his name (his authorship is disputed), but what is clear is that this oath and other ancient oaths and the ethical systems that they imply are as old as (or older than) the profession itself. In addition, as medical care and the societies surrounding it have developed, so have the ethical systems that inform it. Therefore, these ethics began with the rise of the desire to fashion a system that viewed reality from the anonymous perspective of a "reasonable person," which is the standard still used in the present. This move- ment led toward creating a normative view that is theoretically objective:

> One finds already in the Pre-Socratics the notion of a canonical viewpoint transcending cultures and open to all. Heraclitus (fl. 504 B.C.) held, for example, that "Thought is common to all. Men must speak with understanding and hold fast to that which is common to all as a city holds fast to its law, and much more strongly still." (Engelhardt, 1996, p. 4)

It is from this basis that subsequent ethicists developed a complex paradigm now know as *natural law*, which was a system of thinking that did not rely on overt religious or cultural beliefs, but rather drew its inspiration from the idea that the "natural" world had a predetermined order. Natural law has taken many forms over the 23 centuries of its development and has had a diverse multitude of proponents (religious and secular). Its enduring resilience has stemmed from several factors: the appeal to universal reason allows it to transcend time and geography while retaining an ability to analyze contemporary questions; its core formulations reflect a basic humanism that is genuinely egalitarian; and it has the potential for being used by both the powerful and the weak, adding an authentic check against trends toward domination and subjectivity. A basic distillation of the natural law philosophy suggests that only two simple questions are the basis of formulating all natural law arguments: "What does it mean to be a person?" and "What does it mean to be a person in society?" It presupposes not only that these questions can be answered but that reasonable people (regardless of their culture, time period, or personal experiences) will be able to come to a consensus on their answers.

All peoples, including healers, were required to refrain from "unnatural" acts and to direct their energies toward upholding and preserving natural relationships. This ancient system is still very influential today (explicitly and implicitly) for many thinkers, especially within Christian groups (and particularly within Roman Catholicism). The most commonly used term in contemporary medical ethics that is derived from natural law is the *principle of double effect*. This principle is engaged when two effects follow, one good and one evil, from an essentially good act or at least a morally neutral act. If the evil effect is unintended and not a direct result of the act, and if the good effect is proportionate to the evil effect, then the act itself is morally legitimate (McCormick, 1978).

Casuistry Versus Principlism

Two other important traditions form the foundation of contemporary medical ethics, and they can be seen as in tension. They begin with Plato and Aristotle: Plato emphasized *episteme*, a scientific form of knowledge, and Aristotle thought that *phronesis*, or practical reasoning or prudence, was most important. Plato argued against the Sophists' belief that each situation needed to be examined on its own merits, in its unique context. Plato disagreed, believing that moral knowledge was a "sub-species of formally demonstrable, or 'geometrical,' knowledge," (Jonsen & Toulmin, 1988, p. 62) treating ethics much more like a science than an art. In doing so, he depends on the existence of universal principles by which all situations can be judged, based on a timeless and unchangeable vision of the Good. Aristotle departed from his teacher on this point, believing that

Agents are compelled at every step to think out for themselves what the circumstances demand, just as happens in the arts of medicine and navigation. . . . Prudence is not concerned with universals only; it must also take cognizance of particulars, because it is concerned with conduct, and conduct has its sphere in particular circumstances. (Jonsen, 2001, p. 104)

Aristotle's position was exactly opposite of Plato's: instead of creating universal principles

to apply generally, Aristotle thought that each situation is unique and requires a unique ethical insight. In theory, Plato's descendents (to the present) generally tend toward ethical systems that are rely on deductive reasoning based on abstract principles (and are therefore named *principlists*), whereas Aristotle's descendents tend toward ethical systems that emphasize inductive reasoning based on clinical particularities (and are often described as *casuists*). In practice, most modern clinicians and ethicists utilize a hybrid approach, and very few individuals strictly follow only one of these systems; however, for the sake of clarity, they are discussed separately in this chapter.

Casuistry

Cicero, the great rhetorician, described early casuist methodology in his work, *On Duty* (106–43 B.C.). In it he "notes that general moral duties must be interpreted by considering 'what is needful in each case' " (as cited in Jonsen & Toulmin, 1988, p. 79) After Cicero, the next major casuistic development occurred in the writing of the *Penitentials* beginning in the sixth century. These writings were attempts by leaders of the Christian Church (at that time, this was the major venue in the West for such intellectual pursuits) to create paradigm cases by which priests could offer guidance appropriate to the context of the sin to parishioners who came for confession. In addition, these cases could be used by the church members to judge their own actions without aide of a priest-confessor, which would be an avenue of their own personal development of conscience. This is a change within the church thinking from a binary view of sin and faithfulness to an understanding that sins fell on a spectrum of seriousness, which was determined by situational features or context. This new approach required from each individual the application of prudence and practical reason in each circumstance. It was the intention of the authors of the *Penitentials* to aide this process of discernment. Later, Aquinas and Hegel both proposed ideas and ethics that were context dependent and required practical reasoning to discern the best course of action.

Casuistry reached its peak of influence during the 16th to 17th centuries, referred to as the period of *High Casuistry* (Jonson and Toulmin, 1988). During this period, casuistry was championed by many groups, especially the Jesuits, a new religious order within Roman Catholicism whose members held powerful positions both within the church hierarchy and within the rising apparatuses of secular governments. Because of their positions of authority within secular institutions, the Jesuits were faced with problems that could not as easily be brought under classical church law. Casuistry emerged as a favorite approach for them because a case-sensitive approach allowed for flexibility within the complexities of an increasingly multicultural world.

The longevity of casuistry gives evidence that this system of thought is a powerful method within the field of ethics. The Aristotelian emphasis on particularity has also generated a long history outside of ethics—the development of English common law (which forms the basis for American law) is based on this style of thinking, and the skills recognized in medicine as *clinical expertise* draw on this ancient tradition—however, it has long passed its zenith of influence. Although casuistry has had an important history and its legacy remains subtly influential, it is not generally thought of (or taught) explicitly in most contemporary professional education programs in health care.

Principlism

Within the contemporary discussions of bioethical issues in Western liberal society, there is no doubt that the dominating system of thought is based on Plato's *episteme*. Contemporary mainstream bioethics is founded on two assumptions. First, ethics is brought to focus at points of tension or conflict, usually represented through use of real or theoretical problematic situations, relying on only minimal conceptions of what constitutes health, society, and common interest:

Standard bioethics, by which I mean the family of secular approaches that are dominant in the English-speaking world, is a product of modernity, and the moral task of modernity is to resolve conflicts between competing interests in order to secure social cooperation without appeal to robust views of the good. The agenda of standard bioethics, at the risk of oversimplification, follows accordingly: for every new issue that arises in biomedical research and care its task is to safeguard individual autonomy, calculate potential risks and harms, and determine whether or not a just distribution will follow. (McKenny, 1997, p. 8)

Second, the moral dilemmas that are described are best resolved by objective application of universal principles by thoughtful and preferably disinterested actors. Although there is much debate and discussion about what constitutes a moral dilemma, what are the universal principles that ought to be applied, and how these general principles become relevant for the particularities of each individual situation, there has been consensus in the overall approach of principle-driven bioethics. This rise to preeminence and the lasting reign of principlism as the dominant paradigm is due in large part to its clarity and ease of use in communication (to other professionals, students, and the general public). In addition, its deductive nature suggests its similarity to empirical sciences and therefore it is often seen as "more true" than inductive or "softer" sciences. Most important, it is often tremendously helpful in confused situations with many conflicting actors and several important outcomes in the balance. Previously, the dominant paradigm in medicine was based on benevolent paternalism, a system that often neglected to account for the differing perspectives of the many individuals involved in a situation and too heavily relied on rigid structures of authority. Although it has been criticized by many different groups, principlism has supplanted the old paternalism and now is the primary method that is currently taught at professional schools for health care clinicians.

The most influential text used for teaching the system, *Principles of Biomedical Ethics* by Beauchamp and Childress (now in its fifth edition), has certainly evolved with time and in response to critics; however, the central claims remain the same:

The common morality contains a set of moral norms that includes principles that are basic for biomedical ethics. . . . Most classical ethical theories include these principles in some form, and traditional medical codes presuppose at least some of them. . . . The four clusters [of moral principles] are (1) *respect for autonomy* (a norm of respecting the decision-making capacities of autonomous persons), (2) *nonmaleficence* (a norm of avoiding the causation of harm), (3) *beneficence* (a group of norms for providing benefits and balancing benefits against risks and costs), and (4) *justice* (a group of norms for distributing benefits, risks, and costs fairly). (2001, p. 12; italics in original)

In theory, these four principles ought to be weighed equally when they are seen as being in conflict in any given dilemma. In reality, given the underlying assumptions of the liberal society into which they have been promoted, the first principle, autonomy, consistently and effectively trumps all of the others. This has been so obviously the case that Beauchamp and Childress felt compelled in their most recent edition to highlight that this state of affairs was not their original attempt: "Although we begin our discussion of principles of biomedical ethics with respect for autonomy, our order of presentation does not imply that this principle has priority over all other principles" (2001, p. 57).

Their frustrations with the current use of their system, and the problems that ensue from this interpretation, suggest that their system may be "inadequate" to the contemporary situation. Ironically, this inadequacy is not due to the fact that their system has assumptions that are different from those of the larger society (the problem with the earlier systems that they criticize), but rather because it fits all too well into the orientations and desires of the larger society. In other words, their proposals were initially an important corrective to a system that had lost its vitality, but now it seems that their system has become a product of society (rather than a corrective to it). In addition, whereas principlism has clearly shown remarkable skill at abstracting generalities from particulars, it has proven much less adept when working in the opposite direction (i.e., when attempting to provide guidance regarding particular situations by drawing on generalities). The current situation has become one in which principlism reigns because it suits the needs and purposes of teachers, journals, and

institutions while offering little succor to actual patients, family members, and clinicians. This reality has begun to be addressed, even in the journals that benefit from principlism's dominance, as noted by Frank (1998):

I want to advance the stronger claim that in these books we can find the beginnings of a yet-unarticulated ethic. Not an ethic of medicine and professional behavior, but an ethic of illness that addresses both the professional provision of treatment and the experience of being ill. This ethic may exemplify what Australian philosopher and physician Paul Komesaroff calls "microethics." Joining those who have objected to principlist formulations of ethics, Komesaroff writes, "The job of the clinician cannot be formulated in terms of broad principles, bioethical or otherwise, but only as a series of practical tasks" (Komesaroff, 1995, p. 62). These tasks include settling upon "the most appropriate way to approach the patient, to talk with him, to allay his fears, and to establish the common ground on which mutual decisions can be taken" (Komesaroff, p. 63). Thus instead of a principlist bioethics that is "unable to provide an adequate account of day-to-day decision making in medicine, as a result of which it cannot provide any substantial guidance for medical practice" (p. 65), Komesaroff calls for a microethics concerned with "what happens in every interaction between every doctor and every patient" (Frank, 1998, p. 68).

Finally, the greatest problem with principlism, especially regarding the purposes of this chapter, is that it fails to include appropriate provisions for individuals who are unable to exercise independent autonomy and therefore is inadequate for anyone interested in a bioethic that considers individuals with disabilities, especially those whose disability affects their cognition. "People or potential people with intellectual disability are most likely to be rendered, even on biological determination alone, profoundly irrelevant or disqualified within bioethical conversations because they are deemed incapable of being rational, competent, independent beings" (Clapton, 2002, p. 1). Clearly, this is inadequate. To use an example that will take on particular importance in the ensuing discussion, one of the classic texts of contemporary bioethics states that individuals are assumed to have

Personal autonomy, [which] is, at a minimum, self-rule that is free from both controlling interference by others and from limitations. . . . The autonomous individual acts freely in accordance with a self-chosen plan, analogous to the way an independent government manages its territories and sets its policies. (Beauchamp & Childress, 2001, p. 58)

Liberal theorists also came to realize that the society must promote egalitarianism (to enable more widespread competence in decision making) as a secondary principle to support the primary goal, which remains focused on personal freedoms, defined as exercises in choice.

It is critical to note that this framework is based on the definition that *personhood is determined by an ability to choose*. This conception will encounter its greatest difficulties in those situations in which ability to choose becomes disenabled or is intrinsically limited:

People with mental disabilities are lacking to a greater or lesser extent the powers of reason and free will. Since these are the powers that bring substance to the core values of the liberal view on public morality, mentally disabled people never acquire full moral standing in this view. This is because its moral community is constituted by "persons" and these, in turn, are constituted by the powers of reason and free will. (Reinders, 2000, pp. 15–16)

Over time, liberal society has responded to these criticisms regarding membership and has greatly expanded its definition of *citizen*; however, it has not been able to expand this definition beyond the strict limits that are inherent in its conception of citizens as competent choice makers and therefore sees any who do not fit into this rubric as, by definition, defective and needing to be fixed.

In addition, one of liberal society's foundational assumptions is that individuals are inherently in competition, and this is a good that should be encouraged. Consequently, it is particularly adept at helping to referee disputes that arise within a competitive, pluralistic community comprising articulate individuals who are included within liberal society's definition of citizenship. Another consequence is that liberal society has not been fertile ground for the growth of a communitarian spirit and in fact has specifically sought to define itself as distinct from systems that show these tendencies. Because of its primary and exalted emphasis on individual liberties, it has no room for defining or promoting a *common good*. Rather, the tradi-

tional emphasis on individual liberty has led to the liberal convention that any person is free to act in any way that does not impinge on the freedom of another individual or group of individuals, like the image of protecting the boundaries of a country.

PROPOSAL OF "EXCEPTIONAL ETHICS"

Scholarly examinations of the role of differentness, especially focusing on the differentness due to disability, started in the latter half of the 20th century (Davis, 1997; Linton, 1998). Recently, these preliminary investigations have developed into an emerging discipline within the academic community:

Over the last three decades, two intellectual disciplines have emerged alongside paediatric rehabilitation. The first is Disability Studies (DS), a multidisciplinary approach to understanding disabilities, including but not limited to aesthetics, anthropology, archeology, economics, education, ethics, law, literature, philosophy, and history. Greater than the sum of its parts, DS encompasses these diverse methodologies to describe better the social and personal implications of disabilities. Centers and research units for DS have arisen around the globe, with scholars generating many challenging insights. (Schalick, 2001, p. 91)

Although a journal has arisen within the field of disability studies relating to religion and spirituality (*Journal of Religion, Disability & Health* published by Haworth Pastoral Press; http://www.haworthpress.com/store/product.asp?sku=J095) and there are several articulate voices within the field whose interests are in ethics (e.g., Asch, 1989), there has not yet been an attempt to formulate a theory of bioethics from within disability studies; however, there has begun to be an emerging sense that a new type of bioethics needs to be constructed: one that does not characterize individuals with disabilities as problems that need solutions but rather as helpful teachers with important insights, especially with insights into the shortcomings of contemporary bioethics. As Clapton noted, "I argue that the relationship between bioethics and intellectual disability must be confronted to shift ethical understanding from the presumed tragedy of impaired bodies, to consider the impact of impaired theorizing'' (2002, p. 4).

Defining the Terms

When attempting to construct a new paradigm for bioethics, the importance of language cannot be overstated. Therefore, the first step will be to attempt to offer a workable definition of the term *exceptional*. It is important to note that there are many terms that could be chosen to describe the individuals whose perspective will ground and center the endeavor. Definitions of *differentness* and *otherness* not only can be crucial to the ethical systems of cultures, but can also play a huge role in shaping and structuring every aspect of the society, especially influencing aesthetics and art, ideas regarding family unit structure, taboos regarding incest, and customs surrounding all the many daily transactions between individuals. Of course, the language that has often surrounded discussions of otherness has frequently been cast in particularly negative images, displaying undercurrents of fear, anger, confusion, and even disgust or hatred. Within the field of disability studies, one of the most important initial tasks has been to point out terminology of derision (e.g., *defective child*) and replace it with more appropriate usage (e.g., *child with an anomaly*). Unfortunately, terms that initially do not carry negative meanings can become so imbued with unpleasant and unwanted connotations with usage that their original meanings are almost entirely obscured. Therefore, it must be recognized that any term chosen now may eventually come to have currently unforeseen connotations or implications in the future.

Forming an Ethical System

It is the underlying goal of this chapter to begin the process of seeing the work of ethics not as impeded by the difficulties of accounting for differentness, but rather as enhanced by the adoption of a perspective centered on otherness. The concept of *exceptionality* is a familiar one to most English speakers and generally carries positive (or neutral) overtones. It was introduced into the field of disability studies in the address by Allen C. Crocker to the Society

of Developmental and Behavioral Pediatrics on September 28, 1997:

> Most of us handle variation, or exceptionality, on what might be called a "dose-related" basis. In some measured element, whether it be something like IQ, or height, or visual acuity, or whatever number you wish to use, if the individual under discussion deflects by one standard deviation, we commonly refer to this as a "borderline" state. We react to it good-naturedly, and very often take the person to lunch. If, on the other hand, the individual varies by two standard deviations, we now acknowledge by convention, in most of our fields, that this is abnormality. Our response there, very often, is that our service mode kicks in and we begin to think of how we are going to affect or ally ourselves with that person in a more lasting way. If the individual we are discussing varies by four or five standard deviations, in this arbitrary item that we are referring to, this is what might be called "assertive abnormality." Here is where we very commonly become personally uncertain. This is true low incidence, and it will be with that area that a great deal of the matter in discussion will be concerned. (Crocker, 1998, p. 300)

Several significant points are contained within this proposal. First, it must be remembered that all attempts to differentiate between individuals, *by the very nature of the task*, ignore shared humanity. Therefore, every measurement ought to be considered as arbitrary and incomplete. Of course, the reification of abstract classification systems is so common that it can be imperceptible for those who operate within the conceit. The use of the conjoined term *defective child* instantly causes the hearer to focus on *defective*, which implies differentness, rather than *child*, which points to the overwhelming majority of facets of the individual that are shared with the hearer. Second, through the process of dividing peoples through these arbitrary distinctions, the entrenched classifications diminish the likelihood of sharing across boundaries. In essence, some current paradigms sharply restrict ideas of personhood and emphasize competition, while the new model hopes both to encourage the rediscovery of broad diversity within the conception of "people" and to stimulate renewed forms of basic human cooperation.

Third, by choosing the term *exceptional*, an emphasis is placed on those individuals who are "assertively abnormal." The simple fact is that they are rare and therefore *necessarily require* a recalibration of expectations and assumptions. This shift will be required whenever they are encountered within statistical comparisons, whenever they resist definition by law or public policy, and whenever they bump up against personal attitudes that had been formed in their absence. By definition, a system of ethics that is centered on exceptionality will need to be flexible and dynamic and will find unusual confrontations to be enriching rather than detracting: "We and the parents, faced with difference in a young person, are obliged to reset our priorities, our reference frame, and to use new vision" (Crocker, 1998, p. 300). Health care is increasingly faced with conflicts that have "never been seen before" and therefore needs an ethical framework with just this type of adaptability. Simply stated, individuals with disabilities prophetically remind all observers that *it is in the times of vulnerability and being served that strong bonds between people are formed.* For example, who can doubt the love of a parent, spouse, or friend who has served during times of illness, suffering, old age, or infancy? Ironically, exceptional people are blessed with the paradoxical talents of both asserting their uniqueness and insisting on their connectedness within their very nature.

COMPARING METHODS

Principlist's Approach to an Ethical Dilemma

There has been both a substantial and ongoing increase in the basic understandings of human genetics, including the Human Genome Project, as well as tremendous changes in the technology that surrounds the augmentation, manipulation, and diagnostic techniques of human reproduction. Because of this combination of scientific knowledge and technical expertise, there is a rapidly increasing sense of both real and potential control over the initiation, progress, and outcomes of human reproduction. One aspect of this is the increasing ability of potential parents to screen themselves and their gametes for irregularities, including changes in DNA patterns that are consistent with clinically relevant human disorders. Simply put, there are more and more

inherited conditions whose precise gene is known, allowing laboratories to identify (at increasingly early stages) the presence of the irregularity. Coupling this knowledge with the use of either abortion or prevention of implantation, it is (at least theoretically) possible that conditions with known gene sequences can therefore be avoided. The condition most often cited in this discussion is Down syndrome.

This possibility has generally been promoted within Western societies as a sign of tremendous progress and has been widely celebrated. In the most extreme form of exuberance over the possibility of scientific control over intrinsic features of human existence, some authors have already begun arguing that, in the near future, parents who do not avail themselves of this technology will be considered negligent parents:

This reasoning leads me to state with precision the moral norm I want to defend: In the absence of adequate justifying reasons, a child is morally wronged when he/she is knowingly, deliberately, or negligently brought into being with a health status likely to result in significantly greater disability or suffering, or significantly reduced life options relative to the other children with whom he/she will grow up. It is this reasonably expected health condition and the level of life prospects of others in the child's birth cohort, not the state of nonexistence, that is the appropriate benchmark for assessing harm in reproductive decision making. I am also now in a position to state the specific obligations of parents (and, by extension, those who assist them in effecting their reproductive choices) to their children. I contend that: Parents have a *prima facie* obligation not to bring a child into being deliberately or negligently with a health status likely to result in significantly reduced life options relative to the other children with whom he/she will grow up. (Green, 1997, p. 10)

In a similar vein, Brock has coined the term *wrongful handicap* and has also embraced a future dominated by choice and control:

The Human Genome Project will produce information permitting increasing opportunities to prevent genetically transmitted harms, most of which will be compatible with a life worth living, through avoiding conception or terminating a pregnancy. Failure to prevent these harms when it is possible for parents to do so without substantial burdens or costs to themselves or others are what I call "wrongful handicaps." (1995, p. 269)

Of course, these conclusions are based on liberal society's very narrow definition of personhood, which emphasizes choice and believes that disability is a problem, as well as very narrow conceptions of a "life worth living." Although they are extreme examples, they do point to the mood and direction of the discussion in this issue, which emphasizes control and equates all differentness with needless suffering.

Having looked at the mainstream (a.k.a., principlism) approach, the next step is to trace how the new exceptional ethic might respond. Preliminary work in this area has already begun to take shape. There are voices from many perspectives, including feminism (Asch & Geller, 1996), disability studies (International League of Societies for Persons with Mental Handicaps, 1994), philosophy (Reinders, 2000), and theology (Hauerwas, 1986), that have called into question both the underlying assumptions of this project of technological advance and the potential outcomes thought to be possible. The next section briefly reviews three texts that are part of this movement.

Short Literature Review

Prenatal Testing and Disability Rights (Parens & Asch, 2000) was the product of a 2-year Hastings Center project to "explore the disability rights critique of prenatal testing for genetic disability" (p. ix). Because it is an official publication of the largest and best-known bioethics center in the country, it carries significant weight in the field. In creating the panel who eventually became the chapter authors, the Hastings Center employed a cross-section of academics from diverse disciplines and with different life experiences (with and without personal disabilities). It is a text worth reading, and it is too complex to summarize quickly except to say that the only major point on which all participants agreed was that widespread ignorance and discrimination against people with disabilities exists and is an important factor to consider in ethical deliberations on this topic.

Testing Women, Testing the Fetus, by Rayna Rapp, was published in 2000 after a long and often difficult process of data collection. Rapp is a feminist activist and anthropologist, who herself underwent amniocentesis and ultimately chose an abortion after her child was diagnosed with Down syndrome. It was this personal experience that stimulated this research. She employed the common technique in qualitative research of participant observation. Ultimately in this research, the sites studied included medical school classes, labs, prenatal testing centers, and meetings of individuals with disabilities, and interviews with many, diverse women were conducted. This complex and rich ethnographic study is worth reading for anyone in this field, and I think that it is fair to summarize it with the following quotation: "At once conscripts to techno-scientific regimes of quality control and normalization, and explorers of the ethical territory its presence produces, contemporary pregnant women have become our moral philosophers of the private" (2000, p. 306).

Michael Berube is both a literature professor and the father of Jamie, born in 1991 with Down syndrome. His autobiographical book, *Life as We Know It,* is a bestseller in the field of neurodevelopmental disabilities. In it, he argues persuasively that there are some areas of human life in which individuals must be free from political coercion and must be given the private legal space to make exceedingly difficult life-and-death decisions. For him, a larger concern than the abortion issue is the risk that children with disabilities like his Jamie will come to be regarded by society as unproductive citizens and therefore unaffordable luxuries. By writing about Jamie, he hopes to correct that notion, arguing that such children can become productive; this is a way of making Jamie's claims on society loudly and clearly.

Interwoven with this story of Jamie's physical and cognitive development in the first 4 years of his life are Berube's discussions of the changing laws concerning the rights of individuals with disabilities and the various ways in which children with disabilities are educated. He gives an especially lucid picture of the variability and inconsistency with which individual states handle special education and of the incentives for school districts to segregate students by mental or physical ability. By raising questions about what it means to be human and by showing us that his son is indeed fully human, Berube helps us to understand what it is to be a person with Down syndrome:

> Representations matter. Our world, as William Wordsworth once put it, is that which our eyes and ears half create and half perceive; and it is because Wordsworth is right that we need to deliberate the question of how we will represent the range of human variation to ourselves. How we understand people with Down syndrome will become part of what it means to have Down syndrome. (1996, p. 206)

CONCLUSION

Ethical inquiry is frequently misunderstood as the pursuit of the "right" answers to tough questions. Medical ethics is often erroneously thought to have started in the 20th century. Instead, ethics represents an area of thought and debate as old as civilization itself, which attempts to help people live together more happily and together draw deeper meaning from their lives. Currently, medical ethics in the Western world is dominated by paradigms that emphasize a very limited understanding of personhood, centered on individual liberties. People with intellectual disabilities are poorly served by these systems. An exceptional ethic would change this situation for the better by emphasizing the universality of dependence and the need for vulnerability for growth and full self-actualization. It would mandate respect for all humans and would not seek limits on personhood; however, this respect would not imply general answers to questions that necessarily depend on contextual details. It would, it is hoped, be hopeful and encouraging.

REFERENCES

Asch, A. (1989). Reproductive technology and disability. In S. Cohen & N. Taub (Eds.), *Reproductive laws for the 1990s* (pp. 69–124). Clifton, NJ: Humana Press.

Asch, A., & Geller, G. (1996). Feminism, bioethics, and genetics. In S.M. Wolf (Ed.), *Feminism and bioethics* (pp. 318–350). New York: Oxford University Press.

Beauchamp, T.L., & Childress, J.F. (2001). *Principles of biomedical ethics* (5th ed.). New York: Oxford University Press.

Berube, M. (1996). *Life as we know it.* New York: Vintage Books.

Brock, D.W. (1995). The non-identity problem and genetic harms: The case of wrongful handicaps. *Bioethics, 9,* 269–275.

Clapton, J. (2002). Tragedy and catastrophe: Contentious discourse of ethics and disability. *Newsletter of the Network on Ethics and Intellectual Disability,* 6(2), 1, 3–4.

Crocker, A.C. (1998). Exceptionality. *Developmental and Behavioral Pediatrics, 19,* 300–305.

Davis, L.J. (Ed.). (1997). *The disabilities studies reader.* London: Routledge.

Engelhardt, H.T. (1996). *The foundations of bioethics* (2nd ed.). New York: Oxford University Press.

Frank, A.W. (1998). First-person microethics: Deriving principles from below. *Hastings Center Report,* 28(4), 37–42.

Green, R.M. (1997). Parental autonomy and the obligation not to harm one's child genetically. *Journal of Law, Medicine & Ethics, 25,* 5–15.

Hauerwas, S.M. (1986). Suffering the retarded: Should we prevent retardation? In *Suffering presence: Theological reflections on medicine, the mentally retarded, and the church* (pp. 159–81). Notre Dame, IN: University of Notre Dame Press.

International League of Societies for Persons with Mental Handicaps. (1994). *Just technology? From principles to practice in bioethical issues.* Toronto, Ontario: Roeher Institute.

Jonsen, A.R. (2001). Casuistry. In J. Sugarman & D.P. Sulmasy (Eds.), *Methods in medical ethics* (pp. 104–125). Washington, DC: Georgetown University Press.

Jonsen, A.R., & Toulmin, S. (1988). *The abuse of casuistry.* Berkeley: University of California Press.

Komesaroff, P.A. (1995). From bioethics to microethics: Ethical debate and clinical medicine. In P.A. Komesaroff (Ed.), *Troubled bodies: Critical perspectives on postmodernism, medical ethics, and the body.* Durham, NC: Duke University Press.

Linton, S. (1998). *Claiming disability: Knowledge and identity.* New York: New York University Press.

McCormick, R.A. (1978). The principle of double effect. In *How brave a new world?* (pp. 431–447). Washington, DC: Georgetown University Press.

McKenny, G.P. (1997). *To relieve the human condition: Bioethics, technology, and the body.* Albany, NY: State University of New York Press.

Parens, E., & Asch, A. (Eds.). (2000). *Prenatal testing and disability rights.* Washington, DC: Georgetown University Press.

Rapp, R. (2000). *Testing women, testing the fetus.* New York: Routledge.

Reinders, H.S. (2000). *The future of the disabled in liberal society: An ethical analysis.* Notre Dame, IN: University of Notre Dame Press.

Schalick, W.O. (2001). Children, disability and rehabilitation in history. *Pediatric Rehabilitation, 4,* 91–95.

36

Legislative Directives and Trends

ANN W. COX

At the midpoint of the first decade of the 21st century, individuals with developmental disabilities, their families, and the professionals who support them are emerging from a four-decade period of restructuring in the field of developmental disabilities. Since the 1960s, the theories that provided the rationale for practice in the field have changed. Beliefs, theories, and practices continually, but gradually, are revised. This occurs within an overall conceptual framework, or paradigm, that provides stability around which change emerges (Kuhn, 1970).

As paradigm change proceeds and becomes more accepted, the concepts and theories that influence practice commensurate with the older paradigm gradually shift or are replaced with different and newer theories, concepts, and practices. This gradual process is influenced by new knowledge and by new ways of thinking. Research in the field of developmental disability indeed both is framed by a prevailing paradigm and drives a paradigm toward change or shifts in practice (Bradley, 1994; Hagner, 2000; Kuhn, 1970).

An abundance of evidence supports a paradigm shift in the field of developmental disabilities. For example, our understanding of the resilience of the human condition has moved us from a focus on the deficit model toward one that celebrates strengths and abilities—one that is tolerant of and, indeed celebrates, the diversity among us (Hagner, 2000). From the basic sciences, the mapping of the genes located on the human genome, only a dream in the past, is now complete. Proteomics and pharmacogenetics are rapidly emerging as methodologies on which effective treatments for many diseases will be based (Natvig, 2005).

Less obvious is the way a paradigm shift begins to influence the way in which disability is viewed. Advocates and providers now describe disability as a natural experience for which accommodation is required. Thus, the words used to address individuals with disability and their needs have gradually changed. Today, it is considered "best" practice to use person-first language, to talk more about supports than services, and to emphasize individual and family choice and control in decision making.

In addition to new ways to involve and respect the desires of those with disabilities and their families, federal and state policies have changed as a result of this evolving paradigm. Legislation and legislative mandates that guarantee civil rights and protections for people with disabilities, that require active participation by the family and individual with disabilities in decision making, and that redirect resources to community programs have influenced professional practices. Each flurry of new or amended legislation has been sparked either by new knowledge, strong grass roots advocacy, legal action, or some combination of these factors. Health professionals have contributed to and supported much of this progression and continue to shape the direction of services and supports for children and adults with disabilities.

By understanding the evolution of legislation related to developmental disabilities in the United States, the practitioner gains a perspective as to the genesis of current developmental disability policy, legislative mandates, and insight into future directions (van Dyck, 2003). So, then, how have paradigms associated with the field of developmental disabilities changed? How have these theoretical shifts influenced or been influenced by legislation? What mandates have been associated with key legislation? And what lies ahead?

PARADIGM AND LEGISLATIVE PARALLELS

Paradigms typically undergo a gradual shift. These shifts or phases are times when both paradigms thrive together and have adherents of each competing view. Over time, more and more people in leadership positions are persuaded of the new paradigm's value. The old paradigm is eventually supported by only a handful of people who remain resistant to change and then is abandoned entirely (Hagner, 2000).

As with paradigm shifts, legislation and its accompanying mandates evolve. This occurs in response to political, economic, scientific, and philosophical changes. Interesting parallels can be seen between the paradigm phases in the field of developmental disabilities and developmental disability legislation during these times. Figure 36.1 depicts these phases of change that have occurred as the developmental disability paradigm has shifted, the general periods of time in which these phases influenced practice, and the seminal legislation that occurred during these time periods.

A discussion of the phases of change in the evolution of the developmental disabilities paradigm and the federal legislation passed during these phases is provided in the next sections. The legislation that is presented during each of these phases either has supported the basic assumptions of the prevailing paradigm or has elements that signal shifting beliefs. The mandates that accompany the legislation and that influence practice are summarized in this discussion.

BENCHMARK LEGISLATION IN THE EARLY 20TH CENTURY

Prior to the developmental disabilities paradigm shift, which roughly began in the 1960s, two legislative benchmarks of the early 20th century set the tone for the federal government's role in providing services and income assistance for individuals with disabilities for the next several decades. These two legislative initiatives, the Social Security Act (SSA) of 1935 (PL 74-271) and the Vocational Rehabilitation Act of 1943 (PL 78-113), were the first federal legislation to address unmet needs of children and adults with developmental disabilities.

Social Security Act of 1935

An early legislative benchmark was the passage of the SSA and its many provisions in 1935. Although originally focusing on the needs of people with physical disabilities, subsequent amendments to the SSA in 1950 (PL 81-734) expanded its program Aid to the Permanently and Totally Disabled to allow people with severe intellectual disabilities to qualify for income maintenance. The SSA Amendments of 1956 (PL 84-880) authorized payments for adults with disabilities that began in childhood, including those with intellectual disabilities (Kastner & Walsh, 2005). Children with disabilities seldom qualified for assistance under this program until much later.

Title V of the SSA provided services that targeted the reduction of infant mortality and improved the health of mothers and children. The program emphasized reducing the incidence of intellectual and other disabilities caused by complications associated with childbearing. One component, the state Crippled Children's Service (CCS) program, or Part 2 of Title V, provided medical and related health services to "handicapped" children. The CCS program was the first U.S. program of medical care for children with disabilities and was funded through federal grants-in-aid to the states (van Dyck, 2003).

Children who were originally eligible for medical services through the CCS program were underserved children younger than 21 years of age with an organic disease, defect, or condition that might hinder growth and development. Initially, children with intellectual disabilities were not served through the CCS program; however, in 1946 children with cerebral palsy and epilepsy became eligible, and by the late 1950s amendments to the act allowed

Paradigms	Legislation/policy	1960s	1970s	1980s	1990s	2000s
		Facilities paradigm Institutional reform (separate from community) ------>	**Program paradigm** Deinstitutionalization (physically in community) ------>		**Support paradigm** Community membership (part of the community) ------>	
	Social Security Act of 1935 (PL 74-271)					
	Title V (MCH state grants and Crippled Children's Services)------------------------			1981: MCH Block Grant		
	1965: Title XVIII (Medicare)--1972: SSDI-----					
	1965: Title XIX (Medicaid)--1971: ICFs/MR--1974: SSI----1981: HCBS Waivers--1989: EPSDT--1990: SSI eligibility redefined for children					
	CSHCN------------------------1989: CSHCN expanded and changed direction------					
	1997: Title XXI (SCHIP)--2001: CMS systems change					
	Vocational Rehabilitation Act of 1943 (PL 113)------------------------1973: Rehabilitation Act (PL 93-112, Section 504)					
	1961: President's Panel on Mental Retardation					
	1963: MRFs and CMHCs Construction Act (PL 88-164)------1975: **DD Assistance and Bill of Rights Act (PL 94-103)** ------------2000: Amendments (PL 106-402)--					
	1978: Independent Living Centers------------1992 (PL 102-569)--1998 (PL 105-220, Section 508)--					
	1965: **Elementary and Secondary Education Act (PL 89-10)** ----1975: special education----1987: early intervention--1990: IDEA----1997: IDEA amendments---- (PL 94-142) (PL 99-457) (PL 101-476) (PL 105-17)					
	1988: Tech Act (PL 100-407)					
	1990: **Americans with Disabilities Act (PL 101-336)**					
	2001: No Child Left Behind Act (PL 107-110)----					
	2004: IDEA 2004 (PL 108-446)--------					
	1999: Olmstead Decision					
	2001: New Freedom Initiative					

Figure 36.1. Legislative directives and themes in the modern era of services and supports. (*Note:* The paradigm terminology is derived from the work of Thomas Kuhn [1970], as applied by Bradley [1994] and Hagner [2000].) (*Key:* CMHC, Community Mental Health Centers; CMS, Centers for Medicare & Medicaid Services; CSHCN, children with special health care needs; EPSDT, Early Periodic Screening, Diagnosis, and Treatment; HCBS, Home and Community-Based Services; ICFs/MR, Intermediate Care Facilities for the Mentally Retarded; IDEA, Individuals with Disabilities Education Act; IDEA 2004, Individuals with Disabilities Education Improvement Act; MCH, Maternal and Child Health; MRFs, Mental Retardation Facilities; SCHIP, State Children's Health Insurance Program; SSDI, Social Security Disability Income; SSI, Supplemental Security Income.)

expansion of services, at state option, to children with other disabilities.

Vocational Rehabilitation Act

In 1943, the original Vocational Rehabilitation Act of 1918 (PL 65-178) was amended to include, for the first time, services for individuals with intellectual disabilities. The services provided through this program included training, guidance, placement, and prosthetic appliances, all emphasizing reentry into employment. The Rehabilitation Act, as it has come to be known, has been reauthorized and amended and remains an active program serving individuals with disabilities today.

Other Pre-1960 Federal Initiatives

Funds also were earmarked for intellectual disability research and training programs and for intellectual disability diagnostic clinics through the Department of Health, Education and Welfare (DHEW). By 1957, 15 intellectual disability diagnostic clinics were in operation throughout the nation. Recommendations of the DHEW Appropriations Subcommittee and activities of the Committee to Study Mental Retardation within DHEW led to revisions in the Hospital Survey and Construction Act of 1946 (Hill-Burton Act; PL 79-725) via the Hospital and Medical Facilities Amendments of 1964 (PL 88-443) that expanded funding for the construction and expansion of public institutions for the "feeble minded." All departments in DHEW earmarked funds for consultation, training, and research benefiting children with intellectual disabilities. This expansion in services for children with intellectual disabilities was the result of advocacy by parent organizations such as the Association for Retarded Children (now The Arc of the United States) and the United Cerebral Palsy Association (now United Cerebral Palsy) (Biehl, 1996; Kastner & Walsh, 2005).

As the 1950s drew to a close, federal involvement in the field was directed toward 1) supporting schools, separate from public education, for children with intellectual disabilities; 2) creating more humane conditions in residential institutions; and 3) developing ad-

ditional residential capacity within institutions, with some community capacity through specialized health services.

PHASE I: INSTITUTIONAL REFORM AND THE FACILITIES PARADIGM, 1960s TO MID-1970s

Valerie Bradley (1994) described the developmental disability paradigm shift that began in the 1960s in terms of phases. In the first phase, called the *era of institutional reform,* the governing norms were primarily custodial, and the objective was to separate people who were sick and vulnerable from the rest of society. The basic assumptions during this period were that people with disabilities were dependent and in need of custodial care, frequently in separate residential facilities, because of permanent deficits in abilities. These beliefs are reflected in the legislation of the time (Table 36.1). The predominance of institutionalization began to wane, and, in the mid-1970s, the era ended with the advent of developmental/behavioral models. These models grew out of a body of research showing the inadequacies of institutional care and supported the shift toward institutional reform, deinstitutionalization, and specialized programming (Bradley, 1994, 1978).

Initiatives and Legislation During Phase I

In 1961 and only 9 months into his term as president, John F. Kennedy established the President's Panel on Mental Retardation, thus beginning what some have coined the *modern era of federal concern for individuals with disabilities* (Braddock & Parish, 2002). Concerned about the plight of children and adults with intellectual disabilities and encouraged by parent advocates, the Panel's work resulted in 95 broad-based recommendations that ultimately formed the basis of today's federal assistance programs in the field. Issues related to health, education, employment, residential services, prevention, research, and training were addressed through congressional earmarks and special provisions.

In 1963, Congress passed Title I of the Mental Retardation Facilities and Community

Table 36.1. Facilities paradigm: separate from the community

Assumptions	Related legislation
Custodial approach	Social Security Act of 1935 (PL 74-271)
	Title V: Crippled Children's Services program (1935; PL 74-271)
	Title XVIII: Medicare (1965; PL 89-97)
Deficit model	Social Security Disability Income (1972; PL 92-336)
	Title XIX: Medicaid (1965; PL 89-97)
	Intermediate Care Facilities for the Mentally Retarded (1971; PL 92-5)
Dependent	Supplemental Security Income (implemented in 1974 as part of PL 92-336)
	Vocational Rehabilitation Act of 1943 (PL 78-113); Rehabilitation Act of 1973, Section 504 (PL 93-112)
Segregated	Elementary and Secondary Education Act of 1965 (PL 89-10)
	Mental Retardation Facilities and Community Mental Health Centers (1963; PL 88-164)
	Developmental Disabilities Services and Facilities (1970; PL 91-517)

Note: The assumptions that underpin efficacy for the facilities paradigm included a *custodial approach* related to the belief 1) that developmental disabilities represent a *deficit* in function that could not be altered; 2) that, because of this deficit, individuals with disabilities were and would remain *dependent* on others; and 3) that, for their protection and safety, individuals with developmental disabilities should be separated (*segregated*) from the rest of society.

Related legislation refers to legislation that was passed during the prevailing paradigm.

Mental Health Centers Construction Act (PL 88-164) and authorized funds to support the development of several hundred specialty facilities for the diagnosis, treatment, education, training, and care of children with intellectual disabilities. Attention to the other recommendations of the Panel resulted in 1) substantial increases for the Title V Maternal and Child Health (MCH) program of the SSA and expansion of the related CCS program; 2) construction of clinical centers (known as University Affiliated Facilities) created to demonstrate state-of-the-art services and to train health and human service professionals in assessment and management of individuals with intellectual disabilities; and 3) construction of research facilities (known as Mental Retardation Research Centers) intended to study the prevention of intellectual disabilities and associated conditions.

Social Security Act Reauthorization and Amendments
Both Title XVIII (Medicare) and Title XIX (Medicaid) of the SSA were passed in 1965 (PL 89-97). In 1971 (PL 92-5), funding for Intermediate Care Facilities for the Mentally Retarded (ICFs/MR) was added to Medicaid legislation and enabled states to obtain federal funding for institutional services for people with intellectual disabilities (Silverstein, 2000). Social Security Disability Income (SSDI) was passed as an amendment to Medicare (Title XVIII) via the SSA Amendments of 1972 (PL 92-336), creating a new income funding source for working individuals who become disabled. In 1974, Medicaid created the Supplemental Security Income (SSI) program, addressing first the needs of low-income adults with disabilities, then those of eligible children with disabilities. Income assistance and reimbursement for health-related services in institutional and community-based care settings became available for those individuals with disabilities who met eligibility criteria.

Vocational Rehabilitation Act Amendments
The 1973 reauthorization of the Vocational Rehabilitation Act (the Rehabilitation Act of 1973, PL 93-112) included civil rights provisions prohibiting discrimination (Section 504) against individuals with disability in programs receiving federal funding. Although significant, the full power of the civil rights protections of Section 504 was seldom felt by those with disabilities until the passage of the Americans with Disabilities Act of 1990 (PL 101-336), almost two decades later.

Education
In 1965, the Office of Education within the U.S. DHEW created the Division for the Education of Handicapped Chil-

dren. In response to advocacy by parents of children with intellectual disabilities who were living in state residential centers, amendments to the Elementary and Secondary Education Act of 1965 (ESEA; PL 89-10) assured education for children in state mental health and intellectual disability hospitals/institutions. By 1970, resource demonstration centers were established, as a state option, to address community program needs in early childhood education, in educating children with severe disabilities, and for students who are both deaf and blind.

Developmental Disabilities Assistance and Bill of Rights Act

The concept of developmental disability was first defined in federal law in 1970 and again with the Developmental Disabilities Assistance and Bill of Rights Act of 1975 (PL 94-103). Initially this legislation supported the Mental Retardation Research Centers (Part A), University Affiliated Facilities (Part B), and Community Facilities (Part C) found in Title I of the Mental Retardation Facilities and Community Mental Health Centers Construction Act of 1963. The Developmental Disabilities Services and Facilities Construction Act of 1970 (PL 91-517) extended the scope of the program to include individuals with categorically defined conditions such as cerebral palsy and epilepsy, which were viewed as closely related to intellectual disabilities. The term *developmental disability* was substituted to describe this broad category of conditions in 1975.

Summary

Early legislation during this period addressed the needs of individuals with disabilities within the prevailing facilities paradigm. By the late 1960s, both the exposed deterioration of institutions and limitations to the custodial approach led to a reappraisal of the efficacy of institutionalization. A parade of federal court cases and class action suits were brought on behalf of plaintiffs living in institutions (Willowbrook, Partlow, Pennhurst, and others) that spelled out the accounts of abuse of institutional care. Subsequently some residential institutions were closed, others were reformed, and many were downsized. The number of individuals living in institutions peaked in 1967 and has declined steadily since (Braddock & Parish, 2002).

The end of the preeminence of the institutional era (not necessarily the end of institutionalization), which was characterized by segregated, custodial, and dependent care following a deficit model, occurred with the widespread acceptance of the developmental and behavioral models of care (Bradley, 1994). These developmental and behavioral models were characterized by community-based approaches that fostered physical integration through programs in the community. Instead of large congregate-care residential programs, people with developmental disabilities moved to smaller group homes and sheltered workshops. Thus, the prevailing paradigm had shifted toward a programs orientation.

PHASE II: DEINSTITUTIONALIZATION AND THE PROGRAMS PARADIGM, MID-1970s TO 1980s

This shift ushered in the second phase, the era of deinstitutionalization and community development (beginning in the mid-1970s). The transition from Phase I to Phase II encompassed movement from a facilities paradigm to a programs paradigm and was marked by the creation of special education classes, group homes, and sheltered workshops that were physically located in the community (Table 36.2). People with disabilities, however, remained socially segregated in that they lived, went to school, recreated, and worked solely with others with developmental disabilities, just in smaller, community-based settings or specialized programs (Bradley, 1994).

Legislation During Phase II

Social Security Act Amendments   By the early 1980s, Medicaid introduced an assortment of optional services especially designed for individuals with disabilities through waiver programs. Waiver options were devised as a way to stem the increasing costs of institutional care and to allow Medicaid coverage for indi-

Table 36.2. Program paradigm: physically in the community

Assumptions	Related legislation
Developmental/behavioral models	Social Security Act Amendments of 1981 (PL 97-123)
	Title V: Maternal and Child Health Block Grant
	Title XIX: Medicaid
Physically integrated	Home and Community-Based waiver and other waivers
	Rehabilitation Act Amendments of 1978 (PL 95-602)
	Independent Living Centers
Community based	Developmental Disabilities Assistance and Bill of Rights Act of 1975 (PL 94-103) and Amendments of 1978 (PL 95-602)
	University Affiliated Programs
	State Protection and Advocacy Agencies
Socially segregated	State Developmental Disability Councils
	Education for All Handicapped Children Act of 1975 (PL 94-142)

Note: The programs paradigm espoused the *developmental model,* which assumed that all people, regardless of the severity of their disabilities, could grow and develop, and the *behavioral model,* which assumed that behavior occurs because it is reinforced. This conceptual switch from the custodial approach allowed practitioners to treat rather than simply care for individuals with disabilities through alternative service modalities that were *physically integrated and community based,* yet *socially segregated,* and to maximize the person's potential for growth and development through application of specialized services.

Related legislation refers to legislation that was passed during the prevailing paradigm.

viduals living in the community but who would otherwise be eligible for institutional care. Among these were the Home and Community-Based waivers, the Katie Beckett waiver (Tax Equity and Fiscal Responsibility Act [TEFRA] option), the Medically Needy waiver option, and the Working Disabled waiver option. These programs continued to support the shift that was occurring in the field by providing income, services, and resources through specialized community-based programs.

The SSA Title V MCH state grant program and the CCS program were combined in 1981 (via PL 97-123) into the MCH Block Grant program. The *block grant* was a new funding mechanism used by the federal government to fund a bundle of specific services carried out by states. The MCH Block Grant program consolidated seven categorical child health programs into a single program of formula grants to states (van Dyck, 2003). The term *crippled children* was changed to the more inclusive, person-first term *children with special health care needs,* and the "direct service" aspect of the program began to shift toward providing greater coordination of care.

Rehabilitation Act Amendments In 1978, rehabilitation services were expanded to include support for Independent Living Ser-

vices for persons with significant disabilities and individualized written rehabilitation plans. Eligibility remained tied to the Social Security Administration definition of *disability*: a person with a physical or mental impairment that is expected to keep him or her from doing any "substantial" work for at least a year, or a condition that is expected to result in his or her death. The independent living movement, championed by self-advocates, pushed for implementation of the stalled Section 504 regulations of the Rehabilitation Act of 1973. They were eventually successful, but only after 4 years of activism (Hagner, 2000).

Developmental Disability Act The Developmental Disabilities Assistance and Bill of Rights Act of 1975 extended services to children and adults with developmental disabilities and required states to develop a plan for deinstitutionalization and institutional reform, consistent with the prevailing paradigm. In 1978, the Act was revised (Rehabilitation, Comprehensive Services, and Developmental Disabilities Act Amendments of 1978, PL 95-602) and the definition of developmental disabilities shifted from diagnostic categories to that of functional impairments. Also, the emphasis shifted from facility construction to development of programs in communities. Consistent with this trend, University Affiliated

Facilities were renamed University Affiliated Programs and addressed the interdisciplinary training of health and human services professionals, provision of direct services, provision of technical assistance, and dissemination of program accomplishments and research findings. Regulations regarding State Protection and Advocacy Agencies shifted the emphasis of this program from planning to providing priority services. State-level Developmental Disability Planning Councils, with a required majority membership of individuals with disabilities or family members, were established in each state. This required composition was intended to assure greater consumer advocacy in state planning, a trend that has continued in subsequent federal legislation.

Education for All Handicapped Children Act

Initially enacted in 1975, the purpose of Title VI, Part B, of the Education for All Handicapped Children Act (PL 94-142) was to guarantee a free appropriate public education for "handicapped" children (6–21 years of age) by assisting states and local schools to provide specially designed instruction and related services. Special instruction became known as *special education*, and related services included transportation, developmental, corrective, and other supported services to assist the child to benefit from special education. The instructional centerpiece of this state education grant program was the requirement that all eligible children must have an individualized education program (IEP). School health services were included under the definition of *related services*, whereas services provided by a physician, except for diagnosis, were not. Federal funds were allocated to states to assist with implementation of this program on the basis of a formula involving the number of children identified and served; however, the promised level of federal support to states for implementation (40% of the cost) was never achieved.

Summary

Consistent with the prevailing paradigm, specialized community programs expanded and funding mechanisms were modified to allow individuals with disabilities to remain in their communities during the programs paradigm phase. For the first time, public education for all "handicapped" children was mandated; however, although physically in their communities, people with disabilities remained socially isolated in special education classes, sheltered workshops, and specialized programs. A shift was about to occur from the program paradigm to a support paradigm that embraced full community membership.

PHASE III: COMMUNITY MEMBERSHIP AND THE SUPPORT PARADIGM, MID-1980s TO TODAY

The third phase, roughly beginning in the mid-1980s and known as the *era of community membership*, was marked by an emphasis on functional supports to enhance inclusion and quality of life as defined by physical as well as social integration (Table 36.3). This phase was characterized by an emphasis on user choice and control in decisions, individualized and person-centered intervention plans, and inclusive practices (Bradley, 1994). Thus, the field was thrust into another modification or shift in paradigms, one that stressed a support approach rather than a programs approach. Self-determination, choice, and control are the underlying assumptions of the supports paradigm. Shifts from specialized services to services provided within the framework of what everyone else gets became the underlying theme that remains today. This shift to a supports paradigm is evolving. Today, the service structures and funding mechanisms are only beginning to change.

Legislation During Phase III

Social Security Act Amendments

Early Periodic Screening, Diagnosis, and Treatment (EPSDT) was added as a mandated benefit of Medicaid (Title XIX) in 1989 (Omnibus Budget Reconciliation Act of 1989, PL 101-239) and required that all eligible children receive an array of medically necessary services. These services included periodic screening, including a comprehensive health and developmental history, physical examination, immunizations, laboratory tests, and health education; vision services; dental services; hearing services; and other care and treatment to correct or ameliorate physical and mental conditions. A chal-

Table 36.3. Supports paradigm: part of the community

Assumptions	Related legislation
Individual support model	Social Security Act Amendments of 1989 (PL 101-239)
	Title V, CSHCN program expanded and redirected
	Title XIX, Medicaid
Community connections	EPSDT mandated for Medicaid recipients
	SSI expansion for children (1990; *Sullivan v. Zebley*)
	Ticket to Work and Work Incentives Improvement Act (1999; PL 106-170)
	New Freedom Initiative (Exe. Order 13217, 2001)
	Independence Plus Waivers
	Rebalancing Initiative
	Title XXI, Children's Health Insurance Program (1997; PL 105-33)
Person centered	Rehabilitation Act Amendments of 1998 (PL 105-220)
	Section 508
	Developmental Disabilities Assistance and Bill of Rights Act Amendments of 2000 (PL 106-402)
	Education for All Handicapped Children Act Amendments (1986, PL 99-457)
Self-determined	Part H, Early Intervention (birth to three) (1986; PL 99-457)
	Preschool special education mandated (1987)
	Technology-Related Assistance for Individuals with Disabilities Act of 1988 (PL 100-407)
	Individuals with Disability Education Act (IDEA) of 1990 (PL 101-476)
Inclusion	Transition planning required at age 14 (1997; PL 105-17)
	Individuals with Disabilities Education Improvement Act (2004, PL 108-446)
	No Child Left Behind Act of 2001 (PL 107-110)
	New Freedom Initiative (2001)
	Americans with Disabilities Act of 1990 (PL 101-336)

Note: The supports paradigm is based on an *individual support model* that embraces the notion that each individual requires functional supports through a formal and informal network to meet day-to-day demands and to enhance social presence and relationships in communities with friends and family (*community connections*). The support paradigm is achieved through *person-centered* approaches that make the person the subject rather than the object of intervention; that support individual, informed choice and control of the person's life (*self-determined*); and that strive toward *inclusion* of the person with a disability in all elements of community life.

Related legislation refers to legislation that was passed during the prevailing paradigm.

Key: CSHCN, children with special health care needs; EPSDT, Early Periodic Screening, Diagnosis, and Treatment; SSI, Supplemental Security Income.

lenge to implementation is that Medicaid reimburses this array of health services to providers at a reduced fee. The fee reduction has contributed to fewer health practitioners accepting Medicaid reimbursement, thus reducing access to care.

In 1990 and following a Supreme Court decision (*Sullivan v. Zebley*), the Social Security Administration reinterpreted disability eligibility regarding children, allowing more children with disabilities to qualify for SSI and, in many cases, Medicaid. The new eligibility criteria stated that the disability must limit the child's ability to function like other children of the same age to such a degree that the impairment is comparable to one that would classify an adult as having a disability. Disability determination remains a state responsibility.

The State Children's Health Insurance Program (SCHIP) was created by the Balanced Budget Act of 1997 (PL 105-33) to give states the option of offering low-cost health insurance for children, up to age 19, who are uninsured. SCHIP became Title XIX of the Social Security Act in 1997. Limited disability-related services such as physical, occupational, or speech therapy and specialty medical care may be provided. Approximately one half of states used SCHIP to expand access to the full range of Medicaid benefits, including EPSDT. The other half created a new benefits package that did not offer the same range of services covered under Medicaid (Kastner & Walsh, 2005).

Rehabilitation Act Amendments In 1998, Congress amended the Rehabilitation

Act to require federal agencies to make their electronic and information technology accessible to people with disabilities (PL 105-220). Under Section 508 (29 U.S.C. 794d), agencies must give employees with disabilities and members of the public access to information that is comparable to the access available to others. Section 508 was not widely applied until 2001, however.

Developmental Disabilities Assistance and Bill of Rights Act Reauthorization

In 2000, the Developmental Disabilities Assistance and Bill of Rights Act was reauthorized (PL 106-402) to ensure access to appropriate community-based services, individualized supports, and other means of assistance to promote independence, self-determination, and inclusion in society. Federal assistance was provided to state protection and advocacy agencies, state councils on developmental disabilities, and the national network of University Centers for Excellence in Developmental Disabilities Education, Research, and Service (formerly known as University Affiliated Programs), and through projects of national significance. Discretionary programs provided funds for family support, and for direct care worker training.

Education Legislation in the 1980s and 1990s

A number of significant amendments to the Education for All Handicapped Children Act occurred in the 1980s and 1990s. The first occurred in 1986 with the passage of Part H of the Education of the Handicapped Act Amendments (PL 99-457), which allowed states to design and offer early intervention (birth to 3) services, with federal funding, for infants, toddlers, and their families. Characteristics of this discretionary program included a state-determined eligibility definition, entitlement to an array of services by the fifth year of participation in each state, interagency participation, service coordination, family-centered approaches, and transition services. The individualized family service plan (IFSP) drives the intervention services provided by the program.

In 1987, preschool (3–5 years) special education services became a mandatory component of PL 94-142. Previously, incentives were provided for states to serve children 3–5

years of age, but some states elected not to participate.

In 1990, Part B (special education) and Part H (early intervention) of the ESEA were reorganized within federal legislation, collectively referred to as the Individuals with Disability Education Act (IDEA; PL 101-476); however, regulations established for special education and early intervention services within this Act remain distinct elements of separate programs, now called Part B and Part C. The 1997 amendments to IDEA (PL 105-17) required the addition of transition planning from school to adult services, especially work, for each student with an IEP. Also, the provision of services in the *least restrictive environment* was required to foster integrated education with typically developing students.

Also during this phase, the Technology-Related Assistance for Individuals with Disabilities Act of 1988 (PL 100-407; the "Tech Act"), was passed to increase the access to, availability of, and funding for assistive technology. This Act, administratively housed within the U.S. Department of Education, required amendments to other important legislation (e.g., IDEA, the Rehabilitation Act) that ultimately would extend access to technology to children as well as adults. Today, the technology needs of children with disabilities are addressed through IEPs and IFSPs (Biehl, 1996).

Americans with Disabilities Act

The Americans with Disabilities Act (ADA; PL 101-336), the most comprehensive civil rights legislation on behalf of people with disabilities, was passed and signed into law in 1990. It established a three-prong definition of a person with a disability similar to the definition in the Rehabilitation Act. The ADA is a bold and comprehensive law affecting employment, transportation, services provided by state and local governments, services and accommodations offered by private businesses, and telecommunication access for people with communication impairments. The ADA is often referred to as an unfunded mandate, meaning that no federal funding is attached to the requirements of the act.

Medical Home Initiative

Not a law but still an important initiative regarding comprehensive services for children with special health care needs, the Medical Home Initiative strives to ensure equity in access to care. Children with special health care needs have chronic physical, developmental, behavioral, and/or emotional conditions that required specialized health services. The medical home initiative is an approach to health care in which a well-trained primary health care provider partners with the family to establish regular ongoing health care that emphasizes often-neglected health promotion and primary care in a manner typical of all children. The Maternal and Child Health Bureau implemented the national Medical Home Initiative in 1994 in collaboration with the American Academy of Pediatrics.

Summary

A significant shift in practice occurred from institutional to community-based care for individuals with developmental disability and from segregated to inclusive services during the last half of the 20th century. This shift has given rise to concerns about the quality and consistency of health care that is available and accessible as more and more individuals with developmental disabilities strive to achieve self-determined lives within the community. The shift toward a supports paradigm that began in the mid-1980s is likely to take several decades to achieve.

EARLY 21st CENTURY: SUPPORTS PARADIGM CONTINUES

Olmstead Decision

On June 22, 1999, the U.S. Supreme Court ruled in *Olmstead v. L.C.* that unjustified institutional isolation of people with disabilities is a form of discrimination and a violation of the ADA. The ADA integration mandate states that services should be provided "in the most integrated setting appropriate to the needs" of people with mental and physical disabilities. This historic pronouncement makes attainable a goal long sought by people with disabilities and their advocates. The Olmstead Executive Order, issued in 2001, charged six federal agencies to assist states with Olmstead implementa-

tion. These agencies included the Department of Health and Human Services (DHHS), Department of Justice, Department of Education, Department of Housing and Urban Development, Department of Labor, and the Social Security Administration (U.S. DHHS, 2002).

Initiatives and Supportive Legislation

New Freedom Initiative   The New Freedom Initiative was announced in February 2001 as President Bush's disability agenda. The goals are to increase access to assistive technology, expand education opportunities, integrate Americans with disabilities into the workforce, and promote full access to community life. This is to be accomplished by reducing barriers to community living in areas such as 1) health care structuring and financing, 2) housing shortages, 3) direct care services and supports, 4) caregiver and family support, 5) transportation, 6) employment, 7) education and transition services, 8) access to technology, and 9) accountability and legal compliance (U.S. DHHS, 2002). Several recent pieces of legislation support implementation of this initiative, although full implementation lags far behind early hopes.

No Child Left Behind Act   The No Child Left Behind Act (NCLB; PL 107-110) is the nation's latest general education law. It was passed in 2001 and replaces ESEA. The purpose of NCLB is to ensure that all children have a fair, equal, and significant opportunity to obtain a high-quality education. One of the purposes of NCLB is to raise expectations for students with disabilities and to hold school districts accountable for the achievement of these students; thus students with disabilities were included in the accountability system of NCLB.

The reauthorization of IDEA in 2004, now called the Individuals with Disabilities Education Improvement Act (IDEA 2004; PL 108-446), contains language that further supports the provisions of NCLB within special education policy. New requirements of IDEA 2004 include provisions for "highly qualified" personnel, accountability tied to achieving standards of learning, local annual yearly progress in attainment of outcomes, and statewide improvement in achievement with increased graduation rates (Council for Exceptional Children, 2004). Regulations regarding the implementation of IDEA 2004 have not been released.

Rehabilitation Act Amendments By executive order in June 2001, Section 508 of the Rehabilitation Act, which was amended in 1998, was applied to the federal government broadly. This section requires all electronic and information technology used by the federal government to be useable by people with disabilities. The goal is to improve services for individuals with disabilities and to provide a more inclusive, better-equipped workplace for federal employees with disabilities.

Medicaid-Related Initiatives

Ticket to Work and Work Incentives Improvement Act The Social Security Administration administers the Ticket to Work and Work Incentives Improvement Act of 1999 (PL 106-170), which provides incentives to work for the more than 7.5 million Americans with disabilities receiving benefits under federal disability programs. Many states have enacted legislation for Medicaid buy-in programs that ensure health coverage when a person with a disability works and would otherwise lose Medicaid benefits when SSI ends.

Independence Plus Waiver Initiative The Independence Plus Initiative, announced in 2002, is intended to give states new opportunities within Medicaid to allow individuals with disabilities to have greater involvement, control, and choice in identifying, gaining access to, and managing the services they obtain to meet their personal assistance needs.

Real Choice Systems Change Grants for Community Living These grants were awarded to 48 states, the District of Columbia, and two territories in 2001 and 2002. The intent is to revamp the Medicaid state system and to realign its funding provision to better support community living for people with disabilities.

"Money Follows the Person" Rebalancing Initiative This initiative was created to "level the playing field" between institutional and community-based services. This market-based approach allows services and supports to move with the person from the institution to the community to minimize disruption and support successful transition.

Shifts in Theory and Practice

As the 21st century begins, several important theoretical and practical shifts have occurred, and legislation has been implemented that supports these changes. Practitioners in the field of developmental disabilities have witnessed changes in their practice and in services since the 1960s. As early as 1992, Smith and Luckasson articulated the importance of these shifts in contributing to the new definition of *mental retardation* developed by the American Association on Mental Retardation (now the American Association on Intellectual and Developmental Disabilities). Subsequently Luckasson and Spitalnik (1994) developed a striking list of changes in practice that have resulted from the developmental disabilities paradigm shift. Of course, none of this is static. What has been achieved in communities throughout the nation is variable. A summary of some of the important changes in the field are as follows (Luckasson & Spitalnik, 1994; Smith & Luckasson, 1992):

- Custodial care has given way to teaching functional skills for community living.

- The perception that a child with developmental disabilities is a risk to the family's health and integrity gradually has yielded to a celebration of all families and the provision of supportive services to enhance an entire family's well-being.

- Denial of the need for medical care has changed to a recognition that access to specialty and primary health care are essential.

- Segregation in geographically isolated residential institutions has been replaced by a presumption that individuals with developmental disabilities should live in their neighborhoods.

- The belief that children with disabilities should be excluded from schools has been replaced by public instruction in regular schools and classrooms with peers without disabilities.

- Idleness has been replaced first with adult day programs and segregated workshops, then with supported employment and meaningful regular jobs.

- Individuals and family members, once excluded from the planning process, have assumed greater participation and control of the decision-making process.

- Practitioners have moved from independent practice to interdependent and collaborative partnerships with individual, families, and other providers.

BACKING INTO THE FUTURE

The title given to this final section was taken from a chapter written by Thomas Reischl, who recounts the wisdom of the Maori culture of New Zealand. The indigenous Maori believed that moving forward into the future should be done with a keen awareness of the past, as captured by their phrase *backing into the future* (Reischl, 2000, p. 278). Walking backward into the future means looking both to the past and to the future. It allows one to be open to a greater variety of understandings and possibilities because of the focus on meaningful experiences of the past and of lessons that have been learned, while retaining a vision for the future (Reischl, 2000). This phrase is particularly relevant as we begin the 21st century.

Trends in public policy in the early part of the 21st century that will influence the availability and delivery of an array of support services for people with disabilities are emerging. First, there has been a gradual, yet constant, shift toward block granting federal funds for mandated services to states. While freeing states to determine how to implement legislative mandates within basic criteria determined by the federal government, block granting inevitably will lead to greater diversity among states in their service system. One might suggest, as do many proponents of states rights,

that this is good policy; however, it does result in variation among states in what and how services and supports are provided and to whom. The risk is that the mandates achieved through years of advocacy by individuals with disabilities, their families, and practitioners may be lost.

Second, as federal budget deficits approach several trillion dollars, there is an overall decrease in federal discretionary spending for research, training, and innovation and in federal regulatory spending for implementation of mandatory services in the field. Furthermore, health care cost containment strategies have resulted in fewer and less comprehensive services with greater copayments for individuals and less reimbursement for health care providers at the community level. It is now common for practitioners in private practice to deny acceptance of Medicaid as payment for their services. Because the major payer of health care for children and adults with developmental disabilities is Medicaid, this trend has and will continue to have profound effects on the availability of community-based primary and specialty health care (Crowley & Elias, 2003).

Third, health disparities among children and adults with disabilities have been described in several recent national reports (Agency for Healthcare Research and Quality, 2003; U.S. DHHS, 2000, 2005; U.S. Public Health Service, 2002). Even with fragmented data, studies suggest that obesity, osteoporosis, arthritis, high blood pressure, and high cholesterol levels disproportionately affect children and adults with disabilities compared with individuals without disabilities. The development of these secondary conditions is largely preventable in children and adults with disabilities, just as it is in individuals without disabilities. In addition to the high cost of health care contributing to limited accessibility, the health care delivery system 1) lacks trained primary health care providers, 2) contains too few highly qualified specialty health care providers distributed across all areas of the country, and 3) consists of a minimally diverse workforce to address the needs of individuals with disabilities from underrepresented groups. These factors make it even more difficult to make meaningful progress toward increasing access and reducing the health disparities that exist.

Finally, community inclusion and self-determination for children and adults with disabilities is really only in its infancy. The entrenchment of the programs paradigm, which is how agencies manage services and provide funding, will need to undergo significant reorganization and change in order to create mechanisms that are consistent with implementing a supports paradigm. It will take many decades for the supports paradigm to become the usual way things are. In the meantime, there is real risk that, under the guise of community inclusion, needed supports will go unheeded, individualized approaches will be considered "special treatment," enabling legislation will be eroded, and inequities will continue.

CONCLUSION

As we walk backward into the future, practitioners need to be mindful of where the field has been and where it is headed. If the vision of community inclusion and self-determination that is embodied in the supports paradigm is to be achieved, then practitioners must not sit idly by as mandates erode and funding shrinks. Movement from centralized to decentralized application of mandates means that local- and state-level advocacy is more important than ever.

The challenges faced by people with disabilities extend beyond traditional health care practice to supports provided by an array of other people (family, friends, other practitioners and providers). Thus, it becomes imperative that health care providers partner with colleagues in other human services (social services, education, rehabilitation) and with self-advocates and families to intervene when policy leads to barriers rather than access, when restrictive legislation excludes rather than includes, when inequities challenge civil rights, and when the absence of effective legislation limits full participation.

REFERENCES

Agency for Healthcare Research and Quality. (2003). *National healthcare disparities report.* Washington, DC: Author.

Americans with Disabilities Act of 1990, PL 101-336, 42 U.S.C. §§ 12101 *et seq.*

Balanced Budget Act of 1997, PL 105-33, 111 Stat. 251.

Biehl, R.F. (1996). Legislative mandates. In A.J. Caputo & P.J. Accardo (Eds.), *Developmental disabilities in infancy and childhood, Vol. I: The spectrum of developmental disabilities* (2nd ed., pp. 513–518). Baltimore: Paul H. Brookes Publishing Co.

Braddock, D., & Parish, S. (2002). An institutional history of disability. In D. Braddock (Ed.), *Disability at the dawn of the 21st century and the state of the states* (pp. 3–61). Washington, DC: American Association on Mental Retardation.

Bradley, V. (1978). *Deinstitutionalization of developmentally disabled persons: A conceptual analysis and guide.* Baltimore: University Park Press.

Bradley, V. (1994). Evolution of a new service paradigm. In V.J. Bradley, J.W. Ashbaugh, & B.C. Blaney (Eds.), *Creating individual supports for people with developmental disabilities: A mandate for change at many levels* (pp. 11–32). Baltimore: Paul H. Brookes Publishing Co.

Council for Exceptional Children. (2004). *The new IDEA: CEC's summary of significant issues* (pp. 1–32). Arlington, VA: Author.

Crowley, J.S., & Elias, R. (2003). *Medicaid's role for people with disabilities.* Washington, DC: The Kaiser Commission on Medicaid and the Uninsured.

Developmental Disabilities Assistance and Bill of Rights Act Amendments of 2000, PL 106-402, 114 Stat. 1677 (2000).

Developmental Disabilities Assistance and Bill of Rights Act of 1975, PL 94-103, 42 U.S.C. §§ 6000 *et seq.*

Developmental Disabilities Services and Facilities Construction Act of 1970, PL 91-517, 42 U.S.C. §§ 6000 *et seq.*

Education for All Handicapped Children Act of 1975, PL 94-142, 20 U.S.C. §§ 1400 *et seq.*

Education of the Handicapped Act Amendments of 1986, PL 99-457, 20 U.S.C. §§ 1400 *et seq.*

Elementary and Secondary Education Act of 1965, PL 89-10, 20 U.S.C. §§ 6301 *et seq.*

Hagner, D. (2000). Supporting people as part of the community. In J. Nisbet & D. Hagner (Eds.), *Part of the community: Strategies for including everyone* (pp. 15–42). Baltimore: Paul H. Brookes Publishing Co.

Hospital and Medical Facilities Amendments of 1964, PL 88-443, 42 U.S.C. 291 *et seq.*

Hospital Survey and Construction Act of 1946, PL 79-725, 42 U.S.C. §§ 291 *et seq.*

Individuals with Disabilities Education Act Amendments of 1997, PL 105-17, 20 U.S.C. §§ 1400 *et seq.*

Individuals with Disabilities Education Act of 1990, PL 101-476, 20 U.S.C. §§ 1400 *et seq.*

Individuals with Disabilities Education Improvement Act of 2004, PL 108-446, 20 U.S.C. §§ 1400 *et seq.*

Kastner, T.A., & Walsh, K.K. (2005). Economic and policy issues. In W. Nehring (Ed.), *Core curriculum for specializing in intellectual and developmental disability* (pp. 421–436). Sudbury, MA: Jones & Bartlett.

Kuhn, T.S. (1970). *The structure of scientific revolutions* (2nd ed.). Chicago: University of Chicago Press.

Luckasson, R., & Spitalnik, D. (1994). Political and programmatic shifts of the 1992 AAMR definition of mental retardation. In V.J. Bradley, J.W. Ashbaugh, & B.C. Blaney (Eds.), *Creating individual supports for people with developmental disabilities: A mandate for change at many levels* (pp. 81–95). Baltimore: Paul H. Brookes Publishing Co.

Mental Retardation Facilities and Community Mental Health Centers Construction Act of 1963, PL 88-164, 42 U.S.C. §§ 2670 *et seq.*

Natvig, D.A. (2005). Genetic concepts. In W. Nehring (Ed.), *Core curriculum for specializing in intellectual and developmental disability* (pp. 58–80). Sudbury, MA: Jones & Bartlett.

No Child Left Behind Act of 2001, PL 107-110, 20 U.S.C. §§ 6301 *et seq.*

Olmstead v. L.C., 119 S. Ct. 2176 (1999).

Omnibus Budget Reconciliation Act of 1989, PL 101-239, 42 U.S.C. §§ 1396 *et seq.*

Omnibus Budget Reconciliation Act of 1990, PL 101-508, 42 U.S.C. §§ 651 *et seq.*

Rehabilitation Act Amendments of 1978, PL 95-602, 29 U.S.C. §§ 701 *et seq.*

Rehabilitation Act Amendments of 1998, PL 105-220, 29 U.S.C. §§ 701 *et seq.*

Rehabilitation Act of 1973, PL 93-112, 29 U.S.C. §§ 701 *et seq.*

Rehabilitation, Comprehensive Services, and Developmental Disabilities Act Amendments of 1978, PL 95-602, 29 U.S.C. 700 *et seq.*

Reischl, T. (2000). Witnessing the possible for people with disabilities. In J. Nisbet & D. Hagner (Eds.), *Part of the community: Strategies for including everyone* (pp. 265–280). Baltimore: Paul H. Brookes Publishing Co.

Silverstein, R. (2000). Disability policy framework: A guidepost for analyzing public policy. Washington, DC: Center for the Study and Advancement of Disability Policy and the Arc of the United States.

Social Security Act Amendments of 1950, PL 81-734, 42 U.S.C. §§ 101 et seq.

Social Security Act Amendments of 1956, PL 84-880, 42 U.S.C. §§ 101 et seq.

Social Security Act Amendments of 1965, PL 89-97, 42 U.S.C. §§ 101 *et seq.*

Social Security Act Amendments of 1971, PL 92-5, 42 U.S.C. §§ 101 *et seq.*

Social Security Act Amendments of 1972, PL 92-336, 42 U.S.C. §§ 101 *et seq.*

Social Security Act Amendments of 1981, PL 97-123, 42 U.S.C. §§ 101 *et seq.*

Social Security Act of 1935, PL 74-271, 42 U.S.C. §§ 301 *et seq.*

Smith, D., & Luckasson, R. (1992). *Introduction to special education: Teaching in an age of challenges.* Needham Heights, MA: Allyn & Bacon.

Sullivan v. Zebley, 493 U.S. 521 (1990).

Technology-Related Assistance for Individuals with Disabilities Act of 1988, PL 100-407, 29 U.S.C. §§ 2201 *et seq.*

Ticket to Work and Work Incentives Improvement Act of 1999, PL 106-170, 20 U.S.C. §§ 411 *et seq.*

U.S. Department of Health and Human Services. (2000). *Healthy people 2010* (2nd ed.). Washington, DC: Author.

U.S. Department of Health and Human Services. (2002). *New freedom initiative: Fulfilling America's promise to people with disabilities.* Washington, DC: Author.

U.S. Department of Health and Human Services. (2005). *The Surgeon General's call to action to improve the health and wellness of persons with disabilities.* Washington, DC: Author.

U.S. Government Accountability Office. (2005). *Federal disability assistance: Wide array of programs needs to be examined in light of 21st century challenges.* Washington, DC: Author.

U.S. Public Health Service. (2002). *Closing the gap: A national blueprint for improving the health of individuals with mental retardation.* Washington, DC: Author.

van Dyck, P.C. (2003). A history of child health equity legislation in the United States. *Pediatrics, 112,* 727–730.

Vocational Rehabilitation Act of 1943, PL 78-113, 29 U.S.C. §§ 3141 *et seq.*

Vocational Rehabilitation Act of 1918, PL 65-178, 17 U.S.C. §§ 486A *et seq.*

37

International Adoption

CECILIA T. DAVOLI

Out-of-country adoption of children has been a growing phenomenon over the past several decades, both in the United States and throughout the world. Based on estimates from orphan visas issued by the U.S. Immigration and Naturalization Service, more than 22,000 international adoptions occurred in 2005. This is in contrast to about half that number a decade earlier. International adoption can be a long and costly process, which usually involves a waiting period with an unpredictable timetable. Children are adopted from throughout the world, with the majority of adoptions occurring from Eastern Europe, China, and South America.

Prospective parents pursue international adoption for a variety of reasons. In many cases, there has been an antecedent period of infertility, with resultant "older" first-time parents. Many individuals have the perception that there are decreasing numbers of children available for adoption in the United States, despite the fact that there are a tremendous number of children in the U.S. foster care system. Single individuals may choose to adopt internationally due to difficulty meeting regulations involved in domestic adoption. Many parents adopt due to altruism, including those who are specifically seeking a child with special needs.

PREADOPTION ISSUES

Children who are adopted internationally often have the same risk factors for developmental delay as U.S. children in the adoption/foster care systems (Table 37.1). Malnutrition is usually related to inadequate calories/nutrients being available to a child, combined with psychosocial failure to thrive. If it is pres-ent, iron deficiency anemia is an independent risk factor for cognitive deficits. Chinese adoptees, more than 95% of whom are female, are at greater risk for having an elevated lead level (Miller & Hendrie, 2000). Among children from Eastern Europe, fetal alcohol spectrum disorders are more prevalent due to alcohol abuse rates that are higher than in other regions of the world. The orphanage stay itself is a unique risk factor that predisposes a child to long-term effects of institutionalization, including potential difficulty with bonding after adoption. There is no consistent documentation in orphanage medical records regarding whether a specific risk factor applies to an individual child.

One factor that is developmentally protective is being a "favored child" by the orphanage caregivers. This child usually receives more affection and individual attention, resulting in better growth and development in comparison with age peers in the same orphanage. Another protective factor is being raised in a foster home rather than an orphanage prior to adoption (Miller, Chan, Comfort, & Tirella, 2005). Foster placement is very common in many South American countries and in Korea.

Prospective parents are usually given medical records and/or pictures of the child they are considering for adoption. Orphanage medical records are often scanty with missing data and may be as brief as one paragraph (Jenista, 2000). Medical terminology on international records does not always translate directly into Western definitions of the same terms (Table 37.2). Often, the accuracy of the information cannot be verified, although there does not appear to be any direct attempt to

Table 37.1. Risk factors for developmental delay in international adoptees

Maternal/prenatal factors

Poverty/malnutrition

Substance abuse (alcohol, drugs)

Smoking

Lack of prenatal care

Mental illness

Cognitive impairment

Chronic disease

Perinatal factors

Preeclampsia/eclampsia

Traumatic/difficult delivery

Prematurity

Infection

Postnatal factors

Malnutrition (lack of adequate calories and/or protein)

Iron deficiency anemia

Psychosocial impact of orphanage stay

Toxic exposure (e.g., lead)

Lack of adequate medical care

Illness/injury

Neglect

Abuse (physical, emotional, sexual)

hide information or mislead parents/adoption agencies.

In some countries, a videotape is made of the child, often by an orphanage or agency worker. There is no standardized format for these videotapes, which are usually of less than 10 minutes' duration. Because the children are frequently fully clothed, it can be challenging to assess both physical appearance and normalcy of motor skills. Many children appear apprehensive because the filming is often done by an unfamiliar adult in an unfamiliar room.

Table 37.2. Medical terms used frequently on orphanage medical records

Perinatal encephalopathy

Hypertension-hydrocephalic syndrome

Spastic paraparesis

Pyramidal insufficiency

Oligophrenia

Microsomia

Functional cardiopathy

Extra chorda in left ventricle

Open oval window

Convergent squint

Hypermetropia

In some cases, there are serial film segments done at several times in the child's life, which allows for some assessment of developmental progress. Although a videotape review can be fairly predictive for children who manifest little or no developmental delay postadoption, it does not appear to be as accurate in predicting moderate to severe delay (Boone, Hostetter, & Weitzman, 2003).

POSTADOPTION ISSUES

A comprehensive medical evaluation is an important initial assessment that should be done for every child after adoption (Mitchell & Jenista, 1997). This evaluation is usually done through the primary care site or may be coordinated in conjunction with an adoption medicine specialist. In addition to a thorough physical examination, special care should be taken to document scars, lesions, and injection sites. A comprehensive laboratory evaluation will screen for conditions that may need medical treatment, such as iron deficiency anemia, Vitamin D deficiency, or infectious diseases (Reeves, Bachrach, Carpenter, & Mackenzie, 2000) (Table 37.3).

Table 37.3. Postadoption medical evaluation

Complete blood count with differential

Chemistry panel, including electrolytes

Liver function tests

Thyroid function tests

Venous lead level

Metabolic screening tests

Calcium, magnesium, phosphorus

Vitamin D level

Urinalysis

Purified protein derivative (PPD) for tuberculosis

Hepatitis B panel (surface antigen, surface antibody, core antibody)

Hepatitis C antibody

Human immunodeficiency virus (HIV) test

Venereal Disease Research Laboratory (VDRL) to evaluate for syphilis

Stool for ova and parasites (three samples)

Immunization titers (if not reimmunizing from baseline)

Dental evaluation

Vision screen

Hearing screen

Developmental screen

Growth failure is common in international adoptees, usually due to a combination of prenatal factors, malnutrition, psychosocial failure to thrive, and lack of exposure to sunlight. Many adoptees will manifest retardation of linear growth and delayed bone age. There appears to be transient, reversible diminished response to growth hormone for many children during their orphanage stay. Postadoption catch-up growth is usually immediate and rapid for weight, somewhat slower for height, and less predictable for head circumference. Although most children will experience catch-up growth with normal nutritional intake alone, some children require supplemental formula or other calorie expanders. Because of all these factors, postadoption growth parameters should be tracked at every medical encounter, both well and sick visits. Head circumference measurements should be taken and double-checked for every child at every visit, regardless of age. If the expected catch-up growth does not occur, potential etiologies include inadequate caloric intake, functional or structural swallowing abnormalities, malabsorption, thyroid or growth hormone dysfunction, renal tubular acidosis, gastrointestinal parasites, and syndromes (acquired or genetic). Further evaluation by subspecialists is sometimes required.

Infectious diseases are the most common issues needing follow-up and treatment among international adoptees, so screening for them is imperative (Saiman et al., 2001). Because many children are adopted from countries in which tuberculosis is endemic, evaluation with purified protein derivative (PPD) should be done on every child. A positive reaction (induration of 10 mm or greater) merits further evaluation and appropriate treatment, even if the child has previously received the bacille Calmette-Guérin (BCG) vaccination. Gastrointestinal pathogens/parasites can be difficult to diagnose/eradicate and may spread to other family members. Because they are endemic in many areas of the world, vertical transmission of Hepatitis B and C is common. Horizontal transmission of other diseases such as chicken pox and cytomegalovirus (CMV) occurs easily due to the fact that an orphanage is an institutional setting.

Orphanage immunization records need to be interpreted judiciously (Schulte et al., 2002). In many cases, there will be inadequate immunity to infectious diseases for which there is documentation of immunization. Improper storage or dilution of vaccines is one possible cause for inadequate immunity. Per the current Centers for Disease Control and Prevention (CDC) guidelines, reimmunization from baseline *or* evaluation of titers needs to be undertaken for almost all adoptees. In Korea and some South American countries, immunization practices are more consistent with those in the United States, so adoptees from those areas may not need reimmunization.

Feeding/swallowing disorders are common among international adoptees. Many children have only been exposed to pureed or mashed foods and may need slower transition to higher-texture foods after adoption. Children with language delay that is more profound than would be expected for an international adoptee may also have significant difficulty with chewing and swallowing. Some children will have a voracious appetite in the first few months after adoption, usually related to preadoption malnutrition and inadequate intake due to rationing. This usually self-corrects once the child has achieved his or her genetic weight potential. Older children may engage in food-hoarding behavior. Again, this usually resolves over a period of months/years as the child learns to trust that there will always be adequate food available to him or her. In extreme cases of feeding/swallowing disorders, or if symptoms show no evidence of resolution, professional assistance may be necessary.

Almost all male adoptees who are being raised in an orphanage setting are uncircumcised. Regardless of whether they have another son, prospective parents usually need instruction and demonstration regarding care of the uncircumcised penis. In addition, they should be encouraged to discuss and ask questions about circumcision before and after the adoption. At this time, the American Academy of Pediatrics does not consider circumcision to be a medically necessary procedure, except for boys with recurrent urinary tract infections. If the parents desire circumcision, it is an elective procedure that need not be undertaken immediately after adoption. In most cases, it is preferable to wait until the child has gone through a period of adjustment and bonding before having surgery. An older boy should have acquired enough English to be able to understand and ask questions about what will happen when he is circumcised. In many cases, parents choose to have circumcision done at the time of another scheduled surgery. Because there are many uncircumcised boys and men in the United States, many parents defer circumcision until their son is older and can make his own decision about the procedure.

DEVELOPMENTAL ISSUES

Although not every child will require a comprehensive developmental assessment, each adoptee should undergo some type of developmental screening (Miller, 2000). In addition to identifying children in need of close monitoring and/or early intervention services, developmental screening/evaluation results can be educational for parents. With a better understanding of their child's skill levels, they can set appropriate expectations for their child's behavior and select appropriate toys/activities.

Ideally, a baseline developmental assessment occurs between 2 and 4 weeks after adoption. This allows for time zone readjustment, primary care site visit, initiation of comprehensive medical assessment, initial evaluation/treatment of infectious diseases, and parental observation of the child's progress since adoption. Most international adoptees will have a developmental quotient around 60% (of typical development) during the first weeks to month after adoption. Catch-up development usually starts within the first few days after adoption and proceeds steadily. In general, catch-up development will be quicker in younger adoptees but is not necessarily "slow" in older children.

Expressive language is almost universally delayed in international adoptees and is related to a variety of factors (Glennen & Bright, 2005). Regardless of the cause, expressive language development is often the last skill to "catch-up" for many children. In the orphanage, there are usually few caregivers and many children, which results in less opportunity for

interactive language with an individual child. Orphanages usually group children by age, so younger children have less opportunity to mingle with those who might serve functionally as "older siblings" and model the next stage of language development. A child may have orphanage-related language delay superimposed on central language delay. A child with this developmental profile will not experience language catch-up development as quickly as other adoptees and is at risk for later manifestation of language-related problems such as specific learning disabilities in reading and/or spelling.

Postadoption, children begin to switch languages almost immediately after joining their new family. It is recommended that parents use talking, reading, and music to help encourage/enhance their child's language development. Videotapes and television have not been proven to be of as much benefit as interactive language. In many cases, sign language can be used as a communication bridge during the transition from mother tongue to second language. In bilingual adoptive households, catch-up language development will not be slowed substantially, even if both languages are "new" to the child.

Developmental catch-up in motor skills is more predictable and consistent. Postadoption gross motor skills usually improve as nutritional health and muscle mass improve and the child is given increased freedom to explore the environment. In the absence of a permanent motor disability, this usually occurs fairly quickly and steadily. Most international adoptees would walk independently between 15 and 18 months of age if left in the orphanage. Children adopted when they are younger than 1 year often catch-up to walk between 12 and 15 months of age, but there should not be concern if their gross motor development progresses as it would have in the orphanage. Fine motor skills improve with exposure to toys and finger feeding. Handedness is usually established in a typically developing child at 18–24 months of age; as with any child, asymmetry in an adoptee's hand function before then is reason for concern.

International adoptees younger than school age usually qualify for and benefit from early intervention services. By definition, these children are "at risk" for developmental delay, and many of them manifest the minimum 25% delay that qualifies them automatically for services. In addition to providing therapeutic interventions and monitoring development, therapists can often provide new parents with concrete guidance about how to encourage their child's development. Older children can benefit from English as a Second Language (ESL) services/classes. Regardless of whether they were adopted as younger children, many international adoptees manifest learning disabilities and/or attention/behavior problems during the school-age years (Juffer & van Ijzendoorn, 2005). In most cases, these disabilities are probably related to a combination of perinatal, genetic, and orphanage factors.

Parental counseling and ongoing emotional support are of paramount importance because many first-time parents are simultaneously confronting postadoption issues and catch-up development along with normal stages of child development. This means that night terrors and toddler tantrums may be superimposed on adoption-related behaviors such as self-stimulatory rocking, food texture sensitivity, and tantrums due to communication delay. Although the tendency is to attribute all behaviors to the child's orphanage stay, many of the behaviors are better tolerated by parents and addressed more appropriately if understood in the context of typical child development.

Some children merit heightened concern and closer developmental monitoring. If the developmental quotient immediately after adoption is lower than 60%, or if it remains the same (60%) over the first 3–6 months after adoption, the child may have delay that is unrelated to the orphanage stay. In addition, children with dysmorphic features or persistent abnormal behaviors may have an underlying developmental disability. Any concerns voiced by parents or primary care providers should be addressed quickly because astute parents are often the first to notice that something is amiss. Conversely, many parents believe that orphanage-related delay may still "catch-up" multiple years after adoption. Prolonged lag in a child's development can be a manifestation of a long-

term disability, and the parents may need additional guidance and support to help them understand their child's symptoms.

Children with suspected or diagnosed fetal alcohol spectrum disorders such as fetal alcohol syndrome (FAS) and fetal alcohol effects (FAE) will need more specialized monitoring and intervention. FAS and FAE are less common in Asia, where there is less alcohol use, and more common in Eastern Europe and Russia. Specific physical criteria are required for diagnosis of FAS, and diagnosis of FAE requires a history of alcohol use during pregnancy. In many cases, the behavioral symptoms can be quite challenging and may require subspecialty management assistance. Please refer to Chapter 12 in this volume for a detailed discussion of FAS and FAE.

Family/child adjustment issues are very child dependent. Although younger children should theoretically have less difficulty with making the transition to their new home/family, this is often not the case for a specific child. In many cases, there is a "honeymoon period" during the first few postadoption months, during which the child may appear to be making the transition with little or no difficulty. Soon thereafter, the child may begin to "test the boundaries" of his or her new environment, and problem behaviors can develop. "Bonding" is a process rather than an instantaneous occurrence. A small percentage of children manifest significant difficulty with formation of lasting, loving relationships with others, including their adoptive parents. This often results from neglect, abuse, or trauma during the first 2 years of life. Although it is helpful to observe how a child interacts with orphanage caregivers, bonding with those individuals does not guarantee bonding with new parents. If it occurs, this reactive attachment disorder (RAD) often requires prolonged counseling and subspecialty management (Faber, 2000).

CONCLUSION

Children who have been adopted internationally comprise a globally diverse group who manifest a wide variety of reversible and long-term disabilities in the early postadoption period. Most international adoptees do well in the long run, despite the many medical and developmental challenges that confront them initially. To be most helpful to these children and their parents, a clinician can become familiar with the common patterns of postadoption delay and catch-up development, as well as the interventions and resources that can be of assistance.

REFERENCES

Boone, J.L., Hostetter, M.K., & Weitzman, C.C. (2003). The predictive accuracy of pre-adoption video review in adoptees from Russian and Eastern European orphanages. *Clinical Pediatrics, 42,* 585–590.

Faber, S. (2000). Behavioral sequelae of orphanage life. *Pediatric Annals, 29*(4), 242–248.

Glennen, S., & Bright, B.J. (2005). Five years later: Language in school-age internationally adopted children. *Language in School-Age IA Children, 26*(1), 86–101.

Jenista, J.A. (2000). Preadoption review of medical records. *Pediatric Annals, 29*(4), 212–215.

Juffer, F., & Van Ijzendoorn, M.H. (2005). Behavior problems and mental health referrals of international adoptees. *JAMA, 293*(20), 2501–2515.

Miller, L.C. (2000). Initial assessment of growth, development, and the effects of institutionalization in internationally adopted children. *Pediatric Annals, 29*(4), 224–232.

Miller, L.C., Chan, W., Comfort, K., & Tirella, L. (2005). Health of children adopted from Guatemala: Comparison of orphanage and foster care. *Pediatrics, 115*(6), 710–717.

Miller, L.C., & Hendrie, N.W. (2000). Health of children adopted from China. *Pediatrics, 105*(6), 76–82.

Mitchell, M.A., & Jenista, J.A. (1997). Health care of the internationally adopted child. Part 1: Before and at arrival into the adoptive home. *Journal of Pediatric Health Care, 11,* 51–60.

Reeves, G.D., Bachrach, S., Carpenter, T.O., & Mackenzie, W.G. (2000). Vitamin D–deficiency rickets in adopted children from the former Soviet Union: An uncommon problem with unusual clinical and biochemical features. *Pediatrics, 106,* 1484–1488.

Saiman, L., Aronson, J., Zhou, J., Gomez-Duarte, C., San Gabriel, P., Alonso, M., et al. (2001). Prevalence of infectious diseases among internationally adopted children. *Pediatrics, 108,* 608–612.

Schulte, J.M., Maloney, S., Aronson, J., San Gabriel, P., Zhou, J., & Saiman, L. (2002). Evaluating acceptability and completeness of overseas immunization records of internationally adopted children. *Pediatrics, 109,* 22–26.

38

Supports for Families of Children with Disabilities

PETER A. BLASCO,
CHRIS PLAUCHÉ JOHNSON,
AND SANDRA A. PALOMO-GONZALEZ

Families' lives are altered inexorably as a consequence of having children, and parents are called on to undertake additional tasks if a child has special health or educational needs. Although it may be true that much personal growth and insight is gained through the adjustment to and acceptance of raising a child with special needs, most parents would gladly forego those benefits in exchange for less hardship. They often must coordinate evaluations and treatment among a variety of professionals, and they must sort through diagnostic and treatment decisions based on these frequently discrepant inputs. If they have extensive need for support services, they must have skills in case management, care coordination, and personnel management (Case-Smith, 2004). Parents must know the law and advocate for the best interests of their child in multiple service systems that can be exceedingly bureaucratic and often terribly impersonal. They can expect to encounter greater financial stress, more frequent disruptions of family routines, more marital challenges, and reduced social and leisure activities (Singhi et al., 1990). In the midst of all this, parents must maintain their own health, stamina, optimism, and joy for life. Sometimes their best efforts still fall short of satisfactory, and the results are achieved to the detriment of spouses and other children. In the absence of adequate supports,

parents and their child with special needs may languish, and the child may become at risk for placement outside the home.

Children are more likely to reach their maximum potential when they are nurtured by caring and skilled parents who find happiness and fulfillment in their caregiving roles (Clayton, 2000; Rosenau, 2005a, 2005b). The supports needed to promote this process are defined by disability advocates as "providing whatever it takes for families of children with disabilities to live as much like other families as possible" (Agosta & Melda, 1995; Agosta, 2004).

What can physicians do to help families cope with hardships and achieve the balance between challenges and resources? This chapter provides an outline of potential support activities and resources and offers practical suggestions on how to obtain them.

ROLE OF PHYSICIANS

Most parents do not see their doctor as a social worker. In general, they assert that it is the physician's responsibility to help fit the medical care plan and priorities into the overall management picture. They look for guidance and support from their physicians, mainly in the form of collaborative and sometimes creative problem solving rather than ultimate decision conferring (Galil et al., 2006). To partner successfully, physicians must listen to families as

The authors wish to express their heartfelt thanks to Celia Shapland, RN; Linda Kratz; Jill Rinehart; Peggy Mann Rinehart; and Patricia Mulhearn Blasco, Ph.D., for their critical review and suggestions for this chapter.

they describe their needs, know how to obtain both community-based supports and legislated publicly funded systems, and educate and empower colleagues who care for children with disabilities within the context of a medical home.

Parents want to be assured that their physicians know the facts and keep up to date about the latest developments. This is only one aspect of competency. Complaints about physician performance rarely relate to medical content but instead to issues of communication and resource counseling. Good communication skills are just as important as knowledge of the content. In the long term, parents remember the manner in which information is provided much better than the content itself (Hostler, 1991; Sharp, Strauss, & Lorch, 1992).

Good communication skills are founded on sensitivity, patience, and especially good listening skills. The stage is firmly set for the parent–professional partnership during the initial contacts, when parents get a sense of the physician's respect for their expertise, not just their utility as informants. Klein (1993) set forth the challenge of integrating the concepts and techniques of the ideal professional–parent relationship into day-to-day practice in a way that fits with each clinician's personal style, the demands and constraints of the practice setting, and the unique needs of each family. Without bidirectional and positive parent–professional communication, parents feel adrift in a sea of uncertain and unclear information (Korsch, 1984). The critical importance of the first contact to establishing the parent–professional relationship cannot be overstated. In many instances, the first meeting will be a difficult one involving bad news and possibly complicated by added agendas (Table 38.1).

Physicians should have a designed approach to "breaking the news" counseling. Residents and fellows should formally rehearse and discuss the elements of such counseling. Many authors have addressed this issue at length (e.g., Kaminer & Cohen, 1988; Klein, 1993), offering guidelines for difficult counseling sessions (Table 38.2). This interpretive process involves 1) the preparatory stage, which consists of structuring information into well-organized units that make sense, and 2) the

Table 38.1.   Added agendas complicating first encounter

One or both parents have been uneasy about the child's development for some time and have become increasingly frustrated with being put off by such admonitions as "wait and see" or "he'll grow out of it."

One parent believes the child is normal but is being pressured by the other parent or by extended family members to have the child evaluated.

For a variety of reasons, one parent comes to the clinic against his or her will.

A child has already been diagnosed, but the parents are concerned that he or she has not made adequate progress; in this instance, an accurate diagnosis implies to the parents that effective treatment is automatically available.

The parents are dissatisfied with previous evaluations and/or diagnoses.

The parents are seeking a second opinion (openly or covertly) and have withheld or concealed previous evaluation results in order to get an "unbiased" opinion.

Well-read and intelligent parents have researched their child's condition and want to match the physician's expertise against their own.

Professional parents focus on discussions of technicalities and debate trivial and theoretical points, bypassing broader and more meaningful concepts or issues.

Marital separation or strife produces automatic conflicting viewpoints regarding almost everything, including the child.

A long-standing developmental problem has been acutely exacerbated by a crisis (e.g., school expulsion, parent burnout).

translating stage, which involves adapting the information and knowledge base into language and concepts that are understandable to parents and that take into account the educational, cultural, and ethnic characteristics of the family. The presentation should be empathetic as well as informative to foster an emotional connection between the physician and the parent. Despite the great utility of the problem-oriented approach, an important caveat is the repeated plea from parents for the physician not to always focus on the negative.

Person-first language refers to acknowledging the actuality of the individual before the disability. This practice emphasizes personhood, not limitations (e.g., a *child with mental retardation or intellectual disabilities*, as opposed to a *mentally retarded child*). It also emphasizes sensitivity to words and jargon (e.g., *physical disability* instead of *crippled; uses a wheelchair* instead of *wheelchair bound*). In some situations where repetition of the same phrase becomes

Table 38.2. Guidelines for presenting bad news to parents

Advance preparation

Attitude—upbeat, positive, and collaborative

Preparation—facts and structure

Participants—*both* parents, limited numbers

Time—unlimited setting

   Quiet and private location

   Comfortable seating arrangement

   Equitable, eye-level dynamics

   Ability to take/use notes

Discussion mechanics

Opening social amenities

Restatement of the problem and the parents' perception

Review of the evaluation and its validity

Sequential review of problems/diagnoses

Expectation for questions and allowance of space for comments and responses

Discussion of etiology

Discussion of prognosis

Referrals for further evaluation/consultation

Recommendations for treatment

Parting/conclusion

Empathy/encouragement

Refocus on *present* situation and *immediate* plans

Open-door policy

Follow-up

Written documentation of the interpretive session

Sources: Blasco (1988); Kaminer and Cohen (1988); Klein (1993); Sharp et al. (1992).

clumsy, uniform adherence to person-first syntax can result in stilted or excessively wordy prose. Although there may be justifiable exceptions to person-first language in written and verbal presentations, there are no exceptions to its fundamental concept.

Many developmental pediatricians evaluate children in multidisciplinary clinics in which residents, medical students, and allied health care students are in attendance. In this setting, a useful educational approach is the *teaching physical examination* (Wilson & Hostler, 1986). If the pediatrician directs the examination findings to the parents or, where appropriate, to the child, in a manner that conveys respect for their expertise, the accompanying students and residents will be taught that technique at the same time the parents are receiving the proper information. Furthermore, the instructor provides a good role model, conveying the importance of patient education and good patient care, and the patient is not put on display.

Copies of clinic notes, discharge summaries, or separate summary letters sent to parents ensure that the information presented is indeed transmitted and retained. Because the parents' ability to be effective advocates depends on how well professionals share information, additional copies for human services agencies and school programs should be provided either directly (with appropriate permission per Health Insurance Portability and Accountability Act of 1996 [HIPAA] guidelines) or indirectly through the family on their request.

Strengths and Needs of the Family

Although parents of children with disabilities or chronic illness experience greater stress, research suggests that they experience no more dysfunction or marital maladjustment than controls (Cappelli, McGrath, Daniels, Manion, & Schillinger, 1994; Frey, Greenberg, & Fewell, 1989; Sabbeth & Leventhal, 1984). Psychological and physical health of caregivers is influenced by caregiving demands and child behavior (Raina et al., 2005). Physicians and other health care professionals can assist families to effectively meet their children's needs while also addressing the needs of the entire family. There is evidence to suggest that primary care physicians are not often helpful in this regard. In a survey study of parents whose children were entered into early intervention programs, only half of the parents identified their pediatrician as helpful in terms of providing information about support resources (O'Sullivan, Mahoney, & Robinson, 1992) (see Table 38.4 later in the chapter). Behavior problems and school problems were also identified as areas in which more assistance was greatly desired. Similarly, Liptak and Revell (1989) demonstrated a considerable mismatch between parents' and physicians' priorities for services (Table 38.3). This was in striking contrast with the degree of satisfaction that families expressed regarding their child's overall medical health care.

Empowerment Parents must be empowered with the encouragement and skills to become more effective service coordinators and advocates. Parents cannot do this unless they are given extensive information regarding the medical, developmental, and psychoeduca-

Table 38.3. Parents' and physicians' ranking of service priorities

Services	Ranking	
	Parents	Physicians
Information regarding community resources	1	14
Financial information or help	2	5
Parent support groups	3	3
Recreational opportunities	4	13
Psychological services	5	9
Vocational counseling	6	8
Summer camp	7	19
Dental treatment	8	16
Respite care	9	1
Help with behavior problems	10	4
Day care	21	2

Reproduced with permission from *Pediatrics,* Vol. 84, Pages 465–471, Copyright ©
1989 by the AAP.

tional interventions their children are receiving. To empower themselves, parents often ask questions, seek professional literature, attend continuing medical education and parent conferences, and join parent support and advocacy groups to learn as much as possible about their child's disability and advocate for public supports and funding. Generally, parents believe that physicians fail to provide adequate information regarding disease processes, treatment, or prognoses (Liptak & Revell, 1989).

Fathers and Extended Family as Resources   Fathers are stereotyped as being chronically absent from the health care and educational activities surrounding their children with disabilities, an unfair generalization. Involving fathers from the start allows clinicians to validate for children the importance of their father, and, at the same time, relieve mothers of the task of transmitting clinical information. Fathers are usually responsive to this approach, often reporting that it is the first time they have not felt left out by health professionals (Klein, 1982). Pediatricians—particularly developmental subspecialists who may be more likely to have access to fathers—and especially male physicians may be in the best positions to make a special connection with fathers and address their unique concerns. A program to specifically involve fathers in physical therapy has been successfully piloted (Revell, 1990). A national support organization has been established for

fathers (Table 38.4), and some communities have developed fathers' groups.

Extended family members can be tremendously helpful to parents in relieving the demands of physical care and providing psychological and emotional support. Individuals who are uneasy about having a relative with disabilities can be won over or at least positively influenced by being encouraged to participate in medical and therapeutic interactions.

Recognizing the Needs of Siblings   The birth or recognition that a child has a disability or chronic illness has a profound effect on siblings. From the typically developing sibling's perspective, having a brother or sister with a disability is a mixed blessing, and the child's reactions to the sibling with a disability can affect the overall adjustment and development of self-esteem in both children. The large volume of research on siblings is contradictory and confusing, in part because there are so many variables to be considered. In general, however, studies support effects that are mostly negative in the short term and positive in the longer term. Most publications have either assumed or focused on short-term negative impacts on siblings of children with disabilities. A number of excellent studies have noted positive long-term effects enabling siblings to become more flexible, adaptable, tolerant adults who tend to achieve better relationships (Cleveland & Miller, 1977). A few themes con-

Table 38.4. Resources for families of children with disabilities

Specific neurodevelopmental disabilities organizations

American Foundation for the Blind (AFB): http://www.afb.org

The Arc of the United States: http://www.thearc.org

Brain Injury Association of American (BIAA) (formerly the National Head Injury Foundation): http://www.biausa.org

Children and Adults with Attention Deficit Disorder (CHADD): http://www.chadd.org

Epilepsy Foundation: http://www.epilepsyfoundation.org

The International Dyslexia Association (formerly the Orton Dyslexia Society): http://www.interdys.org

Learning Disabilities Association of America (LDA): http://www.ldanatl.org

National Association for the Deaf (NAD): http://www.nad.org

National Down Syndrome Congress (NDSC): http://www.ndsccenter.org

National Organization of Parents of Blind Children (NOPBC): http://www.nfb.org/nfb/Parents_and_Teachers.asp

National Spinal Cord Injury Association (NSCIA): http://www.spinalcord.org

Spina Bifida Association of America (SBAA): http:www.sbaa.org

United Cerebral Palsy (UCP): http://www.ucp.org

Generic support and information organizations

Beach Center on Disability: http://www.beachcenter.org

DisabilityInfo.gov: http://www.disabilityinfo.gov

Easter Seals (formerly the National Easter Seals Society): http://www.easterseals.com

Exceptional Children's Assistance Center (ECAC): http:www.ecac-parentcenter.org

Family Network on Disabilities of Florida, Inc.: http://www.fndfl.org

Federation for Children with Special Needs (FCSN): http://www.fcsn.org

National Dissemination Center for Children with Disabilities (NICHCY): http://www.nichcy.org

National Organization for Rare Disorders (NORD): http://www.rarediseases.org

Ohio Coalition for the Education of Children with Disabilities (OCECD): http://www.ocecd.org

PACER Center (Parent Advocacy Coalition for Educational Rights): http://www.pacer.org

PEAK Parent Center: http://www.peakparent.org

Statewide Parent Advocacy Network (SPAN): http://www.spannj.org

Technical Assistance Alliance for Parent Centers (formerly the Technical Assistance for Parents Program) National Technical Assistance Center: http://www.taalliance.org

Adaptive clothing and equipment

AbleApparel: http://www.ableapparel.com

Access to Recreation: http://www.accesstr.com

Special Clothes: http://www.Special-Clothes.com

Tranquility Incontinence Products: http://www.tranquilityproducts.com

Advocacy and awareness organizations

Family Voices: http:www.familyvoices.org

HEATH Resource Center: http://www.heath.gwu.edu

Architectural access

The American Institute of Architects (AIA): http://www.aia.org

U.S. Access Board: http://www.access-board.gov

Arts

Partners for Youth with Disabilities (PYD) Access to Theatre (ATT): http://www.pyd.org/mentoring_programs/access_to_theatre.htm

VSA Arts: http://www.vsarts.org

Assistive technology

ABLEDATA: http://www.abledata.com

AbilityHub.com: http://www.abilityhub.com

(continued)

Table 38.4. *(continued)*

Augmentative communication

United States Society For Alternative And Augmentative Communication (USSAAC): http://www.ussaac.org

Camps

American Camp Association (ACA): http://www.acacamps.org

Discover Camp: http://ncaonline.org/discover

Communicable diseases

Centers for Disease Control and Prevention National Prevention Information Network (NPIN): http://www.cdcnpin.org/scripts/index.asp

Cookbooks/food

Cooking Made Easy: http://www.cookingmadeeasy.org

Visual Recipes: A Cookbook for Non-Readers: http://www.drlbooks.com

Fathers

The Father's Network: http://www.fathersnetwork.org

Legal services/estate planning

Americans with Disabilities Act Home Page, U.S. Department of Justice: http://www.ada.gov

Disability Rights Education & Defense Fund (DREDF): http://www.dredf.org

Disabled and Alone: http://www.disabledandalone.org

National Disability Rights Network (formerly the National Association of Protection and Advocacy Systems): http://www.napas.org

Special Needs Alliance: http://www.specialneedsalliance.com

Peer support programs

Best Buddies International: http://www.bestbuddies.org

Parent to Parent of the United States (P2P USA): http://www.p2pusa.org

Winners On Wheels (WOW): http://www.wowusa.com

Publications

Exceptional Parent Magazine: http://www.eparent.com

Paul H. Brookes Publishing Co.: http://www.brookespublishing.com

Woodbine House: http://www.woodbinehouse.com

Respite

ARCH National Respite Network and Resource Center: http://www.archrespite.org

Service dogs

Assistance Dogs International: http://www.adionline.org

Siblings

Sibling Support Project: http://www.siblingsupport.org

Sports/recreation

Kids Enjoy Exercise Now (KEEN): http://www.keenusa.org

The National Center on Physical Activity and Disability (NCPAD): http://www.ncpad.org

National Disability Sports Alliance (NDSA): http://www.ndsaonline.org

National Miracle League Association: http://www.miracleleague.com

Palaestra: Forum of Sport, Physical Education, & Recreation for Those with Disabilities: http://www.palaestra.com

Special Olympics: http://www.specialolympics.org

United States Association of Blind Athletes (USABA): http://www.usaba.org

Wheelchair Sports, USA: http://www.wsusa.org

Toys/play

National Lekotek Center: http://www.lekotek.org

Travel

Mobility International USA (MIUSA): http://www.miusa.org

National Park Service, U.S. Department of the Interior: http://www.nationalparks.org/parkspass/default.asp

Society for Accessible Travel & Hospitality (SATH): http://www.sath.org

Travelin' Talk Network (TTN): http://www.travelintalk.net

Vans

The National Mobility Equipment Dealers Association (NMEDA): http://www.nmeda.org

Wheelchair Getaways: http://www.wheelchairgetaways.com

Additional resources

Maternal and Child Health (MCH) Library: http://www.mchlibrary.info/knowledgepaths/kp_community.html

Office of Disability Employment Policy (ODEP), U.S. Department of Labor: http://www.dol.gov/odep

---

sistently appear that are noteworthy for the medical practitioner trouble-shooting for family problems. One is the identification of risk factors for short-term adjustment difficulties:

- *Gender*—male

- *Age*—younger than the sibling with disabilities

- *Age spacing*—closer in age

- The innate personality characteristics of the sibling principals (Simeonsson & Bailey, 1986)

Some of the negative impacts on siblings follow logically from the alterations to normal family functioning necessitated by the special requirements of a child with disabilities. Assisting the parents in identifying the conflicts underlying sibling problems is a valuable support activity. In addition, physicians and other care providers can have a positive influence on siblings simply by validating their concerns, fears, and other issues related to the child with disabilities. Such concerns include

1. *Overidentification*—worrying that they, too, have or will acquire a disability; this is a close kin to genuine empathy.

2. *Embarrassment at the brother's or sister's appearance or behavior*—Over time, this can strengthen a child by prompting in personal and concrete terms the realization that not everyone is the same. By modeling acceptance of, and concern for, the child with disabilities, the physician can powerfully influence the sibling without disabilities. In turn, the sibling becomes a good model for peers—and often for adults as

well. The virtues of tolerance and understanding the needs of others are fostered.

3. *Guilt*—The sibling can live a normal life and his or her brother or sister cannot. Younger children, because of their egocentric perspective, may imagine themselves to be at fault for the disability. Accurate, age-appropriate information about the disabling condition is a prerequisite for the development of healthy sibling relationships.

4. *Isolation*—Wanting to tell friends but being afraid of the reaction; this can be addressed via special activities (e.g., sibling groups, workshops, camp experiences) from which enduring relationships and many insights may evolve. It can be converted from a threat against to an incentive for open communication, particularly with relatives and special friends.

5. *Fears about the future*—Siblings may worry about their brother's or sister's future as well as their own. Who will provide care? This can become a stimulus for teaching the concepts of goal setting and advance planning.

6. *Resentment*—Siblings can be jealous of the reduced amount of parents' time they receive and family financial resources. Frustration may be translated into direct rebellion against parents, teachers, or other authority figures. Adjusting to this unfair situation is an important part of personal growth.

7. *Caregiving*—Siblings are typically the best equipped and most convenient babysitters.

Such caregiving can foster responsibility; however, if caregiving demands are excessive, siblings are deprived of time to themselves, and if the demands are made too early, siblings may be robbed of their own childhood. The concept of "quality time" for siblings comes in here.

8. *Pressure to achieve*—Parental sense of loss experienced when one child has a disability can lead to unrealistically high expectations for the remaining siblings. Similarly, self-induced pressure to please or ease the burden on parents can heighten anxiety and inhibit communication.

For physicians, it is most important to acknowledge the sibling's problem or concern first, let the child expand on it or just reflect for a few minutes, and then gently move into redirection.

Although many specific issues come up, the most frequent is that of *perceived unfairness.* When one child demands so much more attention, time, patience, and financial resources, the other sibling is easily shortchanged (Scheiber, 1989). The pediatrician's role in helping the parents and siblings come to grips with this reality revolves around helping each child feel important and positive about him or herself. Physicians might include siblings in interpretive counseling sessions and thereby model for the family the value of open communication and honesty.

Ethical Dilemmas   Parents often look to their physicians for guidance when difficult decisions must be addressed (Table 38.5; see also Chapter 35, this volume). A structured approach to the decision-making process is a practical first step toward effectively addressing emotionally charged issues (Fost, 1981). This method demands a clear delineation of facts, as opposed to beliefs and anecdotal experiences, and clear identification of the principles involved. Finally, it is important for all parties to know the law as it applies to the situation at hand.

Family-Centered Care

Traditionally, the health care system, in its many facets, has neither supported families nor

Table 38.5.   Ethical dilemmas involving people with disabilities

1. Survival
   Syndromes (selective nontreatment of, e.g., Down syndrome, spina bifida)
   Resuscitation/Do-Not-Resuscitate (DNR) orders
   Medical treatment (e.g., antibiotics, chemotherapy)
   Assisted ventilation
   Tube feeding
   Prenatal diagnosis and abortion

2. Behavior modification (How far do you go?)

3. Health care
   Deinstitutionalized individuals
   HIV (e.g., genuine concern for blood drawing, surgery)

4. Schooling
   Inclusion (Should all children be in inclusive schools/classrooms?)
   Costs (How do you set priorities for limited resources?)
   HIV (safety for others)

5. Employment: Competitive versus supported versus sheltered

6. Institutionalization and deinstitutionalization issues

7. Aging: issues of active programming (Does anyone ever get to "retire" from the sheltered workshop or from behavior modification?)

8. Sexuality and reproduction
   Sterilization versus hygiene/pregnancy
   Opportunities for sex, marriage, childbearing
   Abortion

9. Research on individuals with disabilities (Who can give "informed" consent and for whose good is the study?)

10. Confidentiality and truth telling

Key: HIV, human immunodeficiency virus.

valued the contributions of the family to the well-being of the child. In the past, health care providers were accustomed to authority and control, but more recently providers of care to children with disabilities have embraced the family's role as partners in the health care process (Weil, 1986).

Family-centered care places the family, as opposed to the hospital staff, at the center of the health care universe (Brewer, McPherson, Magrab, & Hutchins, 1989; Hostler, 1991; Shelton, Jeppeson, & Johnson, 1987). The concept was considered revolutionary in the 1990s in terms of attitude about and delivery of services. The key elements of the family-centered process include collaboration with the family as a whole, basing care in the community where the child lives, coordinating care among all levels and disciplines, and establishing appropriate financing mechanisms to support these concepts (Hostler, 1994).

Developmental pediatricians and general pediatricians with a special interest in chronic conditions remain at the forefront of the family-centered care movement. The goal is to ensure that the best supports are made available to the parents of children with any chronic illness or disability. The emphasis in the Americans with Disabilities Act (ADA) of 1990 (PL 101-336) and the early childhood Part H legislation (see Chapter 36, this volume) has been on community-based, family-centered care rather than disease-specific care.

Practice Issues Unique to Children with Disabilities

The complexity of managing some children with developmental disabilities, along with the financial disincentives, lies at the heart of many primary providers' reluctance to accept such children into their practices. Better knowledge and open communication with the neurodevelopmental pediatrician and other specialists in developmental disabilities will facilitate the day-to-day medical care of these children. A number of aspects of medical care specific to this population can present challenges for physicians, especially within the context of managed care restrictions.

Providing a Medical Home for Children with Disabilities The *medical home* philosophy has dominated directives adopted by the American Academy of Pediatrics (AAP Task Force on the Definition of the Medical Home, 1992, updated 2002) and federal funding sources. It implies the essential importance of quality community services to achieve successful family-centered care. Although medical center-based interdisciplinary clinics are needed for comprehensive evaluations, academic pediatricians must address the need for continuing education programs for community

physicians (AAP, 2004). Instruction in nonmedical as well as medical support services should also be included in medical school and residency programs' curricula. General pediatricians and family physicians can then provide better service coordination as well as up-to-date medical care to children and adults with special needs within their own communities. Adults with significant medical conditions living in the community frequently encounter problems gaining access to medical services. There is a need to improve the service delivery system for these individuals (Hayden, Kim, & DePaepe, 2005).

School personnel have urged increased pediatrician input into the educational domain. School staff, like families, need extra support from physicians, especially early intervention and early childhood teachers and therapists. Children whose disabilities come to light before age 3 are likely to be the most medically needy, a very different population from what most special educators encounter in older children (e.g., learning disabilities, attention deficit disorders). In addition to major medical and neurodevelopmental problems (syndromes, seizures, technology dependency), a proportion of these infants have infectious or related etiologies (congenital infections, acquired immunodeficiency syndrome [AIDS]) that can provoke high levels of anxiety for early interventionists, caregivers, and families of other children in center-based programs. Physicians, especially developmental pediatricians, are relied on for information regarding the child's disability or specific syndrome, its cause, and its prognosis, as well as information regarding restrictions from specific interventions and prescriptions for adaptive equipment and/or medications that might be needed to allow the child to receive maximum benefit from therapy. Legislation creates the foundation for a cooperative relationship between medicine and education. To address the health care needs of children with chronic illness or disabilities in the school environment, the use of a formal document—the individual health plan—has been suggested in the Individuals with Disabilities Education Improvement Act of 2004 (PL 108-446) to chronicle the student's needs, clarify roles and responsibilities, and set up lines of communication.

Literature for Parents Parents frequently ask for literature about a new diagnosis. Of the vast amount of literature available for parents about specific disabilities, little has been reviewed critically for quality of content, suitability for parents, or readability by individuals with differing educational backgrounds. Much of this literature is poorly written, misleading, or otherwise unacceptable. In a study critically reviewing literature for parents of children with cerebral palsy, 58% of parent materials were deemed inappropriate to the topic or unacceptable in terms of content (Blasco, Baumgartner, & Mathes, 1983). Undoubtedly, similar problems occur with the quality and appropriateness of literature about other disabling conditions. This experience underscores the need for professionals who deal with children with disabilities to be familiar with the literature or Internet resources generally available and to be prepared to recommend the best materials to families (Anselmo, Lash, Stieb, & Haver, 2004).

Exceptional Parent magazine, written largely by parents, is a forum for sharing information relevant to children with special needs. This publication is practical in nature and inexpensive. Annual focus issues pinpoint relevant topics such as income tax, camps, adaptive equipment, and advocacy and support organizations. An introductory first issue is free to parents. Waiting room subscriptions are available to pediatricians at reduced rates (see also Table 38.4).

Equipment The amount and variety of adaptive equipment and assistive devices available for mobility, communication, and self-help issues can be overwhelming for parents. It is always necessary for the developmentalist to monitor the equipment recommended by therapists and especially by vendors. Experienced clinicians should offer guidance so that children do not end up with expensive but inadequate or ill-matched systems, especially in the most difficult situations (e.g., when a seating system and mobility device must also accommodate an augmentative or alternative communication system). A team approach is essential, whereby knowledgeable individuals from multiple disciplines work in concert with the parents and primary care physician to make complicated decisions about expensive devices.

Dental Care Very few dentists receive training to deal with the special challenges of children with disabilities, and thus access to dental care is a real problem for them due to developmental and behavioral issues. Often children lack understanding and the ability to cooperate. Spasticity and movement disorders may challenge the dentist when trying to perform certain interventions. The issue of restraints becomes a logistical concern. Finally, there may be specific medical precautions (e.g., antibiotic prophylaxis and latex allergy in children with spina bifida and shunts). Pediatricians can help families by recommending resources, in particular the names of dentists who are willing and able to treat patients with disabilities. Developmental pediatricians can assist dentists in their states or local communities by providing training for working with children and adults with special needs (American Dental Association, 2002; Mouradian, Porter, Keegan, & Cantillion, 2001; Perlman, Fenton, & Friedman, 2003). A guide has been developed to assist dental professionals in planning care for children with disabilities (Isman, Newton, Bujold, & Baer, 2000).

Complementary and Alternative Medicine Parents of children with chronic disorders, including many of the neurodevelopmental disabilities, are more likely to use complementary and alternative medicine (CAM). In fact, more than 50% of children with autism, cerebral palsy, or attention-deficit/hyperactivity disorder use CAM (Hyman & Levy, 2005). Thus, both developmental and primary pediatricians should have some knowledge of the popular CAM interventions used in their regions for various disabilities (AAP, 2001a, re-affirmed 2005). The challenge lies in balancing parents' desires to use CAM and the general lack of evidence that the nonstandard treatment is effective. Furthermore, some CAM treatments can have harmful side effects of which physicians must be aware (Cohen & Kemper, 2005) (see Chapter 34 in this volume for an in-depth discussion of CAM).

Administrative and Bureaucratic Detail Both generalist and subspecialist practitioners may fail to appreciate the tremendous support they provide to parents through simple administrative actions (e.g., writing the Letter of Medical Necessity to the insurance company for therapy services or equipment, filling out school physical examination forms or medical eligibility forms for benefits, signing the application for handicapped motor vehicle tags, writing the prescription for therapy services). This is a great deal of bureaucratic paperwork that is often aggravating, time consuming, and mostly unreimbursable, yet it is important that it be completed promptly and courteously and that we avoid giving parents the message that it is a nuisance. Developing a prototype letter to keep on hand and adapt for each circumstance is one way to save some time.

Insurance, Billing, and Reimbursement The effect of health insurance coverage on obtaining medical care for children identified as "disabled" by their schools was examined by Butler, Singer, Palfrey, and Walker (1987). It was found that 1) insurance coverage was a predictor of whether a child with developmental disabilities was seen by a physician in the past year, 2) Hispanic children were less likely than Caucasian or African American children to be insured, and 3) parents of publicly insured children paid for 5% of physician visits out of pocket, whereas parents of privately insured children paid for 30% of visits. Thus, insurance coverage is a significant predictor of physician use, although it only pays for a portion of the care. Prior to 1990, 25% of all children with disabilities had no insurance or only part-year insurance coverage in any given calendar year (Newacheck & McManus, 1988). Among adolescents with disabilities, one in seven (14%) remains uninsured (Newacheck, 1989). Progress has been made in the last 10–15 years in the advent of State

Children's Health Insurance Programs (SCHIP). Modest improvements in coverage and decreases in uninsured status are reported, but access to care and service use have only shown minimal change (Davidoff, Kenney, & Dubay, 2005). In addition, families of children with disabilities, especially those from lower income families, experience higher out-of-pocket expenditures (Newacheck & Kim, 2005).

Issues related to hospital and clinic billing and insensitivity on the part of billing personnel come up repeatedly in parent discussions. Very few parents receive professional advice to help them manage the complex billing and reimbursement systems. Every billing entity should have a representative whose primary function is to advocate for parents and patients.

Financial Management Nobody expects physicians to be financial counselors, but there are some things clinicians can do to help set struggling families on the right track. Worley, Rosenfeld, and Lipscomb (1991) described a program designed at Duke University to teach financial management skills to parents of children with developmental disabilities. They were able to demonstrate money-saving behaviors and other financially sound practices among intervention families compared with controls, and many of the participant families were in considerable debt. Their program includes a section for practicing physicians entitled Advice to Pediatricians to Help Families . . . Save Money.

Partnership Endeavors *Networking* refers to interactions among parents and professionals, generally through large group structures such as The Arc of the United States (formerly the Association for Retarded Citizens) or United Cerebral Palsy (UCP) to help inform and support parents. UCP publishes a newsletter, *The Networker.* Equipment clearinghouses, special babysitting and respite care services, and other resources are typically discovered via these networks. Political and other legislative activities may also be included in network functions. Getting parents linked with local relevant parent support groups is the essential first step toward fruitful networking activities. Parents have become more vocal and invested in relating to professionals as advisors, and advisory boards to hospitals and to specific programs regarding patient care, communication and sensitivity issues, issues of logistics, and advocacy—especially relating to finances and legal rights—have arisen.

An exciting endeavor that has evolved in collaboration between medical center programs and parent groups is the concept of the Parents As Teachers program (Widrick et al., 1991). This program links residents or medical students with volunteer families who have a child with disabilities. The intent of the program is to get the trainee out of the clinic and onto the "turf" of the family to get a realistic and nonmedical view of daily life with the child who is chronically ill or has disabilities. It affords people with hard-earned expertise the chance to pass their important messages on to the next generation of physicians or professionals, who surely will encounter similar situations.

Establishing such a program requires 1) a training director who can structure the Parents As Teachers program into the broader perspective of medical training and who can organize the logistics of directing the trainees, and 2) a parent group or council that can organize the necessary number of volunteer families to participate in the program. Key elements appear to be a solid orientation to the goals and expectations of the program, several substantial visits (2–4 hours each) outside of the clinic setting, and a debriefing session involving program directors, individual families, and individual trainees to discuss and expand on the specific experiences and any insights gained (Blasco, Kohen, & Shapland, 1999).

Summary

Rarely can all of the needs of the child with developmental disabilities be met in the context of the traditional 15- to 20-minute follow-up appointment. This is especially difficult in the context of family-centered care, whereby issues beyond purely medical concerns such as impacts on the parents, siblings, school, and community are addressed. A professional strategy to improve reimbursement for the extra

time and effort this requires is to revert to the disease-centered approach and ask the family to return for multiple appointments, each one concentrating on a specific need and therapeutic modality. This is not very family friendly, although it is sometimes critical for fiscal survival. There is no satisfactory solution to this dilemma; billing codes for counseling time have helped. Green (1991) argued that levels of primary care vary according to the complexity of the patient and family (analogous to primary, secondary, and tertiary levels of inpatient care). As with the inpatient setting, these should be reimbursed in a hierarchical fashion. Advocacy for fair and appropriate reimbursement schemes and personal resistance to fragmentation of care are ongoing issues for the conscientious practitioner.

CHALLENGES OF PARENTING A CHILD WITH DISABILITIES

At the onset of their parenting journey, families of children with disabilities desperately seek information about their child's condition. Parents look for guidance from their pediatrician and from developmental experts. They also seek information from the Internet, public library, early intervention/education professionals, and from other families who face similar challenges. They may discover a parent support group that can provide information about their child's condition. In a survey of parents of children with disabilities in New York, "more information" ranked second in importance on their wish list of needs (Liptak & Revell, 1989).

During the child's preschool years, most parents experience some degree of frustration and burnout. They may feel overburdened by the extra care and supervision that is required, and they may question their ability and stamina to continue to raise their children with disabilities at home. The eventual recognition and acknowledgement that they do indeed need support often corresponds to a crisis or transition when there is disruption of routine daily activities (Brett, 2004). Breaks are important to all parents. Parents of typically developing children can take breaks without much effort since they can usually enlist the help of neighbors, friends and relatives to babysit their child.

Children with disabilities may need baby sitters or temporary caregivers with special training or expertise. Simply defined, *respite* is any temporary relief provided by trained personnel to the primary caregivers of an individual with disabilities or chronic illness. These trained professionals and/or paraprofessionals are usually "strangers" to the family despite their specialized care experience. Usually found in the employ of disability-related agencies, they are more expensive and sometimes more difficult to obtain.

During the child's elementary and middle school years, most parents of typically developing children expect to provide less direct caregiving as their children mature and can perform more tasks by themselves. Also, portions of child care responsibilities may be assumed by the parents of the child's friends, camp counselors, scout leaders, church youth group managers, and so forth. Such opportunities for help may not be readily available to parents of children with disabilities, increasing the risk for parent burn-out.

During adolescence, typically developing teenagers exert more independence, and parents eventually find themselves relieved of almost all direct care responsibilities. Parents' anticipated freedom becomes a reality, and they may again pursue educational or employment goals and/or engage in hobbies or recreation activities that positively affect their own health, self-esteem, spousal relationships, and self-reliance. Parents of a teenager with a disability may not experience this "typical" decline in direct care-providing responsibilities, nor will they get the opportunity to temporarily change course (Parish, Seltzer, Greenberg, & Floyd, 2004). More important, their teenagers may never become independent, such that they may never be able to experience that "freedom" that unfolds later in life. In addition, older children with disabilities are usually physically bigger, making care tasks (e.g., transferring, bathing, toileting) more difficult, especially for aging parents.

Families may have fluctuating needs. There are *critical periods* during the journey when parents of children with disabilities, who otherwise are coping fairly well, might need extra support. These usually represent times of major transitions when the child's "differences" become more obvious. Early in the child's life, these include the periods when the diagnosis is first made, when a younger sibling developmentally "passes" the child with disabilities, and when the child with disabilities first enrolls in "special" education. Later critical periods include the onset of puberty (especially when it is associated with physiological abnormalities and/or the appearance of inappropriate sexual behaviors), graduation from high school (especially in the absence of appropriate vocational opportunities and/or community supports), and transition from pediatric to adult providers of health care. Coping skills are also challenged when the teenager is excluded from typical rites of adolescent passage (e.g., social and athletic events, dating, driving).

Ultimately, when extended family, financial assets, appropriate health care and community services and/or public supports are not available or when there is fear, lack of knowledge or lack of skills, parents may cope less well and some may consider an out-of-home placement. To prevent this, parents may need professional assistance to find the help needed to continue the parenting journey.

LEVELS OF SUPPORTS

Supports that are multifaceted, easy to access, and matched to the family's needs can play a significant role in mediating stress and enhancing coping skills for families of children with disabilities (Brett, 2004; see Table 38.6). In the past, supports provided by state and/or community agencies were dictated by bureaucrats who designed services that met the requirements of a grant or policy rather than the actual needs of the family. More progressive legislation has placed parents in leadership roles where they have had a hand in developing and writing policies. At the grass roots level, these efforts have increasingly resulted in greater parent choice in determining their own family's needs and menu of supportive services.

Resources available to families of children with disabilities can be divided into three broad categories of supports: natural, informal, and formal (Figure 38.1) (Cooley, 1994; Johnson & Blasco, 1997). In Figure 38.1, the center two

Table 38.6. Menu of family support services

Core services

Respite and child care
  Respite
  Child care
  Sitter care

In-home assistance
  Homemaker services
  Attendant care
  Home health care
  Chores

Environmental adaptation
  Adaptive equipment
  Assistive technology
  Home modification

Recreation
  Recreation camp

Support
  Family counseling
  Family support groups

Parent training
  Financial
  Advocacy techniques

Information and legal assistance
  Information and referral
  Advocacy

Other needs
  Special diet
  Special clothing
  Special equipment or supplies
  Health insurance
  Transportation
  Vehicle modification
  Rent assistance
  Utilities

Traditional developmental services

Evaluation/assessment
Medical and dental care
Nursing services
Behavior management
Individual counseling
Speech therapy
Occupational therapy
Physical therapy
Skill training

Financial assistance

Discretionary cash
Allowances
Subsidies
Vouchers

Service coordination

From Human Services Research Institute. (1990). *Family support services in the United States: An end of decade status report* (p. 40). Cambridge, MA: Author.

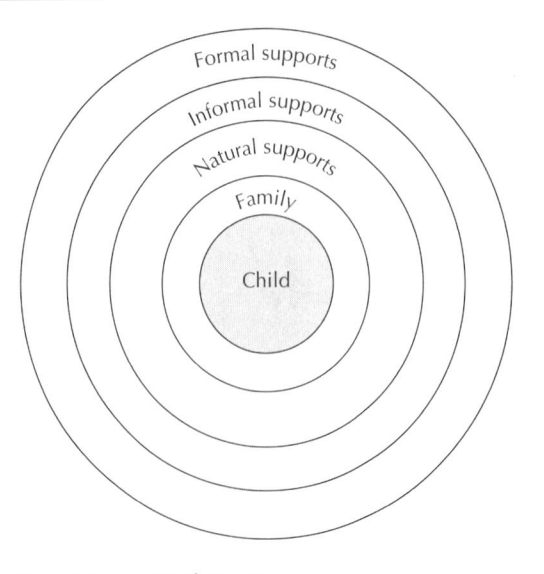

Figure 38.1. Types of support.

rings represent the nuclear family. The next ring is *natural supports*—extended family members, neighbors, church members, and friends. Extended family members, in particular, can be tremendously helpful to parents and siblings both in relieving the demands of physical caregiving and in providing psychological and emotional support. The next ring represents *informal supports,* which includes social networking with other families of children with disabilities through parent support groups and community agencies that provide mother's day out services, respite, social events and recreational activities. Informal supports also include products and equipment that facilitate daily caregiving efforts and access to community events. Finally, the outer ring represents those *formal supports* that are publicly funded and state administered, such as special education programs, accessible transportation, Medicaid, In-Home and Community-Based Waiver Services, Supplemental Security Income benefits, and other financial subsidies.

*Natural support*s are usually free or swapped out and may be adequate for some families; however, at the time of a crisis, even the most resilient families may need to temporarily gain access to *informal* and *formal support* systems. A new crisis can be as simple as denied access to the usual child care arrangement due to acute illness or as complex as the death of a parent or other key caregiver. In order to sustain and enhance caregiving efforts during their parenting journey (in times of crisis as well as throughout typical times), parents of children with disabilities should have access to an array of both formal and informal supports. Support should begin with the closest and most natural resources and proceed outward toward publicly funded programs.

Natural Supports

Immediate family members, friends, and neighbors are usually the primary assets on which parents depend, especially in the beginning. Families that are more mobile tend to have less natural support available. For example, military families, who are typically reassigned to a new location every 3–5 years, are regularly stripped of their natural supports, especially when they are assigned to overseas locations. Families who move multiple times within the same metropolitan area to dodge creditors often lose touch with sources of natural supports. In addition, families who, for various reasons, have been ''abandoned'' by their kinfolk also lack natural supports. In any of these situations, the family may eventually become entirely dependent on (formal) government subsidy programs.

Prayer, worship services, and social activities sponsored by churches can be of tremendous support to many families. In a growing number of communities, churches have developed specialized religious education programs for children with disabilities. A few have also adopted programs that provide a mother's day out or other forms of relief for parents of children with disabilities.

Informal Supports

Informal supports include community-based *services* and commercial *products* that assist parents in their caregiving roles. This category is characterized by the widest spectrum of possibilities. Contact information, including web sites and telephone numbers, are provided in Table 38.4.

Services Availability, eligibility criteria, and access to family support services vary from state to state. Some nonprofit organizations provide support services free of charge; others may apply a sliding fee scale so that all families can afford the services. Community programs may receive government grants or enter into contractual agreements with state agencies that enable them to provide services free to families or for small co-pays. Approximately 20 states provide cash subsidies directly to parents so that they can purchase necessary services or products (Parish, Pomeranz-Essley, & Braddock, 2003).

Advocacy and Support Groups Advocacy and support groups follow a fairly well-structured sequence of objectives (Bergen, 1993). Each physician should keep four or five key telephone numbers readily accessible for referring families to support resources. Parent training programs are most often developed by advocacy and support groups. Their purpose is to support the family as active partners with professionals and agency personnel (collaborators, decision makers, problem solvers). Whereas most advocacy groups are chiefly directed at parents, support groups exist for parents, children with disabilities, and siblings.

Parent groups are places where parents of children with disabilities can share information and provide one another with guidance and support. Numerous organizations were developed by parents for parents. For example, through Parent to Parent, trained, veteran parents are matched in a one-to-one relationship with parents new to the program. Every state has at least one Parent Training and Information Center to support the family as collaborators, decision makers, problem solvers, and active partners with health professionals and agency personnel (contact the PACER Center; see Table 38.4.). Many large national organizations (e.g., The Arc of the United States, Beach Center on Disability) address generic ''process of care'' issues that are important to parents of children with all types of disabilities (e.g., special education, public supports, health insurance). Other organizations are disability-specific (e.g., Spina Bifida Association of America, United Cerebral Palsy) and engage in a broad range of activities that include providing informational materials about the disorder, matching and networking families, publishing newsletters, holding regular meetings, making referrals to local resources, putting on conferences, advocacy efforts, and maintaining a research registry. Equipment clearinghouses, adaptive sporting opportunities, respite care services, and other resources are typically discovered via these networks. A more recent type of parent support is the Internet, especially for parents whose child has a rare disorder and no local support group exists.

Children's groups allow children with various disabilities to benefit from socializing with other children facing similar physical and educational challenges. For example, Winners on Wheels (WOW) is a program that brings together children ages 6–18 who use wheelchairs so that they can talk about shared experiences. Youth with disabilities may also benefit from support programs (e.g., Best Buddies International) that pair them with their peers without disabilities.

Sibling groups allow siblings of children with disabilities the opportunity to discuss issues and share experiences that take place within their families. Sibshops, for example, are agency-based programs that offer peer support and education to school-age siblings in a relaxed, recreational setting.

Respite Care All parents benefit from occasional breaks from the day-to-day challenges of raising children. *Respite*—periodic breaks in caregiving that are provided by professionally trained personal care attendants or respite care providers—has become a critical and immensely valuable part of the comprehensive services now available to children with disabilities. Providers can range from volunteers with training or with expertise gained from personal experience (e.g., via a family member) to registered nurses, and there are several types:

- *Center-based respite*—Children are cared for in hospitals, nursing homes, residential schools, and, more recently, camps, specialized "respite houses," and certain church and private child day care facilities for a contracted period of time ranging from a few hours to one month. The mean duration is about 48 hours, usually occurring over a weekend. Most agencies providing such care operate on a sliding fee scale.

- *In-home respite*—A trained respite caregiver is paid to come into the person's home and provide assistance with daily living activities. The parents may remain at home and relax or work on household projects, leave the home to enjoy local recreational activities, or even leave town on vacation. If a nurse is needed, this can be expensive, costing up to $40 per hour. Otherwise, the cost ranges from $7 to $12 per hour depending on community salary standards.

- *Family co-op respite*—Families of children with developmental disabilities network with each other to provide reciprocating respite. Usually participating families have children who require similar specialized skills. No money is passed between participants; they simply trade (barter) weekends or other periods of time whereby they care for each other's child, usually in the host family's home.

- *Emergency respite*—Families can obtain respite services on short notice. Besides providing a quick "break," another goal of emergency respite is to help parents cope more appropriately during periods of stress and to prevent child abuse.

- *Faith-based respite programs*—As part of their charitable mission, churches are beginning to partner with parent advocacy groups and offer respite in religious education facilities.

Service Dogs The facilitated assistance dog differs from the traditional service dog in that an adult caregiver and the child receive extensive training in how to work as a team to care for the service animal. The adult, however, is responsible for the dog's handling and maintenance. Facilitated service animals are trained to meet the child's needs. For example, the hearing/signal alert dog alerts the child with hearing impairments to sounds such as alarm clocks, telephones and smoke alarms. Although social dogs may be trained to help with physical tasks, their primary functions are to offer emotional support and to assist the child in developing social relationships. Some nonprofit organizations provide financial assistance for the service animal's placement and training; however, the family should be prepared to pay $1,000 or more annually for food and veterinary care. Caregivers will also likely invest up to 10 hours per week feeding, grooming and providing general care for the service animal (Nattrass, Davis, O'Brien, Patronek, & MacCollin, 2004).

Recreation and Leisure Programs

Schools, municipal programs, and national recreational programs offer a spectrum of recreational activities that are accessible to children with disabilities. Many national sports programs to ensure that individuals with disabilities, of all ability levels, have access to traditional *competitive sports.* Special Olympics is the oldest program and provides year-around training and sports competition for children and adults with intellectual disabilities in 26 summer and winter sports. The National Disability Sports Alliance (NDSA) provides athletic opportunities for individuals with physical disabilities including spinal cord injury, amputation, visual impairment, cerebral palsy and traumatic brain injury. The National Center on Physical Activity and Disability is an excellent source for information about all types of recreational activities and adaptive sports.

Some athletic programs for young people with disabilities forego traditional competition in favor of *noncompetitive athletics* designed primarily to build self-esteem and provide children with opportunities to take part in recreational activities and team sports. Through Kids Enjoy Exercise Now Foundation (KEEN), children and young adults with severe and profound physical and intellectual disabilities enjoy social outings and participate in activities such as tennis, swimming, basketball, soccer and fitness training. The Miracle League is a baseball league created for children with a full range of disabilities. Unlike regular baseball, the adaptive league is arranged so everyone bats and everyone scores.

Recreational therapy (e.g., hippotherapy, hydrotherapy) often gets shortchanged when the topic of therapy is covered, but all children should have access to physical activities in the least restrictive environment. Advocates have outlined detailed programs for treatment of acute injuries as well as more chronic neuro-developmental syndromes. The emotional benefits in terms of recreational enjoyment and self-esteem enhancement are more readily apparent in these programs compared with traditional therapy; however, the benefits of riding a horse, for example, exist in terms of balance and tone improvements and are similar to those with the therapy ball that is used in more traditional physical therapy exercises (Cherng et al., 2004; Liptak, 2005).

The U.S. Congress has designated VSA Arts as the coordinating arts organization for individuals with disabilities. An international nonprofit organization, VSA arts was founded in the 1970s to ensure that people with disabilities have full inclusion in *dance, music, and art.* Programs include training institutes, artist-in-residence projects, arts camps, and an awards program to recognize emerging artists. Another innovative arts program is the integrated Partners for Youth with Disabilities Access to Theatre (ATT) program in Boston, Massachusetts. ATT engages youth with and without disabilities interested in poetry, singing, acting and directing to work collaboratively as peers to create theatrical productions.

Summer camp experiences can be enormously valuable to all children. Although the main benefit is simply having fun, organized camping can promote emotional maturity and independence. Group living fosters communication and provides unique opportunities to openly express feelings and to develop relationships. *Discover Camp* is a resource guide that offers practical suggestions for parents choosing a camp program for their child with a disability for the first time. Although a growing number of camps are now serving children with mild and moderate disabilities, most camps are not yet staffed or equipped to accept children with the full spectrum of severe disabilities. There are a few, however, that have recruited large teams of medical volunteers and trained staff. Examples include Camp CAMP in Texas, Camp Courageous in Iowa, and Trail's Edge Camp (specifically for children who use ventilators) in Michigan. The American Camp

Association (ACA), the licensing and accreditation agency for all camps nationwide, has adopted a fairly strict policy to ensure access. Parents should be aware, however, that many camps are not accredited by the ACA and, thus, are not bound by such criteria.

Travel   The ADA now mandates accessibility in hotels, parks, and public transportation. Hotels offering airport shuttle services should have a wheelchair-accessible van. Some travel agencies specialize in making travel arrangements for individuals with disabilities. Another travel resource is the Society for Accessible Travel and Hospitality, a nonprofit membership organization that promotes accessible travel for individuals with disabilities in the United States and abroad.

The National Park Service was the first federal agency to make accessibility a high priority. A general guidebook to accessibility covering more than 350 *national parks* is available: *The Complete Guide to America's National Parks.* Children with disabilities and their families may receive special discounts to *theme parks* and often receive special attention, such as separate and much shorter waiting lines for various attractions. Disney theme parks publish accessibility guidebooks that are available at the theme parks or by calling ahead.

The *Travelin' Talk Network* is dedicated to helping individuals with disabilities enjoy their vacations (Molnar, 1991). The Network was created by a wheelchair user as an informal network of individuals with disabilities and other interested people to serve as a safety net for travelers with disabilities. The premise is simple, yet effective. There are more than 1,000 Network members, most with disabilities, located in every state. Members agree to serve as a resource for other members with disabilities to facilitate travel. When one member travels to another location, he or she can call a member in the destination city in advance for information about weather, local accommodations, accessible activities and more. In the event of an emergency while on the road, one can call a member in the local area for assistance and referrals. All members pay a one-time membership fee.

Products   Although services dominate most discussions about informal supports, various products can be very important to families and can significantly affect the quality of their lives. Some products are needed for safety reasons; others promote independence or facilitate the parent's caregiving efforts. Among parents who received cash subsidies as part of their state's publicly funded family support program, 40% indicated they used the money to purchase diapers, 62% purchased adapted toys, and 36% purchased special foods (Agosta & Melda, 1995).

Clothing   An array of adaptive clothing is on the market for individuals with disabilities. Adaptive items include shirts with Velcro closures, wide-cut trousers with elasticized waistbands for individuals who use wheelchairs, and sneakers specially sized to accommodate orthotics. Jackets and shirts with openings in the back can reduce lifting and make it easier for caregivers to dress a child in a wheelchair. Above all, adaptive clothing should be designed to maintain the child's dignity. Shirts for children who require gastrostomy-tube feedings often utilize discreet openings, for example, behind the shirt pocket, to facilitate feeding. For the older child, the bandana or kerchief is a functional, age-appropriate alternative to the traditional bib.

Adaptive clothing costs may be a reimbursable item covered by insurance. Like adaptive equipment, specialized clothing can promote independence, helping make the case for insurance coverage. Parents should document the need for the adaptive clothing and seek a prescription for each specific item from their physician.

Toys   Parents or caregivers may need assistance when selecting toys for children with disabilities to ensure accessibility. With 36 play centers nationwide, the National Lekotek Center is a nonprofit organization dedicated to ensuring that children with disabilities have access to play. The National Lekotek Center works in partnership with Toys "R" Us and the United Parents' Syndicate on Disabilities to develop the annual *Toy Guide for Differently Abled Kids.* Each item in the catalog has been evaluated by the National Lekotek Center in terms of its educational, developmental and entertainment value. Likewise, *Exceptional Parent* publishes an Annual Toy Review. Although the toys included in the issue are available for all children and have not been adapted or modified, they have been recommended as safe and educational for children with special needs by a panel of parents and professionals.

Cookbooks, Diets, and Feeding Supports Feeding is one of the most important and rewarding caregiving activities parents provide, but it can be one of the most frustrating and stressful when a child with disabilities is not gaining weight and thriving or has feeding difficulties, swallowing and choking problems, food overselectivity, and reflux or habitual vomiting after meals. In some children with disabilities who have oral motor problems or swallowing problems, calorie-rich food thickeners such as Thick-it can facilitate oral feedings and decrease choking and gagging. Clothing catalogues often feature special bibs and other products that can facilitate feeding.

Cookbooks for families of children with disabilities are beginning to appear on the bookstands. Some feature recipes that are fiber rich to help children who do not ambulate have regular bowel movements. Others address specific nutritional challenges associated with a particular disability such as Down syndrome (Medlen, 2002). Adaptive cookbooks (e.g., *Cooking Made Easy, Visual Recipes*) have been created for individuals with disabilities; they utilize simple text and photos to depict step-by step instructions.

Adaptive Sporting and Mobility Equipment and Vehicles Due in part to the growth and availability of adaptive sports and recreational equipment, the number of individuals with disabilities participating in physical activity and sports has increased dramatically since the 1990s. A lightweight sports wheelchair that is easy to maneuver facilitates mobility and is often used by those in competitive games. Bicycles, likewise, are available with modifications for competitive and recreational purposes. Flotation vests, head floats, and hydraulic lifts to facilitate pool transfers are commonly used in water sports and swimming. Other adaptive equipment includes golf clubs shortened for individuals who use wheelchairs.

Adaptive vans enhance mobility and independence for those with physical impairments. Modifications vary according to the needs of the individual, from simple pedal extensions or manual hand controls to more complex adaptations, such as automatic or semi-automatic lifts that facilitate van exit and entry for wheelchair users. The National Mobility Equipment Dealers Association is a trade organization dedicated to ensuring quality transportation options for individuals with disabilities.

Formal Supports

Formal supports include publicly funded programs that, among others, provide financial assistance (e.g., Supplemental Security Income [SSI] benefits, food stamps), special education, medical assistance (Medicaid), vocational training, and residential/living services. For the most part, publicly funded supports exist because of federal legislation, which is then interpreted and legislated at the state level. Implementation of state laws is largely influenced by budgetary restrictions. Many formal programs benefiting families of children with disabilities depend on a combination of both state and federal funds. Depending on the particular "funding formula" and local budgetary constraints, states vary a great deal in what they offer.

Public programs are governed by federal rules and state policies established for each program. State agencies can directly provide services or can contract out services to both private for profit and not-for-profit local organizations; however, they always retain oversight and quality control tasks in-house. Because of the budget deficits during 2002–2004, many states redefined family support programs and are combining them with other programs and or moving them to other state agencies to decrease administrative overhead (Agosta, 2004). In so doing, many of the opportunities for families and advocates to participate in policymaking have been minimized. Agency personnel and advocates are currently striving to break down the barriers of isolated agency funding "silos" and to work toward collaboration and cooperation. More so now than ever, it takes persistence to track multiple changes in contact people, telephone numbers, eligibility criteria, and benefits.

Financial Supports   Supplemental Security Income (SSI) benefits are a "needs-based" benefit (i.e., based on income and assets) for low income families. Eligibility during childhood depends on a disability severity criterion and a financial criterion for the family. If the child meets both criteria, the family will receive a monthly stipend; in most states, the child will automatically become eligible for Medicaid. Some families, depending on their financial circumstances, may also be eligible for food stamps and subsidized housing. A helpful parent handout can be found in the "ABC's of SSI" (Winston, 2004). Many older teens with disabilities first become eligible for SSI benefits (and Medicaid) at their 18th birthday when they are legally adults and their parents' income and financial assets are no longer considered in the eligibility process.

Life insurance companies frequently deny applications for coverage or drastically escalate premiums for children with disabilities, regardless of severity. The lack of a life insurance policy can have a significant impact on the individual's ability in adulthood to finance personal opportunities such as self-employment and buying a home. Several large insurance agencies have created specialized divisions and have trained agents in issues specific to the needs of families with children with disabilities. MassMutual, for example, has developed the SpecialCare program (http://www.massmutual.com) whereby representatives are trained in aspects of tax and estate planning specific for children with disabilities. MetLife has created the Division of Estate Planning for Special Kids (MetDESK), which is committed to helping families through the maze of legal and financial future planning for children with special needs (http://www.metlife.com/desk).

Educational Supports   The possible roles for the physician under the federal early intervention statutes have been outlined by the AAP Committee on Children with Disabilities (2001b) in the policy statement entitled "Role

of the Pediatrician in Family-Centered Early Intervention Services." For a more detailed discussion of early intervention programs see Chapter 26, this volume. The pediatrician also plays an important role in the development of the individualized education program (IEP) as outlined in the AAP Policy Statement entitled, "The Pediatrician's Role in Development and Implementation of an IEP and/or IFSP" (AAP Committee on Children with Disabilities, 1992, affirmed in 1999).

Residential and Daily Living Supports

In addition to supports provided through SSI, health care programs, and school programs, children with disabilities may be eligible for additional support services (in-home nursing care, respite, medical equipment, home modifications for accessibility). These supports are funded by a combination of federal and state funds. States vary a great deal in the degree of funding allocated for these additional support services. Some states have policies that guarantee all children with disabilities will live in family settings, but most states still allocate a majority of spending to institutional settings.

Institutions are state-operated organizations that house hundreds to thousands of individuals in segregated settings. Due to legislation promoting community inclusion, most states are in the process of closing large institutions. *ICF/MRs* are facilities staffed with shift workers, and individuals with disabilities have limited choice or control over their lives. Individuals live in architecturally "typical housing" in more community-based, inclusive settings. ICF/MRs vary in size from small (3–6 people), to medium (7–15 people), to large (more than 16 people). The smallest ICF/MRs are often called "group homes"; however, another type of *group home* (always fewer than six clients) exists where the funding stream is different. In this type of support the family and/or individual with disabilities can choose the group home, there is more client autonomy, and, instead of shift workers, full-time or part-time attendants may also live in the home. The degree of true community inclusion and "normalcy" among all the various group homes vary a great deal.

Funding is available to families raising their children with disabilities in their own homes. The funding for in-home supports is of two types: waiver options and cash subsidies. The most common funding mechanism is called Home and Community-Based Services, or HCBS, Waivers. Eligibility depends on the severity of the child's disability and the circumstances it imposes on the family.

States have developed different mechanisms to distribute their limited resources; some use a combination of options. The options include, but are not limited to:

- First come–first serve waiting lists
- Urgency of need
- Time-limited supports
- Lottery system
- Family council systems

It is clear that the movement away from congregate care is proceeding with the use of HCBS (Medicaid) Waivers and changes in state policies and funding streams. Every state must now have some degree of relevant and directly applicable family support potentially available to families raising children with disabilities at home. The AAP strongly supports the goal of universal home care for all children with special needs (Johnson & Kastner, 2005). The Johnson and Kastner report (2005) introduced permanency planning principles and family-based options for children with disabilities.

Because each state has organized their services and access mechanisms differently, pediatricians and families must learn their own state's idiosyncrasies. To do this, one can contact the state or county offices of the Departments of Health and Human Services, Department of Mental Health and Mental Retardation or Developmental Disabilities Council. Local parent advocacy organizations, The Arc, early intervention administrators and/or school district special education coordinators are often knowledgeable about these various programs and their respective eligibility requirements.

PERMANENCY PLANNING

Permanency planning principles have been employed successfully within the child protective services system for 30 years. The goal of permanency planning is for the child to have an enduring, safe, secure, nurturing family home with parents who have made a long-term commitment to raise him or her and maintain a life-long relationship into adulthood. Permanency goals are met when 1) a child returns to live with his birth family after whatever problems that led to placement have been ameliorated, 2) the child is adopted, or 3) the child lives with foster parents who have made a psychological long-term commitment even though they are not in a position to adopt. Permanency planning is directed at creating the supports necessary around any of the above families so that a child can enjoy the developmental benefits of family life with consistent nurturing adults.

An innovative family-based strategy being developed to move children out of institutions is the use of *support families*. Support families are recruited and trained to share parenting with the birth/adoptive family or, in some cases, they care for the child on a permanent basis with periodic visits to the birth family according to the coping abilities and desires of that family. Support families, as long as they receive adequate levels of support, have been readily recruited from the community (Rosenau, 2005a, 2005b). This model encourages interaction between the birth and support families. The arrangement, unlike traditional foster care or adoption, allows birthparents to retain their parenting rights and to continue their relationship with their child even though they are not able to provide full-time direct care. When the birth family's parenting efforts fall short and they feel overwhelmed, they may express (or hint) a need to seek an out-of-home placement. Introducing the possible option of support families and helping them gain access to agencies that facilitate such an arrangement can be an enormous service, and an enormous relief, to a struggling family.

Whether the child leaving the institution is cared for by the birth family, an adoptive family, or a combination including a support family, family supports are vital in preserving the stamina and optimism of all involved. Unfortunately, in many states, when a child with disabilities leaves the institution, the funding does NOT follow the child to provide supports for the families involved. Revising policies so that funding follows the child instead of being tied to the institution is critical to moving children out of institutions and into family homes (Rosenau, 2005a, 2005b).

SAFEGUARDING PUBLICLY FUNDED SUPPORTS AND RIGHTS

Publicly funded programs may increase or decrease as a result of changing legislation that is usually budget driven. Individual families may lose supports due to specific circumstances, which parents may not be aware of. For example, public supports like Medicaid and SSI are "needs based" and available to the child with disabilities if the family meets certain financial criteria. Although a child with disabilities may have qualified for public supports on medical and financial grounds, a change in his or her family's "worth" may cause a loss of benefits. Parents and professionals should be knowledgeable about policies that govern public supports in order to guarantee that they are appropriately provided and also are safeguarded for the future.

When access to or loss of an entitled benefit occurs, the family can seek assistance from their state protection and advocacy (P&A) agency. These federally mandated agencies are funded by two federal programs: Protection and Advocacy for People with Developmental Disabilities and Protection and Advocacy for Individual Rights. P&A agencies provide a unique and effective resource for disability rights advocacy and education, and the services are usually free of charge to families. Contact information for state offices can be found in the *Exceptional Parent Resource Guide* or one can contact the National Disability Rights Network listed in Table 38.4.

Older teenagers and adults may lose public supports if their personal income or assets increase such that they exceed eligibility criteria. Parents and other relatives must take this into consideration when writing a will and/or choosing beneficiaries for a life insurance policy (Brunetti, 1995). In addition, funds received from a court settlement for personal injury or medical malpractice can also make a

child with disabilities ineligible for public supports. One option is to develop a long-term financial plan that includes a *special needs trust* (SNT) (Brunetti, 1996). The SNT must contain a statement that the inheritance or court settlement may only be spent on items and services that are not otherwise covered by federal subsidies. A guidebook on managing the SNT looks particularly helpful (Jackins et al., 2004). The usual simple will or a conventional trust leaving property or cash to a child with disabilities could be the worst thing parents can do if the assets disqualify the child from receiving public supports. Siblings' inheritances may be similarly at risk.

SUPPORTS FOR OLDER ADOLESCENTS WITH DISABILITIES

Transition is defined as the passage from child-centered activities to adult-oriented activities. Transition occurs in three main aspects of life: 1) from pediatric health care to adult-oriented health care, 2) from school to work, and 3) from home to community. Because of the many barriers that mitigate against teenagers making the transition to providers of adult health care, teen transition has recently become a top priority in the national public health policy arena (Blum, 2002; AAP Committee on Children with Disabilities, 2002). At age 18, a teenager with disabilities may become eligible for Medicaid for the first time because at that time, his or her own income, and not that of the parents, determines eligibility. In addition, when teenagers turn 18 years old, they become their own legal guardians regardless of cognitive abilities. Thus, legally, their parents can no longer make decisions about their health care. If parents feel the adult child is incapable of making such decisions, then they need to seek legal guardianship.

Pediatricians can help families prepare for these transitions during the childhood years by emphasizing the importance of children with disabilities 1) learning as much as possible about their own disability, 2) taking responsibility for their own self-care, and later, 3) becoming active in the decision-making processes regarding their own health care. Simply informing the family about available educational, vocational, and independent living options is an important first step.

Guardianship

If parents and professionals working with a teenager with disabilities do not feel that the individual is capable of making responsible decisions, a formal team evaluation should be done to determine the need for guardianship (Lacey, 2004). Procedures and terminology vary from state to state. It is wise to do this in a proactive manner, well before the child's 18th birthday. If an adult child needs a surgical procedure, the parents will not be allowed to provide *informed consent* unless they have completed the formal guardianship process. This could come up in a crisis situation if the adult child needs a procedure immediately or in the event of trauma or another life-threatening disorder. If guardianship turns out to be in the individual's best interests, then legal services should be sought to help the parents navigate the legal/judicial system in order to file a petition in a probate court and to designate a legal guardian for the individual.

Guardianship should be pursued cautiously because it contradicts the values of self-determination and rights that should be protected in the adult with milder deficits. If the older teenager or adult has some degree of understanding and decision-making skills, less restrictive options exist:

- Powers of attorney
- Representative payee
- Special Needs Trust (SNT) Trustee

These three options do not require court action; the decision-making is kept within the family unit.

Personal Care Attendants and Job Coaches

Personal care attendant (PCA) services are available to older teenagers and young adults who live in an apartment or home but need some degree of assistance. If the individual qualifies and is approved for funding, the local provider agency will conduct a standardized home assessment and determine the number of hours of assistance for which the individual qualifies. The individual with disabilities then recruits, interviews, hires, and supervises a personal care attendant who can help with daily living activities, personal hygiene, household chores, transportation, and shopping. Some individuals with disabilities who are relatively independent at home may require ongoing attendant services at the work place in order to accomplish required duties or may benefit from a temporary job coach to teach new skills needed to work independently at a new job. Some individuals will need support both at home and at the work place, and a PCA may also function as job coach if qualified. The theoretical availability and the reality of finding and retaining some of these services can be distressingly discrepant. A common complaint about PCA services is the lack of trained, experienced, and competent attendants. Rapid turnover of personal care attendants has also been a considerable problem.

PROVIDING RELIEF ALWAYS: HOW THE DEVELOPMENTAL PEDIATRICIAN CAN MAKE AN IMPACT

Families of children with disabilities usually have needs that require greater physician time and attention than those of the typically developing child. Although support activities and support services may at first appear to be overwhelming in number and complexity, physicians can be tremendously helpful in two broad and straightforward ways. First, through the direct activities such as honing one's skill at presenting bad news and having a strategy for addressing sibling issues, physicians can make the lives of parents, siblings, and children with disabilities easier. Most of these direct services are part of the usual repertoire of almost all pediatricians and family physicians.

Second, there is an extensive list of available public and private support resources to which the physician can help the family gain access. Matching a family's or patient's needs to a precise program is often very difficult, and resource guides typically offer no insight to program quality. Parents benefit from the knowledge of an insider who knows what quality services are available in the community and how to obtain them. This is where advocacy and support groups come in. They can provide valuable service to physicians in terms of identifying the best resources. A compendium of resources is provided in Table 38.4. It covers some special topics (e.g., architects, siblings) and emphasizes national organizations that can assist the clinician and/or family in finding the needed regional resources.

Attitudes, legislation, and services since the 1950s have benefited children with disabilities and their families, although existing services cannot be expected to meet the needs of all families at all times. Developmental pediatricians are ideally positioned to both provide relief to families currently in their care and to make a positive impact on other families with whom they may not be directly involved through the training of medical students, pediatrics residents, and practicing pediatricians. Physicians can strive to foster the these aptitudes, capacities, and endeavors.

- Listening to what *parents* feel they need in the way of supports (Liptak & Revell, 1989; Brett, 2004)

- Being knowledgeable about existing family supports and making parents aware of them; a common reason why parents do not obtain supports is because they did not know they exist.

- Meeting with local and state leaders associated with funding, provider agencies, local or state early intervention program, the special education department in the local school districts, and/or the municipal, county, or state health and human services departments

- Promoting parent–professional relationships and partnering with them in medical decision making

- Serving as a consultant or advisor for community organizations and public programs such as early intervention programs, schools, and group homes; physicians can provide in-service training for staff regarding different aspects of caring for a child

with disabilities and provide technical support to increase staff comfort level and to increase access for families of children with disabilities. They can encourage other professionals with expertise in children with disabilities to serve on boards and advisory councils, and to assist with technical support and/or training.

- Advocating for increased breadth and depth of supports in all communities both to prevent out-of-home placements or, when they are absolutely necessary, to support family-based options; physicians can join forces with families, seasoned disability advocates, and state and national representatives to address issues regarding supports for families of children with disabilities. They can stay abreast of pending legislation such as the Family Opportunity Act and the Lifespan Respite Care Act (Johnson & Kastner, 2005) that may potentially expand options and services for families of children with disabilities.

- Conducting research on the effects of existing support programs; the goals are to demonstrate efficacy, educate legislators and public officials, and develop and implement innovative programs.

CONCLUSION

Families of children with disabilities, just like all families, need support along their parenting journey. Early in the journey, they will need information and opportunities to meet other parents of children with the same or similar disability. Later, they will need assistance with navigating the school system. Anywhere along the way, they might need respite. As the child matures into an adolescent, a whole new set of supports evolve that center around independence issues, sexuality, and acceptance/inclusion in social activities. Toward the end of the journey, parents become primarily concerned about their adult child's life without them. The physician's job is to provide whatever it takes and strive to relieve always. Because of this, families of children with disabilities will usually require greater physician time and attention than families of typically developing, well children. Support activities and services may at first appear to be overwhelming in number and complexity, and physicians can be tremendously helpful in helping parents with children with disabilities connect with the services that will best suit their family's needs.

REFERENCES

Agosta, J. (2004). Family support is dead! Long live family support. *TASH Connections, 30*(September/October), 12–15.

Agosta, J., & Melda, K. (1995). Supporting families who provide care at home for children with disabilities. *Exceptional Children, 62*, 271–282.

American Academy of Pediatrics Committee on Children with Disabilities. (1992; reaffirmed in 1999). Pediatricians' role in the development and implementation of an individual education plan (IEP) and/or an individual family service plan (IFSP). *Pediatrics, 89*, 124–127.

American Academy of Pediatrics Committee on Children with Disabilities. (2001a; reaffirmed 2005). Counseling families who choose complementary and alternative medicine for their child with chronic illness or disability. *Pediatrics, 107*, 598–601.

American Academy of Pediatrics Committee on Children with Disabilities. (2001b). Role of the pediatrician in family-centered early intervention services. *Pediatrics, 107*(5), 1155–1157.

American Academy of Pediatrics Committee on Children with Disabilities. (2002). A consensus statement on health care transitions for young adults with special health care needs. *Pediatrics, 110*, 1304–1306.

American Academy of Pediatrics Committee on Children with Disabilities. (2004). Providing a primary care medical home for children and youth with cerebral palsy. *Pediatrics, 114*, 1106–1113.

American Academy of Pediatrics Task Force on Definition of the Medical Home. (1992). The medical home. *Pediatrics, 90*, 774.

American Dental Association. (2002). *Resolution 66H. Access to oral health care for persons with special needs.* Adopted, New Orleans, October 2002.

Americans with Disabilities Act of 1990 (ADA), PL 101-336, 42, U.S.C. §§ 12101 *et seq.*

Anselmo, M.A., Lash, K.M., Stieb, E.S., & Haver, K.E. (2004). Cystic fibrosis on the Internet: A survey of site adherence to AMA guidelines. *Pediatrics, 114*, 100–103.

Bergen, B.B. (1993). Reaching out. *Exceptional Parent, 23*(6), 20–22.

Blasco, P.A., (1988). Breaking the news about retardation. *Contemporary Pediatrics, 5*(8), 9–12.

Blasco, P.A., Baumgartner, M.C., & Mathes, B.C. (1983). Literature for parents of children with cerebral palsy. *Developmental Medicine and Child Neurology, 25*, 642–647.

Blasco, P.A., Kohen, H., & Shapland, C. (1999). Parents-as-teachers: Design and establishment of a training programme for paediatric residents. *Medical Education, 33*, 695–701.

Blum, R.W. (2002). Improving transition for adolescents with special health care needs from pediatric to adult-centered health care. *Pediatrics, 110*(6 Suppl.), 1301–1335.

Brett, J. (2004). The journey to accepting support: How parents of profoundly disabled children experience support in their lives. *Pediatric Nursing, 16*, 14–18.

Brewer, E.J., McPherson, M., Magrab, P.R., & Hutchins, V.L. (1989). Family-centered, community-based, coordinated care for children with special health care needs. *Pediatrics, 83*, 1055–1061.

Brunetti, F.L. (1995). Estate planning: Getting started. *Exceptional Parent, 25*(12), 41–44.

Brunetti, F.L. (1996). Estate planning: Trusts for children with disabilities. *Exceptional Parent, 26*(12), 50–51.

Butler, J.A., Singer, J.D., Palfrey, J.S., & Walker, D.K. (1987). Health insurance coverage and physician use among children with disabilities: Findings from probability samples in five metropolitan areas. *Pediatrics, 79*, 89–98.

Cappelli, M., McGrath, P.J., Daniels, T., Manion, I., & Schillinger, J. (1994). Marital quality of parents of children with spina bifida: A case-comparison study. *Journal of Developmental and Behavioral Pediatrics, 15*, 320–326.

Case-Smith, J. (2004). Parenting a child with a chronic medical condition. *American Journal of Occupational Therapy, 58*, 551–560.

Cherng, R., Liao, H., Leung, H.W.C., et al. (2004). The effectiveness of therapeutic horseback riding in children with spastic CP. *Adaptive Physical Activity Quarterly, 21*, 103–121.

Clayton, M. (2000). Health and social policy: Influences on family-centered care. *Pediatric Nursing, 12*(8), 31–33.

Cohen, M.H., & Kemper, K.J. (2005). Complementary therapies in pediatrics: A legal perspective. *Pediatrics, 115*, 774–780.

Cleveland, D., & Miller, C. (1977). Attitudes and life commitments of older siblings of mentally retarded adults: An exploratory study. *Mental Retardation, 15*, 38–41.

Cooley W. (1994). The ecology of support of caregiving families. *Journal of Developmental and Behavioral Pediatrics, 15*, 117–120.

Davidoff, A., Kenney, G., & Dubay, L. (2005). Effects of the state children's health insurance program expansions on children with chronic health conditions. *Pediatrics, 116*, e34–e42.

Fost, N. (1981). Counseling families who have a child with a severe congenital anomaly. *Pediatrics, 67*, 321–324.

Frey, K.S., Greenberg, M.T., & Fewell, R.R. (1989). Stress and coping among parents of handicapped children: A multidimensional approach. *American Journal on Mental Retardation, 94,* 240–249.

Galil, A., Backner, Y.G., Merrick, J., Flussen, H., Lubetzky, H., Heiman, N., et al. (2006). Physician–parent communication as predictor of parent satisfaction with child development services. *Research in Developmental Disabilities, 27*(3), 233–242.

Green, M. (1991). On making a difference. *Pediatrics, 87,* 712–718.

Hayden, M.F., Kim, S.H., & DePaepe, P. (2005). Health status, utilization patterns, and outcomes of persons with intellectual disabilities: A review of the literature. *Mental Retardation, 43*(3), 175–195.

Health Insurance Portability and Accountability Act of 1996, PL 104–191, 42 U.S.C. §§201 *et seq.*

Hostler, S.L. (1991). Family-centered care. *Pediatric Clinics of North America, 38,* 1545–1560.

Hostler, S.L. (Ed.). (1994). *Family-centered care: An approach to implementation.* Charlottesville: University of Virginia, Kluge Children's Rehabilitation Center.

Human Services Research Institute. (1990). *Family support services in the United States: An end of decade status report.* Cambridge, MA: Author.

Hyman, S.L., & Levy, S.E. (Eds.) (2005). Introduction: Novel therapies in developmental disabilities—hope, reason, and evidence. *Mental Retardation and Developmental Disabilities Research Reviews, 11*(2), 107–109.

Individuals with Disabilities Education Improvement Act of 2004, PL 108-446, 20 U.S.C. §§ 1400 *et seq.*

Isman, B.A., Newton, R.N., Bujold, C., & Baer, M.T. (2000). *Planning guide for dental professionals serving children with special health care needs.* Los Angeles: University of Southern California University Affiliated Program.

Jackins, B.D., Blank, R.S., Macy, P.M., Orello, H.H., & Shulman, K.W. (2004). *Special needs trust administration manual: A guide for trustees.* Brookline, MA: People with Disabilities Press at iUniverse.

Johnson, C.P., & Blasco, P.A. (1997). Community resources for children with special healthcare needs. *Pediatric Annals, 26,* 11–16.

Johnson, C.P., & Kastner, T., & the American Academy of Pediatrics Committee on Children with Disabilities. (2005). Helping families raise children with special health care needs at home. *Pediatrics, 115,* 507–511.

Kaminer, R.K., & Cohen, H.J. (1988). How do you say, "Your child is retarded"? *Contemporary Pediatrics, 5*(5), 36–49.

Klein, S.D. (1982). The role of the family in helping the child with learning disabilities. In M. Davis & J.C. Whitener (Eds.), *The role of vision in multidisciplinary approaches to children with learning disabilities* (pp. 114–115). Springfield, IL: Charles C. Thomas.

Klein, S.D. (1993). The challenge of communicating with parents. *Journal of Developmental and Behavioral Pediatrics, 14,* 184–191.

Korsch, B.M. (1984). What do patients and parents want to know? What do they need to know? *Pediatrics, 74*(Suppl.), 917–919.

Lacey, R.P. (2004). Does my child need a guardian? *Exceptional Parent, 34*(7), 57–59.

Liptak, G.S. (2005). Complementary and alternative therapies for cerebral palsy. *Mental Retardation and Developmental Disabilities Research Reviews, 11,* 156–163.

Liptak, G.S., & Revell, G.M. (1989). Community physician's role in case management of children with chronic illness. *Pediatrics, 84,* 465–471.

Medlen, J.E.G. (2002). *The Down syndrome nutrition handbook: A guide to promoting healthy lifestyles.* Bethesda: Woodbine House.

Molnar, M. (1991). Questions to ask before hitting the vacation trail. *Mainstream, 15*(6), 11–13.

Mouradian, W., Porter, A., Keegan, C., & Cantillon, K. (2001). *Promoting oral health of children with neurodevelopmental disabilities and other special health care needs.* Seattle: University of Washington, Center on Human Development and Disability.

Nattrass, K., Davis, B.W., O'Brien, S., Patronek, G., & MacCollin, M. (2004). In puppy love: How an assistance dog can enhance the life of a child with a disability. *Contemporary Pediatrics, 21,* 57–62.

Newacheck, P.W. (1989). Adolescents with special health needs: Prevalence, severity, and access to health services. *Pediatrics, 84,* 872–881.

Newacheck, P.W., & Kim, S.E. (2005). A national profile of health care utilization and expenditures for children with special health care needs. *Archives of Pediatrics and Adolescent Medicine, 159,* 10–17.

Newacheck, P.W., & McManus, M.A. (1988). Financing health care for disabled children. *Pediatrics, 81,* 385–394.

O'Sullivan, P., Mahoney, G., & Robinson, C. (1992). Perceptions of pediatricians' helpfulness: A national study of mothers of young disabled children. *Developmental Medicine and Child Neurology, 34,* 1064–1071.

Parish, S.L., Pomeranz-Essley, A., & Braddock, D. (2003). Family support in the United States: Financing trends and emerging initiatives. *Mental Retardation, 41,* 174–187.

Parish, S.L., Seltzer, M.M., Greenberg, J.S., & Floyd, F. (2004). Economic implications of caregiving at midlife: Comparing parents with and without children who have developmental disabilities. *Mental Retardation, 42,* 413–426.

Perlman, S., Fenton, S.J., & Friedman, C. (Eds.). (2003). *Oral health care for persons with disabilities.* Boston: Exceptional Parent.

Raina, P., O'Donnell, M., Rosenbaum, P., Brehaut, J., Walter, S.D., Russell, D., et al. (2005). The health and well-being of caregivers of children with cerebral palsy. *Pediatrics, 115,* e626–e636.

Revell, E.O. (1990). Including fathers in early therapeutic intervention. *Developmental Medicine and Child Neurology, 32*(Suppl. 62), 32.

Rosenau, N. (2005a). *A family for every child: Family-based alternatives for children with disabilities.* Austin, TX: Every Child.

Rosenau, N. (2005b). *A guide to choosing a support family: Family-based alternatives for children with disabilities.* Austin, TX: Every Child.

Sabbeth, B.F., & Leventhal, J.M. (1984). Marital adjustment to chronic childhood illness: A critique of the literature. *Pediatrics, 73,* 762–768.

Scheiber, K. (1989). Developmentally delayed children: Effects on the normal sibling. *Pediatric Nursing, 15,* 42.

Sharp, M.C., Strauss, R.P., & Lorch, S.C. (1992). Communicating medical bad news: Parents' experiences and preferences. *Journal of Pediatrics, 121,* 539–546.

Shelton, I.L., Jeppson, E.S., & Johnson, B.H. (1987). *Family-centered care for children with special health care needs.* Washington, DC: Association for the Care of Children's Health.

Simeonsson, R.J., & Bailey, D.B. (1986). Siblings of handicapped children. In J.J. Gallagher & P.M. Vietze (Eds.), *Families of handicapped persons: Research, programs, and policy issues.* Baltimore: Paul H. Brookes Publishing Co.

Singhi, P.D., Goyal, L., Pershad, D., Singhi, S., & Walia, B.N. (1990). Psychosocial problems in families of disabled children. *British Journal of Medical Psychology, 63*(Pt. 2), 173–182.

Weil, W.B. (1986). Review of "neglect of chronically ill children." *American Journal of Diseases of Children, 140,* 628.

Widrick, G., Whaley, C., DiVenere, N., Vecchione, E., Swartz, D., & Stiffler, D. (1991). The Medical Education Project: An example of collaboration between parents and professionals. *Children's Health Care, 20*(2), 93–100.

Wilson, D.D., & Hostler, S.L. (1986). *The teaching physical exam: A manual.* Charlottesville: University of Virginia, Children's Rehabilitation Center.

Winston, N.A. (2004). ABCs of SSI. *Exceptional Parent, 34,* 56–58.

Worley, G., Rosenfeld, L.R., & Lipscomb, J. (1991). Financial counseling for families of children with chronic disabilities. *Developmental Medicine and Child Neurology, 33,* 679–689.

Index

Page numbers followed by "*f*" indicate figures; those followed by "*t*" indicate tables.